PSYCHODYNAMIC DIAGNOSTIC MANUAL

Second Edition

PDM-2

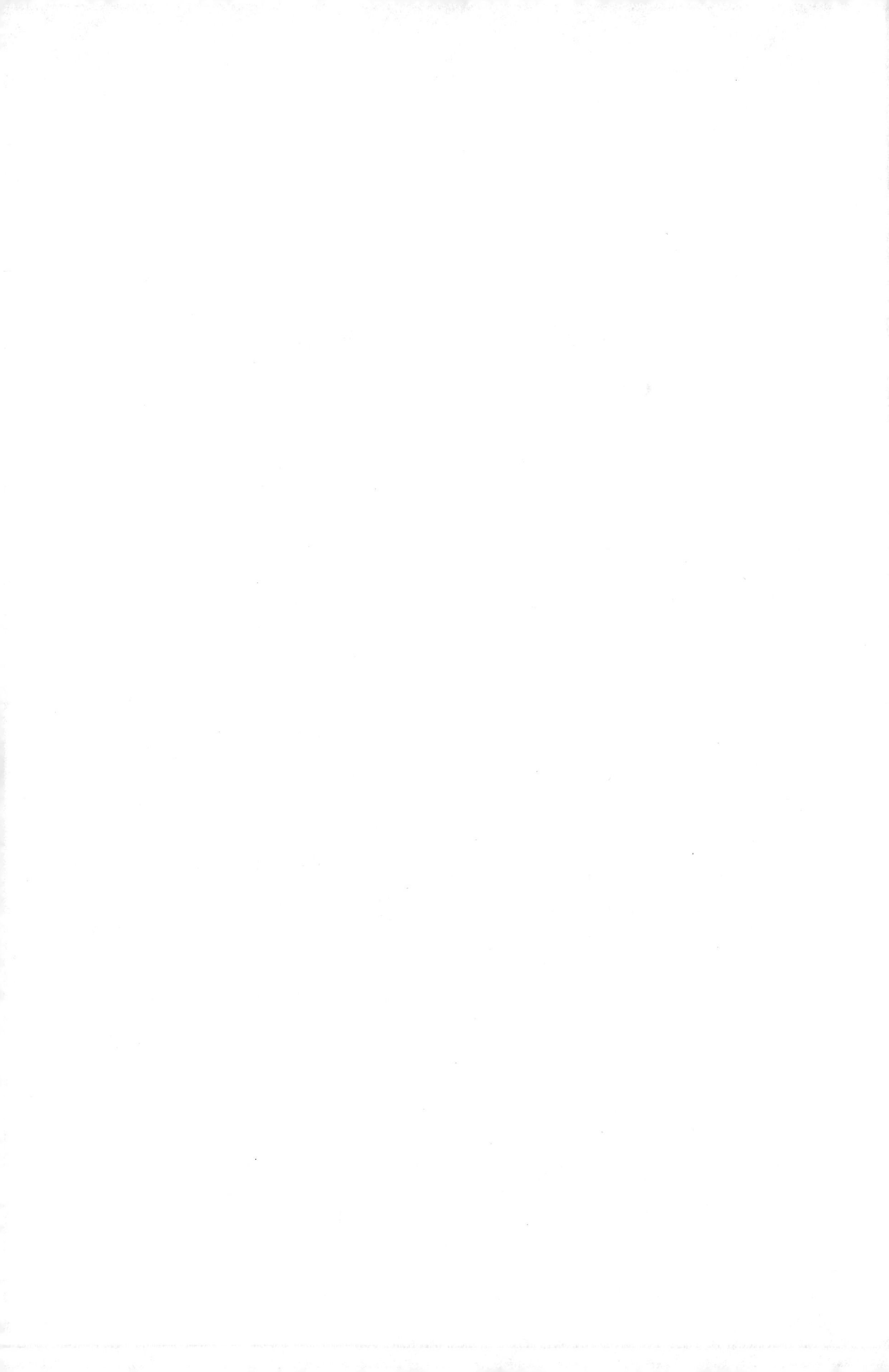

Psychodynamic Diagnostic Manual

Second Edition

PDM-2

Edited by

Vittorio Lingiardi
Nancy McWilliams

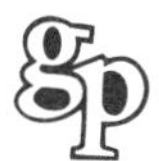

THE GUILFORD PRESS
New York London

Published by The Guilford Press
A Division of Guilford Publications, Inc.
370 Seventh Avenue, Suite 1200, New York, NY 10001
www.guilford.com

Printed in the United States of America

This book is printed on acid-free paper.

Last digit is print number: 9 8 7 6 5 4 3

Library of Congress Cataloging-in-Publication Data

Names: Lingiardi, Vittorio, 1960– editor. | McWilliams, Nancy, editor.
Title: Psychodynamic diagnostic manual : PDM-2 / edited by Vittorio Lingiardi, Nancy McWilliams.
Other titles: PDM-2
Description: Second edition. | New York : The Guilford Press, [2017] | Includes bibliographical references and index.
Identifiers: LCCN 2016049804| ISBN 9781462530540 (pbk. : alk. paper) | ISBN 9781462530557 (hardcover : alk. paper)
Subjects: | MESH: Mental Disorders—diagnosis | Mental Disorders—classification | Case Reports
Classification: LCC RC455.2.C4 | NLM WM 141 | DDC 616.89001/2—dc23
LC record available at *https://lccn.loc.gov/2016049804*

In memory of
Sidney J. Blatt,
Stanley Greenspan,
Robert S. Wallerstein

About the Editors

Vittorio Lingiardi, MD, is Full Professor of Dynamic Psychology and past Director (2006–2013) of the Clinical Psychology Specialization Program in the Department of Dynamic and Clinical Psychology of the Faculty of Medicine and Psychology, Sapienza University of Rome, Rome, Italy. His research interests include diagnostic assessment and treatment of personality disorders, process–outcome research in psychoanalysis and psychotherapy, and gender identity and sexual orientation. He has published widely on these topics, including articles in *The American Journal of Psychiatry*, *Contemporary Psychoanalysis*, *The International Journal of Psychoanalysis*, *Psychoanalytic Dialogues*, *Psychoanalytic Psychology*, *Psychotherapy*, *Psychotherapy Research*, and *World Psychiatry*. Dr. Lingiardi is a recipient of the Ralph Roughton Paper Award from the American Psychoanalytic Association. From 2013 to 2016, he served on the technical committee for the eligibility of the training programs of the psychotherapy private schools of the Italian Ministry of Education, University and Research.

Nancy McWilliams, PhD, ABPP, is Visiting Professor in the Graduate School of Applied and Professional Psychology at Rutgers, The State University of New Jersey, and has a private practice in Flemington, New Jersey. She is on the editorial board of *Psychoanalytic Psychology* and has authored three classic books on psychotherapy, including the award-winning *Psychoanalytic Diagnosis, Second Edition: Understanding Personality Structure in the Clinical Process*. Dr. McWilliams is an Honorary Member of the American Psychoanalytic Association and a former Erikson Scholar at the Austen Riggs Center in Stockbridge, Massachusetts. She is a recipient of the Leadership and Scholarship Awards from Division 39 (Psychoanalysis) of the American Psychological Association (APA) and the Hans H. Strupp Award from the Appalachian Psychoanalytic Society, and delivered the Dr. Rosalee G. Weiss Lecture for Outstanding Leaders in Psychology for APA Division 42 (Psychologists in Independent Practice). She has demonstrated psychodynamic psychotherapy in three APA educational videos and has spoken at the commencement ceremonies of the Yale University School of Medicine and the Smith College School for Social Work.

Chapter Editors

Robert F. Bornstein, PhD, Derner Institute of Advanced Psychological Studies, Adelphi University, Garden City, New York

Franco Del Corno, MPhyl, DPsych, President, Society for Psychotherapy Research—Italy Area Group, Italy

Francesco Gazzillo, PhD, Department of Dynamic and Clinical Psychology, Faculty of Medicine and Psychology, Sapienza University of Rome, Rome, Italy

Robert M. Gordon, PhD, ABPP, Institute for Advanced Psychological Training, Allentown, Pennsylvania

Vittorio Lingiardi, MD, Department of Dynamic and Clinical Psychology, Faculty of Medicine and Psychology, Sapienza University of Rome, Rome, Italy

Norka Malberg, PsyD, Yale Child Study Center, New Haven, Connecticut

Johanna C. Malone, PhD, Department of Psychiatry, Massachusetts General Hospital and Harvard Medical School, Cambridge, Massachusetts

Linda Mayes, MD, Yale Child Study Center and Office of the Dean, Yale School of Medicine, New Haven, Connecticut

Nancy McWilliams, PhD, Graduate School of Applied and Professional Psychology, Rutgers, The State University of New Jersey, Piscataway, New Jersey

Nick Midgley, PhD, Research Department of Clinical Education and Health Psychology, University College London, London, United Kingdom

Emanuela Mundo, MD, Residency Program in Clinical Psychology, Faculty of Medicine and Psychology, Sapienza University of Rome, Rome, Italy

John Allison O'Neil, MD, Department of Psychiatry, McGill University and St. Mary's Hospital, Montréal, Québec, Canada

Daniel Plotkin, MD, Department of Psychiatry and Biobehavioral Sciences, David Geffen School of Medicine, University of California at Los Angeles, Los Angeles, California

Larry Rosenberg, PhD, Child Guidance Center of Southern Connecticut, Stamford, Connecticut

Jonathan Shedler, PhD, University of Colorado School of Medicine, Denver, Colorado

Anna Maria Speranza, PhD, Department of Dynamic and Clinical Psychology, Faculty of Medicine and Psychology, Sapienza University of Rome, Rome, Italy

Mario Speranza, MD, PhD, Department of Psychiatry, Versailles General Hospital, and Faculty of Medicine and Health Sciences, University of Versailles Saint Quentin en Yvelines, Versailles, France

Sherwood Waldron, MD, Psychoanalytic Research Consortium, New York, New York

Consultants

Consultants who are also Chapter Editors appear in the "Chapter Editors" list.

Allan Abbass, MD, Halifax, Nova Scotia, Canada

John S. Auerbach, PhD, Gainesville, Florida

Fabia E. Banella, MA, Rome, Italy

Tessa Baradon, MA, London, United Kingdom

Jacques Barber, PhD, Garden City, New York

Kenneth Barish, PhD, Hartsdale, New York

Thomas Barrett, PhD, Chicago, Illinois

Mark Blais, PsyD, Boston, Massachusetts

Corinne Blanchet-Collet, MD, Paris, France

Anthony Bram, PhD, ABAP, Lexington, Massachusetts

Line Brotnow, MSc, Paris, France

Emanuela Brusadelli, PhD, Milan, Italy

Giuseppe Cafforio, DPsych, Aosta, Italy

Mark Carter, MA, MSc, London, United Kingdom

Irene Chatoor, MD, Washington, D.C.

Richard Chefetz, MD, Washington, D.C.

Manfred Cierpka, MD, Heidelberg, Germany

John F. Clarkin, PhD, White Plains, New York

Antonello Colli, PhD, Urbino, Italy

Christine A. Courtois, PhD, Washington, D.C.

Jacques Dayan, MD, PhD, Rennes, France

Martin Debbané, PhD, Geneva, Switzerland

Ferhan Dereboy, MD, Aydin, Turkey

Kathryn DeWitt, PhD, Stanford, California

Diana Diamond, PhD, New York, New York

Jack Drescher, MD, New York, New York

Karin Ensink, PhD, Québec City, Québec, Canada

Janet Etzi, PsyD, Philadelphia, Pennsylvania

Giovanni Foresti, MD, PhD, Pavia, Italy

Sara Francavilla, DPsych, Milan, Italy

Glen O. Gabbard, MD, Houston, Texas

Michael Garrett, MD, Brooklyn, New York

Federica Genova, PhD, Rome, Italy

Carol George, PhD, Oakland, California

William H. Gottdiener, PhD, New York, New York

Brin Grenyer, PhD, Sydney, Australia

Salvatore Gullo, PhD, Rome, Italy

George Halasz, MS, MRCPsych, Melbourne, Australia

Nakia Hamlett, PhD, New Haven, Connecticut
Alexandra Harrison, MD, Cambridge, Massachusetts
Mark J. Hilsenroth, PhD, Garden City, New York
Leon Hoffman, MD, New York, New York
Per Høglend, MD, Oslo, Norway
Steven K. Huprich, PhD, Wichita, Kansas
Marvin Hurvich, PhD, New York, New York
Lawrence Josephs, PhD, Garden City, New York
Horst Kächele, MD, PhD, Berlin, Germany
Richard Kluft, MD, Bala Cynwyd, Pennsylvania
Guenther Klug, MD, Munich, Germany
Brian Koehler, PhD, New York, New York
Melinda Kulish, PhD, Boston, Massachusetts
Jonathan Lachal, MD, PhD, Paris, France
Michael J. Lambert, PhD, Provo, Utah
Douglas W. Lane, PhD, Seattle, Washington
Alessandra Lemma, MA, MPhil, DClinPsych, London, United Kingdom
Howard Lerner, PhD, Ann Arbor, Michigan
Marianne Leuzinger-Bohleber, PhD, Frankfurt, Germany
Karin Lindqvist, MSc, Stockholm, Sweden
Henriette Loeffler-Stastka, MD, Vienna, Austria
Loredana Lucarelli, PhD, Cagliari, Italy
Patrick Luyten, PhD, Brussels, Belgium
Eirini Lympinaki, MSc, Athens, Greece
Janet A. Madigan, MD, New Haven, Connecticut
Sandra Maestro, MD, Pisa, Italy
Steven Marans, PhD, New Haven, Connecticut
Matthias Michal, MD, Mainz, Germany
Robert Michels, MD, Ithaca, New York
Hun Millard, MD, New Haven, Connecticut
Kevin Moore, PsyD, Philadelphia, Pennsylvania
Seymour Moscovitz, PhD, New York, New York
Filippo Muratori, MD, Pisa, Italy
Laura Muzi, PhD, Rome, Italy
Ronald Naso, PhD, Stamford, Connecticut
John C. Norcross, PhD, Clarks Summit, Pennsylvania
Massimiliano Orri, PhD, Paris, France
J. Christopher Perry, MPH, MD, Montréal, Québec, Canada
Humberto Persano, MD, PhD, Buenos Aires, Argentina
Eleonora Piacentini, PhD, Rome, Italy
Piero Porcelli, PhD, Castellana Grotte (Bari), Italy
John H. Porcerelli, PhD, Bloomfield Hills, Michigan
Timothy Rice, MD, New York, New York
Judith Rosenberger, PhD, LCSW, New York, New York
Babak Roshanaei-Moghaddam, MD, Tehran, Iran
Jeremy D. Safran, PhD, New York, New York
Ionas Sapountzis, PhD, Garden City, New York
Lea Setton, PhD, Panama City, Panama
Golan Shahar, PhD, Beersheba, Israel
Theodore Shapiro, MD, New York, New York
Caleb Siefert, PhD, Dearborn, Michigan
George Silberschatz, PhD, San Francisco, California
Gabrielle H. Silver, MD, New York, New York
Steven Spitz, PhD, New York, New York
Miriam Steele, PhD, New York, New York
Michelle Stein, PhD, Boston, Massachusetts
Matthew Steinfeld, PhD, New Haven, Connecticut
William Stiles, PhD, Miami, Ohio
Danijela Stojanac, MD, New Haven, Connecticut
John Stokes, PhD, New York, New York
Annette Streeck-Fischer, MD, PhD, Berlin, Germany
Karl Stukenberg, PhD, Cincinnati, Ohio
Guido Taidelli, MD, Milan, Italy
Annalisa Tanzilli, PhD, Rome, Italy
Pratyusha Tummala-Narra, PhD, Boston, Massachusetts
Kirkland Vaughans, PhD, Garden City, New York
Fred Volkmar, MD, New Haven, Connecticut
Charles H. Zeanah, MD, New Orleans, Louisiana
Alessandro Zennaro, PhD, Turin, Italy
Alessia Zoppi, PhD, Urbino, Italy

PDM-2 Honorary Scientific Committee

John S. Auerbach, PhD

Anthony W. Bateman, MA, FRCPsych

Sidney J. Blatt, PhD (deceased)

Eve Caligor, MD

Richard A. Chefetz, MD

Marco Chiesa, MD, FRCPsych

John F. Clarkin, PhD

Reiner W. Dahlbender, MD

Jared DeFife, PhD

Diana Diamond, PhD

Jack Drescher, MD

Peter Fonagy, PhD, FBA

Glen O. Gabbard, MD

John G. Gunderson, MD

Mark J. Hilsenroth, PhD

Mardi J. Horowitz, MD

Steven K. Huprich, PhD

Elliot L. Jurist, PhD

Horst Kächele, MD, PhD

Otto F. Kernberg, MD

Alessandra Lemma, MA, MPhil, DClinPsych

Marianne Leuzinger-Bohleber, PhD

Henriette Loeffler-Stastka, MD

Karlen Lyons-Ruth, PhD

Patrick Luyten, PhD

William A. MacGillivray, PhD

Robert Michels, MD

Joseph Palombo, MA

J. Christopher Perry, MPH, MD

John H. Porcerelli, PhD

Jeremy D. Safran, PhD

Allan N. Schore, PhD

Arietta Slade, PhD

Mary Target, PhD

Robert J. Waldinger, MD

Robert S. Wallerstein, MD (deceased)

Drew Westen, PhD

PDM-2 Sponsoring Organizations

American Academy of Psychoanalysis and Dynamic Psychiatry

American Association for Psychoanalysis in Clinical Social Work

American Psychoanalytic Association

Association Européenne de Psychopathologie de l'Enfant et de l'Adolescent

Confederation of Independent Psychoanalytic Societies

Division of Psychoanalysis (39), American Psychological Association

International Association for Relational Psychoanalysis & Psychotherapy

International Psychoanalytical Association

International Society of Adolescent Psychiatry and Psychology

Italian Group for the Advancement of Psychodynamic Diagnosis

Acknowledgments

The Editors express their gratitude to the Erikson Institute at the Austen Riggs Center in Stockbridge, Massachusetts, for supporting Nancy McWilliams in the final phases of editing this manual. They also thank Marie Sprayberry and Laura Specht Patchkofsky of The Guilford Press for their outstanding work as copy editor and production editor, respectively.

Brief Contents

PART III. CHILDHOOD

PART IV. INFANCY AND EARLY CHILDHOOD

PART V. LATER LIFE

PART VI. ASSESSMENT AND CLINICAL ILLUSTRATIONS

Extended Contents

PART II. ADOLESCENCE

PART III. CHILDHOOD

PART IV. INFANCY AND EARLY CHILDHOOD

PART VI. ASSESSMENT AND CLINICAL ILLUSTRATIONS

Purchasers can download and print select materials from this book as well as Web-only case illustrations and PDM-2 profiles at *www.guilford.com/PDM2supplements* for personal use or use with clients (see copyright page for details).

Introduction

Vittorio Lingiardi, MD **Nancy McWilliams, PhD**

The first edition of the *Psychodynamic Diagnostic Manual* (PDM; PDM Task Force, 2006) was published in an era of critical change in psychiatric nosology. This period began with the publication of the *Diagnostic and Statistical Manual of Mental Disorders*, third edition (DSM-III; American Psychiatric Association, 1980), which embraced a shift from a psychoanalytically influenced, dimensional, inferential diagnostic system to a "neo-Kraepelinian," descriptive, symptom-focused, multiaxial classification relying on present-versus-absent criteria sets for identifying discrete mental disorders.

This change was made deliberately, in part to remove psychoanalytic bias from the manual now that other theoretical orientations (e.g., behavioral, cognitive, family systems, humanistic, biological) had arisen. It was also intended to make certain kinds of outcome research easier: Discrete traits could be identified by researchers with little clinical experience, whereas the previous classifications (DSM-I and DSM-II) had required significant clinical training to diagnose inferentially many syndromes. DSM-IV (American Psychiatric Association, 1994) continued the neo-Kraepelinian trend, which has been further elaborated and expanded with DSM-5 (American Psychiatric Association, 2013). Each succeeding edition has included more disorders.

At the same time, the psychodynamic community needed to respond to those of its members who question the usefulness of any diagnostic system and who value qualitative methodologies and clinical reports over quantitative research. The perception that analysts as a group devalue both diagnosis and systematic research has caused many to dismiss its theories and applications on the basis of an assumed lack of empirical evidence. Among the goals of the first PDM was to call attention to how much careful research supports psychoanalytic concepts and approaches.[1]

Like its predecessor, PDM-2 has been influenced by the power and clinical utility of psychodynamic diagnostic formulations such as Shapiro's (1965) *Neurotic Styles*, Kernberg's (1984) object relations model of personality pathology, McWilliams's (e.g., 2011a) contributions on diagnosis and case formulation, and the work of many psychoanalytic researchers. As in the first edition, we offer a diagnostic framework that characterizes an individual's full range of functioning—the depth as well as the surface of emotional, cognitive, interpersonal, and social patterns. We try to promote integration between nomothetic understanding and idiographic knowledge useful for case formulation and treatment planning, emphasizing individual variations as well as commonalities. We hope that this conceptualization will bring about improvements in the diagnosis and treatment of mental problems, and will permit a fuller understanding of the development and functioning of the mind.

This diagnostic framework attempts a systematic description of healthy and disordered *personality functioning*; individual profiles of *mental functioning* (including, e.g., patterns of relating to others, comprehending and expressing feelings, coping with stress and anxiety, regulating impulses, observing one's own emotions and behaviors, and forming moral judgments); and *symptom patterns*, including differences in each individual's personal, subjective experience of symptoms and the related experience of treating clinicians.

Notwithstanding the advantages of the DSM and *International Classification of Diseases* (ICD) systems, often their classifications do not meet the needs of clinicians. Accordingly, PDM-2 adds a needed perspective on symptom patterns depicted in existing taxonomies, enabling clinicians to describe and categorize personality patterns, related social and emotional capacities, unique mental profiles, and personal experiences of symptoms. In focusing on the full range of mental functioning, PDM-2 aspires to be a "taxonomy of people" rather than a "taxonomy of disorders," and it highlights the importance of considering *who one is* rather than *what one has*. Our ability to reduce the gap between a diagnostic process and mental illness in all its complexity, and also the gap between science and practice, depends on communication and collaboration among researchers and clinicians. Hence PDM-2 is based on clinical knowledge as well as process–outcome research and other empirical work.

The rapidly advancing neuroscience field can be only as useful as our understanding of the basic patterns of mental health and pathology, and of the functional nature of disorders. Describing such patterns accurately should eventually permit a greater understanding of etiology. Research on brain development suggests that patterns of

[1]The tension between research-oriented scholars and some in the psychoanalytic community continued after the publication of the first PDM. In 2009, Irwin Hoffman critiqued the document, suggesting that the "privileged status" accorded to systematic empirical research on psychoanalytic process and outcome is "unwarranted epistemologically" and "potentially damaging," and that virtually any use of categorization in relation to patients is a "desiccation" of human experience. Hoffman viewed the PDM as merely giving lip service "to humanistic, existential respect for the uniqueness and limitless complexity of any person" (p. 1060). In response, Eagle and Wolitzky (2011) argued that human experience is not "desiccated" when researchers view it through a diagnostic lens and try to measure it; they suggested that a constructive way to bridge the gap between science and analytic work is to do better, more creative, and more ecologically valid research. Their position is shared by the authors of this document and by several psychodynamic authors involved in this discussion (for varying views, see, e.g., Aron, 2012; Fonagy, 2013; Hoffman, 2012a, 2012b; Lingiardi, Holmqvist, & Safran, 2016; Safran, 2012; Vivona, 2012).

emotional, social, and behavioral functioning involve many areas working together rather than in isolation, with important consequences for clinical psychological models of illness and psychotherapeutic change (Buchheim et al., 2012; Kandel, 1999; Schore, 2014). Outcome studies point to the importance of dealing with the full complexity of emotional and social patterns. Numerous researchers (e.g., Høglend, 2014; Norcross, 2011; Wampold & Imel, 2015) have concluded that the nature of the therapeutic relationship, reflecting interconnected aspects of mind and brain operating together in an interpersonal context, predicts outcome more robustly than any specific treatment approach or technique per se.

Westen, Novotny, and Thompson-Brenner (2004) found that treatments focusing on isolated symptoms or behaviors (rather than on personality, emotional themes, and interpersonal patterns) are not effective in sustaining even narrowly defined changes. In recent years, several reliable ways of measuring complex patterns of personality, emotion, and interpersonal processes—the active ingredients of the therapeutic relationship—have been developed. These include, among others, the Shedler–Westen Assessment Procedure (SWAP-200, Westen & Shedler, 1999a, 1999b; SWAP-II, Westen, Waller, Shedler, & Blagov, 2014), on which we have drawn extensively; the Structured Interview of Personality Organization (STIPO), developed by Kernberg's group (Clarkin, Caligor, Stern, & Kernberg, 2004); the Operationalized Psychodynamic Diagnosis (OPD) system (OPD Task Force, 2008; Zimmermann et al., 2012); and Blatt's (2008) model of anaclitic and introjective personality configurations.

Two pertinent topics are the range of problems for which psychodynamic approaches are suitable, and the effectiveness of short- and long-term psychodynamic psychotherapies (Abbass, Town, & Driessen, 2012; Levy, Ablon, & Kächele, 2012; Norcross & Wampold, 2011). A number of recent reviews (e.g., de Maat et al., 2013; Fonagy, 2015; Leichsenring, Leweke, Klein, & Steinert, 2015) suggest that some psychodynamic treatments are more effective than short-term, manualized forms of cognitive-behavioral treatment (CBT), and that improvement after psychodynamic intervention tends to continue after the therapy ends (Shedler, 2010). In addition to alleviating symptoms, psychodynamically based therapies may improve overall emotional and social functioning.

Like its predecessor, PDM-2 has been a collaborative effort among organizations of psychoanalytically oriented mental health professionals. The manual follows the format of denoting, for each chapter, two or three Editors and a pool of Consultants (clinicians and/or researchers with expertise relevant to that domain). The task of the Chapter Editors, according to guidelines we provided on how to structure each chapter, was to plan and write their respective chapters, coordinating and integrating the texts, documents, critiques, and other materials provided by the Consultants. Final approval of chapters lay with us, the manual's overall Editors.

Rationale for the PDM-2 Classification System

A clinically useful classification of mental disorders must begin with a concept of healthy psychology. Mental health is more than simply the absence of symptoms. Just as healthy cardiac functioning cannot be defined as an absence of chest pain, healthy mental functioning is more than the absence of observable symptoms of psychopathology. Attempts to depict deficiencies in mental health must consider deficits in many different capacities, including some that are not overt sources of dysfunction. For example, as frightening as anxiety attacks can be, an inability to perceive and respond accurately to the emotional cues of others—a far more subtle and diffuse problem—can be a more fundamental difficulty than periodic episodes of panic. A deficit in reading emotional cues can pervasively compromise relationships and thinking, and may itself be a source of anxiety.

That a concept of health is foundational for defining disorder may seem self-evident, but our diagnostic procedures have not always proceeded accordingly. In recent decades, psychological problems have been defined primarily on the basis of observable symptoms and behaviors, with overall personality functioning and adaptation mentioned only secondarily. But there is increasing evidence that to understand symptoms, we must know something about the person who hosts them (Westen, Gabbard, & Blagov, 2006), and that both mental health and psychopathology involve many subtle features of human functioning (e.g., affect tolerance, regulation, and expression; coping strategies and defenses; capacities for understanding self and others; quality of relationships).

In the DSM and ICD systems, the whole person has been less visible than the disorder constructs on which researchers can find agreement. In descriptive psychiatric taxonomies, symptoms that may be etiologically or contextually interconnected are described as "comorbid," as if they coexist more or less accidentally in the one person, much as a sinus infection and a broken toe might coexist (see Borsboom, 2008). Assumptions about discrete, unrelated, comorbid conditions are rarely justified by clear genetic, biochemical, or neurophysiological distinctions between syndromes (Tyrer, Reed, & Crawford, 2015). The cutoff criteria for diagnosis are often arbitrary decisions of committees rather than conclusions drawn from the best scientific evidence.

Oversimplifying mental phenomena in the service of consistency of description (reliability) and capacity to evaluate treatment (validity) may have compromised the laudable goal of a more scientifically sound understanding of mental health and pathology. Ironically, given that current systems were expected to increase them, reliability and validity data for many DSM disorders are not strong (see Frances, 2013; Hummelen, Pedersen, Wilberg, & Karterud, 2015). The effort to construct an evidence-based diagnostic system may have led to a tendency to make overly narrow observations, overstep existing evidence, and undermine the critical goal of classifying states of mental health and disorder according to their naturally occurring patterns.

We worry that mental health professionals have uncritically and prematurely adopted methods from other sciences, instead of developing empirical procedures appropriate to the complexity of the data in our field. It is time to adapt the methods to the phenomena rather than vice versa (Bornstein, 2015). Only an accurate description of psychological patterns can guide vital research on etiology, developmental pathways, prevention, and treatment. As the history of science attests (and as the American Psychological Association stated in its 2012 guidelines), scientific evidence includes and often begins with sound descriptions—that is, naturalistic observations such as case studies. Insufficient attention to this foundation of scientific knowledge, under the pressure of a narrow definition of what constitutes evidence (in the service of rapid quantification and replication), would tend to repeat rather than ameliorate the problems of current systems.

Efforts to complement current classifications with a fuller description of mental health and illness must begin with a consensus of experts, based on disciplined clinical observations informed by accurate appraisal of existing and emerging research

(Kächele et al., 2006; Lingiardi, Gazzillo, & Waldron, 2010; Lingiardi, McWilliams, Bornstein, Gazzillo, & Gordon, 2015; Lingiardi, Shedler, & Gazzillo, 2006). Clinically experienced observers make highly reliable and valid judgments if their observations and inferences are quantified with psychometrically sophisticated instruments (Westen & Weinberger, 2004).

We attempt to maintain a healthy tension between the goals of capturing the complexity of clinical phenomena (functional understanding) and developing criteria that can be reliably judged and employed in research (descriptive understanding). It is vital to embrace this tension by pursuing a stepwise approach in which complexity and clinical usefulness influence operational definitions and inform research, and vice versa. As clinicians and researchers, we strongly believe that a scientifically based system begins with accurate recognition and description of complex clinical phenomena and builds gradually toward empirical validation.

Oversimplification, and favoring what is measurable over what is meaningful, do not operate in the service of either good science or sound practice. We are learning that when therapists apply manualized treatments to selected symptom clusters without addressing the complex person with the symptoms, and without attending to the therapeutic relationship, results are short-lived and remission rates are high. Fundamental psychological capacities involving the depth and range of relationships, feelings, and coping strategies do not show evidence of long-term change (Diener, Hilsenroth, & Weinberger, 2007; McWilliams, 2013; Westen, Novotny, & Thompson-Brenner, 2004). In some studies, these critical areas were not even measured—a contributing factor to "the outcome problem" (e.g., Strupp, 1963; Wampold, 2013; Westen et al., 2004).

Process-oriented research has shown that essential characteristics of the psychotherapeutic relationship as conceptualized by psychodynamic models (the therapeutic alliance, transference and countertransference phenomena, and stable characteristics of patient and therapist; see Betan, Heim, Zittel Conklin, & Westen, 2005; Bradley, Heim, & Westen, 2005; Colli, Tanzilli, Dimaggio, & Lingiardi, 2014; Fluckinger, Del Re, Wampold, Symonds, & Horvath, 2012) are more predictive of outcome than any designated treatment approach is.

Although depth psychologies have a long history of examining human functioning in a searching and comprehensive way, the diagnostic precision and usefulness of psychodynamic approaches have been compromised by at least two problems. First, in attempts to capture the range and subtlety of human experience, psychoanalytic accounts of mental processes have often been expressed in competing theories and metaphors, which have at times inspired more disagreement and controversy than consensus (Bornstein & Becker-Materro, 2011). Second, there has been difficulty distinguishing between speculative constructs on the one hand, and phenomena that can be observed or reasonably inferred on the other. Whereas the tradition of descriptive psychiatry has had a tendency to reify "disorder" categories, the psychoanalytic tradition has tended to reify theoretical constructs.

Recently, however, psychodynamically based treatments, especially for personality disorders (e.g., Bateman & Fonagy, 2009; Clarkin, Levy, Lenzenweger, & Kernberg, 2007), have been the subject of several meta-analyses attesting to their efficacy (see Fonagy, 2015; Leichsenring et al., 2015; Shedler, 2010). Moreover, since several empirical methods to quantify and analyze complex mental phenomena have been developed, depth psychology has been able to offer clear operational criteria for a more comprehensive range of human social and emotional conditions. The current challenge is to systematize these advances with clinical experience.

PDM-2 diagnoses are "prototypic"; that is, they are not based on the idea that a diagnostic category can be accurately described as a compilation of symptoms ("polythetic" diagnosis). Some PDM-2 sections refer to categories of psychopathology used in currently prevailing taxonomies. But unlike the DSM and ICD systems, the PDM-2 system highlights patients' *internal experience* of those conditions. Because mental health professionals deal daily with individuals' subjectivity, they need a fuller description of their patients' internal lives to do justice to understanding their distinctive experiences. Evidence suggests that when making diagnoses, clinicians tend to think in terms of prototypes, even as they speak in terms of categories (Bornstein, 2015). This manual attempts to capture the gestalt of human complexity by combining the precision of dimensional systems with the ease of categorical applications. It uses a multidimensional approach, as follows, to describe the intricacies of the patient's overall functioning and ways of engaging in the therapeutic process.

- *Personality Syndromes—P Axis.* The major organizing principles of the P Axis are the level of personality *organization* (i.e., a spectrum of personality functioning from healthy, through neurotic and borderline, to psychotic levels) and personality *style* or pattern (i.e., clinically familiar types that cross-cut levels of personality organization). In the Adulthood section (Part I), because symptoms or problems often cannot be understood, assessed, or treated without an understanding of the personality patterns of the individual who has them, we have placed this dimension first. A person who fears relationships and avoids feelings will experience depression in markedly different ways from one who is fully engaged in relationships and emotions.
- *Profile of Mental Functioning—M Axis.* The second dimension offers a detailed description of overall mental functioning (i.e., the capacities involved in overall psychological health or pathology). It takes a more microscopic look at inner mental life, systematizing and operationalizing such capacities as information processing; impulse regulation; reflecting on one's own and others' mental states; forming and maintaining relationships; experiencing, expressing, and understanding different emotions; regulating self-esteem; using coping strategies and defenses; adaptation and resiliency; forming internal standards; and giving coherence and meaning to personal experience.
- *Symptom Patterns: The Subjective Experience—S Axis.* The third dimension takes as its starting point the DSM and ICD categories and depicts the affective states, cognitive processes, somatic experiences, and relational patterns most often associated with each. The S Axis presents symptom patterns in terms of patients' most common personal experiences of their difficulties, and also in terms of clinicians' typical subjective responses to them. In addition, this axis includes descriptions of psychological experiences (e.g., conditions related to gender identity, sexual orientation, and minority status) that may require clinical attention.

The order of these axes varies by section. In adults, personality is evaluated before mental functioning, whereas the assessment of children, adolescents, and the elderly starts with their mental functioning. Our rationale for this inconsistency is that by adulthood, personality (Axis P) has become quite stable and usually requires primary clinical focus, whereas in children and adolescents, developmental issues (Axis M) typically take precedence in clinical evaluations over emerging personality patterns. Late in the life cycle, adaptation to various aspects of aging (Axis M) may again be more important to assess than personality trends. The multiaxial approach for the

Infancy and Early Childhood section (Part IV/Chapter 10) differs from the others because of the unique qualities of the first 3 years. It focuses on functional emotional developmental capacities, regulatory–sensory processing capacity, relational patterns and disorders, and other medical and neurological diagnoses.

Updating and Refining the Original PDM

The first edition of the PDM had three sections: (I) Adult Mental Health Disorders; (II) Child and Adolescent Mental Health Disorders (which included Infancy and Early Childhood Disorders); and (III) Conceptual and Research Foundations. Except with infants and preschoolers, clinicians were asked to assess each patient's level of personality organization and prevalent personality styles or disorders (P Axis); level of overall mental functioning (M Axis); and subjective experience of symptoms (S Axis).

The original PDM met with considerable success in the United States and Europe. On January 24, 2006, *The New York Times* reported positively on it. The manual also received some welcome in the clinical literature, as in a 2011 special issue of the *Journal of Personality Assessment* (see Bornstein, 2011; Huprich & Meyer, 2011; McWilliams, 2011b) and several favorable book reviews (e.g., Michels, 2007). In 2009, Paul Stepansky called the first PDM a "stunning success." In the decade after its publication, several national symposia were held on the manual. An Italian translation was published in 2008. PDM's influence has also been documented in Germany, Spain, Portugal, Turkey, France, and New Zealand (Del Corno & Lingiardi, 2012). In some countries (e.g., New Zealand), PDM diagnosis is accepted by governmental authorities who fund treatment. Gordon (2009) found that diverse psychotherapists evaluated the first PDM favorably, regardless of theoretical orientation. Participants in his study emphasized the value of its jargon-free language and usefulness in helping nonpsychodynamic clinicians to formulate a clinically relevant diagnosis.

In *The Pocket Guide to the DSM-5 Diagnostic Exam*, Nussbaum (2013) states:

> ICD-10 is focused on public health, whereas the *Psychodynamic Diagnostic Manual* (PDM) focuses on the psychological health and distress of a particular person. Several psychoanalytical groups joined together to create PDM as a complement to the descriptive systems of DSM-5 and ICD-10. Like DSM-5, PDM includes dimensions that cut across diagnostic categories, along with a thorough account of personality patterns and disorders. PDM uses the DSM diagnostic categories but includes accounts of the internal experience of a person presenting for treatment. (pp. 243–244)

In October 2013, the American Psychoanalytic Association noted:

> No two people with depression, bereavement, anxiety or any other mental illness or disorder will have the same potentials, needs for treatment or responses to efforts to help. Whether or not one finds great value in the descriptive diagnostic nomenclature exemplified by the DSM-5, psychoanalytic diagnostic assessment is an essential complementary assessment pathway which aims to provide an understanding of each person in depth as a unique and complex individual and should be part of a thorough assessment of every patient. Even for psychiatric disorders with a strong biological basis, psychological factors contribute to the onset, worsening, and expression of illness. Psychological factors also influence how every patient engages in treatment; the quality of the therapeutic alliance has been shown to be the strongest predictor of outcome for illness in all modalities. For

> information about a diagnostic framework that describes both the deeper and surface levels of symptom patterns, as well as an individual's personality and emotional and social functioning, mental health professionals are referred to the *Psychodynamic Diagnostic Manual.* (apsa.org, October 2013, quoted in Lingiardi & McWilliams, 2015, p. 238)

Given the success of the first edition, and in response to feedback about its strengths and weaknesses, we decided to revise the original PDM to enhance its empirical rigor and clinical utility (see Clarkin, 2015; Gazzillo et al., 2015; Huprich et al., 2015; Lingiardi et al., 2015; Lingiardi & McWilliams, 2015). The PDM-2 project would never have been achieved without Stanley Greenspan (1941–2010), our Magellan who showed us the way; Nancy Greenspan, a devoted caretaker of her late husband's legacy, who gave the project her unfailingly helpful support; and Robert S. Wallerstein (1921–2014), our Honorary Chair until his death. One of his last letters mentioned his hopes for this manual: "I am happy that PDM will have an enduring life. . . . I do give you my very best wishes for a really successful job in continuing the legacy of PDM."

PDM-2 is based on more systematic and empirical research than that which informed the first edition, especially as such research influences more operationalized descriptions of the different disorders. (Each chapter of the manual includes a Bibliography, which provides not only the references specifically cited in the chapter text, but additional references on the topics covered in that chapter.) Seven task forces have helped to draft its six sections: (I) Adulthood, (II) Adolescence, (III) Childhood, (IV) Infancy and Early Childhood, (V) Later Life, and (VI) Assessment and Clinical Illustrations. Although this second edition preserves the main structure of the first PDM, it is characterized by several important changes and innovations.

In light of research since 2006 supporting the clinical utility of this concept, the P Axis now includes a psychotic level of personality organization. This axis has been integrated and reformulated according to theoretical, clinical, and research indications, including empirically sound measures such as the SWAP-200, SWAP-II, and SWAP-200—Adolescents. A borderline personality typological description has been added, while a dissociative personality type is no longer included (instead, the section on dissociative symptoms has been expanded). In the M Axis for Adulthood, we have increased the number of mental functions from 9 to 12. An assessment procedure with a Likert-style scale is associated with each mental function. The S Axis is integrated more closely with the DSM-5 and ICD-10 systems. In addition, we give a fuller explanation of the rationale for the description of "affective states," "cognitive patterns," "somatic states," and "relationship patterns." This chapter more thoroughly depicts both the common subjective experiences of the patient and the likely countertransference reactions of the clinician.

In PDM-2, we have separated the section on Adolescence (ages 12–19) from the section on Childhood (ages 4–11) because it seems clinically naive to use the same levels and patterns for describing the respective mental functioning of, say, a 4-year-old and a 14-year-old. We have retained the recommendation to assess first on the M Axis, thus guiding the application of the P and S Axes. The section on Infancy and Early Childhood includes more detailed discussion of developmental lines and homotypic–heterotypic continuities of early infancy, childhood, adolescent, and adult psychopathology. We improve the definitions of the quality of primary relationships, emphasizing the evaluation of family systems and their characteristic relational patterns, including attachment patterns and their possible connections to both psychopathology and normative development.

An innovation in PDM-2 is the section on Later Life—the first time such a focus has appeared in any major diagnostic manual. Given the paucity of psychodynamic studies on this life stage and its implications for psychological treatments, much of this section is based on clinical observation.

Finally, PDM-2 contains an Assessment and Clinical Illustrations section. The Psychodiagnostic Chart–2 (PDC-2) and the Psychodynamic Diagnostic Prototypes were derived from the original PDM; other measures were derived from prior studies. (The PDC-2 and versions of the PDC for different age groups are included in the Appendix to this manual.) The chapter within this section on Clinical Illustrations and PDM-2 Profiles is intended to help readers improve their formulations. Illustrative clinical vignettes appear elsewhere, but this final chapter includes five clinical cases illustrated according to the PDM-2 approach.

A substantial part of the first PDM involved articles solicited from leading psychodynamic scholars. In PDM-2, we have chosen instead to integrate the voluminous empirical literature that supports psychodynamic therapy into the sections to which the respective studies apply.

Although psychodynamic practitioners will be more familiar with PDM-2 concepts than clinicians of other orientations will be, we hope that this volume will be of interest to therapists trained in other traditions, including biological, CBT, emotion-focused, family systems, and humanistic approaches. Future clinical practice is likely to be characterized by both diversity and integration of approaches. Consequently, we considered retitling PDM as the *Psychological Diagnostic Manual*, the *Practitioner's Diagnostic Manual*, or the *Psychotherapist's Diagnostic Manual*—but our publisher felt that because the title *Psychodynamic Diagnostic Manual* is already a "brand," we would be confusing our readers. This may be, but we nevertheless emphasize both our respect for alternative terminologies and conceptualizations, and our effort to be helpful to therapists of diverse conceptual systems and therapeutic traditions. We believe that a more thorough diagnostic formulation can inform any treatment plan seeking to take the whole person into account. And we think that even fondly held ideas must be subject to potential disconfirmation. Hence we hope that this manual will be tested and improved in the years to come, as empirical researchers continue to investigate our assumptions, and clinicians continue to report on their applicability.

As teachers and supervisors, we realize every day how many young colleagues feel lost in a biomedical diagnostic world, and how keenly they feel the lack of a more psychologically articulated system. Without the dynamic, relational, and intersubjective aspects of diagnosing, the process stops making sense and becomes routinized and boring. It not only stresses clinicians' professional identities, but also dims or distorts their abilities to detect and describe patients' clinically salient characteristics and mental functioning, resulting in jeopardizing the clinical relationship. One of our prime motives is thus to be useful to beginning therapists.

BIBLIOGRAPHY

Abbass, A., Town, J., & Driessen, E. (2012). Intensive short-term dynamic psychotherapy: A systematic review and meta-analysis of outcome research. *Harvard Review of Psychiatry, 20*(2), 97–108.

American Psychiatric Association. (1980). *Diagnostic and statistical manual of mental disorders* (3rd ed.). Washington, DC: Author.

American Psychiatric Association. (1994). *Diagnostic and statistical manual of mental disorders* (4th ed.). Washington, DC: Author.

American Psychiatric Association. (2013). *Diagnostic*

and statistical manual of mental disorders (5th ed.). Arlington, VA: Author.

American Psychological Association. (2012). Recognition of psychotherapy effectiveness. Retrieved from *www.apa.org/about/policy/resolution-psychotherapy.aspx*.

Aron, L. (2012). Rethinking "doublethinking": Psychoanalysis and scientific research—An introduction to a series. *Psychoanalytic Dialogues, 22*(6), 704–709.

Bateman, A. W., & Fonagy, P. (2009). Randomized controlled trial of outpatient mentalization-based treatment versus structured clinical management for borderline personality disorder. *American Journal of Psychiatry, 166*(12), 1355–1364.

Betan, E., Heim, A. K., Zittel Conklin, C., & Westen, D. (2005). Countertransference phenomena and personality pathology in clinical practice: An empirical investigation. *American Journal of Psychiatry, 162*(5), 890–898.

Blatt, S. J. (2008). *Polarities of experience: Relatedness and self-definition in personality development, psychopathology, and the therapeutic process*. Washington, DC: American Psychological Association.

Bornstein, R. F. (2011). From symptom to process: How the PDM alters goals and strategies in psychological assessment. *Journal of Personality Assessment, 93*(2), 142–150.

Bornstein, R. F. (2015). Personality assessment in the diagnostic manuals: On mindfulness, multiple methods, and test score discontinuities. *Journal of Personality Assessment, 97*, 446–455.

Bornstein, R. F., & Becker-Materro, N. (2011). Reconnecting psychoanalysis to mainstream psychology: Metaphor as glue. *Psychoanalytic Inquiry, 31*, 172–184.

Borsboom, D. (2008). Psychometric perspectives on diagnostic systems. *Journal of Clinical Psychology, 64*, 1089–1108.

Bradley, R., Heim, A. K., & Westen, D. (2005). Transference patterns in the psychotherapy of personality disorders: Empirical investigation. *British Journal of Psychiatry, 186*, 342–349.

Buchheim, A., Viviani, R., Kessler, H., Kaëchele, H., Cierpka, M., Roth, G., . . . Taubner, S. (2012). Changes in prefrontal–limbic function in major depression after 15 months of long-term psychotherapy. *PLoS ONE, 7*(3), 1–8.

Clarkin, J. F. (2015). A commentary on "The *Psychodynamic Diagnostic Manual* Version 2 (PDM-2): Assessing patients for improved clinical practice and research." *Psychoanalytic Psychology, 32*(1), 116–120.

Clarkin, J. F., Caligor, E., Stern, B. L., & Kernberg, O. F. (2004). *Structured Interview of Personality Organization (STIPO)*. Unpublished manuscript, Personality Disorders Institute, Weill Cornell Medical College, New York.

Clarkin, J. F., Levy, K. N., Lenzenweger, M. F., & Kernberg, O. F. (2007). Evaluating three treatments for borderline personality disorder: A multiwave study. *American Journal of Psychiatry, 164*, 922–928.

Colli, A., Tanzilli, A., Dimaggio, G., & Lingiardi, V. (2014). Patient personality and therapist response: An empirical investigation. *American Journal of Psychiatry, 171*, 102–108.

Del Corno, F., & Lingiardi, V. (2012). The *Psychodynamic Diagnostic Manual* (PDM) in the U.S.A. and in Europe: Between commercial success and influence on professionals and researchers. *Bollettino di Psicologia Applicata, 265*, 5–10.

de Maat, S., de Jonghe, F., de Kraker, R., Leichsenring, F., Abbass, A., Luyten, P., . . . Dekker, J. (2013). The current state of the empirical evidence for psychoanalysis: A meta-analytic approach. *Harvard Review of Psychiatry, 21*(3), 107–137.

Diener, M. J., Hilsenroth, M. J., & Weinberger, J. (2007). Therapist affect focus and patient outcomes in psychodynamic psychotherapy: A meta-analysis. *American Journal of Psychiatry, 164*(6), 936–941.

Eagle, M. N., & Wolitzky, D. L. (2011). Systematic empirical research versus clinical case studies: A valid antagonism? *Journal of the American Psychoanalytic Association, 59*(4), 791–817.

Fluckinger, C., Del Re, A. C., Wampold, B. E., Symonds, D., & Horvath, A. O. (2012). How central is alliance in psychotherapy?: A multilevel longitudinal meta-analysis. *Journal of Consulting Psychology, 59*(1), 10–17.

Fonagy, P. (2013). There is room for even more doublethink: The perilous status of psychoanalytic research. *Psychoanalytic Dialogues, 23*, 116–122.

Fonagy, P. (2015). The effectiveness of psychodynamic psychotherapies: An update. *World Psychiatry, 14*(2), 137–150.

Frances, A. (2013). *Saving normal: An insider's revolt against out-of-control psychiatric diagnosis, DSM-5, Big Pharma, and the medicalization of ordinary life*. New York: Morrow.

Gazzillo, F., Lingiardi, V., Del Corno, F., Genova, F., Bornstein, R. F., Gordon, R. M., & McWilliams, N. (2015). Clinicians' emotional responses and *Psychodynamic Diagnostic Manual* adult personality disorders: A clinically relevant empirical investigation. *Psychotherapy, 52*(2), 238–246.

Gordon, R. M. (2009), Reactions to the *Psychodynamic Diagnostic Manual* (PDM) by psychodynamic, CBT and other non-psychodynamic psychologists. *Issues in Psychoanalytic Psychiatry, 31*, 55–62.

Hoffman, I. Z. (2009). Doublethinking our way to "scientific" legitimacy: The dessiccation of human experience. *Journal of the American Psychoanalytic Association, 57*(5), 1043–1069.

Hoffman, I. Z. (2012a). Response to Eagle and Wolitzky. *Journal of American Psychoanalytic Association, 60*, 105–120.

Hoffman, I. Z. (2012b). Response to Safran: The development of critical psychoanalytic sensibility. *Psychoanalytic Dialogues, 22*(6), 721–731.

Høglend, P. (2014). Exploration of the patient–therapist relationship in psychotherapy. *American Journal of Psychiatry, 7*, 1056–1066.

Hummelen, B., Pedersen, G., Wilberg, T., & Karterud, S. (2015). Poor validity of the DSM-IV schizoid personality disorder construct as a diagnostic category. *Journal of Personality Disorders, 29*(3), 334–346.

Huprich, S. K., McWilliams, N., Lingiardi, V., Bornstein, R. F., Gazzillo, F., & Gordon, R. M. (2015). The *Psychodynamic Diagnostic Manual* (PDM) and the PDM-2: Opportunities to significantly affect the profession. *Psychoanalytic Inquiry, 35*, 60–73.

Huprich, S. K., & Meyer, G. J. (2011). Introduction to the JPA special issue: Can the *Psychodynamic Diagnostic Manual* put the complex person back at the center stage of personality assessment? *Journal of Personality Assessment, 93*, 109–111.

Kächele, H., Albani, C., Buchheim, A., Hölzer, M., Hohage, R., Mergenthaler, E., . . . Thomä, H. (2006). The German specimen case, Amalia X: Empirical studies. *International Journal of Psychoanalysis, 87*, 809–826.

Kandel, E. R. (1999). Biology and the future of psychoanalysis: A new intellectual framework for psychiatry revisited. *American Journal of Psychiatry, 156*, 505–524.

Kernberg, O. F. (1984). *Severe personality disorders: Psychotherapeutic strategies.* New Haven, CT: Yale University Press.

Leichsenring, F., Leweke, F., Klein, S., & Steinert, C. (2015). The empirical status of psychodynamic psychotherapy—An update: Bambi's alive and kicking. *Psychotherapy and Psychosomatics, 84*, 129–148.

Levy, R., Ablon, J. S., & Kächele, H. (2012). *Psychodynamic psychotherapy research: Evidence-based practice and practice-based evidence.* New York: Springer.

Lingiardi, V., Gazzillo, F., & Waldron, S. (2010). An empirically supported psychoanalysis: The case of Giovanna. *Psychoanalytic Psychology, 27*(2), 190–218.

Lingiardi, V., Holmqvist, R., & Safran, J. D. (2016). Relational turn and psychotherapy research. *Contemporary Psychoanalysis, 52*, 275–312.

Lingiardi, V., & McWilliams, N. (2015). The *Psychodynamic Diagnostic Manual*—2nd edition (PDM-2). *World Psychiatry, 14*(2), 237–239.

Lingiardi, V., McWilliams, N., Bornstein, R. F., Gazzillo, F., & Gordon, R. M. (2015). The *Psychodynamic Diagnostic Manual Version 2* (PDM-2): Assessing patients for improved clinical practice and research. *Psychoanalytic Psychology, 32*(1), 94–115.

Lingiardi, V., Shedler, J., & Gazzillo, F. (2006). Assessing personality change in psychotherapy with the SWAP-200: A case study. *Journal of Personality Assessment, 86*(1), 36–45.

McWilliams, N. (2011a). *Psychoanalytic diagnosis: Understanding personality structure in the clinical process* (2nd ed.). New York: Guilford Press.

McWilliams, N. (2011b). The *Psychodynamic Diagnostic Manual*: An effort to compensate for the limitations of descriptive psychiatric diagnosis. *Journal of Personality Assessment, 93*, 112–122.

McWilliams, N. (2013). Psychoanalysis and research: Some reflections and opinions. *Psychoanalytic Review, 100*(6), 919–945.

Michels, R. (2007). Review of "Psychodynamic diagnostic manual." *International Journal of Psychoanalysis, 88*(4), 1105–1108.

Norcross, J. C. (Ed.). (2011). *Psychotherapy relationships that work* (2nd ed.). New York: Oxford University Press.

Norcross, J. C., & Wampold, B. E. (2011). What works for whom: Tailoring psychotherapy to the person. *Journal of Clinical Psychology, 67*(2), 127–132.

Nussbaum, A. M. (2013). *The pocket guide to the DSM-5 diagnostic exam.* Arlington, VA: American Psychiatric Association.

OPD Task Force. (Eds.). (2008). *Operationalized psychodynamic diagnosis—OPD-2: Manual of diagnosis and treatment planning.* Cambridge, MA: Hogrefe & Huber.

PDM Task Force. (2006). *Psychodynamic diagnostic manual.* Silver Spring, MD: Alliance of Psychoanalytic Organizations.

Safran, J. D. (2012). Doublethinking or dialectical thinking: A critical appreciation of Hoffman's "doublethinking" critique. *Psychoanalytic Dialogues, 22*(6), 710–720.

Schore, A. N. (2014). The right brain is dominant in psychotherapy. *Psychotherapy, 51*(3), 388–397.

Shapiro, D. (1965). *Neurotic styles.* New York: Basic Books.

Shedler, J. (2010). The efficacy of psychodynamic psychotherapy. *American Psychologist, 65*(2), 98–109.

Stepansky, P. E. (2009). *Psychoanalysis at the margins.* New York: Other Press.

Strupp, H. H. (1963). The outcome problem in psychotherapy revisited. *Psychotherapy: Theory, Research, and Practice, 1*, 1–13.

Tyrer, P., Reed, G. M., & Crawford, M. J. (2015). Classification, assessment, prevalence, and effect of personality disorder. *Lancet, 385*, 717–726.

Vivona, J. (2012). Between a rock and hard science: How should psychoanalysis respond to pressures for quantitative evidence of effectiveness? *Journal of the American Psychoanalytic Association, 60*(1), 121–129.

Wampold, B. E. (2013). The good, the bad and the ugly: A 50-year perspective on the outcome problem. *Psychotherapy, 50*(1), 16–24.

Wampold, B. E., & Imel, Z. E. (2015). *The great psychotherapy debate: The evidence for what makes psychotherapy work* (2nd ed.). New York: Routledge.

Westen, D., Gabbard, G., & Blagov, P. (2006). Back to the future: Personality structure as a context for psychopathology. In R. F. Krueger & J. L. Tackett (Eds.), *Personality and psychopathology: Building bridges* (pp. 335–384). New York: Guilford Press.

Westen, D., Novotny, C. M., & Thompson-Brenner, H. (2004). The empirical status of empirically supported psychotherapies: Assumptions, findings, and reporting in controlled clinical trials. *Psychological Bulletin, 130*, 631–663.

Westen, D., & Shedler, J. (1999a). Revising and assessing Axis II: Part 1. Developing a clinically and empirically valid assessment method. *American Journal of Psychiatry, 156*, 258–272.

Westen, D., & Shedler, J. (1999b). Revising and assessing Axis II: Part 2. Toward an empirically based and clinically useful classification of personality disorders. *American Journal of Psychiatry, 156*, 273–285.

Westen, D., Waller, N. G., Shedler, J., & Blagov, P. S. (2014). Dimensions of personality and personality pathology: Factor structure of the Shedler–Westen Assessment Procedure–II (SWAP-II). *Journal of Personality Disorders, 28*, 281–318.

Westen, D., & Weinberger, J. (2004). When clinical description becomes statistical prediction. *American Psychologist, 59*, 595–613.

Zimmermann, J., Ehrenthal, J. C., Cierpka, M., Schauenburg, J., Doering, S., & Benecke, C. (2012). Assessing the level of structural integration using *Operationalized Psychodynamic Diagnosis* (OPD): Implications for DSM-5. *Journal of Personality Assessment, 94*(5), 522–532.

PART I

Adulthood

CHAPTER 1

Personality Syndromes
P Axis

CHAPTER EDITORS

Nancy McWilliams, PhD **Jonathan Shedler, PhD**

CONSULTANTS

Allan Abbass, MD
John F. Clarkin, PhD
Ferhan Dereboy, MD
Glen O. Gabbard, MD
Brin Grenyer, PhD
Steven Huprich, PhD
Robert Michels, MD
Judith Rosenberger, PhD, LCSW

Introduction

A model of personality is ultimately a form of map. Its purpose is to help users find their bearings, orient themselves with respect to recognizable landmarks, and navigate. Different maps serve different purposes (e.g., road maps, topographical maps, political maps). The purposes of the P-Axis "map" of PDM-2 are to deepen clinical practitioners' understanding of their patients and to help them navigate the terrain of treatment.

Other personality maps, such as those included in the *Diagnostic and Statistical Manual of Mental Disorders* (currently DSM-5; American Psychiatric Association, 2013) and the *International Classification of Diseases* (currently ICD-10; World Health Organization, 2000), serve different purposes. They have advantages and disadvantages, but clinical practitioners generally do not feel that they provide a level of psychological understanding sufficient to guide clinical treatment (e.g., Spitzer, First, Shedler, Westen, & Skodal, 2008). The P-Axis map is intended expressly for this purpose.

A fundamental difference between the DSM and ICD maps and the P-Axis map is that the former are taxonomies of *disorders*, whereas the latter is an effort to represent kinds of *people* (for further discussion of differences and of the rationale for the PDM-2 system, see Appendix 1.1 at the end of this chapter). It aims to promote clinical case formulation—that is, to help clinicians understand an individual's difficulties in the larger context of personality functioning. Such an understanding can inform decisions about whether and when psychotherapy may be helpful, and how to conduct it most effectively for a particular person. Case formulation is also clinically helpful for patients who are *not* in psychotherapy—for example, in helping clinicians understand and address treatment nonadherence, manage trauma or grief, or work effectively in rehabilitation settings. Although the concepts we present here may be most familiar to clinicians with psychodynamic backgrounds, our goal is to provide information that can deepen the understanding and enhance the effectiveness of clinicians of any theoretical orientation (Lingiardi & McWilliams, 2015).

The major organizing principles of the P Axis are (1) *level* of personality organization and (2) personality *style* or *type*. The former is a spectrum describing severity of personality dysfunction that ranges from healthy, through neurotic and borderline, to psychotic levels of personality organization. The latter represents clinically familiar personality styles or types that cross-cut levels of personality organization. The concept of personality style does not inherently connote either health or pathology, but rather core psychological themes and organizing principles. By locating an individual patient with respect to level of organization and personality style, a clinician can begin to develop a case formulation psychologically rich enough to guide effective treatment.

Conceptualizing Personality

Personality is more about who one *is* than about what disorder one *has*. It comprises considerably more than what is readily observable via behavior alone; it subsumes a range of internal psychological processes (motives, fantasies, characteristic patterns of thought and feeling, ways of experiencing self and others, ways of coping and defending, etc.). Irrespective of overt "presenting problems," many patients come to realize, as they participate in therapy, that their difficulties are inextricably tied up with who they are. They need their clinicians to comprehend something psychologically systemic that helps them understand why they are repeatedly vulnerable to certain kinds of suffering. Psychological problems are often complexly intertwined with personality, may be the flip side of a person's strengths, and need to be appreciated in the context of the whole person, as well as the larger relational and cultural contexts in which the person is embedded. (Note that our use of the term "personality" subsumes what has historically been termed "character." See Appendix 1.2 at the end of this chapter for definitions of "personality," "character," "temperament," "traits," "type," "style," and "defense.")

For purposes of psychotherapy aimed at shifting something psychologically fundamental, understanding a person's overall psychological makeup and developmental trajectories may ultimately be more important than classifying symptoms or mastering specific techniques (American Psychological Association, 2012; Norcross, 2011). Consequently, a skilled therapist conducting a clinical interview not only assesses the patient's current symptoms and mental status, and evaluates the sociocultural context of the immediate problem, but also tries to get a feel for the patient's personality, including strengths, weaknesses, and major organizing themes. In psychotherapy outcome studies, investigators are starting to attend to the role of personality differences (e.g., Blatt, 1990, 1992, 1993, 2008; Duncan, Miller, Wampold, & Hubble, 2010; Gabbard, 2009a, 2009b; Horowitz et al., 1996; Roth & Fonagy, 2005; Westen, Novotny, & Thompson-Brenner, 2004)—an emphasis that is crucial to clinical practitioners, but notably absent from most empirical research.

Personality Styles versus Personality Disorders

There is no hard and fast distinction between a personality *type* or *style* and a personality *disorder*. All people have personality styles. The term "disorder" is a linguistic convenience for clinicians, denoting a degree of extremity or rigidity that causes significant dysfunction, suffering, or impairment. One can have, for example, a narcissistic personality *style* without having narcissistic personality *disorder*.

An essential consideration in diagnosing personality disorder is evidence that the person's psychology causes significant distress to self or others, is of long duration, and is so much a part of the person's experience that he or she cannot remember, or easily imagine, being different. Some individuals with personality pathology are unaware of, or unconcerned with, their problematic patterns and come to treatment at the urging of others. Some come on their own, often seeking treatment not for personality patterns but for some more specific, circumscribed distress: anxiety, depression, eating disorders, somatic symptoms, addictions, phobias, self-harm, trauma, and relationship problems, among others.

It is crucial to differentiate personality from symptom syndromes, organic brain syndromes, and psychotic spectrum disorders. Ritualized behavior, for example, may indicate an obsessive–compulsive disorder unrelated to personality, or may be one piece of evidence for a pervasive obsessive–compulsive personality disorder, or may express a psychotic delusion, or may be the result of an organic brain syndrome.

It is also vital to evaluate whether what appears to be a personality disorder is a response to ongoing situational stress. For example, a man who had no notable psychological problems before leaving his homeland, but who has moved into a society whose language he does not speak, may appear paranoid, dependent, or otherwise disturbed in personality functioning (Akhtar, 2011). Under sufficient strain or trauma, any of us can look borderline or even psychotic. Hence it is not possible to diagnose a personality disorder without considering other possibilities that might explain the patient's behavior.

Finally, individuals from cultures unfamiliar to the interviewer can be misunderstood as having personality disorders. Boundaries between normality and pathology are not fixed and universal; they vary, depending on cultural systems (Alarcón & Foulks, 1995a, 1995b; Kakar, 2008; Kitayama & Markus, 1999; Lewis-Fernández et al., 2014; Tummala-Narra, 2016).

Level of Personality Organization (Severity of Disturbance)

The Continuum of Personality Health

The recognition that personality health–disturbance is a dimension or continuum has evolved over decades of clinical observation and research. At the healthy end of the continuum are people who show good functioning in all or most domains. They usually can engage in satisfying relationships, experience and understand a relatively full range of age-expected feelings and thoughts, function relatively flexibly when stressed by external events or internal conflict, maintain a relatively coherent sense of personal identity, express impulses in a manner appropriate to the situation, conduct themselves in accordance with internalized moral values, and neither suffer undue distress nor impose it on others.

At the severely disturbed end of the continuum are people who respond to distress in rigidly inflexible ways, for example, by relying on a restricted range of costly or maladaptive defenses, or have major and severe deficits in many of the domains described in the Summary of Basic Mental Functioning: M Axis (e.g., self–object differentiation, affect regulation, attention, and learning; see Chapter 2, Table 2.1, pp. 118–119).

Historical Context of Levels of Personality Organization

By the end of the 19th century, psychiatric classification distinguished between two general types of problems: (1) "neurosis," a term that may refer to either minor or major psychopathology in which the capacity to perceive reality is intact; and (2) "psychosis," in which there is significant impairment in reality testing. In the ensuing decades, as clinicians slowly appreciated that many people suffer not from isolated symptoms but from issues that pervade their lives more totally, they also began to distinguish between "neurotic symptoms" and "neurotic character," or what we now call "personality disorder."

Throughout the 20th century, clinical writers began describing individuals who seemed too disturbed to be considered neurotic and yet too anchored in reality to be considered psychotic. Slowly, a "borderline" group was identified (Frosch, 1964; Knight, 1953; Main, 1957; Stern, 1938). The concept of a disturbance on the "border" between psychosis and neurosis was subsequently investigated empirically (e.g., Grinker, Werble, & Drye, 1968; Gunderson & Singer, 1975) and elaborated theoretically (e.g., Adler, 1985; Hartocollis, 1977; Kernberg, 1975, 1983, 1984; Masterson, 1972, 1976; Stone, 1980, 1986).

Patients construed as psychologically organized on that border often fared badly in the kinds of treatments that were usually helpful to healthier patients. They would unexpectedly develop intense, problematic, and often rapidly shifting attitudes toward their therapists. Some who did not show psychotic tendencies outside therapy developed intractable "psychotic transferences" (e.g., they might experience their clinicians as omnipotently good or malevolently evil, or as exactly like persons from their past, and could not be persuaded otherwise).

A consensus gradually evolved that personality syndromes exist on a continuum of severity, from a comparatively healthy to a severely disturbed level. This continuum has been conventionally, if somewhat arbitrarily, divided into "healthy," "neurotic," "borderline," and "psychotic" levels of personality organization.

Note that the term "borderline," when used by psychodynamic clinicians to denote a *level of personality organization*, has a different meaning from the term "borderline" as it used in the DSMs, in which only one specific variant of borderline personality organization has been labeled borderline personality disorder (for a discussion of subtypes and differences from complex trauma, see Lewis, Caputi, & Grenyer, 2012; Lewis & Grenyer, 2009). Our use of the term "borderline" is thus broader than that of the DSMs and more consistent with the clinical observations that gave rise to the term and its widespread professional adoption.

Although each personality style can, in principle, exist at any level of organization, some personality styles are more likely to be found at the healthier (e.g., neurotic) end of the severity spectrum, and some at the sicker (e.g., borderline, psychotic) end. For example, patients with hysterical or obsessional personality styles are more likely to be organized at a neurotic level of severity; those with paranoid or psychopathic styles are more likely to be organized at a borderline level.

The distinction between *level* of organization and personality *style* permits, for example, the identification of "quiet borderline" patients (Sherwood & Cohen, 1994), such as schizoid individuals who are psychologically organized at the borderline level of severity. In contrast, the DSM diagnosis of borderline personality disorder essentially conflates borderline organization with histrionic personality disorder (and in the process renders the diagnostic categories of borderline personality disorder and histrionic personality disorder essentially empirically indistinguishable; see Shedler & Westen, 2004). We do refer, however, to research on borderline personality disorder that is based on the DSMs' definitions, given the extensive empirical literature on the DSM-defined syndrome that has accrued since its inclusion in DSM-III in 1980.

Kernberg addressed the problem of discrepant uses of the term "borderline" by distinguishing between borderline personality *disorder* (the DSMs' concept) and borderline personality *organization* (the psychoanalytic concept). We adopt his solution here by describing a borderline level of personality organization, and additionally including borderline personality as a diagnosable P-Axis personality style or type. We recognize that the inclusion of borderline personality as a P-Axis personality style is an imperfect and inelegant solution, and is not fully consistent with the conceptual framework that we lay out in this chapter. However, given the extensive literature that exists on the DSMs' construct of borderline personality disorder and its widespread clinical acceptance, we also felt it was necessary to include it.

Recent Findings on Level of Organization

Research indicates that some problems of patients in the borderline range have a genetic component. Twin studies suggest that in both men and women, genetic influences account for about 40% of the variance in the severity of borderline traits (e.g., Distel et al., 2008; Leichsenring, Leibing, Kruse, New, & Leweke, 2011; Torgersen et al., 2008). Indeed, genetic interpersonal hypersensitivity has been put forward as an endophenotype marker (Gunderson, 2007). Neuroimaging studies have revealed the functional neuroanatomy of borderline disorders that are associated with the hypersensitivity, intolerance for aloneness, and attachment fears typical of patients in this broad diagnostic group (Buchheim et al., 2008; Fertuck et al., 2009; King-Casas et al., 2008).

Whereas past generations of psychoanalytic thinkers tended to view level of severity with fixation at, or regression to, a particular developmental challenge or stage, contemporary theorists understand personality pathology as reflecting a confluence of factors, including genetic heritability, temperament, early life experiences (e.g., trauma, neglect), and early attachments, among other factors. For a discussion of "biopsychosocial" models of personality, see, for example, Leichsenring and colleagues (2011) or Paris (1993).

As suggested by the findings of Clarkin, Kernberg, and their colleagues (e.g., Clarkin et al., 2001; Clarkin, Levy, Lenzenweger, & Kernberg, 2004, 2007; Clarkin, Yeomans, & Kernberg, 1999), and Greenspan and his colleagues (e.g., Greenspan & Shanker, 2004), we recommend evaluating where an individual's personality lies on the severity dimension by assessing the following domains, elaborated in Chapter 2:

1. Capacity for regulation, attention, and learning
2. Capacity for affective range, communication, and understanding
3. Capacity for mentalization and reflective functioning
4. Capacity for differentiation and integration (identity)
5. Capacity for relationships and intimacy
6. Capacity for self-esteem regulation and quality of internal experience
7. Capacity for impulse control and regulation
8. Capacity for defensive functioning
9. Capacity for adaptation, resiliency, and strength
10. Self-observing capacities (psychological mindedness)
11. Capacity to construct and use internal standards and ideals
12. Capacity for meaning and purpose

Chapter 2 describes a way of evaluating an individual's mental functioning that is helpful for locating his or her personality in the healthy, neurotic, borderline, or psychotic range.

Healthy Level of Organization

Psychopathology expresses the interaction of stressors and individual psychology. Some people who become symptomatic under stress have overall healthy personalities, as assessed by the Summary of Basic Mental Functioning: M Axis (see Chapter 2, Table 2.1, pp. 118–119). They may have certain favored ways of coping, but they have enough flexibility to accommodate adequately to challenging realities (though not necessarily to severe trauma, which can damage even people who may seem quite resilient; see Boulanger, 2007). We all have a characteristic style or flavor or type of personality, or a stable mixture of styles. For example, the fact that one has a consistently pessimistic outlook is not a sufficient criterion for diagnosing depressive personality disorder.

Neurotic Level of Organization

Despite having many capacities at the high end of the M Axis, individuals with neurotic-level personality organizations are notable for their relative rigidity (Shapiro, 1965, 1981, 1989, 2002). That is, they tend to respond to certain stresses with a relatively restricted range of defenses and coping strategies. Common personality styles and disorders at this point on the severity continuum are depressive personality, hysteric personality (in evolving clinical language, "hysteric" has been used to denote a constellation of dynamics at the higher-functioning ranges, while "histrionic" has denoted those dynamics in the borderline and psychotic ranges), phobic personality, and obsessive–compulsive personality.

The pattern of suffering of an individual in one of these clusters tends to be restricted to a specific area, such as loss, rejection, and self-punitiveness in depressive personality; issues of gender, sexuality, and power in hysteric–histrionic personality; and control issues in obsessive–compulsive personality. Individuals at the neurotic level of organization frequently experience their problems as involving inner discord or conflict. For example, they may feel sexual temptation, experienced as a wish in conflict with an internal prohibition, or they may find themselves recurrently angry and judgmental while simultaneously feeling that they are "overreacting."

The maladaptive defensive patterns of individuals in the neurotic range may be limited to the area of their particular difficulty. For example, in contrast to patients organized at a borderline level of severity who use defenses that tend to distort reality more globally (e.g., denial, splitting, projective identification, omnipotent control, severe dissociation), the rigid or problematic defenses of neurotic-level patients are more likely to concern one area—problems with authority, for example, rather than problems in all relationships. Outside their areas of difficulty, persons at the neurotic level may have a satisfactory work history, maintain good relations with others, tolerate dysphoric affects without taking impulsive or ill-considered actions, and be able and ready to collaborate in a therapy relationship.

Neurotic-level patients often have some perspective on their recurrent difficulties and can imagine how they would like to change, and they usually form adequate working alliances with their clinicians. In initial interviews, therapists tend to react to them comfortably, respectfully, sympathetically, and with the expectation of a collaborative partnership.

Borderline Level of Organization

People with borderline personality organization have difficulties with affect regulation and are consequently vulnerable to extremes of overwhelming affect, including episodes of intense depression, anxiety, and rage. They may have recurrent relational difficulties; severe problems with emotional intimacy; problems with work; and problems with impulse regulation, including vulnerability to substance abuse and other addictive behaviors (gambling, shoplifting, binge eating, sexual compulsion, addiction to video games or the internet, etc.). In periods of distress (e.g., when an attachment relationship is threatened), they are also at greater risk for self-harm, including self-mutilation, sexual risk taking, accumulation of inordinate debt, and other self-destructive activities (Bourke & Grenyer, 2010, 2013; Clarkin et al., 1999; Yeomans, Clarkin, & Kernberg, 2015).

Such behavior can reflect desperate efforts to regulate unbearable affect, failures in impulse regulation, or both. Generally speaking, individuals with personality pathology severe enough to warrant a DSM personality disorder diagnosis function at a borderline level of organization, irrespective of the specific DSM personality disorder diagnosis (e.g., Yeomans et al., 2015). The borderline level of personality organization can be divided into a higher level (toward the border with the neuroses), describing patients whose overall personality presentation is closer to a neurotic personality organization (Caligor, Kernberg, & Clarkin, 2007), and a lower level (toward the border with the psychoses), describing patients with more severe deficits (Clarkin et al., 2006; Kernberg, 1984). Patients with higher versus lower borderline levels of personality organization may require different therapeutic approaches—that is, more exploratory (i.e., interpretive, insight-oriented) treatments for higher-level patients, and more supportive, capacity-building treatments for lower-level borderline patients.

Clinicians whose descriptions of patients were studied with the Shedler–Westen Assessment Procedure (SWAP; Lingiardi, Shedler, & Gazzillo, 2006; Shedler, 2015; Westen & Shedler, 1999a, 1999b, 2007; Westen, Shedler, Bradley, & DeFife, 2012) have emphasized the affect and impulse regulation problems of individuals with borderline personality organization. They comment on the extremity and rawness of these clients' emotions, and also on their reliance on defenses that many scholars have termed "primitive," "immature," or "costly" (see, e.g., Cramer, 2006; Kernberg, 1984; Kramer, de Roten, Perry, & Despland, 2013; Laughlin, 1979; Perry & Cooper, 1989; Perry & Presniak, 2013; Perry, Presniak, & Olson, 2013; Vaillant, Bond, & Vaillant, 1986). Given that neurotic-level individuals may also use primitive defenses under stress, it is arguable that what differentiates borderline from neurotic-level psychology may have more to do with the absence of mature defenses than with the presence of immature ones (McWilliams, 2011).

The most commonly noted costly or primitive defenses are splitting and projective identification. "Splitting" is the tendency to compartmentalize positive and negative perceptions and feelings, and consequently to view self and others in caricatured, black-or-white, all-good or all-bad categories (e.g., as heroes and rescuers, villains and abusers, or coldly indifferent witnesses to abuse). Splitting may involve viewing certain people as "all good" and others as "all bad," or may involve alternating contradictory perceptions of the same person (e.g., Gairdner, 2002; Main, 1957).

A consequence of splitting is a failure to integrate disparate aspects of identity into a coherent whole. Consequently, patients whose personalities are organized at a borderline level show "identity diffusion": Their attitudes, values, goals, and feelings about self are unstable and changing, and their self-perceptions can oscillate between polarized extremes. Such patients may look quite different on different occasions, as different compartmentalized aspects of identity emerge. For example, when feeling good, they may appear blithely indifferent to the fact that they were suicidally depressed the prior week; when depressed, they may appear to have no access whatever to any positive feelings or self-perceptions.

"Projective identification" involves failing to recognize a disturbing aspect of one's own personality, misattributing it to another person (e.g., the clinician), and then treating that person accordingly—until eventually evoking from the other person the feelings and attitudes that they have projected with such conviction. Clinicians on the receiving end of such projective identifications may feel such intense pressure to conform to the projections that their experience is one of having their minds taken over or "colonized" by something alien (Gabbard, 2009a).

Other defenses characteristic of persons in the borderline range include "denial" (ignoring or disregarding things that are disturbing, as if they did not exist); "withdrawal" (into fantasy); indiscriminate forms of "introjection" (sometimes called "introjective identification"—the wholesale "taking in" of someone else's characteristics, attitudes, and even mannerisms); "omnipotent control" (treating another as an extension of oneself, with little recognition that the other person is a separate human being); "acting out" (repetitively living out an internal drama that cannot be remembered, felt, or conceptualized); "somatization" (developing physical symptoms under stress); severe "dissociation" (incongruous disconnections between different aspects of experience, or shifts of self-states without any sense of the continuity of experience); "primitive idealization" (seeing another as all-good and larger than life, as a small child might see an admired adult); and "primitive devaluation" (seeing another as completely worthless, with no redeeming qualities whatever). Vaillant's (1992) research adds hypochondriacal concerns and passive aggression to the list of psychologically costly defenses that may signal a more severe personality disorder.

The division of defenses into "primitive" or "immature" versus "mature" or "higher-order," despite still being somewhat underresearched, has become common in the literature on severe personality disorders and in empirical research on psychological defenses (e.g., Cramer, 2006, 2015; Di Giuseppe, Perry, Petraglia, Janzen, & Lingiardi, 2014; Drapeau, De Roten, Perry, & Despland, 2003; Hibbard & Porcerelli, 1998; Lingiardi, Lonati, Fossati, Vanzulli, & Maffei, 1999; Perry, 1990, 1993; Perry & Kardos, 1995; Perry, Kardos, & Pagano, 1993; Porcerelli, Cogan, Kamoo, & Miller, 2010; Porcerelli & Hibbard, 2004). (See the discussion of defenses in Appendix 1.2 at the end of this chapter for more on this topic.)

In contrast to the benign compassion that patients with neurotic-level personality disorders tend to elicit in clinicians, patients with borderline organization, especially those at the lower level, evoke intense emotions that clinicians may struggle to contain and manage. Often these are negative—fear, confusion, helplessness, or hostility, for example; yet powerful rescue fantasies, sexual desire, and wishes to cure the patient by love are also common (Betan, Heim, Zittel Conklin, & Westen, 2005; Bourke & Grenyer, 2010; Colli, Tanzilli, Dimaggio, & Lingiardi, 2014; Dahl, Røssberg, Bøgwald, Gabbard, & Høglend, 2012; Gazzillo et al., 2015; Lingiardi, Tanzilli, & Colli, 2015b; Røssberg, Karterud, Pedersen, & Friis, 2007). Patients with severe personality disorders tend to evoke strong tendencies in their therapists to *act*, often in ways incongruent with their professional roles. Clinicians may find themselves wanting to attack these patients or to cross professional boundaries to "save" them (Groves, 1978; Guthiel, 2005; Kernberg, 1984).

Psychotic Level of Organization

The traditional conceptualization of psychosis involves a break with reality. Some patients who have never had a diagnosed psychotic illness, or who have had episodes of psychosis from which they seem to recover quickly and completely, may nonetheless have psychotic features such as overgeneralized, concrete, or bizarre thinking; socially inappropriate behaviors; pervasive and severe annihilation anxiety; and the unshakable conviction that their own attributions about someone are correct, regardless of anything the other person may say or do. People with the most severe personality disorders may impute their own thoughts and feelings to others, become convinced of the rightness of their most erroneous perceptions, and act on the basis of these perceptions. In response to terrifying anxieties, they may use primitive defenses such as psychotic denial, autistic withdrawal, distortion, delusional projection, fragmentation, and concretization (Berney, De Roten, Beretta, Kramer, & Despland, 2014; Vaillant, 1971).

A psychotic level of personality organization implies identity diffusion, poor differentiation between representations of self and others, poor discrimination between fantasy and external reality, reliance on primitive defenses, and severe deficits in reality testing. An example of a person with psychotic personality organization would be a man who stalks his love object in the conviction that this person "really" loves him, despite all of the person's protestations to the contrary. Such behavior demonstrates both a deficit in reality testing and a lack of differentiation between self and other.

Seasoned therapists have long reported that they understand their most disturbed patients to be organized at a psychotic level, even when those patients have never had a diagnosed psychotic illness. Clinical explorations that assume a psychotic range of functioning include the writings of Bion (1967), Kernberg (1984), McWilliams (2015), Rosenfeld (1987), Steiner (1993, 2011), and others. In contrast, researchers have tended to think about psychosis in the framework of a medical model, as a discrete illness. Since the publication of the first PDM, the clinical utility of conceptualizing a psychotic range of personality functioning has gained additional research support (see Lingiardi, McWilliams, Bornstein, Gazzillo, & Gordon, 2015a). We note in this connection that DSM-5 includes schizotypal personality disorder in both its "personality disorders" and its "schizophrenia spectrum and other psychotic disorders" chapters, suggesting that a similar clinical presentation may reflect a personality syndrome *or* a psychotic illness, or some combination of both (see also Chapter 3 of this manual on the S Axis).

Examples of individuals who may be usefully understood as functioning in the psychotic range include anorexic patients who are dangerously close to starvation, but who believe they are overweight; people with extreme compulsions (e.g., severe hoarding) who cling to their rituals and experience annihilation anxiety when asked to consider *not* acting on their compulsions; somatizing patients who regard their own bodies as sadistic persecutors; dissociative patients who cannot distinguish past trauma from present reality; patients with severe factitious disorders; and individuals who suffer from recurrent and severe paranoid reactions, even in the absence of hallucinations or frank delusions. In all these instances, the patients' "fixed ideas" are so absolute as to approach delusional proportions. Attempts to question the fixed beliefs often lead patients to react with anxiety and hostility or to experience their clinicians as dangerous.

Clinical Implications of the Severity Dimension for Psychotherapy

For seasoned therapists, a patient's location on the severity dimension has important implications for treatment focus, level of therapist activity, explicitness of limit setting, frequency of sessions, and other aspects of intervention. Sometimes this adaptation to a patient is intuitive, and sometimes it reflects the therapists' training to the effect that there is a continuum from exploratory to supportive treatment that correlates roughly with the level-of-organization dimension. The addition to PDM-2 of both a chapter on assessment tools (see Chapter 15) and a discussion of "Most Relevant Assessment Tools" for each capacity of the M Axis (see Chapter 2) has, among other aims, the goal of making it easier for clinicians to evaluate each patient's overall level of functioning, along with particular strengths and weaknesses in more specific domains.

Certain inferences typically follow from an evaluation of the level of severity of personality disturbance. First, some caveats: We offer general recommendations for which many exceptions exist; they are not "rules." These ranges lack clearly demarcated boundaries, and as many clinical writers have noted, even psychologically healthy individuals can look borderline or psychotic when they are seriously misunderstood or under severe stress. Ignorance of cultural differences can lead therapists to pathologize individuals whose behavior is unfamiliar but congruent with their own cultural norms. Finally, the unique qualities of a given patient may obviate common clinical wisdom about the implications of severity levels.

Individuals who are psychologically organized in the neurotic-to-healthy range tend to be helped by psychodynamic and psychoanalytic therapies that emphasize self-understanding and insight (Grenyer, 2012; National Health and Medical Research Council, 2012; National Institute for Health and Clinical Excellence, 2009; Project

Air Strategy, 2015; Zanarini, 2009). They may also be helped by other approaches because their capacity to form a therapeutic alliance improves prognosis in any treatment: It will increase the likelihood of their taking medication as prescribed when receiving pharmacological treatment, or the likelihood of their doing homework assignments for cognitive-behavioral treatment (CBT), or their willingness to experience and express the feelings evoked in emotion-focused therapy.

For those with a personality disorder, longer-term or open-ended therapy may provide significant help (Caligor et al., 2007). There is also evidence that short-term, highly focused psychodynamic treatments can have a beneficial effect (Abbass, 2015; Abbass et al., 2014; Abbass, Town, & Driessen, 2011; Town, Abbass, & Hardy, 2011), especially for those with prior long-term psychotherapy (Grenyer, Deane, & Lewis, 2008). A therapist can ordinarily develop a reliable working alliance rather quickly with a neurotic-level patient and feel a sense of partnership with the person's self-observing capacity. Regressive responses tend to be contained within the therapy hour; that is, these patients may become aware of powerful and primitive feelings toward others, including their therapists, but at the end of a session can usually "pull themselves together" and resume normal functioning.

Transferences of less disturbed patients exist in the context of a person's capacity to consider that certain reactions to a therapist *are* transferences. Thus they are usually addressable by the clinician without risking intolerable damage to the patient's self-esteem. For example, an anxious woman experiences her therapist *as if* he or she were her mother; when the therapist points out such reactions, she feels more interested than hurt. Countertransference with higher-functioning people tends to be mild and is usually experienced by their therapists as more interesting than emotionally disruptive (see also Gazzillo et al., 2015). Because less disturbed patients generally have adequate tolerance of anxiety and ambiguity, open-ended exploration tends to facilitate discovery, mastery, and progress, supporting their sense of agency and counteracting their chagrin about whatever they discover. Investigation of historical antecedents of their current feelings and behavior usually contributes to motivation and change.

Patients in the borderline range need therapeutic relationships that take into account their extreme anxiety, intense reactivity, potential for disorganizing regression, lack of self- and object constancy, and the profound fears that coexist with their deep needs for attachment. Patients in the borderline range are helped by clear limits and structure, and they usually need relatively actively engaged clinicians so they can develop a sense of the clinicians as "real persons" (hence neither the psychoanalytic couch nor long silences are usually helpful). Although patients with borderline psychologies suffer painfully and may thus evoke from clinicians a wish to respond to their neediness with increased availability and special adaptations to their pain, efforts by therapists to extend themselves or make exceptions to an established treatment frame (e.g., to offer unusually long or frequent sessions, or to schedule appointments outside normal work periods, or to be available at any hour for emergencies) are usually counterproductive. Deviations from the therapy frame may induce unmanageable regressions and painful levels of emotional disorganization in patients, and may lead therapists to feel depleted or overburdened. In short, the treatment frame provides the safety and security needed for both parties to engage in the work of therapy.

Whatever treatment frame (in terms of session frequency, cost, length, etc.) is adopted by the two parties, the therapist should maintain it consistently and help the patient express negative feelings about its constraints. Many clinicians employ specific contractual agreements about self-destructive acts, in which an ongoing treatment relationship is contingent on a patient's ability to keep self-harming behaviors under control. A clinician must also be capable of sustaining his or her commitment to treatment over a long period. Patients with borderline organization may be exquisitely sensitive to shifts in the tone of their therapists and may become terrified that they will be abandoned. Their most disturbing symptoms may come back at times of separation from their clinicians—and, ironically, during treatment crises caused by their beginning to change for the better and to feel trust and hope in the therapeutic relationship (see also Bion, 1967; Grotstein, 2009; Rosenfeld, 1987).

The transferences of such patients tend to be intense and difficult for the patients to see *as* transferential. For example, a man sees his therapist as alternately negligent and controlling. When the clinician suggests that he is reacting as if the clinician had qualities like those of his mother, he may conclude, "Yes, it's just my bad luck to have gotten a therapist exactly like her." Often a borderline patient's nonverbal behavior and a therapist's countertransference reactions give more useful information than the patient's verbal communications. Investigation of historical antecedents of the current behavior of a patient with borderline personality organization may not foster change; in fact, it may be used to rationalize not changing (e.g., "How could I possibly be different, given my screwed-up background?!"). Thus treatment should generally focus on the here-and-now, especially the ways in which the patient experiences the clinician (Grenyer, 2012; Stern et al., 1998).

Therapies that are helpful to patients with borderline organization tend to be active and structured, and to include affective expressiveness from both patients and clinicians (McCarthy, Mergenthaler, Schneider, & Grenyer, 2011). Because such patients often know that they provoke strong reactions in other people, and because they tend to interpret neutral stimuli with a negative attributional bias (Daros, Zakzanis & Ruocco, 2013), therapists who try to appear nonreactive can be experienced as insincere or dangerously out of touch.

Clinical theorists who have developed specific therapies for patients in the borderline range (including those with DSM-diagnosed borderline personality disorder) include Peter Fonagy, John Gunderson, Otto Kernberg, Marsha Linehan, Giovanni Liotti, James Masterson, Russell Meares, Jeffrey Young, and their colleagues. Although their specific recommendations differ, all advise giving primary attention to the therapeutic relationship, contracting against self-destructive behaviors, clarifying and respecting boundaries, educating patients about issues such as trauma and emotional regulation, keeping the focus on current challenges, and developing self-reflective capacities. All are sensitive to the special vulnerability of people in this group to issues of separation; all note the need for therapists to tolerate strong countertransferences (especially feelings of helplessness and being overwhelmed); and most emphasize the importance of clinicians' having ongoing consultation and support.

Patients whose personalities are organized at the psychotic level need their clinicians to be especially respectful, conversational, and down-to-earth. Patience is also critical: For patients in this range, language may be impoverished, and narrative history reporting may be impaired (Carter & Grenyer, 2012). In traditional psychoanalytic thinking, individuals whose personalities were conceptualized as at a psychotic level of organization were seen as needing supportive rather than exploratory therapy—that is, treatments *supporting* ego functions and defenses, rather than seeking to loosen ego defenses (Federn, 1952). But, realistically, there are supportive elements in exploratory work and exploratory elements in supportive therapeutic relationships; and in the clinical literature, efforts to demarcate the differences between supportive and exploratory therapies have been problematic (see Appelbaum, 2005, 2008; Hellerstein, Pinsker, Rosenthal, & Klee, 1994; Pinsker, 1997; Rockland, 1989).

We have observed, however, that clinicians experienced in working with patients with psychotic tendencies tend to answer questions, rather than acting blank or abstinent; to give advice; to normalize and contextualize patients' distressing experiences; to identify triggers of their worst states of mind; to educate them about elements of emotion, cognition, and behavior about which they may be confused; and to disclose elements of their own personalities and experiences that may make patients feel both more fully understood and less "crazy." They take pains to be experienced as "real persons" who are concerned, nonhumiliating, plain-spoken, and friendly (Atwood, 2011; Garrett & Turkington, 2011; Karon & VandenBos, 1981; Lotterman, 1996, 2015; Silver, 1989, 2003; Sullivan, 1962).

Such therapists are also attuned to the extreme degree of anxiety (e.g., annihilation anxiety) with which patients at the psychotic level may suffer (see, e.g., Hurvich, 2003; Porges, 2011). They may need to monitor medication compliance and find ways of reinforcing basic self-care. They identify their patients' strengths and build on them, rather than encouraging an opening-up, uncovering attitude that may terrify these fragile persons. Their overall stance is authoritative enough that the patients feel safe in their care and reassured that the clinicians will not be destroyed by the patients' pathology. At the same time, the clinicians convey profound respect and a deeply egalitarian attitude, so that the patients' humiliation about symptoms (or even about simply needing help) can be minimized. They emphasize safety, and they focus on the issues of most concern to their patients, not necessarily those that strike the therapists themselves as most troubling (Garrett, 2012; Sullivan, 1953, 1962).

Further Comments on Personality Styles and Disorders

There are many ways to distinguish psychologically between one person and another. All of them are, of course, oversimplifications. Any clinician who gets to know a patient intimately finds that over time, that person no longer seems to fit a clear-cut diagnostic construct; the person's individuality eventually becomes more salient. This is especially true for individuals at the healthier end of the severity spectrum, who commonly show mixes of personality styles. "Purer" examples of personality style are seen primarily at the "sicker" end of the severity continuum. Nevertheless, it is clinically valuable to consider the predominant personality style or styles that best characterize a person. Such an understanding can contextualize presenting complaints and symptoms and provide a preliminary map of the major "terrain features" of the person's internal landscape. The personality styles or syndromes (or "disorders," where degree of dysfunction warrants the term) included in the P Axis represent a synthesis of empirical research, clinical knowledge, and theory accrued over generations of clinical observation.

We cannot emphasize enough that the syndromes we describe are *not* distinct categories to which a patient does or does not "belong." Rather, the descriptions are best understood as prototypes or "ideals" that an individual may approximate to a greater or lesser extent (see Shedler, 2015; Westen et al., 2012). In other words, personality syndromes are "fuzzy sets" or continua lacking clear-cut boundaries, and the degree to which any personality syndrome applies is always a dimension ranging from inapplicable or irrelevant to highly applicable.

Because the syndromes included in the P Axis exist on a spectrum of severity from relatively healthy through severely disturbed, we generally avoid superimposing the term "disorder" on the descriptions and refer instead to personality "styles," "patterns," "types," or "syndromes," using these terms interchangeably. That said, some of the syndromes are more commonly found in the healthier ranges of personality organization and others in the more disturbed ranges, as we have noted previously. For example, psychopathic individuals, whose defensive operations include omnipotent control, projection, denial, and splitting (Meloy, 1997), are found mainly at the borderline and psychotic levels of personality organization (Gacono & Meloy, 1994). Personality syndromes characterized by less "costly" defenses (e.g., intellectualization in obsessive–compulsive personality) may be more commonly found in the neurotic range. Borderline personality disorder is a special case, as the syndrome is inherently linked to the borderline level of organization and necessarily indicates a level of dysfunction that warrants the term "disorder" (see the discussion on page 53).

Internalizing and Externalizing Spectra

Some personality syndromes are more similar to one another than to others. Various schemes exist to organize psychological syndromes and symptoms into superordinate constructs (e.g., the DSM has grouped personality pathology into "Clusters" A, B, and C). Based on both clinical and empirical recognitions, we list the P-Axis syndromes (with the exception of borderline personality disorder) in an order consistent with two empirically identified superordinate groupings or spectra, "internalizing" and "externalizing" (Westen et al., 2012). We consider first those personalities that are generally considered more internalizing (depressive, dependent, anxious–avoidant and phobic, obsessive–compulsive, somatizing, and schizoid) and subsequently those seen as more externalizing (hysteric–histrionic, narcissistic, paranoid, psychopathic, and sadistic).

Generally speaking, patients with internalizing-spectrum personality pathology suffer inwardly. They tend to blame themselves for their difficulties and are chronically vulnerable to depression or anxiety. Patients with externalizing-spectrum personality pathology are more likely to impose suffering on others (although some, notably those with hysteric–histrionic and narcissistic personalities, may experience a deep level of inner suffering as well). They tend to blame others for their difficulties and are more prone to anger and aggression. Borderline personality disorder cannot be readily subsumed under either spectrum. In contrast to either patients with stable internalizing or stable externalizing styles, patients with borderline personality disorder may be better described as "stably unstable" (Schmideberg, 1959), often oscillating between emotions characteristic of both internalizing and externalizing pathology (e.g., depression, anxiety, rage). (For further discussion of internalizing and externalizing spectra, see Westen et al., 2012.)

Consistent Personality Themes, Inconsistent Behavior

Clinical experience and research findings suggest that particular unconscious themes underlie personality styles and syndromes (e.g., Silberschatz, 2005; Weiss, 1993; Weiss, Sampson, & the Mount Zion Psychotherapy Research Group, 1986). These themes can produce behaviors that may *appear* inconsistent, but amount to different ways of expressing the same theme. For example, an obsessive–compulsive man, unconsciously preoccupied with the issue of control of aggression, may be either compulsively prompt or regularly late, fastidiously neat in most areas yet improbably messy in some, ingratiatingly compliant or stubbornly oppositional—depending on how, at the moment, he tries to solve the problem of feeling controlled by others. (See also the discussions of the terms "personality" and "character" in Appendix 1.2 at the end of this chapter.)

A woman with hysterical personality dynamics, unconsciously preoccupied with sexuality, gender, and their relationship to power, may be either promiscuous or inhibited or both (e.g., highly seductive, but unresponsive or unsatisfied in actual sexual involvements because of unconscious fear or envy of her male partner's perceived power). A person with a paranoid personality may alternate between feeling moved to attack others and being terrified of attack by others. Traits (e.g., neatness, sexual expressiveness, provocativeness in the examples above) often coexist with their seeming opposites. Personality distinctions have more to do with differences in underlying themes, schemas, or inner conflicts than with differences in behaviorally evinced traits, which may represent particular expressions of unconscious preoccupations (McWilliams, 2012).

P-Axis Personality Syndromes

Depressive Personalities (Including Comments on Hypomanic Manifestations and Masochism)

Depressive personality may be the most common personality syndrome encountered in clinical practice (Shedler & Westen, 2004). Individuals with depressive personalities find little pleasure in life's activities and are chronically vulnerable to painful affect, especially depression, guilt, shame, and feeling of inadequacy. They appear conflicted about experiencing pleasure, and appear to squelch or inhibit positive feelings such as joy, excitement, and pride. Predominant psychological themes center on internally arising attacks on the self (e.g., "aggression turned inward"), rejection and loss, or both.

Individuals with depressive personalities may be highly self-critical or self-punitive, holding themselves to unrealistic standards and blaming themselves when things go wrong. They may fear rejection or abandonment, feel alone even in the presence of others, or have a pervasive sense that someone or something necessary for their well-being has been lost to them forever. Individuals with depressive personalities are often unaware of underlying anger and hostility. Depression, self-criticism, or self-punitiveness often defend against an awareness of underlying aggression (for further description, see Westen et al., 2012).

Individuals with depressive personalities may or may not experience depressive mood states that reach the intensity of a diagnosable mood disorder. In addition, not all individuals who are chronically vulnerable to depressive symptoms have depressive personalities, organized around the motifs outlined above. Research has made it clear that there are multiple personality pathways to depression as a symptom syndrome (Huprich, DeFife, & Westen, 2014).

Some investigators who study affective disorders view the phenomena we discuss in this section primarily in terms of chronic mood disorder (e.g., recurring major depression and/or chronic subsyndromal depression; e.g., Gwirtsman, Blehar, McCullough, & Kocsis, 1997). Although mood disorders and depressive personality commonly co-occur, depressive personality can be differentiated from mood disorders per se (see this chapter's Appendix 1.2 for discussion). Personality is more constant, whereas mood disorders tend to be episodic, with acute periods and remissions. In the former, a clinician is struck by ingrained and repetitive personality themes that intensify under stress. In the latter, the clinician is more impressed by vegetative symptoms (e.g., psychomotor retardation, appetite change, sleep disturbances, decreased sexual interest), the intensity of dysphoric affect, and the relative incongruence between the severity of mood disturbance and overall psychological functioning. Whereas antidepressant medications may help alleviate suffering in some patients with mood disorders per se, they tend to be ineffective in ameliorating the self-punitiveness or rejection sensitivity of many people with depressive personality styles.

Blatt and his colleagues (Blatt, 2008; Blatt & Bers, 1993) distinguished between two kinds of depressive affect: "introjective" (called "melancholic" by early psychoanalysts), characterized by self-criticism, self-punitiveness, and guilt; and "anaclitic," characterized by sensitivity to loss and rejection, and feelings of emptiness, inadequacy, and shame.

Introjectively depressive individuals berate themselves for real or imagined shortcomings, and they respond to setbacks with the conviction that they are somehow to blame (a tendency that cognitive therapists have described in terms of "attributional style"; e.g., Peterson & Seligman, 1984). This readiness to blame themselves may be a residue of the familiar tendency of children in difficult family situations to deny that their caregivers are negligent, abusive, or fragile (ideas that are too frightening), but instead to ascribe their suffering to their own badness—something they can try to control. Thus introjectively inclined depressive people work hard to be "good," but rarely succeed to their satisfaction.

Anaclitically depressive individuals are notable for their distress and disorganization in the face of loss and separation. Their psychologies are organized around themes of relationship, affection, trust, intimacy, and warmth, or the lack thereof. They feel empty, lonely, incomplete, helpless, and weak rather than perfectionistic or excessively self-critical. They often complain of existential despair and the feeling that life is hollow and meaningless. Shedler (2015) and Westen and colleagues (2012) empirically identified a depressive personality syndrome in which both introjective and anaclitic features may be salient.

Countertransference to patients with depressive personalities, especially those at higher (e.g., neurotic) levels of organization, tends to be positive. Therapy sessions often feel cooperative and collaborative; patient and therapist often develop warm feelings toward one another; and clinicians often report feeling good about themselves and the work. They view these patients as "good" patients. The clinical challenge is recognizing that the positive feelings may stem from the very patterns the patient must change if the treatment is to have lasting benefit. More specifically, the therapist may feel good because the patient is recreating a pattern of subordinating his or her needs to those of others (in this case, those of the therapist), accepting responsibility and blame for the inevitable disappointments and frustrations that arise in the course of treatment, or defending against awareness of dissatisfaction or anger in the therapy relationship.

In treating a patient with a depressive personality, it is vital for the clinician to recognize and welcome the patient's negative feelings, especially hostility and criticism. Where self-critical and self-punitive (introjective) themes are salient, patients benefit from insight into the ways in which they defend against angry and critical feelings toward others and direct them against themselves. Where preoccupations with rejection and loss (anaclitic themes) are salient, patients benefit from the experience of having their perceived inadequacies and "badness" accepted within a relational context. Where preoccupation with loss predominates, patients may need their clinicians' help to mourn what has been lost, before they are able to invest emotionally in what life can offer in the present. Patients with depressive personalities thus benefit from both the interpretive and relational aspects of psychotherapy.

Hypomanic Defenses against Depressive Affect

The clinical literature also describes a phenomenon that has traditionally been termed "hypomanic personality," in which driven, obligatory optimism and energy defend against underlying depressive themes. The term "hypomanic" easily gives rise to confusion because the same term has been used to refer to different things: a defensive style (in the psychoanalytic literature) and one pole of bipolar mood disorder (in the psychiatric literature more generally).

The hypomanic personality, as traditionally conceived, is characterized by mild mood inflation, high energy, conspicuous absence of guilt, inflated self-esteem, vulnerability to substance abuse, and interpersonal wit and charm in the context of rather superficial relationships (Akhtar, 1992). The fact that these qualities are the polar opposites of those of depressive individuals has led some to propose that such a clinical presentation *necessarily* reflects a bipolar diathesis, but we suggest that careful assessment may point to a bipolar etiology for *some* patients, and to a personality style for others. Where the behavior reflects a defensive style and not a subclinical bipolar mood disorder, interpretation leading to insight into its defensive function (e.g., "It seems like you use a lot of energy trying to avoid feeling sadness") may pave the way to new solutions to old psychological problems. If instead it is an expression of a bipolar mood disorder, such interventions will accomplish little.

Therapists initially tend to find patients with hypomanic personalities captivating, but they may soon feel confused, overstimulated, irritatingly "entertained," and distanced. Individuals with hypomanic personalities tend to be resistant to exploratory psychotherapy. In fact, they are hard to keep in treatment because of their tendency to bolt from relationships that elicit their feelings of dependency. They become unconsciously terrified of being abandoned and may seek to master that fear by abandoning the other. Hypomanic personalities may exist at all levels of functioning. Depending on other psychological factors and circumstances, hypomanic defenses can be extremely "costly" or highly adaptive (or both).

Many therapists, after diagnosing a hypomanic personality style in a patient, call to the patient's attention the lifetime pattern of abrupt flight from relationships that usually pervades the person's history. They then try to preempt a similar flight from therapy by negotiating an agreement that the person will keep coming for a given number of sessions after any abrupt, unilateral decision by the patient to stop treatment. Therapy tends to be both slow and fraught with outbreaks of intense negative affect and worrisome enactments.

Differentiating Depressive from Masochistic Personality Dynamics

The psychoanalytic literature is rich in accounts of patients who behave in ways that seem strikingly antithetical to their own well-being and who appear unconsciously drawn to pain and suffering ("masochism"). On the surface, masochistic dynamics may resemble depressive personality dynamics because of the salience of emotional pain in the clinical presentation. However, masochistic and depressive dynamics are different phenomena and often require different treatment approaches.

"Masochism" is not a unitary construct. The term has been used to refer to a range of phenomena that have different psychological origins and serve different psychological functions, with the common denominator of an apparent (unconscious) investment in suffering. Because masochism may be associated with a range of personality styles (e.g., Huprich & Nelson, 2014), we decided to provide a brief review and discussion of the concept but not include it here as a diagnosis or unitary syndrome. A comprehensive discussion is beyond the scope of this chapter. Rather, we simply note some variants that have been described in the clinical literature, and provide citations for readers who wish to explore the topic in more depth.

On the basis of their frequent involvements (with intimates and with clinicians) in alternating dominance–submission or abuser–abused interactions, some writers (e.g., Brenner, 1959; Kernberg, 1991) have linked masochistic personalities with sadistic dynamics. Others have connected them with other types of personality dynamics: narcissistic (e.g., Cooper, 1988; Glickauf-Hughes, 1997), dependent (Bornstein, 1993; Waska, 1997), and paranoid (Bak, 1946; Nydes, 1963). Below, we briefly describe a version of masochistic dynamics associated with dependent personality themes, another associated with narcissistic themes, and still another associated with a more paranoid orientation. All may involve disavowed sadistic elements.

The more anaclitic version of masochistic dynamics, which overlaps with dependent personality, applies to patients who subordinate their needs to those of others and appear to view suffering as a precondition for maintaining an attachment relationship. The attachment relationship may be experienced as desperately needed; fear of losing the attachment overrides the patient's concerns for his or her own safety and welfare. Beneath overt submissiveness, there is often an undercurrent of disavowed aggression, which the patient expresses in passive–aggressive ways that tend to trigger or provoke mistreatment from others (for empirical evidence, see the description of "dependent–victimized personality" offered by Westen et al., 2012). At the more disturbed levels of personality organization, the patient may rely on projective identification to defend against awareness of his or her own sadism, while simultaneously inducing the other person to enact it.

The more introjective version of masochistic dynamics applies to patients who equate self-renunciation and suffering with virtue. In other words, the person's self-esteem is tied to self-deprivation or suffering: The more self-deprivation, the greater the person's sense of importance and virtue. This pattern includes patients who self-righteously seek to demonstrate that their suffering makes them morally superior to others (Reich's [1933/1972] "masochistic character" or Reik's [1941] "moral masochist"). Such "moral masochism" is not uncommon in people drawn to the so-called helping professions, who attend to others' needs while neglecting their own. Disavowed sadism may be revealed through intolerance (or outright aggression) toward others who do not share their moral values.

Another variant applies to patients who appear to hold the (unconscious) conviction that the world owes them compensation in proportion to their suffering (the "aggrieved pattern" of Millon & Grossman, 2007). To the extent that suffering secures imagined compensation and reward, such patients may be deeply invested in defeating their clinicians' efforts to help (cf. the "help-rejecting complainer" of Frank et al.,

1952). The attitude that contemporary therapists tend to call "victim entitlement" ("I've had a terrible life, so the world owes me") often evokes irritated, judgmental, and even sadistic countertransferences. Clinicians can be helpful to the extent that they keep a focus on these patients' need to grieve for past misfortunes and their capacity to take responsibility for current choices, irrespective of their difficult histories. In the context of a solid alliance, a clinician can help a patient recognize the negative consequences of efforts to convince the world that they have been wronged and to extract compensation in proportion to their grievances.

The more paranoid version of masochistic dynamics involves the conviction that something terrible is bound to happen. For example, some patients who experienced a childhood caregiver as envious and retaliatory may become paralyzed with anxiety, expecting to be attacked for any personal success. Unconsciously, they may seek to "get it over with" by provoking the attack they anticipate as inevitable. This pattern is identifiable by the relief that follows the self-destructive enactment. The pattern needs to be identified and worked through patiently in treatment, as such a patient can only slowly tolerate the anxiety behind the urge toward self-destructive action.

Patients with depressive personality dynamics generally benefit from their clinicians' sympathetic care and concern. In contrast, it is generally unwise to be too explicitly sympathetic or generous when dealing with masochistic dynamics. Explicit compassion and generosity may reinforce a patient's unconscious conviction that suffering is the best or only route to connection, or may provoke self-destructive enactments in a patient who experiences guilt for accepting care that feels undeserved. Instead, tactful confrontation about the patient's own contributions to his or her difficulties can stimulate curiosity about the meaning of self-defeating patterns.

Finally, patients with masochistic personality dynamics may hold the unconscious conviction that their clinicians are interested in them only because they are suffering; such belief s can pose a powerful barrier to getting well. A clinician can help a patient become aware of such unconscious expectations, as well as help the patient recognize and feel that the clinician's (and others') interest and attention are not contingent on his or her suffering.

KEY FEATURES

Contributing constitutional–maturational patterns: Possible genetic predisposition to depression.

Central tension/preoccupation: Self-criticism and self-punitiveness, or preoccupation with relatedness and loss (or both).

Central affects: Sadness, guilt, shame.

Characteristic pathogenic belief about self: "There is something essentially bad or inadequate about me," "Someone or something necessary for well-being has been irretrievably lost."

Characteristic pathogenic belief about others: "People who really get to know me will reject me."

Central ways of defending: Introjection, reversal, idealization of others, devaluation of self.

Dependent Personalities

Some people come to therapy because their personalities are characterized centrally by excessive dependency needs. Because individuals with severely dependent psychologies may find themselves unable to leave relationships that are exploitive or even abusive, such phenomena have sometimes been called "self-defeating" or "masochistic" (see the previous discussion of masochistic dynamics). The categories of "inadequate" and "infantile" personality in earlier taxonomies connote roughly the same construct as our use of the term "dependent personality."

Individuals who are characterologically overdependent are found at all levels of severity. They define themselves mainly in relation to others, and seek security and satisfaction predominantly in interpersonal contexts ("I am fine as long as everything is OK with my husband"). Psychological symptoms may appear when something goes wrong in a primary attachment relationship. At the neurotic level, people with dependent personality may seek treatment in midlife or later, after a bereavement or divorce, or after retirement confronts them with the absence of a context in which rules and expectations are clear. At the borderline and psychotic levels, dependent patients may become dysregulated when expected to depend on their own resources and may use costly defenses, such as somatization and acting out, in desperate bids to elicit care.

Overly dependent individuals may feel ineffectual when left to themselves. They tend to regard others as powerful and effective. Organizing their lives with a view to maintaining nurturing relationships in which they are submissive, they may feel contented when they have successfully developed such a relationship and acutely distressed when they have not. Emotional preoccupations include performance anxiety and fears of criticism and abandonment (Bornstein, 1993). People with dependent personalities tend to feel weak and powerless, to be passive and nonassertive, and to be easily influenced by others. They often appear naive. They may feel worthless and have difficulties in expressing anger. In therapy, which they may enter readily, they may be compliant to a fault. They tend to idealize their therapists, ask for advice, and seek reassurances that they are "good patients." In attempts to become special, they may try to "read" their therapists and meet the clinicians' assumed needs. Some insist, even after being informed about professional boundaries, on offering favors and bringing gifts.

Bornstein (1993, 2005) has conducted the only comprehensive empirical examination of pathological dependency known to us. His findings suggest that it may arise from any or all of the following: overprotective and/or authoritarian parenting, gender role socialization, and cultural attitudes about achievement versus relatedness. Participants in his studies demonstrated "relationship-facilitating self-presentation strategies" such as ingratiation, supplication, exemplification, self-promotion, and intimidation. Although popular prejudice assumes that female patients are more likely than males to be excessively dependent, Bornstein notes that women may simply be more willing to acknowledge dependent longings.

Contemporary feminist psychoanalysts (see, among others, Benjamin, 1988, 1995; Chodorow, 1994, 1999; Dimen, 2003; Dimen & Goldner, 2002, 2012) have criticized Freudian theories about female sexuality for normalizing the devaluation of femininity and the normal relational orientation of women. They argue that this masculinist bias has fueled cultural prejudice toward women and gender stereotypes. In addition to being sensitive to this issue, clinicians should recognize that different cultures have different conceptions of how much dependency is "too much." A diagnosis of dependent personality *disorder* should always consider the cultural context.

Clinicians' countertransference with excessively dependent patients, especially those who are notably self-defeating, is typically benign at first, then increasingly characterized by irritation and a sense of burden. A patient with a dependent personality may devise unconscious tests (Bugas & Silberschatz, 2000; Weiss, 1993) to see whether the clinician supports the patient's nascent strivings toward autonomy, or basks in the patient's invitation to take on the role of expert and advisor. It is important that the clinician resist seduction into the role of expert authority, encourage the patient toward autonomous functioning, and contain the patient's anxieties that arise in the process. Although clinicians treating patients with dependent personalities may be tempted to collude in avoiding negative affect, if they make room for the patients' anger and other more aggressive feelings, they may facilitate the patients' ultimate sense of personal agency and pride in accomplishment.

An important variant of dependent psychology is a passive–aggressive pattern, in which the patient's relationships are characterized by hostile dependency. Passive–aggressive individuals define themselves in relation to others, but with a negative valence (e.g., "I'm the husband of that bitch"). Because they locate themselves psychologically in opposition to others, it is hard for them to conceive of and to pursue their own autonomous goals. Like paranoid patients, they may attack to preempt expected attacks by others, but do so indirectly. Their indirect, underlying aggression often triggers mistreatment from others, perpetuating a vicious cycle: Underlying anger and resentment lead to passive–aggressive behavior, triggering aggression and mistreatment from others, which in turn fuel more anger and resentment. This self-perpetuating pattern reinforces the core conviction that anger must not be experienced or expressed directly.

It is therapeutically challenging to connect with a person who responds passive–aggressively to efforts to connect. The clinician needs a sense of humor as a counterpoise to the feelings of impatience and exasperation that the patient is likely to evoke. Negative feelings arise quickly in treatment, and power struggles are a risk to avoid. Sometimes stunningly naive about the hostility they exude, passive–aggressive patients need help naming their negative feelings and differentiating verbal from behavioral expressions of anger. To avoid activating their oppositionality, which may take the form of sabotaging any outcome their clinicians seems to desire, the clinicians should take care not to seem highly invested in their progress. Instead, clinicians need to take their provocations and inconsistencies in stride, keeping the therapy focused on the price the patients pay for passive–aggressive acts.

Finally, there is a counterdependent version of dependent psychology. Bornstein (1993) describes a continuum from maladaptive dependency (submissiveness) through healthy interdependency (connectedness) to inflexible independence (unconnected detachment). Some individuals at the inflexibly independent end of that spectrum have powerful dependent longings that they keep out of awareness via denial and reaction formation. They thus have what amount to dependent personality dynamics masked by denial and pseudoindependence. In their relationships, they may define themselves as the ones on whom *others* depend, and they may pride themselves on being able to take care of themselves.

Counterdependent individuals may look askance at expressions of need and may regard evidence of emotional vulnerability in themselves or others with scorn. It is probable that their childhood attachment style would have been measured as avoidant.

Often they have some secret area of dependency (on a substance, a partner, a mentor, an ideology); some have a tendency toward illness or injury that gives them a "legitimate" reason to be cared for by others. Like counterphobic individuals, counterdependent individuals seldom seek psychotherapy but may be pushed into it by partners who feel starved for genuine emotional intimacy. In treatment, they need help to accept their dependent needs as normal aspects of being human before they can develop a healthy balance between connectedness and separateness. Therapists who tolerate their defensive protestations about their independence long enough to develop a therapeutic alliance report that when the counterdependent defenses are given up, a period of mourning for early and unmet dependent needs then ensues, followed by more genuine autonomy.

KEY FEATURES

Central constitutional–maturational patterns: Unknown.

Central tension/preoccupation: Keeping versus losing relationships.

Central affects: Pleasure when securely attached; sadness and fear when alone.

Characteristic pathogenic belief about self: "I am inadequate, needy, impotent" (including its conscious converse in passive–aggressive and counterdependent individuals).

Characteristic pathogenic belief about others: "Others are powerful, and I need (but may resent) their care."

Central ways of defending: Regression, reversal, avoidance, somatization.

Anxious–Avoidant and Phobic Personalities

Many individuals currently diagnosed with Generalized Anxiety Disorder as defined in the DSMs are perhaps better understood as having a personality style in which anxiety is the psychologically organizing experience. As with depressive personalities, this construct is controversial, as some scholars prefer to locate any chronic anxiety on a wide spectrum of the psychiatric symptomatologies rather than a personality spectrum (see also the discussion of the anxiety disorders in Chapter 3 on the S Axis, pp. 164–168). Although avoidant personality disorder does appear in the DSMs, the work of Shedler and Westen (2004) suggests that there is a somewhat broader spectrum in which anxiety dominates the personality. In the first PDM, we described phobic personalities as separate from anxious personalities, but in response to the research based on the SWAP (e.g., Shedler, 2015; Westen et al., 2012), and in an effort to emphasize overall continuities rather than artificially discrete subtypes of personality configuration, we are including anxious, avoidant, and phobic in one general anxiety cluster and depicting specific differences here.

Characterological anxiety is found in the neurotic through the borderline ranges. At the psychotic level, individuals with anxiety-driven psychologies become so filled with dread that they depend on primitive externalizing defenses. The overall psychologies of such patients may be better understood as overlapping with the paranoid area.

In the higher-functioning ranges, patients with an anxious personality structure appear at first to be either hysterical (hence the old diagnosis of "anxiety hysteria") or obsessional, depending on how they attempt to deal with their pervasive sense of fear. Unlike individuals with hysterical or obsessional psychologies, however, they are chronically aware of their anxiety because their efforts at defense fail to keep their apprehensiveness out of consciousness. Phobic and avoidant patients attach these anxieties to specific objects or situations, from which they try to stay away; other characterologically anxious individuals experience a free-floating, global sense of anxiety, with no idea what frightens them.

Phobic and avoidant patients can be shy and reserved, tend to feel inferior and inadequate, indecisive, and inhibited, and may have difficulties in recognizing and describing their feelings. Contemporary cognitive theorists emphasize how such patients show difficulties in identifying their anxiety-charged thoughts, connecting them to their environmental triggers, mastering them, and assuming a "decentered" perspective on the anxiety-inducing situations.

Long clinical experience has identified several different kinds of anxiety that seem universal among human beings, including "separation anxiety" (fear of losing an attachment object), "castration anxiety" (fear of damage to the body, especially sexual mutilation), "moral anxiety" (dread of violating one's core values), and "annihilation anxiety." Annihilation anxiety can involve either a terror of fragmentation and consequent loss of the sense of self (cf. Kohut's [1977] concept of "disintegration anxiety") or a terror of destruction based on prior traumatic experience. In contrast to patients in whom one of these types of anxiety tends to predominate, these different subjective experiences of anxiety may *all* be discernible in patients whose anxiety is incapacitating enough for them to be diagnosed with a personality disorder.

In general, the more disturbed the anxious person's level of personality organization, the more likely it is that annihilation anxiety dominates the clinical picture (Hurvich, 2003). Research confirms that these characterological anxieties have a developmental trajectory, impede treatment progress, and, most important, require a deeper form of therapy than the traditional exposure therapies that are often cited as "empirically supported" approaches to treating anxiety (Boulanger, 2007; Kirsten, Grenyer, Wagner, & Manicavasagar, 2008).

The proximal source of characterological anxiety may lie in affective dysregulation (Schore, 2003) and consequent failure to have developed coping strategies or defenses that mitigate normal developmental fears. Individuals with anxious personalities often report having had primary caregivers who, because of the caregivers' own anxiety, could not adequately comfort them or convey a sense of security or support a sense of agency. Mikulincer and Shaver (2012, 2016) note that most people with characterological anxiety would probably have been identifiable in early childhood as having an anxious attachment style. Their research suggests that despite the continuity of attachment style across the lifespan, insecure attachment styles may slowly change toward more secure attachment in the context of a long, devoted relationship, particularly intensive psychotherapy (cf. Sroufe, 2005).

Countertransference with chronically anxious patients may include a responsive anxiety, including, with those at the borderline or psychotic level, a degree of annihilation anxiety intense enough to make their therapists feel overwhelmed and hence impelled to step outside the therapeutic role to "do" something to offer relief to the patients. Preliminary research findings suggest that clinicians working with anxious patients tend to develop both parental and disengaged feelings, while specifically phobic patients tend to elicit mainly parental affects (Colli et al., 2014; Gazzillo et al., 2015; Gordon et al., 2016). In therapy, anxious patients may connect in a submissive, apprehensive way, asking for relief. Because of the unbearable nature of anxious affect, they often come to treatment already addicted to antianxiety drugs. Although clinicians may be tempted to offer chemical relief based on countertransferential parental feelings, the risk of addiction suggests that for people with characterological anxiety, one should prescribe anxiolytic medications with great caution.

Especially in characterologically phobic patients, who may want to believe that as long as they keep away from certain dangers they are safe, there tends to be a degree of magical thinking that their therapists will have a formula to resolve the anxiety without the patients' having to face it. Anxious patients tend to feel small, inadequate, and threatened when alone, and they deal with such feelings by trying to elicit protection from those to whom they impute power. It is vital that their clinicians not act out a rescue fantasy, but, instead, encourage phobic patients toward graduated exposures to feared objects and situations (Sadock & Sadock, 2008; Weinberger, 2014).

A therapist should maintain confidence in a patient's own capacities to tolerate and reduce anxiety. It is important also to try to help the patient give words to previously inchoate states of feeling (Stern, 1997). Many anxious patients are both verbally and behaviorally avoidant, changing the subject whenever anything disturbing enters their consciousness. When they make sweeping proclamations of danger, they should be pressed for details ("And then what would happen?") and asked for specific fantasies. Once there is a secure therapeutic alliance, phobic patients need to face what they fear. Exposure and response prevention treatments, as well as education in mindfulness and meditative disciplines (Wallin, 2007), may be useful adjuncts to understanding, naming, and mastering previously unformulated emotional states.

Relatively infrequently, therapists see characterologically counterphobic patients. Their rarity in clinical caseloads may be due to their avoidance of vulnerable acts such as asking for help. They may, however, come for treatment when urged by a partner or in the aftermath of traumatic events. Counterphobic individuals are psychologically organized around defenses against their fears. They may seek out dangerous situations, thrive on risk, and have a reputation for unnerving calm in the face of peril. Having disowned and projected their own anxieties, they evoke anxious countertransferences in therapists, who see the realistic dangers in their risk taking. It is critical to work slowly with them and to tolerate their bravado for some time before beginning to push them to acknowledge even normal fear, much less neurotic anxiety. In all patients for whom anxiety is pervasive, there may be a period in treatment in which they suffer a depressive reaction to giving up some of the magical ideas that accompany their anxiety-driven psychology.

KEY FEATURES

Contributing constitutional–maturational patterns: Possible anxious or timid disposition.

Central tension/preoccupation: Safety versus danger.

Central affects: Fear.

Characteristic pathogenic belief about self: "I am in constant danger that I must somehow elude."

Characteristic pathogenic belief about others: "Others arc sources of either unimagined dangers or magical protection."

Central ways of defending: Symbolization, displacement, avoidance, rationalization; inchoate anxieties may mask more upsetting specific anxieties (i.e., anxiety itself may be defensive).

Obsessive–Compulsive Personalities

Individuals with obsessive–compulsive personalities are emotionally constricted and regimented. They prefer to operate as if emotions were irrelevant and to defend against threatening emotions and desires through rigidity, regimentation, and intellectualization. They tend to be excessively concerned with rules, procedures, order, organization, schedules, and so on, and may be excessively devoted to work and "productivity" to the detriment of leisure and relationships. They rely on intellectualization as a defense and tend to see themselves as logical and rational, uninfluenced by emotion. Asked how they *feel*, they are likely to describe what they *think*. They tend to think in abstractions or become preoccupied with details. Beneath an "orderly" and regimented exterior, they are preoccupied with underlying issues of control, and caught in an unconscious conflict between feeling that they must submit to others' demands (which elicits rage and shame) or rebel and defy them (which elicits anxiety and fear of retaliation). Rigidity, order, and intellectualization defend against awareness of the underlying conflict and the emotions that accompany it.

Central to an obsessive–compulsive psychology is a resistance to feeling "out of control." This issue may originate in early struggles with caregivers/authority figures. Freud (1913) became impressed with the similarity of the stubborn, punctilious, and hoarding tendencies of the obsessive–compulsive adult to a resistant child's response to toilet training—a leap that captured the imagination of his contemporaries and gave us the word "anal" as a descriptor of this psychology. He associated a tendency toward this character style with high levels of temperamental aggressiveness, which may make toilet training a struggle, but which also may intensify any situation in which a child is required to exert control over impulses and desires (eating, sexuality, general obedience). Parents with controlling tendencies may contribute to this character style and to its characteristic conflicts between giving versus withholding, generosity versus selfishness, and compliant submission versus oppositional defiance.

People with obsessive–compulsive personalities, evocatively described by Reich (1933/1972) as "living machines," seem to have identified with caregivers who expected them to be more grown-up than was possible at their age. They regard expressions of most affects as "immature," they overvalue rationality, and they suffer humiliation when they feel they have acted childishly. Only when an emotion is logically defensible or morally justified—for example, righteous anger—do they find it acceptable.

Psychoanalytic scholarship (Fisher & Greenberg, 1985; Salzman, 1980; Shapiro, 1965) suggests that people with obsessive–compulsive personality styles fear that their impulses, especially their aggressive urges, will get out of control. Most obsessive thoughts and compulsive actions involve efforts to undo or counteract impulses toward destructiveness, greed, and messiness. Because guilt over unacceptable wishes is severe, the conscience of a pathologically obsessive–compulsive person is famously rigid and punitive. Self-criticism is harsh; such individuals hold themselves (and others) to ideal standards. They follow rules literally, get lost in details, and postpone making decisions because they want to make the perfect one. They are scrupulous to a fault, but may have trouble relaxing, joking, and being intimate.

Although obsessive and compulsive qualities express similar unconscious preoccupations and hence appear together, some people exhibit obsessional features with little compulsivity, while others exhibit compulsive features with little obsessionality. Obsessive people are chronically "in their heads": thinking, reasoning, judging, doubting. Compulsive souls are chronically "doing and undoing": cleaning, collecting, perfecting. Obsessive patients are ruminative and cerebral; their self-esteem may depend on *thinking*. Compulsive individuals tend to be busy, meticulous, perfectionistic; their self-esteem depends on *doing*.

In therapy, an individual with an obsessive–compulsive personality may try hard to be cooperative but covertly resist the therapist's efforts to explore the patient's affective world. The patient may become subtly oppositional, expressing unconscious opposition by coming late, forgetting to pay, and prefacing responses to the therapist's comments with "Yes, but . . ." The person may interrupt and talk over the therapist. To the clinician, the relationship may feel subtly (on not so subtly) like an ongoing power struggle. As the patient insists on tendentious argument rather than more authentic emotional engagement, the therapist may become impatient and exasperated. Effective therapy requires sustained and patient exploration of those aspects of personality that individuals with obsessive–compulsive personalities otherwise spend inordinate energy trying to subdue.

KEY FEATURES

Contributing constitutional–maturational patterns: Possible aggressivity, irritability, orderliness.

Central tension/preoccupation: Submission to versus rebellion against controlling authority.

Central affects: Anger, guilt, anxiety, shame, fear.

Characteristic pathogenic belief about self: "Most feelings are dangerous and must be controlled."

Characteristic pathogenic belief about others: "Others are less precise and in control than I am, so I have to control what they do and resist being controlled by them."

Central ways of defending: Isolation of affect, reaction formation, intellectualizing, moralizing, undoing.

Schizoid Personalities

The term "schizoid" may be among the more confusing in the clinical literature because the same term has been used to describe markedly different psychologies. Individuals who receive a DSM diagnosis of schizoid personality disorder are most often characterized by severe deficits in basic psychological resources and capacities. Some may have subsyndromal schizophrenia spectrum disorders in which "negative symptoms" predominate (e.g., affective flattening, impoverished speech and thought). There is evidence (e.g., Lenzenweger, Clarkin, Kernberg, & Foelsch, 2001) that the more schizotypal the patient's presentation, the more grave the level of severity (we view schizotypy as a trait common in schizoid psychologies and not as a type of personality). Westen and colleagues (2012) empirically identified a grouping of patients in a clinical sample that they labeled "schizoid–schizotypal," characterized by "pervasive impoverishments, and peculiarities in, interpersonal relationships, emotional experience, and thought processes" (p. 280).

Although this deficit-based version of "schizoid" may be more familiar to clinicians, psychoanalytic writers have observed and described a different psychology to which they have also applied the term "schizoid." Individuals with this version of a schizoid personality style are not characterized by the kind of *inner* impoverishment of thought and feeling that is typically associated with the DSM diagnosis, and their psychological makeup may be better understood (at least in part) as conflict-based rather than solely deficit-based. Here we focus on the less familiar personality syndrome described by psychoanalytic writers, and simply note that the term "schizoid" has been used differently in the broader clinical (especially psychiatric) literature.

Individuals with schizoid personality styles easily feel in danger of being engulfed, enmeshed, controlled, intruded upon, overstimulated, and traumatized—dangers that they associate with becoming involved with other people (Klein, 1946). They may appear notably detached, or they may behave in a socially appropriate way while privately attending more to their inner world than to the surrounding world of human beings (Fairbairn, 1952). Some schizoid individuals withdraw into solitary environments and even hermit-like reclusiveness; others retreat in more psychological ways to the fantasy life in their minds (Winnicott, 1971).

Although seriously schizoid individuals, especially those with schizotypy, may appear indifferent to social acceptance or rejection, to the extent of having eccentricities that serve to put others off, this apparent indifference may have more to do with establishing a tolerable level of space between themselves and others than with ignorance of social expectations; in this way, they differ significantly from individuals on the autism spectrum (Ridenour, 2014). The clinical literature is mixed about whether to view schizoid psychology from the perspective of conflict (between closeness and distance needs) or from that of deficit (developmental arrest that precluded the achievement of interpersonal relatedness). We suspect that both kinds of schizoid psychologies can be found across the health-to-illness spectrum, with the more conflicted version characterizing schizoid individuals in the higher-functioning ranges.

Schizoid individuals are often seen as loners and tend to be more comfortable by themselves than with others. At the same time, they may feel a deep yearning for closeness and have elaborate fantasies about emotional and sexual intimacy (Doidge, 2001; Guntrip, 1969; Seinfeld, 1991). They can be startlingly aware of features of their inner lives that tend to be unconscious in individuals with other kinds of personality, and they consequently may be perplexed when they find that others are unaware of aspects of themselves that, to the schizoid persons, seem obvious. Although some schizoid people seem content in their isolation, there is often a longing for intimacy that their avoidant defenses conceal (Shedler & Westen, 2004).

The DSM generalization that people diagnosed as schizoid rarely experience strong emotions is not supported by clinical experience or research (Shedler & Westen, 2004). Some schizoid individuals feel pain of an intensity so excruciating as to require their defensive detachment in order to endure it. They may seldom feel strong pleasurable emotions, however. Moreover, if they have a low-level borderline or a psychotic personality organization, they may show signs of thought disorder, persecutory anxieties, and concrete thinking.

Schizoid individuals may do well in therapies that both allow emotional intimacy and respect their need for sufficient interpersonal space (Khan, 1974; Ridenour, 2014). They may communicate their concerns most intimately and comfortably via metaphor and emotionally meaningful references to literature, the arts, and areas in which they have a passionate solo interest, whether in abstract realms such as theology or in more prosaic pursuits such as video games. In some cases, particularly those in which their schizoid qualities seem to express a core deficit in relating rather than a conflict around relating, they may not be consciously aware of the psychological meaning of these communications. People with this type of schizoid psychology—in particular, those at a borderline level of personality organization—may show evidence of severe deficits in making sense of their own and other people's behaviors.

KEY FEATURES

Contributing constitutional–maturational patterns: Highly sensitive, shy, easily overstimulated; possibly vulnerable to psychosis.

Central tension/preoccupation: Fear of closeness versus longing for closeness.

Central affects: General emotional pain when overstimulated; affects so powerful that these persons feel they must suppress them.

Characteristic pathogenic belief about self: "Dependency and love are dangerous."

Characteristic pathogenic belief about others: "The social world is impinging, dangerously engulfing."

Central ways of defending: Withdrawal, both physically and into fantasy and idiosyncratic preoccupations.

Somatizing Personalities

Psychiatrists and other physicians are more likely than other therapists to have recurrently somatizing patients in their caseloads. A cluster of individuals whose problems are chronically expressed in bodily difficulties did not emerge from the research conducted by Shedler (2015) and Westen and colleagues (2012) using the SWAP instrument, perhaps because it was conducted mainly by sampling from the caseloads of psychologists and psychiatrists (i.e., patient populations that have identified their difficulties as mental, rather than medical, health problems). In the first PDM, we posited a somatizing personality disorder, and we retain our sense of the value of this construct—but, as with depressive psychologies, some scholars see this kind of clinical presentation as outside the personality spectrum. However, for many patients psychosomatic pathologies are still a major source of concern and the "preferential" means through which they express their painful experiences, which is why we thought it important to devote some reflections to this specific group of patients. Somatization and somatic preoccupations are common throughout the severity dimension but become particularly difficult to treat in the borderline range, where illness may interfere gravely with the continuity of treatment, and in the psychotic range, where psychotic preoccupations may be expressed as somatic delusions.

There is scant empirical literature on characterological somatization. Investigation of the psychological aspects of a person's chronic and medically confounding bodily complaints is complicated by the likelihood that some individuals diagnosed as defensively somatizing have an undiagnosed illness, such as an autoimmune or infectious disease, that explains their physical preoccupations. Clinically, it is hard to tell whether the self-involved, complaining style common among those with inexplicable, intractable ailments represents preexisting personality characteristics or the psychological consequences of chronic physical discomfort (MacKinnon & Michels, 1971; MacKinnon, Michels, & Buckley, 2006).

Notwithstanding this problem, clinical experience suggests the existence of a personality tilt toward expressing dysphoria in bodily complaints (McDougall, 1989). Some somatizing patients may present a confusing combination of hypochondriacal preoccupations, diagnosable physical illness known to be stress-related, and bodily symptoms that express ideas and affects too painful to put into words ("conversion reactions"). Often a somatizing patient consults a psychotherapist reluctantly and in desperation, at the urging of a series of defeated medical specialists. The patient who is "sent" to therapy in this way may arrive in a resentful, defensive state of mind. Addiction to prescribed pain medications is a common complication.

Although there is some overlap between the two kinds of suffering, individuals who somatize should be differentiated from those with hypochondriasis—a more severe condition characterized by excessive concern with the body; exaggerated fears of physical illness; a low threshold of physical discomfort; rituals related to bodily concerns; and the substitution of a preoccupation with the body for meaningful, in-depth relationships with other individuals. In intensive psychotherapy, patients with hypochondriacal tendencies may become paranoid when the therapist tries to explore transference reactions.

Somatizing patients are notable for their "alexithymia" (McDougall, 1989; Sifneos, 1973), or the inability to express emotions verbally. Although the connection between somatization and difficulty putting feelings into words is not necessarily present in all somatizing patients, clinicians have reported this observation frequently. It is also inferable from research with toddlers and young children. Greenspan (1992), for example, found that children who cannot verbalize feelings tend either to act out or to somatize. Marty and M'Uzan (1963) described somatizing patients as using *la pensée opératoire* or "operational thinking," meaning that they were strikingly devoid of fantasy, incapable of symbolic expression, and invested more in "things" than in products of the imagination. Their preoccupations tend to be concrete and repetitive (Joyce, Fujiwara, Cristall, Ruddy, & Ogrodniczuk, 2013).

Presumably, early caregivers of somatizing patients failed to foster a capacity to represent feelings, leaving their bodies to convey what their minds could not (cf. van der Kolk, 1994). Their alexithymia makes talk therapy difficult, but also vital for their improvement. Although they may have once received some secondary gain from the sick role, the pain they suffer is real and debilitating, and in adulthood there is very little that is rewarding about their psychology, unless they are invested in maintaining a legally disabled status.

Their sense of self tends to be fragile; they may feel unentitled and powerless. Individuals who somatize chronically often report that they feel repeatedly *unheard*—no doubt partly because listeners tune out defensively as their efforts to help are frustrated, but possibly also because of early experiences with caregivers who failed to respond to their communications. With professionals, they may act both helpless and oppositional. The unvoiced hatred that interviewers often feel from somatizing patients, especially those in the borderline range, may result from their repeated experience of being treated as annoying complainers and given the message "It's all in your head." In addition, their inner working model of relatedness may require them to be ill as a condition of being cared about by someone important to them.

Common countertransferences to somatizing patients may include feelings of futility, impatience, and irritation. Boredom, inner deadness, and disengagement are also not uncommon. Treatment of individuals with somatizing tendencies is difficult and requires patience with their inarticulateness and negativity. Empathic acknowledgment that their suffering is real is critical; otherwise, they may feel accused of malingering. Because any movement toward emotional expression is stressful for them, they frequently become ill and cancel appointments just when their therapists begin to see progress. Central to their improvement is their therapists' tactful encouragement to feel, name, and accept their emotional states.

KEY FEATURES

Contributing constitutional–maturational patterns: Possible physical fragility, early sickliness; some clinical reports of early physical and/or sexual abuse.

Central tension/preoccupation: Integrity versus fragmentation of bodily self.

Central affects: Global distress; inferred rage; alexithymia prevents acknowledgment of emotion.

Characteristic pathogenic belief about self: "I am fragile, vulnerable, in danger of dying."

Characteristic pathogenic belief about others: "Others are powerful, healthy, and indifferent."

Central ways of defending: Somatization, regression.

Hysteric–Histrionic Personalities

Individuals with hysteric–histrionic personality styles are preoccupied with gender, sexuality, and their relation to power. Unconsciously, they see their own sex as weak, defective, or inferior, and the opposite sex as powerful, exciting, frightening, and enviable (Horowitz, 1991, 1997; McWilliams, 2011). With respect to outward behavior, they typically come across as flamboyant, attention-seeking, and seductive (although a subset may, paradoxically, strike clinicians as curiously naive, conventional, and inhibited). Before DSM-III introduced the diagnosis of histrionic personality disorder, most psychoanalytic thinkers used the term "hysteric" for neurotically organized people with these personality dynamics, and "histrionic" or "hysteroid" for those in the borderline and psychotic ranges. The DSM diagnosis of borderline personality disorder essentially depicts hysteric–histrionic personality organized at a borderline level of severity (cf. Zetzel, 1968).

Individuals with hysteric–histrionic personalities tend to seek power via seductiveness toward persons of the overvalued gender ("pseudohypersexuality"). Such use (or misuse) of sexuality has a defensive function, serving to ward off feelings of weakness, defectiveness, or fearfulness, and to gain a sense of power or conquest over the exciting (but envied and frightening) overvalued gender. Sexual intimacy, however, is a source of conflict because of unconscious shame about one's gendered body and fears of being damaged by the more powerful other. People with hysteric–histrionic psychologies often flaunt their sexuality in an exhibitionistic way, in an unconscious effort to counteract unconscious shame and fear (although some are sexually avoidant or unresponsive). Many observers have noted that hysteric–histrionic psychologies are more common in cultures with strict, hierarchical gender roles. Cultural factors influence the nature of hysterical expression. For example, in Western societies, hysteric–histrionic individuals are more likely to dramatize, while those in cultures that try to control the sexuality of people of their gender are apt to be inhibited—as were the "hysterics" with whom Freud originally worked in post-Victorian Vienna.

Clinical experience suggests that heterosexual individuals who grow up disappointed by a same-sex parent and overstimulated by an opposite-sex parent may develop hysteric–histrionic personality styles. Thus women with hysteric–histrionic personality dynamics tend to describe their mothers as cold, depressed, or inept, and their fathers as larger than life. An opposite-sex caregiver may have been seductive or sexually inappropriate, sometimes to the point of molestation.

Patients with hysteric–histrionic personalities fear overstimulation, much as schizoid patients do, but from inside rather than from outside. Their own feelings and desires evoke anxiety. The dread of being overwhelmed by affect may be expressed in a self-dramatizing way of speaking, as if emotion is being unconsciously derided by being exaggerated. Cognitive style may be impressionistic (Shapiro, 1965), as these persons prefer not to look too closely at details for fear of seeing and knowing too much. Medically inexplicable physical symptoms expressing dissociated conflicts (conversion) may be present. Behavior, especially sexual behavior, may be impulsive or driven, yet regarded by these persons as unrelated to identifiable internal states. Like narcissistic individuals, patients with hysteric–histrionic personalities may compete for attention that reassures them of their value, but their exhibitionistic and competitive qualities are limited to the realm of sexuality and gender. Outside that arena, they may be capable of warm and stable attachments.

When both parties are heterosexual, high-functioning (neurotic-level) female patients with hysteric personality dynamics may charm and captivate male therapists, at least initially, but annoy female therapists (although this pattern is not universal). For neurotic-level male patients with these dynamics, the reverse is true. As treatment progresses, clinicians' own conflicts and discomfort around issues of gender, power, and sexuality may emerge. Therapists whose gender is devalued may feel irritated and demeaned; those whose gender is overvalued may initially feel narcissistically inflated (but may later come to feel manipulated or played). At the borderline level, histrionic patients tend to evoke fear and exasperation, as their intense unconscious anxiety impels them to act out rather than talk. With a therapist of the gender they see as powerful, they may be flagrantly seductive in ways therapists experience as alarming and disturbing.

A patient with hysteric–histrionic personality dynamics can benefit from both the relational and interpretive (exploratory) aspects of psychotherapy. The therapy relationship constitutes a new and different kind of relationship, one in which a therapist of the overvalued gender is neither seductive nor seducible, and a therapist of the undervalued gender is neither competitive with the patient nor powerless and ineffectual. The dependability and emotional availability of the therapist, and the safety and stability of the therapeutic frame, provide a context for self-examination and interpretation in which the patient can gain insight into conflicts around gender, power, and sexuality. Neurotically organized patients with hysteric–histrionic personality styles respond well to the interpretive or insight-oriented aspects of therapy; treatment of patients organized at the at the borderline level may require more deliberate handling of boundary issues, confrontation about destructive enactments, and explicit psychoeducation.

KEY FEATURES

Contributing constitutional–maturational patterns: Possible sensitivity, sociophilia.

Central tension/preoccupation: Gender and power; unconscious devaluation of own gender/envy and fear of opposite gender.

Central affects: Fear, shame, guilt (over competition).

Characteristic pathogenic belief about self: "There is something problematic with my gender and its meaning."

Characteristic pathogenic belief about others: "The world is best understood in terms of gender binaries and gender conflicts."

Central ways of defending: Repression, regression, conversion, sexualization, acting out.

Narcissistic Personalities

Individuals with problematic narcissistic preoccupations exist along a continuum of severity, from the neurotic through the psychotic level of organization. Toward the neurotic end of the spectrum, narcissistic individuals may be socially appropriate, personally successful, charming, and (although somewhat deficient in the capacity for intimacy) reasonably well adapted to their family circumstances, work, and interests. In contrast, people with narcissistic personalities at the more pathological levels, whether or not they are personally successful, suffer from identity diffusion (often concealed by a grandiose self-presentation), lack an inner-directed morality, and may behave in ways that are highly destructive and toxic to others. Kernberg (1984) characterizes the most problematic type of narcissistic individual as suffused with "malignant narcissism" (i.e., narcissism blended with sadistic aggression)—a condition that he places on a continuum with the frankly psychopathic personality (Meltzer, 1973; Rosenfeld, 1987).

The characteristic subjective experience of narcissistic individuals is a sense of inner emptiness and meaninglessness that requires recurrent infusions of external affirmation of their importance and value. Narcissistic individuals who succeed in extracting such affirmation in the form of status, admiration, wealth, or success may feel an internal elation, behave in a grandiose and arrogant manner, evince a sense of entitlement, and treat others (especially those perceived as of lower status) with contempt. When the environment fails to provide such evidence, narcissistic individuals may feel depressed, ashamed, and envious of those who succeed in attaining the status that they lack. They often fantasize about unlimited success, beauty, glory, and power, and their lack of real pleasure in either work or love can be painful to witness. Given these considerations, they would belong on the introjective end of Blatt's (2008) continuum because their patterns reflect attempts to establish and maintain a sense of self and their preoccupations with issues of autonomy, control, self-worth, and identity.

The DSMs' narcissistic personality disorder describes the more grandiose or arrogant version of narcissistic personality (first described by Reich, 1933/1972, as the "phallic narcissistic character"). It omits from consideration the many persons who come to therapists feeling shy and ashamed, avoiding relationships, and looking diffident. Although often less successful than arrogant individuals with this psychology, they are internally preoccupied with grandiose fantasies.

Rosenfeld (1987) distinguished between the "thick-skinned" and "thin-skinned" narcissist; Akhtar (1989) between the "overt" and "covert" (shy) patient; Gabbard (1989) between the "oblivious" and the "hypervigilant" types; Masterson (1993) between the "exhibitionistic" and "closet" types; and Pincus and colleagues (Pincus, Cain, & Wright, 2014; Pincus & Roche, 2011) between the "grandiose" and "vulnerable" ones. Russ, Shedler, Bradley, and Westen (2008) identified three subtypes of narcissistic patients, labeled "grandiose/malignant," "fragile," and "high-functioning/exhibitionistic"; they described the last subtype as notable for grandiosity, attention seeking, and seductive or provocative attitudes, but also for significant psychological strengths. Patients with narcissistic concerns who are not in a position to act arrogantly may demand that the therapist teach them how to be "normal" or "popular," complaining that they want what more fortunate people have. Narcissistic individuals frequently have hypochondriacal preoccupations and somatic complaints.

Recently, attachment and mentalization in patients with comorbid narcissistic and borderline personality disorders have been extensively addressed by Diamond and colleagues (2013, 2014). This literature suggests that narcissistic people have insecure attachment styles (both attachment anxiety and avoidance) that may result from early relationships with others that are confusing, unpredictable, and full of hidden agendas (cf. Diamond et al., 2014; Fossati, Feeney, Pincus, Borroni, & Maffei, 2015; Kealy, Ogrodniczuk, Joyce, Steinberg, & Piper, 2013; Miller, 1979/1981). Under such circumstances, children may respond by divesting themselves of meaningful emotional investment in others and becoming preoccupied instead with their selves and their bodily integrity.

Individuals with narcissistic personalities spend considerable energy evaluating their status relative to that of others. They tend to defend their wounded self-esteem through a combination of idealizing and devaluing others (Bradley, Heim, & Westen, 2005). When they idealize someone, they feel more special or important by virtue of their association with that person; when they devalue someone, they feel superior. Therapists who work with such individuals tend to feel unreasonably idealized, unreasonably devalued, or simply disregarded. Effects on the therapists may include boredom, detachment, distraction (daydreaming, inability to focus attention or to track therapeutic dialogue), mild irritation, impatience, and the feeling that they are invisible (Colli et al., 2014). They may also, especially if the wounds to these patients' self-esteem are apparent, have parental feelings (Gazzillo et al., 2015; Gordon et al., 2016). Gabbard (2009b) noted that a narcissistic patient, especially one of the grandiose and overt type, can be experienced "as speaking 'at' instead of 'to' the therapist, leaving him/her unable to emotionally invest in the therapeutic relationship and to be a real 'participant observer' " (p. 528).

The clinical literature on narcissistic personality disorder includes diverse speculations about etiology and consequently diverse treatment recommendations. Kohut (1971, 1977) emphasized empathic attunement and exploration of the therapist's inevitable empathic failures, and described periods in treatment when the patient idealizes the analyst, treating him or her as a perfect and all-powerful parent figure (the "idealizing transference"). He felt that during these times, the primary challenge for the therapist is to resist the temptation to confront this pattern too quickly. Kernberg (1975, 1984), on the other hand, has recommended the tactful but systematic exposure of defenses against shame, envy, and normal dependency. Contemporary practitioners are more likely to adopt an integrated approach to working with narcissistic individuals—confronting defenses when they are salient, and empathically attuning to underlying hurt and vulnerability when those feelings are accessible.

Narcissistic envy can create a subtle fear of progress in therapy (because improvement would reveal that there was originally something to improve), whereas the idealization puts pressure on the therapist to be brilliant (but not so brilliant as to threaten the patient's intelligence by comparison). Progress may thus be slow, but any improvement for a patient with a narcissistic psychology is valuable for both the patient and those who relate to him or her. Like persons whose character structure is more psychopathic, narcissistic people may be easier to help in therapy in midlife or later, when their investments in beauty, fame, wealth, and power have been disappointed, and when they have run into realistic limits on their grandiosity.

KEY FEATURES

Contributing constitutional–maturational patterns: No clear data.

Central tension/preoccupation: Inflation versus deflation of self-esteem.

Central affects: Shame, humiliation, contempt, envy.

Characteristic pathogenic belief about self: "I need to be perfect to feel OK."

Characteristic pathogenic belief about others: "Others enjoy riches, beauty, power, and fame; the more of those I have, the better I will feel."

Central ways of defending: Idealization, devaluation.

Paranoid Personalities

Individuals who are so recurrently or chronically paranoid that they have a diagnosable personality disorder are found mainly in the borderline and psychotic ranges. Paranoid psychologies are characterized by unbearable affects, impulses, and ideas that are disavowed and attributed to others, and are then viewed with fear and/or outrage. They occupy the introjective, self-definition end of Blatt's continuum from relatedness to self-definition.

Projected feelings may include hostility, as in the common paranoid conviction that one is being persecuted by hostile others; dependency, as in the sense of being deliberately rendered humiliatingly dependent by others; and attraction, as in the belief that others have sexual designs on the self or on the people to whom one is attached (e.g., in the common phenomenon of paranoid jealousy or the syndrome of erotomania). Other painful affects, such as hatred, envy, shame, contempt, disgust, and fear, may also be disowned and projected. Although paranoia is described in somewhat one-dimensional ways in the DSMs, persons with paranoid psychologies may have complex subjective experiences organized around their terror to trust.

Because pathologically paranoid individuals tend to have histories marked by felt shame and humiliation (Gilbert, Boxall, Cheung, & Irons, 2005; Meissner, 1978), they expect to be humiliated by others and may attack first in order to spare themselves the agony of waiting for the inevitable attack from outside. Their expectation of mistreatment creates the suspiciousness and hypervigilance for which they are noted—attitudes that tend to evoke the hostile and humiliating responses they fear. Their personality is defensively organized around the themes of danger and power (either the persecutory power of others or the megalomanic power of the self).

Paranoid patients tend to have more or less mild thought disorders and trouble conceiving that thoughts are different from actions—a belief that may stem from childhoods in which they were (or felt) criticized for their real or presumed attitudes, as if feelings are equivalent to action. Some clinical reports (Bonime, 1979; Stern, 1989) suggest that they have experienced a parent as seductive or manipulative and are consequently alert to the danger of being seduced and exploited by the therapist and others. They may exist in anxious conflict between feeling panicky when alone (afraid that they will be damaged by an unexpected attack, and/or afraid that their destructive fantasies will damage or have already damaged others) and anxious in relationships (afraid that they will be used and destroyed by the agendas of others). Finally, paranoid people have severe difficulties putting themselves in others' shoes and examining experiences from such a perspective; that is, they have problems in "cognitive decentration" (Dimaggio & Semerari, 2004).

Clinical experience attests to the rigidity of the pathologically paranoid person (Shapiro, 1981). A therapist's countertransference may be strong, mirroring feelings that the paranoid person disowns and projects, such as helplessness, fright, and a sense of being criticized when the patient expresses only the angry aspects of his or her emotional reaction and shows no fear or vulnerability. Such reactions also occur in other people interacting with paranoid individuals.

The clinical literature emphasizes the importance of maintaining a patient, matter-of-factly respectful attitude; the communication of a sense of strength (lest a paranoid patient worry unconsciously that his or her negative affects could destroy the therapist); a willingness to respond with factual information when the patient raises questions (lest the patient feel evaded or toyed with); and attending to the patient's private conviction that aggression, dependency, and sexual desire—and the verbal expressions of any of these strivings—are inherently dangerous. It is best not to be too warm and solicitous, as such attitudes may stimulate a terror of regression and fuel suspicions about why the therapist is "really" being so nice.

KEY FEATURES

Contributing constitutional–maturational patterns: Possibly irritable/aggressive.

Central tension/preoccupation: Attacking versus being attacked by humiliating others.

Central affects: Fear, rage, shame, contempt.

Characteristic pathogenic belief about self: "I am in constant danger."

Characteristic pathogenic belief about others: "The world is full of potential attackers and users."

Central ways of defending: Projection, projective identification, denial, reaction formation.

Psychopathic Personalities

We prefer the earlier term "psychopathic" (Cleckley, 1941; Hare, 1991; Meloy, 1988, 1997) to the current "antisocial." Many people with psychopathic personalities are not obviously antisocial; that is, they are not observably at odds with social norms. In fact, many people with psychopathic personalities are able to pursue their agendas in contexts of social approval and even admiration. In some occupations, psychopathic behavior is rewarded (e.g., in the world of high-stakes finance, as journalistic coverage of the events leading to the 2008–2009 U.S. economic collapse exposed). Although many psychopathic individuals run into trouble with authorities, some are quite adept at evading accountability for the damage they do to others.

Once referred to as having "moral insanity" (Prichard, 1835), individuals with psychopathic personalities are commonly found in the borderline to the psychotic range of severity (Gacano & Meloy, 1994). Their characteristic orientation is toward seeking power for its own sake. They take pleasure in duping and manipulating others (Bursten, 1973). Deutsch's (1955) classic concept of the "impostor" fits within the psychopathic realm. Although the stereotype of antisocial personality involves aggression and violence, clinical writings over many decades (beginning with Henderson, 1939) have also noted more passive, parasitic versions of psychopathy, such as the person who operates a scam or Ponzi scheme within a relational matrix.

Psychopathic people feel anxiety less frequently and intensely than others (Ogloff & Wong, 1990; Zuckerman, 1999). People with diagnosed antisocial personality disorder have a higher-than-normal craving for stimulation and may seek it addictively (Raine, Venables, & Williams, 1990; Vitacco & Rogers, 2001). Psychopathic individuals lack the empathy and the moral center of gravity that, in people of other personality types, tames the striving for power and directs it toward socially valuable ends.

Psychopathic individuals may be charming and even charismatic, and they may read others' emotional states with great accuracy (Dolan & Fullam, 2004). They may be hyperacutely aware of their surroundings, but think and act from a self-referential stance and for egoistic purposes. Their own emotional life tends to be impoverished, and their expressed affect is often insincere and intended to manipulate. Their affective connection to others is minimal; they typically lose interest in people they see as no longer useful. They cannot describe their emotional reactions with any depth or nuance. Their indifference to the feelings and needs of others, including their characteristic lack of remorse after harming others, may reflect a grave disorder of early attachment. Neglect, abuse, addiction, chaotic undependability in caregivers, and profoundly bad fits between a child's temperament and those of responsible adults have been associated with later psychopathy, but there also appear to be temperamental contributing factors.

Therapists working with psychopathic individuals may find themselves feeling initially charmed and then deeply disturbed. They lack the usual sense of emotional connection and may find themselves feeling uncharacteristically apprehensive, jittery, or even "under the thumb" of their psychopathic patients—all countertransferences that are highly informative. Recent empirical studies have identified clinicians' emotional reactions of being criticized and overwhelmed while working with psychopathic patients (Colli et al., 2014; Gazzillo et al., 2015). Any known history of violence in a patient that coexists with these distressing emotional reactions should impel a therapist to give first consideration to issues of his or her own safety.

Treatment in which therapists persistently try to reach out sympathetically may come to grief with psychopathic patients, who regard kindness as signs of weakness. It is possible, however, to have a therapeutic influence on many psychopathic individuals if their clinicians convey a powerful presence, behave with scrupulous integrity, and recognize that these patients' motivations revolve primarily around the desire for power. The prospects for any therapeutic influence are better if a psychopathic individual has reached midlife or later, and has thus felt a decline in physical power and encountered limits to omnipotent strivings.

KEY FEATURES

Contributing constitutional–maturational patterns: Possible congenital aggressiveness, high threshold for emotional stimulation.

Central tension/preoccupation: Manipulating versus fear of being manipulated.

Central affects: Rage, envy.

Characteristic pathogenic belief about self: "I can do whatever I want."

Characteristic pathogenic belief about others: "Everyone is selfish, manipulative, dishonorable, and/or weak."

Central ways of defending: Reaching for omnipotent control.

Sadistic Personalities

Sadistic personality organization is found mainly at the borderline or psychotic level and is organized around the theme of domination. Internally, the sadistic person may experience deadness and affective sterility, which are relieved by inflicting pain and humiliation—in fantasy and often in reality. The diagnosis of sadistic personality disorder was listed as a provisional category in DSM-III-TR but disappeared in DSM-IV; yet, as Meloy (1997, p. 631) noted, "burning the map does not eliminate the territory." The reasons for the removal of this syndrome from the DSM are not clear, but may have included a concern that there is considerable overlap between sadistic and antisocial psychopathology. Yet, despite the fact that sadism and psychopathy are highly related (Holt, Meloy, & Strack, 1999), they are not identical. Not all psychopathic people are notably sadistic, nor are all sadistic people psychopathic.

Except for studies of criminal sexual sadism, there has been very little empirical research on sadistic personality patterns or disorders. Millon (1996) offers one of the few comprehensive accounts in the literature. Sadistic individuals are seen mainly in forensic settings, in which professionals may confront numerous people whose overriding motivation involves controlling, subjugating, and forcing pain and humiliation on others. Sadistic personality is readily recognizable. Meloy (1997) cites the man who smiles broadly and shamelessly while recounting his battering of his wife, and the child "who does not angrily kick a pet, but instead tortures animals with detached pleasure" (p. 632). In the search for total control over another—a project Fromm (1973, p. 323) called the turning of "impotence into omnipotence"—the sadistic person always chooses as a target those who are subordinate, weaker, and comparatively powerless (Shapiro, 1981).

Only a fraction of those who abuse others are characterologically sadistic. Although many people strike out when they feel provoked or attacked, sadistic people tend to inflict their tortures with a dispassionate calm (perhaps originally a defense against being overwhelmed by rage). Thus forensic scientists distinguish between "affective" (catathymic) and "predatory" violence (e.g., Serin, 1991). The hallmark of sadism is the emotional detachment or guiltless enthusiasm with which domination and control are pursued. This detachment, which may include the systematic, step-by-step preparation of a sadistic scenario, has the effect (and probably expresses the intent) of dehumanizing the other (Bollas, 1995). Although it is likely that all individuals with sadistic personality disorder are sadistic in their preferred expressions of sexuality, many people whose sexual fantasies or enactments involve sadistic themes are not sadistic generally and so cannot be considered to have the personality syndrome.

Professionals interviewing sadistic individuals typically report feelings of visceral disturbance, vague uneasiness, intimidation, "creepiness," and being overwhelmed by strong negative feelings. Meloy (1997) mentions goose bumps, the feeling of one's hair standing on end, and other atavistic reactions to a predator–prey situation. Because sadistic individuals are mendacious (Stone, 1993) and may enjoy tormenting their interviewers by lying or by withholding verbal descriptions of their sadistic preoccupations, such countertransferences may be a prime indication of underlying sadism. A therapist should always take seriously disturbing reactions of this sort, as indicating the need for more thorough assessment and a treatment plan that takes into account the person's possible dangerousness.

We know of no reports of successful psychotherapy for characterological sadism. Stone (1993, 2009), who has carefully analyzed biographical accounts of murderers, considers the sadistic individuals he has studied to be beyond the reach of therapy. The attachment deficit manifested by treating other beings as objects to toy with rather than subjects to respect may preclude developing the capacity for a therapeutic alliance. In addition, the pleasure in sadistic acts, especially orgiastic pleasure in sexual sadism, may be so reinforcing that efforts to reduce the sadistic pattern are futile. Still, accurate diagnosis of sadistic personality has significant implications for making recommendations to judicial officers, reducing opportunities for harm, helping people affected by sadistic persons, and allocating resources realistically.

KEY FEATURES

Contributing constitutional–maturational pattern: Unknown.

Central tension/preoccupation: Suffering indignity/inflicting such suffering.

Central affects: Cold hatred, contempt, pleasure (sadistic glee).

Characteristic pathogenic belief about self: "I am entitled to hurt and humiliate others."

Characteristic pathogenic belief about others: "Others exist as objects for my domination."

Central ways of defending: Detachment, omnipotent control, reversal, enactment.

Borderline Personalities

In the first PDM, we used the term "borderline" to refer only to a clinically inferred level of personality organization. Since its publication, the concept of a specific borderline *type* of personality disorder, defined by DSM criteria, has become so pervasive that we now follow Kernberg's solution of discriminating between borderline personality *organization* and borderline personality *disorder*. In addition, Shedler (2015) and Westen, Shedler, Bradley, and DeFife (2012) have found that clinicians identify a construct of borderline-dysregulated personality disorder that overlaps with both the DSM diagnostic construct of borderline personality disorder and Kernberg's concept of borderline organization.

In attachment research, scholars have identified a relevant disorganized/disoriented or "type D" insecure attachment style (e.g., Fonagy, Target, & Gergely, 2000; Liotti, 2004; Liotti, Pasquini, & Cirricone, 2000; Main & Solomon, 1986). This pattern is characterized by chronic, long-term difficulties in tolerating and regulating affect, and involves regarding attachment figures (such as therapists) as both objects of safety and objects of fear, causing them to be treated with confusing combinations of desperate clinging, hostile attack, and dissociative-like states of detachment. Neuroscientific research (Fertuck, Lenzenweger, Hoermann, & Stanley, 2006; van der Kolk, 2003) indicates that early trauma can damage the capacities for executive control (and thus affective regulation).

Efforts to understand the psychologies of people with borderline personalities span decades and have been undertaken from many perspectives. The concept has always been seen as complex and multifaceted. Scholars have viewed borderline personality in terms of reliance on splitting, projective identification, and other highly costly defenses (Kernberg, 1967, 1984); problems in psychiatric management (Gunderson & Singer, 1975; Main, 1957; Skodol, Gunderson, et al., 2002a; Skodol, Siever, et al., 2002b); disorganized attachment (Fonagy et al., 2000; Holmes, 2004; Liotti, 2004); inability to mentalize (to recognize internal states in self and others that underlie behaviors) and regulate affect (Fonagy, Gergely, Jurist, & Target, 2002); and inability to experience continuity of self and others (Bromberg, 1998; Chefetz, 2015; Meares, 2012).

In regard to etiology, there is evidence for a genetic vulnerability (Kernberg & Caligor, 2005; Paris, 1993; Siever & Davis, 1991; Stone, 1980; Torgersen, 2000), for origins in an early attachment disorder (Guidano & Liotti, 1983), for developmental arrest (Bateman & Fonagy, 2004; Fonagy et al., 2002; Masterson, 1972, 1976, 1988), and for the effects of severe relational trauma (Meares, 2012). The relative weight of each of these factors varies from person to person. Individuals with borderline personality disorder are notoriously difficult patients, partly because they may challenge ordinary therapeutic limits and evoke intense countertransference reactions, and partly because they require modification of the treatment models in which many therapists are trained.

Patients with borderline personality disorder feel emotions that easily spiral out of control and reach extremes of intensity, compromising their capacity for adaptive functioning. They tend to catastrophize, and they consequently require the presence of another person to help regulate their affect and be soothed. When the relationship with this other person becomes closer, however, they feel easily controlled or engulfed, and at the same time feel a deep fear of being rejected and abandoned. This inner turmoil disposes them to misunderstand the attitudes and behaviors of others as signs of present or future rejection and abandonment.

Such patients tend to have difficulties in connecting their own actions and feelings with what they think and with what is happening. They have trouble understanding other people's behaviors, intentions, desires, and emotions (i.e., failures in mentalization), often misinterpreting them via projection, or taking it for granted that others think and feel as they do. They have difficulties in putting themselves in other people's shoes and taking their perspectives. As a consequence, they tend to see other people in a binary (good or bad) and egocentric way. They may be naive, with a tendency to develop stereotypical explanations of their own and other people's behaviors, intentions, and desires; or they may be unduly suspicious, developing interpretations of these experiences that are so convoluted that they lose connection with the experiences themselves.

They additionally have difficulties in feeling a sense of continuity in their own experience. They may shift from one affect to another, from one self-representation to another, and from one self-state to another, without noticing the inconsistencies between these different affects, representations, and states. As a consequence, they may feel disoriented by their own behavior and may disorient people who are interacting with them. They tend to stir up in others emotions similar to those they are experiencing and/or emotions that they disavow in themselves.

They tend to feel an inner "void" and may enter into dissociated, trance-like states of consciousness. They may use self-mutilating behavior to soothe themselves. Often they report that these self-harming acts make them feel alive or reconnected with their bodies. They may make suicide threats or gestures for this reason, or, alternatively, to attract other people's attention or to manipulate them (or both). They may behave sexually or aggressively when their attachment needs are stirred up. They may often (but not always) be impulsive, and they tend to have trouble making and maintaining long-lasting, gratifying close relationships and stable, satisfying work lives.

The general recommendations in this manual for working with individuals in the borderline range of severity apply to those with diagnosable borderline personality disorder. To our knowledge, all approaches to helping an individual with borderline personality disorder emphasize the centrality of the working alliance and the importance of repairing it when it is damaged; the critical role of boundaries and the therapist's willingness to tolerate the patient's rage and hurt when boundaries are maintained; the discouragement of regression; the expectation of intensity; the inevitability of either–or dilemmas; the importance of the patient's sense of the therapist as an affectively genuine person; and the development of capacities for self-reflection, mentalization, or mindfulness. They also emphasize the need for ongoing clinical supervision and consultation.

Interestingly, psychoanalytic theorists who have written about the treatment of borderline personality disorder emphasize how their treatments deviate from standard psychoanalytic treatments (e.g., Bateman & Fonagy, 2004; Clarkin et al., 2006; Kernberg, 1989; Masterson, 1976, 1983), and cognitive-behavioral therapists emphasize how their treatments deviate from standard CBT (e.g., Linehan, 1993; Young, Klosko, & Weishaar, 2003).

KEY FEATURES

Contributing constitutional–maturational patterns: Congenital difficulties with affect regulation, intensity, aggression, capacity to be soothed.

Central tension/preoccupation: Self-cohesion versus fragmentation; engulfing attachment versus abandonment despair.

Central affects: Intense affects generally, especially rage, shame, and fear.

Characteristic pathogenic belief about self: "I don't know who I am; I inhabit dissociated self-states rather than having a sense of continuity."

Characteristic pathogenic belief about others: "Others are one-dimensional and defined by their effects on me, rather than by a sense of their complex individual psychology."

Central ways of defending: Splitting, projective identification, denial, dissociation, acting out, and other primitive defenses.

BIBLIOGRAPHY

Abbass, A. A. (2015). *Reaching through resistance: Advanced psychotherapy techniques*. Kansas City, MO: Seven Leaves Press.

Abbass, A. A., Kisely, S. R., Town, J. M., Leichsenring, F., Driessen, E., de Maat, S., . . . Crowe, E. (2014). Short-term psychodynamic psychotherapies for common mental disorders. *Cochrane Database of Systematic Reviews, 7*, CD004687.

Abbass, A., Town, J., & Driessen, E. (2011). The efficacy of short-term psychodynamic psychotherapy for depressive disorders with comorbid personality disorder. *Psychiatry, 74*(1), 58–71.

Achenbach, T., & Edelbrock, C. (1978). The classification of child psychopathology: A review and analysis of empirical efforts. *Psychological Bulletin, 85*, 1275–1301.

Adler, G. (1985). *Borderline psychopathology and its treatment*. New York: Aronson.

Ainsworth, M., Blehar, M. C., Waters, E., & Wall, S. (1978). *Patterns of attachment: A psychological study of the Strange Situation*. Hillsdale, NJ: Erlbaum.

Akhtar, S. (1989). Narcissistic personality disorder: Descriptive features and differential diagnosis. *Psychiatric Clinics of North America, 12*, 505–529.

Akhtar, S. (1992). *Broken structures: Severe personality disorders and their treatment*. Northvale, NJ: Aronson.

Akhtar, S. (1999). *Immigration and identity: Turmoil, treatment, and transformation*. Lanham, MD: Jason Aronson.

Akhtar, S. (Ed.). (2009). *Freud and the Far East: Psychoanalytic perspectives on the people and culture of China, Japan, and Korea*. Lanham, MD: Jason Aronson.

Akhtar, S. (2011). *Immigration and acculturation: Mourning, adaptation, and the next generation*. Lanham, MD: Jason Aronson.

Alarcón, R. D., & Foulks, E. F. (1995a). Personality disorders and culture: Contemporary clinical views (Part A). *Cultural Diversity and Mental Health, 1*, 3–17.

Alarcón, R. D., & Foulks, E. F. (1995b). Personality disorders and culture: Contemporary clinical views (Part B). *Cultural Diversity and Mental Health, 1*, 79–91.

Allport, G. W. (1937). *Personality: A psychological interpretation*. New York: Holt.

American Psychiatric Association. (1980). *Diagnostic and statistical manual of mental disorders* (3rd ed.). Washington, DC: Author.

American Psychiatric Association. (1987). *Diagnostic and statistical manual of mental disorders* (3rd ed., rev.). Washington, DC: Author.

American Psychiatric Association. (1994). *Diagnostic and statistical manual of mental disorders* (4th ed.). Washington, DC: Author.

American Psychiatric Association. (2000). *Diagnostic and statistical manual of mental disorders* (4th ed., text rev.). Washington, DC: Author.

American Psychiatric Association. (2013). *Diagnostic and statistical manual of mental disorders* (5th ed.). Arlington, VA: Author.

American Psychological Association. (2012). Recognition of psychotherapy effectiveness. Retrieved from *www.apa.org/about/policy/resolution-psychotherapy.aspx*.

Anstadt, T., Merten, J., Ullrich, B., & Krause, R. (1997). Affective dyadic behavior, core conflictual relationship themes and success of treatment. *Psychotherapy Research, 7*, 397–417.

Appelbaum, A. (2005). Supportive psychotherapy. In J. M. Oldman, A. E. Skodol, & D. S. Bender (Eds.), *Textbook of personality disorders* (pp. 335–346). Washington, DC: American Psychiatric Association.

Appelbaum, A. (2008). Supportive psychotherapy for borderline patients. *Social Work in Mental Health, 6*, 145–155.

Aron, L. (1991). Working through the past—working toward the future. *Contemporary Psychoanalysis, 27*, 81–108.

Atwood, G. E. (2011). *The abyss of madness*. New York: Routledge.

Bak, R. (1946). Masochism in paranoia. *Psychoanalytic Quarterly, 15*, 285–301.

Bakan, D. (1966). *The duality of human existence: Isolation and communion in Western man.* Boston: Beacon Press.

Bateman, A., & Fonagy, P. (2004). *Psychotherapy for borderline personality disorder: Mentalization-based treatment.* New York: Oxford University Press.

Beck, A. T. (1983). Cognitive therapy of depression. New perspectives. In P. J. Clayton & J. E. Barrett (Eds.), *Treatment of depression: Old controversies and new approaches* (pp. 265–290). New York: Raven Press.

Bender, D. S., Morey, L. C., & Skodol, A. E. (2011). Toward a model for assessing level of personality functioning in DSM-5: Part I. A review of theory and methods. *Journal of Personality Assessment, 93,* 332–346.

Benjamin, J. (1988). *The bonds of love: Psychoanalysis, feminism, and the problem of domination.* New York: Pantheon.

Benjamin, J. (1995). *Like subjects, like objects: Essays on recognition and sexual difference.* New Haven, CT: Yale University Press.

Berney, S., de Roten, Y., Beretta, V., Kramer, U., & Despland, J. N. (2014). Identifying psychotic defenses in a clinical interview. *Journal of Clinical Psychology, 70,* 428–439.

Betan, E., Heim, A. K., Zittel Conklin, C., & Westen, D. (2005). Countertransference phenomena and personality pathology in clinical practice: An empirical investigation. *American Journal of Psychiatry, 5,* 890–898.

Bion, W. R. (1967). *Second thoughts.* London: Karnac.

Blatt, S. J. (1990). Interpersonal relatedness and self-definition: Two personality configurations and their implications for psychopathology and psychotherapy. In J. L. Singer (Ed.), *Repression and dissociation* (pp. 299–336). Chicago: University of Chicago Press.

Blatt, S. J. (1992). The differential effect of psychotherapy and psychoanalysis with anaclitic and introjective patients: The Menninger Psychotherapy Research Project revisited. *Journal of the American Psychoanalytic Association, 40,* 691–724.

Blatt, S. J. (1993). Different kinds of folks may need different kinds of strokes: The effect of patients' characteristics on therapeutic process and outcome. *Psychotherapy Research, 3,* 245–259.

Blatt, S. J. (2004). *Experiences of depression: Theoretical, clinical and research perspectives.* Washington, DC: American Psychological Association.

Blatt, S. J. (2006). A fundamental polarity in psychoanalysis: Implications for personality development, psychopathology, and the therapeutic process. *Psychoanalytic Inquiry, 26,* 494–520.

Blatt, S. J. (2008). *Polarities of experience: Relatedness and self-definition in personality development, psychopathology, and the therapeutic process.* Washington, DC: American Psychological Association.

Blatt, S. J., & Auerbach, J. S. (1988). Differential cognitive disturbances in three types of "borderline" patients. *Journal of Personality Disorders, 2,* 198–211.

Blatt, S. J., & Bers, S. A. (1993). The sense of self in depression: A psychodynamic perspective. In Z. V. Segal & S. J. Blatt (Eds.), *The self in emotional distress: Cognitive and psychodynamic perspectives* (pp. 171–210). New York: Guilford Press.

Blatt, S. J., & Blass, R. B. (1990). Attachment and separateness: A dialectic model of the products and processes of psychological development. *Psychoanalytic Study of the Child, 45,* 107–127.

Blatt, S. J., & Luyten, P. (2010). Reactivating the psychodynamic approach to classify psychopathology. In T. Millon, R. F. Krueger, & E. Simonsen (Eds.), *Contemporary directions in psychopathology. Scientific foundations of the DSM-V and ICD-11* (pp. 483–514). New York: Guilford Press.

Blatt, S. J., & Zuroff, D. C. (1992). Interpersonal relatedness and self-definition: Two prototypes for depression. *Clinical Psychology Review, 12,* 527–562.

Blatt, S. J., Zuroff, D. C., Hawley, L. L., & Auerbach, J. S. (2010). Predictors of sustained therapeutic change. *Psychotherapy Research, 20,* 37–54.

Bollas, C. (1995). *Cracking up: The work of unconscious experience.* New York: Hill & Wang.

Bollas, C. (2012). *China on the mind.* London: Routledge.

Bonime, W. (1979). Paranoid psychodynamics. *Contemporary Psychoanalysis, 15,* 514–527.

Bornstein, R. F. (1993). *The dependent personality.* New York: Guilford Press.

Bornstein, R. F. (2005). *The dependent patient: A practitioner's guide.* Washington, DC: American Psychological Association.

Boulanger, G. (2007). *Wounded by reality: Understanding and treating adult onset trauma.* Mahwah, NJ: Analytic Press.

Bourke, M. E., & Grenyer, B. F. S. (2010). Psychotherapists' response to borderline personality disorder: A core conflictual relationship theme analysis. *Psychotherapy Research, 20,* 680–691.

Bourke, M. E., & Grenyer, B. F. S. (2013). Therapists' accounts of psychotherapy process associated with treating patients with borderline personality disorder. *Journal of Personality Disorders, 27,* 735–745.

Bowlby, J. (1969). *Attachment and loss: Vol. 1. Attachment.* London: Hogarth Press.

Bradley, R., Heim, A., & Westen, D. (2005). Transference patterns in the psychotherapy of personality disorders: Empirical investigation. *British Journal of Psychiatry, 186,* 342–349.

Brenner, C. (1959). The masochistic character: Genesis and treatment. *Journal of the American Psychoanalytic Association, 7*, 197–226.

Bromberg, P. M. (1998). *Standing in the spaces: Essays on clinical process, trauma and dissociation*. Hillsdale, NJ: Analytic Press.

Bucci, W. (1997). *Psychoanalysis and cognitive science*. New York: Guilford Press.

Buchheim, A., Erk, S., George, C., Kachele, H., Kircher, T., Martius, P., . . . Walter, H. (2008). Neural correlates of attachment trauma in borderline personality disorder: A functional magnetic resonance imaging study. *Psychiatry Research: Neuroimaging, 163*, 223–235.

Bugas, J., & Silberschatz, G. (2000). How patients coach their therapists in psychotherapy. *Psychotherapy: Theory, Research, Practice, Training, 37*(1), 64–70.

Bursten, B. (1973). *The manipulator: A psychoanalytic view*. New Haven, CT: Yale University Press.

Caligor, E., Kernberg, O. F., & Clarkin, J. F. (2007). *Handbook of dynamic psychotherapy for higher level personality pathology*. Washington, DC: American Psychiatric Association.

Carter, P., & Grenyer, B. F. S. (2012). Expressive language disturbance in borderline personality disorder in response to emotional autobiographical stimuli. *Journal of Personality Disorders, 26*(3), 305–321.

Chefetz, R. A. (2000). Disorder in the therapist's view of the self: Working with the person with dissociative identity disorder. *Psychoanalytic Inquiry, 20*, 305–329.

Chefetz, R. A. (2015). *Intensive psychotherapy for persistent dissociative processes: The fear of feeling real*. New York: Norton.

Chodorow, N. J. (1994). *Femininities, masculinities, sexualities: Freud and beyond*. Lexington: University Press of Kentucky.

Chodorow, N. J. (1999). *The reproduction of motherhood* (2nd ed.). Berkeley: University of California Press.

Cierpka, M., Grande, T., Rudolf, G., von der Tann, M., Stasch, M., & OPD Task Force. (2007). The operationalized psychodynamic diagnostics system: Clinical relevance, reliability and validity. *Psychopathology, 40*, 209–220.

Clarkin, J. F., Foelsch, P. A., Levy, K. M., Hull, J. W., Delaney, J. D., & Kernberg, O. F. (2001). The development of a psychodynamic treatment for patients with borderline personality disorder: A preliminary study of behavioral change. *Journal of Personality Disorders, 15*, 487–495.

Clarkin, J. F., Levy, K. N., Lenzenweger, M., & Kernberg, O. F. (2004). The Personality Disorders Institute/Borderline Personality Research Foundation randomized control trial for borderline personality disorder: Rationale, methods, and patient characteristics. *Journal of Personality Disorders, 18*, 51–72.

Clarkin, J. F., Levy, K. N., Lenzenweger, M. F., & Kernberg, O. F. (2007). Evaluating three treatments for borderline personality disorder: A multiwave study. *American Journal of Psychiatry, 164*, 922–928.

Clarkin, J. F., Yeomans, F. E., & Kernberg, O. F. (1999). *Psychotherapy for borderline personality: Focusing on object relations*. Washington, DC: American Psychiatric Association.

Cleckley, H. (1941). *The mask of sanity: An attempt to clarify some issues about the so-called psychopathic personality*. St. Louis, MO: Mosby.

Colli, A., Tanzilli, A., Dimaggio, G., & Lingiardi, V. (2014). Patient personality and therapist response: An empirical investigation. *American Journal of Psychiatry, 171*, 102–108.

Compton, W. M., & Guze, S. B. (1995). The neo-Kraepelinian revolution in psychiatric diagnosis. *European Archives of Psychiatry and Clinical Neuroscience, 245*, 196–201.

Cooper, A. M. (1988). The narcissistic–masochistic character. In R. A. Glick & D. I. Meyers (Eds.), *Masochism: Current psychological perspectives* (pp. 189–204). Hillsdale, NJ: Analytic Press.

Cramer, P. (2006). *Protecting the self: Defense mechanisms in action*. New York: Guilford Press.

Cramer, P. (2015). Defense mechanisms: 40 years of empirical research. *Journal of Personality Assessment, 97*, 114–122.

Czubak, K. (2014). Attachment styles and personality disorders. *Personality and Individual Differences, 60*(Suppl.), S51.

Dahl, H. (1988). Frames of mind. In H. Dahl, H. Kachele, & H. Thomae (Eds.), *Psychoanalytic process research strategies* (pp. 51–66). New York: Springer-Verlag.

Dahl, H. S. J., Røssberg, J. I., Bøgwald, K. P., Gabbard, G. O., & Høglend, P. A. (2012). Countertransference feelings in one year of individual therapy: An evaluation of the factor structure in the Feeling Word Checklist–58. *Psychotherapy Research, 22*, 12–25.

Daros, A. R., Zakzanis, K. K., & Ruocco, A. C. (2013). Facial emotion recognition in borderline personality disorder. *Psychological Medicine, 43*, 1953–1963.

Davis, K. L., & Panksepp, J. (2011). The brain's emotional foundations of human personality and the Affective Neuroscience Personality Scales. *Neuroscience and Biobehavioral Reviews, 35*, 1946–1958.

Deutsch, H. (1955). The impostor: Some forms of emotional disturbance and their relationship to schizophrenia. *Psychoanalytic Quarterly, 11*, 301–321.

Diamond, D., Levy, K. N., Clarkin, J. F., Fischer-Kern,

M., Cain, N. M., Doering, S., . . . Buchheim A. (2014). Attachment and mentalization in female patients with comorbid narcissistic and borderline personality disorder. *Personality Disorders, 5*, 428–433.

Diamond, D., Yeomans, F. E., Stern, B., Levy, K. N., Hörz, S., Doering, S., . . . Clarkin, J. F. (2013). Transference focused psychotherapy for patients with comorbid narcissistic and borderline personality disorder. *Psychoanalytic Inquiry, 33*, 527–551.

Di Giuseppe, M. G., Perry, J. C., Petraglia, J., Janzen, J., & Lingiardi, V. (2014). Development of a Q-sort version of the Defense Mechanism Rating Scales (DMRS-Q) for clinical use. *Journal of Clinical Psychology, 70*, 452–465.

Dimaggio, G., & Semerari, A. (2004). Disorganized narratives: the psychological condition and his treatment. How to achieve a metacognitive point of view order to chaos. In L. Angus & J. McLeod (Eds.), *Handbook of narrative psychotherapy: Practice, theory and research* (pp. 263–282). Thousand Oaks, CA: SAGE.

Dimen, M. (2003). *Sexuality, intimacy, power.* Hillsdale, NJ: Analytic Press.

Dimen, M., & Goldner, V. (Eds.). (2002). *Gender in psychoanalytic space.* New York: Other Press.

Dimen, M., & Goldner, V. (2012). Gender and sexuality. In G. O. Gabbard, B. E. Litowitz, & P. Williams (Eds.), *Textbook of psychoanalysis* (2nd ed., pp. 133–154). Arlington, VA: American Psychiatric Publishing.

Distel, M. A., Trull, T. J., Derom, C. A., Thiery, E. W., Grimmer, M. A., Martin, N. G., . . . Boomsma, D. I. (2008). Heritability of borderline personality disorder features is similar across three countries. *Psychological Medicine, 38*, 1219–1229.

Doi, T. (1981). *The anatomy of dependence: The key analysis of Japanese behavior* (2nd ed.). Tokyo: Kodansha International.

Doidge, N. (2001). Diagnosing *The English Patient*: Schizoid fantasies of being skinless and being buried alive. *Journal of the American Psychoanalytic Association, 49*, 279–309.

Dolan, R., & Fullam, R. (2004). Theory of mind and mentalizing ability in antisocial personality disorders with and without psychopathy. *Psychological Medicine, 34*, 1093–1102.

Dozier, M., Stovall-McClough, K. C., & Albus, K. E. (2008). Attachment and psychopathology in adulthood. In J. Cassidy & P. R. Shaver (Eds.), *Handbook of attachment: Theory, research, and clinical applications* (2nd ed., pp. 718–744). New York: Guilford Press.

Drapeau, M., De Roten, Y., Perry, J. C., & Despland, J. N. (2003). A study of stability and change in defense mechanisms during a brief psychodynamic investigation. *Journal of Nervous and Mental Disease, 191*, 496–502.

Duncan, B. L., Miller, S. D., Wampold, B. E., & Hubble, M. A. (Eds.). (2010). *The heart and soul of change: Delivering what works in therapy* (2nd ed.). Washington, DC: American Psychological Association.

Fairbairn, W. R. D. (1952). *An object-relations theory of the personality.* New York: Basic Books.

Federn, P. (1952). *Ego psychology and the psychoses.* New York: Basic Books.

Feighner, J. P., Robins, E., Guze, S. B., Woodruff, R. A., Winokur, G., & Munoz, R. (1972). Diagnostic criteria for use in psychiatric research. *Archives of General Psychiatry, 26*, 57–63.

Fertuck, E., Bucci, W., Blatt, S. J., & Ford, R. Q. (2004). Verbal representation and therapeutic change in anaclitic and introjective patients. *Psychotherapy: Theory, Research, Practice, Training, 41*, 13–25.

Fertuck, E. A., Jekal, A., Songa, I., Wyman, B., Morris, M. C., Wilson, S. T., . . . Stanley, B. (2009). Enhanced "reading the mind with the eyes" in borderline personality disorder compared to healthy controls. *Psychological Medicine, 39*, 1979–1988.

Fertuck, E. A., Lenzenweger, M. F., Hoermann, S., & Stanley, B. (2006). Executive neurocognition, memory systems, and borderline personality disorder. *Clinical Psychology Review, 26*, 346–357.

Fisher, S., & Greenberg, R. P. (1985). *The scientific credibility of Freud's theories and therapy.* New York: Columbia University Press.

Fonagy, P., Bateman, A. W., Lorenzini, N., & Campbell, C. (2014). Development, attachment, and childhood experiences. In J. M. Oldham, A. E. Skodol, & D. Bender (Eds.), *Textbook of personality disorders* (2nd ed., pp. 55–78). Washington, DC: American Psychiatric Association.

Fonagy, P., Gergely, G., Jurist, E., & Target, M. (2002). *Affect regulation, mentalization, and the development of the self.* New York: Other Press.

Fonagy, P., Target, M., & Gergely, G. (2000). Attachment and borderline personality disorder: A theory and some evidence. *Psychiatric Clinics of North America, 23*, 103–122.

Fonagy, P., Target, M., Gergely, G., Allen, J. G., & Bateman, A. W. (2003). The developmental roots of borderline personality disorder in early attachment relationships: A theory and some evidence. *Psychoanalytic Inquiry, 23*, 412–459.

Fossati, A., Feeney, J., Pincus, A., Borroni, S., & Maffei, C. (2015). The structure of pathological narcissism and its relationships with adult attachment styles: A study of Italian nonclinical and clinical adult participants. *Psychoanalytic Psychology, 32*, 403–431.

Frank, J. D., Margolin, J., Nash, H. T., Stone, A. R., Varon, E., & Ascher, E. (1952). Two behavior patterns in therapeutic groups and their apparent motivation. *Human Relations, 5*, 289–317.

French, T. (1958). *The integration of behavior: Vol. 3.*

The reintegrative process in a psychoanalytic treatment. Chicago: University of Chicago Press.

Fromm, E. (1973). *The anatomy of human destructiveness.* New York: Fawcett.

Frosch, J. (1964). The psychotic character: Clinical psychiatric considerations. *Psychiatric Quarterly, 38,* 91–96.

Freud, S. (1913). The disposition to obsessional neurosis. *Standard Edition, 12,* 311–326.

Gabbard, G. O. (1989). Two subtypes of narcissistic personality disorder. *Bulletin of the Menninger Clinic, 53,* 527–539.

Gabbard, G. O. (2009a). *Textbook of psychotherapeutic treatments.* Washington, DC: American Psychiatric Association.

Gabbard, G. O. (2009b). Transference and countertransference: Developments in the treatment of narcissistic personality disorder. *Psychiatric Annals, 39,* 129–136.

Gacono, C., & Meloy, J. R. (1988). The relationship between cognitive style and defensive process in the psychopath. *Criminal Justice and Behavior, 15,* 472–483.

Gacono, C., & Meloy, J. R. (1994). *Rorschach assessment of aggressive and psychopathic personalities.* Hillsdale, NJ: Erlbaum.

Gairdner, W. (2002). The ailment: 45 years later. *Clinical Child Psychology and Psychiatry, 7,* 288–294.

Garrett, M. (2012). Cognitive behavioral therapy for psychosis. In H. L. McQuistion, W. E. Sowers, J. M. Ranz, & J. M. Feldman (Eds.), *The American Association of Community Psychiatrists handbook of community psychiatry* (pp. 153–162). New York: Springer.

Garrett, M., & Turkington, D. (2011). CBT for psychosis in a psychoanalytic frame. *Psychosis, 3,* 1–13.

Gazzillo, F., Lingiardi, V., Del Corno, F., Genova, F., Bornstein, R. F., Gordon, R., & McWilliams, N. (2015). Clinicians' emotional responses and *Psychodynamic Diagnostic Manual* adult personality disorders: A clinically relevant empirical investigation. *Psychotherapy, 52*(2), 238–246.

Gilbert, P., Boxall, M., Cheung, M., & Irons, C. (2005). The relation of paranoid ideation and social anxiety in a mixed clinical population. *Clinical Psychology and Psychotherapy, 12*(2), 124–133.

Glickauf-Hughes, C. (1997). Etiology of the masochistic and narcissistic personality. *American Journal of Psychoanalysis, 57,* 141–148.

Gordon, R. M., Gazzillo, F., Blake, A., Bornstein, R. F., Etzi, J., Lingiardi, V., . . . Tasso, A. F. (2016). The relationship between theoretical orientation and countertransference awareness: Implications for ethical dilemmas and risk management. *Clinical Psychology and Psychotherapy, 23*(3), 236–245.

Gordon, R. M., & Stoffey, R. W. (2014). Operationalizing the *Psychodynamic Diagnostic Manual*: A preliminary study of the Psychodiagnostic Chart (PDC). *Bulletin of the Menninger Clinic, 78*(1), 1–15.

Grant, B., Chou, S., Goldstein, R., Huang, B., Stinson, F., Saha, T., . . . Ruan, W. (2008). Prevalence, correlates, disability, and comorbility of DSM-IV borderline personality disorder: Results from the wave 2 National Epidemiologic Survey on alcohol and related conditions. *Journal of Clinical Psychiatry, 69,* 533–545.

Greenspan, S. I. (1992). *Infancy and early childhood: The practice of clinical assessment and intervention with emotional and developmental challenges.* Madison, CT: International Universities Press.

Greenspan, S. I., & Shanker, S. (2004). *The first idea: How symbols, language, and intelligence evolve from primates to humans.* Reading, MA: Perseus Books.

Grenyer, B. F. S. (2012). The clinician's dilemma: Core conflictual relationship themes in personality disorders. *ACPARIAN (Australian Clinical Psychologist), 4,* 20–26.

Grenyer, B. F. S., Deane, F. P., & Lewis, K. (2008). Treatment history and its relationship to outcome in psychotherapy for depression. *Counselling and Psychotherapy Research, 8,* 21–27.

Grinker, R. R., Werble, B., & Drye, R. C. (1968). *The borderline syndrome: A behavioral study of ego functions.* New York: Basic Books.

Group for the Advancement of Psychiatry. (2002). *Cultural assessment in clinical psychiatry.* Washington, DC: American Psychiatric Association.

Grotstein, J. (2009). *". . . But at the same time and on another level . . . "* London: Karnac.

Groves, J. E. (1978). Taking care of the hateful patient. *New England Journal of Medicine, 298*(16), 883–887.

Guidano, V., & Liotti, G. (1983). *Cognitive processes and emotional disorders: A structural approach to psychotherapy.* New York: Guilford Press.

Gunderson, J. G. (2007). Disturbed relationships as a phenotype for borderline personality disorder. *American Journal of Psychiatry, 164,* 1637–1640.

Gunderson, J. G., & Singer, M. T. (1975). Defining borderline patients: An overview. *American Journal of Psychiatry, 133,* 1–10.

Guntrip, H. (1969). *Schizoid phenomena, object relations and the self.* New York: International Universities Press.

Guthiel, T. G. (2005). Boundary issues and personality disorders. *Journal of Psychiatric Practice, 11,* 88–96.

Gwirtsman, H. E., Blehar, M. C., McCullough, J. P., & Kocsis, J. H. (1997). Standardized assessment of dysthymia: Report of a National Institute of Mental Health conference. *Psychopharmacology Bulletin, 33,* 3–11.

Hare, R. (1991). *The Hare Psychopathy Checklist:*

Revised manual. Toronto, ON, Canada: Multi-Health Systems.

Hartocollis, P. (Ed.). (1977). *Borderline personality disorders: The concept, the syndrome, the patient*. New York: International Universities Press.

Hellerstein, D. J., Pinsker, H., Rosenthal, R. N., & Klee, S. (1994). Supportive therapy as the treatment model of choice. *Journal of Psychotherapy Practice and Research, 3*, 300–306.

Henderson, D. K. (1939). *Psychopathic states*. London: Chapman & Hall.

Herman, J. L., Perry, J. C., & van der Kolk, B. A. (1989). Childhood trauma in borderline personality disorder. *American Journal of Psychiatry, 146*, 490–495.

Hibbard, S., & Porcerelli, J. C. (1998). Further validation of the Cramer Defense Mechanisms Manual. *Journal of Personality Assessment, 70*, 460–483.

Hillenbrand, L. (2003, July 7). A sudden illness. *The New Yorker*, pp. 56–65.

Hilsenroth, M., Callahan, K., & Eudell, E. (2003). Further reliability, convergent and discriminant validity of overall defensive functioning. *Journal of Nervous and Mental Disease, 191*, 730–737.

Hirschfeld, R. M. A. (1991). Depressive illness: Diagnostic issues. *Bulletin of the Menninger Clinic, 55*, 144–155.

Holmes, J. (2004). Disorganized attachment and borderline personality disorder: A clinical perspective. *Attachment and Human Development, 6*, 181–190.

Holt, S., Meloy, J. R., & Strack, S. (1999). Sadism and psychopathy in violent and sexually violent offenders. *Journal of the American Academy of Psychiatry and the Law, 27*, 23–32.

Horney, K. (1950). *Neurosis and human growth: The struggle toward self-realization*. New York: Norton.

Horowitz, L., Gabbard, G. O., Allen, J. G., Frieswyk, S. H., Colson, D. B., Newsom, G. E., & Coyne, L. (1996). *Borderline personality disorder: Tailoring the psychotherapy to the patient*. Washington, DC: American Psychiatric Association.

Horowitz, M. J. (1991). *Hysterical personality style and the histrionic personality disorder*. Northvale, NJ: Aronson.

Horowitz, M. J. (1997). Psychotherapy for histrionic personality disorder. *Journal of Psychotherapy Practice and Research, 6*, 93–104.

Horowitz, M. (1998). *Cognitive psychodynamics: From conflict to character*. New York: Wiley.

Huprich, S. K. (1998). Depressive personality disorder: Theoretical issues, clinical findings, and future research questions. *Clinical Psychology Review, 18*, 477–500.

Huprich, S. K. (2014). Malignant self-regard: A self-structure enhancing the understanding of masochistic, depressive, and vulnerably narcissistic personalities. *Harvard Review of Psychiatry, 22*, 295–305.

Huprich, S. K., DeFife, J., & Westen, D. (2014). Refining a complex diagnostic construct: Subtyping dysthymia with the Shedler–Westen Assessment Procedure–II. *Journal of Affective Disorders, 152–154*, 186–192.

Huprich, S. K., McWilliams, N., Lingiardi, V., Bornstein, R. F., Gazzillo, F., & Gordon, R. M. (2015). The *Psychodynamic Diagnostic Manual* (PDM) and the PDM-2: Opportunities to significantly affect the profession. *Psychoanalytic Inquiry, 35*(9), 60–73.

Huprich, S. K., & Nelson, S. M. (2014). Malignant self-regard: Accounting for commonalities in vulnerably narcissistic, depressive, self-defeating, and masochistic personality disorders. *Comprehensive Psychiatry, 55*, 989–998.

Hurvich, M. (2003). The place of annihilation anxiety in psychoanalytic theory. *Journal of the American Psychoanalytic Association, 51*, 579–616.

Joyce A. S., Fujiwara, E., Cristall, M., Ruddy, C., & Ogrodniczuk, J. S. (2013). Clinical correlates of alexithymia among patients with personality disorder. *Psychotherapy Research, 23*, 690–704.

Jung, C. G. (1971). *The collected works of C. G. Jung: Vol. 6. Psychological types* (H. B. Baynes, Trans.). London: Routledge. (Original work published 1921)

Kagan, J. (1994). *Galen's prophecy: Temperament in human nature*. New York: Basic Books.

Kakar, S. (2008). *Culture and psyche: Selected essays*. London: Oxford University Press.

Karon, B. P., & VandenBos, G. R. (1981). *Psychotherapy of schizophrenia: The treatment of choice*. New York: Aronson.

Kealy, D., Ogrodniczuk, J. S., Joyce, A. S., Steinberg, P. I., & Piper, W. E. (2013). Narcissism and relational representations among psychiatric outpatients. *Journal of Personality Disorder, 27*, 1–5.

Kendler, K. S., Prescott, C. A., Myers, J., & Neale, M. C. (2003). The structure of genetic and environmental risk factors for common psychiatric and substance use disorders in men and women. *Archives of General Psychiatry, 60*, 929–937.

Kernberg, O. F. (1967). Borderline personality organization. *Journal of the American Psychoanalytic Association, 15*, 641–685.

Kernberg, O. F. (1975). *Borderline conditions and pathological narcissism*. New York: Aronson.

Kernberg, O. F. (1983). Object relations theory and character analysis. *Journal of the American Psychoanalytic Association, 31*, 247–271.

Kernberg, O. F. (1984). *Severe personality disorders: Psychotherapeutic strategies*. New Haven, CT: Yale University Press.

Kernberg, O. F. (1988). Clinical dimensions of masochism. *Journal of the American Psychoanalytic Association, 36*, 1005–1029.

Kernberg, O. F. (1989). *Psychodynamic psychotherapy of borderline patients*. New York: Basic Books.

Kernberg, O. F. (1991). The psychopathology of hatred. *Journal of the American Psychoanalytic Association, 39*(Suppl.), 209–238.

Kernberg, O. F. (1992). Psychopathic, paranoid, and depressive transferences. *International Journal of Psycho-Analysis, 73*, 13–28.

Kernberg, O. F. (2014). An overview of the treatment of severe narcissistic pathology. *International Journal of Psychoanalysis, 95*, 865–888.

Kernberg, O. F., & Caligor, E. (2005). A psychoanalytic theory of personality disorders. In M. F. Lenzenweger & J. F. Clarkin (Eds.), *Major theories of personality disorders* (2nd ed., pp. 114–156). New York: Guilford Press.

Khan, M. R. (1974). *The privacy of the self.* London: Karnac.

King-Casas, B., Sharp, C., Lomax-Bream, L., Lohrenz, T., Fonagy, P., & Read Montague, P. (2008). The rupture and repair of cooperation in borderline personality disorder. *Science, 321*, 806–810.

Kirsten, L. T., Grenyer, B. F. S., Wagner, R., & Manicavasagar, V. (2008). Impact of separation anxiety on psychotherapy outcomes for adults with anxiety disorders. *Counselling and Psychotherapy Research, 8*, 36–42.

Kitayama, S., & Markus, H. R. (1999). Yin and yang of the Japanese self: The cultural psychology of personality coherence. In D. Cervone & Y. Shoda (Eds.), *The coherence of personality: Social cognitive bases of personality consistency, variability, and organization* (pp. 242–302). New York: Guilford Press.

Klein, M. (1946). Notes on some schizoid mechanisms. *International Journal of Psychoanalysis, 27*, 99–110.

Klerman, G. L. (1978). The evolution of a scientific nosology. In J. C. Shershow (Ed.), *Schizophrenia: Science and practice* (pp. 99–121). Cambridge, MA: Harvard University Press.

Knight, R. (1953). Borderline states in psychoanalytic psychiatry and psychology. *Bulletin of the Menninger Clinic, 17*, 1–12.

Kohut, H. (1971). *The analysis of the self: A systematic approach to the psychoanalytic treatment of narcissistic personality disorders.* New York: International Universities Press.

Kohut, H. (1977). *The restoration of the self.* New York: International Universities Press.

Kramer, U., de Roten, Y., Perry, J. C., & Despland, J. (2013). Beyond splitting: Observer-rated defense mechanisms in borderline personality disorder. *Psychoanalytic Psychology, 30*, 3–15.

Krueger, R. F. (1999). The structure of common mental disorders. *Archives of General Psychiatry, 56*, 921–926.

Laughlin, H. P. (1979). *The ego and its defenses* (2nd ed.). New York: Aronson.

Leary, T. (1957). *Interpersonal diagnosis of personality: A functional theory and methodology for personality evaluation.* New York: Ronald Press.

Leichsenring, F., Leibing, E., Kruse, J., New, A., & Leweke, F. (2011). Borderline personality disorder. *Lancet, 377*, 74–84.

Lenzenweger, M. F., Clarkin, J. F., Kernberg, O. F., & Foelsch, P. A. (2001). The Inventory of Personality Organization: Psychometric properties, factorial composition, and criterion relations with affect, aggressive dyscontrol, psychosis proneness, and self-domains in a nonclinical sample. *Psychological Assessment, 13*, 577–591.

Levy, K., & Blatt, S. J. (1999). Attachment theory and psychoanalysis. *Psychoanalytic Inquiry, 19*, 541–575.

Levy, K. N., Edell, W. S., & McGlashan, T. H. (2007). Depressive experiences in inpatients with borderline personality disorder. *Psychiatric Quarterly, 78*, 129–143.

Lewis, K., Caputi, P., & Grenyer, B. F. S. (2012). Borderline personality disorder subtypes: A factor analysis of the DSM-IV criteria. *Personality and Mental Health, 6*(3), 196–206.

Lewis, K., & Grenyer, B. F. S. (2009). Borderline personality or complex posttraumatic stress disorder?: An update on the controversy. *Harvard Review of Psychiatry, 17*(5), 322–328.

Lewis-Fernández, R., Aggarwal, N. K., Bäärnhielm, S., Rohlof, H., Kirmayer, L. J., Weiss, M. G., . . . Lu, F. (2014). Culture and psychiatric evaluation: Operationalizing cultural formulation for DSM-5. *Psychiatry: Interpersonal and Biological Processes, 77*, 130–154.

Linehan, M. M. (1993). *Cognitive-behavioral treatment of borderline personality disorder.* New York: Guilford Press.

Lingiardi, V., Gazzillo, F., & Waldron, S. (2010). An empirically supported psychoanalysis: The case of Giovanna. *Psychoanalytic Psychology, 27*(2), 190–218.

Lingiardi, V., Lonati, C., Fossati, A., Vanzulli, L., & Maffei, C. (1999). Defense mechanisms and personality disorders. *Journal of Nervous and Mental Disease, 187*, 224–228.

Lingiardi, V., & McWilliams, N. (2015). The *Psychodynamic Diagnostic Manual*—2nd edition (PDM-2). *World Psychiatry, 14*(2), 237–239.

Lingiardi, V., McWilliams, N., Bornstein, R. F., Gazzillo, F., & Gordon, R. (2015a). The *Psychodynamic Diagnostic Manual* version 2 (PDM-2): Assessing patients for improved clinical practice and research. *Psychoanalytic Psychology, 32*, 94–115.

Lingiardi, V., Shedler, J., & Gazzillo, F. (2006). Assessing personality change in psychotherapy with the SWAP-200: A case study. *Journal of Personality Assessment, 86*(1), 36–45.

Lingiardi, V., Tanzilli, A., & Colli, A. (2015b). Does

the severity of psychopathological symptoms mediate the relationship between patient personality and therapist response? *Psychotherapy, 52*(2), 228–237.

Liotti, G. (1999). Disorganization of attachment as a model for understanding dissociative psychopathology. In J. Solomon & C. George (Eds.), *Attachment disorganization* (pp. 291–317). New York: Guilford Press.

Liotti, G. (2004). Trauma, dissociation, and disorganized attachment: Three strands of a single braid. *Psychotherapy: Theory, Research, Practice, Training, 41*, 472–487.

Liotti, G., Pasquini, P., & Cirricone, R. (2000). Predictive factors for borderline personality disorders: Patients' early traumatic experiences and losses suffered by attachment figures. *Acta Psychiatrica Scandinavica, 102*, 282–289.

Lotterman, A. (1996). *Specific techniques for the psychotherapy of schizophrenic patients*. New York: International Universities Press.

Lotterman, A. (2015). *Psychotherapy for people diagnosed with schizophrenia: Specific techniques*. New York: Routledge.

Luborsky, L., & Crits-Cristoph, P. (1996). *Understanding transference* (2nd ed.). Washington, DC: American Psychological Association.

Luyten, P., & Blatt, S. J. (2013). Interpersonal relatedness and self-definition in normal and disrupted personality development: Retrospect and prospect. *American Psychologist, 68*, 172–183.

Luyten, P., Blatt, S. J., & Mayes, L. C. (2012). Process and outcome in psychoanalytic psychotherapy research: The need for a (relatively) new paradigm. In R. A. Levy, J. S. Ablon, & H. Kächele (Eds.), *Psychodynamic psychotherapy research: Evidence-based practice and practice-based evidence* (pp. 345–359). New York: Springer.

Lyons-Ruth, K. (1999). The two-person unconscious: Intersubjective dialogue, enactive relational representation, and the emergence of new forms of relational organization. *Psychoanalytic Inquiry, 19*, 576–617.

MacKinnon, R. A., & Michels, R. (1971). *The psychiatric interview in clinical practice*. Philadelphia: Saunders.

MacKinnon, R. A., Michels, R., & Buckley, P. J. (2006). *The psychiatric interview in clinical practice* (2nd ed.). Washington, DC: American Psychiatric Association.

Main, M. (1995). Recent studies in attachment: Overview, with selected implications for clinical work. In S. Goldberg, R. Muir, & J. Kerr (Eds.), *Attachment theory: Social, developmental, and clinical perspectives* (pp. 407–474). Hillsdale, NJ: Analytic Press.

Main, M., & Solomon, J. (1986). Discovery of an insecure disorganized/disoriented attachment pattern: Procedures, findings and implications for classification of behaviour. In M. W. Yogman & T. B. Brazelton (Eds.), *Affective development in infancy* (pp. 95–124). Norwood, NJ: Ablex.

Main, T. F. (1957). The ailment. *British Journal of Medical Psychology, 30*, 129–145.

Malan, D. H. (1976). *The frontier of brief psychotherapy*. New York: Plenum Press.

Markon, K. E., Krueger, R. F., & Watson, D. (2005). Delineating the structure of normal and abnormal personality: An integrative hierarchical approach. *Journal of Personality and Social Psychology, 88*, 139–157.

Markus, H. R., & Kitayama, S. (1991). Culture and the self: Implications for cognition, emotion, and motivation. *Psychological Review, 98*, 224–253.

Marty, P., & M'Uzan, M. de. (1963). La pensé opératoire. *Revue Française de Psychoanalyse, 27*(Suppl.), 345–356.

Masterson, J. F. (1972). *Treatment of the borderline adolescent: A developmental approach*. New York: Wiley.

Masterson, J. F. (1976). *Psychotherapy of the borderline adult: A developmental approach*. New York: Wiley-Interscience.

Masterson, J. F. (1983). *Countertransference and psychotherapeutic technique: Teaching seminars on psychotherapy of borderline adult*. New York: Other Press.

Masterson, J. F. (1988). *Search for the real self*. New York: Free Press.

Masterson, J. F. (1993). *The emerging self: A developmental, self and object relations approach to the treatment of closet narcissistic disorder of the self*. New York: Brunner/Mazel.

McAdams, D. P. (1988). *Power, intimacy, and the life story: Personological inquiries into identity*. New York: Guilford Press.

McCarthy, K. L., Mergenthaler, E., Schneider, S., & Grenyer, B. F. S. (2011). Psychodynamic change in psychotherapy: Cycles of patient–therapist interactions and interventions. *Psychotherapy Research, 21*, 722–731.

McCrae, R. R., & Costa, P. T., Jr. (2003). *Personality in adulthood: A five-factor theory perspective* (2nd ed.). New York: Guilford Press.

McDougall, J. (1989). *Theaters of the body: A psychoanalytic approach to psychosomatic illness*. New York: Norton.

McWilliams, N. (2011). *Psychoanalytic diagnosis: Understanding personality structure in the clinical process* (2nd ed.). New York: Guilford Press.

McWilliams, N. (2012). Beyond traits: Personality as intersubjective themes. *Journal of Personality Assessment, 94*, 563–570.

McWilliams, N. (2015). More simply human: On the universality of madness. *Psychosis: Psychological, Social and Integrative Approaches, 7*, 63–71.

Meares, R. (2012). *A dissociation model of borderline personality disorder*. New York: Norton.

Meissner, W. (1978). *The paranoid process.* New York: Aronson.

Meloy, J. R. (1988). *The psychopathic mind. Origins, dynamics, and treatment.* New York: Aronson.

Meloy, J. R. (1997). The psychology of wickedness: Psychopathy and sadism. *Psychiatric Annals, 27,* 630–633.

Meltzer, D. (1973). *Sexual states of mind.* London: Karnac.

Mikulincer, M., & Shaver, P. R. (2012). An attachment perspective on psychopathology. *World Psychiatry, 11,* 11–15.

Mikulincer, M., & Shaver, P. R. (2016). *Attachment in adulthood: Structure, dynamics, and change* (2nd ed.). New York: Guilford Press.

Miller, A. (1981). *Prisoners of childhood: The drama of the gifted child and the search for the true self.* New York: Basic Books. (Original work published 1979)

Millon, T. (1996). *Disorders of personality: DSM-IV and beyond.* New York: Wiley.

Millon, T., & Grossman, S. (2007). *Moderating severe personality disorders: A personalized psychotherapy approach.* Hoboken, NJ: Wiley.

Morse, J. Q., Robins, C. J., & Gittes-Fox, M. (2002). Sociotropy, autonomy, and personality disorder criteria in psychiatric patients. *Journal of Personality Disorders, 16,* 549–560.

National Health and Medical Research Council. (2012). *Clinical practice guideline for the management of borderline personality disorder.* Melbourne, Australia: Author.

National Institute for Health and Clinical Excellence. (2009). *Borderline personality disorder: Treatment and management.* London: British Psychological Society and Royal College of Psychiatrists.

Norcross, J. C. (2011). *Psychotherapy relationships that work* (2nd ed.). New York: Oxford University Press.

Nurnberg, G. H., Raskin, M., Levine, P. E., Pollack, S., Siegel, O., & Prince, R. (1991). The comorbidity of borderline personality disorder and other DSM-III Axis II personality disorders. *American Journal of Psychiatry, 148,* 1371–1377.

Nussbaum, A. M. (2013). *The pocket guide to the DSM-5 diagnostic exam.* Washington, DC: American Psychiatric Association.

Nydes, J. (1963). The paranoid–masochistic character. *Psychoanalytic Review, 50,* 215–251.

Ogloff, J., & Wong, S. (1990). Electrodermal and cardiovascular evidence of a coping response in psychopaths. *Criminal Justice and Behavior, 17,* 231–245.

Ouimette, P. C., Klein, D. N., Anderson, R., Riso, L. P., & Lizardi, H. (1994). Relationship of sociotropy/autonomy and dependency/self-criticism to DSM-III-R personality disorders. *Journal of Abnormal Psychology, 103,* 743–749.

OPD Task Force (Ed.). (2008). *Operationalized psychodynamic diagnosis—OPD-2: Manual of diagnosis and treatment planning.* Cambridge, MA: Hogrefe & Huber.

Panksepp, J. (1998). *Affective neuroscience: The foundation of human and animal emotions.* New York: Oxford University Press.

Panksepp, J. (2001). The long-term psychobiological consequences of infant emotions: Prescriptions for the twenty-first century. *Neuro-Psychoanalysis, 3,* 149–178.

Panksepp, J., & Biven, L. (2012). *The archeology of mind: Neuroevolutionary origins of human emotions.* New York: Norton.

Paris, J. (1993). *Borderline personality disorder: Etiology and treatment.* Washington, DC: American Psychiatric Association.

Paris, J. (2012). *The bipolar spectrum: Diagnosis or fad?* New York: Routledge.

Perry, J. C. (1990). *The Defense Mechanism Rating Scale manual* (5th ed.). Cambridge, MA: Author.

Perry, J. C. (1993). Defenses and their affects. In N. E. Miller, L. Luborsky, J. P. Barber, & J. P. Docherty (Eds.), *Psychoanalytic treatment research: A handbook for clinical practice* (pp. 274–306). New York: Basic Books.

Perry, J. C. (2001). A pilot study of defenses in adults with personality disorders entering psychotherapy. *Journal of Nervous and Mental Disease, 189,* 651–660.

Perry, J. C. (2014). Anomalies and specific functions in the clinical identification of defense mechanisms. *Journal of Clinical Psychology, 70,* 406–418.

Perry, J. C., & Cooper, S. H. (1989). An empirical study of defense mechanisms. *Archives of General Psychiatry, 46,* 444–452.

Perry, J. C., & Høglend, P. (1998). Convergent and discriminant validity of overall defensive functioning. *Journal of Nervous and Mental Disease, 186,* 529–535.

Perry, J. C., & Kardos, M. E. (1995). A review of Defense Mechanism Rating Scales. In H. R. Conte & R. Plutchik (Eds.), *Ego defenses: Theory and measurement* (pp. 283–299). New York: Wiley.

Perry, J. C., Kardos, M. E., & Pagano, C. J. (1993). The study of defenses in psychotherapy using the Defense Mechanism Rating Scales—DMRS. In U. Hentschel, G. J. W. Smith, W. Ehlers, & G. Draguns (Eds.), *The concept of defense mechanisms in contemporary psychology: Theoretical, research and clinical perspectives* (pp. 122–132). New York: Springer.

Perry, J. C., & Presniak, M. D. (2013). Conflicts and defenses in narcissistic personality disorder. In J. S. Ogrodniczuk (Ed.), *Understanding and treating pathological narcissism* (pp. 147–166). Washington, DC: American Psychological Association.

Perry, J. C., Presniak, M. D., & Olson, T. R. (2013). Defense mechanisms in schizotypal, borderline, antisocial, and narcissistic personality disorders.

Psychiatry: Interpersonal and Biological Processes, 76, 32–52.

Peterson, C., & Seligman, M. E. (1984). Causal explanations as a risk factor for depression: Theory and evidence. *Psychological Review, 91*, 347–374.

Pincus, A. L. (2005). A contemporary integrative interpersonal theory of personality disorders. In M. F. Lenzenweger & J. F. Clarkin (Eds.), *Major theories of personality disorder* (2nd ed., pp. 282–331). New York: Guilford Press.

Pincus, A. L., Cain, N. M., & Wright, A. G. C. (2014). Narcissistic grandiosity and narcissistic vulnerability in psychotherapy. *Personality Disorders: Theory, Research, and Treatment, 5*, 439–443.

Pincus, A. L., & Roche, M. J. (2011). Narcissistic grandiosity and narcissistic vulnerability. In W. K. Campbell & J. D. Miller (Eds.), *Handbook of narcissism and narcissistic personality disorder* (pp. 31–40). Hoboken, NJ: Wiley.

Pinsker, H. (1997). *A primer of supportive psychotherapy*. Hillsdale, NJ: Analytic Press.

Porcerelli, J. C., & Hibbard, S. (2004). Projective assessment of defense mechanisms. In M. Hersen, M. J. Hilsenroth, & L. D. Segal (Eds.), *Comprehensive handbook of psychological assessment: Vol. 2. Personality assessment* (pp. 466–475). Hoboken, NJ: Wiley.

Porcerelli, J. H., Cogan, R., Kamoo, R., & Miller, K. (2010). Convergent validity of the Defense Mechanisms Manual and the Defensive Functioning Scale. *Journal of Personality Assessment, 92*, 432–438.

Porges, S. W. (2011). *The polyvagal theory: Neurophysiological foundations of emotions, attachment, communication and self-regulation*. New York: Norton.

Prichard, J. C. (1835). *A treatise on insanity*. London: Gilbert & Piper.

Project Air Strategy. (2015). *Treatment guidelines for personality disorders* (2nd ed.). Wollengong, Australia: New South Wales Health and Illawarra Health and Medical Research Institute. Retrieved from *www.projectairstrategy.org/content/groups/public/@web/@ihmri/documents/doc/uow189005.pdf.*

Raine, A., Venables, P., & Williams, M. (1990). Relationships between central and autonomic measures of arousal at age 15 and criminality at age 24. *Archives of General Psychiatry, 47*, 1003–1007.

Reich, W. (1972). *Character analysis*. New York: Farrar, Straus & Giroux. (Original work published 1933)

Reik, T. (1941). *Masochism in modern man*. New York: Farrar & Rinehart.

Ridenour, J. M. (2014). Psychodynamic model and treatment of schizotypal personality disorders. *Psychological Assessment, 13*, 577–591.

Rockland, L. H. (1989). *Supportive therapy: A psychodynamic approach*. New York: Basic Books.

Roland, A. (1988). *In search of self in India and Japan: Toward a cross-cultural psychology*. Princeton, NJ: Princeton University Press.

Rosenfeld, H. (1987). *Impasse and interpretation*. London: Routledge.

Rosenstein, D. S., & Horowitz, H. A. (1996). Adolescent attachment and psychopathology. *Journal of Consulting and Clinical Psychology, 64*, 244–253.

Røssberg, J. I., Karterud, S., Pedersen, G., & Friis, S. (2007). An empirical study of countertransference reactions toward patients with personality disorders. *Comprehensive Psychiatry, 48*, 225–230.

Roth, A., & Fonagy, P. (2005). *What works for whom?: A critical review of psychotherapy research* (2nd ed.). New York: Guilford Press.

Russ, E., Shedler, J., Bradley, R., & Westen, D. (2008). Refining the construct of narcissistic personality disorder: Diagnostic criteria and subtypes. *American Journal of Psychiatry, 165*, 1473–1481.

Sadock, B. J., & Sadock, V. A. (2008). *Kaplan & Sadock's concise textbook of clinical psychiatry* (3rd ed.). Philadelphia: Lippincott Williams & Wilkins.

Salzman, L. (1980). *Treatment of the obsessive personality*. New York: Aronson.

Samuel, D. B., & Widiger, T. A. (2008). A meta-analytic review of the relationships between the five-factor model and DSM-IV-TR personality disorders: A facet level analysis. *Clinical Psychology Review, 28*, 1326–1342.

Sanders, J. L. (2011). A distinct language and an historic pendulum: The evolution of the *Diagnostic and Statistical Manual of Mental Disorders. Archives of Psychiatric Nursing, 25*, 394–403.

Saulsman, L. M., & Page, A. C. (2004). The five-factor model and personality disorder empirical literature: A meta-analytic review. *Clinical Psychology Review, 23*, 1055–1085.

Schmideberg, M. (1959). The borderline patient. In S. Arieti (Ed.), *American handbook of psychiatry* (Vol. 1, pp. 398–416). New York: Basic Books.

Schore, A. N. (2003). *Affect dysregulation and disorders of the self*. New York: Norton.

Seinfeld, J. (1991). *The empty core: An object relations approach to psychotherapy of the schizoid personality*. Northvale, NJ: Aronson.

Serin, R. (1991). Psychopathy and violence in criminals. *Journal of Interpersonal Violence, 6*, 423–431.

Shapiro, D. (1965). *Neurotic styles*. New York: Basic Books.

Shapiro, D. (1981). *Autonomy and rigid character*. New York: Basic Books.

Shapiro, D. (1989). *Psychotherapy of neurotic character*. New York: Basic Books.

Shapiro, D. (2002). *Dynamics of character: Self-regulation in psychopathology*. New York: Basic Books.

Shedler, J. (2015). Integrating clinical and empirical perspectives on personality: The Shedler–Westen Assessment Procedure (SWAP). In S. K. Huprich (Ed.), *Personality disorders: Toward theoretical and empirical integration in diagnosis and assessment.* Washington, DC: American Psychological Association.

Shedler, J., & Westen, D. (2004). Refining personality disorder diagnosis: Integrating science and practice. *American Journal of Psychiatry, 161,* 1350–1365.

Sherwood, V. R., & Cohen, C. P. (1994). *Psychotherapy of the quiet borderline patient: The as-if personality revisited.* Northvale, NJ: Aronson.

Shira, G., & Gardner, W. L. (1999). Are there "his" and "hers" types of interdependence?: The implications of gender differences in collective versus relational interdependence for affect, behavior, and cognition. *Journal of Personality and Social Psychology, 77,* 642–655.

Siever, L. J., & Davis, K. L. (1991). A psychobiological perspective on the personality disorders. *American Journal of Psychiatry, 148,* 1647–1658.

Sifneos, P. (1973). The prevalence of "alexithymia" characteristics in psychosomatic patients. *Psychotherapy and Psychosomatics, 22,* 255–262.

Silberschatz, G. (Ed.). (2005). *Transformative relationships: The control–mastery theory of psychotherapy.* New York: Routledge.

Silver, A.-L. (Ed.). (1989). *Psychoanalysis and psychosis.* Madison, CT: International Universities Press.

Silver, A.-L. (2003). The psychotherapy of schizophrenia: Its place in the modern world. *Journal of the American Academy of Psychoanalysis and Dynamic Psychiatry, 31,* 325–341.

Singer, J. A. (2005). *Personality and psychotherapy: Treating the whole person.* New York: Guilford Press.

Skodol, A. E., Bender, D. S., & Morey, L. C. (2013). Narcissistic personality disorder in DSM-5. *Personality Disorders: Theory, Research, and Treatment, 5,* 422–427.

Skodol, A. E., Gunderson, J. G., Pfohl, B., Widiger, T. A., Livesley, W. J., & Siever, L. J. (2002a). The borderline diagnosis: I. Psychopathology, comorbidity, and personality structure. *Biological Psychiatry, 51,* 936–950.

Skodol, A. E., Siever, L. J., Livesley, W. J., Gunderson, J. G., Pfohl, B., & Widiger, T. A. (2002b). The borderline diagnosis: II. Biology, genetics, and clinical course. *Biological Psychiatry, 51,* 951–963.

Sperling, M. B., Sharp, J. L., & Fishler, P. H. (1991). On the nature of attachment in a borderline population: A preliminary investigation. *Psychological Reports, 68,* 543–546.

Spiegel, H., & Spiegel, D. (1978). *Trance and treatment: Clinical uses of hypnosis.* New York: Basic Books.

Spitzer, R. L., First, M. B., Shedler, J., Westen, D., & Skodal, M. D. (2008). Clinical utility of five dimensional systems for personality diagnosis: A "consumer preference" study. *Journal of Nervous and Mental Disease, 196,* 356–374.

Sroufe, L. A. (2005). Attachment and development: A prospective, longitudinal study from birth to adulthood. *Attachment and Human Development, 7,* 349–367.

Sroufe, L. A., Carlson, E. A., Levy, A. K., & Egeland, B. (1999). Implications of attachment theory for developmental psychopathology. *Development and Psychopathology, 1,* 1–13.

Steiner, J. (1993). *Psychic retreats: Pathological organizations in psychotic, neurotic, and borderline patients.* London: Routledge.

Steiner, J. (2011). *On seeing and being seen.* London: Routledge.

Stern, A. (1938). Psychoanalytic investigation and therapy in borderline group of neuroses. *Psychoanalytic Quarterly, 7,* 467–489.

Stern, D. N. (1985). *The interpersonal world of the infant: A view from psychoanalysis and developmental psychology.* New York: Basic Books.

Stern, D. N. (1997). *Unformulated experience: From dissociation to imagination in psychoanalysis.* Hillside, NJ: Analytic Press.

Stern, D. N., Sander, I. W., Nahum, J. P., Harrison, A. M., Lyons-Ruth, K., Morgan, A. C., . . . Tronick, E. Z. (1998). Non-interpretive mechanisms in psychoanalytic therapy: The "something more" than interpretation. *International Journal of Psycho-Analysis, 79,* 903–921.

Stern, E. M. (1989). *Psychotherapy and the grandiose patient.* New York: Hawthorn Press.

Stone, M. H. (1980). *The borderline syndromes: Constitution, personality, and adaptation.* New York: McGraw-Hill.

Stone, M. H. (Ed.). (1986). *Essential papers on borderline disorders: One hundred years at the border.* New York: New York University Press.

Stone, M. H. (1993). *Abnormalities of personality: Within and beyond the realm of treatment.* New York: Norton.

Stone, M. H. (2009). *The anatomy of evil.* Amherst, NY: Prometheus Books.

Sullivan, H. S. (1953). *The interpersonal theory of psychiatry.* New York: Routledge.

Sullivan, H. S. (1956). *Clinical studies in psychiatry.* New York: Norton.

Sullivan, H. S. (1962). *Schizophrenia as a human process.* New York: Norton.

Thomas, A., Chess, S., & Birch, H. G. (1968). *Temperament and behavior disorders in children.* New York: New York University Press.

Tomkins, S. (1995). Script theory. In E. V. Demos (Ed.), *Exploring affect: The selected writings of Silvan Tomkins* (pp. 312–388). New York: Cambridge University Press.

Torgersen, S. (2000). Genetics of patients with

borderline personality disorder. *Psychiatric Clinics of North America, 23*, 1–9.

Torgersen, S., Czajkowski, N., Jacobson, K., Reichborn-Kjennerud, T., Roysamb, E., Neale, M. C., & Kendler, K. S. (2008). Dimensional representations of DSM-IV cluster B personality disorders in a population-based sample of Norwegian twins: A multivariate study. *Psychological Medicine, 38*, 1617–1625.

Town, J. M., Abbass, A., & Hardy, G. (2011). Short-term psychodynamic psychotherapy for personality disorders: A critical review of randomized controlled trials. *Journal of Personality Disorders, 25*(6), 723–740.

Trull, T. J. (2012). The five-factor model of personality disorder and DSM-5. *Journal of Personality, 80*, 1697–1720.

Trull, T. J., Widiger, T. A., & Frances, A. (1987). Covariation of criteria sets for avoidant, schizoid, and dependent personality disorders. *American Journal of Psychiatry, 144*, 767–771.

Tummala-Narra, P. (2016). *Psychoanalytic theory and cultural competence in psychotherapy*. Washington, DC: American Psychological Association.

Vaillant, G. E. (1971), Theoretical hierarchy of adaptive ego mechanisms: A 30-year follow-up of 30 men selected for psychological health. *Archives of General Psychiatry, 24*, 107–118.

Vaillant, G. E. (1992). *Ego mechanisms of defense: A guide for clinicians and researchers*. Washington, DC: American Psychiatric Press.

Vaillant, G. E., Bond, M., & Vaillant, C. O. (1986). An empirically validated hierarchy of defense mechanisms. *Archives of General Psychiatry, 42*, 597–601.

van der Kolk, B. (1994). The body keeps the score: Memory and the evolving psychobiology of posttraumatic stress. *Harvard Review of Psychiatry, 1*, 253–265.

van der Kolk, B. (2003). The neurobiology of childhood trauma and abuse. *Child and Adolescent Psychiatric Clinics of North America, 12*, 293–317.

Vitacco, M. J., & Rogers, R. (2001). Predictors of adolescent psychopathy: The role of impulsivity, hyperactivity, and sensation seeking. *Journal of American Academy of Psychiatry and the Law, 29*, 374–382.

Wachtel, P. L. (1997). *Psychoanalysis, behavior therapy, and the relational world: Psychotherapy integration*. Washington, DC: American Psychological Association.

Wachtel, P. L. (2008). *Relational theory and the practice of psychotherapy*. New York: Guilford Press.

Wachtel, P. L. (2011). *Inside the session: What really happens in psychotherapy*. Washington, DC: American Psychological Association.

Wallin, D. (2007). *Attachment in psychotherapy*. New York: Guilford Press.

Waska, R. T. (1997). Precursors to masochistic and dependent character development. *American Journal of Psychoanalysis, 57*, 253–267.

Weinberger, J. (2014). Common factors are not so common and specific factors are not so specified: Toward an inclusive integration of psychotherapy research. *Psychotherapy, 51*, 514–518.

Weiss, J. (1993). *How psychotherapy works: Process and technique*. New York: Guilford Press.

Weiss, J., Sampson, H., & the Mount Zion Psychotherapy Research Group. (1986). *The psychoanalytic process: Theory, clinical observations, and empirical research*. New York: Guilford Press.

West, M., & Keller, A. (1994). Psychotherapy strategies for insecure attachment in personality disorders. In M. B. Sperling & W. H. Berman (Eds.), *Attachment in adults: Clinical and developmental perspectives* (pp. 313–330). New York: Guilford Press.

Westen, D., Novotny, C. M., & Thompson-Brenner, H. (2004). The empirical status of empirically supported psychotherapies: Assumptions, findings, and reporting in controlled clinical trials. *Psychological Bulletin, 130*, 631–663.

Westen, D., & Shedler, J. (1999a). Revising and assessing Axis II: Part I. Developing a clinically and empirically valid assessment method. *American Journal of Psychiatry, 156*, 258–272.

Westen, D., & Shedler, J. (1999b). Revising and assessing Axis II: Part II. Toward an empirically based and clinically useful classification of personality disorders. *American Journal of Psychiatry, 156*, 273–285.

Westen, D., & Shedler, J. (2007). Personality diagnosis with the Shedler–Westen Assessment Procedure (SWAP): Integrating clinical and statistical measurement and prediction. *Journal of Abnormal Psychology, 116*, 810–822.

Westen, D., Shedler, J., Bradley, B., & DeFife, J. A. (2012). An empirically derived taxonomy for personality diagnosis: Bridging science and practice in conceptualizing personality. *American Journal of Psychiatry, 169*, 273–284.

Westen, D., Waller, N. G., Shedler, J., & Blagov, P. S. (2014). Dimensions of personality and personality pathology: Factor structure of the Shedler–Westen Assessment Procedure–II (SWAP-II). *Journal of Personality Disorders, 28*, 281–318.

Westen, D., & Weinberger, J. (2004). When clinical description becomes statistical prediction. *American Psychologist, 59*, 595–613.

Widiger, T. A., & Costa, P. T. (2002). Five-factor model personality disorder research. In P. T. Costa & T. A. Widiger (Eds.), *Personality disorders and the five-factor model of personality* (2nd ed., pp. 59–87). Washington, DC: American Psychological Association.

Winarick, D. J., & Bornstein, R. F. (2015). Toward resolution of a longstanding controversy in personality disorder diagnosis: Contrasting correlates of schizoid and avoidant traits. *Personality and Individual Differences, 79*, 25–29.

Winnicott, D. W. (1971). *Playing and reality.* New York: Routledge.

World Health Organization. (2000). *The ICD-10 classification of mental and behavioural disorders: Diagnostic criteria for research.* Geneva: Author.

Yeomans, F. E., Clarkin, J. F., & Kernberg, O. F. (2015). *Transference-focused psychotherapy for borderline personality disorder: A clinical guide.* Washington, DC: American Psychiatric Association.

Young, J. E., Klosko, J. S., & Weishaar, M. E. (2003). *Schema therapy: A practitioner's guide.* New York: Guilford Press.

Young-Bruehl, E., & Bethelard, F. (2000). *Cherishment: A psychology of the heart.* New York: Free Press.

Zanarini, M. C. (2009). Psychotherapy of borderline personality disorder. *Acta Psychiatrica Scandinavica, 120*, 373–377.

Zetzel, E. (1968). The so-called good hysteric. *International Journal of Psycho-Analysis, 49*, 256–260.

Zimmerman, M., Rothschild, L., & Chelminski, I. (2005). The prevalence of DSM-IV personality disorders in psychiatric outpatients. *American Journal of Psychiatry, 162*, 1911–1918.

Zuckerman, M. (1999). *Vulnerability to psychopathology: A biosocial model.* Washington, DC: American Psychological Association.

APPENDIX 1.1

Comparison of PDM-2 with Other Diagnostic Systems

As noted at the beginning of this chapter, the PDM-2 classification system serves different purposes from those of the American Psychiatric Association's DSM system and the World Health Organization's ICD system. It is intended to provide a deeper clinical understanding for purposes of case formulation and treatment planning, especially when psychotherapy is a reasonable treatment recommendation.

The DSM and ICD systems have been geared to the reliability of their designated categories for research purposes; for purposes of comparing researched populations across different samples, sites, and theoretical frameworks within which researchers operate; for billing and insurance reimbursement purposes, to distinguish between what is and is not covered by insurance programs; for epidemiological purposes; and for selected treatment purposes (e.g., to facilitate psychopharmacological decision making). Our diagnostic approach is geared toward individualized case formulation and treatment planning for therapies that attempt to address the full range and depth of a person's psychological experience.

The DSM and ICD taxonomies continue to offer a largely categorical (present–absent) approach to diagnosis. PDM-2 diagnoses, in contrast, are meant to refer to spectra or continua. Some personality patterns or syndromes exist on a spectrum that ranges from a "normal" or healthy level of functioning, through neurotic and borderline ranges, into thought-disordered functioning and frank psychosis. Others, such as paranoid and sadistic psychologies, are found mainly in the borderline and psychotic ranges.

Clinical theorizing has viewed many conditions, including personality patterns (the P Axis) and overall mental functioning (the M Axis), as existing on continua rather than as mutually exclusive categories. For example, hysterical and obsessional styles have sometimes been construed as two ends of a polarity (Shapiro, 1965; Sullivan, 1956). A spectrum that runs from schizoid to paranoid psychologies can be described (Klein, 1946); another has been described as connecting depressive and masochistic orientations (Kernberg, 1988). Narcissistic and psychopathic personalities can be formulated on a continuum of severity of incapacity to care about others (Gacono & Meloy, 1988; Kernberg, 1992, 2014; Meloy, 1988). Interestingly, in response to critiques of prior DSMs to the effect that personality disorders are dimensional, the members of the DSM-5 Personality and Personality Disorders Work Group attempted to reclassify personality pathology via a dimensional trait model. Although their recommendations were eventually rejected (perhaps because trait models, even dimensional ones, may fail to capture *thematic* personality differences; see McWilliams, 2012), they survive in an appendix of DSM-5.

As there are numerous lenses through which types and disorders of personality can be viewed, theorists and researchers have suggested many different ways to conceptualize them. In academic personality psychology, there is a vast literature on the "five-factor model" (Markon, Krueger, & Watson, 2005; McCrae & Costa, 2003; Singer, 2005; Widiger & Costa, 2002), which focuses on the factor-analytically derived traits of extraversion, neuroticism, openness to experience, agreeableness, and conscientiousness. The "alternative DSM-5 model" for personality disorders relies heavily on that model (Samuel & Widiger, 2008; Saulsman & Page, 2004; Trull, 2012). Diagnosis involves (1) an assessment of the level of impairment in personality functioning (including disturbances in self or interpersonal functioning); and (2) an evaluation of pathological personality traits (organized in five broad domains—negative affective, detachment, antagonism, disinhibition, and psychoticism—with 25 trait "facets"). This approach allows one to derive a personality pathology classification that includes antisocial, avoidant, borderline, narcissistic, obsessive–compulsive, and schizotypal disorders, or, in cases in which a personality disorder is considered present but the criteria for any specific psychopathological picture are not met, a diagnosis of personality disorder—trait specified (PD-TS).

Our classification system, which has been influenced by both scientific researchers and observant practitioners, derives more from the clinical psychological and psychiatric traditions. It is a dimensional system, but in contrast to the DSM-5 alternative model, it emphasizes groupings that reflect underlying psychological themes and tensions rather than discussed discrete, variable-centered (vs. person-centered) trait dimensions. In the clinical literature, such themes have been variously discussed as "internalized object relations" (Fairbairn, 1952), "repetitive structures" (French, 1958), "inner working models" (Bowlby, 1969), "nuclear conflicts" (Malan, 1976), "representations of internalizations that have been generalized" (Stern, 1985), "fundamental and repetitive emotional structures" (Dahl, 1988), "internal relational models" (Aron, 1991), "nuclear scenes" (Tomkins, 1995), "emotion schemas" (Bucci, 1997), "core conflictual relationship themes" (Luborsky & Crits-Cristoph, 1996), "implicit relational knowing" (Lyons-Ruth, 1999), "personal schemes" (Horowitz, 1998), and "individual schemas" (Young et al., 2003).

The DSM system is intended to be noninferential: It is constructed to put symptoms and attributes that people have in common into the same diagnostic compartments, without imputations of underlying mental processes or meaning. In fact, the intent of the framers of recent editions of DSM, beginning with DSM-III, was to be atheoretical—that is, to describe phenomena without assuming any overarching theory of mental functioning (American Psychiatric Association, 1980, 1987, 1994, 2000, 2013). Moreover, because DSM-III was intended to be more useful to researchers in psychopathology than its predecessors had been, its syndromes were described in terms of noninferential, present-versus-absent criteria sets that can be easily noted by a nonclinician.

This "neo-Kraepelinian" model (Compton & Guze, 1995; Feighner et al., 1972; Klerman, 1978; Sanders, 2011) has made it easier for mental health professionals to talk across differences of theoretical orientation, and it has made randomized controlled trials of different approaches to specific categories of psychopathology easier to conduct. But it has not been so useful to therapists, who have typically preferred more dimensional, inferential, and contextual diagnostic approaches. Our intent, in the various dimensions that constitute our nosological array, is to describe human problems dimensionally and to infer meanings, as best we can discern them, of observed phenomena: symptoms, behaviors, traits, affects, attitudes, thoughts, fantasies, and so on—the full range of human mental functioning.

One classification system cannot capture all the ways in which human beings vary along clinically relevant dimensions. But because of its significance for therapeutic choices, we have put primary emphasis here on what Kernberg (1984) has called the "severity dimension" in personality pathology. Readers interested in other psychodynamic ways of construing individual differences in personality and psychopathology are encouraged to look into *Operationalized Psychodynamic Diagnosis* (OPD; Cierpka et al., 2007; OPD Task Force, 2008), which includes axes for traditional DSM and ICD categories and other axes to capture the severity of relationship, conflict, and structural characterological psychopathology from a psychodynamic perspective.

In recent editions of DSM, some personality syndromes and disorders known to therapists have been omitted because they are not commonly seen in ordinary clinical practice (e.g., individuals with sadistic or counterdependent personalities, respectively, tend to avoid mental health treatment) and/or because there has been little empirical investigation of them (e.g., although depressive personality disorder is common, it was excluded from DSM-III and subsequent editions on the basis of insufficient research; see Hirschfeld, 1991; Kernberg, 1984). Rather than omitting underresearched disorders, we include those on which there is broad clinical agreement in the hope that future research will refine our formulations. In PDM-2, we have also tried to synthesize and simplify—thus resisting the temptation to keep generating ever more diagnostic entities, as seems to have happened in DSM-5. Accordingly, we have been less definitive and categorical about variants and subtypes of personality.

DSM categories of personality attempt to describe distinct clusters of symptoms and attributes, but "in nature," their discrete disorders frequently overlap in part with the clusters of symptoms and attributes of other DSM categories. Thus it has been conventional in recent decades to put an individual's difficulties into two (or more) illness categories and to describe the person as suffering from two (or more) "comorbid" illnesses. In contrast, we emphasize, for each individual, one coherent and meaningful organization of personality, which can represent a unique set of recurrent concerns or a particular admixture of the defining characteristics of two or more personality organizations and symptom patterns. Robert Michels (personal communication to the P-Axis chairs, July 14, 2014) describes an image that may speak for many scholars of personality:

> I think of a multidimensional conceptual space of personality and personality disorders with each individual a point. Many points are distributed diffusely, but there are some clusters—these are the specific types. I would emphasize, however, that many (most?) individuals are near but not in a cluster, while others are not near any cluster. It is clinically helpful to identify a nearby cluster if there is one, but important to recognize that there often is not.

Although psychodynamically oriented practitioners will be more familiar with PDM concepts than clinicians of other theoretical orientations, we hope that this volume will be of use to a broad range of clinicians. We wish to emphasize both our respect for alternative terminologies and conceptualizations and our effort to be helpful to therapists of diverse conceptual systems and therapeutic traditions.

APPENDIX 1.2

Definitions of Relevant Terms and Concepts

For purposes of our classification, it may be useful to define the boundaries of the word "personality," especially in comparison to "character" and "temperament." Similarly, we attempt a conceptual comparison of the terms "style," "trait," and "type," and comment on the meaning of "defense" as it has been used in clinical practice and research. We emphasize that these concepts, and the nuances that differentiate them, are products of Western intellectual and medical traditions; as such, they have some limitations that we address later.

Personality

We define "personality" as relatively stable ways of thinking, feeling, behaving, and relating to others. In this context, "thinking" encompasses not only one's belief systems and ways of making sense of self and others, but also one's moral values and personal ideals. Each of us has a set of individual assumptions and templates by which we try to understand our experience; a set of values and ways of pursuing what we see as valuable; a personal repertoire of familiar emotions and ways of handling them; and some characteristic patterns of behaving, especially in our personal relationships. "Personality" denotes one person's type of adaptation and lifestyle—the pattern that has resulted from the convergence of constitutional factors, development, and social and cultural experience. Some of these processes are conscious and experienced as voluntary; others are unconscious, automatic, and not readily accessible via introspection (in currently popular terminology, they are "implicit").

We use the terms "personality" and "character" (see below) essentially synonymously, but the terms have different etymologies. "Personality" derives from *persona*, the social mask in theater (see, e.g., Allport, 1937); "character" has traditionally referred to etched mental structure. In other words, "personality" historically referred to observed phenomenology, "character" to the inferred mental interior. With the advent of DSM-III and its disavowal of theory, the term "personality" largely supplanted the term "character" in the clinical literature. We follow contemporary convention in using "personality" as the umbrella term, subsuming the historical concepts of both "personality" and "character."

Although the term implies significant components of stability and continuity, personality is not fixed and immutable; it evolves throughout the lifespan. Moreover, what we describe as "stable" is often not continually expressed in behavior. Rather, what are stable are the underlying psychological patterns and organizing themes, the expression of which is contingent on specific circumstances. For example, individuals with narcissistic personality pathology may become enraged and aggressive *in response to feeling slighted*, but may be cooperative, affable, and even empathic when feeling secure and appreciated. Likewise, individuals with a borderline personality organization may engage in self-harm (such as self-cutting and parasuicidality) *when an attachment relationship is threatened*, but may function relatively stably when feeling secure in an attachment relationship. In other words, what are stable are not necessarily behaviors per se, but psychological propensities that may be activated or dormant at a given juncture. The study of personality thus requires attention to both nomothetic elements (individual differences in traits, features, ways of acting, etc., that can be meaningfully studied and discussed vis-à-vis a *population*) and idiographic ones (psychological features, experiences, and meanings that apply to a *specific individual*, and that cannot meaningfully be described vis-à-vis a population).

Temperament

"Temperament" refers to constitutional components of the personality—in particular, to the relatively stable dispositions that are present from birth (Kagan, 1994; Thomas, Chess, & Birch, 1968). Most of these aspects of self-experience and self-expression are genetically or epigenetically determined, but some immutable aspects of temperament may result from intrauterine events with lifelong consequences, such as prenatal exposure to high levels of maternal stress hormones (Panksepp, 2001).

Character

"Character" derives from the ancient Greek *kharássein* ("to engrave, to trace, to inscribe"). This term indicates the set of distinctive characteristics of an individual, his or her "brand." The term was widely used by early psychoanalysts (e.g., Abraham) in reference to the theory of psychosexual development and fixation (oral, anal, phallic, or genital character). Reich (1933/1972) used the term as we would generally use "personality" today. In contemporary, everyday usage, however, "character" tends to imply either morality, as in "She is a person of the finest character," or eccentricity, as in "He is quite a character!" The latter usage notably implies uniqueness, rather than inclusion in a cluster.

Traits

"Traits" are relatively narrow-band psychological attributes that can be studied on a population basis, such that individuals can be located on a continuum (i.e., described as "low" or "high" on a trait) relative to a population or normative reference sample. Concepts such as "agreeableness" or "conscientiousness" are examples of traits. The five-factor model is widely used, especially in academic psychology, as a trait-based method of understanding people and locating them on well-researched dimensions relative to other people. Traits occur in a wide spectrum of social and personal contexts. The concept of "trait" varies with theoretical context and usually denotes stability. Recent cognitive-interactionist voices have urged the elimination of the essentialism once suggested by the term, and have asked that we consider such phenomena as "under construction"—in other words, as variable moderators of the personality that mediate one's relationship with the environment. Despite the variability of their manifestations in different populations, some trait concepts emerge reliably in transcultural research.

Type of Personality

The term "type" may describe a complex but recognizable configuration of multiple interrelated psychological and behavioral characteristics that describes clusters of people. The term connotes a recognizable general pattern of functioning without implying psychopathology. Jung (1921/1971, p. 612) defined "type" as the "characteristic pattern of a general *attitude* that recurs in many individual shapes." In everyday language, this connotation is preserved in the notion of "Type A" versus "Type B" individuals (Horney, 1950; Leary, 1957) or in expressions such as "He's the controlling type."

Style of Personality

"Style" is similar to "type," in that it deliberately avoids imputing psychopathology to a recognizable pattern. It is often used to denote a type of personality that is not problematic enough to warrant the term "disorder." For example, a woman with an obsessional "style" has relatively adaptive traits and defenses that, in their extreme and maladaptive forms, characterize obsessive personality disorder. In other words, she has an obsessive personality, but not an obsessive personality disorder. The term "style" has been used extensively, including in several editions of DSM, to describe a more or less stable and "everyday" configuration of the personality of an individual.

Shapiro (1965), whose work originally popularized this usage, noted the "styles of functioning as a matrix for specific traits or symptoms" which are "presumably, slow to change, and, therefore, guarantee not only an individual's consistency, but also his relative stability over long periods of time" (p. 4). More recently, probably because of its nonpathologizing connotation, the notion of "style" has also been applied to measured attachment patterns (e.g., "This child has an avoidant attachment style").

Defenses

The term "defenses" refers to the characteristic ways in which we protect ourselves from psychological threats and aversive affect states, and attempt to maintain psychological equilibrium and homeostasis in the face of challenges and hardships. In contrast to "coping" mechanisms, defenses operate in a mostly automatic manner, partially or wholly out of awareness. In the historical context of psychoanalytic drive or conflict theory, defenses arise from inner or intrapsychic conflict: the interplay of needs, impulses, or desires on the one hand and prohibitions or painful realities that oppose them on the other.

Everyone has a repertoire of defensive processes, which may be more or less adaptive versus costly. There are more "mature" or adaptive defenses (such as humor, altruism, sublimation, and suppression) that contribute to effective functioning, and less adaptive defenses (such as denial, acting out, projective identification, and splitting) that are psychologically costly and may significantly disrupt effective functioning. The less mature defenses involve conspicuous levels of distortion of self, others, or external reality (Cramer, 2015; Perry, 1990, 2014; Vaillant, 1992).

"Defensive style" is intertwined with personality. Pervasive, rigid, and/or intense use of maladaptive defenses underlies both symptom formation and personality disturbances severe enough to be termed "disorders" (Hilsenroth, Callahan, & Eudell, 2003; Kramer et al., 2013; Lingiardi et al., 1999; Perry, 2001; Perry & Høglend, 1998; Perry & Presniak, 2013; Perry et al., 2013).

The Anaclitic–Introjective Polarity (Relatedness vs. Self-Definition)

The "anaclitic–introjective" (or "relatedness vs. self-definition") dimension refers to the two-polarities model of personality proposed by Blatt and colleagues (Blatt, 2008; Blatt & Blass, 1990; Blatt & Luyten, 2010), in which personality evolves through a dialectic interaction between these two fundamental psychological coordinates. It overlaps conceptually with the dimension of extraverted/extratensive/externalizing–introverted/introtensive/internalizing and many similar polarities (e.g., Jung's [1921/1971] introversion–extraversion, Bakan's [1966] and Pincus's [2005] communion–agency, Beck's [1983] sociotropic–autonomous dimension, McAdams's [1988] relationship–independence,

Spiegel & Spiegel's [1978] Nietzsche-inspired Dionysian–Apollonian dimension, and Westen et al.'s [2012] internalizing–externalizing personality disorders).

More specifically, relatedness and self-definition are involved in the development of the capacity to establish and maintain, respectively, (1) reciprocal, meaningful, and satisfying relationships and (2) a coherent, realistic, differentiated, and positive sense of self. These two developmental processes influence each other; well-functioning personality organization expresses comfort at both ends of the spectrum. In contrast, personality pathology is characterized by a defensive and exaggerated emphasis on one developmental dimension at the expense of the other. The various personality disorders can be organized into two basic configurations: one focused around issues of relatedness ("anaclitic") and the other focused around issues of self-definition ("introjective") (Luyten & Blatt, 2013). This conceptualization seems to have influenced the alternative DSM-5 model for personality disorders discussed in Appendix 1.1, whose criterion A for the diagnosis of personality disorder is moderate or severe impairment in self and interpersonal functioning (Bender, Morey, & Skodol, 2011).

Blatt's polarity has been found to discriminate between patients at all levels of psychological health and to have vital implications for the understanding and treatment of depression, personality disorders, and other psychopathologies (Blatt, 2004, 2008; Blatt & Zuroff, 1992; Fertuck, Bucci, Blatt, & Ford, 2004; Morse, Robins & Gittes-Fox, 2002; Ouimette, Klein, Anderson, Riso, & Lizardi, 1994). For example, there is emerging research evidence that supportive–expressive therapies work better with patients with anaclitic psychologies, at least initially, whereas interpretive interventions are preferable for those with introjective personality structures (Blatt, 2006; Blatt, Zuroff, Hawley, & Auerbach, 2010).

CHAPTER 2

Profile of Mental Functioning

M Axis

CHAPTER EDITORS

Vittorio Lingiardi, MD **Robert F. Bornstein, PhD**

CONSULTANTS

Janet Etzi, PhD
Alessandra Lemma, MA, MPhil, DClinPsych
Laura Muzi, PhD
J. Christopher Perry, MPH, MD
Caleb Siefert, PhD
Alessandro Zennaro, PhD

Introduction

This chapter describes 12 categories of basic mental functions that can help clinicians capture the complexity and individuality of each patient. We provide descriptions of different levels of psychological functioning and adaptation, ranging from more compromised to more functional, along with descriptors that allow a clinician to rate a patient in each capacity. Clinical utility demands that both adaptive and maladaptive functioning be taken into account in order to plan the most effective and well-rounded therapeutic interventions, anticipate challenges that may arise during treatment, delineate therapeutic goals, and evaluate treatment progress.

While the P Axis encourages clinicians to think about both overall functioning and specific personality patterns/disorders, the M Axis encourages them to consider and assess particular areas of mental functioning. The P Axis captures the level of personality functioning and a patient's fit within a prototype, and the M Axis complementarily fleshes out the specific functions that contribute to the patient's personality organization. Consider, for example, two patients, both of whom have borderline organizations. One may have a borderline organization because of his or her cognitive schemas and/or frequent use of immature defenses, whereas the other has a borderline organization associated with poor interpersonal functioning, poor self-integration, and use of midlevel defenses. Even though both have an ostensibly similar personality organization, the M Axis helps the clinician flesh out at a granular level the mechanisms that contribute to and shape the overarching organization for each patient.

The M-Axis domains are built on a wide range of psychodynamic, cognitive, and developmental models, as well as on research related to these frameworks. The inclusion of multiple models allows for an in-depth approach to personality, clinical symptoms, and the therapeutic process. Although DSM diagnoses have been useful for research purposes, and provide a common vocabulary for mental health professionals, they are not written to encourage further thinking about an individual's overall personality functioning, the underlying psychological dynamics, or the therapeutic process and therapeutic relationship.

Compared to those in the first edition of the manual, the PDM-2 labels and descriptions of mental functioning included in this chapter have been revised and reformulated in a clinician-friendly, empirically grounded, and assessment-relevant way. We have also introduced an assessment procedure (see Table 2.1, pp. 118–119) whereby a clinician can indicate on a 5-point scale the level at which each mental function is articulated in a patient (descriptors for key characteristics of levels of functioning 5, 3, and 1 are provided for *each* mental function). Moreover, the M Axis explicitly conceptualizes personality and mental functioning as resulting from the integration of nature (temperament, genetic predisposition, basic underlying traits) and nurture (learning, experience, attachment style, cultural and social context). We try to make this integration clear in our descriptions of different mental capacities, clarifying the complex nature of what is being conceptualized in each domain, so that the work of streamlining the assessment of such complex phenomena might continue.

The 12 M-Axis capacities are conceptualized with two fundamental questions in mind: (1) Which processes are being assessed in each capacity? (2) How can these processes be systematically and practically assessed to facilitate psychotherapy? In addition, to provide a better understanding of the underlying constructions of the capacities, we link each description to relevant clinical and empirical literature.

Although the PDM-2 M Axis articulates mental functioning in 12 distinct capacities, it is important to recognize that—although conceptually distinct—these capacities are not completely separate. Mental functioning should be conceptualized as a unified, integrated set of processes—a totality, a *unicum*—that operationally can be divided into contiguous categories, in the Aristotelian sense. As the ensuing definitions illustrate, these 12 capacities cover a variety of areas and a broad array of psychological processes. By necessity, some overlap exists. Despite the inherent overlap among certain capacities, each category highlights a critical, unique feature of mental functioning that cannot be completely accounted for by other capacities. Although no profile or set of scores can capture the full richness of each person's mental life—as Virginia Woolf wryly observed, "It is no use trying to sum people up"—the following 12 crucial areas can be schematically grouped into four domains:

- Cognitive and affective processes
  1. Capacity for regulation, attention, and learning
  2. Capacity for affective range, communication, and understanding
  3. Capacity for mentalization and reflective functioning

- Identity and relationships
  4. Capacity for differentiation and integration (identity)
  5. Capacity for relationships and intimacy
  6. Capacity for self-esteem regulation and quality of internal experience
- Defense and coping
  7. Capacity for impulse control and regulation
  8. Capacity for defensive functioning
  9. Capacity for adaptation, resiliency, and strength
- Self-awareness and self-direction
  10. Self-observing capacities (psychological mindedness)
  11. Capacity to construct and use internal standards and ideals
  12. Capacity for meaning and purpose

Definitions of the 12 M-Axis Capacities

The *capacity for regulation, attention, and learning* includes fundamental processes that enable human beings to attend to and process information (both internal and external), regulate their attentional focus, divide their attention as needed to carry out multiple tasks simultaneously, filter extraneous information from consciousness when appropriate, and learn from their experiences.

The *capacity for affective range, communication, and understanding* reflects a person's ability to experience, express, and comprehend the full range of pre-representational and representational patterns of affects in ways that are appropriate for a particular situation and consistent with the expectations and norms of the person's cultural milieu. This capacity also reflects the individual's ability to symbolize affectively meaningful experience (i.e., to represent it mentally rather than in somatic or behavioral form) and to verbalize affect states appropriately. Impairments in this domain, when pronounced, may be reflected in alexithymic tendencies in the patient.

The *capacity for mentalization and reflective functioning* concerns the individual's ability to infer and reflect on his or her own mental states as well as those of others, and to use this capacity in personal and social interactions. Mentalization is a form of mental activity that is considered imaginative (because when we mentalize, we are "imagining" what others think or feel); it is primarily preconscious (typically occurring outside the focus of attention) and aimed at understanding and interpreting the behavior of self and others in terms of mental states (e.g., needs, desires, feelings, beliefs, goals, intentions, and motivations). This capacity enables the individual to use ideas to experience, describe, and express internal life; to regulate affects and develop a coherent sense of self; and to make accurate inferences regarding others' mental states. Mentalization is supported by several related cognitive skills, including an understanding of emotional states and the ability to think implicitly about others' states of mind. The construct of reflective functioning represents the operationalization of the capacity to mentalize—the way, in other words, that we measure mentalization.

The *capacity for differentiation and integration* involves the ability to distinguish self from other, fantasy from reality, internal representations from external objects and circumstances, and present from past and future, and to make connections between these elements without confounding them. It specifically reflects the ability to construct and maintain a differentiated, realistic, coherent, complex representation of self (identity) and others, and to connect these pools of representations.

The *capacity for relationships and intimacy* reflects the depth, range, and consistency (i.e., stability) of the person's relationships and ability to adjust interpersonal distance–closeness as needed for different relationships, in line with cultural expectations. Healthy interpersonal relatedness reflects not only the degree to which the individual has stable, mutually satisfying relationships, but also the quality of the person's internalized object relations—mental representations of self, other people, and self–other interactions. This capacity includes the person's sexuality as reflected in awareness of desires and emotions, ability to engage in pleasurable sexual fantasies and activities, and ability to blend sexuality with emotional intimacy. Just as "quality of internal experience" is an index of confidence and self-esteem, "capacity for relationships and intimacy" is an index of relatedness.

The *capacity for self-esteem regulation and quality of internal experience* captures the level of confidence and self-regard that characterizes an individual's relationship to self, others, and the larger world. Optimal functioning in this capacity involves balance, with self-confidence and self-esteem based on reality-based perceptions of one's positive features and accomplishments, being neither unrealistically high nor unrealistically low. This capacity also includes the degree to which the individual experiences a sense of internal control, self-efficacy, and agency.

The *capacity for impulse control and regulation* reflects the individual's ability to modulate impulses and express them in adaptive, culture-appropriate ways. Deficiencies in this capacity may lead to unmodulated expression of impulses (impulsivity) or rigid overcontrol of impulses (inhibition), with concomitant affective constriction. High functioning in this capacity involves the ability to tolerate frustration, when appropriate or necessary, and to recognize and describe impulses as a means of self-regulation.

The *capacity for defensive functioning* highlights the ways the individual attempts to cope with and express wishes, affect, and other inner experience, along with the ability to modulate anxiety resulting from internal conflict, external challenge, or threat to self without excessive distortion in self-perception and reality testing, and without making excessive use of acting out. High functioning in this area enables the person to use defenses effectively, with only modest distortion in reality testing; lower functioning in this area involves a less effective defense style and greater distortion.

The *capacity for adaptation, resiliency, and strength* reflects the person's ability to adjust to unexpected events and changing circumstances, and the ability to cope effectively and creatively when confronted with uncertainty, loss, stress, and challenge. Such adjustment is not equivalent to uncritical or conformist adaptation to expectations, but reflects a mindful choice about how best to respond. This capacity may include individual strengths, such as empathy and sensitivity to others' needs and feelings, capacity to recognize alternative viewpoints, and appropriate assertiveness. When optimal, it enables one to transcend obstacles and turn setbacks into opportunities for growth and positive change.

Self-observing capacities (psychological mindedness) concern the individual's ability to observe his or her own internal life mindfully and realistically and use this information adaptively. This capacity also reflects the degree to which the person can be introspective—the degree to which he or she shows an inherent interest in better self-understanding.

The *capacity to construct and use internal standards and ideals* is an index of the personal sense of morality. The capacity to formulate internal values and ideals reflects a consideration of one's self in the context of one's culture, and the ability to make mindful decisions based on a set of coherent, flexible, and internally consistent underlying moral principles. High functioning in this domain requires that one's moral reasoning be based not only on a set of cohesive core principles, but also on an awareness of the impact of one's moral decisions on others.

The *capacity for meaning and purpose* reflects the individual's ability to construct a personal narrative that gives coherence and meaning to personal choices, a sense of directedness and purpose, a concern for succeeding generations, and a spirituality (not necessarily expressed as traditional religiosity) that imbues one's life with meaning. High functioning for this capacity entails the ability to think beyond immediate concerns to consider the broader implications of one's attitudes, beliefs, and behaviors.

Empirically Grounded Assessment of M-Axis Capacities

A growing body of research demonstrates that it is possible to assess these 12 components of mental functioning. To facilitate clinically useful diagnosis and case conceptualization, assessment of M-Axis capacities must yield *practically applicable* results with utility for diagnostic formulation, treatment planning, and treatment implementation, usable by clinicians across orientations. Thus, for each capacity, we provide a list of well-validated clinical tools that can aid in assessment. In general, we favor clinician-rated and performance-based assessment measures, but in many cases self-reports can complement and enrich the data obtained via clinician-rated and performance-based scales.

These lists of well-validated assessment tools include the following, among others:

- The Adult Attachment Interview (AAI; George, Kaplan, & Main, 1985; Main, Goldwyn, & Hesse, 2002), the Adult Attachment Projective (AAP; George & West, 2012; George, West, & Pettem, 1997; Jones-Mason, Allen, Hamilton, & Weiss, 2015), and the Reflective Functioning Scale (RFS; Fonagy, Target, Steele, & Steele, 1998).
- The Defense Mechanism Rating Scales (DMRS; Perry, 1990).
- The Object Relations Inventory (ORI) and the Differentiation–Relatedness Scale (D-RS) (Blatt & Auerbach, 2001; Blatt, Auerbach, & Levy, 1997; Blatt, Stayner, Auerbach, & Behrends, 1996; Diamond, Blatt, Stayner, & Kaslow, 1991; Huprich, Auerbach, Porcerelli, & Bupp, 2016).
- The Severity Indices of Personality Problems–118 (SIPP-118; Verheul et al., 2008).
- The Shedler–Westen Assessment Procedure–200 (SWAP-200; Westen & Shedler, 1999a, 1999b), and the related Personality Health Index (PHI, which provides a single overall index of personality functioning) and RADIO Index (which delineates an individual's strengths and difficulties within five key domains of personality functioning: reality testing, affect regulation and tolerance, defensive organization, identity integration, and object relations; see Waldron et al., 2011).
- The Social Cognition and Object Relations Scale (SCORS; Stein, Hilsenroth, Slavin-Mulford, & Pinsker, 2011; Westen, 1995; Westen, Lohr, Silk, & Kerber, 1985).
- The Structured Interview of Personality Organization (STIPO; Clarkin, Caligor, Stern, & Kernberg, 2004; Stern et al., 2010).
- The Wechsler Adult Intelligence Scale—Fourth Edition (WAIS-IV; Wechsler, 2008).

In addition to these measures, the Rorschach Inkblot Test, scored and interpreted by using Exner's Comprehensive System (Exner, 2003) or the Rorschach Performance Assessment System (Meyer, Viglione, Mihura, Erard, & Erdberg, 2011), allows the clinician to assess various components of personality, psychological capacities, and cognitive performance. A description of the Rorschach can be found in Chapter 15 of this manual (pp. 930–932). Administration requires at least 1 hour; scoring and interpretation require approximately 2 additional hours. Despite its relevance for the assessment of most of the 12 M-Axis capacities, we have opted not to include specific descriptions of the most relevant Rorschach categories for each mental capacity because its administration, scoring, and interpretation are quite complex and require considerable formal training and experience.

To obtain a more nuanced and detailed picture of a patient's functioning in each capacity, these empirically validated assessment instruments can and should be integrated with information obtained in other ways (e.g., clinical interview, life history records, reports from individuals who are familiar with the patient). For a broader array of assessment instruments and strategies for integrating information derived from these instruments, see Chapter 15.

1. Capacity for Regulation, Attention, and Learning

The capacity for regulation, attention, and learning encompasses the range of constitutional and maturational contributions to an individual's overall psychological functioning, as manifested in the domains of auditory processing and language, visual–spatial processing, motor planning and sequencing, and sensory modulation. Other processes involved in this capacity include executive functioning, attention, intelligence, processing of affective and social cues, and memory in its various forms (short- and long-term, semantic, autobiographical/episodic, and implicit/nondeclarative). Taken together, these mental functions enable people to attend to and process internal and external information, regulate the experience of self and the environment, filter extraneous input from consciousness when appropriate, and learn from their experiences to enhance adaptation and coping.

In rating this capacity, one should note that variations in genetic predisposition, temperament, and neurobiological substrates of regulation, attention, and learning are modified by a person's social and emotional context throughout development, beginning with early child–caregiver interactions. The individual develops characteristic predispositions and biases in attention and executive functioning as a result of these (and other) early experiences, and these predispositions and biases will be evident in how he or she interacts with others and the external environment later in life. Moreover, this capacity can be influenced by affect states the individual is experiencing at the moment (anxiety, distress, fear, etc.), so performance may vary across situations and settings.

This capacity differs somewhat from others on the M Axis, in that ratings of the patient's functioning in this domain are strengthened by (and in some cases require) external corroboration. Although the clinician's initial conclusions about the patient's capacity for regulation, attention, and learning may be based primarily on self-report and referral data, when difficulties are documented in the patient's file, in life history records, or by knowledgeable informants (e.g., a sibling or partner), confidence in the accuracy of the patient's report is increased.

Rating Scale

For this and each of the other M-Axis capacities, a 5-point rating scale, in which each mental function can be assessed from 5 to 1, is provided in Table 2.1 at the end of the chapter. Descriptions of the anchor points for levels 5, 3, and 1 for each capacity are provided in the text.

5. The individual is appropriately focused, well organized, and able to adapt and learn from experience, even under stress. There is a good ability to express thoughts, affects, and other inner experiences, both verbally and nonverbally. Memory, attention, and executive function are all functioning at a high level, and well integrated.
3. The individual is generally focused, organized, and able to adapt and learn when motivated. When not fully engaged, the person may show a moderate decline from customary functioning. Even when functioning optimally, the individual at this level can attend and focus only for relatively short periods and to a limited degree. Under stress, there may be a significant decline, with emergence of problems in language, information processing, and/or executive function.
1. The individual's attention is fleeting, and he or she is generally incapable of remaining focused, organized, and attentive. The person may have difficulty adapting to the environment and learning from experience, and may be self-absorbed, lethargic, or passive. Learning capacity is severely limited by one or more processing difficulties. Verbal expressions may be compromised, impoverished, or peculiar.

Most Relevant Assessment Tools

A broad array of assessment tools are relevant to assessing regulation, attention, and learning. Among the most important are measures of (1) intelligence; (2) working memory and autobiographical/episodic memory; (3) neuropsychological functioning; (4) learning capacity and learning disability (e.g., focus, concentration); (5) attention regulation and its deficits (including indices of dissociative symptoms); and (6) executive function (sequencing, attentional filtering, etc.).

Formal assessment of regulation, attention, and learning differs somewhat from evaluating other M-Axis capacities, in that many clinicians are not fully trained in administering and interpreting cognitive and neuropsychological tests. Moreover, many such measures are revised and updated frequently, requiring continued retraining. We recommend that clinicians with appropriate background and experience administer and score cognitive and neuropsychological tests that fall within their areas of competence. When more specialized interpretation is required, a patient should be referred to an appropriately trained neuropsychologist for more advanced assessment.

The tests described below are examples of measures that may be useful in assessing regulation, attention, and learning; they are not meant to constitute a comprehensive or definitive list.

Wechsler Adult Intelligence Scale—Fourth Edition

The Wechsler Adult Intelligence Scale—Fourth Edition (WAIS-IV; Wechsler, 2008) is the most widely used intelligence test. Normed on individuals ages 16–90, it includes verbal comprehension, with subtests of similarities (abstract, associative, and categorical reasoning, and verbal concept formation), vocabulary (word knowledge, language development, long-term memory), information (factual knowledge) and comprehension (judgment, knowledge of conventions, standards of behavior); perceptual reasoning, with subtests of block design (nonverbal concept formation and reasoning), matrix reasoning (broad visual intelligence, classification, and spatial ability), visual puzzles (nonverbal reasoning), picture completion (visual perception and organization, concentration, visual recognition), and figure weights (analogical reasoning, inductive and deductive logic, quantitative reasoning); working memory, with subtests of digit span (rote learning, memory, attention, mental manipulation, visual–spatial imaging), arithmetic (attention and concentration, mental alertness, short-term memory, numerical reasoning, long-term memory) and letter–number sequencing (attention and concentration, memory span, short-term auditory memory); and processing speed, with subtests of symbol search (attention and concentration), coding (learning, visual–motor coordination, visual perception), and cancellation (attention and concentration). Administration requires about an hour; coding and summarizing take about 2 hours.

Modified Mini-Mental State Examination

The Modified Mini-Mental State Examination (3MS; Teng & Chui, 1987) is a brief mental status exam that extends the original Mini-Mental State Examination (MMSE; Folstein, Folstein, & McHugh, 1975). It provides a brief screening assessment of key areas of cognitive functioning, including attention, short-term memory, orientation, and some basic executive tasks. The 3MS is not intended to serve as a replacement for more extensive neuropsychological testing batteries; rather, it provides clinicians with an easy way to screen for areas of gross cognitive impairment.

Montreal Cognitive Assessment

The Montreal Cognitive Assessment (MoCA; Nasreddine et al., 2005) is a 10-minute, 30-point, validated cognitive screening test developed to detect mild cognitive impairment in patients scoring between 24 and 30 points on the MMSE. Compared to the MMSE, the MoCA uses more numerous and demanding tasks to assess executive function, higher-level language abilities, memory, and complex visual–spatial processing.

Conners Continuous Performance Test

The Conners Continuous Performance Test (CPT; Conners, 2008; Conners & Multi-Health Systems Staff, 2000) is a task-oriented computerized test tapping constructs associated with distractibility, selective attention, and impulse control. By indexing the respondent's performance in areas of inattentiveness, impulsivity, sustained attention, and vigilance, the Conners CPT can be useful in helping diagnose attention-deficit/hyperactivity disorder (ADHD) and other neurological conditions related to attention. The Conners CPT 3 provides objective information about an individual's performance in attention tasks, complementing information obtained from rating scales.

Wisconsin Card Sorting Test

The Wisconsin Card Sorting Test (WCST; Berg, 1948; Grant & Berg, 1948) is a widely used neuropsychological measure of multiple cognitive skills usually referred to as "executive functions," with particular attention to decision making and problem solving. The participant's task is to sort two sets of 64 response cards on the basis of shapes, colors, and numbers, which change during the course of sorting. Participants must infer the correct sorting principles through limited feedback from the experimenter, who says only whether the sorting is correct or incorrect. Scores may be tallied along several dimensions, but the number of categories achieved and the number of perseverative errors are the most commonly reported outcomes (Rhodes, 2004).

Barkley Deficits in Executive Functioning Scale

The Barkley Deficits in Executive Functioning Scale (BDEFS; Barkley, 2014) evaluates dimensions of adult executive functioning. The 89-item version assesses executive problems within five domains: time management problems, organizational problems, self-restraint problems, self-motivation problems, and emotion regulation problems. Participants rate each item on a 1–4 Likert scale (never, sometimes, often, very often).

Rivermead Behavioural Memory Test—Third Edition

The Rivermead Behavioural Memory Test—Third Edition (RBMT-3; Wilson, Cockburn, Baddeley, & Hiorns, 1989; Wilson et al., 2008) tests short-term and long-term memory for verbal and spatial information, as well as prospective memory (i.e., remembering to do something in the future), visual memory, and memory of faces. It has the following subtests: names, belonging, appointment, pictures, immediate story, delayed story, faces, immediate route, delayed route, immediate message, delayed message, orientation, and date. The RBMT-3 includes new subtests designed to assess the ability to acquire skills and adds a separate measure of implicit memory. Because it simulates everyday tasks, the RBMT-3 is regarded as an "ecological memory battery." Some studies have found it a valid and reliable tool to detect memory deficits in patients with different neuropsychological profiles, including those with brain injury (Makatura, Lam, Leahy, Castillo, & Kalpakjian, 1999), epilepsy (Pérez & Godoy, 1998), Alzheimer's disease (Cockburn & Keene, 2001), and age-related brain changes (Ostrosky-Solis, Jaime, & Ardila, 1998). Retest stability and interrater reliability are good (Wilson et al., 1989).

Benton Visual Retention Test

The Benton Visual Retention Test (BVRT; Benton, 1974) is a well-established neurodiagnostic instrument that assesses visual recall, perception, and constructional ability (Strauss, Sherman, & Spreen, 2006). Performance involves visual–motor response, visual–spatial perception and retention, visual and verbal conceptualization, and immediate memory span (Lezak, Howieson, Bigler, & Tranel, 2012). There are multiple administration formats for the BVRT, each measuring a different aspect of perceptual–motor functioning (Strauss et al., 2006). All formats use cards containing geometric and abstract figures, which the examinee must either construct or recognize. Both the most frequently used and the lesser-used format test visual memory. Each card is exposed for 10 seconds, after which the examinee draws the figure(s) from immediate memory. In the multiple-choice format (BVRT-MC), stimulus cards are used with four-choice response cards to measure recognition memory.

Behavioural Assessment of the Dysexecutive Syndrome

The Behavioural Assessment of the Dysexecutive Syndrome (BADS; Wilson, Alderman, Burgess, Emslie, & Evans, 1996) is designed to predict "everyday problems arising from the dysexecutive syndrome" (Wilson et al., 1996, p. 4) and to evaluate disorders of planning, organization, problem solving, and attention. The dysexecutive syndrome is a major area of cognitive deficit that may impede functional recovery and the ability to respond to rehabilitation programs. Four subtests measure problem solving, organizing, and planning; conventional scheduling system; supervisory attention system; and assessing real-life behaviors. It is designed to find both general and specific executive deficits. The significant correlation of the BADS and most of its subtests with the standard executive tests indicates that it has adequate concurrent validity. In terms of construct validity, it is comparable to standard executive tests in discriminating between individuals with and without brain damage (Norris & Tate, 2000).

Stroop Color and Word Test

The Stroop Color and Word Test (Golden & Freshwater, 2002; Jensen & Rohwer, 1966; Stroop, 1935) is used to determine a person's capacity to direct attention toward relevant information while inhibiting irrelevant information. The time between presentation of the stimulus and behavioral response is measured. There are several test variants in common clinical use, with differences in number of subtasks, type and number of stimuli, times for the task, and scoring procedures. The most widely used version consists of three trials, each with 100 items, presented across 5 columns of 20 items.

2. Capacity for Affective Range, Communication, and Understanding

The second capacity reflects the ability to experience, comprehend, and express affects in a way that is appropriate to a particular situation and consistent with one's cultural milieu. Clinicians should consider all three of this capacity's components. "Affective range" is the capacity to experience a wide range of affects and emotions, including positive as well as negative states, in varying degrees of intensity. "Affective communication" is the ability to communicate affective experience effectively and adaptively to other people through different modalities (i.e., verbal, nonverbal). It includes the quality of expression, intentional or unintentional, of inner emotional experiences (i.e., if the expression of affects and emotions is appropriate in quality and intensity to the situation at hand; if the affects are particularly variable or labile). "Affective understanding" is the ability to recognize one's own emotions and to read and interpret others' emotional communications (verbal, nonverbal) in adaptive, empathic, responsive, and relationship-facilitating ways. Very low functioning in this domain can lead to difficulties in identifying, differentiating, and communicating feelings, a lack of imagination, and a constricted, externally oriented thinking style (i.e., alexithymic tendencies).

This capacity, largely influenced by early infant–caregiver interactions, is related to social cognition insofar as it allows a person to understand, act on, and benefit from interpersonal interactions. Some individuals may be relatively strong in one component but weak in another. Individual differences in this capacity can be due in part to cultural background, norms, and experience. In general, these unique patterns should be captured in the narrative characterizing the person.

Rating Scale

5. Individuals at this level can use, express, communicate, and understand a wide range of subtle emotions effectively. They can decipher and respond to most emotional signals flexibly and accurately, even under stress (e.g., safety vs. danger, approval vs. disapproval, acceptance vs. rejection, respect vs. disdain). Affective communication almost always seems appropriate in quality and intensity to the situation experienced in the moment.

3. Individuals at this level seem to experience and communicate a constricted range of emotional states, and/or show difficulty experiencing specific affects (e.g., anger). They decipher others' emotional states with difficulty and may respond to emotional signals in a dysregulated and asynchronous way, especially when challenged or stressed. Or they may express emotions in an inadequate way, disproportionate to situations and social expectations.

1. Individuals at this level show mostly fragmented, chaotic emotional expressions, or convey little emotion at all (e.g., they may be unable to show facial expression, modulate vocal tone, or maintain body posture appropriate to the situation). Low functioning in this capacity may involve distortion of others' emotional signals (e.g., misreading cues and therefore feeling suspicious, mistreated, unloved, angry, etc.), and/or difficulty identifying feelings and distinguishing them from bodily sensations. Affective responses may be perceived by others as odd or incongruous.

Most Relevant Assessment Tools

Shedler–Westen Assessment Procedure–200

The Shedler–Westen Assessment Procedure–200 (SWAP-200; Westen & Shedler, 1999a, 1999b) is described in Chapter 15. Along with the Personality Health Index (PHI) and the RADIO Index, the SWAP-200 is useful for M-Axis assessment (Porcerelli, Cogan, & Bambery, 2011). The capacity for affective range, communication, and understanding is covered by the following items: 12. Emotions tend to spiral out of control, leading to extremes of anxiety, sadness, rage, excitement, etc.; 57. Tends to feel guilty; 74. Expresses emotion in exaggerated and theatrical ways; 106. Tends to express affect appropriate in quality and intensity to the situation at hand; 126. Appears to have a limited or constricted range of emotions; 131. Has difficulty allowing self to experience strong pleasurable emotions (e.g., excitement, joy, pride); 144. Tends to see self as logical and rational, uninfluenced by emotion; prefers to operate as if emotions were irrelevant or inconsequential; 157. Tends to become irrational when strong emotions are stirred up; may show a noticeable decline from customary level of functioning; and 191. Emotions tend to change rapidly and unpredictably.

Social Cognition and Object Relations Scale

The Social Cognition and Object Relations Scale (SCORS; Stein, Hilsenroth, Slavin-Mulford, & Pinsker, 2011; Westen, 1995; Westen, Lohr, Silk, & Kerber, 1985) contains multiple scales on which cognitive and affective dimensions of object relations are rated based on narrative data (such as the Thematic Apperception Test; Stein et al., 2014). The original SCORS has four scales; the first revision, a Q-sort version (SCORS-Q; Westen, 1995), has five; and the most recent, the SCORS Global Rating Method (SCORS-G; Stein et al., 2011), has eight. Particularly relevant to this capacity is the scale assessing "affective quality of representations," which can be used to code affective components of respondent narratives related to affective communication. Clinicians rate examinees' narratives and note their expectations of how others will affect them emotionally, how others experience the respondent emotionally, and how they typically conceptualize the affective experiences of others.

Affective Regulation and Experience Q-sort-Questionnaire Version

The Affective Regulation and Experience Q-sort-Questionnaire Version (AREQ-QV; Westen, Muderrisoglu, Fowler, Shedler, & Koren, 1997) is a 98-item questionnaire in which experienced clinicians rate patients on components of affective experience and regulation. Written to minimize jargon, enabling reliable description of subtle processes across judges, items were derived from research and theoretical literatures and from the item content of self-report questionnaires on affect. They assess explicit cognitive coping strategies, behavioral strategies for regulating affects (e.g., drug use), and implicit affect regulation strategies (defenses) in relatively straightforward, behavioral language (Zittel-Conklin, Bradley, & Westen, 2006).

Affective Communication Questionnaire

The Affective Communication Questionnaire (ACQ; Meehan, 2004; Meehan, Levy, & Clarkin, 2012) is a 28-item self-report measure asking therapists to rate patients on how much they felt enlivened and engaged by them, the nature of affect in sessions, and the degree to which patients imbued language with affect. Each statement is rated from 1 (not true) to 5 (very true), reflecting how well it characterized the therapeutic work. Items were derived from clinical and empirical literatures on implicit communication of affect in therapy (i.e., Bucci, 1997; Kernberg, 1984). Designed to evaluate co-created affective experience, and written to be unambiguous to therapists of all orientations, the ACQ evaluates how both patient and therapist feel, think, and act.

Levels of Emotional Awareness Scale

The Levels of Emotional Awareness Scale (LEAS; Lane & Garfield, 2005; Lane, Quinlan, Schwartz, Walker, & Zeitlin, 1990) is a written-performance tool assessing the ability to give complex descriptions of emotional experience in self and others; the scale differentiates between explicit (conscious) and implicit (unconscious) levels of emotional awareness (Lane & Schwartz, 1987). Respondents are asked to describe their anticipated feelings and those of another person in each of 20 two-person scenarios of emotion-evoking interactions. A glossary links affect-related words to appropriate levels. The LEAS has a maximum score of 100; scores between 0 and 20 indicate level 1, and scores between 81 and 100 indicate level 5. Normative data from a U.S. community sample demonstrated good psychometric properties (Lane et al., 1990). Since hand scoring is time-consuming, Barchard, Bajgar, Duncan, and Lane (2010) have developed and validated a computer scoring system. Using the 4 items of the original 20 with the highest discrimination, Subic-Wrana, Beutel, Brahler, and Stobel-Richter (2014) created a short form. Internal consistency of this version of the LEAS was adequate (Cronbach's alpha of .67) and correlated strongly with the original 20-item version (*r* = .85).

Positive and Negative Affective Schedule—Expanded Form

The Positive and Negative Affective Schedule—Expanded Form (PANAS-X; Watson & Clark, 1994) is a 60-item self-report questionnaire, an expanded version of the original PANAS (Watson, Clark, & Tellegen, 1988; see also Leue & Beaducel, 2011). The PANAS-X measures two original higher-order scales (PA—Positive Affect and NA—Negative Affect) and 11 specific affects: fear, sadness, guilt, hostility, shyness, fatigue, surprise, joviality, self-assurance, attentiveness, and serenity. Test items consist of single mood descriptors. Respondents rate the extent to which they have had these feelings within a specified period, using a scale from 1 (very slightly or not at all) to 5 (very much). Research supports the PANAS-X as a measure of short-term affect and notes its sensitivity to fluctuations in external and internal conditions (Hussong & Hicks, 2003).

State–Trait Emotion Measure

The State–Trait Emotion Measure (STEM; Levine et al., 2011) evaluates five positive and five negative emotions: affection, anger, anxiety, attentiveness/energy, contentment, envy, guilt/shame, joy, pride, and sadness. The definitions of these emotions are based on numerous sources. Several potential situations are provided within which each emotion might arise. Respondents are asked to state the extent to which they felt each emotion both at a particular time (state) and generally (trait) on a 10-point scale, with anchors denoting levels of intensity. Higher-order emotions are measured by summing positive and negative emotions, respectively, for state and trait indicators. Cronbach's alpha reliabilities for summed scales are .83 (state) and .86 (trait) for the positive emotions and .63 (state) and .65 (trait) for the negative emotions.

Affective Neuroscience Personality Scales

The Affective Neuroscience Personality Scales (ANPS; Davis & Panksepp, 2011; Davis, Panksepp, & Normansell, 2003) is a 112-item self-report measure of behavioral correlates of six primary neural affective systems identified in animal models (play, seeking, care, fear, anger, and sadness), plus a seventh construct (spirituality) without an a priori neural basis. Each subscale consists of 14 items in the form of statements representing facets of primary affective tendencies. A number of filler items check validity and social desirability. Psychometric properties are good (Davis et al., 2003), and the ANPS has been validated clinically (Savitz, van der Merwe, & Ramesar, 2008).

Empathy Quotient

The Empathy Quotient (EQ; Baron-Cohen & Wheelwright, 2004) is a 60-item questionnaire (there is also a shorter, 40-item version) assessing empathy in adults. Explicitly designed for clinical applications, it is sensitive to lack of empathy as a feature of psychopathology. Responses are given on a 4-point scale from "strongly agree" to "strongly disagree." Participants receive 0 for a "nonempathic" response, whatever the magnitude, and for an "empathic response" a 1 or 2, depending on the strength of the reply. Items are augmented by 20 filler items that distract respondents from a relentless focus on empathy. Preliminary studies suggest good reliability and validity (Allison, Baron-Cohen, Wheelwright, Stone, & Muncer, 2011; Lawrence, Shaw, Baker, Baron-Cohen, & David, 2004).

Emotion Regulation Questionnaire

The Emotion Regulation Questionnaire (ERQ; Gross & John, 2003) is a 10-item self-report measure of habitual expressive suppression (4 items) and reappraisal (6 items) strategies for emotion regulation. Items are rated on a Likert scale from 1 (strongly disagree) to 7 (strongly agree). Sample questions include "I control my emotions by changing the way I think about the situation I'm in" (reappraisal) and "I control my emotions by not expressing them" (suppression). Internal consistency has been adequate and consistent across studies (Melka, Lancaster, Bryant, & Rodriguez, 2011; Spaapen, Waters, Brummer, Stopa, & Bucks, 2014; Wiltink et al., 2011).

Difficulties in Emotion Regulation Scale

The Difficulties in Emotion Regulation Scale (DERS; Gratz & Roemer, 2004) is a 36-item self-report measure providing a comprehensive assessment of overall emotion dysregulation and six specific dimensions: nonacceptance of negative emotions, difficulties engaging in goal-directed behaviors when distressed, difficulties controlling impulsive behaviors when distressed, limited access to effective emotion regulation strategies, lack of emotional awareness, and lack of emotional clarity. Items are rated from 1 (almost never, 0–10%) to 5 (almost always, 91–100%), yielding a total from 36 to 180, with higher scores indicating greater degrees of impairment in emotion regulation. The DERS has excellent internal consistency and good test–retest reliability (Fowler et al., 2014). It is used extensively in psychiatric research as a predictor of psychopathology, in treatment trials as a mediator variable, and as a primary outcome variable.

3. Capacity for Mentalization and Reflective Functioning

"Mentalization"—the ability to infer and reflect on one's own and others' mental states—is a form of mental activity considered to be imaginative (because when we mentalize, we are "imagining" what others think or feel). Mentalization is primarily preconscious, typically occurring outside the focus of attention, and aims at understanding and interpreting the behavior of self and others in terms of mental states (e.g., needs, desires, feelings, beliefs, goals, intentions, and motivations). This capacity enables individuals to use ideas to experience, describe, and express internal life; to regulate their own affects and develop a coherent sense of self; and to make accurate inferences regarding the mental states of others. It allows them to distinguish between internal and external reality and between mental and emotional processes and real-world interactions. Mentalization is supported by several cognitive skills, including understanding of emotional states and the ability to think implicitly about others' states of mind. Allen, Fonagy, and Bateman (2008) have described mentalization as a means through which we "keep in mind the mind," "understand misunderstandings," "see [ourselves] from the outside and the other from the inside," and "[attribute] a quality of mind to things or develop a mental perspective" (p. 3). The construct of *reflective functioning* represents the operationalization of the capacity to mentalize—the way, in other words, that we measure mentalization.

The capacity for mentalization and reflective functioning reflects the ability to symbolize affectively meaningful experience (i.e., to organize experience via mental representation rather than somatically or behaviorally), and to use this experience effectively both for self-regulation and in interpersonal interactions. It may be apparent in verbal behavior but can also be manifested in more subtle and indirect ways, nonverbally and via the body. The capacity to represent experience—a crucial aspect of mentalization—enables individuals to use ideas to experience, describe, and express internal life and to make accurate inferences regarding the mental states of others.

The foundation for mentalization and reflective functioning is laid early in life, as dyadic interactions with caregivers are encoded and internalized. The "psychological self" develops as a child experiences a caregiver who thinks of the child as an individual with mental states. Thus the capacity to develop a mentalizing stance depends greatly on parental mentalizing capacities. The parents must be able to take the child's perspective and, appreciating the inherent separateness of minds populated by different contents, treat the child as a "psychological agent" whose actions are motivated by mental states. This parental capacity includes the ability to make sense of the infant's powerful affect states and other aspects of his or her nonverbally expressed internal world.

Parents who cannot reflect empathically on the inner experience of their child and respond accordingly deprive the child of a nuclear psychological experience necessary to build a cohesive sense of self. Highly maladaptive caregiving (e.g., a mother with borderline personality organization) can foster severe distortions in mentalizing ability, including hypermentalization (overinterpretive mental state reasoning) or vulnerability to breakdowns in mentalizing capacity, especially under stress. Attuned caregiving, in contrast, fosters the elaboration, differentiation, and integration of affective self-states, setting the stage for the capacity to experience one's own and others' subjectivity. Awareness that other people accurately attend to and respond to one's experience gradually builds in the infant the ability to reflect on these experiences through using language (i.e., private and shared symbols), and ultimately increases the capacity for mentalization.

Rating Scale

5. Individuals at this level can comprehend and reflect on internal mental states (e.g., emotions, thoughts, desires, and needs) and understand, even when challenged or distressed, internal experiences that underlie others' actions and reactions. They are highly capable of distinguishing inner from outer reality; have psychological insight into their own motives, affects, and behaviors; and can think about self and others in subtle and sophisticated ways. They also show a capacity to construct representations of internal mental states using both overt and subtle cues (e.g., arousal, behavior, context). Emotions are experienced and represented in complex and nuanced ways, in the context of social-emotional relationships and behavior patterns. Internal representations are used to modulate and inhibit impulses and to allow adaptive, appropriate expression of impulses.

3. Individuals at this level are generally able to understand and reflect on their own behavior and reactions in terms of mental states (e.g., needs, desires, feelings); to infer others' internal experiences from behavioral and contextual cues; and to construct and use internal representations to experience a cohesive sense of self and others. In situations of conflict or intensity, however, there is a notable decline from usual levels of awareness of mental states of self and others, with difficulties in perceiving and representing emotions in the moment. They may have a limited ability to elaborate on a feeling in its own right, and tend toward external justifications; wishes and feelings may be acted out (i.e., in impulsive behavior) or somatized (e.g., "My stomach hurts").

1. Individuals at this level are unable to infer, understand, or reflect upon their own affective experiences or to symbolize others' mental states. They have severe difficulties distinguishing between internal and external reality and between mental and emotional processes and real-world interactions; it seems that what exists in the mind must exist "out there," and vice versa. They often misunderstand, misinterpret, or are confused by others' actions and reactions, and are generally unable to represent emotions as they are being experienced. They remain embedded in the affect, unable to express the experience in words or to regulate affective states effectively. When functioning in this capacity is extremely low, there is no experience of connection between internal experiences and possibilities for self-observation; especially under stress, the self may be experienced as incoherent, depleted, or altogether absent.

Most Relevant Assessment Tools

Reflective Functioning Scale

The Reflective Functioning Scale (RFS; Fonagy, Target, Steele, & Steele, 1998) is a quantified index of the ability to mentalize applied to transcripts of the Adult Attachment Interview (AAI; George, Kaplan, & Main, 1985). AAI questions are divided into two groups: (1) "permit questions," which allow the speaker to demonstrate reflective capacities, and (2) "demand questions," which require a reflective response. Answers are evaluated by whether they contain markers of an appreciation of mental functioning. Statements must be specific (not generic), refer to identifiable mental states, involve an example that relates to the attachment, and refer to self–other interactions. Reflective functioning is rated on a scale with scores from –1 to +9. The RFS can also be used to measure reflective functioning in parents, via the Parent Development Interview (PDI; Aber, Slade, Berger, Bresgi, & Kaplan, 1985; Slade, 2005), a semi-structured clinical interview examining parents' representations of their children, of themselves as parents, and of their relationships with their children.

Shedler–Westen Assessment Procedure–200

In the SWAP-200 (Westen & Shedler, 1999a, 1999b), mentalization and reflective functioning are covered by the following items: 29. Has difficulty making sense of other people's behavior; often misunderstands, misinterprets, or is confused by others' actions and reactions; 41. Appears unable to describe important others in a way that conveys a sense of who they are as people; descriptions of others come across as two-dimensional and lacking in richness; 87. Is quick to assume that others wish to harm or take advantage of him or her; tends to perceive malevolent intentions in others' words and actions; 105. Tends to avoid confiding in others for fear of betrayal; expects things s/he says or does will be used against him or her; 148. Has little psychological insight into own motives, behavior, etc.; is unable to consider alternate interpretations of his/her experiences; 183. Is psychologically insightful; is able to understand self and others in subtle and sophisticated ways.

SWAP Insight Scale

The authors of the SWAP Insight Scale (SIS; Lehmann & Hilsenroth, 2011) identified six SWAP-200 items as optimal in assessing patient insight, with a Cronbach's alpha of .78. The construct validity of the SIS was based on independent videotape ratings of the Capacity for Dynamic Process Scale, specifically the items "appears introspective" and "manifests insight." Authors also examined the relationship between SIS ratings and independent clinical videotape ratings of the SCORS-G, specifically ratings of "complexity of representations" and "social causality." Results showed significant positive correlations between SIS scores and all five criterion measures; partial correlations showed that even when the effects of global psychiatric severity were controlled for, the SIS was significantly related to independent clinical videotape ratings of patients' insight. Relevant SIS items include the following: 75 (R). Tends to think in concrete terms and interpret things in overly literal ways; has limited ability to appreciate metaphor, analogy, or nuance; 82. Is capable of hearing information that is emotionally threatening (i.e., that challenges cherished beliefs, perceptions, and self-perceptions) and can use and benefit from it; 89. Appears to have come to terms with painful experiences from the past; has found meaning in and grown from such experiences; 111. Has the capacity to recognize alternative viewpoints, even in matters that stir up strong feelings; 148 (R). Has little psychological insight into own motives, behavior, etc.; is unable to consider alternate interpretations of his/her experiences; 183. Is psychologically insightful; is able to understand self and others in subtle and sophisticated ways.

Parental Embodied Mentalizing

Parental Embodied Mentalizing (PEM; Shai & Belsky, 2011; Shai & Fonagy, 2013) is a coding system for video-recorded parent–infant interaction, designed to assess the parental capacity for embodied mentalizing and parental ability to repair dyadic interactive misattunement. "Parental embodied mentalizing" is described as a parent's capacity to (1) implicitly conceive, comprehend, and extrapolate the infant's mental states (such as wishes, desires, or preferences) from the infant's whole-body kinesthetic expressions and (2) adjust his or her own kinesthetic patterns accordingly. The PEM focuses exclusively on the quality of dynamic, moment-to-moment changes in whole-body kinesthetic patterns during parent–infant dyadic interactions. Assessment involves considering several kinesthetic qualities reflecting mental states that an observer can reliably interpret: "Directionality" refers to the direction of movement in relation to the individual's body center; "tension flow" to sequences of fluency and restraint of the muscles reflecting pleasure or distress/discomfort; and "tempo" to the pulse of movement within a time unit.

4. Capacity for Differentiation and Integration (Identity)

The capacity for differentiation and integration involves the ability to distinguish self from other, fantasy from reality, internal objects and representations from external objects and circumstances, and present from past and future, and to delineate connections between these elements without confounding them. It reflects the ability to construct and maintain a differentiated, realistic, coherent, and nuanced representation of self (identity) and other people, and to connect these internalized representations in a manner that facilitates adaptation and functioning.

A core feature of the capacity for differentiation and integration is the ability to construct and maintain a realistic and coherent *identity* in relation to another. High levels of this capacity imply that a person can organize and manage complex role demands and affects; low levels imply constriction and oversimplification of experience or confusion between self and others, fantasy and reality, and past, present, and future. High levels of the capacity typically result in openness to novel experience and the accompanying ability to shift flexibly or adjust in a complex, ambiguous environment.

Rating Scale

5. Individuals at this level can appreciate the separateness and relatedness of different affect states, motives, and wishes of self and others, even when these are nuanced and ambiguous, and can organize experience and social-emotional demands over time (i.e., past, present, future) and across contexts with contrasting role demands (e.g., relating to a spouse versus a parent). They can interact with an increasingly complex and demanding environment while using defenses and coping resources with adequate stability, flexibility, and spontaneity.

3. Individuals at this level can differentiate and integrate experience, but with some constriction and oversimplification, especially under stress. Strong emotions or wishes, both general and context specific, can lead to the temporary fragmentation or polarization (all-or-nothing extremes) of internal experience. Capacities for differentiation and integration are limited to a few emotional realms (e.g., superficial relationships). Challenges outside these areas often lead to diminished functioning and impaired coping.

1. At this level, internal experience is fragmented or rigidly compartmentalized and oversimplified most of the time; in extreme cases, it may be detached from external context, and self and other may be confused. There is little ability to move through a range of emotional states either autonomously or in interactions with others without intense anxiety (sometimes expressed as guilt or shame), acting out, or reliance on maladaptive defenses (e.g., severe splitting and dissociation), with concomitant impairment in reality testing.

Most Relevant Assessment Tools

Differentiation–Relatedness Scale

The Differentiation–Relatedness Scale (D-RS; Blatt, Stayner, Auerbach, & Behrends, 1996; Diamond, Blatt, Stayner, & Kaslow, 1991) identifies two fundamental dimensions of self–other representations: "differentiation of self from others," implying a perception of self as consolidated, integrated, and individualized; and "mature relationality," understood as the ability to integrate one's self with others within interpersonal relationships. These two independent yet interrelated lines of psychological development are each evaluated with a global score from 1 to 10. A score of 1 or 2 indicates lack of differentiation between self and other. Increasing points acknowledge the use of mirroring (3), self–other idealization or denigration (4), and oscillation between idealization and denigration poles (5). A more differentiated and related sense of self and other is captured in 6 and 7. Scores of 8 and 9 indicate that self and other are empathically related, with increasing acknowledgment of mutually reinforcing relationships. A score of 10 indicates an integrated construction of self and other in empathic and reciprocal relationships; these representations reflect conscious acknowledgment that the relationship between self and other is evolving through an intersubjective process.

Scales of Psychological Capacities

The Scales of Psychological Capacities (SPC; DeWitt, Hartley, Rosenberg, Zilberg, & Wallerstein, 1991; Wallerstein, 1996) is a set of expert-rated scales designed to measure a series of constructions defined as "psychological abilities." The third ability, "organization of the self," may help evaluate the capacity for differentiation and integration. Subscales rate the range from integrity to fragmentation in the sense of agency and from integrity to fragmentation in the integration of self.

Object Relations Inventory

The Object Relations Inventory (ORI; Blatt, Auerbach, & Levy, 1997; Blatt et al., 1996; Huprich, Auerbach, Porcerelli, & Bupp, 2016) is designed to evaluate relationships with others and their internal representations. It consists of three tools that can be applied to the answers provided to performance-based tests (narrative and Rorschach), as well as to reports of preconscious memories and dream tales. The clinician assesses the conceptual level of the descriptions of self and other; levels of differentiation–relationality in those descriptions; and thematic qualitative dimensions in the descriptions of meaningful others.

Shedler–Westen Assessment Procedure–200

In the SWAP-200 (Westen & Shedler, 1999a, 1999b), differentiation and integration are covered by the following items: 10. Feels some important other has a special, almost magical ability to understand his/her innermost thoughts and feelings (e.g., may imagine rapport is so perfect that ordinary efforts at communication are superfluous); 15. Lacks a stable image of who s/he is or would like to become (e.g., attitudes, values, goals, or feelings about self may be unstable and changing); 38. Tends to feel s/he is not his/her true self with others; tends to feel false or fraudulent; 47. Is unsure whether s/he is heterosexual, homosexual, or bisexual; 89. Appears to have come to terms with painful experiences from the past; has found meaning in, and grown from such experiences; 92. Is articulate; can express self well in words.

Social Cognition and Object Relations Scale

The SCORS (Stein, Hilsenroth, Slavin-Mulford, & Pinsker, 2011; Westen, 1995; Westen, Lohr, Silk, & Kerber, 1985) taps areas demonstrated to be useful for assessing the capacity for differentiation and integration (identity), such as "identity and coherence of self" and "complexity of representation of people."

Severity Indices of Personality Problems–118

The Severity Indices of Personality Problems–118 (SIPP-118; Verheul et al., 2008) is a self-report questionnaire covering core components of personality functioning. It consists of 118 items assessed on a 4-point Likert scale (from 1 = fully disagree to 4 = fully agree), relative to five clinically relevant higher-order domains. Particularly significant for this capacity is the identity integration domain.

Adult Attachment Interview

The Adult Attachment Interview (AAI; George, Kaplan, & Main, 1985) is a semistructured interview assessing attachment "states of mind." Sharing a "state of mind" means narrating a history of internal working models in their conscious aspects, but also in connection with deeper experiences not fully accessible to consciousness. Central tasks include producing and reflecting on relationships in one's attachment history, while maintaining a coherent, cooperative conversation with the interviewer. The coding system (Main, Goldwyn, & Hesse, 2002) includes scales relevant for assessing differentiation and integration issues: "Coherence of transcript" and "coherence of mind" assess ability to organize thoughts and feelings about attachment experiences without resorting to splitting, idealization, and denial, and test the coherence of the internal representations of childhood memories. Relevant interview questions include "I'd like you to try to describe your relationship with your parents as a young child, if you could start from as far as you can remember"; "In general, how do you think your overall experiences with your parents have affected your adult personality?"; "Were there many changes in your relationship with your parents after childhood?"; "What is your relationship with your parents like for you now as an adult? Here I am asking about your current relationship."

Mutuality of Autonomy Scale

The Mutuality of Autonomy Scale (MOA; Urist, 1977; Urist & Shill, 1982), one of the most widely used and well-validated scoring systems measuring quality and structure of implicit mental representations, is a scale derived from the Rorschach Inkblot Test. It derives levels or stages of relatedness based on a sense of individual autonomy and capacity to establish and sustain mutuality. Every Rorschach response that includes a relationship between animate or inanimate objects is scored on a 7-point Likert scale; scores cover a range from healthy relationships marked by capacity for mutuality and respect of the other's autonomy (scores of 1–2) to unhealthy, increasingly malevolent relationships with lack of boundaries (scores of 5–7). Reliability and clinical utility of the MOA have been well established (Bombel, Mihura, & Meyer, 2009; Graceffo, Mihura, & Meyer, 2014), including by a recent meta-analysis confirming the criterion validity of its scores as measures of object relations (Monroe, Diener, Fowler, Sexton, & Hilsenroth, 2013).

5. Capacity for Relationships and Intimacy

The fifth capacity reflects two key areas for adaptively relating to others. First, it captures the depth, range, and consistency (i.e., stability) of the person's interpersonal relationships. Healthy relatedness reflects not only the degree to which an individual has stable, mutually satisfying relationships with others, but also the quality of internalized object relations—mental representations of self, other people, and self–other interactions. When object relations are developmentally mature, affectively positive, and capable of evolving over time, individuals typically show a good capacity for relationships and intimacy. Conversely, when object relations are developmentally primitive (i.e., lacking in nuance), negatively toned, and rigid (i.e., incapable of changing in response to new experiences), individuals typically show an impairment in this domain.

The second component of the capacity for relationships and intimacy reflects a person's ability to adjust interpersonal distance and closeness in response to situational demands, based on each specific relationship and consistent with cultural expectations. When a person functions well in this component, stability in relationships is balanced with spontaneity, allowing the individual to adjust interpersonal behaviors and attitudes flexibly yet reliably, depending on interpersonal and intrapersonal demands and circumstances. Adaptive functioning in this capacity also implies that the individual is capable of reciprocity and mutuality, particularly in long-term relationships; in other words, he or she is capable of accepting support from others and providing support to others as situations demand.

This capacity includes the person's sexuality as reflected in an awareness of his or her desires and emotions, the ability to engage in pleasurable sexual fantasies and activities, and the ability to blend sexuality with emotional intimacy. Just as "self-esteem regulation and quality of internal experience" is an index of vitality and self-regard, "capacity for relationships and intimacy" is an index of relatedness—the ability to develop and sustain relationships by engaging in a wide array of behaviors, including sexual behaviors, that are relationship-promoting in nature.

Depth of relatedness varies across relationships. Adaptive functioning in adulthood involves navigating and facilitating connections that differ in levels of intimacy (e.g., casual acquaintances, professional relationships, friendships, close friendships, romantic relationships). Although there are individual differences in interpersonal desires and needs, adaptive functioning in this capacity typically entails depth and stability in core relationships (long-term friendships and romantic relationships); cultivation of relational networks of varying levels of closeness; and adaptive adjustment of one's interpersonal behavior, including limit setting.

Rating Scale

5. Individuals at this level have a deep, emotionally rich capacity for intimacy, caring, and empathy, even when feelings are intense or when they are under stress. An individual can adjust to changing social-emotional demands and can adjust as circumstances change, providing support to others and accepting support from others on the basis of situational needs.

3. At this level, the person's capacity for intimacy, caring, and empathy is present but may be disrupted by strong emotions such as anger, shame, or separation anxiety. In

such situations, the person may withdraw, act out, or become overly needy, clingy, and dependent. The individual finds it difficult to adjust to situational demands, and there are some deficits in either the ability to accept support from others or the ability to provide others with support.

1. Individuals at this level appear superficial, self-focused, and need-oriented, lacking in intimacy and empathy. They are indifferent to the needs of others, and appear aloof, withdrawn, socially isolated, and detached. Interactions tend to be one-way and lacking in mutuality, characterized by marked deficits in the ability to support others or accept support from them.

Most Relevant Assessment Tools

Core Conflictual Relationship Theme

The Core Conflictual Relationship Theme (CCRT) measure (Luborsky & Crits-Christoph, 1998) is a clinically founded, systematic instrument describing schemes of interpersonal relatatedness based on reports of therapeutic sessions. The CCRT describes the relational scheme or conflict, using three components: (1) the subject's desires, needs or intentions; (2) others' answers or pending answers; (3) answers of self (i.e., the reactions to other people's answers, which can include emotions, behaviors, symptoms, etc.). Related to the CCRT is the Central Relationship Questionnaire (CRQ; Barber, Foltz, & Weinryb, 1998; McCarthy, Gibbons, & Barber, 2008), a self-report instrument that measures central relationship patterns. Also related to the CCRT is the Relationship Anecdotes Paradigms (RAP) interview (Luborsky, 1998), which can be applied to almost any sample of people and can elicit narratives to use as data for similar purposes as the narratives drawn from therapy.

Karolinska Psychodynamic Profile

The Karolinska Psychodynamic Profile (KAPP; Weinryb, Rossel, & Asberg, 1991a, 1991b), derived from Kernberg's (1984) structural interview, proposes a measure of mental procedures as manifested in the perception of self and in interpersonal relationships. Its 18 subscales depict levels of functioning, conceptualizing a complex reality that includes the quality of interpersonal relationships, more specific aspects of personality functioning, differentiation of affects in experience and expression, the body as a factor in self-respect, sexuality as a specific aspect of interpersonal relationships, and individuals' impressions of their own personality and social meaning.

Object Relations Technique

The Object Relations Technique (ORT; Del Corno & Lang, 2006; Knafo, 2010; Phillipson, 1955) is a performance-based method for adults and adolescents ages 14 and over. It investigates types and levels of relationship on the assumption that they express attempts to reconcile unconscious fantasies of primary object relations (product of the relationships with primary objects, always actively seeking gratification) with conscious experiences of object relations acquired from experience.

Object Relations Inventory

The ORI (Blatt, Auerbach, & Levy, 1997; Blatt, Stayner, Auerbach, & Behrends, 1996; Huprich, Auerbach, Porcerelli, & Bupp, 2016), as noted earlier, evaluates object relations and their representations. It consists of three tools that can be applied to the answers provided to performance-based tests and to reports of preconscious memories and dream tales. Clinicians evaluate conceptual level of the descriptions of self and other, levels of differentiation–relationality in such descriptions, and their thematic qualitative dimensions.

Adult Attachment Interview and Adult Attachment Projective

The AAI (George, Kaplan, & Main, 1985) and the Adult Attachment Projective (AAP; George, West, & Pettem, 1997; Jones-Mason, Allen, Hamilton, & Weiss, 2015) are methodologies that assess inner working models (IWMs) of attachment. IWMs contain implicit rules for how one "lives in relationships" (Slade, 1999); they are "maps" (mental representations) of self and others that enable members of an attachment dyad (e.g., parent–child, romantic couple) to foresee, interpret, and engage appropriately in mutual interactions. Secure attachment (assessed by the AAI or the AAP) is linked to the capacity to update one's IWMs and to approach close relationships in flexible, creative, and nondefensive ways.

Shedler–Westen Assessment Procedure–200

In the SWAP-200 (Westen & Shedler, 1999a, 1999b), relationships and intimacy are addressed by the following items: 5. Tends to be emotionally intrusive; tends not to respect others' needs for autonomy, privacy, etc.; 11. Tends to become attached quickly or intensely; develops feelings, expectations, etc., that are not warranted by the history or context of the relationship; 17. Tends to be ingratiating or submissive (e.g., may consent to things s/he does not agree with or does not want to do, in the hope of getting support or approval); 18. When romantically or sexually attracted, tends to lose interest if other person reciprocates; 23. Tends to become involved in romantic or sexual "triangles" (e.g., is most interested in partners who are already attached, sought by someone else); 26. Tends to get drawn into or remain in relationships in which s/he is emotionally or physically abused; 32. Is capable of sustaining a meaningful love relationship characterized by genuine intimacy and caring; 58. Has little or no interest in having sexual experiences with another person; 65. Seeks to dominate an important other (e.g., spouse, lover, family member) through violence or intimidation; 77. Tends to be overly needy or dependent; requires excessive reassurance or approval; 94. Has an active and satisfying sex life; 98. Tends to fear s/he will be rejected or abandoned by those who are emotionally significant; 153. Interpersonal relationships tend to be unstable, chaotic, and rapidly changing; 158. Appears afraid of commitment to a long-term love relationship.

Social Cognition and Object Relations Scale

The SCORS (Stein, Hilsenroth, Slavin-Mulford, & Pinsker, 2011; Westen, 1995) contains several scales useful for assessing adaptive and maladaptive functioning in clinical contexts. Clinicians' ratings are based on respondent narratives, either those provided by a test or method (e.g., an "early memories" protocol) or those based on clinical data. The SCORS-G (Stein et al., 2011) taps several areas demonstrated to be useful for assessing interpersonal functioning, including complexity of representations; emotional investment in relationships, understanding of social causality, and experience and management of aggressive impulses.

Structural Analysis of Social Behavior

The Structural Analysis of Social Behavior (SASB; Benjamin, 1996; Benjamin, Rothweiler, & Critchfield, 2006) assesses interpersonal and intrapsychic interactions in terms of three dimensions: (1) focus (other, self, introject); (2) affiliation–hostility (love–hate), and (3) interdependence–independence (enmeshment–differentiation). Self-ratings on the Intrex questionnaires produce scores ranging from 0 (does not apply at all/never) to 100 (applies perfectly/all the time).

Inventory of Interpersonal Problems—Circumplex

The Inventory of Interpersonal Problems—Circumplex (IIP-C; Alden, Wiggins, & Pincus, 1990; Horowitz, Alden, Wiggins, & Pincus, 2000) is a 64-item self-report inventory for identifying problematic aspects of relational functioning. Items are organized in two sets: things the respondents do too much and things that respondents find hard to do. Each item is rated on a scale from 0 (not at all) to 4 (extremely). The IIP-C provides eight subscales (domineering, vindictive, cold, socially avoidant, nonassertive, exploitable, overly nurturant, intrusive). The psychometric adequacy of the tool is well established (see also Gurtman, 1996; Hilsenroth, Menaker, Peters, & Pincus, 2007).

Experiences in Close Relationships

The Experiences in Close Relationships (ECR) inventory (Brennan, Clark, & Shaver, 1998) is a 36-item self-report measure designed to assess patterns of adult attachment separate from idiosyncratic influences of individuals' current circumstances. Respondents use a 7-point, partly anchored, Likert-type scale from 1 (disagree strongly) to 7 (agree strongly). Participants rate how well each statement describes their typical feelings in romantic relationships. A factor analysis by Brennan and colleagues (1998) identified two relatively orthogonal continuous attachment dimensions labeled "anxiety" (18 items) and "avoidance" (18 items). Higher scores on the anxiety and avoidant subscales indicate higher levels of attachment anxiety and attachment avoidance, respectively. The instructions allow for valid responses from respondents not currently in a romantic relationship. Although the ECR appears to be highly reliable and valid, and has been used widely, its length (36 items) may be problematic in some applications. Wei, Russell, Mallinckrodt, and Vogel (2007) accordingly introduced the 12-item ECR—Short Form; they found that, whether this was administered alone or as part of the original 36-item version, it retained psychometric properties similar to those of the original ECR.

6. Capacity for Self-Esteem Regulation and Quality of Internal Experience

The sixth capacity reflects the level of confidence in and regard for an individual's relationship to self, other people, and the larger world. These qualities initially emerge from relationships with primary caregivers: Experiences of well-being, self-respect, vitality, and realistic self-esteem are internalized in infancy when caregivers co-construct affectively attuned interactions, resulting in the infant's sense of self as worthy, and a belief that his or her life is meaningful and valued by others.

Optimal functioning in this capacity involves balance, with self-esteem that is neither unrealistically high nor unrealistically low, and confidence that varies realistically from one situation to another. Good capacity for self-esteem regulation "expresses the feeling that one is 'good enough.' The individual simply feels that he is a person of worth. . . . He does not necessarily consider himself superior to others" (Rosenberg, 1989, p. 31). This capacity includes the degree to which the individual has a sense of internal control, self-efficacy, and ability to organize and implement a course of action. Thus a critical component is a sense of "agency"—the subjective awareness of a capacity to initiate, execute, and control one's actions effectively.

Rating Scale

5. Individuals at this level maintain a stable sense of well-being, confidence, vitality, and realistic self-esteem in varying contexts and even under stress. Their self-confidence is appropriate to internal and external situations. They show a reality-based trust in their capacity to deal with a wide range of challenges, including novel situations.

3. At this level, the individual's sense of well-being, confidence, vitality, and self-esteem is generally adequate, but may be easily disrupted by strong emotions and stressful situations. Expressed self-esteem may be moderated by inner feelings of vulnerability and inadequacy, resulting in diminished confidence in dealing with certain tasks.

1. Individuals at this level have feelings of depletion, emptiness, and incompleteness, and/or excessive self-involvement. Self-esteem is either unrealistically low or irrationally inflated, and may oscillate between these poles. There may be discrepancies between internal experience and external behavior (e.g., overcompensations for underlying feelings of vulnerability) and between implicit and explicit self-esteem; both are associated with diminished adaptation and resilience.

Most Relevant Assessment Tools

Rosenberg Self-Esteem Scale

The Rosenberg Self-Esteem Scale (RSES; Rosenberg, 1989; see also Donnellan, Ackerman, & Breechen, 2016; McKay, Boduszek, & Harvey, 2014), a Likert-type scale of 10 items, is used widely to assess global self-esteem. Respondents indicate the level of agreement with each item on a scale from 1 (strongly disagree) to 4 (strongly agree). Totals thus range from 10 to 40, with higher scores reflecting more positive evaluations of self.

Shedler–Westen Assessment Procedure–200

In the SWAP-200 (Westen & Shedler, 1999a, 1999b), self-esteem regulation is covered by the following items: 4. Has an exaggerated sense of self-importance; 36. Tends to feel helpless, powerless, or at the mercy of forces outside his/her control; 54. Tends to feel s/he is inadequate, inferior, or a failure; 63. Is able to assert him- or herself effectively and appropriately when necessary; and 199. Tends to be passive and unassertive.

Adult Attachment Interview and Adult Attachment Projective

In the AAI (Main, Cassidy, & Hesse, 2002) and the AAP (George, West, & Pettem, 1997; Jones-Mason, Allen, Hamilton, & Weiss, 2015), typically secure IWMs are related to a representation of the attachment figure as loving and protective, and a representation of self as worthy of love and care. Insecure IWMs may entail representations of the other as rejecting, neglecting, or unloving, and the self as unworthy of care. A key feature is how acceptable or unacceptable the subject feels in an attachment relationship. The quality of this aspect of internal experience varies from secure to insecure states of mind.

Scales of Psychological Capacities

The SPC (DeWitt, Hartley, Rosenberg, & Zilberg, 1991; Wallerstein, 1996) constitutes a semistructured, clinician-rated interview designed to measure both personality structure and changes in personality organization resulting from intensive, long-term psychoanalytic psychotherapy. A 7-point Likert-type scale is used to rate 38 aspects of psychological functioning, culminating in a comprehensive description of personality and mental functioning. The "capacities" are low-level constructs, readily inferable from observable behaviors that include reportable mental states and feelings. Particularly relevant to this capacity are the SPC scales of self-coherence, self-esteem, assertion, and trust.

Core Self-Evaluations Scale

The Core Self-Evaluations Scale (CSES; Gardner & Pierce, 2010; Judge, Erez, Bono, & Thoresen, 2003) is a 12-item self-report instrument for measuring "core self-evaluation," understood as a higher-order personality trait that accounts for variance in four specific traits: self-esteem, generalized self-efficacy, locus of control, and neuroticism (Judge, Erez, & Bono, 1998). Judge and colleagues (2003) found that these tend to load on a single factor, suggesting that they are features of a common latent construct. Sample CSES items include "I am confident I get the success I deserve in life" and "When I try, I generally succeed," each of which is assessed by a 5-point Likert-type scale.

7. Capacity for Impulse Control and Regulation

The next capacity reflects an individual's ability to modulate impulses and express needs, motives, and urges in flexible, adaptive, culture-appropriate ways. Deficiencies in this capacity appear as unmodulated impulsivity or rigid overcontrol of impulses, with concomitant affective constriction. "Impulsivity" has been defined variously as presence of affective lability or instability (e.g., difficulties in anger management), tendency to behave rashly when distressed or emotionally overwhelmed, difficulty in premeditation and planning (failure to think about consequences of behavior before acting), lack of perseverance (failure to persist in tasks or obligations), or difficulty tolerating delay of gratification. These features may be accompanied by self-destructive actions or impulsive aggression toward others, often related to an attempt to express, externalize, or control anger, anxiety, and psychic pain that cannot be expressed verbally. Overcontrol of impulses can include rigid restraint of affects, denial of aggressive urges and feelings, inflexibility, or a harsh need to control self and others.

Diverse personality styles and disorders are rooted in part in variations in this capacity, ranging from borderline and histrionic pathology at the undercontrolled/dysregulated end of the spectrum to obsessive traits and obsessive–compulsive personality disorder at the overcontrolled end.

At a neurophysiological level, inhibitory control is a function of the orbital prefrontal region, primarily in the right hemisphere of the brain. The emotion-generating and emotion-processing "right brain" develops within the crucible of the primary caregiver's moment-by-moment affectively attuned interactions with the infant (Schore, 2003). Early encoding of arousal modulation by the baby's caregiver becomes the foundation for the adult's capacity to regulate impulses. Trauma, neglect, or inability to form a stable infant–caregiver bond may lead to difficulties in self-concept, attachment, and development of IWMs, impairing the ability to function in this domain.

Rating Scale

5. At this level, the person can express impulses appropriately, in a manner appropriate to the situation at hand and to the cultural milieu. Impulse control is flexible and effective; urges and affects are expressed in a modulated and adaptive manner, in a way that strengthens interpersonal ties.

3. The person is somewhat able to control and regulate impulses, but may encounter difficulties in certain affect- and conflict-laden situations (e.g., with a romantic partner, a supervisor at work, or family members). Individuals at this level may show a characteristic pattern of overcontrol (rigidity) or undercontrol (dysregulation) across many situations.

1. The person is unable to control or regulate impulses appropriately, leading to profound difficulties in social, sexual, and professional relationships. Impulse control may be so weak that the individual is incapable of modulating anger and other strong affects; alternatively, impulse control may be so rigid that impulses remain almost completely unexpressed.

Most Relevant Assessment Tools

Shedler–Westen Assessment Procedure–200

In the SWAP-200 (Westen & Shedler, 1999a, 1999b), impulse control and regulation are covered by the following items: 109. Tends to engage in self-mutilating behavior (e.g., self-cutting, self-burning); 119. Tends to be inhibited or constricted; has difficulty allowing self to acknowledge or express wishes and impulses; 134. Tends to act impulsively, without regard for consequences; 142. Tends to make repeated suicidal threats or gestures, either as a "cry for help" or as an effort to manipulate others; 166. Tends to oscillate between undercontrol and overcontrol of needs and impulses (i.e., needs and wishes are expressed impulsively and with little regard for consequences, or else disavowed and permitted virtually no expression); 192. Tends to be overly concerned with rules, procedures, order, organization, and schedules.

Barratt Impulsiveness Scale—Version 11

The Barratt Impulsiveness Scale—Version 11 (BIS-11; Patton, Stanford, & Barratt, 1995; Weinstein, Crocker, Ayllon, & Caron, 2015) is a 30-item self-report questionnaire assessing general impulsivity and various subfacets of impulsivity. Ratings are made on a 4-point Likert scale ranging from 1 (rarely/never) to 4 (almost always/ always). Patton and colleagues found evidence for separate inattentive, motor, and nonplanning factors of impulsivity; others have found that responses to the BIS-11 better fit a two-factor solution reflecting cognitive and behavioral aspects of impulsivity (Reise, Moore, Sabb, Brown, & London, 2013).

Urgency, Premeditation, Perseverance, and Sensation-Seeking Impulsive Behavior Scale

The Urgency, Premeditation, Perseverance, and Sensation-Seeking (UPPS) Impulsive Behavior Scale (Whiteside & Lynam, 2001) is a 44-item inventory designed to measure pathways to impulsive behavior. Based on the five-factor model of personality (Costa & McCrae, 1992), it assesses four facets of personality: urgency, (lack of) premeditation, (lack of) perseverance, and sensation seeking. "Urgency" refers to the tendency to experience and act on strong impulses, frequently under conditions of intense affect (e.g., "I have trouble resisting my cravings"). Lack of "premeditation" denotes the inability to think and reflect on the consequences of an act before engaging in it; it is reflected in a tendency to disagree with items such as "I usually make up my mind through careful reasoning." Lack of "perseverance" refers to the inability to remain focused on a task (e.g., "I tend to give up easily"). "Sensation seeking" has two aspects: (1) a tendency to enjoy and pursue exciting activities and (2) an openness to trying new experiences that may be risky (e.g., "I'll try anything once"). The UPPS Impulsive Behavior Scale has excellent internal consistency and convergent validity (Whiteside & Lynam, 2001). Its subscales make unique contributions to different disorders, suggesting that these capture aspects of impulsivity not assessed in other impulsivity measures (Whiteside, Lynam, Miller, & Reynolds, 2005).

Brief Self-Control Scale

The Brief Self-Control Scale (BSCS; Tangney, Baumeister, & Boone, 2004) is a self-report tool measuring dispositional self-regulatory behaviors, using 13 items rated on a 5-point Likert scale, ranging from 1 (not at all like me) to 5 (very much like me). It assesses five domains of self-control: controlling thoughts, controlling emotions, controlling impulses, regulating behavior/performance, and habit breaking. Sample items are "People would say that I have iron self-discipline" and "I often act without thinking through all the alternatives." Preliminary evidence exists for its reliability and construct validity (Lindner, Nagy, & Retelsdorf, 2015; Maloney, Grawitch, & Barber, 2012).

Cognitive Emotion Regulation Questionnaire

The Cognitive Emotion Regulation Questionnaire (CERQ; Garnefski & Kraaij, 2007; Garnefski, Kraaij, & Spinhoven, 2002) is a 36-item multidimensional questionnaire constructed to identify the cognitive coping strategies a person may use after negative experiences. In contrast to questionnaires that do not explicitly differentiate thoughts and actions, this instrument refers exclusively to an individual's thoughts after a negative event. It consists of nine subscales of four items, each referring to what someone might think after experiencing threatening or stressful life events: self-blame, other-blame, rumination, catastrophizing, putting into perspective, positive refocusing, positive reappraisal, acceptance, and planning. Individual cognitive emotion regulation strategies are measured on a 5-point Likert scale ranging from 1 (almost never) to 5 (almost always); subscale scores are obtained by summing the scores on items belonging to a particular subscale (ranging from 4 to 20).

Momentary Impulsivity Scale

The Momentary Impulsivity Scale (MIS; Tomko et al., 2014) is a 9-item self-report measure of momentary impulsivity designed to be used in real-world settings. It is intended to provide information about the variability of impulsivity over time and to permit the examination of potential antecedents (e.g., time of day, presence of stressors, mood, nutrition, amount of sleep, medication) and consequences (e.g., interpersonal conflict, change in mood, health-related concerns) of impulsivity.

8. Capacity for Defensive Functioning

The capacity for defensive functioning highlights the way an individual attempts to manage motives, affects, urges, conflicts, memories, thoughts, and other potentially anxiety-related inner experiences, along with the individual's response to anxiety resulting from external challenge or threat to the self. High functioning in this area means that the person uses defenses effectively, with minimal distortion in reality testing; lower functioning involves the use of less adaptive defenses with greater distortion.

As discussed in Chapter 1, "defenses" are automatic psychological responses to internal or external stressors and emotional conflicts. They protect an individual against excessive anxiety, manage conflictual wishes, affects, ideas, memories, and other inner experiences, and adapt to the external world. They occur partly or wholly out of awareness. People vary in the degree to which they have insight about their defenses, with more psychologically minded people having greater insight. Although individuals tend to use the same defenses across different stressors, defenses may vary as a function of the motives or conflicts active at the time and of the person's mood and anxiety level. Most can be adaptive in at least some situations, but they differ with respect to the overall level of adaptiveness; commonly used defenses form a hierarchy of adaptation. Defenses overlap with conscious coping strategies.

Rating Scale

5. Adaptive defenses predominate, along with some neurotic-level defenses, allowing the individual to experience a broad range of affects, to be aware of salient ideas and motives, and to interact with others and the world in adaptive—even creative—ways. When neurotic-level defenses (e.g., isolation, intellectualization, repression, displacement) are used by a person functioning at this level, they do not significantly impair functioning, as the individual will typically revert to more adaptive defenses (e.g., altruism, affiliation, anticipation, humor, self-assertion, suppression, and sublimation) when anxiety, conflict, and stress diminish.
3. Individuals at this level often experience conflict when under stress, and tend to see problems as external, minimizing or ignoring internal sources. As a result, they may distort reality to some degree, especially when feeling threatened. They may seem defensive and may disavow aspects of internal experience through denial, rationalization, or projection. Or they may mask negative experiences (e.g., powerlessness, disappointment, shame) by devaluing or idealizing self or others, or by maintaining an illusion of omnipotence. They may use some neurotic defenses, but at times of greatest stress may revert to immature defenses (e.g., passive–aggressive responses, acting out).
1. The individual is overwhelmed, for no evident reason, by fears of dissolution or annihilation of the self, physical harm, or death. External reality may be grossly distorted, anxiety uncontained, and adaptation impaired. Common defenses include delusional projection, distortion, psychotic denial, fragmentation, concretization, and apathetic withdrawal. These may either repel others or induce them to take control to help the individual contain affect and manage anxiety. At times of low conflict and minimal stress the individual may use midlevel defenses (e.g., rationalization, denial), ultimately reverting to lower-level defenses when conflict and stress increase.

Most Relevant Assessment Tools

Defense Mechanism Rating Scales

The Defense Mechanism Rating Scales (DMRS; Perry, 1990) is a quantitative, observer-rated method to identify and assess defensive patterns that occur in the clinical session. It defines 30 defenses and describes how to discriminate each from others that are similar (see Chapter 15). Seven defense levels are arranged hierarchically, characterized in ascending order of health (psychotic defenses, action defenses, major image-distorting defenses, disavowal defenses and autistic fantasy, minor image-distorting defenses, other neurotic defenses, hysterical defenses, obsessional defenses, high adaptive defenses). Three levels of scoring (individual defense score, defense-level score, and overall defensive functioning or ODF) are calculated by multiplying the instances of each by its level (1–7) on the overall 7-point hierarchy, summing the results for all defenses, and dividing by the total number of defenses identified. Both convergent and discriminant validity for the overall hierarchy are good (Hilsenroth, Callahan, & Eudell, 2003; Perry & Høglend, 1998), and interrater reliability has ranged from acceptable to very good (Perry & Bond, 2012). Recently, six psychotic defenses have been added (see scale point 1 above), scored at level 0, making the ODF scale 0–7 (Berney, de Roten, Beretta, Kramer, & Despland, 2014).

Defensive Functioning Scale

The Defensive Functioning Scale (DFS; American Psychiatric Association, 1994) was a provisional axis in DSM-IV. It is modeled on the DMRS and includes four additional psychotic defenses. An ODF score can be calculated. It has good reliability and correlates with other measures of symptoms and functioning (Hilsenroth et al., 2003).

Defense Mechanism Rating Scales Q-Sort

The DMRS Q-Sort (Di Giuseppe, Perry, Petraglia, Janzen, & Lingiardi, 2014) is based on DMRS definitions, functions, and discriminations (see above). It includes 150 low-inference statements, five for each defense mechanism, that describe personal mental states, relational dynamics, verbal and nonverbal expressions, behaviors and coping skills, and distorting perceptions. Ratings using a forced distribution in the 150 items are sorted into seven ordinal columns, corresponding to the level of descriptiveness of the statement, and evaluated in terms of intensity or frequency (from 1, not used at all, to 7, rigidly or always used). It provides three levels of quantitative scores (proportional score for each defense, proportion of defensive functioning for each level, and ODF score) and a qualitative profile of a person's most relevant defensive manifestation (DPN).

Vaillant Q-Sort

The Vaillant Q-Sort (Roston, Lee, & Vaillant, 1992) is composed of 51 items involving 15 defenses, divided into three levels of maturity. Some statements are derived from the Haan Q-sort instrument (Haan, 1977), while others describe defenses introduced by Vaillant. Psychotic defenses are not included. Following a fixed distribution, each item is assigned to one of the nine ordinal columns according to its descriptiveness. Items in the first four columns are considered the most representative of the individual's defensive functioning. This tool provides scores for each defense for the three levels of defensive functioning and a global score for defense maturity.

Defense-Q

The Defense-Q (Davidson, Johnson, & Woody, 1995) is an observer-rated Q-sort designed to assess the relative use of 25 defense mechanisms and overall ego strength. Each defense is sorted into seven piles from least to most characteristic. The number of defenses in each category is predetermined. There is a three-item scale to assess ego strength, scored with a 7-point Likert scale that provides a single index of this function. Internal consistency of these items ranges from .71 to .89 (Davidson & MacGregor, 1996). The authors found that the averaged coder reliability across all participants for each defense individually, the averaged coder reliability across all defenses for each participant, and reliability across all participants and all defenses for each coder were good.

Defense Style Questionnaire

The Defense Style Questionnaire (DSQ; Bond, Gardner, Christian, & Sigal, 1983) is a widely used self-report questionnaire for assessing defenses (see Bond, 2004) that evaluates conscious derivatives of defense in everyday life. It was developed on the assumption that defenses tend to group into clusters, or "defense styles." The original factor-analytical study of the DSQ (Bond et al., 1983) identified four styles: maladaptive, image-distorting, self-sacrificing, and adaptive. Successive studies only partially confirmed this factor structure (San Martini, Roma, Sarti, Lingiardi, & Bond, 2004; Thygesen, Drapeau, Trijsburg, Lecours, & de Roten, 2008), often finding three styles: maladaptive, neurotic, and mature. Reliability varies significantly among different versions of the instrument.

Response Evaluation Measure–71

The Response Evaluation Measure–71 (REM-71; Steiner, Araujo, & Koopman, 2001) is a 71-item, self-administered instrument for assessing defenses in adults and adolescents, based on a model of defenses considered as unconscious, unplanned reactions at the interface between innate temperament traits and learned coping strategies. It was developed to overcome the psychometric limitations of existing measures such as the DSQ, excluding defenses close to DSM definitions of disorders and psychiatric syndromes (e.g., consumption of substances) and those related to coping strategies (e.g., anticipation). Items were worded to avoid ambiguous meanings and overtly pathological wording. Each defense is represented by a minimum of three and a maximum of four items. The REM-71 was administered to 1,875 nonclinical participants drawn from two suburban high schools and from a public waiting area of a local airport (1,038 female subjects; mean age = 21.0 years, *SD* = 11.9, range = 13–89), who were also assessed with a simple screening measure covering demographic variables and satisfaction with life. Two factors emerged, paralleling Vaillant's theoretical model of mature and immature defenses; the latter were significantly associated with psychological distress (Prunas, Preti, Huemer, Shaw, & Steiner, 2014). Internal consistency of the questionnaire items was good.

Shedler–Westen Assessment Procedure–200

In the SWAP-200 (Westen & Shedler, 1999a, 1999b), defensive functioning is covered by the following items: 45. Tends to idealize certain others in unrealistic ways; sees them as "all good," to the exclusion of commonplace human defects; 76. Manages to elicit in others feelings similar to those he or she is experiencing (e.g., when angry, acts in such a way as to provoke anger in others; when anxious, acts in such a way as to induce anxiety in others); 78. Tends to express aggression in passive and indirect ways (e.g., may make mistakes, procrastinate, forget, become sulky, etc.); 79. Tends to see certain others as "all bad," and loses the capacity to perceive any positive qualities the person may have; 100. Tends to think in abstract and intellectualized terms, even in matters of personal import; 116. Tends to see his/her own unacceptable feelings or impulses in other people instead of in him- or herself; 152. Tends to repress or "forget" distressing events, or to distort memories of distressing events beyond recognition; 154. Tends to elicit extreme reactions or stir up strong feelings in others; 165. Tends to distort unacceptable wishes or feelings by transforming them into their opposite (may express excessive concern or affection while showing signs of unacknowledged hostility; disgust about sexual matters while showing signs of interest or excitement).

Adult Attachment Interview

The AAI (George, Kaplan, & Main, 1985) coding system (Main, Goldwyn, & Hesse, 2002) includes some subscales that evaluate defensive processes (related to the concept of "defensive exclusion"; Bowlby, 1980) typical of "dismissing" individuals and aimed at keeping actual childhood attachment experiences of rejection or neglect out of conscious awareness. "Idealization of parent" evaluates the discrepancy between interviewees' probable experience with attachment figures and their positive generalized or "semantic" descriptions; "insistence on lack of recall" focuses on subjects' direct references to their own inability to remember childhood experience; "dismissing derogation" denotes the cool, disdainful devaluation of attachment relationships/experiences and their importance. Other subscales give information about mechanisms typical of "preoccupied" individuals. These mechanisms are often called "cognitive disconnection" (George & West, 2012), and they reflect the failure of defenses to cope with cognitions and affects about childhood attachment difficulties, making the interviewee overwhelmed or compulsively focused on past events or past relationships. "Involving/preoccupying anger" evaluates a particular form of speech (e.g., run-on/grammatically entangled sentences, incongruous extensive discussion of apparently unimportant recent parental offenses) that can be used when anger toward a particular attachment figure is implied or expressed; "passivity or vagueness of discourse" refers to a deep absorption into childhood memory revealed by an inability to find words, understand meaning, or focus on a topic, and statements that may include vague expressions, nonsense words, or childish language. Finally, "unresolved loss" and "unresolved abuse" assess disorganization and/or disorientation in thinking or discourse that can result in recourse to primitive defensive processes (e.g., freezing, absorption, dissociation).

9. Capacity for Adaptation, Resiliency, and Strength

The capacity for adaptation, resiliency, and strength reflects the ability to adjust to unexpected events and changing circumstances, along with the ability to cope effectively and creatively when confronted with uncertainty, loss, stress, and challenge. "Adaptation" reflects the ability to cope with changing and uncertain circumstances, whereas "resiliency" denotes the ability to thrive when faced with adverse (even traumatic) events. "Strength," a less formal term, is the capacity for adaptation and resiliency considered together.

Clinicians rating this capacity should note that a person's ability to adapt does not reflect uncritical or conformist adaptation to social expectations, but may involve unusual and creative ways of dealing with challenges. This capacity may also include individual domain-specific strengths, such as empathy, sensitivity to others' needs and feelings, ability to recognize alternative viewpoints, and ability to be appropriately assertive. An individual with optimal adaptation, resiliency, and strength can transcend obstacles and turn setbacks into opportunities for growth and positive change.

The ability to adapt to a complex social-emotional environment and to accommodate one's dynamically shifting internal states is based in part on unconscious affective and conscious cognitive processes. It includes the capacity to manage a wide range of emotional experiences and situations that are novel, inherently ambiguous, and fluid in nature.

Rating Scale

5. High levels of resiliency and adaptation imply good capacity to transition among positive and negative affect states, even in the face of considerable stress. Individuals functioning at this level can adapt to complex social-emotional contexts and novel situations, and can manage shifting emotional states without decreased clarity of thought or compromised interpersonal functioning.
3. An individual at this level can shift between positive and negative affect states, as long as these are mild to moderate; when affect is intense, the person functions less well. The individual is somewhat able to adapt to complex social-emotional contexts and novel situations, but may experience some impairment in thought processes and interpersonal functioning when challenged.
1. Cognitively mediated defenses and regulatory mechanisms are severely lacking, leading to reliance on primitive defenses like splitting and projective identification, along with fragmentary affect states and periods of dissociation. Individuals functioning at this level are unable to manage complex social-emotional situations and experience uncontrolled, vacillating emotional states that significantly impair both thought processes and interpersonal functioning.

Most Relevant Assessment Tools

Shedler–Westen Assessment Procedure–200

In the SWAP-200 (Westen & Shedler, 1999a, 1999b), adaptation, resiliency, and strength are covered by the following items: 2. Is able to use his/her talents, abilities, and energy effectively and productively; 19. Enjoys challenges; takes pleasure in accomplishing things; 32. Is capable of sustaining a meaningful love relationship characterized by genuine intimacy and caring; 37. Finds meaning in belonging and contributing to a larger community (e.g., organization, church, neighborhood); 59. Is empathic; is sensitive and responsive to other people's needs and feelings; 63. Is able to assert him- or herself effectively and appropriately when necessary; 82. Is capable of hearing information that is emotionally threatening (i.e., that challenges cherished beliefs, perceptions, and self-perceptions) and can use and benefit from it; 89. Appears to have come to terms with painful experiences from the past; has found meaning in, and grown from such experiences; 101. Generally finds contentment and happiness in life's activities; 111. Has the capacity to recognize alternative viewpoints, even in matters that stir up strong feelings; 179. Tends to be energetic and outgoing; 183. Is psychologically insightful; is able to understand self and others in subtle and sophisticated ways; 196. Is able to find meaning and satisfaction in the pursuit of long-term goals and ambitions; 200. Is able to form close and lasting friendships characterized by mutual support and sharing of experiences.

Health–Sickness Rating Scale

The Health–Sickness Rating Scale (HSRS; Luborsky, 1962) is widely used to evaluate overall mental health. The scale consists of a continuum; a score of 100 represents an ideal state of complete functional integration, resilience in the face of stress, and happiness and social effectiveness, whereas a score of 0 denotes virtually no adaptation or independent functioning (i.e., if unattended, the patient would die; Luborsky, 1975). Reliability of the HSRS is well established (Luborsky, 1962, 1975).

Ways of Coping Questionnaire

The Ways of Coping Questionnaire (WCQ; Folkman & Lazarus, 1988) is probably the instrument most frequently used to assess basic coping strategies. It is a 50-item self-report tool based on Folkman and Lazarus's (1988) view that coping has two major functions: "the regulation of distressing emotions (emotion-focused coping)" and "doing something to change for the better the problem causing the distress (problem-focused coping)" (p. 19). The WCQ uses a 4-point Likert scale from 0 to 3. Factor analysis has supported the construction of eight scales, each corresponding to a specific coping dimension: (a) confrontive coping, (b) distancing, (c) self-controlling, (d) seeking social support, (e) accepting responsibility, (f) escape–avoidance, (g) planful problem solving, and (h) positive reappraisal.

COPE Inventory

The COPE Inventory (Carver, Scheier, & Weintraub, 1989) is a 60-item self-report measure to assess coping strategies. To assess a broader range of coping styles that Lazarus and Folkman considered, they developed a tool with 15 scales and four dimensions. One factor corresponded closely to problem-focused coping; a second was defined mainly by emotion-focused strategies (restraint, originally considered a problem-focused strategy, also loaded on this factor); a third involved seeking social support for advice or to express emotions, and a fourth concerned attempts to avoid dealing with the problem or the associated emotions. Participants indicate on a 4-point scale how frequently they use each coping strategy from "usually do not do this at all" to "usually do this a lot."

Ego Resiliency Scale–89

The Ego Resiliency Scale–89 (ER89; Block & Kremen, 1996) is a 14-item self-report scale that measures ego resiliency via subjective self-ratings on a 4-point Likert scale. In Block and Block's (1980) personality model, the construct of "ego resiliency" refers to an individual's capacity for flexible and resourceful adaptation to external and internal stressors. More recently, Block and Kremen (1996) identified ego resiliency as "trait resilience"—that is, the individual ability to self-regulate dynamically and appropriately, allowing prompt adaptation to changing circumstances. Letzring, Block, and Funder (2005) supported the unidimensionality, internal consistency, and construct validity of the scale. A revised version of this scale, the ER89-R (Alessandri, Vecchione, Caprara, & Letzring, 2012; Vecchione, Alessandri, Barbaranelli, & Gerbino, 2010) is a 10-item inventory in which participants indicate the degree to which they agree with each statement on a scale ranging from 1 (does not apply at all) to 7 (applies very strongly).

Connor–Davidson Resilience Scale

The Connor–Davidson Resilience Scale (CD-RISC; Connor & Davidson, 2003) is a self-report, 25-item instrument that measures resilience, conceptualized as the capacity to change and cope with adversity. Responses use a 5-point Likert scale, with higher scores indicating greater resilience. The CD-RISC has been used with clinical and non-clinical populations as a measure of psychological resources in moderating childhood maltreatment and adult psychiatric symptoms (Campbell-Sills, Cohan, & Stein, 2006) and as an indicator of successful resilience training (Davidson et al., 2005).

Adult Attachment Interview and Adult Attachment Projective

In the AAI (George, Kaplan, & Main, 1984) and the AAP (George, West, & Pettem, 1997), the assessment of free/autonomous versus insecure "state of mind" with respect to attachment can inform about a person's ability to use interpersonal support (in more or less adaptive ways) when faced with adverse or traumatic events, to handle and find meaning in such experiences (e.g., when an individual is able to give a coherent narrative of difficult attachment experiences), and to use solitude as a spur to thinking sincerely about self and the others ("internalized secure base"; George & West, 2012).

Most stimuli ask the interviewee to tell a story of an imagined stressful situation, followed by questions that seek memories of the person's attachment behavior during childhood adversity: "When you were upset as a child, what would you do?"; "When you were upset emotionally when you were little, what would you do? Can you think of a specific time that happened?"; "Can you remember what would happen when you were hurt, physically? Again, do any specific incidents (or, do any other incidents) come to mind?"; "What is the first time you remember being separated from your parents? How did you respond?"; "Did you ever feel rejected as a young child? Of course, looking back on it now, you may realize it wasn't really rejection, but what I'm trying to ask about here is whether you remember ever having felt rejected in childhood. How old were you when you first felt this way, and what did you do? Were you ever frightened or worried as a child?"

10. Self-Observing Capacities (Psychological Mindedness)

The term "self-observing capacities," or "psychological mindedness," refers to individuals' ability and proclivity to observe their own internal life mindfully and realistically; to see relationships among disparate aspects of their own thoughts, feelings, and behaviors; and to infer accurately the inner needs, motives, and experiences of others. It involves the ability to discern patterns among these concepts to make sense of internal experience and the ability to use this information effectively in interpersonal interactions.

Psychological mindedness is related to self-consciousness and self-awareness, and reflects the degree to which individuals are motivated to introspect and to seek insight—that is, the degree to which they take an inherent interest in understanding themselves more deeply. The self-observing capacities can play a key role in organizing one's emotional experiences and evaluating internal affective shifts by reflecting on them coherently. They enables an individual to pause and reflect even when an experience is intense or uncomfortable. Self-observing capacities are related to theory of mind, mentalizing ability, and intersubjectivity; low levels of psychological mindedness are related to alexithymia.

"Alexithymia" encompasses a cluster of characteristics that are the obverse of several key features of psychological mindedness: lack of emotional awareness, paucity of inner experiences, minimal interest in dreams, concrete thinking, and externalized style of living. It is a narrower construct, predominantly focused on the emotional domain, whereas psychological mindedness encompasses cognitive, emotional, and behavioral dimensions of human experience.

Rating Scale

5. Individuals at this level are highly motivated to observe and understand themselves in relation to others and to reflect on the full range of their own and others' experiences and feelings (including subtle variations in feelings). They understand psychological constructs. In this range, a person can reflect in present and past, with a long-term view of self, values, and goals, and can appreciate complex patterns and relationships among feelings, thoughts, and behaviors across the full range of age-expected experiences in the context of new challenges.
3. At this level, individuals seem somewhat motivated and able to recognize and reflect on meanings that underlie overt words and actions, have some degree of insight into their own and others' motives and intentions, and can see links between past and present. Under stress, capacity for self-awareness, self-reflection, and self-examination may fluctuate or deteriorate, as may awareness of others' subjective experience.
1. These individuals seem poorly motivated or unable to reflect on feelings, thoughts, and actions, both present and past. They may not conceptualize psychological constructs. Self-awareness is lacking and typically consists of polarized affect states or simple emotional reactions without an appreciation of subtle variations in feelings. Awareness of others' subjectivity is deficient, and there is a tendency toward fragmentation. The person is unable to reflect on specific emotional experiences or affect states even when called upon to do so, and in the face of intense affect may use primitive defenses, act out impulsively, or dissociate.

Most Relevant Assessment Tools

Psychological Mindedness Scale

The Psychological Mindedness Scale (PMS; Conte et al., 1990; Shill & Lumley, 2002) is a self-administered, 45-item questionnaire developed to assess suitability for psychodynamic psychotherapy, characterized by versatility, simple scoring, promising psychometric properties, and attention to the capacity for self-observation and insight (Conte & Ratto, 1997). In a preliminary communication, Conte and colleagues (1990) reported good internal reliability and specific predictive validity for psychotherapy outcome with psychiatric patients. An examination of construct validity revealed a five-factor structure accounting for 38% of total variance (Conte, Ratto, & Karasu, 1996). The factors were (a) willingness to try to understand self and others; (b) openness to new ideas and capacity to change; (c) access to feelings; (d) belief in the benefits of discussing one's problems; and (e) interest in the meaning and motivation of own and others' behavior.

Balanced Index of Psychological Mindedness

The Balanced Index of Psychological Mindedness (BIPM; Nyklíček & Denollet, 2009) is a self-report, 14-item questionnaire using a 5-point Likert scale from "strongly disagree" (1) to "strongly agree" (5). Reflecting Hall's (1992) model, it has two subscales of seven items each: (a) interest in one's internal psychological phenomena and (b) insight into these phenomena. Internal consistency and test–retest reliability are adequate (Giromini, Brusadelli, Di Noto, Grasso, & Lang, 2015); high correlations with related constructs such as self-consciousness, emotional intelligence, and alexithymia (negative) (Nyklíček, Poot, & van Opstal, 2010) established convergent and discriminant validity.

Psychological Mindedness Assessment Procedure

The Psychological Mindedness Assessment Procedure (PMAP; McCallum & Piper, 1990) is a video-recorded interview measure of psychological mindedness consisting of two simulated patient–therapist interactions. In the first scenario, a recently divorced woman tells her therapist about an unexpected encounter with her ex-husband. In the second, the patient recounts starting an argument with her boyfriend. Examinees are asked for their understanding of the patient's problem. Responses are scored according to psychodynamic ideas of psychological mindedness: Higher scorers can identify an internal experience of the patient (criterion for the lowest levels of the scale), appreciate the conflicted nature of the patient's feelings (criterion for the midpoint), and identify the patient's efforts to defend herself against these feelings (criterion for the highest levels).

Shedler–Westen Assessment Procedure–200

In the SWAP-200 (Westen & Shedler, 1999a, 1999b), self-observing capacities are covered by the following items: 25. Has difficulty acknowledging or expressing anger; 82. Is capable of hearing information that is emotionally threatening (i.e., that challenges cherished beliefs, perceptions, and self-perceptions) and can use and benefit from it; 100. Tends to think in abstract and intellectualized terms even in matters of personal import; 119. Tends to be inhibited or constricted; has difficulty allowing self to acknowledge or express wishes and impulses; 148. Has little psychological insight into own motives, behavior; is unable to consider alternate interpretations of his/her experiences; 183. Is psychologically insightful; is able to understand self and others in subtle and sophisticated ways.

Toronto Alexithymia Scale–20

The Toronto Alexithymia Scale–20 (TAS-20; Bagby, Parker, & Taylor, 1994a; Bagby, Taylor, & Parker, 1994b) is a 20-item self-report measure using a Likert scale from 1 (strongly disagree) to 5 (strongly agree). Higher scores indicate higher levels of alexithymia. The TAS-20 has three subscales that assess (1) difficulty identifying feelings and distinguishing them from the bodily sensations that accompany states of emotional arousal (seven items); (2) difficulty describing feelings to others (five items); and (3) externally oriented style of thinking (eight items). The validity and reliability of the TAS-20 among adults have been largely supported (Bagby et al., 1994b).

Toronto Structured Interview for Alexithymia

The Toronto Structured Interview for Alexithymia (TSIA; Bagby, Taylor, Dickens, & Parker, 2005; Keefer, Taylor, Parker, Inslegers, & Bagby, 2015) is a 24-question interview addressing four areas: (1) difficulty identifying feelings and distinguishing between feelings and the bodily sensations of emotional arousal; (2) difficulty describing feelings to others; (3) restricted imaginal processes (paucity of fantasies); and (4) stimulus-bound, externally oriented cognitive style. Each question is scored on a Likert scale ranging from 0 to 2. Higher total scores indicate greater alexithymia.

Psychological Mindedness Scale of the California Psychological Inventory

The Psychological Mindedness (PM) scale of the California Psychological Inventory (CPI; Gough, 1975) is a widely used, 434-item self-report measure of psychological characteristics relevant to daily life, especially social life (Gough & Bradley, 1992). It is commonly scored by using 20 "folk scales" and three "vector scales." The folk scales assess qualities (e.g., social presence and flexibility) relevant to social functioning. Each vector scale assesses a theme (e.g., norm-favoring vs. norm-doubting) common to several folk scales. Individuals with high scores on psychological mindedness show interest in why people do what they do; they are good judges of how people feel and think. Low scorers are less abstract and tend to focus on *what* people do rather than *why* they do it.

11. Capacity to Construct and Use Internal Standards and Ideals

The next capacity indexes one's personal sense of morality, including moral beliefs and associated emotions and motives. The capacity to formulate internal values and ideals reflects a consideration of self in the context of one's culture and the ability to make mindful decisions based on a set of coherent, internally consistent underlying moral principles. This capacity is related theoretically to the psychoanalytic construct of the "superego," the mental agency concerned with self-approval and disapproval based on approximating one's ego ideal.

Emotional interactions with caregivers influence the internalization of ideals, and consequently the development of moral competencies, ethical actions, and empathy. Schore (2003) posits that internal standards develop from early shame experiences: When a shame experience becomes humiliation because of a caregiver's lack of attunement or inability to repair disruptions, secure attachment is compromised, along with the construction of flexible, integrated, and realistic internal standards. Neuroscientific studies, including research on mirror neurons, support the importance of early relational experiences: The neural network underlying moral decisions appears to overlap with the network representing others' intentions (i.e., theory of mind; see also Lagattuta & Weller, 2014) and the network representing others' vicariously experienced emotional states (i.e., empathy).

Internal standards and ideals internalized early in life through interactions with caregivers are elaborated and refined in later interactions with peers and models (e.g., teachers, mentors), and by immersion in the values, norms, and expectations of one's culture. In rating this capacity, clinicians should consider the flexibility with which individuals interpret their own and others' behaviors. High functioning requires that an individual's moral reasoning be based not only on a set of cohesive core principles, but also on awareness of the impact of one's decisions on others.

Rating Scale

5. The individual's internal standards seem flexible and integrated with a realistic sense of the person's capacities, values, ideals, and social contexts. Internal standards support meaningful striving and feelings of authenticity and self-esteem. Feelings of guilt are balanced with a measure of self-compassion, and so are used as signals for reappraising one's behavior. Others are viewed with a balance of compassion, empathy, and objective criticism.
3. Internal standards and ideals are somewhat rigid and inflexible, or variable and inconsistent across contexts, driven more by the person's needs, desires, and feelings than by a coherent set of moral guidelines. They are not fully integrated with a realistic sense of one's capacities, values, and ideals or with social contexts. The individual's self-esteem oscillates, and feelings of guilt are experienced more as paralyzing self-criticism than as signals for reappraising behavior.
1. Internal standards and ideals seem either absent or rigid and inflexible, based on harsh, punitive expectations. The person lacks a realistic sense of his or her capacities, values, and ideals, and is unintegrated with the social context and cultural milieu. The moral sense seems to have either an insignificant or a tyrannical role in organizing self-experience and in how the person interprets behavior of self and others. Feelings of guilt, if present at all, are not balanced with compassion and objective criticism; self and others are often viewed as "totally bad" or "totally good."

Most Relevant Assessment Tools

Prosocial Reasoning Objective Measure

The Prosocial Reasoning Objective Measure (PROM; Carlo, Eisenberg, & Knight, 1992) is a paper-and-pencil structured interview evaluating levels of prosocial moral reasoning (hedonistic, needs-oriented, approval-oriented, stereotyped, or internalized). Seven stories of moral dilemmas show conflicts among needs, wills, and desires of protagonists. After reading each, the examinee states how the protagonist should act. Six motives are introduced for each decision; subjects assess the importance of each motive. Test–retest reliability ranged from .70 to .79, while Cronbach's alpha ranged from .56 to .78. The PROM has been translated into, and validated in, several languages.

Psychopathy Checklist—Revised

The Psychopathy Checklist—Revised (PCL-R; Hare, 2003) is a 20-item, clinician-rated measure of psychopathy in research, clinical, and forensic settings. Based on a semistructured interview and an extensive review of life records, items are scored on a 3-point scale (0 = not present, 1 = somewhat present, and 2 = definitely present). According to the four-factor model of psychopathy (Hare & Neumann, 2008), 18 of the 20 items can be seen as representing four underlying constructs or first-order factors: deceitful and manipulative (interpersonal factor); emotional detachment (affective factor); reckless, impulsive, and irresponsible (lifestyle factor); and propensity to violate social norms (antisocial factor). The interpersonal and affective components, on the one hand, and the lifestyle and antisocial components, on the other, load on two second-level factors (Hare & Neumann, 2008). The PCL-R has shown good reliability and validity, and is the most widely used instrument for the assessment of psychopathic personality traits (Hare, 1999; Patrick, 2006).

Moral Foundations Questionnaire

The Moral Foundations Questionnaire (MFQ; Graham et al., 2011) is a 30-item self-report measure of degree to which individuals endorse each of five intuitive systems posited by moral foundations theory: harm/care, fairness/reciprocity, ingroup/loyalty, authority/respect, and purity/sanctity (see also Shweder, Much, Mahapatra, & Park, 1997). It has two 15-item subscales: The first measures the relevance ascribed to each foundation on a 7-point response scale (anchored by 1 = not at all relevant and 7 = extremely relevant); a sample item is "whether or not some people were treated differently than others." The second is made up of concrete moral judgment items; participants indicate on a 7-point scale whether they agree or disagree with a range of moral statements; a sample item is "Chastity is an important and valuable virtue."

Levenson's Self-Report Psychopathy Scale

Levenson's Self-Report Psychopathy Scale (LSRP; Levenson, Kiehl, & Fitzpatrick, 1995) is a 26-item self-report instrument widely used for assessing psychopathic traits in nonforensic and forensic populations. It consists of two positively correlated scales: primary psychopathy (16 items), and secondary psychopathy (10 items). Agreement with each item is assessed via a Likert-type scale from 1 (strongly disagree) to 5 (strongly agree). Research indicates adequate reliability for the two subscales (Levenson et al., 1995), and there is emerging evidence for the tool's factor structure and convergent and discriminant validity (Brinkley, Diamond, Magaletta, & Heigel, 2008; Lynam, Whiteside, & Jones, 1999; Salekin, Chen, Sellbom, Lester, & MacDougall, 2014).

Shedler–Westen Assessment Procedure–200

In the SWAP-200 (Westen & Shedler, 1999a, 1999b), internal standards and ideals are covered by the following items: 3. Takes advantage of others; is out for number one; has minimal investment in moral values; 15. Lacks a stable image of who s/he is or would like to become (e.g., attitudes, values, goals, or feelings about self may be unstable and changing); 20. Tends to be deceitful; tends to lie or mislead; 31. Tends to show reckless disregard for the rights, property, or safety of others; 39. Appears to gain pleasure or satisfaction by being sadistic or aggressive toward others (whether consciously or unconsciously); 57. Tends to feel guilty; 91. Tends to be self-critical; sets unrealistically high standards for self and is intolerant of own human defects; 113. Appears to experience no remorse for harm or injury caused to others; 120. Has moral and ethical standards and strives to live up to them; 114. Tends to be critical of others; 163. Appears to want to "punish" self; creates situations that lead to unhappiness, or actively avoids opportunities for pleasure and gratification; 164. Tends to be self-righteous or moralistic.

12. Capacity for Meaning and Purpose

The final capacity reflects the ability to construct a narrative that gives cohesion and meaning to personal choices. It includes a feeling of individuation, a concern for succeeding generations, a capacity for psychological growth, and a spirituality (not necessarily traditional religiosity) that imbues one's life with direction and purpose. It involves the ability to think beyond immediate concerns and grasp the broader implications of one's attitudes, beliefs, values, and behaviors.

Individuals functioning at a high level of this capacity show a strong sense of direction and purpose; a coherent personal philosophy that guides decisions; comfort with personal choices, including those that do not produce expected outcomes; acceptance of alternative viewpoints, even when these conflict with their own; a well-developed capacity for mentalization, reflected in sensitivity to others' attitudes, values, thoughts, and feelings; the ability to transcend immediate concerns and grasp "the big picture"; and a childlike curiosity, wonder, and freshness of perspective.

Rating Scale

5. Individuals at this level show a clear, unwavering sense of purpose and meaning, along with an intrinsic sense of agency and the ability to look outside the self and transcend immediate situational concerns. Subjectivity and intersubjectivity are highly valued. New situations and relationships are approached with an open, fresh perspective.

3. At this level, individuals show some sense of purpose and meaning, along with periods of uncertainty and doubt. Looking outside the self requires effort. There is some sense of connectedness with other people and the world. The broader implications of attitudes and beliefs are grasped, and alternative perspectives are accepted in certain conflict-free domains.

1. Individuals at this level show lack of direction, aimlessness, and little or no sense of purpose. When asked, they are unable to articulate a cohesive personal philosophy or set of life goals. Subjectivity and intersubjectivity have little or no importance. Whether or not they are aware of their lack of direction, they experience pervasive isolation, meaninglessness, alienation, and anomie.

Most Relevant Assessment Tools

Dispositional Flow Scale–2

The Dispositional Flow Scale–2 (DFS-2; Jackson & Ecklund, 2002) is a 36-item, self-administered questionnaire designed to tap centeredness, living in the moment, and "flow" (the feeling of being in harmony with self and surroundings, an intrinsically rewarding state of immersion and enjoyment in an activity requiring deep concentration). Grounded in Csikszentmihalyi's (1990) nine-dimensional concept of flow, the scales measure challenges–skills balance, action–awareness merging, clear goals, unambiguous feedback, concentration on task, sense of control, loss of self-consciousness, time transformation, and autotelic experience (sense of purpose and curiosity). Summing these obtains a global score for dispositional flow. Evidence supporting the construct validity of the DFS-2 is compelling (see Johnson, Kaiser, Skarin, & Ross, 2014).

Personal Orientation Inventory

The Personal Orientation Inventory (POI; Shostrom & Knapp, 1966), a forced-choice self-report test, assesses qualities of Maslow's self-actualization. Twelve subscale scores tap a range of traits, including inner-directedness, existentiality, spontaneity, self-acceptance, and capacity for intimacy. Evidence of construct validity is strong; POI scores predict knowledgeable informants' ratings of an individual's degree of self-actualization, capacity to benefit from psychotherapy, and success in Peace Corps training (see Burwick & Knapp, 1991; Fogarty, 1994).

Qualitative and Structural Dimensions of Self-Descriptions

Qualitative and Structural Dimensions of Self-Desriptions (QSDSD; Blatt, Bers, & Schaffer, 1993) is a scoring system using open-ended descriptions of the self. It enables clinicians to generate ratings of self-attributions and complexity of self-representation and to track changes in these areas over time (see Bers, Blatt, Sayward, & Johnston, 1993; Blatt, Auerbach, & Levy, 1997). It can also be used as a prompt for discussing the patient's goals, aspirations, and feelings about past, present, and future events.

Relational Humility Scale

The Relational Humility Scale (RHS; Davis et al., 2011) is a 16-item questionnaire yielding three subscale scores: global humility, accurate view of self, and superiority (inversely related to the other two subscales). Scores predict the individual's behavior in several areas related to meaning and purpose, including empathy, forgiveness, self-direction (agency), warmth, and conscientiousness. The RHS has good internal consistency, test–retest reliability, and convergence with scores on measures of related constructs.

Temperament and Character Inventory—Revised

The Temperament and Character Inventory—Revised (TCI-R; Cloninger, 1999) includes 240 items tapping four temperament dimensions (novelty seeking, harm avoidance, reward dependence, persistence) and three character domains (self-directedness, cooperativeness, self-transcendence). Subscales relevant to meaning and purpose include self-acceptance, enlightened second nature, compassion, pure-hearted conscience, transpersonal identification, and spiritual acceptance.

Values in Action

The Values in Action (VIA) measure (Peterson & Seligman, 2004) includes 24 subscales, a number of which tap traits germane to a sense of meaning and purpose (e.g., capacity for love, hope/optimism, integrity/authenticity, perspective/wisdom,

TABLE 2.1. Summary of Basic Mental Functioning: M Axis

To obtain a rating of a patient's overall mental functioning, a clinician should add up the 1–5 point ratings assigned to each capacity (Table 2.1a), yielding a single numerical index of overall functioning ranging from 12 to 60. This total permits provisionally assigning a patient to one of the categories outlined in Table 2.1b, which provides brief qualitative descriptions of seven levels of mental functioning. Schematically, *healthy* mental functioning corresponds to M1; *neurotic* to M2 and M3; *borderline* to M4, M5, and M6 (from high to low, from moderate impairments to significant defects); and *psychotic* to M7.

TABLE 2.1a. M-Axis Functioning: Total Score

M-Axis capacities	Rating scale				
1. Capacity for regulation, attention, and learning	5	4	3	2	1
2. Capacity for affective range, communication, and understanding	5	4	3	2	1
3. Capacity for mentalization and reflective functioning	5	4	3	2	1
4. Capacity for differentiation and integration (identity)	5	4	3	2	1
5. Capacity for relationships and intimacy	5	4	3	2	1
6. Capacity for self-esteem regulation and quality of internal experience	5	4	3	2	1
7. Capacity for impulse control and regulation	5	4	3	2	1
8. Capacity for defensive functioning	5	4	3	2	1
9. Capacity for adaptation, resiliency, and strength	5	4	3	2	1
10. Self-observing capacities (psychological mindedness)	5	4	3	2	1
11. Capacity to construct and use internal standards and ideals	5	4	3	2	1
12. Capacity for meaning and purpose	5	4	3	2	1
	Total score = ____				

TABLE 2.1b. Levels of Mental Functioning

Level; range	Heading	Description
		Healthy
M1; 54–60	Healthy/optimal mental functioning	Optimal or very good functioning in all or most mental capacities, with modest, expectable variations in flexibility and adaptation across life contexts.
		Neurotic
M2; 47–53	Good/appropriate mental functioning with some areas of difficulty	Appropriate level of mental functioning, with some specific areas of difficulty (e.g., in three or four mental capacities). These difficulties can reflect conflicts or challenges related to specific life situations or events.
M3; 40–46	Mild impairments in mental functioning	Mild constrictions and areas of inflexibility in some domains of mental functioning, implying rigidities and impairments in areas such as self-esteem regulation, impulse and affect regulation, defensive functioning, and self-observing capacity.

(continued)

TABLE 2.1b. *(continued)*

Level; range	Heading	Description
		Borderline
M4; 33–39	Moderate impairments in mental functioning	Moderate constrictions and areas of inflexibility in most or almost all domains of mental functioning, affecting quality and stability of relationships, sense of identity, and range of affects tolerated. Functioning begins to reflect the significantly impaired adaptations that are described as "borderline-level" in many psychodynamic writings, and that are found, in increasing severity, in the next two levels.
M5; 26–32	Major impairments in mental functioning	Major constrictions and alterations in almost all domains of mental functioning (e.g., tendencies toward fragmentation and difficulties in self–object differentiation), along with limitation of experience of feelings and/or thoughts in major life areas (i.e., love, work, play).
M6; 19–25	Significant defects in basic mental functions	Significant defects in most domains of mental functioning, along with problems in the organization and/or integration–differentiation of self and others.
		Psychotic
M7; 12–18	Major/severe defects in basic mental functions	Major and severe defects in almost all domains of mental functioning, with impaired reality testing; fragmentation and/or difficulties in self–object differentiation; disturbed perception, integration, and regulation of affect and thought; and severe defects in one or more basic mental functions (e.g., perception, integration, motor, memory, regulation, judgment).

spirituality). Clinicians can administer some or all subscales. Evidence for construct validity and clinical utility of subscale scores is strong.

Shedler–Westen Assessment Procedure–200

In the SWAP-200 (Westen & Shedler, 1999a, 1999b), items tapping meaning and purpose include the following: 37. Finds meaning in belonging and contributing to a larger community (e.g., organization, church, neighborhood, etc.); 50. Tends to feel life has no meaning; 121. Is creative, able to see things or approach problems in novel ways; 149. Tends to feel like an outcast or outsider; feels as if s/he does not truly belong; 151. Appears to experience the past as a series of disjointed or disconnected events; has difficulty giving a coherent account of his/her life story.

Summary of Basic Mental Functioning

We recommend that clinicians summarize basic mental functioning quantitatively (see Table 2.1).

BIBLIOGRAPHY

1. Capacity for Regulation, Attention, and Learning

Aiken, L. R., & Groth-Marnat, G. (2006). *Psychological testing and assessment* (12th ed.). New York: Pearson.

Barkley, R. A. (2014). The assessment of executive functioning using the Barkley Deficits in Executive Functioning Scales. In S. Goldstein & J. A. Naglieri (Eds.), *Handbook of executive functioning* (pp. 245–263). New York: Springer.

Benton, A. L. (1974). *The Revised Visual Retention Test* (4th ed.). New York: Psychological Corporation.

Berg, E. A. (1948). A simple objective technique for measuring flexibility in thinking. *Journal of General Psychology, 39*, 15–22.

Cockburn, J., & Keene, J. (2001). Are changes in everyday memory over time in autopsy-confirmed Alzheimer's disease related to changes in reported behaviour? *Neuropsychological Rehabilitation, 11*, 201–217.

Conners, C. K. (2008). *Conners 3 manual*. North Tonawanda, NY: Multi-Health Systems.

Conners, C. K., & Multi-Health Systems Staff. (2000). *Conners' Continuous Performance Test (CPT II) computer programs for Windows™ technical guide and software manual*. North Tonawanda, NY: Multi-Health Systems.

Conway, F. (Ed.). (2014). *Attention deficit hyperactivity disorder: Integration of cognitive, neuropsychological, and psychodynamic perspectives in psychotherapy*. New York: Routledge.

Folstein, M. F., Folstein, S. E., & McHugh, P. R. (1975). Mini-Mental State: A practical method for grading the cognitive state of patients for the clinician. *Journal of Psychiatric Research, 12*, 189–198.

Golden, C. J., & Freshwater, S. M. (2002). *Stroop Color and Word Test: Revised examiner's manual*. Wood Dale, IL: Stoelting.

Gorman, J. M., & Roose, S. P. (2011). The neurobiology of fear memory reconsolidation and psychoanalytic theory. *Journal of the American Psychoanalytic Association, 59*, 1201–1219.

Grant, D. A., & Berg, E. A. (1948). A behavioural analysis of degree of reinforcement and ease of shifting to new responses in a Weigl-type card sorting problem. *Journal of Experimental Psychology, 38*, 404–411.

Groth-Marnat, G. (Ed.). (2000). *Neuropsychological assessment in clinical practice: A guide to test interpretation and integration*. New York: Wiley.

Groth-Marnat, G. (2009). *Handbook of psychological assessment* (5th ed.). Hoboken, NJ: Wiley.

Hitchcock, C., Nixon, R. D., & Weber, N. (2014). A review of overgeneral memory in child psychopathology. *British Journal of Clinical Psychology, 53*, 170–193.

Hobson, P. (2004). *The cradle of thought: Exploring the origins of thinking*. New York: Oxford University Press.

Hunter, S. J., & Sparrow, E. P. (2012). *Executive function and dysfunction: Identification, assessment and treatment*. Cambridge, UK: Cambridge University Press.

Jensen, A. R., & Rohwer, W. D. (1966). The Stroop Color–Word Test: A review. *Acta Psychologica, 25*, 36–93.

Lezak, M. D., Howieson, D. B., Bigler, E. D., & Tranel, D. (2012). *Neuropsychological assessment* (5th ed.). New York: Oxford University Press.

Makatura, T. J., Lam, C. S., Leahy, B. J., Castillo, M. T., & Kalpakjian, C. Z. (1999). Standardized memory tests and the appraisal of everyday memory. *Brain Injury, 13*(5), 355–367.

Minshew, R., & D'Andrea, W. (2015). Implicit and explicit memory in survivors of chronic interpersonal violence. *Psychological Trauma: Theory, Research, Practice, and Policy, 7*(1), 67–75.

Miyake, A., & Friedman, N. P. (2012). The nature and organization of individual differences in executive functions: Four general conclusions. *Current Directions in Psychological Science, 21*, 8–14.

Nasreddine, Z. S., Phillips, N. A., Bédirian, V., Charbonneau, S., Whitehead, V., Collin, I., . . . Chertkow, H. (2005). The Montreal Cognitive Assessment, MoCA: A brief screening tool for mild cognitive impairment. *Journal of the American Geriatrics Society, 53*, 695–699.

Norris, G., & Tate, R. L. (2000). The Behavioural Assessment of the Dysexecutive Syndrome (BADS): Ecological, concurrent and construct validity. *Neuropsychological Rehabilitation, 10*(1), 33–45.

Ostrosky-Solis, F., Jaime, R. M., & Ardila, A. (1998). Memory abilities during normal aging. *International Journal of Neuroscience, 93*, 151–162.

Pérez, M., & Godoy, J. (1998). Comparison between a "traditional" memory test and a "behavioral" memory battery in Spanish patients. *Journal of Clinical and Experimental Neuropsychology, 20*(4), 496–502.

Polak, A. R., Witteveen, A. B., Reitsma, J. B., & Olff, M. (2012). The role of executive function in posttraumatic stress disorder: A systematic review. *Journal of Affective Disorders, 14*, 11–21.

Porges, S. W. (2011). *The polyvagal theory*. New York: Norton.

Rhodes, M. G. (2004). Age-related differences in performance on the Wisconsin Card Sorting Test: A meta-analytic review. *Psychology and Aging, 19*(3), 482–494.

Schore, A. N. (2012). *The science of the art of psychotherapy*. New York: Norton.

Siegel, D. J. (2012). *The developing mind: How relationships and the brain interact to shape who we are* (2nd ed.). New York: Guilford Press.

Snyder, P. J., Nussbaum, P. D., & Robins, D. L. (Eds.). (2005). *Clinical neuropsychology: A pocket handbook for assessment.* Washington, DC: American Psychological Association.

Stanovich, K. E., & West, R. F. (2014). What intelligence tests miss. *The Psychologist, 27,* 80–83.

Strauss, E., Sherman, E. M. S., & Spreen, O. (2006). *A compendium of neuropsychological tests: Administration, norms, and commentary* (3rd ed.). New York: Oxford University Press.

Stroop, J. R. (1935). Studies of interference in serial verbal reactions. *Journal of Experimental Psychology, 18,* 643–662.

Teng, E. L., & Chui, H. C. (1987). The Modified Mini-Mental State (3MS) Examination. *Journal of Clinical Psychiatry, 48,* 314–318.

Todd, R. M., Cunningham, W. A., Anderson, A. K., & Thompson, E. (2012). Affect-biased attention as emotion regulation. *Trends in Cognitive Sciences, 16,* 365–372.

Verneau, M., van der Kamp, J., Savelsberg, G. J., & de Loose, M. P. (2014). Age and time effects on implicit and explicit learning. *Experimental Aging Research, 40,* 477–511.

Wechsler, D. (2008). *Wechsler Adult Intelligence Scale—Fourth Edition (WAIS-IV).* San Antonio, TX: Pearson.

Wilson, B. A., Alderman, N., Burgess, P. W., Emslie, H., & Evans, J. J. (1996). *Behavioural Assessment of the Dysexecutive Syndrome.* St. Edmunds, UK: Thames Valley Test Company.

Wilson, B., Cockburn, J., Baddeley, A. D., & Hiorns, R. (1989). The development and validation of a test battery for detecting and monitoring everyday memory problems. *Journal of Clinical and Experimental Neuropsychology, 11*(6), 855–870.

Wilson, B. A., Greenfield, E., Clare, L., Baddeley, A., Cockburn, J., Watson, P., . . . Nannery, R. (2008). *The Rivermead Behavioural Memory Test—Third Edition (RBMT-3).* London: Pearson.

2. Capacity for Affective Range, Communication, and Understanding

Allison, C., Baron-Cohen, S., Wheelwright, S. J., Stone, M. H., & Muncer, S. J. (2011). Psychometric analysis of the Empathy Quotient (EQ). *Personality and Individual Differences, 51,* 829–835.

Barchard, K. A., Bajgar, J., Duncan, E., & Lane, R. D. (2010). Computer scoring of the Levels of Emotional Awareness Scale. *Behavior Research Methods, 42,* 586–595.

Baron-Cohen, S., & Wheelwright, S. (2004). The Empathy Quotient: An investigation of adults with Asperger syndrome or high functioning autism, and normal sex differences. *Journal of Autism and Developmental Disorders, 34,* 163–175.

Bates, G. C. (2000). Affect regulation. *International Journal of Psychoanalysis, 81,* 317–319.

Boesky, D. (2000). Affect, language and communication. *International Journal of Psychoanalysis, 81,* 257–262.

Bradley, B., DeFife, J. A., Guarnaccia, C., Phifer, J., Fani, N., Ressler, K. J., & Westen, D. (2011). Emotional dysregulation and negative affects: Association with psychiatric symptoms. *Journal of Clinical Psychiatry, 72,* 685–691.

Bucci, W. (1997). *Psychoanalysis and cognitive science: A multiple code theory.* New York: Guilford Press.

Bucci, W. (2000). Biological and integrative studies on affect. *International Journal of Psychoanalysis, 81,* 141–144.

Bucci, W. (2001). Pathways of emotional communication. *Psychoanalytic Inquiry, 21,* 40–70.

Charles, S. T., & Luong, G. (2013). Emotional experience across adulthood: The theoretical model of strength and vulnerability integration. *Current Directions in Psychological Science, 22,* 443–448.

Conklin, C. Z., Bradley, R., & Westen, D. (2006), Affect regulation in borderline personality disorder. *Journal of Nervous and Mental Disease, 194,* 69–77.

Davis, K. L., & Panksepp, J. (2011). The brain's emotional foundations of human personality and the Affective Neuroscience Personality Scales. *Neuroscience and Biobehavioral Reviews, 35,* 1946–1958.

Davis, K. L, Panksepp, J., & Normansell, L. (2003). The Affective Neuroscience Personality Scales: Normative data and implications. *Neuropsychoanalysis, 5*(1), 57–69.

Ditzfeld, C. P., & Showers, C. J. (2014). Self-structure and emotional experience. *Cognition and Emotion, 28,* 596–621.

Emde, R. M. (2000). Commentary on emotions: Ongoing discussion. *Neuropsychoanalysis, 2,* 69–74.

Fonagy, P., Gergely, G., Jurist, E. L., & Target, M. (2004). *Affect regulation, mentalization and the development of the self.* London: Karnac.

Fowler, J. C., Charak, R., Elhai, J. D., Allen, J. G., Frueh, B. C., & Oldham, J. M. (2014). Construct validity and factor structure of the Difficulties in Emotion Regulation Scale among adults with severe mental illness. *Journal of Psychiatric Research, 58,* 175–180.

Gratz, K. L., & Roemer, L. (2004). Multidimensional assessment of emotion regulation and dysregulation: Development, factor structure, and initial validation of the Difficulties in Emotion Regulation Scale. *Journal of Psychopathology Behaviour Assessment, 26,* 41–54.

Greenberg, L. E., & Safran, J. D. (1987). *Emotion in psychotherapy.* New York: Guilford Press.

Gross, J. J., & John, O. P. (2003). Individual differences in two emotion regulation processes: Implications for affect, relationships, and wellbeing.

Journal of Personality and Social Psychology, 85, 348–362.

Hussong, A. M., & Hicks, R. E. (2003). Affect and peer context interactively impact adolescent substance use. *Journal of Abnormal Child Psychology, 31*, 413–426.

Jurist, E. L. (2005). Mentalized affectivity. *Psychoanalytic Psychology, 22*, 426–444.

Kernberg, O. F. (1984). *Severe personality disorders: Psychotherapeutic strategies.* New Haven, CT: Yale University Press.

Lane, R. D., & Garfield, D. A. S. (2005). Becoming aware of feelings: Integration of cognitive-developmental, neuroscientific, and psychoanalytic perspectives. *Neuro-Psychoanalysis, 7*, 5–30.

Lane, R. D., Quinlan, D. M., Schwartz, G. E., Walker, P. A., & Zeitlin, S. (1990). The Levels of Emotional Awareness Scale: A cognitive-developmental measure of emotion. *Journal of Personality Assessment, 55*, 124–134.

Lane, R. D., & Schwartz, G. E. (1987). Levels of emotional awareness: A cognitive-developmental theory and its application to psychopathology. *American Journal of Psychiatry, 144*, 133–143.

Lawrence, E. J., Shaw, P., Baker, D., Baron-Cohen, S., & David, A. S. (2004). Measuring empathy: Reliability and validity of the Empathy Quotient. *Psychological Medicine, 34*, 911–919.

Le, B. M., & Impett, E. A. (2013). When holding back helps: Suppressing negative emotions during sacrifice feels authentic and is beneficial for highly interdependent people. *Psychological Science, 24*, 1809–1815.

Leue, A., & Beauducel, A. (2011). The PANAS structure revisited: On the validity of a bifactor model in community and forensic samples. *Psychological Assessment, 23*, 215–225.

Levine, E. L., Xu, X., Yang, L. Q., Ispas, D., Pitariu, H. D., Bian, R., Ding, D., . . . Musat, S. (2011). Cross-national explorations of the impact of affect at work using the State–Trait Emotion Measure: A coordinated series of studies in the United States, China, and Romania. *Human Performance, 24*(5), 405–442.

Meehan, K. B. (2004). *Affective Communication Questionnaire.* Unpublished manuscript, Cornell Medical Center, White Plains, NY.

Meehan, K. B., Levy, K. N., & Clarkin, J. F. (2012). Construct validity of a measure of affective communication in psychotherapy. *Psychoanalytic Psychology, 29*(2), 145–165.

Melka, S. E., Lancaster, S. L., Bryant, A. R., & Rodriguez, B. F. (2011). Confirmatory factor and measurement invariance analyses of the Emotion Regulation Questionnaire. *Journal of Clinical Psychology, 67*, 1283–1293.

Porcerelli, J. H., Cogan, R., & Bambery, M. (2011). The mental functioning axis of the *Psychodynamic Diagnostic Manual*: An adolescent case study. *Journal of Personality Assessment, 93*, 177–184.

Porges, S. W. (2011). *The polyvagal theory.* New York: Norton.

Roth, G., Benita, M., Amrani, C., Shachar, B. H., & Hadas, A. (2014). Integration of negative emotional experience versus suppression: Addressing the question of adaptive functioning. *Emotion, 14*, 908–919.

Savitz, J., van der Merwe, L., & Ramesar, R. (2008). Dysthymic and anxiety-related personality traits in bipolar spectrum illness. *Journal of Affective Disorders, 109*, 305–311.

Scherer, K. R., & Ekman, P. (1984). *Approaches to emotion.* Hillsdale, NJ: Erlbaum.

Schore, A. N. (1994). *Affect regulation and the origin of the self: The neurobiology of emotional development.* Hillsdale, NJ: Erlbaum.

Schore, A. N. (2003). *Affect dysregulation and disorders of the self.* New York: Norton.

Spaapen, D. L., Waters, F., Brummer, L., Stopa, L., & Bucks, R. S. (2014). The Emotion Regulation Questionnaire: Validation of the ERQ-9 in two community samples. *Psychological Assessment, 26*, 46–54.

Stein, M., Hilsenroth, M., Slavin-Mulford, J., & Pinsker, J. (2011). *Social Cognition and Object Relations Scale: Global Rating Method* (SCORS-G; 4th ed.). Unpublished manuscript, Massachusetts General Hospital and Harvard Medical School.

Stein, M. B., Siefert, C. J., Stewart, R. V., & Hilsenroth, M. J. (2011). Relationship between the Social Cognition and Object Relations Scale (SCORS) and attachment style in a clinical sample. *Clinical Psychology and Psychotherapy, 18*, 6, 512–523.

Stein, M. B., Slavin-Mulford, J., Siefert, C. J., Sinclair, S. J., Renna, M., Malone, J., . . . Blais, M. A. (2014). SCORS-G stimulus characteristics of select Thematic Apperception Test cards. *Journal of Personality Assessment, 96*(3), 339–349.

Subic-Wrana, C., Beutel, M. E., Brahler, E., & Stobel-Richter, Y. (2014). How is emotional awareness related to emotion-regulation strategies in the general population? *PLoS ONE, 9*, e91843.

Trevarthen, C. (2009). The functions of emotion in infancy: The regulation and communication of rhythm, sympathy, and meaning in human development. In D. Fosha, D. J. Siegel, & M. F. Solomon (Eds.), *The healing power of emotion: Affective neuroscience, development, and clinical practice* (pp. 55–85). New York: Norton.

Tronick, E. (2007). *The neurobehavioral and social-emotional development of infants and children.* New York: Norton.

Watson, D., & Clark, L. A. (1994). *The PANAS-X: Manual for the Positive and Negative Affect Schedule—Expanded Form.* Unpublished manuscript, University of Iowa.

Watson, D., Clark, L. A., & Tellegen, A. (1988). Development and validation of brief measures of positive and negative affect: The PANAS scales.

Journal of Personality and Social Psychology, 54, 1063–1070.

Westen, D. (1995). *Social Cognition and Object Relations Scale: Q-sort for Projective Stories (SCORS-Q)*. Unpublished manuscript, Department of Psychiatry, Cambridge Hospital and Harvard Medical School.

Westen, D., Lohr, N., Silk, K., & Kerber, K. (1985). *Measuring object relations and social cognition using the TAT: Scoring manual*. Unpublished manuscript, University of Michigan.

Westen, D., Muderrisoglu, S., Fowler, C., Shedler, J., & Koren, D. (1997). Affect regulation and affective experience: Individual differences, group differences, and measurement using a Q-sort procedure. *Journal of Consulting and Clinical Psychology, 3*, 429–439.

Westen, D., & Shedler, J. (1999a). Revising and assessing Axis II: I. Developing a clinically and empirically valid assessment method. *American Journal of Psychiatry, 156*, 258–272.

Westen, D., & Shedler, J. (1999b). Revising and assessing Axis II: II. Toward an empirically based and clinically useful classification of personality disorders. *American Journal of Psychiatry, 156*, 273–285.

Wiltink, J., Glaesmer, H., Canterino, M., Wolfling, K., Knebel, A., Kessler, H., . . . Buetel, M. E. (2011). Regulation of emotions in the community: Suppression and reappraisal strategies and its psychometric properties. *GMS Psycho-Social-Medicine, 8*, 1–12.

Zittel-Conklin. C., Bradley, R., & Westen, D. (2006). Affect regulation in borderline personality disorder. *Journal of Nervous and Mental Disease, 194*, 69–77.

3. Capacity for Mentalization and Reflective Functioning

Aber, J. L., Slade, A., Berger, B., Bresgi, I., & Kaplan, M. (1985). *The Parent Development Interview*. Unpublished manuscript.

Allen, J. G., Fonagy, P., & Bateman, A. W. (2008). *Mentalizing in clinical practice*. Washington, DC: American Psychiatric Publishing.

Bateman, A. W., & Fonagy, P. (2012). *Handbook of mentalizing in mental health practice*. Arlington, VA: American Psychiatric Publishing.

Bateman, A. W., & Fonagy, P. (2013). Mentalization based treatment. *Psychoanalytic Inquiry, 33*, 595–613.

Bush, F. N. (2008). *Mentalization: Theoretical considerations, research findings, and clinical implications*. New York: Analytic Press.

Choi-Kain, L., & Gunderson, J. G. (2008). Mentalization: Ontogeny, assessment, and application in the treatment of borderline personality disorder. *American Journal of Psychiatry, 165*, 1127–1135.

Fonagy, P., Gergely, G., Jurist, E. L., & Target, M. (2002). *Affect regulation, mentalization, and the development of the self*. New York: Other Press.

Fonagy, P., Luyten, P., & Strathearn, L. (2011). Borderline personality disorder, mentalization, and the neurobiology of attachment. *Infant Mental Health Journal, 32*, 47–69.

Fonagy, P., Steele, H., Moran, G., Steele, M., & Higgit, A. (1991). The capacity for understanding mental states: The reflective self in parent and child and its significance for security of attachment. *Infant and Mental Health Journal, 13*, 200–217.

Fonagy, P., & Target, M. (1997). Attachment and reflective function: Their role in self-organization. *Development and Psychopathology, 9*, 679–700.

Fonagy, P., Target, M., Steele, H., & Steele, M. (1998). *Reflective functioning manual, version 5.0, for application to adult attachment Interviews*. London: University College London.

Gabbard, G. O. (2005). Reflective function, mentalization, and borderline personality disorder. In B. D. Beitman (Ed.), *Self-awareness deficits in psychiatric patients: Neurobiology, assessment, and treatment* (pp. 213–228). New York: Norton.

George, C., Kaplan, N., & Main, M. (1985). *The Adult Attachment Interview*. Unpublished manuscript, University of California at Berkeley.

Hobson, P. (2004). *The cradle of thought: Exploring the origins of thinking*. New York: Oxford University Press.

Jurist, E. L. (2005). Mentalized affectivity. *Psychoanalytic Psychology, 22*, 426–444.

Jurist, E. L., & Slade, A. (Eds.). (2008). *Mind to mind: Infant research, neuroscience, and psychoanalysis*. New York: Other Press.

Krugman, S. (2013). Mentalization in group: Implicit and explicit. *Group, 37*, 119–133.

Lehmann, M. E., & Hilsenroth, M. J. (2011). Evaluating psychological insight in a clinical sample using the Shedler–Westen Assessment Procedure. *Journal of Nervous and Mental Disease, 199*, 354–359.

Liljenfors, R., & Lars-Gunnar, L. (2015). Mentalization and intersubjectivity: Toward a theoretical integration. *Psychoanalytic Psychology, 32*(1), 36–60.

Müller, C., Kaufhold, J., Overbeck, G., & Grabhorn, R. (2006). The importance of reflective functioning to the diagnosis of psychic structure. *Psychology and Psychotherapy: Theory, Research and Practice, 79*, 485–494.

Schore, A. N. (2012). *The science of the art of psychotherapy*. New York: Norton.

Shai, D., & Belsky, J. (2011). When words just won't do: Introducing Parental Embodied Mentalizing. *Child Development Perspectives, 5*(3), 173–180.

Shai, D., & Fonagy, P. (2013). Beyond words: Parental Embodied Mentalizing and the parent–infant dance. In M. Mikulincer & P. R. Shaver (Eds.), *Mechanisms of social connection: From brain to group* (pp. 185–203). Washington, DC: American Psychological Association.

Siegel, D. J. (2012a). *The developing mind: How relationships and the brain interact to shape who we are* (2nd ed.). New York: Guilford Press.

Siegel, D. J. (2012b). *Pocket guide to interpersonal neurobiology: An integrative handbook of the mind*. New York: Norton.

Slade, A. (2005). Parental reflective functioning: An introduction. *Attachment and Human Development, 7*, 269–281.

Smith, J. D. (2014). Focusing on reflections: Mentalization and mirroring in brief dynamic therapy. *British Journal of Psychotherapy, 30*, 212–228.

4. Capacity for Differentiation and Integration (Identity)

Blatt, S. J., Auerbach, J. S., & Levy, K. N. (1997). Mental representations in personality development, psychopathology and the therapeutic process. *Review of General Psychology, 1*, 351–374.

Blatt, S. J., & Blass, R. B. (1996). Relatedness and self-definition: A dialectic model of personality development. In G. G. Noam & K. W. Fischer (Eds.), *Development and vulnerabilities in close relationships* (pp. 309–338). Hillsdale, NJ: Erlbaum.

Blatt, S. J., Stayner, D., Auerbach, J., & Behrends, R. S. (1996). Change in object and self-representations in long-term, intensive, inpatient treatment of seriously disturbed adolescents and young adults. *Psychiatry, 59*, 82–107.

Blatt, S. J., & Zuroff, D. C. (1992). Interpersonal relatedness and self-definition: Two prototypes for depression. *Clinical Psychology Review, 12*, 527–562.

Bombel, G., Mihura, J. L., & Meyer, G. J. (2009). An examination of the construct validity of the Rorschach Mutuality of Autonomy (MOA) Scale. *Journal of Personality Assessment, 91*(3), 227–237.

DeWitt, K. N., Hartley, D., Rosenberg, S. E., Zilberg, N. J., & Wallerstein, R. S. (1991). Scales of Psychological Capacities: Development of an assessment approach. *Psychoanalysis and Contemporary Thought, 14*, 334–343.

Diamond, D., Blatt, S. J., Stayner, D., & Kaslow, N. (1991). *Self–other differentiation of object representations*. Unpublished research manual, Yale University.

Erikson, E. H. (1956). The problem of ego identity. *Journal of the American Psychoanalytic Association, 4*, 56–121.

Firestone, R. W., Firestone, L., & Catlett, J. (2013). *The self under siege: A therapeutic model for differentiation*. New York: Routledge.

Graceffo, R. A., Mihura, J. L., & Meyer, G. J. (2014). A meta-analysis of an implicit measure of personality functioning: The Mutuality of Autonomy Scale. *Journal of Personality Assessment, 96*, 581–595.

Horowitz, L. M. (2004). *Interpersonal foundations of psychopathology*. Washington, DC: American Psychological Association.

Horowitz, L. M. (2014). *Identity and the new psychoanalytic explorations of self-organization*. New York: Routledge.

Huprich, S. K., Auerbach, J. S., Porcerelli, J. H., & Bupp, L. L. (2016). Sidney Blatt's Object Relations Inventory: Contributions and Future Directions. *Journal of Personality Assessment, 98*(1), 30–43.

Jankowski, P. J., & Hooper, L. M. (2012). Differentiation of self: A validation study of the Bowen theory construct. *Couple and Family Psychology: Research and Practice, 1*, 226–243.

Kernberg, O. F. (1984). *Severe personality disorders*. New Haven, CT: Yale University Press.

Kernberg, O. F. (2005). Identity diffusion in severe personality disorders. In S. Strack (Ed.), *Handbook of personology and psychopathology* (pp. 39–49). Hoboken, NJ: Wiley.

Kernberg, O. F. (2006). Identity: Recent findings and clinical implications. *Psychoanalytic Quarterly, 75*, 969–1004.

Main, M., Goldwyn, R., & Hesse, E. (2002). *Classification and scoring systems for the Adult Attachment Interview*. Unpublished manuscript, University of California at Berkeley.

Monroe, J. M., Diener, M. J., Fowler, J. C., Sexton, J. E., & Hilsenroth, M. J. (2013). Criterion validity of the Rorschach Mutuality of Autonomy (MOA) scale: A meta-analytic review. *Psychoanalytic Psychology, 30*(4), 535–566.

Reniers, R. L., Vollm, B. A., Elliott, R., & Corcoran, R. (2014). Empathy, ToM, and self–other differentiation: An fMRI study of internal states. *Social Neuroscience, 9*, 50–62.

Schore, A. N. (1994). *Affect regulation and the origin of the self: The neurobiology of emotional development*. Hillsdale, NJ: Erlbaum.

Schore, A. N. (2003). *Affect dysregulation and disorders of the self.* New York: Norton.

Siegel, D. J. (2012). *The developing mind: How relationships and the brain interact to shape who we are* (2nd ed.). New York: Guilford Press.

Slotter, E. B., Winger, L., & Soto, N. (2015). Lost without each other: The influence of group identity loss on the self-concept. *Group Dynamics, 19*, 15–30.

Stern, D. (1985). *The interpersonal world of the human infant*. New York: Basic Books.

Summers, F. (2014). Ethnic invisibility, identity, and the analytic process. *Psychoanalytic Psychology, 31*, 410–425.

Urist, J. (1977). The Rorschach test and the assessment of object relations. *Journal of Personality Assessment, 41*, 3–9.

Urist, J., & Shill, M. (1982). Validity of the Rorschach

Mutuality of Autonomy Scale: A replication using excerpted responses. *Journal of Personality Assessment, 46*, 450–454.

Vanheule, S., & Verhaeghe, P. (2009). Identity through a psychoanalytic looking glass. *Theory and Psychology, 19*(3), 391–411.

Verheul, R., Andrea, H., Berghout, C. C., Dolan, C., Busschbach, J. J., van der Kroft, P. J., . . . Fonagy, P. (2008). Severity Indices of Personality Problems (SIPP-118): Development, factor structure, reliability, and validity. *Psychological Assessment, 20*(1), 23–34.

Wallerstein, R. S. (1996). *The Scales of Psychological Capacities, Version 1.* Unpublished manual.

Westen, D., & Heim, A. K. (2003). Disturbances of self and identity in personality disorders. In M. R. Leary & J. P. Tangney (Eds.), *Handbook of self and identity* (pp. 643–664). New York: Guilford Press.

Wilkinson-Ryan, T., & Westen, D. (2000). Identity disturbance in borderline personality disorder: An empirical investigation. *American Journal of Psychiatry, 157*, 528–541.

5. Capacity for Relationships and Intimacy

Alden, L. E., Wiggins, J. S., & Pincus, A. L. (1990). Construction of circumplex scales for the Inventory of Interpersonal Problems. *Journal of Personality Assessment, 55*, 521–536.

Aron, L. (1996). *A meeting of minds: Mutuality in psychoanalysis.* Hillsdale, NJ: Analytic Press.

Aron, L., & Anderson, F. S. (1998). *Relational perspectives on the body.* Hillsdale, NJ: Analytic Press.

Barber, J. P., Foltz, C., & Weinryb, R. M. (1998). The Central Relationship Questionnaire: Initial report. *Journal of Counseling Psychology, 45*, 131–142.

Beebe, B., & Lachmann, F. M. (2002). *Infant research and adult treatment: Co-constructing interactions.* Hillsdale, NJ: Analytic Press.

Benjamin, J. (1995). *Like subjects, love objects: Essays on recognition and sexual difference.* New Haven, CT: Yale University Press.

Benjamin, L. S. (1996). *Interpersonal diagnosis and treatment of personality disorders* (2nd ed.). New York: Guilford Press.

Benjamin, L. S., Rothweiler, J. C., & Critchfield, K. L. (2006). The use of Structural Analysis of Social Behavior (SASB) as an assessment tool. *Annual Review of Clinical Psychology, 2*, 83–109.

Blatt, S. J., Stayner, D. A., Auerbach, J. S., & Behrends, R. S. (1996). Change in object and self representations in long-term, intensive, inpatient treatment of seriously disturbed adolescents and young adults. *Psychiatry, 59*, 82–107.

Bornstein, R. F. (2012). Dependent personality disorder. In T. A. Widiger (Ed.), *The Oxford handbook of personality disorders* (pp. 505–526). New York: Oxford University Press.

Bornstein, R. F., & Languirand, M. A. (2003). *Healthy dependency.* New York: Newmarket Press.

Brennan, K. A., Clark, C. L., & Shaver, P. R. (1998). Self-report measurement of adult attachment: An integrative overview. In J. A. Simpson & W. S. Rholes (Eds.), *Attachment theory and close relationships* (pp. 46–76). New York: Guilford Press.

Cassidy, J., & Shaver, P. R. (Eds.). (2008). *Handbook of attachment* (2nd ed.). New York: Guilford Press.

Cozolino, L. (2006). *The neuroscience of human relationships: Attachment and the developing social brain.* New York: Norton.

Del Corno, F., & Lang, M. (2006). *La diagnosi delle relazioni oggettuali con l'Object Relations Technique [Object relations diagnosis with the Object Relations Technique].* Milan: Raffaello Cortina.

Denckla, C. A., Mancini, A. D., Bornstein, R. F., & Bonanno, G. A. (2011). Adaptive and maladaptive dependency in bereavement: Distinguishing prolonged and resolved grief trajectories. *Personality and Individual Differences, 51*, 1012–1017.

Dimen, M. (2003). *Sexuality, intimacy, power.* New York: Routledge.

George, C., West, M., & Pettem, O. (1997). *The Adult Attachment Projective.* Unpublished manual, Mills College, Oakland, CA.

Gurtman, M. B. (1996). Interpersonal problems and the psychotherapy context: The construct validity of the Inventory of Interpersonal Problems. *Psychological Assessment, 8*, 241–255.

Hilsenroth, M. J., Menaker, J., Peters, E. J., & Pincus, A. L. (2007). Assessment of borderline pathology using the Inventory of Interpersonal Problems Circumplex Scales (IIP-C): A comparison of clinical samples. *Clinical Psychology and Psychotherapy, 14*(5), 365–376.

Horowitz, L., Alden, L., Wiggins, J., & Pincus, A. L. (2000). *Inventory of Interpersonal Problems.* San Antonio, TX: Psychological Corporation.

Kernberg, O. F. (1984). *Severe personality disorders: Psychotherapeutic strategies.* New Haven, CT: Yale University Press.

Jones-Mason, K., Allen, I. E., Hamilton, S., & Weiss, S. J. (2015). Comparative validity of the Adult Attachment Interview and the Adult Attachment Projective. *Attachment and Human Development, 17*(5), 429–447.

Kernberg, O. F. (2012). *The inseparable nature of love and aggression: Clinical and theoretical perspectives.* Washington, DC: American Psychiatric Publishing.

Knafo, D. S. (2010). The O.R.T. (the Object Relations Technique): A reintroduction. *Psychoanalytic Psychology, 27*, 182–189.

Luborsky, L. (1998). The Relationship Anecdotes Paradigm (RAP): Interview as a versatile source of narratives. In L. Luborsky & P. Crits-Christoph (Eds.), *Understanding transference: The Core Conflictual Relationship Theme method* (2nd ed., pp.109–120). Washington, DC: American Psychological Association.

Luborsky, L., & Crits-Christoph, P. (1998). *Understanding transference: The Core Conflictual Relationship Theme method* (2nd ed.). Washington, DC: American Psychological Association.

McCarthy, K. S., Gibbons, M. B. C., & Barber, J. P. (2008). The relation of rigidity across relationships with symptoms and functioning: An investigation with the revised Central Relationship Questionnaire. *Journal of Counseling Psychology, 55*(3), 346–358.

McWilliams, N. (2006). Some thoughts about schizoid dynamics. *Psychoanalytic Review, 93*, 1–24.

Mikulincer, M., & Shaver, P. R. (2016). *Attachment in adulthood: Structure, dynamics, and change* (2nd ed.). New York: Guilford Press.

Mitchell, S. A. (2000). *Relationality: From attachment to intersubjectivity.* Hillsdale, NJ: Analytic Press.

Mitchell, S. A. (2002). *Can love last?: The fate of romance over time.* New York: Norton.

Phillipson, H. (1955). *The object relations technique (plates and manual).* London: Tavistock.

Praeger, K. J. (2014). *The dilemmas of intimacy: Conceptualization, assessment, and treatment.* New York: Routledge.

Schore, A. N. (2012). *The science of the art of psychotherapy.* New York: Norton.

Siegel, D. J. (2012). *The developing mind: How relationships and the brain interact to shape who we are* (2nd ed.). New York: Guilford Press.

Slade, A. (1999). Attachment theory and research: Implications for the theory and practice of individual psychotherapy with adults. In J. Cassidy & P. R. Shaver (Eds.), *Handbook of attachment: Theory, research, and clinical applications* (pp. 575–594). New York: Guilford Press.

Triebwasser, J., Chemerinski, E., Roussos, P., & Siever, L. J. (2013). Schizoid personality disorder. *Journal of Personality Disorders, 26*, 919–926.

Wei, M., Russell, D. W., Mallinckrodt, B., & Vogel, D. L. (2007). The Experiences in Close Relationship Scale (ECR)—Short Form: Reliability, validity, and factor structure. *Journal of Personality Assessment, 88*, 187–204.

Weinryb, R. M., Rossel, R. J., & Asberg, M. (1991a). The Karolinska Psychodynamic Profile: I. Validity and dimensionality. *Acta Psychiatrica Scandinavica, 83*, 64–72.

Weinryb, R. M., Rossel, R. J., & Asberg, M. (1991b). The Karolinska Psychodynamic Profile: II. Interdisciplinary and cross-cultural reliability. *Acta Psychiatrica Scandinavica, 83*, 73–76.

Yoo, H., Bartle-Haring, S., Day, R. D., & Gangamma, R. (2014). Couple communication, emotional and sexual intimacy, and relationship satisfaction. *Journal of Sex and Marital Therapy, 40*, 275–293.

6. Capacity for Self-Esteem Regulation and Quality of Internal Experience

Abramson, L. Y., Seligman, M. E. P., & Teasdale, J. D. (1978). Learned helplessness in humans: Critique and reformulation. *Journal of Abnormal Psychology, 87*, 49–74.

Bandura, A. (2000). Exercise of human agency through collective efficacy. *Current Directions in Psychological Science, 9*, 75–78.

Bandura, A. (1986). The explanatory and predictive scope of self-efficacy theory. *Journal of Social and Clinical Psychology, 4*, 359–373.

Barnett, M. D., & Womack, P. M. (2015). Fearing, not loving, the reflection: Narcissism, self-esteem, and self-discrepancy. *Personality and Individual Differences, 74*, 280–284.

Beebe, B., & Lachmann, F. M. (2014). *The origins of attachment: Infant research and adult treatment.* New York: Routledge.

Beitman, B. D. (Ed.). (2005). *Self-awareness deficits in psychiatric patients: Neurobiology, assessment, and treatment.* New York: Norton.

Blatt, S. J., Auerbach, J. S., & Behrends, R. S. (2008). Changes in the representation of self and significant others in the treatment process: Links between representation, internalization, and mentalization. In E. L. Jurist, A. Slade, & S. Bergner (Eds.), *Mind to mind: Infant research, neuroscience, and psychoanalysis* (pp. 225–263). New York: Other Press.

DeWitt, K. N., Hartley, D. E., Rosenberg, S. E., & Zilberg, N. J. (1991). Scales of psychological capacities: Development of an assessment approach. *Psychoanalysis and Contemporary Thought, 14*, 343–361.

Donnellan, M. B., Ackerman, R. A., & Brecheen, C. (2016). Extending structural analyses of the Rosenberg Self-Esteem Scale to consider criterion-related validity: Can composite self-esteem scores be good enough? *Journal of Personality Assessment, 98*(2), 169–177.

Gardner, D. G., & Pierce, J. L. (2010). The Core Self-Evaluation Scale: Further construct validation evidence. *Educational and Psychological Measurement, 70*(2), 291–304.

Hagememeyer, B., & Neyer, F. J. (2012). Assessing implicit motivation orientation in couple relationships: The Partner Related Agency and Communion Test. *Psychological Assessment, 24*, 114–128.

Horowitz, L. M. (2004). *Interpersonal foundations of psychopathology.* Washington, DC: American Psychological Association.

Horvath, S., & Morf, C. C. (2010). To be grandiose

or not to be worthless: Different routes to self-enhancement for narcissism and self-esteem. *Journal of Research in Personality, 44*(5), 585–592.
Judge, T. A., Erez, A., & Bono, J. E. (1998). The power of being positive: The relation between positive self-concept and job performance. *Human Performance, 11*(2–3), 167–187.
Judge, T. A., Erez, A., Bono, J. E., & Thoresen, C. J. (2003). The Core Self-Evaluation Scale: Development of a measure. *Personnel Psychology, 56*, 303–331.
Kernberg, O. F. (1975). *Borderline conditions and pathological narcissism.* New York: Aronson.
Kohut, H. (1971). *The analysis of the self.* New York: International Universities Press.
Kohut, H. (1977). *The restoration of the self.* New York: International Universities Press.
Koren-Karie, N., Oppenheim, D., Dolev, S., Sher, E., & Etzion-Carasso, A. (2002). Mothers' insightfulness regarding their infants' internal experience: Relations with maternal sensitivity and infant attachment. *Developmental Psychology, 38*, 534–542.
Maxwell, K., & Huprich, S. (2014). Retrospective reports of attachment disruptions, parental abuse and neglect mediate the relationship between pathological narcissism and self-esteem. *Personality and Mental Health, 8*(4), 290–305.
McAdams, D. P., & McLean, K. C. (2013). Narrative identity. *Current Directions in Psychological Science, 22*, 233–238.
McKay, M. T., Boduszek, D., & Harvey, S. A. (2014). The Rosenberg Self-Esteem Scale: A bifactor answer to a two-factor question? *Journal of Personality Assessment, 96*(6), 654–660.
Rosenberg, M. (1989). *Society and the adolescent self-image* (rev. ed.). Middletown, CT: Wesleyan University Press.
Siegel, D. J. (2012). *The developing mind: How relationships and the brain interact to shape who we are* (2nd ed.). New York: Guilford Press.
Silverstein, M. L. (2007) *Disorders of the self: A personality-guided approach.* Washington, DC: American Psychological Association.
Strelan, P., & Zdaniuk, A. (2015). Threatened state self-esteem reduces forgiveness. *Self and Identity, 14*, 16–32.
Zeigler-Hill, V. (2006). Discrepancies between implicit and explicit self-esteem: Implications for narcissism and self-esteem instability. *Journal of Personality, 74*, 120–143.

7. Capacity for Impulse Control and Regulation

Bates, G. C. (2000). Affect regulation. *International Journal of Psychoanalysis, 81*, 317–319.
Berlin, H. A., Rolls, E. T., & Iversen, S. D. (2005). Borderline personality disorder, impulsivity, and the orbitofrontal cortex. *American Journal of Psychiatry, 162*, 2360–2373.
Coffey, S. F., Schumacher, J. A., Baschnagel, J. S., Hawk, L. W., & Holloman, G. (2011). Impulsivity and risk-taking in borderline personality disorder with and without substance use disorders. *Personality Disorders: Theory, Research, and Treatment, 2*, 128–141.
Costa, P. T., & McCrae, R. R. (1992). *Revised NEO Personality Inventory (NEO–PI–R) and NEO Five-Factor Inventory (NEO–FFI) professional manual.* Odessa, FL: Psychological Assessment Resources.
Eretz, G., Pilver, C. E., & Potenza, M. N. (2014). Gender-related differences in the associations between sexual impulsivity and psychiatric disorders. *Journal of Psychiatric Research, 55*, 117–125.
Fonagy, P., Gergely, G., Jurist, E. L., & Target, M. (2002). *Affect regulation, mentalization, and the development of the self.* New York: Other Press.
Gagnon, J., & Daelman, S. (2011). An empirical study of the psychodynamics of borderline impulsivity: A preliminary report. *Psychoanalytic Psychology, 28*, 341–362.
Garavan, H., Ross, T. J., & Stein, E. A. (1999). Right hemisphere dominance of inhibitory control: An event-related functional MRI study. *Proceedings of the National Academy of Sciences USA, 96*, 8301–8306.
Garnefski, N., & Kraaij, V. (2007). The Cognitive Emotion Regulation Questionnaire: Psychometric features and prospective relationships with depression and anxiety in adults. *European Journal of Psychological Assessment, 23*, 141–149.
Garnefski, N., Kraaij, V., & Spinhoven, P. (2002). *Manual for the use of the Cognitive Emotion Regulation Questionnaire.* Leiderdorp, The Netherlands: DATEC.
Garrett, K. J., & Giddings, K. (2014). Improving impulse control: Using an evidence-based practice approach. *Journal of Evidence-Based Social Work, 11*, 73–83.
Grant, J. E., & Potenza, M. N. (Eds.). (2012). *The Oxford handbook of impulse control disorders.* New York: Oxford University Press.
Kernberg, O. F. (1984). *Severe personality disorders.* New Haven, CT: Yale University Press.
Lieb, K., Zanarini, M. C., Schmahl, C., Linehan, M. M., & Bohus, M. (2004). Borderline personality disorder. *Lancet, 364*, 453–461.
Lindner, C., Nagy, G., & Retelsdorf, J. (2015). The dimensionality of the Brief Self-Control Scale: An evaluation of unidimensional and multidimensional applications. *Personality and Individual Differences, 86*, 465–473.
Lynam, D. R., Miller, J. D., Miller, D. J., Bornovalova, M. A., & Lejuez, C. W. (2011). Testing the relations between impulsivity-related traits, suicidality, and

nonsuicidal self-injury: A test of the incremental validity of the UPPS model. *Personality Disorders: Theory, Research, and Treatment, 2*, 151–160.

Maloney, P. W., Grawitch, M. J., & Barber, L. K. (2012). The multi-factor structure of the Brief Self-Control Scale: Discriminant validity of restraint and impulsivity. *Journal of Research in Personality, 46*, 111–115.

Moeller, F. G., Barratt, E. S., Dougherty, D. M., Schmitz, J. M., & Swann, A. C. (2001). Psychiatric aspects of impulsivity. *American Journal of Psychiatry, 158*, 1783–1793.

Patton, J. H., Stanford, M. S., & Barratt, E. S. (1995). Factor structure of the Barratt Impulsiveness Scale. *Journal of Clinical Psychology, 51*, 768–774.

Plutchik, R., & van Praag, H. M. (1995). The nature of impulsivity: Definitions, ontology, genetics, and relations to aggression. In E. Hollander & D. J. Stein (Eds.), *Impulsivity and aggression* (pp. 7–24). New York: Wiley.

Potenza, M. N., Koran, L. M., & Pallanti, S. (2009). The relationship between impulse-control disorders and obsessive–compulsive disorder: A current understanding and future research directions. *Psychiatry Research, 170*, 22–31.

Reise, S. P., Moore, T. M., Sabb, F. W., Brown, A. K., & London, E. D. (2013). The Barratt Impulsiveness Scale–11: Reassessment of its structure in a community sample. *Psychological Assessment, 25*, 631–642.

Schore, A. N. (2003). *Affect dysregulation and disorders of the self.* New York: Norton.

Sher, K. J., Winograd, R., & Haeny, A. M. (2013). Disorders of impulse control. In G. Stricker, T. A. Widiger, & I. B. Weiner (Eds.), *Handbook of psychology: Vol. 8. Clinical psychology* (2nd ed., pp. 217–239). Hoboken, NJ: Wiley.

Tangney, J. P., Baumeister, R. F., & Boone, A. L. (2004). High self-control predicts good adjustment, less pathology, better grades, and interpersonal success. *Journal of Personality, 72*, 271–324.

Tomko, R. L., Solhan, M. B., Carpenter, R. W. Brown, W. C., Jahng, S., Wood, P. K., & Trull, T. J. (2014). Measuring impulsivity in daily life: The Momentary Impulsivity Scale. *Psychological Assessment, 26*, 339–349.

Tragesser, S. L., & Robinson, R. J. (2009). The role of affective instability and UPPS impulsivity in borderline personality disorder features. *Journal of Personality Disorders, 23*, 370–383.

Villemarette-Pittman, N. R., Stanford, M. S., & Greve, K. W. (2004). Obsessive–compulsive personality disorder and behavioral disinhibition. *Journal of Psychology, 138*, 5–22.

Weinstein, K., Crocker, A. G., Ayllon, A. R., & Caron, J. (2015). Impulsivity in an epidemiological catchment area sample of the general population: A confirmatory factor analysis of the Barratt Impulsiveness Scale (version 11a). *The International Journal of Forensic Mental Health, 14*, 120–131.

Whiteside, S. P., & Lynam, D. R. (2001). The five-factor model and impulsivity: Using a structural model of personality to understand impulsivity. *Personality and Individual Differences, 30*, 669–689.

Whiteside, S. P., Lynam, D. R., Miller, J. D., & Reynolds, S. K. (2005). Validation of the UPPS Impulsive Behaviour Scale: A four-factor model of impulsivity. *European Journal of Personality, 19*, 559–574.

8. Capacity for Defensive Functioning

American Psychiatric Association. (1994). *Diagnostic and statistical manual of mental disorders* (4th ed.). Washington, DC: Author.

Beresford, T. (2012). *Psychological adaptive mechanisms: Ego defense recognition in practice and research.* New York: Oxford University Press.

Berney, S., de Roten, Y., Beretta, V., Kramer, U., & Despland, J. N. (2014). Identifying psychotic defences in a clinical interview. *Journal of Clinical Psychology, 70*, 428–439.

Bond, M. (2004). Empirical studies of defense style: Relationships with psychopathology and change. *Harvard Review of Psychiatry, 12*, 263–278.

Bond, M., Gardner, S. T., Christian, J., & Sigal, J. J. (1983). Empirical study of self-rated defense styles. *Archives of General Psychiatry, 40*, 333–338.

Bond, M., & Vaillant, G. (1986). An empirical study of the relationship between diagnosis and defense style. *Archives of General Psychiatry, 43*, 285–288.

Bowlby, J. (1980). *Attachment and loss: Vol. 3. Loss.* New York: Basic Books.

Cramer, P. (2006). *Protecting the self: Defense mechanisms in action.* New York: Guilford Press.

Davidson, K., Johnson, E. A., & Woody, E. Z. (1995). *Defense mechanisms assessment: The Defense-Q.* Unpublished manuscript.

Davidson, K., & MacGregor, M. W. (1996). Reliability of an idiographic Q-sort measure of defense mechanisms. *Journal of Personality Assessment, 66*, 624–639.

Di Giuseppe, M., Perry, C. J., Petraglia, J., Janzen, J., & Lingiardi, V. (2014). Development of a Q-sort version of the Defense Mechanism Rating Scales (DMRS-Q) for clinical use. *Journal of Clinical Psychology, 75*, 452–465.

George, C., & West, M. (2012). *The Adult Attachment Projective Picture System: Attachment theory and assessment in adults.* New York: Guilford Press.

Haan, N. (1977). *Coping and defending: Processes of self-environment organization.* New York: Academic Press.

Hilsenroth, M., Callahan, K., & Eudell, E. (2003).

Further reliability, convergent and discriminant validity of overall defensive functioning. *Journal of Nervous and Mental Disease, 191*, 730–737.

Kramer, U. (2010). Coping and defence mechanisms: What's the difference?: Second act. *Psychology and Psychotherapy: Theory, Research and Practice, 83*, 207–221.

Kramer, U., de Roten, Y., Michel, L., & Despland, J. N. (2009). Early change in defence mechanisms and coping in short-term dynamic psychotherapy: Relations with symptoms and alliance. *Clinical Psychology and Psychotherapy, 16*, 408–417.

Lingiardi, V., Gazzillo, F., & Waldron, S. (2010). An empirically supported psychoanalysis: The case of Giovanna. *Psychoanalytic Psychology, 27*, 190–218.

Lingiardi, V., Lonati, C., Fossati, A., Vanzulli, L., & Maffei, C. (1999). Defense mechanisms and personality disorders. *Journal of Nervous and Mental Disease, 187*, 224–228.

Olson, T. R., Perry, C. J., Janzen, J. I., Petraglia, J., & Presniak, M. D. (2011). Addressing and interpreting defense mechanisms in psychotherapy: General considerations. *Psychiatry, 74*, 142–165.

Perry, J. C. (1990). *The Defense Mechanism Rating Scales manual* (5th ed.). Cambridge, MA: Author.

Perry, J. C. (2001). A pilot study of defenses in psychotherapy of personality disorders entering psychotherapy. *Journal of Nervous and Mental Disease, 189*, 651–660.

Perry, J. C. (2014). Anomalies and specific functions in the clinical identification of defense mechanisms. *Journal of Clinical Psychology, 75*, 406–418.

Perry, J. C., Beck, S. M., Constantinides, P., & Foley, J. E. (2009). Studying change in defensive functioning in psychotherapy, using the Defense Mechanism Rating Scales: Four hypotheses, four cases. In R. A. Levy & J. S. Ablon (Eds.), *Handbook of evidence-based psychodynamic psychotherapy* (pp. 121–153). New York: Humana Press.

Perry, J. C., & Bond, M. (2012). Change in defense mechanisms during long-term dynamic psychotherapy and five-year outcome. *American Journal of Psychiatry, 169*, 916–925.

Perry, J. C., & Høglend, P. (1998). Convergent and discriminant validity of overall defensive functioning. *Journal of Nervous and Mental Disease, 186*, 529–535.

Perry, J. C., & Ianni, F. (1998). Observer-rated measures of defense mechanisms. *Journal of Personality, 66*, 993–1024.

Perry, J. C., Petraglia, J., Olson, T. R., Presniak, M. D., & Metzger, J. (2012). Accuracy of defense interpretation in three character types. In R. Levy, S. Ablon, & H. Kachele (Eds.), *Psychodynamic psychotherapy research: Evidence-based practice and practice-based evidence* (pp. 417–447). New York: Humana Press/Springer.

Prunas, A., Preti, E., Huemer, J., Shaw, R. J., & Steiner, H. (2014). Defensive functioning and psychopathology: A study with the REM-71. *Comprehensive Psychiatry, 35*, 33–37.

Roston, D., Lee, K. A., & Vaillant, G. E. (1992). Q-sort approach to identifying defenses. In G. E. Vaillant (Ed.), *Ego mechanisms of defense: A guide for clinicians and researchers* (pp. 217–232). Washington, DC: American Psychiatric Press.

Roy, C. A., Perry, C. J., Luborsky, L., & Banon, E. (2009). Change in defensive functioning in completed psychoanalyses: The Penn Psychoanalytic Treatment Collection. *Journal of the American Psychoanalytic Association, 57*, 399–415.

San Martini, P., Roma, P., Sarti, S., Lingiardi, V., & Bond, M. (2004). Italian version of the Defense Style Questionnaire. *Comprehensive Psychiatry, 45*, 483–494.

Steiner, H., Araujo, K., & Koopman, C. K. (2001). The Response Evaluation Measure (REM-71): A new instrument for the measurement of defenses in adults and adolescents. *American Journal of Psychiatry, 158*, 467–473.

Thygesen, K. L., Drapeau, M., Trijsburg, R. W., Lecours, S., & de Roten, Y. (2008). Assessing defense styles: Factor structure and psychometric properties of the new Defense Style Questionnaire 60 (DSQ-60). *International Journal of Psychology and Psychological Therapy, 8*, 171–181.

Vaillant, G. E. (1977). *Adaptation to life*. Boston: Little, Brown.

Vaillant, G. E. (1993). *The wisdom of the ego*. Cambridge, MA: Harvard University Press.

9. Capacity for Adaptation, Resiliency, and Strength

Alessandri, G., Vecchione, M., Caprara, G., & Letzring, T. D. (2012). The Ego Resiliency Scale revised: A cross-cultural study in Italy, Spain, and the United States. *European Journal of Psychological Assessment, 28*, 139–146.

Block, J. H., & Block, J. (1980). The role of ego-control and ego-resiliency in the organization of behavior. In W. A. Collins (Ed.), *Minnesota Symposia on Child Psychology* (Vol. 13, pp. 39–101). Hillsdale, NJ: Erlbaum.

Block, J. H., & Kremen, A. M. (1996). IQ and ego-resiliency: Conceptual and empirical connections and separateness. *Journal of Personality and Social Psychology, 70*, 349–361.

Bonanno, G. A. (2004). Loss, trauma, and human resilience: Have we underestimated the human capacity to thrive after extremely aversive events? *American Psychologist, 59*, 20–28.

Bonanno, G. A. (2012). Uses and abuses of the resilience construct: Loss, trauma, and health-related adversities. *Social Science and Medicine, 74*, 753–756.

Bonanno, G. A., Pat-Horenczyk, R., & Noll, J. (2011). Coping flexibility and trauma: The Perceived

Ability to Cope With Trauma (PACT) scale. *Psychological Trauma: Theory, Research, Practice, and Policy, 3*, 117–129.

Bornstein, R. F., & Languirand, M. A. (2003). *Healthy dependency.* New York: Newmarket Press.

Campbell-Sills, L., Cohan, S. L., & Stein, M. B. (2006). Relationship of resilience to personality, coping, and psychiatric symptoms in young adults. *Behaviour Research and Therapy, 44*, 585–599.

Carver, C. S., Scheier, M. F., & Weintraub, J. K. (1989). Assessing coping strategies: A theoretically based approach. *Journal of Personality and Social Psychology, 56*, 267–283.

Charney, D. S. (2004). Psychobiological mechanisms of resilience and vulnerability: Implication for successful adaptation to extreme stress. *American Journal of Psychiatry, 161*, 195–216.

Connor, K. M., & Davidson, J. R. (2003). Development of a new resilience scale: The Connor–Davidson Resilience Scale (CD–RISC). *Depression and Anxiety, 18*, 76–82.

Davidson, J. R., Payne, V. M., Connor, K. M., Foa, E. B., Rothbaum, B. O., Hertzberg, M. A., & Weisler, R. H. (2005). Trauma, resilience, and saliostasis: Effects of treatment on posttraumatic stress disorder. *International Clinical Psychopharmacology, 20*, 43–48.

Denckla, C. A., & Mancini, A. D. (2014). Multimethod assessment of resilience. In C. J. Hopwood & R. F. Bornstein (Eds.), *Multimethod clinical assessment* (pp. 254–282). New York: Guilford Press.

Dickinson, P., & Adams, J. (2014). Resiliency, mental health, and well-being among lesbian, gay, and bisexual people. *International Journal of Mental Health Promotion, 16*, 117–125.

Duckworth, A. L., Peterson, C., Matthews, M. D., & Kelly, D. R. (2007). Grit: Perseverance and passion for long-term goals. *Journal of Personality and Social Psychology, 92*, 1087–1101.

Folkman, S. (Ed.). (2011). *The Oxford handbook of stress, health, and coping.* New York: Oxford University Press.

Folkman, S., & Lazarus, R. S. (1988). *Manual for the Ways of Coping Scale.* Palo Alto, CA: Consulting Psychologists Press.

Hatcher, R. L., & Rogers, D. T. (2012). The IIS-32: A brief Inventory of Interpersonal Strengths. *Journal of Personality Assessment, 94*, 638–646.

Letzring, T. D., Block, J., & Funder, D. C. (2005). Ego-control and ego-resiliency: Generalization of self report scales based on personality descriptions from acquaintances, clinicians and the self. *Journal of Research in Personality, 39*, 395–422.

Luborsky, L. (1962). Clinicians' judgment of mental health: A proposed scale. *Archives of General Psychiatry, 7*, 407–417.

Luborsky, L. (1975). Clinicians' judgment of mental health: Specimen case descriptions and forms for the Health–Sickness Rating Scale. *Bulletin of the Menninger Clinic, 39*, 448–480.

Luthar, S. S. (2006). Resilience in development: A synthesis of research across five decades. In D. Cicchetti & D. J. Cohen (Eds.), *Developmental psychopathology: Vol. 3. Risk, disorder, and adaptation* (pp. 739–795). Hoboken, NJ: Wiley.

Lynn, S. J., O'Donohue, W. T., & Lilienfeld, S. O. (Eds.). (2015). *Health, happiness, and well-being: Better living through psychological science.* Thousand Oaks, CA: Sage.

Masten, A. S. (2001). Ordinary magic: Resilience processes in development. *American Psychologist, 56*, 227–238.

Northoff, G., Bermpohl, F., Schoeneich, F., & Boeker, H. (2007). How does your brain constitute defense mechanisms?: First-person neuroscience and psychoanalysis. *Psychotherapy and Psychosomatics, 76*, 141–153.

Shedler, J. (2010). The efficacy of psychodynamic psychotherapy. *American Psychologist, 65*(2), 98–109.

Skodol, A. E., Bender, D. S., Pagano, M. E., Shea, M. T., Yen, S., . . . Gunderson, J. G. (2007). Positive childhood experiences: Resilience and recovery from personality disorder in early adulthood. *Journal of Clinical Psychiatry, 68*(7), 1102–1108.

Southwick, S. M., Litz, B. T., Charney, D., & Friedman, M. J. (Eds.). (2011). *Resilience and mental health: Challenges across the lifespan.* New York: Cambridge University Press.

Taylor, Z. E., Sulik, M. J., Eisenberg, N., Spinrad, T. L., & Silva, K. M. (2014). Development of ego resiliency: Relations to observed parenting and polymorphism in the serotonin transporter gene during early childhood. *Social Development, 23*, 433–450.

Tedeschi, R. G., & Calhoun, L. G. (2004). Posttraumatic growth: Conceptual foundations and empirical evidence. *Psychological Inquiry, 15*, 1–18.

Vecchione, M., Alessandri, G., Barbaranelli, C., & Gerbino, M. (2010). Stability and change of ego resiliency from late adolescence to young adulthood: A multiperspective study using the ER89–R Scale. *Journal of Personality Assessment, 92*, 1–10.

10. Self-Observing Capacities (Psychological Mindedness)

Appelbaum, S. A. (1973). Psychological-mindedness: Word, concept and essence. *International Journal of Psycho-Analysis, 54*, 35–46.

Bagby, R. M., Parker, J. D. A., & Taylor, G. J. (1994a). The twenty-item Toronto Alexithymia Scale: I. Item selection and cross-validation of the factor structure. *Journal of Psychosomatic Research, 38*, 23–32.

Bagby, R. M., Taylor, G. J., Dickens, S. E., & Parker, J. D. (2005). *The Toronto Structured Interview for Alexithymia Administration and Scoring Guidelines*. Unpublished manuscript.

Bagby, R. M., Taylor, G. J., & Parker, J. D. A. (1994b). The twenty-item Toronto Alexithymia Scale: II. Convergent, discriminant, and concurrent validity. *Journal of Psychosomatic Research, 38*, 33–40.

Beitel, M., & Cecero, J. J. (2003), Predicting psychological mindedness from personality style and attachment security. *Journal of Clinical Psychology, 59*, 163–172.

Beitel, M., Cecero, J. J., & Ferrer, E. (2004), Psychological mindedness and cognitive style. *Journal of Clinical Psychology, 60*, 567–582.

Beitel, M., Cecero, J. J., & Prout, T. (2008). Exploring the relationship among early maladaptive schemas, psychological mindedness and self-reported college adjustment. *Psychology and Psychotherapy, 81*, 105–118.

Beitel, M., Ferrer, E., & Cecero, J. J. (2005). Psychological mindedness and awareness of self and others. *Journal of Clinical Psychology, 61*, 739–750.

Bourne, K., Berry, K., & Jones, L. (2014). The relationships between psychological mindedness, parental bonding and adult attachment. *Psychology and Psychotherapy: Theory, Research, and Practice, 87*, 167–177.

Conte, H. R., Plutchik, R., Jung, B. B., Picard, S., Karasu, B., & Lotterman, A. (1990). Psychological mindedness as a predictor of psychotherapy outcome: A preliminary report. *Comprehensive Psychiatry, 31*, 426–431.

Conte, H. R., & Ratto, R. (1997). Self-report measures of psychological mindedness. In M. McCallum & W. E. Piper (Eds.), *Psychological mindedness: A contemporary understanding* (pp. 1–26). Mahwah, NJ: Erlbaum.

Conte, H. R., Ratto, R., & Karasu, T. B. (1996). The Psychological Mindedness Scale: Factor structure and relationship to outcome of psychotherapy. *Journal of Psychotherapy Practice and Research, 5*, 250–259.

Fonagy, P., Gergely, G., Jurist, E. L., & Target, M. (2002). *Affect regulation, mentalization, and the development of the self*. New York: Other Press.

Fonagy, P., & Target, M. (1997). Attachment and reflective function: Their role in self-organization. *Development and Psychopathology, 9*, 679–700.

Ginot, E. (2012). Self-narratives and dysregulated affective states: The neuropsychological links between self-narratives, attachment, affect, and cognition. *Psychoanalytic Psychology, 29*, 59–80.

Giromini, L., Brusadelli, E., Di Noto, B., Grasso, R., & Lang, M. (2015). Measuring psychological mindedness: Validity, reliability, and relationship with psychopathology of an Italian version of the Balanced Index of Psychological Mindedness. *Psychoanalytic Psychotherapy, 29*, 70–87.

Gough, H. G. (1975). *Manual of the California Psychological Inventory*. Palo Alto, CA: Consulting Psychologists Press.

Gough, H. G., & Bradley, P. (1992). Delinquent and criminal behavior as assessed by the revised California Psychological Inventory. *Journal of Clinical Psychology, 48*, 298–308.

Hall, J. A. (1992). Psychological-mindedness: A conceptual model. *American Journal of Psychotherapy, 46*, 131–140.

Keefer, K. V., Taylor, G. J., Parker, J. D. A., Inslegers, R., & Bagby, M. R. (2015). Measurement equivalence of the Toronto Structured Interview for Alexithymia across language, gender, and clinical status. *Psychiatry Research, 228*, 760–764.

Levenson, L. N. (2004). Inhibition of self-observing activity in psychoanalytic treatment. *Psychoanalytic Study of the Child, 59*, 167–187.

McCallum, M., & Piper, W. E. (1990). The Psychological Mindedness Assessment Procedure. *Psychological Assessment: Journal of Consulting and Clinical Psychology, 2*, 412–418.

McCallum, M., & Piper, W. E. (Eds.). (1997). *Psychological mindedness: A contemporary understanding*. Mahwah, NJ: Erlbaum.

McCallum, M., Piper, W. E., Ogrodniczuk, J. S., & Joyce, A. S. (2003). Relationships among psychological mindedness, alexithymia and outcome in four forms of short-term psychotherapy. *Psychology and Psychotherapy: Theory, Research and Practice, 76*, 133–144.

Miller, A. A., Isaaks, K. S., & Haggard, E. A. (1965). On the nature of the observing function of the ego. *British Journal of Medical Psychology, 38*, 161–169.

Nemiah, J. C., Freyberger, H., & Sifneos, P. E. (1976). Alexithymia: A view of the psychosomatic process. In O. W. Hill (Ed.), *Modern trends in psychosomatic medicine* (Vol. 2, pp. 26–34). London: Butterworths.

Nyklíček, I., & Denollet, J. (2009). Development and evaluation of the Balanced Index of Psychological Mindedness (BIPM). *Psychological Assessment, 21*, 32–44.

Nyklíček, I., Poot, J. C., & van Opstal, J. (2010). Psychological mindedness in relation to personality and coping in a sample of young adult psychiatric patients. *Journal of Clinical Psychology, 66*, 34–45.

Shill, M. A., & Lumley, M. A. (2002). The Psychological Mindedness Scale: Factor structure, convergent validity and gender in a non-psychiatric sample. *Psychology and Psychotherapy: Theory, Research, and Practice, 75*, 131–150.

Taylor, G. J., Bagby, M., & Parker, J. (1989). Psychological-mindedness and the alexithymia construct. *British Journal of Psychiatry, 154*, 731–732.

Trudeau, K. J., & Reich, R. (1995). Correlates of psychological mindedness. *Personality and Individual Differences, 19*, 699–704.

11. Capacity to Construct and Use Internal Standards and Ideals

Bouchard, M. A., & Lecours, S. (2004). Analyzing forms of superego functioning as mentalizations. *International Journal of Psychoanalysis, 85*, 879–896.

Brinkley, C. A., Diamond, P. M., Magaletta, P. R., & Heigel, C. P. (2008). Cross-validation of Levenson's Psychopathy Scale in a sample of federal female inmates. *Assessment, 15*, 464–482.

Carlo, G., Eisenberg, N., & Knight, G. P. (1992). An objective measure of adolescents' prosocial moral reasoning. *Journal of Research on Adolescence, 2*, 331–349.

Cleckley, H. (1976). *The mask of sanity* (5th ed.). St. Louis, MO: Mosby.

Decety, J., & Howard, L. H. (2014). Emotion, morality, and the developing brain. In M. Mikulincer & P. R. Shaver (Eds.), *Mechanisms of social connection: From brain to group* (pp. 105–122). Washington, DC: American Psychological Association.

Dunn, J. (2006). Moral development in early childhood and social interaction in the family. In M. Killen & J. G. Smetana (Eds.), *Handbook of moral development* (pp. 331–350). Mahwah, NJ: Erlbaum.

Eisenberg, N., Duckworth, A. L., Spinrad, T. L., & Valiente, C. (2014). Conscientiousness: Origins in childhood. *Developmental Psychology, 50*, 1331–1349.

Frank, G. (1999). Freud's concept of the superego: Review and assessment. *Psychoanalytic Psychology, 16*, 448–463.

Glenn, A. L., Iyer, R., Graham, J., Koleva, S., & Haidt, J. (2009). Are all types of morality compromised in psychopathy? *Journal of Personality Disorders, 23*, 384–398.

Graham, J., Nosek, B. A., Haidt, J., Iyer, R., Koleva, S., & Ditto, P. H. (2011). Mapping the moral domain. *Journal of Personality and Social Psychology, 101*, 366–385.

Hare, R. D. (1999). *Without conscience: The disturbing world of the psychopaths among us*. New York: Guilford Press.

Hare, R. D. (2003). *The Hare Psychopathy Checklist—Revised* (2nd ed.). Toronto, ON, Canada: Multi-Health Systems.

Hare, R. D., & Neumann, C. S. (2008). Psychopathy as a clinical and empirical construct. *Annual Review of Clinical Psychology, 4*, 217–246.

Hausner, R. (2009). The superego in observing ego functioning. *Psychoanalytic Psychology, 26*, 425–446.

Holmes, J. (2011). Superego: An attachment perspective. *International Journal of Psychoanalysis, 92*, 1221–1240.

Jesperson, K., Kroger, J., & Martinussen, M. (2013). Identity status and moral reasoning: A meta-analysis. *Identity, 13*, 266–280.

Jurist, E. L. (2014). Whatever happened to the superego?: Loewald and the future of psychoanalysis. *Psychoanalytic Psychology, 31*, 489–501.

Kohlberg, L. (1984). *Essays on moral development: Vol. 2. The psychology of moral development*. San Francisco: Harper & Row.

Lagattuta, K. H., & Weller, D. (2014). Interrelations between theory of mind and morality: A developmental perspective. In M. Killen & J. G. Smetana (Eds.), *Handbook of moral development* (2nd ed., pp. 385–407). New York: Psychology Press.

Levenson, M. R., Kiehl, K. A., & Fitzpatrick, C. M. (1995). Assessing psychopathic attributes in a noninstitutionalized population. *Journal of Personality and Social Psychology, 68*, 151–158.

Loewald, H. W. (2007). Internalization, separation, mourning, and the superego. *Psychoanalytic Quarterly, 76*, 1113–1133.

Lynam, D. R., Whiteside, S., & Jones, S. (1999). Self-reported psychopathy: A validation study. *Journal of Personality Assessment, 73*, 110–132.

Narvaez, D., & Lapsley, D. K. (2005). Moral identity, moral functioning, and the development of moral character. In D. M. Bartels, C. W. Bauman, L. J. Skitka, & D. L. Medin (Eds.), *The psychology of learning and motivation* (Vol. 50, pp. 237–274). San Diego, CA: Academic Press.

Patrick, C. J. (Ed.). (2006). *Handbook of psychopathy*. New York: Guilford Press.

Peterson, C., & Seligman, M. E. P. (2004). *Character strengths and virtues*. Washington, DC: American Psychological Association.

Safran, J. D. (2014). A commentary on Elliot Jurist's "Whatever happened to the superego?": Loewald's conceptualization of the superego and the developmental basis of morality. *Psychoanalytic Psychology, 31*, 502–506.

Salekin, R. T., Chen, D. R., Sellbom, M., Lester, W. S., & MacDougall, E. (2014). Examining the factor structure and convergent and discriminant validity of the Levenson Self-Report Psychopathy Scale: Is the two-factor model the best fitting model? *Personality Disorders: Theory, Research, and Treatment, 5*, 289–304.

Schirmann, F. (2013). Invoking the brain in studying morality: A theoretical and historical perspective on the neuroscience of morality. *Theory and Psychology, 23*, 289–304.

Schore, A. N. (2003). *Affect dysregulation and disorders of the self*. New York: Norton.

Shen, Y. L., Carlo, G., & Knight, G. P. (2013). Relations between parental discipline, empathy-related traits, and prosocial moral reasoning: A multicultural examination. *Journal of Early Adolescence, 33*, 994–1021.

Shweder, R. A., Much, N. C., Mahapatra, M., & Park, L. (1997). The "big three" of morality (autonomy, community, and divinity), and the "big three" explanations of suffering. In A. Brandt & P.

Rozin (Eds.), *Morality and health* (pp. 119–169). New York: Routledge.
Spezzano, C., & Gargiulo, G. J. (Eds.). (1997). *Soul on the couch: Spirituality, religion, and morality in contemporary psychoanalysis*. New York: Routledge.

12. Capacity for Meaning and Purpose

Benedik, E. (2009). Representational structures and psychopathology: Analysis of spontaneous descriptions of self and significant others in patients with different mental disorders. *Psychiatria Danubina, 21*, 14–24.
Bers, S. A., Blatt, S. J., Sayward, H. K., & Johnston, R. S. (1993). Normal and pathological aspects of self-descriptions and their change over long-term treatment. *Psychoanalytic Psychology, 10*, 17–37.
Blatt, S. J., Auerbach, J. S., & Levy, K. N. (1997). Mental representations in personality development, psychopathology, and the therapeutic process. *Review of General Psychology, 1*, 351–374.
Blatt, S. J., Bers, S. A., & Schaffer, C. E. (1993). *The assessment of self*. Unpublished manuscript, Yale University, New Haven, CT.
Burwick, S., & Knapp, R. R. (1991). Advances in research using the Personal Orientation Inventory. *Journal of Social Behavior and Personality, 6*, 311–320.
Cloninger, C. R. (1999). *The Temperament and Character Inventory—Revised*. St Louis, MO: Center for Psychobiology of Personality, Washington University.
Csikszentmihalyi, M. (1990). *Flow: The psychology of optimal experience*. New York: Harper & Row.
Davis, D. E., Hook, J. N., Worthington, E. L., Van Tongeren, D. R., Gartner, A. L., Jennings, D. J., & Emmons, R. A. (2011). Relational humility: Conceptualizing and measuring humility as a personality judgment. *Journal of Personality Assessment, 93*, 225–234.
Emmons, R. A., & McCullough, M. E. (Eds.). (2004). *The psychology of gratitude*. New York: Oxford University Press.
Fogarty, G. J. (1994). Using the Personal Orientation Inventory to measure change in student self-actualization. *Personality and Individual Differences, 17*, 435–439.
Greene, R. R., Graham, S. A., & Morano, C. (2010). Erikson's healthy personality, societal institutions, and Holocaust survivors. *Journal of Human Behavior in the Social Environment, 20*, 489–506.
Habermas, T., & Bluck, S. (2000). Getting a life: The emergence of the life story in adolescence. *Psychological Bulletin, 126*, 748–769.
Helm, F. L. (2004). Hope is curative. *Psychoanalytic Psychology, 21*, 554–566.
Hill, P. L., & Turiano, N. A. (2014). Purpose in life as a predictor of mortality across adulthood. *Psychological Science, 25*, 1482–1486.
Jackson, S. A., & Eklund, R. C. (2002). Assessing flow in physical activity: The Flow State Scale–2 and Dispositional Flow Scale–2. *Journal of Sport and Exercise Psychology, 24*, 133–150.
Johnson, J. A., Kaiser, H. N., Skarin, E. M., & Ross, S. R. (2014). The Dispositional Flow Scale–2 as a measure of autotelic personality: An examination of criterion-related validity. *Journal of Personality Assessment, 96*, 465–470.
Liechty, D. (2003). Who in their right mind wants war?: Violence, death, and meaning. *Psychoanalytic Review, 90*, 440–456.
McAdams, D. P. (2013). The psychological self as actor, agent, and author. *Perspectives on Psychological Science, 8*, 272–295.
Midlarsky, E., & Kahana, E. (2007). Altruism, well-being, and mental health at midlife. In S. G. Post (Ed.), *Altruism and health: Perspectives from empirical research* (pp. 56–69). Oxford, UK: Oxford University Press.
Miller, L. (1998). Ego autonomy and the healthy personality: Psychodynamics, cognitive style, and clinical applications. *Psychoanalytic Review, 85*, 423–448.
Park, N., & Peterson, C. (2009). Achieving and sustaining a good life. *Perspectives on Psychological Science, 4*, 422–428.
Peterson, C., & Seligman, M. E. P. (2004). *Character strengths and virtues*. Washington, DC: American Psychological Association.
Shostrom, E. L., & Knapp, R. R. (1966). The relationship of a measure of self-actualisation (POI) to a measure of pathology (MMPI) and to therapeutic growth. *American Journal of Psychotherapy, 20*, 193–202.
Stern, B. L., Caligor, E., Clarkin, J. F., Critchfield, K. L., Horz, S., MacCornack, V., Lenzenweger, M. F., Kernberg, O. F. (2010). Structured Interview of Personality Organization (STIPO): Preliminary psychometrics in a clinical sample. *Journal of Personality Assessment, 92*(1), 35–44.
Tangney, J. P., Stuewig, J., & Mashek, D. J. (2007). Moral emotions and moral behavior. *Annual Review of Psychology, 58*, 345–372.
Waldron, S., Moscovitz, S., Lundin, J., Helm, F. L., Jemerin, J., & Gorman, B. (2011). Evaluating the outcomes of psychotherapies: The Personality Health Index. *Psychoanalytic Psychology, 28*(3), 363–388.
Warner, M. S. (2009). Defense or actualization?: Reconsidering the role of processing, self, and agency within Rogers' theory of personality. *Person Centered and Experiential Psychotherapies, 8*, 109–126.
Wilson, T. D. (2009). Know thyself. *Perspectives on Psychological Science, 4*, 384–389.

CHAPTER 3

Symptom Patterns: The Subjective Experience

S Axis

CHAPTER EDITORS

Emanuela Mundo, MD **John Allison O'Neil, MD**

CONSULTANTS

Richard Chefetz, MD
Christine A. Courtois, PhD
Jack Drescher, MD
Giovanni Foresti, MD, PhD
Michael Garrett, MD
William H. Gottdiener, PhD
Marvin Hurvich, PhD
Richard Kluft, MD
Brian Koehler, PhD
Matthias Michal, MD
Kevin Moore, PsyD
Humberto Persano, MD, PhD
Babak Roshanaei-Moghaddam, MD
Golan Shahar, PhD
Pratyusha Tummala-Narra, PhD

Introduction

This chapter refers mostly to the symptom descriptions of the *Diagnostic and Statistical Manual of Mental Disorders*, fifth edition (DSM-5; American Psychiatric Association, 2013) and of the *International Classification of Diseases*, 10th revision (ICD-10; World Health Organization, 1992), although earlier versions of both systems (particularly the earlier DSMs; American Psychiatric Association, 1968, 1980, 1994, 2000) are referenced as well. The intent is to elaborate on a patient's subjective experience of the symptom pattern. We depict individual subjectivity in terms of affective patterns, mental content, accompanying somatic states, and associated relationship patterns.

To have an overview of the mental health field, it is essential, in addition to simply listing their symptoms, to consider the subjective lived experience of people with psychiatric disorders. Subjective experiences have been particularly neglected, since the usual methodologies of "descriptive" or "categorical" psychiatry are not adequate to reflect the complexity of human subjective experience in pathological and non-pathological conditions that may need attention and/or treatment. People in the same diagnostic category, with similar symptoms, may still vary widely in their subjective experience, and these variations have implications for treatment.

International and North American Taxonomies

We provide both ICD-10 and DSM-5 listings for a number of reasons. PDM-2, like its predecessor (PDM Task Force, 2006), is a collaborative effort of North American and international associations; DSM-5 has adopted a number of ICD-10's innovations; the United States has finally moved from ICD-9 codes to ICD-10 codes for recording DSM diagnoses; finally, ICD-11 is scheduled to appear in 2017, and so familiarity with ICD-10 will prepare the reader for its successor. When ICD changed its first coding character from a number to a letter, it enormously expanded the number of available codes. This is reflected in the replacement of the all-purpose "not otherwise specified" (NOS) of DSM-III and -IV by the "other specified" (last digit 8) and "unspecified" (last digit 9) listings of DSM-5. DSM-5 has also followed a number of ICD-10 reclusterings, such as separating out obsessive–compulsive disorder (OCD) and posttraumatic stress disorder (PTSD) from the anxiety disorders.

PDM-2's S Axis adopts most of this reclustering, but with one major modification: A second level of grouping is introduced. The lower-level groups correspond largely to those of DSM-5. The second level would correspond to what is implicit but unstated in DSM-5 and explicit in ICD-10. We regard the ICD and DSM characterizations of psychological problems as useful starting points for elucidating aspects of mental and emotional suffering. A deeper exploration would be expected to merge some diagnostic categories and differentiate others.

This chapter on symptom patterns is placed third in our overall diagnostic profile for adulthood because such patterns are best understood in the context of a patient's overall personality structure and profile of mental functioning. Symptoms such as anxiety, depression, and/or impulse-control problems may be part of an overall emotional challenge. For example, problems with impulse control and mood regulation are common in patients with the larger developmental deficit of inability to represent (symbolize) a wide range of affects and wishes.

In some instances, notably those in which there has been long-standing psychoanalytic scholarship, we comment on psychodynamic understandings of a given symptom pattern and include general implications for treatment, transference, and countertransference.

Differential Diagnosis of Certain Subjective Experiences

Some symptoms, such as fear, anxiety, and sadness, are universal, and consequently also common in most psychiatric disorders and nonpsychopathological conditions. Others are rarer and specific (e.g., tactile hallucinations), and so a given symptom may be compatible with a very long or very short differential diagnosis. Symptoms may have specific interactions, such as those delusions that derive from hallucinations. These anomalous subjective experiences are most often psychological ("psychogenic," "functional"), but virtually all may be organic in origin, and all may be the result of complex interactions between psychological factors and the biological background. Thus substance-mediated symptoms and symptoms caused by another medical condition should always be considered. Some other examples are the following:

- *Anxiety and depression.* These are the most common unpleasant subjective states and may appear in almost any disorder. When they are relatively monosymptomatic, pronounced, or specific, an anxiety or depressive disorder can be diagnosed. When their absence seems perplexing, then a search for a "primary gain" or for a specific mental functioning (examples include emotional blunting, isolation of affect, *la belle indifférence*, dissociation of affect, etc.) is in order.

- *Insomnia.* This is a frequent condition. Early morning awakening is especially indicative of major depression. Difficulty in falling asleep is common in anxiety disorders (e.g., generalized anxiety disorder), but may also be motivated by a dread of falling asleep because of increased flashbacks while falling asleep or subsequent nightmares in posttraumatic pathology.

- *Somatoform symptoms.* These may be direct bodily expressions of emotional pain, especially in persons not psychologically minded. Symptoms may include tactile posttraumatic flashbacks of real past events, whose origins are murky because autobiographical memory and context are missing. They may be somatic "betrayals" of unacceptable repressed impulses, as in classic conversion disorders. Negative somatoform symptoms, such as conversion anesthesia for sharp pain, commonly accompany self-mutilation and worsen its prognosis.

- *Hallucinations.* These symptoms carry a wide differential diagnosis. These may be (in decreasing order of frequency) auditory, tactile, visual, olfactory, or gustatory. Auditory hallucinations may occur in toxic or epileptic psychosis, schizophrenia, brief psychotic disorder, mania, melancholia, PTSD, dissociative identity disorder (DID), or very severe personality disorders, without calling for another diagnosis. Visual hallucinations may also occur in many of these disorders and in depersonalization disorder (as in out-of-body experience). Tactile hallucinations (negative and positive) are especially common as components of posttraumatic and dissociative psychopathology. Olfactory and gustatory hallucinations are likewise often posttraumatic or dissociative, but may also be organic.

- *Delusions.* These may occur in toxic or epileptic psychosis, schizophrenia, brief psychotic disorder, mania, melancholia, delusional disorder, or very severe personality disorders (transiently), without calling for another diagnosis. Some delusions are paired with hallucinations. Hallucinations of persecutory voices may lead to persecutory delusions. Hallucinating one's own thoughts aloud may lead to the delusion of thought broadcasting. The negative hallucination of feeling unreal or alien may lead to the delusion of being an extraterrestrial. Somatic hallucinations may lead to delusions of infestation. And so on.

- *Amnesia.* This may occur in organic conditions, but also commonly in PTSD, dissociative disorders, and borderline personality disorder (BPD) (transiently).

- *Depersonalization/derealization.* These occur, of course, in the disorder itself, but may also complicate schizophrenia, severe depression, PTSD, panic attacks, DID, and severe personality disorders (transiently).

- *Suicidal ideation, behavior, attempts.* These are typical "cross-sectional" symptoms, attitudes, and behaviors; thus they may be present in many disorders at different times, as most of the psychodynamic and biological literature points out. Suicidal risk should be carefully assessed for any patient, regardless of the "primary diagnosis" or the patient's primary treatment request. In addition, the subjective experience of suicidal thoughts or behavior may vary widely within the same patient in the course of his or her life or treatment, and it should always be considered as one of the primary risk factors for suicidal attempts. Some guidelines for the clinical assessment for suicidal risk (in various clinical conditions) follow:
    - Presence of suicidal or homicidal ideation, intent, or plans
    - Ready access to means for suicide, and the lethality of those means
    - Presence of psychotic symptoms, especially command hallucinations
    - Presence of suicidal or homicidal alters in DID
    - Distinction between suicidal intent and parasuicidal intent (especially regarding self-injury)
    - Presence of serious alcohol or other substance misuse
    - History and seriousness of previous self-harm attempts
    - Family history of, or recent exposure to, suicide
    - Absence of a significant network of supportive relationships and social services

Context of Subjective Experience: Time

Symptoms may indicate what disorder a person has, but a psychodynamic practitioner is also interested in the role symptoms play in the personal experience of a patient's overall life history. Symptoms indicate a diagnosis, but they also tell a story. They express how someone characteristically copes with experience. They have a temporality: Why now? And how does this relate to this person's past and future?

Developmental Context

Even in adults, developmentally relevant aspects of symptom patterns interact with personality variables. A depression in an elderly woman may be experienced quite differently from a depression in a woman in her thirties, and it may consequently call for a different therapeutic approach. A formulation and treatment plan should recognize such age-related differences in addition to the patient's history, individual life/relational events, and social, economic and cultural context.

Temporal Aspects of the Current Condition

Why are these symptoms occurring now, and what do they mean? One technique is to wonder about the first and worst: If a man is depressed, when does he remember being depressed like this for the first time? And is this the most depressed he has ever felt? The first and worst may be extended to thoughts and interpersonal conundrums. Does he remember when he was first concerned about this question? And was he once even more concerned or worried about it than at present? When does he remember being in this sort of interpersonal conflict for the first time? And was it ever more serious than at present?

Bimodal Symptoms

Some symptoms were present at some discrete time in the past and reappear today. What was the trigger? It may have been any item of "unfinished business" (fixation) from a person's past, which becomes reactivated under stressful conditions or specific life events—regression to a point of fixation—especially if the trigger has some thematic affinity to the original item. Sexual molestation in earlier childhood may have been perplexing, but may become more overtly traumatic retrospectively when puberty arrives, and the sexual intent suddenly becomes experientially clear (Freud's *Nachträglichkeit*); or it may have been successfully repressed until a patient's child reaches the age at which the patient was first abused.

Interpersonal Functioning

The family of origin is the original crucible where relationship patterns originate, whether in "objective fact" or in the patient's personal perception. A simple way to elicit the subjective experience of relationship patterns with historical pertinence is to wonder how the patient relates/related to and takes after his or her mother and father. Contrasts sometimes emerge first, but it is worth pursuing identifications, as the most clinically pertinent ones are the ones most regretted: "I *hate* the fact that Mother always put herself first, and I find myself doing the same thing. . . ." Counterintuitive questions may also bear fruit: "How does your boyfriend take after your father?" Even less obvious: "How does your boyfriend take after your mother?"—"Absolutely not at all! What a stupid question! He's everything I always wanted my mother to be!" Siblings: "Who was Mother's favorite? Father's favorite? And then who was the next favorite? Who was most like Mother? Like Father?" And so on. This type of questioning helps bring to light how primary relationships affect the patient's current subjective experience.

Comorbidity

We do not assume that the presence of multiple symptom expressions inevitably constitutes "comorbidity" between different mental health disorders; we believe that more commonly, they are expressions of a basic complex disturbance of mental functioning.

Each person's symptom patterns, while sharing common features with similar patterns in other persons, have a unique signature. The clinical illustrations within each section of this chapter are intended to provide examples of specific patterns of internal experiences of some patients. They are not meant to comprise a definitive or exhaustive listing. The clinician is encouraged to capture each patient's unique subjective experience in a narrative form by considering the applicable descriptive patterns. In some instances, research findings support the observations that follow; in others, in the absence of empirical work on the topic, we have drawn on the combined clinical experience of therapists with expertise in each area covered. For example, clinical expertise has led us to include the "diagnosis" of complex PTSD.

Our approach also includes consideration of the biological contributions to some of these patterns and may even facilitate meaningful exploration of biological correlates for a variety of mental health disorders, as well as the complex interaction between psychological and biological factors. We see mind and brain as in a dialogic relationship.

Psychological Experiences That May Require Clinical Attention

For the purposes of this manual, we have thought it important to make room for a discussion of the subjective experiences of particular groups whose members may come for mental health services because of difficulties associated with certain situations that are not pathological conditions. Consequently, this discussion is added as an appendix to this chapter's main listing of the S Axis. The three groupings are demographic: ethnic, linguistic, and/or religious minorities; lesbian, gay, and bisexual communities; and those with gender incongruence. This last condition—called gender identity disorder in ICD-10 and DSM-IV/DSM-IV-TR, relabeled as gender dysphoria in DSM-5, and called gender incongruence here—is no longer considered by most in the field as a disorder. See the World Professional Association for Transgender Health (WPATH, 2011) for further discussion and standards of care for this population.

Table 3.1 provides an overview of the S Axis, listing the sections and subsections of the various conditions we address in this chapter.

S1 Predominantly Psychotic Disorders

We have provided a concordance (see Table 3.2, pp. 245–250) between the PDM-2 classification and the ICD-10 and DSM-5 classifications of psychotic disorders (apart from psychoses related to mood disorders). The most notable changes from DSM-IV and -IV-TR to DSM-5 are the following:

1. *Schizophrenia.* This is no longer diagnosed by subtype (paranoid, disorganized/hebephrenic, catatonic, undifferentiated, residual).

2. *Catatonia.* This is now an independent specifier to be appended to another mental disorder or to another medical disorder. ICD-10 has no provision for catatonia associated with a mental disorder other than schizophrenia.

3. *Schizotypal personality disorder.* DSM-5 and ICD-10 have yet to decide what to do with this condition. ICD-7, -8, and -9 and DSM-II listed simple schizophrenia; DSM-III recategorized it as schizotypal personality disorder and moved it to the personality disorders. Just as for schizophreniform disorder, this move was intended to reduce the premature diagnosis of schizophrenia. Most researchers in schizophrenia, however, continued to regard it as within the "schizophrenia spectrum." Although ICD-10 retained simple schizophrenia, it ambiguously added schizotypal disorder to its schizophrenia section (despite the two disorders' historically naming the same entity), but not to its personality disorder section. DSM-5 continues to list schizotypal personality disorder as a personality disorder, but now double-lists schizotypal (personality) disorder among the schizophrenia spectrum disorders (note the parentheses

TABLE 3.1. Adult Symptom Patterns: The Subjective Experience—S Axis

S1 Predominantly psychotic disorders
- S11 Brief psychotic disorder (Hysterical psychosis, Bouffée Délirante Polymorphe Aigüe)
- S12 Delusional disorder (Pure paranoia)
- S13 Schizotypal disorder (Simple schizophrenia, Residual schizophrenia)
- S14 Schizophrenia and schizoaffective disorder

S2 Mood disorders
- S21 Persistent depressive disorder (dysthymia)
- S22 Major depressive disorder
- S23 Cyclothymic disorder
- S24 Bipolar disorders
- S25 Maternal affective disorders

S3 Disorders related primarily to anxiety
- S31 Anxiety disorders
  - S31.1 Specific phobias
  - S31.2 Social phobia
  - S31.3 Agoraphobia and panic disorder
  - S31.4 Generalized anxiety disorder
- S32 Obsessive–compulsive and related disorders
  - S32.1 Obsessive–compulsive disorder
  - S32.2 Body dysmorphic disorder (Dysmorphophobia)
  - S32.3 Hoarding disorder
  - S32.4 Trichotillomania and excoriation disorder

S4 Event- and stressor-related disorders
- S41 Trauma- and stressor-related disorders
  - S41.1 Adjustment disorders
  - S41.2 Acute and posttraumatic stress disorders
  - S41.3 Complex posttraumatic stress disorder
- S42 Dissociative disorders
  - S42.1 Depersonalization/derealization disorder
  - S42.2 Dissociative amnesia ± fugue
  - S42.3 Dissociative identity disorder and other specified dissociative disorder–1
- S43 Conversion disorder

S5 Somatic symptom and related disorders
- S51 Somatic symptom disorder
- S52 Illness anxiety disorder (Hypochondriasis)
- S53 Factitious disorders

S6 Specific symptom disorders
- S61 Feeding and eating disorders
- S62 Sleep–wake disorders
- S63 Sexual dysfunctions
- S64 Paraphilic disorders
- S65 Disruptive, impulse-control, and conduct disorders

(continued)

TABLE 3.1. *(continued)*

S7	**Disorders related to addiction and to other medical conditions**		
	S71	Addictions	
		S71.1	Substance-related disorders
		S71.2	Behavioral addictions (Gambling, Internet addiction, Sex addiction)
	S72	Mental disorders due to another medical condition	
		S72.1	HIV-related neurocognitive disorder
SApp	**Appendix: Psychological experiences that may require clinical attention**		
	SApp1	Demographic minority populations (ethnic, cultural, linguistic, religious, political)	
	SApp2	Lesbian, gay, and bisexual populations	
	SApp3	Gender incongruence	

around "personality"), capitulating to the historical "wisdom" of the simple schizophrenia diagnosis. The first PDM made no reference at all to "schizotypal," reflecting the absence of the term in the psychodynamic literature, but did discuss schizoid personality disorder. Finally, PDM-2, supporting the existence of both psychotic personality functioning and major psychotic disorders, includes schizotypal personality in the P Axis and schizotypal disorder in the S Axis. Within the current P Axis, the psychodynamics of schizoid and schizotypal personalities are addressed together, despite the fact that these conditions have never been considered diagnostically related in the past; and schizotypal disorder is mentioned very briefly here, given its historic roots in simple schizophrenia and its current "double listing" in both DSM-5 and ICD-10.

4. *Shared psychotic disorder* (*folie à deux*). This is no longer listed in DSM-5, though it persists in ICD-10.

We focus on the most pertinent groupings: brief psychotic disorder (acute transient psychotic episodes), delusional disorder ("pure paranoia"), and schizophrenia and schizoaffective disorder. Before describing the different diagnostic categories, we offer a methodological premise that may be helpful to the beginning professionals we regard as among our primary audience.

Psychosis prompts a conflicting blend of horror and pity, cruelty and generosity in outside observers. The seeming alien quality of psychotic experience may persuade the clinician to give up trying to empathize with the patient's subjective experience. Clinicians may phobically dismiss subjective experience and seek refuge in the self-reassuring certainty of diagnostic criteria and categorical classification. They would do well to train themselves to delay jumping to premature nosological conclusions, which then impede their capacity to appreciate their patient's subjective experience. Clinicians as participant observers must immerse themselves in the seemingly odd and puzzling experience of the patient so as to rediscover the clinical wisdom embedded in Harry Stack Sullivan's (1962) dictum: "We are all more simply human than otherwise."

S11 Brief Psychotic Disorder (Hysterical Psychosis, Bouffée Délirante Polymorphe Aigüe)

The S11 diagnosis unifies in a single nosological category a wide series of psychotic conditions variously classified in the past, including, among others, benign schizophreniform psychosis, hysterical psychosis, psychogenic psychosis, benign stupor, and acute reactive psychosis.

ICD-10 lists F23, acute and transient psychotic disorder, with four subtypes, two of which are linked to the French diagnosis *bouffée délirante polymorphe aigüe* ("acute polymorphous delusional puff"). Some episodes were reinterpreted as "micropsychotic episodes" in BPD (DSM-5, BPD criterion 9), though this only works in the presence of BPD/emotionally dysregulated borderline personality pattern. As "dissociation" has generally come to replace what had been "hysteria," some prefer to consider brief psychotic disorder as "dissociative psychotic episode."

In order to define the characteristics of this diagnosis, ICD-10 stresses acuteness of onset (2 weeks or less from nonpsychotic premorbid functioning and the current clinical syndrome); the polymorphous features of symptoms (tumultuous, unstable, and rapidly shifting subjective experience); a precipitating stressor (a major life event such as bereavement, loss of work, divorce, financial collapse, car accident, psychic trauma from torture, terrorism, or war, etc.); and complete recovery within 3 months.

DSM-5's brief psychotic disorder describes a condition with abrupt, unexpected onset lasting less than a month and characterized by delusions, hallucinations, formal thought disorder, or grossly disorganized behavior.

What all these named conditions have in common are (1) an acute, rich, polymorphous clinical presentation and (2) a relatively brief and self-limited clinical course. The latter characteristic—clinical course—is critical for differential diagnosis, though even this apparently simple characteristic may be difficult to ascertain exactly.

Onset of symptoms is generally inferred from personal and familiar narratives, which can be biased by many factors, and their apparent remission can be influenced by several misleading factors, including a patient's wish to seal over the psychotic episode and the family's collusion regarding the psychotic episode has ended. Once again, the clinician's flexibility, openness of mind, and professional caution remain essential ingredients for the correct use of this diagnosis.

Brief psychotic disorder is identified by the presence of symptoms of schizophrenia (e.g., delusions, hallucinations, disorganized thinking, speech, or behavior) for at least 1 day but less than 1 month, followed by a return to premorbid levels of functioning. Although brief, this disorder can be severe and presents a high risk for suicide. Personality disorders at the low borderline level of organization may predispose the individual to the development of this condition. Average age of onset is the late 20s to early 30s.

Hysterical psychosis is described in the psychoanalytic literature as occurring usually (but not necessarily) in individuals with "hysterical character" (now called "histrionic" or "dysregulated"), and emerging within the context of specific severe stress and traumatic events, or as a transference reaction in an intensive psychoanalytic therapy (this last situation has been defined as "transference psychosis"). In hysterical psychosis, we may find severe distortions of reality testing, including delusions and even hallucinations, but no signs or symptoms generally attributed to schizophrenia (i.e., formal thought disorders). When this condition occurs in a treatment context, it may be confined there, or it may spill over into the patient's ongoing life outside. It is a psychotic condition that can be addressed psychotherapeutically.

As with any disorder, the clinician ought to be attentive to possible underlying dynamics: Do the symptoms seem to be obscuring or modifying some affective state? Does the transient flight from reality testing seem to be motivated by denial: (a reality from which the patient is fleeing), or rather by wishful thinking (a wished-for reality *to* which the patient is fleeing)?

S12 Delusional Disorder ("Pure Paranoia")

Emil Kraepelin divided the five major psychoses (catatonia, hebephrenia, mania, melancholia, paranoia) into two groups, "manic–depressive insanity" (mania and melancholia) and "dementia praecox" (catatonia, hebephrenia, paranoia), on the basis of clinical course: dementia praecox with a chronic deteriorating course, and manic–depressive insanity with return to a normal state between episodes. But there were some paranoid "leftover" individuals, with clinical courses more seemingly akin to those with manic–depressive insanity than to those with "precocious dementia." Thus those with delusional disorder, or "pure paranoia," have a delusion or a structured system of delusions, but rarely hallucinations (if present, they are related to the primary delusion), never with formal thought disorder, catatonia, wild mood swings, or chronic deteriorating course. In ICD-7, -8, and -9 and in DSM-II, "paranoid states" included (pure) paranoia and involutional paranoid state (also known as involutional paraphrenia), developing in later middle age, but the latter has fallen into disuse and disappeared from current nosologies. The former remains as delusional disorder.

Delusional disorder is diagnosed when an individual has one or more delusions for a month or more that may be nonbizarre (delusions with plausible themes and situations that might conceivably occur; e.g., being followed) or bizarre (entirely implausible beliefs that are under no conditions conceivably true). Other positive symptoms of schizophrenia are not present unless related directly to the delusion(s). Mood episodes, if present, are brief and/or transient. Levels of functioning and behavior vary, and may appear relatively intact in life areas unrelated to the delusion(s). Although functional impairment may be significant, functioning is generally less impaired and disorganized than that of individuals with a diagnosis of schizophrenia.

DSM-5 includes five distinct subtypes of delusional disorder: (1) erotomanic (e.g., the patient believes a prominent person is in love with him or her, and may sometimes get into legal troubles as a result of misdirected amorous pursuits); (2) grandiose (e.g., the patient believes he or she is specially talented and should be famous); (3) jealous (e.g., the patient believes his or her partner is unfaithful); (4) persecutory (e.g., the patient believes he or she is being plotted against, harassed, or having life goals obstructed; such patients may seek legal redress for imagined wrongs); and (5) somatic (e.g., the patient believes his or her body is ugly, disgusting, affected by a severe or terminal disease, or infested by parasites). DSM-5 also includes the obligatory mixed and unspecified subtypes. The persecutory type is most common and may lead to violence against persons delusionally perceived as persecutors. Violence may also occasionally occur in the jealous and erotomanic types. Depending on the subtype, other symptoms commonly observed in those with delusional disorders are ideas of reference, irritable or dysphoric mood, and violent behavior.

Delusional disorder is more common among individuals with personality disorders at the low borderline level of organization. The age at onset varies, ranging from adolescence to late in life. The course of the illness is also variable, ranging from full remissions to repeated relapses over a lifetime.

A shared delusional disorder (*folie à deux*) occurs when two closely related individuals, who generally live together, have identical delusions. Typically, the delusions originate in the person who is more dominant in the relationship and are internalized by the more submissive and/or dependent individual, previously nonpsychotic. The submissive person's delusions often disappear when the relationship is interrupted. Very little is known about the prevalence of this disorder, and many cases likely go unrecognized. The course is variable, often depending on the length and intensity of the relationship within which it occurs.

S13 Schizotypal Disorder (Simple Schizophrenia, Residual Schizophrenia)

Following Kraepelin, whose focus was on the acute presenting syndromes of dementia praecox (catatonia, hebephrenia, paranoia), Eugen Bleuler focused more on the residual nonpsychotic interepisodic symptoms, which were summarized as his "four A's." All three subtypes were characterized by blunted or inappropriate Affect; residual catatonia was seen as Ambivalence (paralysis of decision); residual hebephrenia involved mild loosening of Associations; residual paranoia was characterized as Autism, by which Bleuler meant idiosyncratic thought and social isolation. This constellation formed the basis of the diagnosis of simple schizophrenia: It denoted someone who seemed to have residual (or interepisode) schizophrenia, but in the absence of a history of any acute psychotic episode.

The reader is referred to the discussion of schizoid (and schizotypal) personalities in Chapter 1 on the P Axis for further details.

S14 Schizophrenia and Schizoaffective Disorder

Schizophrenia is a "functional" syndrome of signs and symptoms leading to dysfunction in the context of an observed clinical course. "Functional" implies the absence of any co-occurring medical conditions that may explain the clinical picture. Signs and symptoms are regarded as "positive" (something present that shouldn't be there) and "negative" (something missing that should be present). Positive signs and symptoms include delusions, hallucinations, disorganized speech, and disorganized or catatonic behavior. Negative signs and symptoms include diminished emotional expressiveness, abulia (inability to make decisions), apathy, withdrawal, and anhedonia. The various signs and symptoms lead to significant deterioration in personal, social, and occupational functioning. Signs/symptoms and dysfunction must be present for at least 6 months.

The attention of psychotic individuals is commonly focused on their internal reality at the expense of external reality, such that their affect and gestures appear discordant with external reality and thus socially inappropriate. Other common symptoms of schizophrenia include depression, anxiety, anger, phobias, depersonalization, derealization, sleep–wake pattern disturbances, and social incompetence.

Schizophrenia is best considered a clinical syndrome with different etiologies rather than a single discrete illness. Currently there are no radiological, laboratory, or psychometric tests that are specific for it, even though a few neuroimaging studies have pointed out some modifications common among individuals with a diagnosis of schizophrenia as compared to controls.

The "stress–vulnerability" model of psychosis holds that conditions arise from the interaction of a wide variety of biological, social, and psychological stressors in individuals with varying degrees of predisposing biological, psychological, and/or social vulnerabilities. There is also strong evidence that adverse events occurring during childhood, such as physical or sexual abuse or bullying, predispose to the development of psychosis.

An increased incidence of schizophrenia has also been correlated with perinatal abnormalities and also with atypical craniofacial morphologies consistent with a neurological insult occurring early in life. Incidence in females tends to be slightly lower than in males, and the prognosis is slightly better. Malnutrition in children who survived the Dutch Hunger Winter of 1944–1945 was correlated with an increased incidence of schizophrenia in this group decades later. Schizophrenia has been associated with increased paternal age, maternal diabetes, perinatal hypoxia, urban living, poverty, and Vitamin D deficiency. All these findings suggest that a prenatal or perinatal insult to early brain development may predispose some individuals to psychosis. More than 100 genes show a weak correlation with psychosis, while a small number of genes appear highly correlated with psychosis and schizophrenia, suggesting a familial susceptibility to the disorder. Despite these genetic correlations, most people who develop a schizophrenic illness do not have a positive family history for psychoses.

On the other hand, gene expression is epigenetically modified by environmental factors. As an example, Tienari and colleagues (2002) studied a cohort of adopted-away children with biological mothers diagnosed with schizophrenia, but raised in the different (positive) environment of their adoptive families. In these adoptees, the prevalence of schizophrenia was 1.49% (slightly higher than the 1% incidence in the general population). This finding suggests that sharing genes with a psychotic parent increases the probability of developing schizophrenia. If, however, the adoptees were raised in families rated as "disturbed," the prevalence of psychosis increased to 13.04%, indicating a strong interaction between genes and environmental factors.

The onset of schizophrenia usually occurs between the late teens and mid-30s, and may be either abrupt or insidious. Most patients experience a prodromal phase in which those close to the patients describe them as if they were "slipping away." Contrary to the common misconception that the prognosis of schizophrenia is invariably poor, outcome is highly variable. In a 37-year follow-up of 289 patients, Ciompi (1980) found that approximately 50% of the cases recovered or were only mildly symptomatic by the end of follow-up; the other 50% had moderate to severe symptoms. Patients taking medication frequently relapse when they stop. Long-term follow-up studies, however, indicate that patients with long-term recovery from their symptoms are more likely to have stopped taking antipsychotics than those who continued on them. Two possible explanations for this apparent contradiction are that (1) patients with a better prognosis are able to stop medication without decompensating or (2) for some patients, stopping medication is preferable for their long-term prognosis to remaining on medication for decades. Suicide risk in patients with schizophrenia is high: 20% attempt suicide, and 5% succeed.

Schizophreniform disorder is a DSM-5 diagnostic label intended to minimize the premature diagnosis of schizophrenia and schizoaffective disorder. Descriptively, it is identical to schizophrenia except for its short course (less than 6 months) and less severe impairment in social and occupational functioning. Roughly two-thirds of patients diagnosed with schizophreniform disorder will progress to a final diagnosis of schizophrenia or schizoaffective disorder. Because it is hard to control for the effects of good, timely treatment approaches, these patterns should be interpreted cautiously. Most studies are not able to ascertain whether each case is approached in an optimal manner (e.g., psychosocial/familial support, medication, psychotherapeutic work, reduction of stressors likely to precipitate symptoms). Developing countries have higher prevalence rates of schizophreniform disorder than developed countries.

Schizoaffective disorder is "located" between schizophrenia and bipolar disorder, and is arbitrarily classified with schizophrenia rather than bipolar disorder. Symptoms meeting the criteria for a mood disorder episode (manic, depressive, or mixed) should be present for the majority of the active or residual phase of the disorder, together with symptoms of schizophrenia. Since mania and depression may have psychotic features (hallucinations, delusions, etc.), most often mood-congruent but also mood-incongruent, the patient must experience hallucinations or delusions without mood symptoms for at least 2 weeks in order to "qualify" for the schizophrenic component of the disorder. Onset may occur between adolescence and late in life, but schizoaffective disorder most commonly begins in early adulthood. The condition appears to be less common than schizophrenia. As with schizophrenia, there are indications of a genetic component that predisposes a person to developing schizoaffective disorder.

Recent genetic studies of individuals with schizophrenia, schizoaffective disorder, and bipolar disorder with psychotic symptoms suggest a number of common genes for "psychosis," regardless of the diagnostic category involved. But genes are only part of the story. Neuroscientific research underscores the importance of brain plasticity: Different brain areas change in structure and function, depending on environmental context and life events, including psychotherapeutic treatment. Thus genetic inheritance is one issue, but whether and how this is expressed in psychosis will depend on what happens in a person's life.

The Subjective Experience of Schizophrenic Psychosis

While the previous depictions of the various nonaffective psychotic disorders identify qualities that are observable in those afflicted, they do not capture the internal world of someone suffering from any of these conditions. Psychological treatments presume sufficient overlap between ordinary mental life and psychopathological states to allow the clinician some empathic understanding of the subjective experience of psychosis. Melanie Klein's formulation of the paranoid–schizoid position that dominates early mental life has been found useful in understanding the primitive mental states expressed in both psychotic and nonpsychotic conditions. The subjective experience of psychosis is such that the usual four subcategories—affect, cognition, somatic states, and interpersonal relations—do not suffice.

Ego Boundaries and Experience of Self

A person generally experiences the self as a first-person "I" with a personal point of view embedded in an ongoing experience of the real world. Thoughts, feelings, and perceptions are tacitly felt to be one's own, without the need for metacognitive self-conscious reflection to establish a link between ongoing experience and the self. One's sense of self and experience of the world are seamlessly intertwined. In psychosis, this natural un-self-conscious relationship between one's own internal world and the perceived world is disturbed. The full-bodied first-person "I" fades and is replaced by an uncomfortably insubstantial "lightness of being."

Psychotic individuals often report a variety of anomalous subjective states and disturbances in their first-person experience of the self, in both the prodromal and acute phases of the illness. These disturbances occur along a continuum in multiple domains, may wax and wane, or may remain relatively stable over extended periods. A classic expression is the blurring of ego boundaries. Such boundaries include differences among thoughts, feelings, and perceptions, and the boundaries between self and environment, self and others—the appreciation of where one begins and ends, of what is "me" versus "not me," and so on. The boundary of the self may be so permeable that one's identity merges with someone else's, or one becomes transparent, vulnerable, or an open book, easily invaded by others. Loss of the boundary between thought and perception may lead to hearing one's own thoughts aloud, which invites the delusion that others can hear one's thoughts (thought broadcasting), and read and control one's mind.

Psychotic individuals may lose their sense of personal agency, doubting that they are the originators and authors of their thoughts. In more extreme cases, they may believe that their thoughts are being inserted into their mind by an outside agency. They may say, "I feel like a ghost," or "Do I really exist? Am I really here?" or "It feels like someone else is thinking my thoughts."

As the self fades, a pathological hyperreflexive self-awareness takes hold. Instead of a life where much in daily experience is familiar and can be comfortably taken for granted, now little is automatic or goes unquestioned. All life experience is simultaneously accompanied by a constant referral to a fragmented internal experience. For example, instead of simply enjoying the redness of a rose, a psychotic man might reflexively ask himself, "Why is red called 'red'?" When the natural automaticity of the familiar erodes, the psychological basis for opinion, motivation, and action is lost. Nothing can be assumed; everything has to be considered. The person may feel flooded by choices and unable to make even mundane decisions, such as whether to have coffee or tea with breakfast. In this state of hypertrophied self-awareness, instead of thinking thoughts and feeling emotions, mental activity takes on the quality of perceived objects. Thoughts may take on an uncanny acoustic (or, in the case of verbal hallucinations, auditory) quality, and seem to have a spatial location not ordinarily associated with the ephemeral experience of thinking a thought: "I hear my thoughts as I am thinking them," or "My voice and my thoughts feel alien to me," or "All my thoughts seem to pass through a certain channel in my mind." Whereas a nonpsychotic person might have the repetitive thought "I am a loser," a psychotic person might perceive that thought as a hallucinated "voice" saying, "You are a loser!"

When experienced to a minor degree, this slipping away of the foundation of the self can be accompanied by an ongoing pervasive sense of anxiety, or anxiety that intensifies in the context of interpersonal contact; when felt to a marked degree, it may result in an overwhelming feeling of dread that psychoanalysts have termed "annihilation anxiety." People in psychotic states are preoccupied with the survival of the self rather than worried about the fate of the real people in their lives. They may feel that they are fundamentally different from other human beings owing to some failing in themselves that excludes them from the human community.

It is against this background of a globally altered change in self-experience that the particulars of affect, perception, cognition, and somatic states ought to be interpreted.

Affective States

Affect may appear blunted to observers, or may be obscured internally such that psychotic people may have trouble naming their feelings, but it can at times be intense and overwhelming. What in a nonpsychotic person might be "signal anxiety" that triggers a defense may in psychosis flood the person in a tidal wave of intense anxiety and consequent wishes to withdraw from the world into sleep, not to respond to stimuli while awake (catatonia), or to end one's suffering with suicide. Terror is a core affective experience, both of the disintegration of the self (Bion's [1962] "nameless dread,") and of persecutors believed to intend harm. Overt rage at imagined enemies and suppressed rage over developmental impingements are common, as are despair, intense shame, deep sadness, and terrible loneliness.

Perceptual Changes

Perceptual changes in psychotic subjects may affect various sensory modalities and their subjective interpretation. People in psychotic states may have a derealized experience of the environment, in which the world is apprehended through a veil or fog. At the other extreme, there may be heightened sensory awareness of the outside world and of sensory changes. Colors may appear more vivid, and spatial relationships distorted, such that stepping off a curb into the street may feel like leaping off a cliff. Sounds may be more intense, too high or too low in pitch, or strange. Sounds from the environment may mix with speech perception, such that one is uncertain whether one is hearing the wind or voices whispering. The person's attention may be drawn to fragments of the perceptual frame, such that ambient stimuli that would ordinarily go unnoted are now the focus of attention. At first these sensory changes may not be related to the self, but they inevitably take on personal meaning for the psychotic individual.

Hallucinations occur when a person perceives something that does not exist. A hallucination is a "perception in the absence of a percept." Although visual hallucinations may occur, the most common hallucinations are auditory verbal hallucinations ("voices") perceived as originating outside the boundary of the self. These voices may resemble what happens in dissociative states. In psychosis, however, voices are better understood as arising from a noncohesive self, and not necessarily as the voice of an alternative self. They are commonly critical, threatening, or commanding, causing great distress. Critical voices mock, degrade, and insult the person; threatening ones predict harm or punishment; command hallucinations often instruct self-harm or suicide, and, less often, destruction or harm of others. Locutions are typically in the second person (insulting or commanding), or third-person comments about the patient. Voices are typically felt as omnipotent and omniscient and frighteningly beyond the patient's control.

In a minority of cases, voices depart from these patterns, at which point differential diagnosis becomes more important. Voices that are positive and supportive, telling the person that he or she is special or has religious significance, may be more indicative of mania (see pp. 158–159). Voices capable of conversation (such that talking back alters a voice's message) may be more indicative of dissociative identity disorder (see p. 198), where helpful messages supplying information or advice are more typical, though they may also include the insulting, threatening, and commanding voice of a self-state identified with a perpetrator of earlier abuse (identification with the aggressor).

Cognitive Dysfunctions

Formal Thought Disorder

People suffering from psychosis may have trouble maintaining a focused, organized, goal-directed train of thought. They may experience thought blocking, when no thought seems to come, and at other times may feel swamped by a flood of pressured thoughts. They may have trouble accessing words when they attempt to express thoughts or feelings, and may lose track of the main idea they wish to express. They may express themselves in concrete or idiosyncratic phrases, images, and metaphors not easily understood by others. For example, the answer to the question "What do a bus and a bicycle have in common?" may be concrete, such as "Wheels," or else bizarrely idiosyncratic, such as "They both achieve forward locomotion by an impetus imparted to the rear axle." Such disorders of thought form are indicative of what was previously called hebephrenia or disorganized schizophrenia.

Global Reality Sense, Memory, Orientation

Short-term memory may be impaired. Time may appear to speed up, slow down, or lose its continuity. A patient may report never feeling fully awake, and complain of mental fatigue, clouded thinking, and lack of pleasure. He or she may feel less easily affected by and engaged in life events. Existential orientation to the world may shift. To compensate for this, a new interest in metaphysical, philosophical, or religious themes may take hold, at times accompanied by the belief that the patient is seeing more deeply into events than the average person. These themes are generally idiosyncratic and unshared with others.

Positive Cognitive Symptoms

Disorders of Thought Content

There is a wide spectrum of severity. At the mild end are idiosyncratic beliefs, preoccupations, and magical thinking, which may occur in the prodromal period leading up to frank psychosis. Delusions often arise in the context of the psychotic person's attempts to find an explanation for anomalous experiences, such as hallucinations, or to express sentiments too powerful and conflicted to be easily put into socially consensual language. Early on, there may be a state of "delusional mood," a vague sense or anxious expectation that something is about to happen, that significant change is afoot. This may be followed by a delusion, which brings some cognitive "order" to the emotional chaos by bringing some closure or meaning to particular intrapsychic themes of importance to the patient.

In ideas of reference, an otherwise normal perception is interpreted as having personal significance (e.g., "The man on television told me I was pathetic, and I know he was talking about me because he was looking right into my eyes when he said it!"), and the possibility of benign coincidence dissolves. Nothing is thought to happen by chance. A person might say, "When I walked down the block, it seemed that the cars on the block had been arranged in a special pattern to send a message to me."

Delusional Perceptions

In a delusional perception, an apparently normal perception is interpreted delusionally: While the person's literal perception of an event is congruent with what others perceive (e.g., all people present would affirm that two men indeed entered an elevator together), the person's interpretation of the meaning of the event is radically altered (e.g., the men are FBI agents who have the person under surveillance). They may be quite elaborate, as in this example: "When he looked at me angrily, his eyes were spinning in his head [illusion]; later, his buddies were following me in their cars, and I could tell for sure because as they drove by, the car wheels were spinning—just like his eyes! One of them drove right past me, and I could tell right away—he didn't look at me! He didn't want me to know that he was following me!"

Such delusional beliefs, illogical to others, may provide seemingly logical explanations for events that have puzzled the psychotic person. For example, a man with a disturbance in his self-experience, who reported hearing his own thoughts aloud, concluded that the government had advanced spy technology that could read his thoughts from a distance, and then that spy agents were playing his thoughts back to him through tiny speakers hidden along the sidewalk, so as to drive him mad into revealing what the government thought he knew about a terrorist operation. His delusion flies in the face of common sense, but has a certain internal logic to it.

Insight

Insight in psychosis is a topic in its own right. One view is that this "lack of insight" is similar to anosognosia, the neurological deficit that causes patients to be unaware of their own disability (e.g., patients after stroke who seem to be unaware of their own paralyzed limbs). A second view is that it is simply a component of delusional thinking. A third is that psychosis and insight are independent of each other. Most psychotic patients with positive symptoms of psychosis are also without insight into their condition or else have delusional interpretations of their overall state. Some, however, especially later in the course of their illness, even while hallucinating or experiencing paranoid delusions, may still have intact insight into their condition: They may recognize that the hallucinations and the experienced paranoia are products of their psychosis.

Somatic States

Individuals in psychotic states may report a variety of anomalous body experiences, including the feeling of their minds' being disconnected from their bodies; or parts of their bodies' enlarging or shrinking or feeling lifeless or strange in some way; or sensations of numbness, pressure, pain, heat, or cold; or "electric" sensations. Gastrointestinal and cardiac complaints are common. A person may say, "My guts are rotting," or "My head is exploding," or "The color of my skin has changed." The person may experience an internal impediment to intended motor actions, and, in the extreme, an inability to carry out what would ordinarily be habitual motor actions such as toothbrushing. The erosion of an integrated, central, first-person "I" may result in splits in internal experience that might be described in certain psychoanalytic theory as a fragmentation of the self into a variety of internal psychological objects. A person might report, "The right side of my body is male, and the left side of my body is female," or "There is a cat in my stomach that controls my thoughts."

Hallucinations and delusions are elaborated into a delusional narrative, which often features a beleaguered self assailed by a persecutor. Once a stable, systematized delusion has been established, various feelings of conflict and social alienation arise from the contrast between the person's beliefs and consensual reality. Some psychotic individuals fight to impose their personal reality on the world, in which case they may experience anger toward society for opposing the outcomes they think their beliefs require. Others withdraw into a psychotic world that they struggle to hide from their family and the mental health establishment, in which case they may regard others with suspicion lest they intrude upon their private delusional world. Delusions of omnipotence (feelings of great power and importance that have gone unnoticed by other people or feelings of special powers of prophecy, mind reading, and mind control) and ideas of reference (feelings that everything that happens pertains to oneself) may be both comforting and terrifying, as such power is expected to evoke attacks by envious others.

Relationship Patterns

Owing to their psychological history and current state of mind, psychotic persons have experienced a succession of interpersonal disappointments and failures that leave them feeling socially incompetent. Feelings of being disoriented or "out of synch" with other people may be pervasive. Psychotic individuals have difficulty accurately intuiting what other people are thinking and feeling, often framed as a limitation or aberration in their "theory of mind," and so they have difficulty negotiating social situations. A psychotic person may have deep convictions of being unlikable or toxic and may on that basis be suicidal. Intense self-disgust may lead to the belief that one will inevitably be rejected or abandoned. People in psychotic states assume that their interpersonal needs cannot and will not be met. They may surrender hope of expressing their individuality and attempt to relate to other people in a needy, clinging surrender (e.g., to a family member, therapist, or friend), or may remain avoidant and suspicious. People close to a psychotic person may feel frightened, helpless, or exasperated, as their efforts to calm the person fail, and attempts to persuade him or her of their own version of reality are rejected.

The clinician can understand that the patient is caught in a desperately problematic version of Schopenhauer's "porcupine dilemma," in which too much closeness with other human beings can bring intense pain, and too much distance brings loneliness and social isolation that impoverishes the spirit. Having found that attempts to relate to others have in the past occasioned intense anxiety and repeated interpersonal failures, the psychotic person withdraws from consensual reality and ordinary social contact into a solitary delusional world.

The Subjective Experience of Taking Antipsychotic Medication

Although first- and second-generation antipsychotic medications can ameliorate psychotic symptoms, these drugs may induce subjective changes. Effects are especially pronounced for first-generation antipsychotics, but are generally milder and more varied, and thus less predictable, for second-generation antipsychotics. Single doses of first-generation antipsychotic medication in nonpsychotic volunteers induce flattened mental states akin to the negative symptoms of schizophrenia. They may also exert an emotional numbing effect that induces a relative state of indifference (a state that may be welcomed by psychotic people suffering intense emotional pain). Rather than changing a delusional belief, a person might report being less bothered by the delusional idea: "I still believe it, but I don't think about it as much anymore." This state of relative indifference to psychotic symptoms may be accompanied by a more generally diminished capacity to experience pleasure and may contribute to social withdrawal.

The Subjective Experience of "Recovery"

Over the last few decades, some first-person accounts of people diagnosed with schizophrenia have shed light on the subjective experience of "recovery." This term does not imply the traditional meaning of full clinical remission, but a subjective experience of being relieved of symptoms and severe impairments in social, occupational, and relational areas.

The Subjective Experience of the Therapist

Clinicians' understanding of the inner experience of persons suffering from psychosis emerges from a complex process of emotional exchanges and verbal communications. At the individual level, countertransference experience may vary along a continuum, from immediate and irrational aversion to dedicated and affectionate interest. Early in the last century, Karl Jaspers opined that psychosis was psychologically incomprehensible, and that a clinician could diagnose schizophrenia or dementia praecox if a patient elicited in the clinician a rejecting, distancing reaction to a seemingly alien quality in the patient—a countertransference reaction that Henricus Cornelius Rümke termed the *praecox Gefühl* or "praecox feeling." The opposite reaction has been described under the name of "empathism" (as opposed to the more balanced and spontaneous feeling of empathy) and conceptualized as the result of a reciprocal "narcissistic seduction" within the patient-clinician dyad, or as the effect of a denial of the "hate" that may arise in the countertransference with psychotic individuals.

Similar extreme reactions can be observed at the group level. Psychotic persons are often treated in a group therapy format, most often by a treatment team affiliated with an inpatient facility. If not attended to, "basic-assumption group" functioning may divert the clinical team from the primary patient care task to the institutional group itself, resulting in a collective loss of purpose, the feeling that the group's work is meaningless, discouragement, and staff burnout. To understand the emotional swings that may occur in reaction to psychosis, and how or to what extent these swings may affect clinical judgment, clinicians should consider not only individual transference and countertransference dynamics, but also collective group attitudes that may result in messianic, dependent, or belligerent group dynamics (where the patient group serves as the target for the team's projections of deficits and failures, thus functioning as the team's scapegoat).

The basic emotional and affective disturbances that characterize a psychotic patient's inner experience resonate with a clinician's mental functioning at a deep level. The resulting intense reactions and primitive emotions can be either a precious occasion for learning or a source of personal distress and professional dysfunction. Countertransference reactions, along that continuum between opposite extremes, may include the following:

1. Interplay between the patient's psychotic and nonpsychotic partial components of the self may blur the clinician's own distinction between "normal"

and "psychotic," and stir up the terror of becoming crazy. On the other hand, it may evoke a better understanding of the overlap of psychotic and nonpsychotic elements in our common humanity.

2. The patient's "need–fear" dilemma, which deeply interferes with the patient's ability to be involved in close relationships (the "porcupine dilemma"), may amplify the clinician's ambivalence about intimacy and trigger loathsome or disdainful withdrawal from the patient. On the other hand, it may enhance the clinician's ability to feel comfortable with balancing closeness and distance with the psychotic patient.
3. The ambivalent intertwining in psychosis between love and hate may frighten the clinician and keep him or her at a distance. On the other hand, it may become a field of relational experience where unforeseen opportunities of communication may be created.
4. Difficulties in reaching the patient within his or her internal retreat may evoke a dysfunctional and overconfident feeling that progress and symptom recovery can be readily achieved. On the other hand, it may prompt the clinician's insight into the magnitude of the work needed to engage the patient in individual treatment and in rehabilitation programs.

Psychotic patients' lack of insight may present clinicians with a peculiar countertransference challenge. They may feel confounded by the patients' seeming inability to grasp a reality that appears perfectly obvious to everyone else. Patients often do not realize they are suffering from a mental illness, and delusional beliefs that are patently absurd to others appear literally true to them. Faced with these patients' inability to affirm the obvious, clinicians may take on the role of attempting to represent "consensual reality" to the patients, but at the cost of dispensing with efforts to understand primary gain (e.g., the psychodynamic etiology underlying a delusion that makes it psychologically preferable to the alternative, whatever that might be). One ought to avoid becoming that English speaker who, in trying to communicate with a nonspeaker of English, simply raises his or her voice, speaks in a more insistent tone, and dramatically gesticulates.

In addition to the above-described reactions, other countertransference feelings or attitudes may arise within the relationship with a psychotic patient. As an example, when the clinician is asked to certify the patient's eligibility for government-sponsored support or care programs, the clinician may have difficulty in sorting out the patient's primary psychological inability (which would elicit sympathy—though this is not equivalent to primary gain) from secondary gain (which might elicit a negative countertransference reaction). Secondary gain is often overemphasized, and primary gain is often neglected entirely. The clinician may feel deeply gratified by the intense work with the patient, to the point of having difficulties in recognizing and encouraging the patient's progress, and also in encouraging a reduced frequency of sessions and termination of treatment. Finally, the clinician may notice a diminished interest in the patient as the dramatically interesting flare of the psychosis fades and a more deeply defended "normality," dominated by boring negative symptoms rather than dramatic positive ones, ensues.

Finally, a quite common emotional reaction of clinicians working with psychotic ennui is a deep sense of boredom, sleepiness, difficulty in remaining awake and thinking, and the tendency to fall asleep, with dream-like thoughts and images that come up but are difficult to remember and put together, even after a few moments.

Clinical Illustration

A 21-year-old college student became undone when a man she had been dating broke up with her. She felt devastated, anxious, unable to sleep, and then oppressed by a mounting sense of impending doom. She began to notice strangers looking at her in a way she believed indicated that they knew intimate details of her relationship with her former boyfriend. She feared that other students were in league with him and talking about her, and she began hearing a "voice" telling her she was a loser. Her friends found her suddenly uncommunicative. She felt little need to explain her feelings; she thought people could read her mind. Her roommate escorted her to the emergency room, where she was admitted with a diagnosis of schizophreniform disorder.

S2 Mood Disorders

We have provided a concordance (see Table 3.2, pp. 245–250) between the PDM-2 classification and the ICD-10 and DSM-5 classifications of mood disorders.

DSM-5 divides mood disorders into "depressive disorders" and "bipolar and related disorders." Depressive (or unipolar) disorders are further subdivided into major depressive disorder, persistent depressive disorder (which now includes both dysthymic disorder and chronic major depressive disorder), disruptive mood dysregulation disorder, and premenstrual dysphoric disorder. The bipolar disorders include bipolar I, bipolar II, and cyclothymic disorders. Despite this clear delineation, the clinical presentation of virtually all depressive and bipolar disorders is markedly heterogeneous, and "textbook cases" appear to be quite rare.

S21 Persistent Depressive Disorder (Dysthymia)

DSM-II's depressive neurosis became DSM-III and DSM-IV's dysthymic disorder; in DSM-5 it is now relabeled as persistent depressive disorder (PDD), which is clinically broader and implies more significant clinical impact than former labels.

As mentioned above, while DSM-5's PDD is a relatively homogeneous category, these patients represent a heterogeneous population whose common denominator is the persistence of symptoms. People suffering from PDD experience depressed mood with little to no fluctuation over time. They have low energy and initiative, poor concentration, and difficulty in making decisions. Depressive symptoms include low self-esteem, hopelessness, guilt, and self-reproach.

Chronic depressive symptoms may be masked by physical symptoms such as sleep and appetite disturbance (either decreased or increased), fatigue, headaches, or chronic pain, often the presenting complaints to general practitioners. The depressive symptoms may gradually accumulate over a certain time interval and coalesce into PDD.

Characterological pessimism may predispose to low-grade PDD. Life events, stressors, and failures in parental caregiving and family functioning may also predispose to PDD. Acute symptoms are often precipitated by further external events and cause significant impairment in social, academic, or occupational activities, and on health.

The research literature highlights correlations among brain development, stressful environmental factors, and depressive conditions.

Given this multifactorial pathogenesis, evaluation of depressed patients should always include an assessment of psychological attitudes and/or personality traits, together with family and environmental factors involved in both the precipitation and perpetuation of these long-lasting depressive states. Psychodynamically, these factors are broadly related to loss (and thus with a link to anaclitic depression), which causes feelings of loneliness, helplessness, hopelessness, emptiness, and boredom, as well as abandonment anxiety. Self-criticism and guilt may arise from unconscious conclusions that it was one's badness that caused the loss. Concomitant defense mechanisms are introjection and turning hostility against the self. All mentioned cases of long-standing depressive symptoms are characterized by low self-esteem and disturbances in affect regulation. See also the discussion of depressive personalities (including hypomanic manifestations and masochism) in Chapter 1 on the P Axis.

Given the complex and multifactorial causes of PDD, patients who present with persistent symptoms are not likely to respond adequately to pharmacotherapy; most of them need integrated psychotherapeutic treatment.

S22 Major Depressive Disorder

Depression is common. It is commonly supposed that major depressive disorder (MDD) largely begins during adolescence, but epidemiological evidence suggests that its onset may be as early as the preschool years. In any case, recent studies suggest that the prevalence of MDD markedly increases during adolescence and young adulthood. Symptoms develop over days to weeks. Some people have only one single episode, with a full return to premorbid functioning. More than 50% of those who initially suffer a single major depressive episode, however, eventually develop another.

MDD is not just a form of extreme sadness. It is a disorder that affects both brain and body, including cognition, behavior, the immune system, and the peripheral nervous system. Unlike transient sadness, MDD is considered a disorder because it interferes with ordinary functioning in work, school, or relationships.

Loss of a loved one is a common precipitant of MDD, although it should not be confused with "pathological bereavement." DSM-IV-TR had an exclusion criterion for a major depressive episode if symptoms lasted less than 2 months following the death of a loved one. DSM-5 has omitted this "bereavement exclusion," somewhat controversially, as it could lead to an artifactual increase in the prevalence of depression. DSM-5 argues, however, that bereavement is a major life stressor that may precipitate MDD, and that the resultant clinical syndrome takes precedence over the purported etiology. From a psychodynamic point of view, the presumed causal effect of bereavement on MDD makes sense, especially among individuals prone to depression prior to losing their loved ones.

Although depression might deal a devastating blow to one's functioning, many high-functioning people are severely depressed, and hide their plight behind such behaviors as overworking, alcoholism, and aggressiveness. Such "masked depression," more common among men, suggests psychodynamic notions such as "manic defenses" and "narcissistic rage."

The medical definition of depression is a sustained abnormality in a person's mood, or feelings of despair, hopelessness, and negative cognitions about the self and world. A major depressive episode is defined as a period lasting at least 2 weeks in which a person feels depressed or becomes unable to experience any pleasure, accompanied by some of the following: changes in sleep patterns, changes in appetite, changes in sexual desire, loss of interest in things that were previously interesting, loss of pleasure in life (anhedonia), loss of energy, inability to concentrate, slowing of reflexes and bodily movements (psychomotor retardation), feelings of guilt, and suicidal ideation or planning. Overt behaviors and symptoms include crying spells; loss of interest in previously enjoyable activities; indifference to social interaction; neglect of personal care and physical appearance; passive or withdrawn behavior; restlessness; and slowed movement, thought, and/or speech.

The quality, intensity, and disruptive nature of the symptoms appear to be most relevant clinically. Depression is a condition that can vary in intensity from relatively mild to highly severe, from a subtle experience to a severely disabling clinical disorder. Depression also appears to be a leading cause of suicidality. Finally, a relatively rare "psychotic depression," complicated by delusions (e.g., the belief that one is someone else, or the belief that one must kill oneself to purge the world of evil) and/or hallucinations (e.g., hearing voices that savagely criticize the self or command one to die), may also present itself in the clinic. Thus the reality distortions accompanying depression may vary along a very broad continuum.

A careful assessment for MDD includes screening for medical problems and asking questions about what else may be going on in a person's life that might produce depression-like symptoms. Numerous medical conditions (including cancer, diabetes, hypo- or hyperthyroidism, multiple sclerosis, Parkinson's disease, head trauma, chronic pain, hepatitis, HIV-related conditions, and other infectious diseases) may cause symptoms that resemble depression. Use of steroids or withdrawal from cocaine, alcohol, or amphetamines may also produce depressive reactions. Finally, normal bereavement may resemble depression, except that in normal grief the painful mood state tends to come in waves, between which there is normal functioning; also, the source of pain is subjectively located in a failure of one's world (loss or disappointment in an external reality) rather than a failure or inadequacy of oneself.

Various relatively elusive forms of MDD may be highlighted. "Seasonal affective disorder syndrome" pertains to recurrent depression occurring annually, usually during the winter months. "Agitated depression" pertains to depression accompanied by nervousness and agitation, as opposed to a prototypical "lethargic depression," and may be better classified as belonging to the bipolar disorder spectrum. "Double depression" pertains to the repeated occurrences of major depressive episodes superimposed upon PDD. Finally, "depression with atypical features" is characterized by mood reactivity (mood brightens in response to actual or potential positive events), interpersonal rejection sensitivity resulting in significant social or occupational impairment, and hypocortisolism.

While the first of these conditions might lead a clinician to overlook depression, the last three might persuade the clinician that a patient is "beyond cure." This is particularly the case in patients with double depression, where the acute depressive episode abates, but the patients return to a baseline dysphoric state, feeling demoralized and thinking, "Is this all the treatment can do for me?" Such demoralization may lead to hostile countertransferential reactions.

The Subjective Experience of Depressive Disorders

The subjective experience of individuals with depressive disorders is complex. In addition, the clinical presentation is often "masked" by somatic states. Thus, a clear distinction among affective, cognitive, somatic, and relational patterns appears not to be clinical-friendly. Affective states experienced by individuals with depression include two general psychic orientations that have been described, respectively, as "anaclitic" and "introjective" patterns. Anaclitic depressive patterns, frequently associated with the disruption of the relationship with a primary caregiver, are characterized by feelings of helplessness, weakness, inadequacy, interpersonal guilt, and depletion; fears of being abandoned, isolated, and unloved; struggles to maintain direct physical contact with a need-gratifying person; wishes to be soothed, helped, fed, and protected; difficulty tolerating delay and postponement; difficulty expressing anger and rage (for fear of destroying the other as a source of satisfaction); and valuing caregivers only for their capacity to provide needed gratification. Individuals with strong anaclitic tendencies appear to experience others ("objects") as unreliable and unstable, and their defense mechanisms are characterized by shutting anger down, so as to maintain interpersonal harmony.

Introjective depressive patterns are characterized by harsh, punitive, unrelenting self-criticism; feelings of inferiority, worthlessness, and guilt; a sense of having failed to live up to expectations and standards; fears of loss of approval, recognition, and love from important others; and fears of the loss of acceptance of assertive strivings. Self-esteem suffers badly under such onslaughts. Cognitive patterns may include rationalized conviction of guilt; fantasies of loss of approval, recognition, and love; inability to make decisions; low self-regard; suicidal ideas; and impaired memory. Individuals with strong introjective tendencies appear to experience others ("objects") as punitive and judgmental and to employ "counteractive" defense mechanisms that deny dependency and establish autonomy and separation.

While both anaclitic and introjective tendencies have been implicated in psychopathology in general and depression in particular, self-criticism confers increased risk for a host of psychopathologies as well as for suicidality. Moreover, research indicates that self-criticism specifically increases "active vulnerability." Individuals with strong self-critical tendencies actively generate negative interpersonal conditions (e.g., stressful events, lack of positive events, and an absence of social support), which in turn lead to depression. The occurrence of this process within treatment, consistent with psychodynamic notions of "projective identification" and "externalization," has been empirically tested and corroborated. Thus the treatment of self-critical, depressed individuals is likely to be tumultuous, characterized by therapeutic ruptures and rifts. It is likely to involve strong countertransferential reactions, including therapists' doubting and criticizing themselves.

Another important development in depression research is the line of inquiry attesting to depression's scarring effect. Formulated within the cognitive perspective but consistent with psychodynamic theory, the scarring hypothesis posits that depression adversely affects personality similarly to a scar that forms around a wound. Although initial research failed to confirm this supposition, the past decade has yielded numerous studies attesting to the adverse effect of depression on the self-concept, including on self-criticism and self-esteem. Thus it is the case not only that a pathological self leads to depression, but also that depression, arguably acting as a persecutory object, erodes the self.

Clinical Illustration

A woman in her late 40s, previously an avid reader, presented with apathy and feelings of guilt, unreliability, and failure for having given up her job as a nurse in order to mother her twin sons, now 13 years old. "I know that I had a lot to enjoy in life, and that I've been a good mother for my babies all along. My sons are doing well at school; my relationship with my husband and family is really good; but I still don't feel well within myself, for no good reason." She adds, "I can't read a single page of any of my books. Sometimes I try, but I can't concentrate. And my children—I know I love them, but sometimes I feel as if I have no feelings for them anymore." She ruminated about finding a job, but felt she would not be able to handle both home and work. She said, "I have failed as a woman and as a mother. I should probably accept this and think that I am only a burden on everyone; I have lost my self-respect."

S23 Cyclothymic Disorder

Cyclothymic disorder is diagnosed when persistent mood fluctuations are present and notable, but insufficiently severe or persistent to be classified as bipolar disorder. Cyclothymic disorder can appear as early as adolescence, with an average age at onset similar to that for bipolar disorder (i.e., early 20s), with no gender difference.

The subjective experience of patients with cyclothymic disorder may include being out of control of their unexpected mood variations and subsequent behavior. An additional subjective consequence of the disorder is the experience of an unstable sense of self. People with cyclothymic disorder oscillate between feeling weak and strong, competent and incompetent, and so on. Once they understand that this oscillation stems from the effect of fluctuating moods on their self-state, the confusion is abated. Even though symptom and behavior severity does not appear at first glance as serious as in bipolar disorder, social roles and relational functioning may be affected quite seriously.

S24 Bipolar Disorders

Bipolar disorders—which Kraepelin originally labeled "manic–depressive insanity," later toned down to "manic–depressive illness"—involve fluctuating mood states, generally characterized as hypomanic, manic, depressive, or mixed. While diagnostic criteria for bipolar depression are the same as for MDD, bipolar patients are more likely to exhibit agitated or atypical features during their depressive episodes, which may be understood as the simultaneous presence of some manic features. According to DSM-5, manic episodes last at least 1 week; hypomanic episodes last at least 4 days; major depressive episodes last at least 2 weeks. Bipolar patients are said to exhibit "rapid cycling" if there are four distinct episodes (manic, hypomanic, or major depressive) in a given year (contiguous hypomanic and manic symptoms count as a single episode). Cycling that is faster than this (episodes lasting less than the required times, especially if within the same day) suggests another diagnosis (e.g., switching in a patient with DID), or else mixed states of depressive and manic symptoms co-occurring. Patients falling outside these narrow constraints ought to be treated according to the primary presenting pathology. "Pure" mania is more common in the early years of the illness; mixed states are more common in later years, when euphoria may be replaced with oppressive hostility.

Bipolar disorders are characterized by the presence of at least one episode with manic features (full mania, mixed features, or hypomania), usually in addition to a depressive episode. Manic episodes involve a distinct period in which the person experiences an elevated and/or irritable mood, along with inflated self-esteem, difficulties sleeping, pressured speech, flights of ideas, difficulties concentrating and focusing, psychomotor agitation, and engagement in activities that, while pleasurable, have damaging consequences and risks (e.g., spending money crazily, engaging in promiscuous and health-threatening sexual relations). In full manic episodes, psychotic symptoms may be present, including delusions and hallucinations that are usually congruent with the mood states. Formal thought disorders may also be present.

Diagnosis of bipolar disorder requires longitudinal observation, as the disorder may begin with a major depressive episode. DSM's bipolar I disorder is diagnosed when a patient meets the criteria for both a full manic episode and major depressive episode; bipolar II disorder is identified by the presence and/or history of at least one major depressive episode and the existence and/or history of hypomanic episodes. Average age at onset is in the early 20s, with no gender-related differences. Family studies suggest that bipolar disorder has a strong genetic influence.

Perhaps the greatest challenge in diagnosing bipolar disorders is their similarity in symptoms and phenomenology to some expressions of low-level borderline personality organizations (including psychopathic, narcissistic, and histrionic organizations, as well as diagnoses of BPD). These personality states, characterized by mood lability, are highly prevalent in patients suffering from all forms of bipolar disorders and consequently may complicate diagnosis. A common diagnostic error is to determine that a narcissistic or histrionic personality organization exists when a patient's uncontrolled behavior is driven by hypomanic mood states.

The Subjective Experience of Manic States

Affective States

In manic states, a person may feel intense euphoria or intense irritability, often with transient agitation and hypersensitivity to real and expected insult and rejection. Mania is characterized by excessive energy that may be experienced positively or negatively, as a disruptive and distracting internal pressure, or as infinite power, ability, and creativity. In either case, the internal overreaction may be accompanied by impulsive, risky behavior. Patients experiencing manic states often report increased desire—even desperate cravings—for others, frequently accompanied by intense sexual desire and loss of social inhibition.

Individuals with mania may have feelings of being strained, fragmented, and restless, as well as feelings of utter elation and absolute well-being. Their rapid mood fluctuations are accompanied by equally rapid fluctuations in the experience of self. Thus an individual may feel sullen, useless, and agitated for a time—and, immediately afterward, like a hero, a prophet, or a person with infinite powers and energies. These changes may be sudden, unpredictable, and uncontrollable. There can be feelings of loss when the mania dissipates—a yearning for the emotional intensity, ecstasy, and productivity. Thus many with manic tendencies seek out "upper" drugs (i.e., cocaine or methamphetamines) to intensify or maintain the manic euphoria.

Cognitive Patterns

Cognitive patterns may include fantasies of invincibility and exceptional, unrecognized talent; a sense of ability to succeed at any task; and wishes for fame or adoration. Difficulties in thinking clearly, logically, and linearly are also experienced in severe manic or mixed states. Individuals may be concerned about not being able to hold onto their flighty and pressuring thoughts. They may sometimes feel disoriented and unable to identify which of their racing thoughts are more important; at other times, they may experience the turmoil of thoughts as highly pleasant. They frequently express the contents of their mind without self-censorship or inhibition. Psychoanalytic theory and research have construed these processes as denial and narcissistic defenses. This line of inquiry is consistent with the aforementioned findings that hypomanic mood states are associated with narcissistic (and histrionic) features.

Somatic States

Somatic states may include restlessness, sleeplessness, and increased energy. Some patients in a manic state insist that sleep is literally a waste of time. They may feel full of energy and describe a need to "Never stop!" Sexual desire is frequent and intense. Physical exhaustion following manic states of any intensity may evoke suicidal depression, a serious risk.

Relationship Patterns

Relationship patterns are often unpredictable, chaotic, impulsive, and highly sexualized. Some people with manic features inspire followers and protégés, whose moods are elevated by sharing in the manic persons' grand schemes. In this context, we note that the psychodynamic treatment of bipolar states is likely to be daunting. Therapists may have trouble keeping up with the (hypo-)manic phases and may be bewildered by rapid shifts between these phases and depressed ones. The resultant confusion may spiral into countertransferential hostility.

Clinical Illustration

An energetic 28-year-old woman with a previous diagnosis of MDD began feeling "low" as an intimate relationship was ending. Coffee and "herbal remedies" increased her energies and elevated her mood, but she also needed alcohol to quell excessive agitation. After a sleepless night, she became suddenly irritable and then elated. She became hyperactive and impulsively accepted several dates, on which she felt high sexual arousal. She rapidly changed her whole wardrobe at huge expense. Thinking she had a "special ability" at prophecy, she approached friends and colleagues to predict their futures. Her work functioning decreased significantly, as her hyperactivity was not focused properly. Her family helped her to enter an inpatient program and get medication. At the time, she was unable to sustain a psychotherapeutic relationship.

S25 Maternal Affective Disorders

During pregnancy, a mother normally enters a mental state of "primary maternal preoccupation," which involves heightened sensitivity toward, and intense identification with, her developing baby. With the baby's birth, she develops a new mental organization that has been called the "motherhood constellation." The psychic organization that emerges may be permanent, transient, or (most frequently) permanently evocable. The mother reorganizes her self-identity, putting her baby first and herself second.

The puerperium is a well-recognized time of increased vulnerability to depression. Sociocultural evolution has led to a relative disappearance of the functional extended family that traditionally aided mothers; this support has not been replaced by any other social unit or health structure, although recent research has found that home visits to teenage mothers enhance parenting, reduces maternal risks, and improves child developmental outcomes. Understanding this phase is crucial because difficulties during pregnancy and in the postpartum period have a profound impact on the mother–baby dyad and on the baby's developing mental organization.

Three relevant conditions within the category of maternal affective disorders, in order of severity, are maternity blues, postpartum depression, and puerperal psychosis. Professional consultation is recommended for maternity blues and considered mandatory for postpartum depression and puerperal psychosis.

Maternity Blues

The term "maternity blues" (or "baby blues") denotes a common, relatively mild, transient mood disturbance. Dysphoria or mood swings peak between the third and fifth day after childbirth, with some cultural variation (e.g., symptoms could appear as late as the 10th day after labor). Prevalence varies between 26 and 80%, depending on culture and context (e.g., immigrants vs. nonimmigrants, socioeconomic stressors, high vs. low social support, wanted vs. unwanted pregnancy, good vs. poor vs. nonexistent marital relationship). A family history of depression and a personal history of depression or premenstrual dysphoria are common. Risk factors include stressful events, poor social adjustment, ambivalence in families, economic difficulties, and unplanned pregnancies. Symptoms may include transient tearful episodes, anxiety, headache, fatigue, emotional lability, irritability, depersonalization/derealization, and depressed mood.

Maternity blues is a common enough condition to be seen as within the normal spectrum, and so does not appear in DSM, ICD, or most psychiatric textbooks. Maternity blues may have serious consequences, however, including compromise of emotional closeness and maternal competence (see also Chapter 10). Mothers can be fragile in the postpartum period and generally benefit from family ties, especially if these are not compromised by prior conflicts.

Postpartum Depression

Postpartum depression is a significant health problem affecting 10–20% of new mothers yearly. It involves persistent sadness; frequent crying; emotional lability; poor concentration; memory troubles; feelings of worthlessness, inadequacy, or guilt; irritability; loss of interest in self-care; not feeling up to everyday tasks; loss of energy; anxiety; bizarre thoughts and fears; obsessive thoughts of harm to the baby; feeling overwhelmed; and loss of pleasure in previously enjoyable activities, including sex. Other symptoms include those typical of MDD: psychomotor agitation or retardation, insomnia or hypersomnia, significant decrease or increase in appetite, and somatic symptoms (see below). The mother bonds poorly with her baby, in whom she shows little interest. Thoughts of death or suicide are common, continuing beyond 2 weeks after delivery. Symptoms may occur right after birth and persist up to 1 year after delivery. Women vulnerable to depression prior to delivery tend to have depressions that extend into the postpartum period. Undiagnosed depression during pregnancy is the primary risk factor.

Postpartum depression affects not only mothers but also their children, with immediate and long-term adverse consequences (see also Chapter 10). It leads to insecure attachment patterns and increased risk of untreated emotional problems in children. Clinical decisions must weigh the relative risks and benefits of antidepressant medication and breastfeeding; emotional and practical support to the family should be considered, as well as psychotherapy.

Puerperal Psychosis

Puerperal psychosis (postpartum psychosis) is characterized by polymorphic delusions, alteration of consciousness, and affective symptoms of acute dramatic onset. Delusional themes generally relate to the child: Was he or she exchanged for another child? Was the baby's sex changed? The delusion may be limited to denial—denial of the marriage or relationship, of motherhood, or of the child's existence. Pan-anxiety and ecstasy are also observed, sometimes followed by stupor and other catatonic symptoms. Altered states of consciousness may also occur: Psychotic symptoms may have dreamlike features; there may be agitated somnambulistic features at night. Mother–baby contact is invariably impaired, and breastfeeding is usually interrupted.

Manic or depressive symptoms represent 80% of puerperal psychosis; 40% of mothers admitted to mental hospitals have shown manic features. Symptoms persist from a few days to a few weeks and may last 6 months; they fluctuate and generally have a favorable prognosis. A family history of mood disorder is common. Suicide risk is low, but risk for infanticide is elevated, often reflecting delusions about the child. The mother's despair may spread to her family, and when family support is insufficient, hospitalization is commonly required.

The Subjective Experience of Maternal Affective Disorders

Obstetricians and pediatricians should ask about sadness and dysphoria in recent mothers; while maternity blues are common and not severe, postpartum depression and puerperal psychosis imply serious risks for both mother and child.

Affective States

Affective states in mothers suffering from maternal affective disorders may range, on the depressive spectrum, from transient episodes of tearfulness in maternity blues to frank depressed mood, mixed states, or manic states in postpartum depression and puerperal psychosis. Anxiety symptoms range from fears and mild somatic symptoms in maternity blues to frankly manic agitation in puerperal psychosis. Common feelings include sadness ("I don't know why I feel so sad, I should be happy, but I'm feeling very sad"); loss of interest, especially in the baby; weakness and fatigue; guilt ("I don't know if I'll be a good mother"); extreme anxiety ("I need to rest, but I can't"); and feelings of being overwhelmed ("I'm too exhausted to do anything well").

Cognitive Patterns

Cognitive patterns may include identity disturbances, depersonalization, or obsessions and fears about the baby. Puerperal psychosis involves a more dramatic disruption of consciousness, including delusions, confusion, identity disorganization, stupor.

Mothers may say things like "It's a great responsibility for me . . . If I don't feed him, he could die," or "Delivery was so strange, I feel myself as an animal." In one case, a new mother was smiling into space; beside her a baby was crying inconsolably, but she did not react. Another mother had this delusion: "She isn't my baby; my baby was stolen."

Somatic States

Somatic states may include headaches, chest pains, heart palpitations, anorexia, numbness, and hyperventilation. Depressive or manic states may induce insomnia, anorexia, and psychomotor retardation or agitation, especially at night.

Relationship Patterns

Relating to a newborn requires empathy. Mothers who suffer from maternal affective disorders have difficulty making contact with their babies, and this difficulty often precludes genuine emotional intimacy. New mothers need the support of partners and extended families to cope with their new role. The "motherhood constellation" is based primarily on identification with one's own mother and the quality of one's own mothering in early childhood. The following difficulties in the immediate mother–baby relationship are common, in increasing severity: difficulty breastfeeding, awkward mother–baby relationships, difficulty calming and soothing the baby, rejecting contact with the baby, and denying the baby's reality.

There are also difficulties the new mother may have with her close relations, such as (1) changes in the parental couple, as the baby's needs come first, the mother's come second, and the father's or partner's are felt to come "10th"; (2) in second and subsequent births, conflict with or problems posed by the other children because of their relative neglect; and (3) changing work relationships as the mother's career is interrupted, while the father's or partner's may be barely affected.

The Subjective Experience of the Therapist

All health care professionals start life as babies with variably adequate mothers; many have parented their own babies. Countertransference feelings are inevitably mediated by similarities and differences between the clinical challenges a patient poses and a clinician's own history. Any clinician should be alarmed by an infant at risk. Against this background is the specific countertransference arising from the patient's transference and, in severe cases, the patient's use of primitive defenses. Some clinicians find themselves playing the role of surrogate caregiver, others the role of surrogate partner. A clinician needs insight into what "belongs" to the patient and what "belongs" to him- or herself to maintain professional identity and equanimity.

Clinical Illustration

An adolescent mother was referred for difficulties in breastfeeding and care of her newborn. She had become pregnant after unprotected sex with her boyfriend, who abandoned her on learning of the pregnancy; she was now living with her widowed mother in a small suburban apartment. Difficulties arose as soon as the baby came home. She did not know how to feed him, and he cried every night. The mental health team found sadness, irritability, and threats of self-harm in the mother, as well as anxiety and insomnia in the grandmother. The home was a mess, the baby crying. The mother stated, "I'm not ready to be a mother; it's all my fault. I can't manage the situation at home. . . . Sometimes I'm ready to explode, and I've actually had outbursts." The team referred her to individual and group therapy. These improved the mother–baby relationship and mitigated the grandmother's anxiety and insomnia.

S3 Disorders Related Primarily to Anxiety

The large S3 grouping is borrowed from ICD-10, and explains the contiguity of a number of DSM-5 diagnostic groups and their ICD-10 codes. See the concordance in Table 3.2 (pp. 245–250).

A major change from DSM-IV to DSM-5 is the "promotion" of obsessive–compulsive and traumatic diagnoses from the anxiety disorders to their own groups, in line with ICD-10. Another is folding factitious disorders into the somatic symptom and related disorders. Major differences persist between ICD-10 and DSM-5 for dissociative and somatoform disorders. ICD-10 continues to regard dissociation and conversion as different expressions of the same thing, and not to regard depersonalization as dissociative, in continuity with the dissociative and conversion subtypes of DSM-II's hysterical neurosis and distinct depersonalization neurosis. DSM-5 continues to follow DSM-III, -IV, and -IV-TR in interpreting depersonalization as dissociative and in separating out conversion disorder.

Under the rubric of anxiety disorders, DSM-5 includes specific phobia; social anxiety disorder; panic disorder; agoraphobia; generalized anxiety disorder (GAD); substance/medication-induced anxiety disorder; anxiety disorder due to another medical condition; and other specified and unspecified anxiety disorder. Obsessive–compulsive disorder (OCD) now has its own grouping in DSM-5, following ICD-10, but is included here among the disorders related to anxiety. DSM-5 goes beyond the ICD-10 grouping by moving body dysmorphic disorder and trichotillomania to the obsessive–compulsive grouping, and adding hoarding disorder and excoriation disorder to this grouping. Posttraumatic disorders (PTSD, acute stress disorder) also now have their own grouping, again following ICD-10, and PDM-2 follows this convention (see section S4, below).

S31 Anxiety Disorders

Anxiety is fear in the absence of obvious danger. Psychodynamically oriented clinicians, who have found anxiety lurking behind virtually all psychopathological symptoms, have distinguished carefully between potential danger and present danger; between the evaluation of danger and the response to danger; and between an adaptive response to actual danger (which may or may not include fear/anxiety) and an anxiety response, in which the fight–flight–freeze system is activated in the expectation of disaster. In light of the fact that some individuals suffer pervasive, chronic, and disabling anxieties, with unclear onset of these subjective experiences, we regard many individuals currently diagnosed with GAD as having a personality disorder rather than a symptom syndrome (see the discussion of anxious–avoidant and phobic personalities in Chapter 1 on the P Axis, pp. 36–38; this issue is also addressed in the S31.4 subsection, pp. 170–171).

The psychoanalytic literature identifies different kinds of anxiety, any one of which may be conscious or unconscious. Separation anxiety is the fear of losing a love object. Castration anxiety, a term used generally by some and specifically by others, is fear of damage to the body and sometimes specifically to the genitals. Moral anxiety is fear of the consequences of transgressing one's values. Annihilation anxiety (see below) includes the apprehension of being catastrophically overwhelmed, invaded, and destroyed. Fragmentation anxiety is fear of self-disintegration. Persecutory anxiety and irrational fears of harm to loved ones are understood psychoanalytically as the outcome of denial and projection and projective identification of one's own hostile feelings in the former case, and of omnipotent destructive unconscious fantasies in the latter. In certain contexts and in bearable amounts, some of these anxieties are relatively common, but when they are unremitting or disproportionate, they constitute psychopathology.

Women have twice the risk for anxiety disorders as men. A number of variables may account for this disparity, including hormonal factors, life events such as pregnancy and menopause, cultural pressures on women to meet the needs of others before their own, and more openness in women to reporting anxiety to physicians and therapists.

Maturationally, anxiety evolves from diffuse somatic excitation to pervasive psychic anxiety to a more mature signaling function. "Signal anxiety," a concept similar to "learned expectations" in contemporary learning theory, is a state of arousal signaling that past experience has identified an object or situation as a danger. It involves both anticipation and an attenuated level of affect.

The Subjective Experience of Anxiety

In this section, we address anxiety as the core experience of the different anxiety-related disorders and also as a subjective cross-sectional experience, anxiety possibly being an epiphenomenon of many other clinical conditions. We underscore that the affective states, cognitive patterns, somatic states, and relationship patterns associated with anxiety overlap across different disorders.

Affective States

The affective states are often related to Freud's (1909a, 1909b) four basic danger situations: fear of (1) loss of the object; (2) loss of the object's love; (3) castration; and (4) loss of the approval of one's superego. In less technical terms, these situations translate into fear of (1) loss of a significant other, resulting in feelings of abandonment expressed as anger, anxiety, depression, and/or guilt; (2) loss of love, experienced as rejection, and usually accompanied by rage, anxiety, depression, guilt, and feelings of being unworthy and even unlovable; (3) loss of bodily integrity and functioning; and (4) loss of affirmation and approval by one's own conscience, resulting in anxiety, guilt, shame, or depression.

In addition, there may be fear of loss of self-regulation (e.g., loss of control of one's feelings, thoughts, sensations, movements, actions). Anxiety associated with anticipating these dangers may be controlled or uncontrolled. When out of control, it may spark annihilation concerns. Annihilation anxiety originates very early but can be triggered at any point in life by threats to survival; it may arise without warning, in presymbolic form or in fantasies involving conflict and compromise formation, and may involve particularly recalcitrant resistance.

The study of annihilation anxiety in relation to the basic danger series has both theoretical and clinical advantages, especially for understanding panic, generalized anxiety, and phobias, but also psychoses, dissociative states, sexual problems (including paraphilias), and personality patterns. Fears typical of annihilation anxiety are of being overwhelmed, trapped, invaded, fragmented, merged, and destroyed; many of these relate to conscious and unconscious memories of early childhood experience. At its most severe, annihilation anxiety is experienced as intolerable and may be associated with a breakdown of functioning and sense of loss of self.

Cognitive Patterns

Anxious patients may have a range of cognitive symptoms: poor concentration, difficulty focusing, easy distractibility, and poor memory. Basic fears (e.g., of separation, abandonment, rejection) are common; more severe and complex fears and related thoughts, such as of being devoured or engulfed, of losing mental or bodily control, of falling in space, or of being injured and dying, are less common. Some patients have overwhelming catastrophic anxiety, which compromises their sense of body boundaries and sense of identity. There may be intense worry over losing someone they depend on or of losing financial security. Fear of fear, also referred to as anticipatory anxiety, is common in those with panic attacks; they avoid certain things or places for fear they will have another attack.

Somatic States

Somatic states include tension, sweaty palms, the sense of butterflies in one's stomach or a tight band around one's head, bladder and bowel urgency, and breathing difficulties. Anxiety disorders may be complicated by depersonalization/derealization—the feeling of being disconnected from one's body or from external reality. Anxiety can be associated with varying degrees of autonomic or physiological arousal. More frequently, individuals afflicted by anxiety experience hyperarousal.

Relationship Patterns

Relationship patterns may include expressions of fear of rejection, such as clinging and seeking reassurance; expressions of guilt, such as blaming, guilt assignment, and blame avoidance; and expressions of conflicts about dependency, such as the feeling of being smothered or suffocating, drowning, or choking, and vacillation between pulling others closer and pushing them away.

The Subjective Experience of the Therapist

Countertransferential experiences may vary widely. Clinicians may feel empathic involvement, parental countertransference, and the need to reassure their anxious patients. Or they may feel overwhelmed by the anxiety, as they become objects of projective identification, especially in patients with severe personality disorder or psychosis. In response, they are at risk of defensively disengaging themselves from the relationship. It is common to experience frustration while treating individuals with anxiety or phobias, as reflected in the clinical adage that "Any symptom, behavior pattern, or ideational content that serves in part as a defense against experiencing annihilation anxiety will be highly resistant to change."

Clinical Illustrations

Since anxiety is a cross-sectional experience, we discriminate in the following among clinical conditions that may involve anxiety. Clinical vignettes on specific anxiety disorders as listed at the beginning of this section will follow the specific diagnostic subsections.

Here are some examples of anxiety experienced by individuals at the neurotic or borderline level of organization:

> "My mind is deluged with all sorts of frightening thoughts and images. My body is all nerves. I can't sit down for any period of time; I'm constantly up and down. I feel like I'm going to crack up. At my job, I can't do a thing; I just feel I can't go on."
>
> "I can't stand the fear; I need comfort. Once fear steps in, I can't see anything or do anything. There are so many things I do out of fear. I'm afraid I'll fall apart, lose control, be taken over, be shot down with a machine gun. . . . The fear is always of something extreme happening. I won't get smacked; I'll get bombed. Some people fight or run away. When I'm cornered, I crumble."
>
> "When I get involved [in a relationship], I feel I have no rights, no prerogatives. The other person can make decisions; I can't. They can do what they want; I can't. I feel like I can't maintain my separate existence; I can't be a person when I'm involved in a relationship. It makes me feel panicky."

Examples of anxiety experiences in individuals at a psychotic level of organization, or with delusional thinking, include the following:

> "My brain and body are being eaten away by parasites. That is why I can't think or move my bowels."
>
> "I have faded into nothingness. I am no longer alive."
>
> "*They* have been blowing poison gas through the keyhole. It's destroying me and obliterating my thoughts."

Preliminary Note on Phobias

Although phobias may vary, all phobic experiences are seen by psychodynamic scholars as having the same core mechanism: In line with Freud's "drive–conflict" model, phobias have been described as the simplest form of "psychoneurosis," in which free-floating anxiety is transformed via repression, displacement, and projection into a more specific symptom symbolizing the underlying neurotic conflict. Therein lies the primary gain of a phobia: It carries less anxiety than full consciousness of the conflict.

Phobias have been known for centuries, including by Hippocrates. The term is derived from the Greek φόβος = *phobos* = "fear." In phobias, the emotion is always an irrational fear of a specific object (e.g., blood, insects, heights, flying) or situation (e.g., giving a talk, being blocked in a crowded place), exposure to which elicits anxiety reactions or the idea of which elicits active avoidance. Clinical assessment of patients suffering from phobias includes (1) whether the person has one or many phobias, (2) whether the phobic concern is specific or general, (3) the content of the phobia, (4) the presence of panic attacks associated with the phobic experience and behavior, and (5) the level of psychic functioning reflected in the phobia.

In some phobic individuals, one sees counterphobic behavior: Instead of being avoided, a frightening object or situation is actively pursued, evidently in an unconscious effort to master the fear rather than to endure it passively. Counterphobic repetitions rarely eventuate in mastery of phobic apprehensions, but instead tend to lead to the compulsive repetition of the counterphobic activity. Although this phenomenon has been reliably observed clinically, it has received little empirical investigation, perhaps because it is not a problem for which treatment is ordinarily sought. These factors may explain the absence of counterphobia from the various editions of DSM, despite its being potentially self-destructive and thus warranting clinical attention.

As a psychopathological manifestation, phobia occupies a prominent place in the psychoanalytic literature. From the dynamic–genetic perspective, much literature on it has involved exploring the symbolic meaning and underlying (unconscious) fantasy behind particular phobic symptoms, as a parallel to what one finds in the manifest content of a dream. A number of dynamics have been identified by psychoanalysts, who endorse a spectrum of theoretical positions. Freud emphasized the centrality of phallic–oedipal dynamics, though he also granted that prephallic phobias were more important and more serious. From the structural perspective, phobic symptoms are interpreted with reference to the ego and superego. Some authors have seen phobias as expressions of fears projected from bad internal objects or identifications or of superego failures. Others have understood them as reflecting an underlying conflict over dependency or separation. And still others underscore conflicts over aggression.

In the formation of a phobic symptom, preexisting developmental arrests expedite a regression of various ego functions, with a related increase in primary-process functioning, leading to a confusion between potential danger and actual danger. Fantasy, thought, and action are equated, while internal (instinctual drive) danger and external danger become muddled. This process results in controlled anxiety's reverting to uncontrolled anxiety, and reflects the failure of the ego to limit these responses to a signal level.

Phobic symptoms involve less suffering and better overall adaptation than intense states of free-floating anxiety (i.e., panic attacks). In phobias, defensive measures restrict and focus what is feared, allowing afflicted individuals to remain free of anxiety as long as they avoid specific objects or situations. Clinically, phobias have been found to derive from attempts to moderate anxieties over competition and feared retaliation (oedipal issues), as well as efforts to deal with fears of loss of control (autonomy issues). At a more basic level, they may defend against fears of abandonment by caregivers, represent concerns over body integrity, and involve loss of ego functions. At a still more primitive level, phobias may entail efforts to restore a lost sense of connection with others and to reestablish a lost sense of identity.

S31.1 *Specific Phobias*

The age at onset of specific phobias is usually early (5–9 years), even though it may occur later (ages 20–25 years), at which point the object of the phobia tends to be a situation (e.g., heights, flying, storms) rather than an object (e.g., blood, scars, needles) or a type of animal (e.g., spiders, insects, dogs, horses). Many cases of infantile specific phobias are an exacerbation of evolutionarily based fears specific to primates, such as the fear of darkness and of certain animals.

The general psychiatric/psychological definition of a phobia as fearful avoidance is not sufficient to define a phobia psychoanalytically; it must be a symbolic representation of an underlying neurotic conflict. The adaptive gain of phobia over anxiety neurosis inheres in this advantage: From raw anxiety, a person may attempt to run, but he cannot hide. The phobic person, however, can sometimes escape the anxiety by avoiding the phobic object or situation.

S31.2 *Social Phobia*

Social phobia has been described as fear, anxiety, and/or excessive embarrassment when a person is involved in public encounters (e.g., giving a speech, attending a party where no one is familiar, talking in public, or being looked at). The age at onset is frequently in the teens, or even earlier; the disorder may imply dysfunction at school and poor adjustment in relationships with peers. It frequently co-occurs with depressive symptoms and/or substance misuse secondary to efforts to deal with public situations that trigger anxiety reactions.

S31.3 *Agoraphobia and Panic Disorder*

Both DSM-5 and ICD-10 separate agoraphobia (from Greek αγορά = agora = "marketplace") from panic disorder, based on epidemiological and observational data indicating that agoraphobia may occur without a history of panic attack or panic disorder, with a lifetime prevalence of 1.7%. It is worth noting, however, that the relationship between panic and the onset of agoraphobia has been endorsed by both psychoanalysts and nonpsychoanalytic researchers. Empirical evidence supports the view that most persons with agoraphobia have a prior history of panic attacks, and that they attribute the onset of their agoraphobia to the panic experience.

Agoraphobia is described as the anxiety of being in places or situations from which it would be difficult or embarrassing to escape. Also, it is depicted as fear of being in a place or situation where it would be difficult or embarrassing to seek help if a panic attack were to occur. These places or situations may be either faced with extreme anxiety and distress or actively avoided. The presence of a "phobic partner" (a person who can share the agoraphobic situation and provide reassurance and help) is not infrequent. Fear of being trapped is common: Fears of sitting too far from the door in a church or movie theater, or of being trapped in a crowded mall, are prototypic agoraphobic situations. Fear of being unable to escape is found in transportation fears and fears of crossing bridges (i.e., specific phobias), the common element being that the context prevents easy escape in the event of an emergency. The blocking of this powerful and ethologically ancient action tendency intensifies and prolongs the alarms and potentiates learning. It is probably interference or conflict with this survival-based behavior that is the most important factor in "convincing" the organism not to let this happen again at any cost.

A prominent current view is that panic attacks in phobic conditions (especially agoraphobia) are "spontaneous"—unrelated to psychic events—and based on pure physiology. A psychodynamically oriented therapist, on the other hand, would make the general assumption that agoraphobia and susceptibility to panic attacks might both be based on ego weakness or deficit, and would be interested as well in what specific underlying conflicts and deficits, possibly related to past events, predispose a given patient to develop agoraphobia, and what specific stressors might trigger a panic attack. These issues are amenable to empirical study.

A number of authors have noted close connections between agoraphobic and claustrophobic symptomatology. For Weiss (1964), they are both attempts to deal with "specific threats to the patient's ego unity." Claustrophobia and agoraphobia are considered to be the basic phobias, and reflect in extreme form two major annihilation-related dangers for young children as they go through phases of separation–individuation. Too much closeness can lead to fear of loss of the self through merger or engulfment, and too much distance can lead to feelings of abandonment and its attendant dangers.

The word "panic" owes its origin to the Greek god Pan, the patron of shepherds and god of woods and streams. When disturbed from his nap in a thicket or cave near the road, this apparently benign sprite is alleged to have let out a yell so intense and terrifying that a passerby would be frightened to death. A panic attack is an unpredictable acute anxiety reaction with no known significant stressor or trigger. The attack is frequently described by the person as involving somatic symptoms that resemble those of a heart attack. For this reason, many patients seek help at hospital emergency rooms and may develop secondary illness anxiety disorder (hypochondriasis). The attack typically lasts for 5–20 minutes and is almost always characterized by both somatic and psychic symptoms (e.g., shortness of breath, tachycardia, sweating, dizziness, nausea, the feeling of losing control, fear of dying, derealization, depersonalization).

Panic disorder is diagnosed when panic attacks are recurrent. Usually they are followed by anticipatory anxiety (fear of having another panic attack) and active avoidance of certain situations in which it would be difficult or embarrassing to seek help if a panic attack were to occur. The first panic attack is usually vividly remembered by the sufferer. The age at onset is usually early adulthood (20–24 years), with a lifetime prevalence twice as high in women. Agoraphobia and panic disorder are frequently complicated by depressive symptoms secondary to the primary anxiety disorder, and by substance misuse for self-medication (e.g., alcohol, benzodiazepines).

It is plausible that a panic attack in the background of phobic symptom onset reflects a traumatic factor in phobias. See section S41.2 (pp. 182–190) for further details.

S31.4 *Generalized Anxiety Disorder*

For both DSM-5 and ICD-10, GAD is a specific clinical condition requiring a specific diagnostic label, even though symptoms of this condition do not appear to be specific. Rather, they appear to constitute the "generalization" of an anxiety state experienced by sufferers as both psychic and somatic (e.g., restlessness, fatigue, muscle tension). Patients suffering from GAD usually report hyperarousal and constant exaggerated apprehension in dealing with most everyday activities. As a specific diagnostic condition, GAD has a lifetime prevalence as high as 8% in the general population, presenting in early adulthood or even in childhood, and with a higher prevalence in females than in males (2:1). As stated earlier, considering the fact that anxious individuals suffer pervasive, disabling, and chronic anxieties, we may also regard GAD as a personality pattern/disorder rather than a symptom syndrome (see the discussion in Chapter 1 on the P Axis).

Clinical Illustration

A 31-year-old corporate lawyer was referred by his CEO for his feeling "stressed" at work and for multiple somatic complaints. He began by saying what he had been going through was "pretty scary." He described a recent work experience: "I went to the meeting, and shortly after being there, I felt a wave go through my head. I began to feel dizzy, like I was going to pass out—and I started to breathe fast and feel nauseated." He emphasized that it was a terrible experience, yet added that his recent medical tests had all produced normal results. He began to feel calmer as the day progressed, especially after going home. Several better days followed, marred only by stomach cramps. He still did not feel quite right, describing an ongoing discomfort in social situations, wherein he would feel lightheaded and dizzy in conversation. He speculated about having an "anxiety condition," and mentioned a "phobia for public speaking." He wondered whether his condition was mental or physical, and seemed to be asking for reassurance.

S32 Obsessive–Compulsive and Related Disorders

Obsessive–compulsive disorder (OCD) began as one of the ICD-9/DSM-II neuroses. DSM-III, -IV, and -IV-TR grouped it among the anxiety disorders. ICD-10 elevated it to a specific group of disorders—obsessive–compulsive syndromes—embedded in the F40–48 group "neurotic, stress-related, and somatoform syndromes." DSM-5 has followed ICD-10's lead in "promoting" OCD to its own category, together with other disorders hypothesized to be related to it. Thus DSM-5 "imports" trichotillomania from DSM-IV's impulse-control disorders and body dysmorphic disorder (BDD) from DSM-IV's somatoform disorders; it adds two new diagnoses, hoarding disorder and excoriation disorder. In this way, the obsessive–compulsive and related disorders have become one of the major groupings in the DSM-5 classification.

The psychopathological core of the spectrum of OCD is well known and easily described. "Obsessions" are recurrent thoughts, impulses, or images that impinge upon the affected person's mental functioning; "compulsions" are actions, mental activities, and repetitive behaviors that the patient experiences as "compulsory" and that significantly affect his or her functioning, with a severity that varies widely across different patients and within the life of a given patient. These repetitive behaviors may become more and more inflexible; the subject may not only be forced to perform some action or mental activity, but to do so in a certain rigidly organized sequence (compulsive rituals).

DSM-5's OCD spectrum disorders include BDD, where obsessive thinking is focused on imagined or exaggerated body imperfections; hoarding disorder, where the content of the obsessive thinking and consequent compulsive behavior are related to the urge to accumulate objects of no objective or sentimental value from which one cannot separate (e.g., old newspapers, receipts, garbage); and trichotillomania and excoriation disorder, the compulsive urge to pull hair or pick at skin with a frequency that causes hair loss or observable scars and sometimes bleeding. The psychodynamics underlying these last two diagnostic entities may be different from those underlying obsessive–compulsive disorders.

The subjective experience of obsessive–compulsive problems and related symptoms and disorders is the result of many factors, including age at onset and level of insight. Children between 6 and 9 years old (see Chapter 9 of this manual on the SC Axis, pp. 561–563) frequently develop minor rituals, accompanied by magical thinking, to avoid dire consequences (e.g., "Step on a crack and break your mother's back!"—the horrific temptation is often implied). Ordinarily, such rituals are short-lived and not incapacitating. Although more serious obsessions, compulsions, and rituals are rare, they may persistent for years and extend to other contexts (e.g., contamination, order, and symmetry). From a psychodynamic perspective, obsessive–compulsive symptom formation results from unconscious conflicts, usually between drive and conscience, desire and repulsion, appetite and prohibition, or initiative and guilt. They cause much distress, inclining the sufferer to translate them into some compromise symptom or behavior (e.g., persons experiencing sexual impulses that they see as repulsive may wash their hand repeatedly in order to undo the impulses).

Symptoms may be recognized as a serious problem by the patient, and may be completely ego-dystonic, leading to an active struggle against them. Yet obsessions and compulsions may be experienced as mostly or completely ego-syntonic, and involve passive acceptance of what is considered one's ordinary mental functioning. Quite often, ego-syntonic symptoms are related to poor insight. In such cases, clinicians should consider the differential diagnosis with obsessive–compulsive personality disorder (as defined in DSM) or obsessive–compulsive personality (as defined in Chapter 1 of this manual on the P Axis). The two conditions, though sharing to some extent the same diagnostic "label," are significantly different. While patients may experience specific, ego-syntonic obsessions and compulsions, individuals with obsessive–compulsive personalities do not experience symptoms of OCD. Rather, they have personality traits, attitudes, and general behavior characterized by perfectionism, moral inflexibility, and difficulties in delegating tasks to others. According to recent literature, the co-occurrence of DSM-diagnosed OCD and obsessive–compulsive personality disorder is not frequent.

Other factors help shape the clinical presentation and the subjective experience of OCD and related symptoms: level of personality organization, maturity of defenses, and level of cognitive functioning. Probably more than any other class of symptoms, obsessions and compulsions are present in various diagnostic categories and should be considered to a certain extent as transdiagnostic. They may affect persons with a high level of relational and social functioning, as well as patients with a frankly psychotic structure and functioning. In the latter cases, OCD should be considered a pseudoneurotic façade superimposed on a deeper, hidden, more disturbed mental functioning.

It is valuable to investigate recent losses, stresses, and other possible precipitants of onset of OCD and related disorders, especially those that may have affected a patient's fantasies of control. Conveying the message that hostile and selfish thoughts are understandable and not inherently dangerous may also be of help. Although notably challenging clinically, some obsessions and compulsions remit when the afflicted person can express the feelings connected with difficult experiences—especially normal disappointment, anger, and grief.

S32.1 *Obsessive–Compulsive Disorder*

OCD is the historical prototype for the other diagnoses within its grouping. It may be characterized by prevalent obsessions, compulsions, or both. As noted above, obsessions include ruminations and horrific temptations; compulsions include rituals. The subject unsuccessfully resists either one, resulting in unpleasant repetition. Onset is generally in adolescence or early adulthood and tends to be earlier in males and in those with a tic disorder. To be diagnosed as OCD, symptoms must have been present for at least 2 weeks. Insight is an important consideration: Patients often have sufficient insight to have intact reality testing, but there is a spectrum of insight that at its lower end approaches zero, associated with patients who are quasi- or frankly delusional (approximately 4% of patients with diagnosed OCD). Depression in which recurrent and sometimes intrusive thoughts about death, failure, or inadequacy are frequently present may mimic OCD.

The Subjective Experience of OCD

Affective States

Obsessive and compulsive patients, being heterogeneous in severity, mental functioning, and insight, may experience a range of affective states. Depression is not uncommon, with suicidal ideation and plans related to the sense of being unable to deal with symptoms in everyday life. This complication is more frequent in patients with good insight. Patients diagnosed with OCD and poor insight, contrastingly, may experience a sense of pain and isolation at being considered weird and unacceptable by others, even significant others. When insight is largely absent and close to delusional thinking, a person is likely to project aggression into others, thereby feeling actively isolated by others or in danger from them. When individuals with this disorder are prevented from carrying out their compulsions or rituals, they may become diffusely terrified, irritable, or overtly aggressive. Behind such symptoms, psychoanalytic clinical experience points to a range of unconscious concerns, including potential loss of control (especially with respect to contamination, aggression, and shame).

Cognitive Patterns

Insight is a critical dimension in assessing individuals with obsessions and compulsions. Obsessions may be recognized as a mental dysfunction, something that interferes with the common functioning and flow of thinking, and may be experienced as highly ego-dystonic, disturbing, and intrusive. Ego-syntonic obsessions are usually related to poor insight. Magical thinking in the absence of insight may seem delusional; patients with intact insight tend to find it absurd and shameful. Compulsive activity is often a remnant of the magical thinking of early childhood, when impulses and actions were incompletely differentiated. Thus, individuals with obsessive–compulsive symptoms may be understood as having convicted themselves unconsciously of thought crimes (hostile, selfish cognitions), which continue to haunt them in the form of obsessive images and ideas, motivating attempts to expiate their guilt through rituals that represent the defenses of reaction formation and undoing.

Somatic States

Patients with OCD often present with hyperarousal and somatic anxiety symptoms. In subjects with contamination obsessions and severe cleaning/washing compulsions, it is quite frequent to see health problems (e.g., infections, skin excoriations) due to excessive washing. Some subjects complain of fatigue or restlessness. In addition, even though it is not exactly a somatic state but rather a motor disturbance, it should be noted that patients with obsessions and compulsions may present with co-occurring motor tics (approximately 30% over a lifetime, according to recent epidemiology studies).

Relationship Patterns

Obsessions and compulsions may severely affect quality of life by impairing social and relational functioning. In some severe cases, they intrude into the persons' lives, leading to social isolation. In general, afflicted individuals tend to remain in relationships if they can control the partner. They may also choose significant others who actively reassure them in their symptoms or even become participants in their compulsive rituals.

The Subjective Experience of the Therapist

The internal experience of a person with an obsession has often been intuited as shaped by a struggle between besieging and besieged parts of the mind. Clinicians' experience with patients who have OCD may oscillate between an optimistic, positive, empathic attitude that frames such behavior as normal defenses of daily life and astonished and pessimistic discouragement and doubt in their ability to be of any help in the face of such a "cold, metallic" organization of defenses. Countertransference may be dominated by themes of "control" as patients try to control their lives and behaviors—efforts often deemed as tragically defeated. Whatever strength is expended in efforts to control inner life by throwing rejected thoughts out the window is sabotaged by their quickly and triumphantly reentering via the front door as uncontrolled compulsions. A beleaguered clinician is often left feeling impotent.

Clinical Illustration

A 33-year-old man comes to a therapist after being fired for delays in completing work assignments. He is very anxious about his future, with pessimism not only about finding another job, but also about the future of his marital relationship: His wife is becoming less and less tolerant of what she calls his "manias." When asked about these, he says, "Nothing really serious. I think many people should behave like I do. There are too many contaminants outside, and so I take particular care of my hands and clothes. I wash my hands up to 30 times a day, and clean my desk and computer quite often with special products to remove the dust and to kill all the germs. I know that this is time-consuming, but it is necessary to prevent contamination and diseases."

S32.2 *Body Dysmorphic Disorder (Dysmorphophobia)*

BDD, also known as "body dysmorphia," "dysmorphic syndrome," or "dysmorphophobia," involves recurrent and intrusive thoughts about one's appearance, which is considered defective and worthy of being hidden or fixed with medical or surgical interventions. Many sufferers spend several hours a day attempting to conceal or correct their perceived flaws, which may be really present though exaggerated in severity. Compulsive checking of physical appearance (e.g., at the mirror) and repetitive asking for reassurance are also common.

DSM-5 criteria include the presence of a specific BDD subtype in which the dysmorphic thinking focuses on muscles (i.e., the person's concern is mostly on the inadequate development of muscular body mass). This subtype is mostly seen in male patients. ICD-10 includes BDD and nondelusional dysmorphophobia among somatoform disorders.

BDD is common, with lifetime prevalence of approximately 2%, and no significant differences between males and females. Earlier literature reported gender-based discrepancies about prevalence, which likely arose from inconsistent views among researchers prior to the creation of standardized questionnaires and more clinical assessment. Age at onset is usually adolescence (prompted by the somatic changes of puberty) or early adulthood.

Although its etiology is unknown, BDD is considered to be complex and multifactorial. Current models include aesthetic sensitivity and the self as an aesthetic object, social pressure to appear "perfect," and neurobiological predisposition. From a psychoanalytic perspective, pervasive identification with an uncompromising ego ideal underlies these excessive bodily concerns, with severity in direct proportion to ego-ideal demands, which may be persecutory. The criticized part of the body thus represents a hated part of one's personality.

A second psychoanalytic construct is the "body-self": the body image that develops within the self in the context of the early relationship with the "object of desire," usually the mother. Two distinct versions of the mother-as-mirror have been observed in patients with BDD: She may be felt to be providing a one-way or blank mirror (the "one-way-mirror mother"), or to be more actively distorting and rejecting, looking at the baby with hateful eyes (the "distorting-mirror mother").

The Subjective Experience of BDD

Affective States

Individuals with BDD experience severe distress and frequently develop depressive symptoms of varying severity. In some cases, severe depression may occur, and suicidal risk becomes a critical issue to be carefully assessed in clinical settings. Mood swings are frequent, as the incomplete or unstable sense of self (largely reduced to the body-self) follows the concerns about being ugly and not acceptable to others. Irritability may occur when the person cannot obtain the reassurances he or she is seeking compulsively or when the aesthetic, medical, or surgical interventions do not have the expected outcome.

Cognitive Patterns

As in OCD, assessing insight in BDD is critical. Insight varies along a continuum with two extremes: Symptoms may be recognized as absurd or exaggerated concerns and behaviors (good insight) or may be psychotically denied, with the insistence that such "real" physical problems call for medical or surgical attention. Repetitive thoughts about body parts and defects may become frankly delusional. Anxiety related to dysmorphic symptoms may lead to cognitive deficits, such as poor attention or difficulties in concentrating on issues other than body appearance.

Somatic States

Like patients with OCD, individuals with BDD may experience intense somatic anxiety, hyperarousal, and a wide variety of somatic complaints.

Relationship Patterns

BDD can severely impair social, occupational, and relational functioning. In some cases, concerns about physical appearance eventuate in social isolation. Severe damage to relationships is also common since the affected individuals may be too scared or ashamed by their physical appearance to get involved in close relationships. In some cases, patients' significant others may be used as "special" source of reassurance.

S32.3 *Hoarding Disorder*

As noted earlier, DSM-5 has coined a new entity, hoarding disorder, as one of the obsessive–compulsive and related disorders. The disorder is diagnosed when there is a pattern of compulsive and excessive acquisition of, and inability or unwillingness to separate from, many and various objects that have no objective value or use (e.g., old receipts, empty bottles, broken electrical appliances, empty paper or plastic bags, garbage).

When severe, hoarding may so compromise the home living space that it limits activities such as cleaning, moving around, cooking, and even sleeping. It may endanger the individual and others by creating risks of fire, falling, and contamination. Compulsive hoarding has also been associated with health risks, impaired functioning, economic burdens, and adverse effects on friends and family members. Hoarders may have varying degrees of insight into their dysfunctional behavior, but the emotional attachment to the hoarded objects far exceeds the motivation to discard them.

DSM-5 notes that approximately 80% of those with hoarding disorder are driven to collect, buy, or steal objects, thus warranting a specifier to the diagnosis ("with excessive acquisition"). Researchers have only recently begun to study hoarding, as it had not its own diagnosis in the past and thus was either ignored or clustered with OCD. In addition, because of either lack of insight or shame, subjects with hoarding disorder very rarely seek treatment. Thus the affective, cognitive, relational, and somatic patterns associated with hoarding are still not well enough defined to be described independently from those associated with obsessive and compulsive disorders.

S32.4 *Trichotillomania and Excoriation Disorder*

DSM-IV/-IV-TR and ICD-10 list trichotillomania as an impulse-control disorder. DSM-5 has moved it to the obsessive–compulsive and related disorders. DSM-5 has also coined excoriation disorder, which is unrepresented in ICD-10.

Trichotillomania involves recurrent, compulsive hair pulling, sufficient to cause noticeable hair loss from different body areas (most frequently the scalp, eyebrows, and eyelashes). Individuals may also examine the hair root, twirl a strand, pull it between the teeth, or eat it ("trichophagia"). The subject feels the urge to pull out hair and often actively struggles against this compulsive, repetitive behavior, even though the pulling gives a sense of gratification and/or relief of tension. Despite the overt evidence of their disorder, those afflicted with it typically pull out their hair only in private and deny that they do so. They may go to great lengths to conceal their behavior. This secrecy may reflect deep shame, or may be carried out in a mild dissociative state, or both. Age of onset for trichotillomania is usually before young adulthood, with peaks at 5 to 8 and around age 13. Some individuals have continuous symptoms for decades, while in others the disorder may remit for weeks, months, or years at a time. The prevalence of the disorder is considerably higher in females than in males (10:1).

Excoriation disorder is similar: Individuals afflicted by it feel the urge to pick repetitively at their skin to the extent of inflicting scars and bleeding. As in trichotillomania, they may actively struggle against the compulsive, repetitive behavior, or they may appear unaware of it. Despite scars that are sometimes severe, patients with excoriation disorder may cover the parts of the body that have been picked (usually fingers or arms) and deny their behavior.

Clinical Illustration

A 22-year-old woman with trichotillomania stated, "It started when I was a child; it has been waxing and waning ever since. Sometimes I feel weird, uncomfortable, almost like when you have an itch you need to scratch. It gets worse and worse, and then I just have to pull out my eyebrows to feel relieved and calm. But then it starts up again, and I have to do it again. Sometimes I do it without knowing—until I go to the mirror and see I have almost no eyebrows left. I feel so bad at that point, I know people will notice it, and I try to disguise the damage with makeup."

S4 Event- and Stressor-Related Disorders

In this section, we group DSM-5's new trauma- and stressor-related disorders with another group of disorders historically linked to—and, in much current thinking, closely related to—developmental trauma and neglect: dissociative disorders. We also follow the historical linking of dissociation and conversion, maintained in ICD-10, by including conversion disorder in this grouping. Table 3.2 (pp. 245–250) provides an overview of these diagnoses.

Prefatory Comments

A number of comments are in order to clarify the complex "historical pedigree" of some of these categories of experience.

Dissociation and Conversion

Note that ICD-10's F44 diagnostic group, dissociative (conversion) disorders, bridges two groups in DSM-5: dissociative disorders and somatic symptom and related disorders. We have opted to follow the same line, given that the massive past psychodynamic literature on hysteria (dissociative and conversion) is matched today by a growing literature about psychoform versus somatoform dissociation. The term "conversion" was coined by Freud to designate somatic symptoms arising as a consequence of repression (of both intolerable events and intolerable wishes). Prior to that, such symptoms had been of interest to neurologists and psychiatrists and interpreted as symptoms of hysteria. The generic meaning of conversion covers any "psychogenic" or "functional" symptom that mimics an organic, especially neurological, condition. Altered states of consciousness and such somatoform symptoms were combined in the ICD-7, -8, and -9 and DSM-II diagnosis of hysterical neurosis, dissociative and conversion types. The link remains in ICD-10's dissociative (conversion) disorders. DSM-III, -IV, and –IV-TR separated conversion from dissociation by grouping it among the somatoform disorders, which DSM-5 now calls somatic symptom and related disorders.

Depersonalization/Derealization

Note that ICD-10's depersonalization–derealization syndrome is not one of its dissociative (conversion) disorders. Depersonalization neurosis was a stand-alone diagnosis in ICD-7, -8, and -9 and in DSM-II, distinct from hysterical neurosis. DSM-III reinterpreted it as dissociative; this reinterpretation may well be adopted by ICD-11.

Adjustment Disorders

Adjustment disorders were called transient situational disturbances in ICD-7, -8, and -9 and in DSM-II. One of them, adjustment reaction of adult life, included an example: "Fear associated with military combat and manifested by trembling, running, and hiding." This is the closest that these taxonomies came to categorizing overt trauma, and the example was pretraumatic rather than posttraumatic.

Posttraumatic Stress Disorder (and Acute Stress Disorder)

Astonishingly, posttraumatic stress disorder (PTSD) was absent from ICD-9 and DSM-II, and entered official nosology only with DSM-III in 1980 as a result of lobbying by a group of veterans and their psychiatrists—despite the long history of attention by clinicians to battlefield casualties dating back to the 19th century, and the early recognition, later suppressed, of the psychological sequelae of childhood and relational neglect and abuse. For want of its own category, DSM-III classified PTSD as an anxiety disorder, thereby construing its symptoms as primarily anxiety based. ICD-10 followed suit by adopting PTSD, but also added acute stress reaction and regrouped these two with the adjustment disorders, thereby stressing the "cause" more than the "effect." DSM-IV then modified ICD-10's acute stress reaction, calling it acute stress disorder (ASD) with updated criteria, but keeping it with PTSD as an anxiety disorder.

The clinical course of acute stress reaction/ASD stresses the role of peritraumatic dissociation and dissociative symptoms shortly after the trauma, and a clinical course lasting from 3 days to 1 month after the index trauma. If symptoms persist beyond a month, then PTSD is diagnosed. Thus the "course" relationship of ASD to PTSD is the same as the "course" relationship of schizophreniform disorder to schizophrenia (see section S1, pp. 139–141). Finally, DSM-5 caught up with ICD-10's regrouping by putting adjustment disorders, ASD, and PTSD together, thereby stressing the "cause" more than the "effect." Each step has led to improved criteria for symptoms and clinical course. Because DSM-III's PTSD was largely the creation of the U.S. Veterans Administration, its relatively narrow criteria were most applicable to war veterans (in particular, Vietnam war veterans). DSM-5 has broadened the criteria to a wider spectrum of trauma victims. There is still some way to go, however. Thus, in PDM-2, we include complex PTSD (CPTSD) in subsection S41.3 (pp. 190–194).

Trauma and Dissociation

Another player in the "cause versus effect" dynamic is dissociation. A focus on cause will highlight trauma- and stressor-related disorders, whereas a focus on effect will highlight dissociative disorders. Dissociative disorders are generally interpreted as complex posttraumatic conditions, but the trauma need not be identified—a necessity, given that dissociative amnesia is an effect that removes consciousness of the cause. Certain core symptoms of posttraumatic conditions are interpreted as dissociative, but the trauma needs to be identified, and consequently there is a small literature on "PTSD without the trauma" for cases where the trauma is unknown, or else where it is thought to be the "wrong kind" of trauma. Again, PDM-2's CPTSD helps fill this gap.

Meanings of "Dissociation"

Over the past century and a half, the meanings of the term "dissociation" have greatly evolved, and they continue to evolve. As noted above, dissociation was originally seen as a type of hysteria, related to conversion, and distinct from depersonalization. It included amnesia, fugue, certain altered states (e.g., somnambulism), and multiple personality. DSM-III distanced conversion from dissociation and added depersonalization to it.

DSM-III and -IV also invoked dissociation in the criteria for PTSD and ASD, but with contrasting emphasis. DSM-III PTSD invoked "flashback or dissociative episodes" among its criteria when a dissociative episode involves an especially severe flashback with full, prolonged sensorimotor reliving; this coalesced into "dissociative flashback episodes" in DSM-IV. The "flashback" concept views it as a positive symptom: something present that ought to be absent. On the other hand, DSM-III and -IV's ASD declined to interpret flashbacks as dissociative and instead interpreted numbing, detachment, reduced awareness, derealization, depersonalization, and amnesia as dissociative, thereby interpreting dissociation as a negative symptom—something absent that ought to be present. Finally, in DSM-5, the criteria for both ASD and PTSD interpret all these positive and negative symptoms as dissociative. But semantic confusion persists: DSM-5's PTSD criteria clearly label flashbacks and amnesia as dissociative symptoms, but even when present, they do not qualify for the addendum "*Specify* whether: With dissociative symptoms" (p. 272); only symptoms of depersonalization and derealization qualify for that specifier.

Dissociation also occurs in DSM-5 criterion 9 for borderline personality disorder (BPD), as "Transient, stress-related . . . severe dissociative symptoms" (p. 663), for which the text gives only depersonalization as an example. Patients with dissociative identity disorder (DID) are frequently misdiagnosed as having BPD, through an overgenerous interpretation of this criterion 9, whereas such patients routinely fail to fulfill criteria B, D, and E for general personality disorder, which require a single enduring pattern of personality functioning that is stable, inflexible, and pervasive. Thus any patient with a dissociative disorder who switches cannot, by definition, have a personality disorder. This conclusion is clearly an artifact of faulty criteria, as the various individual self-states of someone with DID will commonly manifest themselves in exaggerated personality traits, and may present as extreme caricatures of personality disorders. Perhaps this anomaly will be addressed in DSM-6.

In summary, there are at least three distinct meanings of "dissociation" as subjective experience:

1. *Dissociation of some of one's mental functions or faculties.* This is closest to the DSM-5 definition: "a disruption of and/or discontinuity in the normal integration of consciousness, memory, identity, emotion, perception, body representation, motor control, and behavior" (p. 291). Examples of "negative" dissociative symptoms involve the withdrawal of something, such as dissociation of memory (amnesia), sensation (conversion anesthesia), or affect (emotional blunting). Examples of "positive" dissociative symptoms involve the intrusion of something, such as the sensory reexperiencing of a trauma (flashback), or any other intrusion of affect, knowledge, sensation (in any modality), or behavior (action, unintended vocalization, etc.). Most of these symptoms may occur within a single consciousness.

2. *Depersonalization/derealization.* These may be interpreted as negative symptoms, the withdrawal of the sense of reality, though DSM-5 considers them positive, as intrusions. This ambiguity goes along with their odd history. They may occur as solitary symptoms, but are common ancillary symptoms in other posttraumatic and dissociative conditions.

3. *Dissociative multiplicity.* This is a plurality of consciousness, most obvious in DID, in which the first two types of dissociation commonly co-occur; thus, there is always the possibility that cases featuring the first two types of dissociation may have covert multiplicity as well. The DSM-5 definition does not really work for multiplicity because once there is more than one self occupying the center of consciousness, there is more than one center of subjective experience and consequently more than one set of symptoms.

S41 Trauma- and Stressor-Related Disorders

To reiterate, DSM-5 follows ICD-10's lead in regrouping ASD, PTSD, and adjustment disorders together under trauma- and stressor-related disorders, so that their listings are now near-identical, according to Table 3.2 (pp. 245–250).

In PDM-2, along with adjustment disorders and ASD/PTSD, we have added CPTSD, as the criteria for PTSD are too narrow to accommodate the wider spectrum of posttraumatic conditions—especially of conditions involving repeated trauma and abuse that interfere with normal childhood development.

S41.1 *Adjustment Disorders*

The diagnosis of adjustment disorders covers a wide range of maladaptive responses to psychological stress, whether acute, chronic, or repeated. Such reactions are considered to be adjustment disorders if they occur within 3 months of the stress and last for no more than 6 months. They may be responses to challenges, such as illness or changes in one's family, or to developmental milestones such as puberty, leaving for college or military service, marriage, changes in employment, retirement, or the development of new interests. Adjustment disorders are described in relation to anxious mood, depressed mood, conduct disturbances, physical complaints, withdrawal, work or academic inhibition, or mixtures of these.

The Subjective Experience of Adjustment Disorders

Affective States

Affective states accompanying an adjustment disorder vary from individual to individual. Often an overriding affective feature is a vague uneasiness deriving from a sense of change or flux. At a deeper subjective level than the presenting anxiety, depression, or behavior change, there may be a pervasive uncertainty and apprehensiveness. Clearly, preexisting personality patterns and affective tendencies further color the subjective experience. It is often helpful to facilitate the patient's detailed descriptions of these more vague, pervasive affects.

Cognitive Patterns

Cognitive patterns include either a focus on the current stress or a marked avoidance of the changes that a patient needs to assimilate. In other words, individuals with adjustment disorders may be preoccupied with what they are facing or may be defensively avoiding it.

Somatic States

Somatic states may accompany the predominant reaction to the stress (depression or anxiety or behavior change) and the general state of tension and apprehensiveness. The nature of the somatic expression depends on the affective response.

Relationship Patterns

Relationship patterns may be characterized by either an expansion of expressions of dependency or attempts to distance from potentially helpful relationships because of shame about an increased sense of neediness.

Clinical Illustration

A 35-year-old woman with a 4-year-old child had just learned that her father required cardiac bypass surgery. She recalled having felt betrayed by her father at 12, when he had divorced her mother. Nonetheless, she had tried to endear herself to him. With the news of his illness, she found herself experiencing waves of anxiety, including nightmares filled with gory details and daytime images of "his heart being cut open and blood gushing all over." She was only partially successful at calming herself by slowing her breathing but continued to function well as a mother, wife, and freelance writer. On becoming more aware of the different feelings she had toward her father, she was able to shift gradually back to feeling calm, organized, and methodical. She was able to return to this level of functioning after four weekly consultations.

S41.2 *Acute and Posttraumatic Stress Disorders*

Historical Background

The entry of psychic trauma into psychiatry and medical sciences began at the end of the 19th century, when Freud and his contemporaries took note of its effects and began to identify different types of traumatic experiences and reactions. Freud (1914) wrote that the effect of trauma on an individual was to alter the foundations and contours of his or her life and to impair the person's ability to live in the present, due to ongoing efforts to reconcile the past trauma and its impact on present and future. He also described the core elements of what makes an event or experience traumatic: it overwhelms the capacity to cope with it and renders a person helpless.

Freud and his colleague Josef Breuer (1895) identified the root of hysteria in women as child sexual abuse, specifically incest. Freud eventually reversed that emphasis to focus on a child's fantasies of sex instead of the reality of sexual abuse. Other contemporaries—notably Pierre Janet (1889) outside the psychoanalytic movement, and Sandor Ferenczi (1949) within it—retained a focus on the trauma of childhood abuse, positing dissociation rather than repression as the main method a child (and later an adult) uses to cope. They observed that if the trauma were not worked through and resolved at some point, its residual effects would often have a lifelong (and negative) influence across various domains. In the early 20th century, the study of psychic trauma was largely limited to understanding and treating the effects of combat exposure during each of the World Wars and the Korean conflict—an effort that was largely abandoned during peacetime when soldiers were encouraged to "get back to normal." This is reflected in the absence of any reference to posttraumatic stress in ICD-7, -8, or -9 or in DSM-II.

Contemporary Research

The episodic focus on trauma changed dramatically in the late 1970s and early 1980s, when a confluence of social issues and movements led to much more sustained attention to trauma and its effects and to the development of the academic field of traumatic stress studies. The Vietnam War, specifically the reactions and symptoms reported by returning soldiers, was the primary social catalyst. Movements for racial equality added racial discrimination and its effects. The women's movement added gender-based violence and sexual assault of women and girls, rekindling a focus on domestic life. These concerns led to a resumption of the study of child abuse (abandoned in the 1930s and 1940s). Various posttraumatic syndromes were named: rape trauma syndrome, battered-women syndrome, post-Vietnam syndrome, and others.

Over the last four decades, clinicians and researchers have resumed the study of trauma and dissociation that had largely been eclipsed by the Freudian concept of repression. Contemporary researchers have found that being overwhelmed has a physiological correlate in that basic brain structures and functions are altered, along with basic physiological responses, in individuals who face trauma and later develop PTSD. They have returned to the teachings of Janet and Ferenczi, identifying the high prevalence of trauma-related distress, developmental impact, and psychopathology in a wide variety of traumatized populations—including combat veterans, but extending to concentration camp survivors and their offspring; victims of childhood physical, sexual, and emotional abuse and neglect; and victims of terror, torture, displacement, refugee status, and human trafficking. Peritraumatic dissociation (at the time of the trauma or shortly thereafter) has been identified as a risk factor for later PTSD. It is hypothesized that dissociation, while protective at the time, compromises one's ability to work through the trauma subsequently, thereby leading to the development of PTSD.

Contemporary Society

The PTSD label is now widely applied to the sequelae of a variety of psychic and physical traumas, so much so that some critics believe that it has lost its focus. Others charge that as it has become more widely accepted and understood, its true impact and highly subjective nature have been lost. In other words, contemporary society now accepts and even expects PTSD in response to a wide array of traumatic experiences, but fails to grasp how traumatized individuals are injured and changed, and how difficult it is to recover from a psychic injury of this type. The pendulum may have swung so far that some have been misled into interpreting PTSD as a normal response to adversity, and yet the impact on the affected individual's life is anything but normal.

PTSD involves an alteration of the self and familiar landmarks. Many traumatized individuals describe having a pretrauma and a posttrauma self, and see the traumatic experience as life-changing. When these individuals make a disclosure of what has happened to them, others' misunderstanding or minimization of the subjective impact can lead to comments and questions that range from the unhelpful (e.g., "Can't you just get over it?" or "Did you ever kill someone in combat?") to the preposterous (e.g., "You must have done something in a past life to have something like that happen to you"). In such circumstances, their posttraumatic alienation gets reinforced rather than ameliorated.

The Trauma

The criteria for ASD and PTSD continue to evolve. Despite ASD's "becoming" PTSD after 1 month, their respective DSM criteria have never easily correlated. The trauma and resulting symptoms have generally broadened from the original DSM-III focus on foreign wars to the domestic scene: civilian trauma on home soil, especially domestic trauma.

The traumatic stressor was originally described as being "outside the range of normal events," a depiction that was too broad and insufficiently specific. DSM-IV narrowed it to a criterion involving an experience and a subjective reaction to it: experiencing, witnessing, or being confronted with an event that involved actual or threated death or serious injury to self or other, together with a response of fear, helplessness, or horror. DSM-5 criterion A has dropped the subjective reaction, added sexual violence to actual or threatened death or serious injury, and further specified the kinds of exposure: (1) direct experiencing, (2) witnessing in person, (3) learning of events happening to close family members or friends, and (4) repeated work-related exposure (in the cases of police and other first responders). This helps "repatriate" the foreign war focus back to the domestic front, and represents a significant resolution of national paranoia: Bad things are not done just by *them over there*, they are also done by *us right here*. Beyond DSM-5, the research literature over the past several decades has identified five types of primary trauma:

- *Type I, impersonal/accidental/disaster/shock trauma*, for which there is no particular causation. This category has recently been expanded to include illness and medical conditions that occur or develop randomly, as well as any ongoing treatment and rehabilitation (often ongoing and physically or emotionally painful) that is required.

- *Type II, interpersonal trauma*, committed by other humans as a means of gratifying their own needs by exploiting those of another. Type II trauma can be a one-time or time-limited occurrence (usually when a stranger is the assailant), but it may also be repeated over months or years when the victim and perpetrator are related in some way and there is the potential for entrapment within the ongoing relationship. The interpersonal dimension of the primary trauma is most important with respect to symptom severity, which is worse when perpetrated by someone known to or related to the victim (or who has a role or relationship that involves nurturance of or protection that is used to dupe the victim)—a pattern called "betrayal trauma."

- *Type III, identity trauma*, based on largely immutable individual characteristics (ethnic/racial group and features, gender, gender identity, and sexual orientation) that are the basis for victimization.

- *Type IV, community trauma*, based on group identity, culture, beliefs, traditions and community membership, the basis of much sectarian and intergroup strife and violence.

- *Type V, ongoing, layered, and cumulative trauma*, based on revictimization and retraumatization.

There are also different types of secondary trauma. Most commonly with Type II trauma, when the victim turns to others for help and it is not forthcoming, or when the victim is shamed or blamed for being victimized, a second injury occurs and is additionally traumatizing. When the one turned to is also in a nurturing role, this second injury becomes a component of betrayal trauma. Type II betrayal trauma prototypically involves a child's parents or parent substitutes, one of whom is abusing and the other negligent. Later in adulthood, when an institution does not respond and instead scapegoats the victim, supports the perpetrator, and covers up the occurrence, *institutional betrayal* is said to occur—the betrayal trauma of adulthood.

Nachträglichkeit, a concept coined by Freud (1914) over a century ago, is another sort of second injury—a generic, repetitive additional effect that crosses the spectrum of trauma and neglect. It was clumsily translated into English by Strachey as "deferred action" (literally, *afterwardsness*), and cleverly translated into French by Rudolphe Loewenstein (1991) as *après coup*, or "aftershock" (or knock, blow, bump, strike, etc.). Loewenstein's analysand, Jacques Lacan, made it a central concept in French psychoanalysis. *Après coup* occurs whenever personal maturation (especially puberty) or new knowledge or life experience occasions a revision of past experience. This revision occasions retraumatization. For example, sexual molestation by a parent at a young age, and one's response to it, may be more confusing than traumatic. But with puberty, the perpetrator's motivation and perverse manipulation may become experientially clear, and the full horror of the earlier events is retraumatizing. Similarly, with maturity, the nonabusing parent, formerly forgiven with lame rationalizations, may be seen more clearly to have been grossly negligent and even complicit in the abuse.

For all these types of trauma, research indicates that the PTSD syndrome remains an *atypical response* in traumatized adults, and that most are able to work through what happened to them after a period of normal posttraumatic responses and reactions that fade over time. Thus, any of the five types of trauma, and the various forms of second injury, may or may not lead to ASD, PTSD, and/or CPTSD (see subsection S41.3, pp. 190–194) in a given individual.

Symptom Variability in ASD/PTSD

Clinicians now acknowledge ASD and PTSD to be highly variable, multifaceted psychophysiological and spiritual conditions that can take different courses at different times (immediate onset, chronic course, delayed expression), varying widely among individuals and circumstances. Both objective severity (ranging from relatively mild to torturous) and impact can differ markedly. Response has been found to be very subjective, depending on the victim's characteristics (including temperament, age, resilience, and gender) and experience (initial reaction, family history and stability, prior history of traumatization, and prior PTSD, among other factors). In fact, research has demonstrated that two individuals who have exactly the same traumatic exposure may have entirely different outcomes or have different forms of PTSD.

Subjective Symptoms

Subjective symptoms have also evolved. The criteria for DSM-III and -IV required three groups of symptoms: reexperiencing, numbing/avoidance, and arousal. DSM-IV's ASD had the same general structure, but teased apart numbing (amnestic–affective–somatic) from avoidance (intentional), and so had four groups of symptoms. DSM-5's PTSD requires symptoms from all four of these groupings, but their definitions have expanded. Reexperiencing includes flashbacks, nightmares, and intrusive memories, but also responses to triggers. Numbing has extended beyond amnesia and emotional numbing to negative beliefs and expectations, as well as to anhedonia and other negative emotions (fear, horror, anger, guilt, shame). Arousal (exaggerated startle, hypervigilance) is now extended to anger and irritability, reckless behavior, and so on. DSM-5's ASD, on the other hand, now has 14 possible symptoms grouped into six clusters: re-experiencing, dysphoria, anhedonia, dissociation (depersonalization, amnesia), avoidance, and arousal. ASD does not require symptoms from all five groupings, but rather 9 symptoms from the total list of 14.

Symptom Alternation

Numbing and reexperiencing (DSM-5's PTSD criteria D and B) are both considered dissociative but are to some extent opposites and generally occur in alternation. Dissociative amnesia and emotional blunting are best viewed as effects of strong dissociative defenses. The offending trauma is successfully removed from memory, and its accompanying affect is erased. The amnesia and blunting are often stronger than necessary, such that many good memories and feelings are dissociated together with the traumatic memories and emotions, leaving sufferers emotionally blunted and with little sense of their own history. Dissociative flashbacks and other intrusions are best interpreted as effects of periodic weakening of dissociative defenses. The offending trauma is suddenly released from its dissociative container and floods the person's senses and emotions. The dissociated good memories and feelings may likewise be liberated during such flashbacks, but are generally overshadowed by the trauma and dysphoria, to which the person attempts to respond by dissociating the material once again. This dynamic leads to the alternation between too much and too little.

Reexperiencing is more often covert than obvious. Full hallucinatory reliving provides its own "narrative context," whereas an isolated visual, auditory, tactile, olfactory, gustatory, or affective flashback may be misinterpreted as either a hallucination indicative of psychosis or a conversion symptom. Isolated affective flashbacks (experienced as affective intrusions of fear, sadness, revulsion, etc.) may also be confused for paranoid or affective pathology.

Avoidance

The person suffering from PTSD attempts to prevent flashbacks, motivating DSM-5's criterion C: active avoidance of triggers. This further complicates the negative criterion D symptoms by increasing social isolation and defensive withdrawal, or specific trigger-focused phobias. A patient with a spider phobia, after some years of therapy, worked through a childhood trauma that began in an outhouse. She was sitting in the dark; the door opened; a man stood there, legs apart, arms up and to either side, a black outline of his central body with appendages against the daytime sky. Then he raped her. Once she had worked through the trauma, the spider phobia resolved (as did several other symptoms connected to the rape). Other strategies to prevent or blunt flashbacks are chemical—the use of alcohol and other intoxicants. These responses explain the high prevalence of comorbid substance-related disorders.

The Subjective Experience of Psychic Trauma and Posttraumatic Stress

Individuals who experience trauma, especially those who go on to develop PTSD, describe themselves in literature and memoirs as having been transformed and their lives demarcated forever into pre- and posttrauma. Trauma has been described by memoirists and clinicians alike as time-distorting, causing time to stand still and to conflate. In the traumatized mind, the past event can overtake the present when a posttraumatic response is evoked by a strong enough trigger (something internal or external to the individual that serves as a reminder of what took place). Victims describe feeling helpless and out of control, at the mercy of outside forces; overwhelmed and disoriented; wrenched from their normal way of being in the world, and losing a sense of ongoing security; challenged to make sense of what happened to them; overcome by loss and grief; terrified; and fearful of injury and death. Many cope through the use of dissociation at the time of the trauma or utilize it in the aftermath to split and avoid painful reminders of the experience. Those who do not develop PTSD usually have some way of understanding and/or working through what happened to them, as well as a fair amount of personal resilience (although it is understood that virtually all individuals have a threshold or "tipping point" beyond which they will be traumatized).

In PTSD, however, a sufferer experiences being out of control and at the mercy of the symptoms in an ongoing or ambient replay of the trauma as the brain and mind struggle to process it. Attempts to master the traumatic experiences, usually unconscious, are common, and involve reenactments, repetition compulsions, and revictimization.

Psychodynamic formulations have emphasized the shock, helplessness, vulnerability, and terror specific to trauma. Traumatic experience may overwhelm mental functioning; interrupt initiative; disturb affective experience, identification, and expression; and interfere with the capacity for symbolization and fantasy. In these ways, it challenges the individual's meaning, personal relevance, and vocation in life. Trauma-related memories and fantasies are more difficult to work through, as psychic trauma alters the sense of self and of the familiar, as well as the quality of interpersonal relationships. Victims often feel different and alienated from "normal people" (i.e., those who have not been traumatized) and come to mistrust others, especially in the wake of interpersonal victimization.

Clinical literature from the time of Freud and Janet has highlighted persistent reexperiencing and repetition of traumatic events through recurring nightmares/flashbacks/reminiscences, as well as through unconsciously or dissociatively driven reenactments of traumatic themes—sometimes in psychotherapy, where it is an important source of information leading to understanding of what the individual is struggling with. The importance of the individual meaning of traumatic experience and the fact that trauma may constitute a psychic organizer of sorts have also received emphasis, in the psychodynamic literature and more generally, as shifts in personal assumptions and meaning making.

Affective States

Affective states include both unmanageably overwhelming feeling reactions expressed in explosions of affect, on the one hand, and their dissociation (numbing) on the other, manifest especially in affective detachment (emotional numbness, blankness, apathy, dissociation of disturbing feelings from the events that gave rise to them) and somatic states (sensory numbness, depersonalization, derealization). Trauma compromises the identification and management of affect in general. Horowitz (1997) and Herman (1992), among others, have identified a host of subjective emotions that accompany severe psychic trauma:

- Fear/terror that the trauma will be repeated; fear of identification with the perpetrator and of becoming similarly destructive; fear of identifying with victims and of defining oneself as a victim.
- Anger and rage directed toward the source of the trauma, and about having been traumatized, resulting in negative identity and self-loathing.
- Sadness and grief.
- Guilt about one's angry or destructive impulses; survivor guilt, especially when others perish, and about actions or passivity which caused survival; guilt over one's believed responsibility for the trauma—a defense against the more terrifying realization that one was helpless (this overlaps with thought content);
- Shame about feeling helpless and empty, and about having been traumatized.
- Self-loathing and contempt, arising from rage, guilt, and shame; the sense of being defective, contaminated, irredeemable;
- Existential despair, a sense that no one can understand, loss of faith in humanity, in God, in the cosmos.

Cognitive Patterns

Traumatic alterations of perception include both reexperiencing (flashbacks, intrusive affects, images, sounds, sensations, ideas, actions) and numbing (depersonalization, derealization, conversion anesthesia). This alternation causes constant shifting in one's perception of reality, which can lead to "realistic" paranoia. The thinking of traumatized individuals is variably affected by the kind of trauma suffered (see above) and the prior personal history, against the background of constitutional temperament. The sense of reality (again, see above) and reality testing may be compromised. Thought content may be dominated by convictions of having been betrayed (especially following interpersonal trauma, betrayal trauma, institutional betrayal, and related secondary injury) or by defensively wishful convictions of the benevolence of abusers or failed protectors (trauma accommodation). There may be the inability to think about the trauma, or an uncompromising avoidance of thinking or talking about the trauma.

There may be either total amnesia for the trauma or partial amnesia for certain components of the trauma. This amnesia typically alternates with hypermnesia, ruminating about nothing but the trauma, and formulating theories about how one could have avoided the trauma (omen formation). Flashbacks may blur past and present, leading to transient disorientation to time and place. Beliefs may develop to counteract the terrifying experience of helplessness: What one did, what one failed to do, and/or something that one fantasized that led to the trauma, concretely or magically—with the concomitant price of relentless self-criticism and the compulsive urge to punish or avenge oneself. There may be a loss of, or substantial interference with, the capacities for ongoing autobiographical as well as traumatic memory, compromising self-reflection, problem solving, and intentional action.

The broad compromising of critical ego functions, sense of reality, judgment, defense, and organization/integration of memory may lead to disorders of the self. There tends to be a decreased ability to integrate experiences, as well as a discontinuity of self and personal experience. Damage to ego functions varies, depending on both the prior stability of specific functions and the patient's particular defenses (flexible or rigid, adaptive or maladaptive).

Somatic States

Somatic states characteristic of posttraumatic disorders (also frequently found in other anxiety conditions) include irritability, physiological hyperarousal, sleep disturbances, nightmares, and efforts at self-medication through substance abuse or behavioral or process addictions (food, sex, shopping, workaholism, self-injury). Psychosomatic complaints are frequent, with some traumatized individuals reexperiencing physical states and reactions that occurred in conjunction with the trauma (partial tactile posttraumatic flashbacks). For example, a woman forced to perform fellatio as part of sexual abuse may feel strong sensations of choking or nausea, which she may or may not connect to the childhood experience; or the reactions may be connected more concretely to eating meat, leading to posttraumatic vegetarianism. Actual physical damage (e.g., war injuries, infertility due to scarring from violent rape) or illness (e.g., gonorrhea or a compromised immune system resulting from a rape) may also be a consequence of the trauma that may lead to intense rage and grief, or, alternatively, may be minimized in ways that suggest unconscious denial of its gravity. A growing body of research suggests the previous lack of recognition of the role of trauma (especially childhood trauma) in later physical illness and somatic response.

Relationship Patterns

Relationship patterns may include changes in relating to others based on decreased trust and increased insecurity, and/or on states of numbness, alienation, fearfulness, withdrawal, chronic rage, and guilt. Traumatized individuals who are highly shamed may fear rejection or keep themselves away from others for fear of contaminating them. Extreme withdrawal is not uncommon. The reality-shifting alternations between reexperiencing and numbing can also lead to guardedness around others based on alienation and mistrust and to associated difficulty in developing intimate relationships with trustworthy others. Dissociation, substance abuse, and other consequences of trauma may be helpful in the short term, but over the longer term significantly interfere with relationships and the ability to be intimate with others.

The Subjective Experience of the Therapist

The subjective experience of the therapist is highly variable and may alternate between extremes, mirroring the patient's alternation between PTSD's reexperiencing and blunting. Ultimately, resolution of reexperiencing requires working through the trauma. The therapist needs to tolerate the patient's doing so. Working through implies accepting rather than trying to ward off the trauma, approaching rather than avoiding trauma memories, and facing the intolerable. Reexperiencing is suffered passively; working through is pursued actively. Purposeful reexperiencing involves exposure to what is most feared, in imagination, in writing, or *in vivo*, so as to transform reexperiencing into narrative. Patient and therapist must face together what brings the most shame, terror, revulsion, and self-blame.

Vicarious Traumatization

Patients often fear that their therapy may affect their therapists in various ways, and these fears are all "realistic": Therapists may indeed suffer secondary traumatization. A therapist may be revolted or terrified by some aspects of the trauma and loath to explore any further; there may be some aspect of a patient's behavior during the trauma that leads to that familiar response of "blaming the victim"; or attention may be diverted toward the external perpetrators, and into questions of justice, law, and punishment, at the cost of setting aside the patient's inner suffering.

Secondary traumatization may be especially likely to occur if the therapist is unprepared to face the gravity of the trauma suffered. Symptoms of secondary traumatization include preoccupation with the patient's issues between sessions, insomnia and dreams of the patient, exaggerated eagerness or reluctance for the next session, and so on. Role reversal may involve the patient's sparing essential details of the trauma and carefully monitoring the therapist's responses to guide what material is "permissible."

A frequent complicating factor concerns the "wounded healer"—an ancient tradition given modern expression by Carl Jung (1963) to denote the healer with a history of suffering that originally motivated his or her work as healer. When the personal histories of therapist and patient intersect, the specific neglect and trauma reported or implied by the patient may selectively trigger the therapist's own unresolved trauma, eliciting reexperiencing, blunting, avoidance, or arousal, and thus further compounding vicarious traumatization. In general, trauma work calls for more supervision and peer support than therapy of most other psychopathologies. On the other hand, traumatized therapists who have successfully worked through their histories may be especially appropriate and effective in the treatment of patients with comparable traumatic histories.

In work with traumatized patients, therapist self-care is especially important. Immersing oneself in a patient's trauma may lead to vicarious traumatization, resulting in emotional exhaustion, stress, irritation, frustration, stressful dreams, or preoccupation. Aside from one's professional obligations, an interesting and developed personal life—one that is lively, meaningful, and nourishing, independent of one's work—is an important remedy to counter professional burnout and to "recharge one's batteries."

Patients with a history of secure attachment and a variety of personal and interpersonal resources who suffer from ASD or PTSD arising from single-incident adult-onset trauma may be able to approach the trauma early in the treatment and without a great deal of resourcing or pretreatment focus. Those with more complex trauma histories are dealt with in the next subsection, on CPTSD.

S41.3 *Complex Posttraumatic Stress Disorder*

CPTSD occurs in neither ICD nor DSM, but it has been proposed for over two decades. DSM-5 criteria for PTSD have broadened toward accommodating this disorder to some extent, but a number of dimensions remain unaddressed. In CPTSD, untoward events that interfere with optimal personal development between birth and adulthood produce adults who are not intact, who are in some way wounded or vulnerable to subsequent stress. Consequently, another name proposed for this disorder is "developmental trauma disorder." Developmental trauma compromises an individual's identity, self-worth, and personality; emotional regulation and self-regulation; and ability to relate to others and engage in intimacy. In many, it leads to ongoing despair, lack of meaning, and a crisis of spirituality.

While PTSD is an atypical response in traumatized adults, developmental trauma may be a very common (and thus the typical) response in traumatized children. Such trauma often goes unrecognized, is misunderstood or denied, or is misdiagnosed by many who assess and treat children. Developmental psychologists have been active in noting that because of a child's immaturity, size, and dependent and developmental status, it takes much less to traumatize a child than an adult. They further report that from infancy on, relational and attachment difficulties on the part of parents and other primary caregivers can be understood as developmental trauma—trauma that is a precursor to an identified set of posttraumatic *and* developmental reactions.

CPTSD is generally associated with a history of chronic neglect, trauma, and abuse over the course of childhood. Neglect in early childhood compromises secure attachment and tends to result in avoidant or resistant/ambivalent attachment—or, most severely, toward the disorganized/disoriented attachment style that leads to significant dissociative pathology. This neglect sets the stage for trauma in early childhood, which further interferes with normal affective maturation and the verbalization of feelings, leading to anhedonia, alexithymia, and intolerance of affective expression.

Children and adolescents are more prone to dissociate than are adults. Dissociation is especially linked to betrayal trauma—the neglect that allows for, or passively tolerates, more active trauma. In the face of betrayal trauma, dissociation may be the child's best life-saving defense in the short term, even if this leads to depersonalization, derealization, and discontinuities of self and personal experience in the long term.

Comorbidity

CPTSD, if it were more widely recognized, would result in a significant reduction of spurious or artifactual comorbidity. Apparent comorbidity is perhaps the single most striking characteristic of CPTSD. There are few rules dictating how a given adult with compromised personal development will manifest this history in his or her subsequent symptomatology. Unlike the more solid syndromes of schizophrenia and bipolar disorder, a patient with significantly compromised development, manifest or covert, may present with some combination of overt or subtle symptoms from a wide variety of disorders. These include depressive, anxiety, obsessive–compulsive, posttraumatic, dissociative, somatoform, eating, sleep–wake, sexual, gender, impulse-control, substance-related, and personality disorders. The astute reader will note that this covers almost the entire nosology, apart from schizophrenia, bipolar disorder, and organic brain syndromes. To repeat, there are few rules. Almost no one will have symptoms from all categories, but anyone with symptoms from two or three categories ought to be questioned about all the others. What results may not be strict diagnostic comorbidity—a very ill patient with very many symptoms may not have enough in any one category to yield a firm "diagnosis"—but it will result in a wider appreciation of the patient's suffering and its roots. With such a patient, the primary temptation may be to identify the disorder one prefers to treat, while turning a "blind eye" to the rest. Treatment focused on the trauma itself, on the other hand, may ameliorate symptoms across these diagnostic groupings.

The Subjective Experience of the Therapist

Emotional reactions of therapists treating CPTSD are highly variable. These may range from the depressive (such as sympathy, sorrow, horror, and guilt) to the paranoid–schizoid (such as fear, rage, disgust, and contempt). Fantasies may range from the maternal/caring/protective toward the victim to the paternal/enraged/punitive against the perpetrator; or else, escaping from this polarity, to fantasies of denial and flight.

The Therapeutic Interaction

The dynamics of the therapeutic interaction have been conceptualized in a variety of ways. Freud introduced acting out: "The patient does not remember anything of what he has forgotten and repressed, but acts it out. He reproduces it not as a memory but as an action; he repeats it, without, of course, knowing that he is repeating it" (1914, p. 150). A patient unconsciously acts out some dyadic component of an old interpersonal drama with the therapist. The therapist unconsciously responds to this drama in emotion, thought, and behavior. If this carries on for some time, then the interpersonal drama is called an "enactment." This sequence may also be conceptualized in Kleinian terms of projective and introjective identification. The trauma and neglect of CPTSD are essentially relational, and so the therapeutic relationship itself becomes the principal vehicle of change. How the therapist feels, thinks, and acts depends on what aspect of the neglect/trauma drama is being played out with the patient.

Trust

Repeated relational trauma and neglect suffered in childhood are generally marked by betrayal by those caregivers who were supposed to have been the most trustworthy. As a consequence, the first issue in therapy is usually trust. The patient's most important developmental lesson may be that one can least afford to trust the people who are supposed to be the most trustworthy. The therapist may well begin therapy as "guilty until proven innocent," and being put in this position may challenge the therapist's personal and professional self-image and prompt a judgmental or defensive response. It is important to understand that such enactments are meaningful communications, to be welcomed as illuminating. In keeping with the oscillation between reexperiencing and blunting, the patient may also oscillate between guarded hypervigilance and naive hypovigilance and tempt the therapist to loosen therapeutic boundaries. This would be an enactment of the pattern of revictimization so common among those with developmental trauma, and a test of trustworthiness in its own right.

Safety

Trust can be fostered only in safety. This includes both maintaining safety within the therapeutic relationship and helping the patient be safe in the real world. Maintaining safety in the therapy is often a balancing act: Insufficient emotional warmth may be experienced by the patient as delinquent neglect, disdain, or repugnance; an excess of emotional warmth may be experienced as the seductive prelude to sexual assault.

Personal History Variables

Traumatized children receive no detailed instruction as to how to defend themselves against or cope with the trauma. In the face of overwhelming trauma, children react spontaneously with some combination of desperation and creativity. For any given patient, the therapist may reflect on what is generic (some variation on the average expectable pattern of reaction) and on what is specific to that child, in those circumstances, with that history. What results is some aspect of psychic structure, which, if properly understood, will be a unique structure for that patient. So a common roadblock obstructing further therapeutic progress in the treatment of a given patient may be the therapist's exaggerated devotion to a particular model of psychic functioning, which happens not to be applicable to this particular patient.

Enactments

The reader is advised to consult the preceding subsection on ASD/PTSD, all of which applies to CPTSD. For posttraumatic conditions arising from prolonged interpersonal dynamics, psychodynamic therapists may find it useful to "locate" themselves and their patients on a triangle analogous to the oedipal one: the drama triangle of Karpman (1968). Davies and Frawley (1994) apply this triangle to bring order to the chaos of traumatic transference–countertransference. Repeated trauma in childhood involves a perpetrator and victim, but also a parent who permits the trauma to occur; is uninvolved, oblivious, and neglectful; or else is paralyzed by fear into inaction. Patient and therapist may find themselves playing any of these roles and their opposites.

We have touched already on the therapist as the untrustworthy potential perpetrator. Reverse enactments may also occur, as therapists find themselves attacked, criticized, and humiliated by these patients—leading either to wishes to stop treatment, or to expressions of gratitude to the patients for effectively conveying what it felt like to be on the receiving end of such abuse. The role of the nonabusing, negligent parent is especially easy to fall into if the patient dwells in avoidance and numbness rather than reexperiencing. More seriously, the nonabusing parent may also be complicit in the abuse, as voyeur. Patients are invited to tell all, but in doing so may transform their therapists into voyeurs, presuming that the clinical material is for their therapists' entertainment and titillation. The opposite dynamic may be acted out instead, with a patient inviting a therapist to be everything the nonabusing parent was not: The patient is needy and wounded; prior therapists were ignorant and incompetent; and the current therapist is wondrously wise, patient, understanding, kind, and lovable. The therapist in such a position can only disappoint.

Trauma wherein one parent is both the "worst" and the "best" parent may be especially difficult for the therapist. Abuse that is overtly sadistic throughout is sometimes less confusing and easier to resolve than abuse that begins with gradual affectionate and gratifying sensuality—seduction—before turning into overt sexual assault. The loving warmth of the seductive phase may be far more gratifying than anything the nonabusing parent has to offer—an œdipal triumph. The point where this turns into sexual trauma will be confusing to the patient. Enacted in therapy, therapists may find themselves seduced by, or seductive toward, the patient, with a focus on the gratifying intimacy to defend against confronting the trauma; a dynamic that also increases the risk of boundary violations and may lead to the familiar pattern of revictimization being played out in the therapy.

Clinical Illustrations

Case 1

A survivor of 9/11 who from her nearby building witnessed the plane crash, the jumping of people from the World Trade Center towers, and the towers' collapse escaped Manhattan with coworkers. Her company immediately set up a temporary office in New Jersey, expecting managers like her to resume responsibilities. She began working there the next day, wearing the same clothes as the day before. This expectation resulted in her splitting from the experience. She began showing a pattern of self-disregard, risk-taking, and substance use, all of which she minimized. She denied any connection with 9/11, yet actively avoided stories about it and found ways to distract herself on that date. Eventually, she became addicted to alcohol and was sent to rehabilitation. Once sober, she began to remember and reexperience the traumatic events and to talk about them with her therapist.

Case 2

An Iraq combat veteran returned from four tours of duty, the last of which involved a traumatic brain injury from an improvised explosive device. His family described him as not the same man who had deployed: He was subject to excruciating headaches, emotional dysregulation and rages, ongoing irritability, guardedness, hypervigilance, and startle responses. He was also profoundly depressed, due to both survivor guilt and recognition of the cost of his injuries to his life. Differential diagnosis and treatment were required for the effects of both the brain injury and the PTSD.

S42 Dissociative Disorders

A concordance between the ICD-10/DSM-5 and the PDM-2 classification of dissociative disorders is shown in Table 3.2 (pp. 245–250). As mentioned earlier, ICD-10 and DSM-5 cluster these disorders differently. ICD-10 remains in line with ICD-7, -8, and -9 and with DSM-II, where dissociation and conversion were different types of hysterical neurosis, and depersonalization was a stand-alone neurosis. DSM-III reinterpreted depersonalization as dissociative and divided dissociation and conversion between the dissociative and somatoform disorders. Here we follow DSM-5 dissociative disorders, and in subsection S43, DSM-5 somatic symptom and related disorders, which include conversion disorder.

S42.1 *Depersonalization/Derealization Disorder*

Depersonalization/derealization disorder is characterized by persistent or recurrent experiences of depersonalization, derealization, or both. During these, reality testing remains intact. Depression and anxiety disorders are the most common comorbid conditions, followed by certain personality patterns (avoidant, borderline, and obsessive–compulsive; see Chapter 1 on the P Axis). The severity of symptoms, however, is independent of the presence or severity of comorbid conditions.

While the prevalence of depersonalization/derealization disorder in the general population is about 1%, this condition is very rarely diagnosed. Because most professionals are unfamiliar with the diagnosis, patients often receive the correct diagnosis only after several years of treatment. Mean age of onset is 16 years; it usually begins before age 25. Both sexes are equally affected. The course is often persistent and unresponsive to nonspecific treatments.

Depersonalization/derealization disorder has wide ranges of symptomatic distress and social impairment, which do not easily correlate. Diagnostic signs are generally entirely absent, and so diagnosis rests entirely on self-disclosure. The extreme emotional pain of sufferers often appears incongruent with their seemingly normal behavior and apparently normal affective or motor expression. Most report that they experience depersonalization and/or derealization permanently during waking hours, and sometimes even while they are dreaming. Symptom intensity may be constant and unwavering or may wax and wane, sometimes triggered by specific situations (e.g., artificial light, social contacts). Sometimes they have no apparent trigger.

Emotional neglect and abuse are significant environmental risk factors. Harm avoidance is considered as a temperamental risk factor. In contrast to DID (see subsection S42.3, below), severe traumatic experiences are rare. Common precipitants of depersonalization and derealization are panic attacks, cannabis intoxication, depressive episodes, and psychosocial stressors.

So far, no drugs have been approved for the treatment of this disorder. First-line treatment is psychotherapy. Early psychodynamic approaches construed symptoms of depersonalization and derealization as specific and complex defenses against emotional experiencing and anxiety, respectively. Fenichel (1945) suggested that the obsessional self-observation in this disorder represents a countercathexis against feelings of anxiety from conflicts, including those around separation–individuation, conflicting identifications, and self-esteem.

The Subjective Experience of Depersonalization and Derealization

Because symptoms of depersonalization are primarily somatic-like, we have changed the usual order of presentation.

Somatic States

The central symptom is the blunting or absence of the global subjective sense of reality—the feeling of being detached from the self, the body, the environment. As an item on the Cambridge Depersonalization Scale (CDS) puts it, "I feel strange, as if I were not real or as if I were cut off from the world" (Sierra & Berrios, 2000). Depersonalization may be a general sense of corporeal blunting; of one's body not being one's own; of being a driver or passenger in a robot; of being located just behind the eyeballs and looking out as if through portholes; of being "me" in a body which is somehow "not me"; and so on. The experience commonly includes the whole body, but may have a "cutoff" line, such that the head feels real, but everything below the neck feels unreal: "Parts of my body feel as if they don't belong to me" (CDS). Other somatic states commonly co-occur (e.g., fullness of the head, lightheadedness, dizziness, visual distortions). Most patients, with prompting, can identify somatic symptoms of anxiety and depression (e.g., muscle tension, butterflies in the stomach, chest pain, lump in the throat) without connecting them to the related emotions. Depersonalization may be mild or severe and when severe may be extremely unpleasant. On the other hand, in the midst of ongoing calamity, depersonalization may induce odd calmness and even serenity, where its defensive function is most obvious.

An out-of-body experience may complicate depersonalization, in which one not only feels that one's body is unreal, but also experiences oneself as spatially separate from the body, which one may see from the outside. Frequent viewing "positions" are behind, to either side, or above, but rarely in front of, one's normal field of vision. An out-of-body experience may also occur in DID, in which case it is generally the host personality that views the body from without, while one of the alter personalities is in the body. This may be corroborated if the therapist gets a report about the subjective experience of the alter in the body for the interval during which the host was having the experience.

Derealization is rarely present in the absence of depersonalization, and so is generally a complication of depersonalization. In derealization, the world feels unreal; it may seem to be a two-dimensional image, a three-dimensional hologram, or a "virtual" world created by computer graphics (like the "holodeck" on *Star Trek*).

Affective States

Depersonalization generally includes emotions. Emotions may be accurately identified but felt to be fake, "as-if," or absent: "I don't feel any feelings any more" (CDS). Depersonalization is quite distinct from depression, but depersonalization may lead to depression, at which point the average clinician may focus on the depression as the more familiar pathology and overlook the depersonalization. Suicidal ideation may complicate chronic or treatment-resistant depersonalization/derealization disorder.

Cognitive Patterns

Cognitive patterns are captured by further items from the CDS: "I have the feeling of not having any thoughts at all, so that when I speak it feels as if my words were being uttered by an automaton"; "My surroundings feel detached or unreal, as if there were a veil between me and the outside world." There is generally no disorder of orientation, memory, or thought. Perception, while globally altered, generally includes no true anesthesia or other negative hallucinatory phenomena. In persons lacking insight, a delusional perception may occur (i.e., a delusional explanation for the feeling of unreality). As with any such dynamic, the content of such a delusion will vary enormously, depending on personal history. Despite the absence of true amnesia, an individual's affective relationship with his or her own past is often changed: "I feel detached from memories of things that have happened to me—as if I had not been involved in them" (CDS).

Relationship Patterns

Relationship patterns are often compromised by depersonalization and derealization. Depersonalized patients may lose relationships because of their inability to express feelings and/or to respond to the emotional needs of others or because relationships without emotion are experienced as meaningless. The self may be experienced as defective, worthless, incompetent, unacceptable, and overly dependent on others, while others may be experienced as disappointing, mistreating, neglecting, or abusive. These negative expectations compromise intentions, authenticity, and openness in relationships, impeding the ability to express wishes, feelings, and thoughts. This dynamic also plays out in therapy, becoming a specific form of resistance in which patients fear being rejected or mortified if they reveal their "true self" or behave in authentic and spontaneous ways. Such maladaptive self- and object representations tend to persist as long as the depersonalization remains present. Nonetheless, a considerable minority of individuals with depersonalization and derealization enjoy positive but constricted relationships, and a smaller minority pursue overstimulation in order to feel alive.

The Subjective Experience of the Therapist

A patient with depersonalization or derealization may be silent, monotonous, emotionally "dead," or concrete, with inevitable consequences for the dyad. The therapist may feel a variety of concomitant dysphoric states: emptiness, unreality, sleepiness, distraction, or boredom. One task is to wonder whether this is simply the therapist's defensiveness against the patient's dysphoria, a reflection of that dysphoria, or one pole of a more complex transference–countertransference enactment.

- *As a defense:* The therapist's own inattention, boredom, sleepiness, and depersonalization may be forms of denial and isolation defending the therapist from a clinical situation devoid of feelings, fantasies, memories, and dreams, in which he or she may feel at a loss about how to interpret such a paucity of clinical material.
- *As a reflection:* The patient's internal states may defend against intolerable impulses, thoughts, feelings, and memories. To the extent that the therapist reflects these feelings and this dynamic, the person's dysphoria may in turn prompt angry or aggressive fantasies in reaction; what is intolerable in the patient is welling up within

the therapist. This is consonant with a schizoid defense against intolerable impulses in the patient.

- *As one pole of a transference–countertransference enactment:* The challenge is to use one's experience to wonder about the therapeutic couple: "Am I feeling like this as a direct reflection of how the patient feels? Or am I feeling and interacting the way the patient experienced his or her mother as being? Or has the patient become the mother to give me the experience of being him- or herself in relation to her?" This dynamic is dominated more by deficit and insecure attachment.

Clinical Illustration

A 24-year-old psychology student consulted a therapist after suffering for 2 years from depersonalization, derealization, and major depression. Onset occurred when she quit medical school, despite her successful performance, and left her hometown to study psychology. Ever since, she had felt as if she had died and was now only a detached observer of herself or living in a dream. Despite adequate social integration and only mild impairment in academics, she felt desperate and disconnected. There was no history of severe childhood adversity, but her parents had been overbearing and had never accepted her interest in psychology.

S42.2 *Dissociative Amnesia ± Fugue*

Dissociative Amnesia without Fugue

Pure dissociative amnesia is the primary symptom of the disorder called dissociative amnesia. The hallmark is a blackout for a specific interval of time—an episode of "lost time"—with no medical explanation. This should not be confused with forgetfulness, such as difficulty remembering certain specific information. Forgetfulness describes someone who remembers reading an article yesterday, but forgets what it was about; amnesia applies to someone who has no memory for the interval of time during which he or she read the article yesterday.

Dissociative amnesia is commonly complicated by disorientation to time. On "emerging" from a dissociative episode of unknown duration, different people experience different levels of disquiet. Some are shaken by the lapse of time. Some grow accustomed to it. A patient explained: "Time, for me, is like a loaf of sliced bread. Various slices are removed, but then I push the two ends together so that I don't really notice it anymore." In any case, the person needs to reorient to time. Many with recurrent dissociative amnesia become quite skillful at hiding their disorientation and finding ways to quickly assess the current time.

Dissociative Amnesia with Fugue

Dissociative fugue was a separate diagnosis in DSM-III and -IV, but DSM-5 has "demoted" it to a specifier for dissociative amnesia because full dissociative fugue is vanishingly rare. The full syndrome is an episode during which one is amnestic for all autobiographical memory, and consequently disoriented in all three spheres: not knowing who one is, where one is, or what time and date it is. On the other hand, semantic and procedural memory remain intact, and so the person remembers how to understand and speak the given language, what words mean, how to tie shoelaces, how to negotiate traffic, and so on.

"Minifugues" (*fuguettes*), on the other hand, are common in dissociative amnesia: When coming out of an amnestic episode, a person may be in a different place from the last-remembered location, without any memory of the passage to that place, and consequently transiently disoriented to time and possibly place. The mildest minifugue may occur in one's own home—for instance, waking in the morning, sitting on the edge of the bed; then a "blank"; then emerging from the blank to the sound of the whistle from the kettle as it comes to a boil, and finding oneself sitting at the kitchen table, having already eaten breakfast.

Between full fugue and *fuguette* are moderate fugues, which suggest the presence of DID. A woman driving to a therapy session remembered reaching the corner where she was to turn left. She blanked out and emerged from this blank exiting a mall, having bought a number of inappropriate items of clothing (black lace undergarments), and having no idea where she had parked the car. She would sometimes fall asleep in bed at night, wake on the living room sofa at 2:00 P.M., and telephone her therapist to apologize for having missed her 10:00 A.M. appointment, only to find out that she had in fact attended, had been on time, and had stayed for the full session (though in one of her other self-states).

The relationship patterns of those suffering from psychogenic amnesia or fugue may be determined by what has been forgotten and/or fled. For example, abuse victims who have forgotten their mistreatment are often vulnerable to revictimization; individuals whose fugue takes them from a position of responsibility may face serious consequences for their flight.

S42.3 Dissociative Identity Disorder and Other Specified Dissociative Disorder–1

Dissociative identity disorder (DID) and other specified dissociative disorder, example 1 (OSDD-1) are put together here because they are essentially the same diagnosis, differing only in degree. The acronym OSDD-1 has replaced its equally ungainly predecessor, DDNOS-1 (dissociative disorders not otherwise specified, example 1). For over three decades, when the scientific literature has mentioned DDNOS, it has invariably meant DDNOS-1 (subclinical DID), as it is more common than DID and also more common than DSM-IV's DDNOS-2 through DDNOS-6. It remains more common than DSM-5's OSDD-2 through OSDD-4.

The first PDM differed from ICD and DSM in recategorizing DID as a personality disorder in its P Axis, where it was called dissociative personality disorder. Here in PDM-2, DID is moved back to the dissociative disorders, bringing it back into harmony with its ICD and DSM classifications.

There was good reason to propose considering DID as a personality disorder. On the surface, in many cases of severe and ongoing dissociative problems, the principal center of consciousness out in the world presents as if with a personality disorder of some kind. The other centers of consciousness—variably called "alter personalities," "alters," "others" (Latin *alter* = English "other"), "ego states," or "self-states"—almost always present with the appearance of personality disorders of their own, and these presentations tend to be narrow and more exaggerated than average, sometimes to the point of caricature. These presentations are "as-if," however, because the more significant the alterity, switching, and exaggeration, the less the person in question satisfies the general criteria for any personality disorder.

At a deeper level, when the creation of new centers of consciousness become someone's primary, habitual response to stress and negative affect, dissociation becomes characterological in the same way that any other defense may become the person's "default" mode of adaptation. The basis of DID is the co-occurrence of a constitutional capacity to go into trance, in an early childhood with such disordered attachment and failed protection that early-onset, severe, repeated traumatization becomes possible, and takes place.

Covert DID and OSDD-1

The most recent scientific estimate (DSM-5's) of the prevalence of diagnosed DID is 1.5% of the general population. This figure is worthy of some contemplation and should guide the clinician toward a careful differential diagnostic assessment. Some examples follow.

- *Schizophrenia*. The so-called first-rank Schneiderian symptoms of schizophrenia, such as the intrusion or withdrawal of voices, emotions, thoughts, knowledge, and behavior, are common in DID/OSDD-1, and so may be misinterpreted as schizophrenic rather than dissociative. The specific hallucination of hearing one's thoughts aloud and its concomitant delusion of thought broadcasting is generally absent, however, in DID, as are delusional perceptions.
- *Brief psychotic disorder*. DID/OSDD-1 ought to be on the differential diagnosis for all presentations of this condition. Recently decompensated multiplicity with rapid switching may manifest themselves with hallucinations and disorganized speech and behavior. This experience may be interpreted by the "host" personality in terms that appear delusional—for example, the conviction that one has been invaded by evil spirits.
- *Bipolar disorder*. Rapid-cycling bipolar disorder is diagnosable when there are at least four mood episodes per year. In DID, switching between alters of abruptly contrasting moods may give the false impression of extremely rapid cycling, closer to four episodes per day or even per hour, and, in extreme cases, four episodes per minute. Such rapidity is beyond the reach of bipolar disorder.
- *PTSD*. Dissociative symptoms (flashbacks, amnesia, emotional blunting, depersonalization, etc.) in PTSD are often present in DID and other dissociative disorders and may distract from the central diagnosis. There is also debate regarding the structure of PTSD itself, with some positing that the alternation between too much (criterion B—reexperiencing) and too little (criterion D—numbing, amnesia) may reflect a switch between two rudimentary self-states created during the trauma, an emotional self-state and an "apparently normal" one, in the terminology of a World War I psychiatrist named Myers. The diagnosis of PTSD, may thus lead to that of DID.
- *Depersonalization*. This may be uncomplicated, as in the pervasive feeling of being unreal. It may also be a symptom of one self-state who remains passively copresent during an executive switch to another self-state. In the event of an out-of-body experience, a freshly created self-state may remain "in the body" undergoing the trauma, allowing the primary self-state to escape to, say, the ceiling.

• *Dissociative amnesia* ± fugue. In some cases, it may emerge that there was a switch to an alter self-state who took over executive control for an amnestic episode or fugue.

• *Conversion disorder.* Somatoform symptoms are common, though of disparate etiology. Only a minority would qualify as classical psychoanalytic conversion (a somatic symptom caused by incomplete repression of an unacceptable wish or impulse). More common are partial tactile posttraumatic flashbacks (or bluntings) of real past events. In both cases, the symptom often originates in a self-state different from the one complaining, through "leakage" caused by incomplete dissociation, just as classical conversion is caused by incomplete repression.

• *Eating disorders.* These may interact with severe and complex dissociative patterns in a numerous ways. A patient, and some of his or her alter self-states, may have no experience of having eaten for months or years; there may be a covert self-state who emerges at night to eat and "keep the body alive," blissfully ignored by "most" of the patient. Vegetarianism may be a generic means of limiting food intake, along with whatever "diet" interferes with eating; however, it may also be a specific avoidance of the experience of having meat in the mouth, which would trigger posttraumatic flashbacks of forced fellatio, a dynamic hidden in an as-yet covert alter self-state. A comparable dynamic may underlie avoidance of creamy foods (e.g., yogurt).

• *Sleep-wake disorders.* Chronic daytime sleepiness may be the result of switching to an alter self-state during the night, for which the presenting patient is amnestic.

• *Gender incongruence.* Severe and complex dissociation commonly involves cross-gender self-states. When someone complains of gender dysphoria, one should rule out a switch to a cross-gendered alter self-state, who may have taken the "host" position.

Explaining Dissociative Multiplicity

In explaining psychopathology, we generally attempt to explain the abnormal with reference to theories we know and accept. Psychodynamic authors have approached dissociative psychopathology from many different starting points. Janet (1889) has been "rediscovered" as a nonpsychoanalytic contributor to understanding dissociative pathology. Hypnoid hysteria has been resurrected from Breuer and Freud's (1895) *Studies on Hysteria*, thereby readmitting altered states of consciousness into psychodynamic explanation. Brenner (2001) explains dissociative multiplicity through Freud's (1904) "Splitting of the Ego in the Process of Defence." Tarnopolsky (2003) explains dissociative multiplicity through Kleinian splitting. A number of authors draw on the work of Fairbairn (1944) or Kohut (1984) to reinstate dissociation within psychoanalytic thought. Bowlby's attachment theory has attracted wide attention as an explanation, especially of attachment deficits in the etiology of severe and complex dissociative disorders. Watkins and Watkins (1997), borrowing the concept of ego state from Paul Federn (1952), developed ego state theory, an explanatory and therapeutic approach that has become a central pillar of the contemporary dissociative community. Ego states have led to a general interest in different states of self, beginning in infancy. This has all coalesced into an overall reconceptualization of psychodynamic thinking into a multiple self-state model of mind. Instead of having to explain how a single mind could give rise to multiplicity, the normal mind is constituted as multiple, and dissociative disorders emerge as a particular exaggeration of that multiplicity—a dramatic variation on the theme.

Putnam (1997) built upon the work of others to describe the origins of this kind of mental organization in the discrete behavioral states of infants. Lacking transitional states, normal infants hop over the gaps between states with shifts so rapid (e.g., cooing calmly to ear-piercing cries of distress) that parents are often surprised. When there is a failure of caregiving adults to facilitate emotional and perceptual bridges of these behavioral states in infants, transitional states do not develop. This deficit may underlie the characteristic emotional lability described in many dissociative adults and borderline adults with dissociative features, who have difficulty anticipating self-state changes and lose control of behavior. Early extreme and repeated stress allows these multiple self-state gaps, which are already there, to become especially visible.

The multiple self-state model of mind, then, arose from theories of infant attachment and relational psychoanalysis and has undergone robust research testing in infant attachment and behavior. A mind chronically brutalized lays bare boundaries and gaps between "different ways of being me" that miss the opportunity to normally associate so as not to know, feel, or sense what has happened. The resulting segregation of emotion, behavior, and experience obstructs the creation of a coherent autobiographical narrative. This process results in biased perception and skewed interpretation of self–other experience: altered subjectivity.

The Subjective Experience in General in Severe Dissociative Disorders

The question of subjective experience immediately becomes more complex in severe dissociative disorders because there is more than one subject per patient. To understand the subjective experience of people with severe dissociative problems, it may be helpful to contrast their situation with the integrated sense of self of more stable individuals. Healthier people generally experience their initiatives, actions, and experiences as their own. They experience their bodies' movements and their sensory perceptions as aspects of themselves, of who they are. They synthesize the information from their various senses (sight, sound, smell, etc.) and from an appreciation of their history and current circumstances into an integrated perception of what they are doing on their own initiative, and/or what is happening to them. Their thoughts and ideas are invested with different affects that help determine their meaning, and these affectively meaningful cognitions are all integrated into a sense of self. Even complex social interactions and their associated affective states are assimilated in connection with themselves in an integrated way. Whether feelings are mixed, ambivalent, or even further conflicted, they are experienced as one's own.

In severe or complex dissociation, the synthesis of input from these varied sources cannot be taken for granted; any or all of them can be severed from experience or experienced as alien, as "not-me." The range of symptomatic expression varies enormously, however, from person to person, and may also vary over time within the same person. This is a key reason why many cases of DID are undetected or misdiagnosed: We see those cases that are sufficiently symptomatic that they seek or are brought to treatment. Some seem to have led relatively "normal" lives until some trauma in adulthood has precipitated decompensation in their adaptive functioning. This underscores a difference from personality disorder in clinical course. It is likely that many cases manage to remain undetected until death intervenes.

The "default" subject, the one who most often deals with real interactions in the real world, often called the "host," may be remarkably without subjective symptoms, apart from inferring that he or she has recurrent intervals of "lost time." Such individuals may discover, to their chagrin, something about their manifest behavior from evidence around the house or from other people who witnessed them during the amnestic interval. The "host" role is just that, and over time the host role may be taken on by different alters.

If the alternate subject, or alter, present during the host's "amnestic interval," appears in a therapy session, he or she may likewise be remarkably without subjective symptoms and may give a coherent account of experience during the interval in question. While the host may be ignorant of other selves, most of the others are usually cognizant of the host, and often of each other, or at least of some subset of the others. More commonly, especially in the clinic, the host does have symptoms; these may include amnesia, depersonalization, derealization, and any variety of "intrusion" symptoms from any of the other self-states. Intrusions (and withdrawals) include hallucinations of others' voices and of their flashbacks, and intrusion and withdrawal of emotions, thoughts, impulses, fears, sensations, and so on. The default subject, with time, may also come to appreciate that the "host" position is a role that others can play. Especially with therapy, different alters may take turns playing the "host" role as the system evolves.

Therapy makes use of the inherently autohypnotic elements of DID. Some patients have elaborated autohypnotic solutions to managing symptoms and multiplicity itself in what has been called the "third reality." Clinicians have borrowed some of these solutions as therapeutic techniques for use in patients with severe and/or complex dissociation.

The Three Realities

Significantly dissociative patients commonly experience three "realities." The first is "objective" reality—the reality that "everyone" agrees on. The second is subjective reality, or what is real for a given individual consciousness—the locus of subjective experience. The third reality is generally experienced by alters, not always by the host: an internal virtual or phantom landscape, sometimes called the "inscape," wherein the various alters experience each other as cohabiting this space, much as different real people experience each other in the first reality.

In patients with DID and related disorders, there is generally a multiplicity of second realities. For an overwhelmed person, the alters serve as vehicles for endorsing and inhabiting more tolerable alternative realities. The primary gain is the sequestering of the burden of an intolerable reality, at the cost of the confusing and often chaotic flux of alters' subjective experiences, perceptions, and understandings of themselves, their lives, and their relationships with significant others. Paradoxically, this confusion may be minimal when dissociative barriers among alters are very strong; with less severe presentations, or with the weakening of barriers that generally occurs in therapy, copresence and "symptom leakage" may increase among self-states to such an extent that a patient may complain "I don't really know who I am right now!"

The third reality, the internal landscape or "inscape," is a feature of the subjective experiences of many patients. Even if the subjective experiences of the various alters yield conflicting perceptions of the first reality, there is generally consensus about this third reality, where alters appear with phantom bodies appropriate to their gender, age, putative personal history, and temperamental characteristics, and which has other characteristics of "real" reality (persistence over time, from visit to visit, commonly over years, and in the "real" consequence of "historical" events that happen there). The clinical advantage of working in the third reality is that it guarantees a certain level of co-presence and immediate sharing across self-states. Such "face-to-face" encounters have proven to be therapeutically useful for negotiation and compromise among host and alters; for the expression, containment, and sharing of posttraumatic memories; and for the integration of self-states.

Specific Subjective Experiences in Severe Dissociative Disorders

Amnesia

As noted, patients typically manifest dissociative amnesia, often with minifugues. "Lost time" occurs most commonly because of an executive switch to another self-state. Subsequent recall may be absent, or else delayed, with sketchy recall, or as if recalling a dream; alternatively, there may be no sensory recall per se, but "second-hand" knowledge of the period in question through a "verbal report" from another self-state. This process may be very upsetting. Further dissociative defenses may then lead to indifference, distracting idle chatter, or amnesia for what has just happened or for what has just been verbally shared.

Affective States

Certain affects may "belong" to a given self-state, and may be relatively absent from all others. Rage may be the prerogative of one; lust of another; fastidious housecleaning yet another. Incomplete switches to another self-state may leave the subject in the role of passive observer of another's perception of reality and behavior, possibly experienced as if it were a nightmare. The inner confusion occasioned by the clash of such simultaneously experienced alternate realities may cause many forms of distress and withdrawal, anxiety and panic, with an intense preoccupation with what is happening, terrifying fear of loss of control, and paralyzing despair.

The loss of "I," a sense of grounding in "me," may be accompanied by sharp anxiety, even to the point of panic—or by its opposite, a strange indifference or calm. It is often helpful to encourage individuals with dissociative disorders to describe their affective experiences in detail and/or to reflect upon their apparent absence. Exploration of such reports—even if fragmentary, seemingly contradictory, or full of numbness or nothingness—may prove a valuable step in reintegrating the different states that constitute a sense of self. As therapy proceeds, it is usually valuable to study the relationship of these accounts to the stressful experiences that may have been their antecedents and the triggers for the onset or mobilization of dissociative defenses.

Perception

Unlike a patient with schizophrenia, a patient with a significant dissociative disorder may often give a description of the hallucinatory voices: name, gender, age, appearance, how and of what they speak, their "function" or purpose in the system, and so on. In addition, the interaction between the person and the voices is typically closer to a normal conversation than one finds in schizophrenia.

Cognitive Symptoms

Patients vary widely in their insight. Interpretation of the presence of intact or defective insight hinges, of course, on what the clinician believes to be the case. If DID and OSDD-1 are regarded as "true" diagnoses, then a patient who claims that the alters are all imaginary and don't really exist will be regarded as in denial by a clinician who "believes in" DID and as intact reality testing by a clinician who doesn't "believe in" DID. There are some common false beliefs that arise in specific self-states (e.g., belief of one or more alters that they do not share the body with others, and that they may commit suicide, or else kill one of the other self-states, without killing "everyone"; that if the body dies, they can migrate to someone else's body; or that therapy ought to be terminated because DID does not exist).

Somatic States

Somatic symptoms are very common and may be dominated by intrusions of posttraumatic reexperiencing. The source may be the patient before one, but such symptoms often constitute "leakage" from another self-state. Partial tactile flashbacks are especially common, resulting in body symptoms that involve pain, unpleasant sensation, or numbness.

Somatic intrusions may also be peculiarly prosaic. For instance, a woman is walking down the department store aisle on her way to the exit. Her left hand reaches out and grabs a brightly colored scarf and stuffs it into her pocket. Alarmed, the woman tries to put the scarf back. Her left arm will not move. She reaches over with her right hand, and has a minor struggle to free the scarf from the left hand. She replaces it on the display table and exits the store immediately. Later on, she discovers that a child alter had seen the scarf, found it pretty, and wanted it.

Relationship Patterns

The relationships of dissociative patients vary widely. They may show a wide range of capabilities to relate. Certain self-states may look after home, spouse/partner, and children; others may look after work. Adaptation may be more apparent than real, as competent functioning may be carried out by a self-state with no life outside the workplace. Disturbed relationships are common and often mimic or recreate some aspect of the traumatic history: Alters may be perceived as perpetrators, exploiters, or rescuers. Sexual trauma often impairs sexual intimacy, which triggers overt flashbacks. The trauma bond may be repeated with subsequent partners, with patterns of masochistic submissiveness and revictimization. The traumatic history that engenders this condition, usually involving abuse by a primary caregiver, creates in its victims a disposition to placate authorities—including therapists, from whom grave mistreatment is unconsciously feared. Patients have little reason to trust clinicians, and clinicians who convey skepticism about amnesia and altered states of consciousness unwittingly discourage patients from revealing the dissociative symptoms from which they suffer.

The Subjective Experience of the Therapist

The overall encounter with a dissociative patient may leave the average therapist feeling completely deskilled—at a loss. Without specific training in the condition, it is common to feel blamed for not being or knowing or doing enough. Because of a vague, disjointed, or contradictory narrative, history taking may engender confusion and a sense of futility. The dissociative structure (self-states and their attributes and relationships) may be so interesting that the clinician becomes immersed in it to the detriment of other therapeutic needs. The trauma history may excite rescue fantasies in the therapist. Patience is needed to tolerate the patient's deep mistrust. Perceived sensitivity to closeness may lead to distancing, which may reenact the negligent, nonabusing parent whose oblivion allowed the abuse to happen. Limits and boundaries may be tested by the patient who presents as "the exception" (Freud, 1925) in many different ways. Child alters may excite the desire to reparent the patient. Claims of childhood traumatization may come with insistent demands to be believed or else with insistent demands that the clinician collude with the patient's denial. The patient may be rocked by seemingly interminable flashbacks or else frozen into protracted affective numbing and amnesia.

Therapists may suffer secondary traumatization to the extent that they are unprepared to confront pervasive emotional and physical neglect in early childhood, together with the early, severe, repeated emotional, physical, and sexual traumatization that this neglect permitted. Countertransference reactions may range from outrage to denial. Supervision with a trusted colleague is often critical.

Clinical Illustrations

Case 1

A woman in her 30s began having panic attacks, severe abdominal pain, and moments of confusion with no organic origin. Evaluators noted that the symptoms had begun after she gave birth to her first child. Then she mentioned traumatic nightmares of abuse when she and her daughter had returned home and panic after a family visit, including an uncle with whom she had always felt uncomfortable. "These dreams must be crazy," she said. "I can't believe things like that could have happened to me." Her husband called her sister, who said that this uncle had abused both siblings, but that her sister had refused to believe it. When the sisters talked, with the husband listening, she spoke as if she had always remembered the abuse, but when her husband tried to discuss what he had heard her say, she had no recall of it.

Case 2

A middle-aged woman went to bed at night and woke to find herself in a teller's booth serving a client. She had no memory of applying for the job or of the 2-week training. She retreated to the washroom. The following day she woke up at home; this happened a few times. She eventually earned a supervisory role for exemplary performance. She remained largely amnestic and feared she would be exposed any moment as a fraud. At the bank, she had two nicknames: "Mother Hen" when working in-house, and "The Shark" when dealing with other financial institutions. Her husband and children knew only the devoted mother. Years later, she was sexually assaulted, and her dissociative structure collapsed. Posttraumatic child alters surfaced, along with hallucinations and flashbacks. She never returned to work, but had 4 years of hospital admissions and heavy antipsychotic medication, all accompanied by a worsening clinical picture, before finally beginning therapy for DID.

S43 Conversion Disorder

ICD-10 and DSM-5 classify conversion disorder according to Table 3.2 (pp. 245–250).

The essence of the medical diagnosis of conversion disorder is that it must be pseudoneurological and psychogenic. The ultimate diagnosis is made by neurology, which then refers the patient to psychiatry; the patient may then be seen by a therapist. The concept of "conversion" has had a checkered history. Freud (1894) coined the word: "In hysteria, the incompatible idea is rendered innocuous by its sum of excitation being transformed into something somatic. For this I should like to propose the name of conversion." Freud originally attributed the "sum of excitation" to external trauma. Not long afterward, however, conversion rapidly became the paradigmatic compromise formation between drive (urge, intent, wish, motive) and defense (repression), and only secondarily between trauma and defense; and a paradigmatic example of primary gain: Better to suffer the symptom than to be conscious of the forbidden wish or impulse. The psychiatric sense of conversion—pseudoneurological—would then be considered as a mere surface phenomenon of a more specific underlying dynamic, repressed drive. Since then, there has been something of a return of the repressed: Repressed wish remains, but repressed trauma has been reinstated.

Hysterical neurosis was present in both ICD-9 and DSM-II, and it had two major types: dissociative type and conversion type. ICD-10 dropped the word "hysterical," but maintained the grouping of the two types in a single category, dissociative (conversion) disorders, despite having its own somatoform disorders category. DSM-III and -IV relabeled conversion hysteria as conversion disorder and moved it to the new category of somatoform disorders. DSM-5 maintains the link to dissociation in its text: "Conversion disorder is often associated with dissociative symptoms, such as depersonalization, derealization, and dissociative amnesia" (p. 320).

These days, repression and conversion continue to be invoked for repressed wishes with somatic expression. Repressed trauma has to share the field with dissociated trauma. Some authors regard all unremembered trauma as dissociated rather than repressed; others maintain the distinction. The difficulty derives from the polysemy of both repression and dissociation: Classically, repression stood for all defenses before other defenses were distinguished, and in recent decades, dissociation has expanded to cover a myriad of distinct psychic operations. The DSM definition of a conversion symptom requires neurological competence to judge its pseudoneurological status. Once faced with such a symptom, one may then wonder whether it is evidence of a repressed wish, or a partial posttraumatic reexperiencing (or blunting), or neither.

In the course of the psychotherapeutic working through of a conversion symptom, there is the opportunity to witness the simultaneity of diagnosis and treatment. This occurs when the patient is able to enunciate the symbolic significance of the symptom, and it then vanishes. Rarely, a clear example of repression and conversion is seen in clinic practice. For example, a woman wakes up with pain and stiffness in the neck and shoulders. Midway in a session, she describes a familiar conversation with her mother: "I wanted to strangle her!" Her arms start to wave rhythmically in front of her. The pain and stiffness have vanished—a sure sign that they were strictly "supratentorial," conversion symptoms nipped in the bud. The primary gain: Better for the patient to have pain and stiffness in those muscle groups needed to strangle her mother than to recall what she said, or, indeed, that she wanted to strangle her.

But the therapy might reveal something entirely different: The identical pain and stiffness could be a partial tactile flashback of having struggled against being pinned down and strangled 30 years ago, with onset during a forgotten posttraumatic nightmare last night, triggered by the appearance of a man on the street who reminded her of her original assailant.

A negative pseudoneurological symptom (e.g., local anesthesia or analgesia or paralysis) may also be a reliving of one's dissociative state at the time of a trauma, and so have the quality of a "negative" PTSD symptom. For instance, a patient in an eating disorders inpatient unit claims to be anesthetic from umbilicus to midthigh. She seems surprised when told that most women have sensation "down there." This is a variant on what has been called *la belle indifférence*—a puzzling emotional minimization of the seriousness of conditions as disabling as blindness, paralysis, or anesthesia.

La belle indifférence is the emotional expression of primary gain: Although the symptom ought to disturb the patient, it is preferable to the alternative, and thus minimally upsetting. This should not be confused with the more generic alexithymia or *pensée opératoire* associated with somatizing personalities or somatic symptom disorders (see Chapter 1 on the P Axis, and section S5 below).

Pseudoneurological symptoms may occur also in the context of DID. If this is the case, the "source" needs to be ascertained before the kind of symptoms can be clarified. Is the symptom coming from the version of the person who is before the therapist in the office, or is it an intrusion from one of that person's alters? In DID, the most common somatoform symptoms are intrusions from an alter, and true conversion symptoms (incompletely repressed impulses) are rare enough that they come as a surprise. Intrusion phenomena are more commonly partial and undisguised revivifications from a traumatized child alter (e.g., oneself being strangled 30 years ago, or oneself in the cellar at age 3), so that psychoanalytic interpretation of symbolic significance may then be in the service of denial rather than insight. For example, if a patient feels "as if I'm being fucked in the head," this may be interpreted as symbolic of some sophisticated interpersonal manipulation, obscuring the more concrete possibility of having endured forced fellatio as a child. Combinations may also occur. A partial somatic (primarily posttraumatic) symptom may have secondary symbolic elaboration, as a compromise formation expressive of a wish–defense conflict.

In conclusion, the classic Freudian concept of repression continues to apply to the history of the conversion concept—both the repression of a trauma that gains somatic expression in a partial posttraumatic flashback (body memory) and the repression of a wish that gains somatic expression in a compromise formation (conversion proper).

S5 Somatic Symptom and Related Disorders

ICD-10 and DSM-5 classify somatic symptom and related disorders according to Table 3.2 (pp. 245–250; note the difference in clustering, and hence in sequence).

As noted just above in the discussion of conversion disorder, ICD-10 and DSM-5 cluster these disorders differently. ICD-10 has a somatoform disorders section that does not include conversion disorder, which remains within its section on dissociative (conversion) disorders. DSM-5 follows DSM-III and -IV in retaining conversion disorder as a somatic symptom (somatoform) disorder, but has now also reclassified factitious disorders with the somatic symptom and related disorders. Somatization disorder, present in DSM-III and -IV, has been dropped. This condition, once called "Briquet's syndrome," followed a tradition of requiring a certain elevated somatic symptom count—at least 14 out of a list of 37 for DSM-III; at least 8 from four groups (pain, gastrointestinal, sexual, and pseudoneurological) for DSM-IV. The large number of symptoms was the factor that had differentiated Briquet's syndrome from conversion hysteria. The new somatic symptom disorder requires only one somatic symptom that is distressing or disruptive. It is also intended to include roughly three out of every four patients formerly diagnosed as having hypochondriasis (all those with actual symptoms). Illness anxiety disorder is now reserved for those with illness anxiety but without actual symptoms.

DSM-5 notes that these disorders all feature prominent somatic symptoms, with distress and impairment. The need for symptoms to be medically unexplained has been dropped, except for conversion disorder. More central are the subjective reactions to the somatic symptom: thoughts, feelings, and behavior. A grouping with such minimal requirements necessarily puts together conditions that are psychologically quite disparate, as least one of which we view as characterological (see the discussion of somatizing personalities in Chapter 1 on the P Axis, pp. 42–44). These conditions are generally encountered, in decreasing frequency, in physicians' offices; then in hospital psychiatric consultation–liaison services (for patients admitted to medical or surgical floors); then in psychiatrists' offices; and, rarely, in the offices of psychologists and other nonmedical therapists.

With a somatic symptom, one should wonder whether it is consciously produced or feigned, as in Munchausen's syndrome and malingering, or unconsciously produced; whether the symptom is an exaggeration of an underlying physical condition or is entirely "psychogenic"; whether it is specific, having some thematic affinity to a psychological issue, as obtains especially in conversion disorder; or whether it is generic, with no such affinity.

Beyond the conditions itemized here, there are some that remain on the border between psychiatry and certain medical specialties because of the severity of complaints, paucity of clear pathophysiology, and lack of effective biological treatments. These include, among others, chronic fatigue syndrome, irritable bowel syndrome, and fibromyalgia. In some cases of these, trauma and neglect during childhood and adolescence figure in the history; in others nothing can be found.

S51 Somatic Symptom Disorder

The diagnosis of somatic symptom disorder is given when there are somatic symptoms about which a patient is highly distressed, most often about prognosis, and for which the patient spends inordinate time and energy pursuing medical treatments. It includes what was formerly called "psychalgia" (pain disorder, in earlier DSMs). The possibility of an underlying organic condition is always there, and the somatic presentation may be a functional exaggeration of this. Dynamically, the assumption is that dysphoria is expressed somatically and that the primary field of play is the body-self. As noted, it includes the majority of patients formerly diagnosed with hypochondriasis.

The tendency to experience, conceptualize, and communicate psychological distress as somatic symptoms, and to seek medical attention for them, is universal. Somatizing patients appear to feel most comfortable providing details of symptoms in physical or somatic terms. Cultural, social, and economic factors are important in the expression and subjective experience of the disorder (e.g., a lower socioeconomic status, immigration from developing countries).

Focus on secondary gain (hypothesized attempts to "profit" from a condition) should not distract from the deeper task of determining primary gain (ways in which somatizing it may spare the patient from some dysphoria). An early classic example of close attention to primary gain is found in Deutsch's "The Associative Anamnesis" (1939), in which gentle, focused, nonconfrontational exploration of the symptom generally leads to significant underlying interpersonal issues (e.g., trauma, losses, disappointments, conflicts) that may be dynamically relevant to the onset and clinical course of somatic symptoms. These ought to be carefully tracked, even as the patient continues to deny a connection between them and the symptoms concerned.

Secondary gain is often also present and, if severe, may interfere with attempts to appreciate primary gain. Secondary gain may eventually be interpreted as a "legitimate" way to get dependency needs met. Primary and secondary gain considerations are generally considered unconscious, whereas conscious secondary gain motivations (e.g., to get off work, to maximize insurance payments) are considered malingering. If the focus is too narrowly on secondary gain, patients may feel accused of malingering.

The Subjective Experience of Somatic Symptom Disorder

Affective States

Patients with somatic symptom disorder may be unable to recognize, name, and express their own affects (alexithymia). However, feelings of vulnerability, helplessness, and sadness, together with excessive somatic concerns and hyperarousal, are also common.

Cognitive Patterns

Accompanying alexithymia is a common cognitive deficit called *la pensée opératoire*. This "operational thinking" is characterized by concrete thinking, which is comfortable with things, but not with feelings, symbolic expression, imagination, or fantasy. The combination of alexithymia and operational thinking may epitomize patients about whom one might conclude are "not psychologically minded." In accordance with their varying degrees of insight, patients may or may not continue to attribute symptoms to an undiagnosed medical disorder despite an adequate or repeated medical workup. Such attribution leads to rumination about bodily symptoms, selective attention to or frequent checking of symptoms, and catastrophic thinking. In turn, such preoccupation leads to a high number of health care visits, seeking care from multiple providers for the same symptoms, requests for repeated unnecessary medical tests, and medical procedures with some risk of iatrogenic complications.

Somatic States

In addition to the somatic symptoms involved, somatic states include the physiological accompaniments of anxiety, such as rapid heartbeat, blood pressure increase, and muscle tensions that give rise to pain. These responses of the autonomic nervous system are part of the "fight-or-flight" reaction.

Relationship Patterns

Preoccupation with the body supplants in-depth relationships with other individuals, including relationships with doctors, such that others are reduced to potential sources of reassurance (which fail to reassure), or else are alienated and distanced. Encounters of these patients with their clinicians generally evoke frustration and disengagement on both sides. Patients may seem desperate to connect with clinicians through their symptoms, perhaps as a repetition of the quality of some attachment failure in childhood. In psychotherapy, patients are often poised to see the therapist as yet another authority who does not really listen or really care. They may feel disbelieved or blamed or become paranoid when the therapist tries to explore meanings beyond the purely medical.

The Subjective Experience of the Therapist

Countertransference feelings are often a reflection of the alexithymia or operatory thinking of the patient: inner deadness and disengagement, leading to boredom, irritation, and futility, especially as the patient proves to be immune to efforts to steer the focus off the worry for somatic symptoms and on other issues.

S52 Illness Anxiety Disorder (Hypochondriasis)

Illness anxiety disorder in DSM-5 supersedes the diagnosis of hypochondriasis in earlier DSMs. Hypochondriasis literally means "under" (*hypo*) "the ribs" (*chondria*), as a patient would typically enter a doctor's office with a hand cradling the right or left side, the source of some feared or imagined illness. As noted above, DSM-5 now reserves this diagnosis for patients with illness anxiety, but without actual symptoms. This overstates matters to some extent: There may well be mild symptoms, often a nonpathological physiological sign or symptom, whose meaning, significance, or cause the patient will misinterpret.

The Subjective Experience of Illness Anxiety Disorder

Affective States

There is general anxiety about one's health, and about illness in general, with particular anxiety regarding prognosis—feeling vulnerable and fearing death. Such fears may be accompanied by depressed affect and a sense of doom. Subjective state varies from preoccupation and hypervigilance to intense anxiety in reaction to what are probably normal variations in internal sensations.

Cognitive Patterns

There is a general cognitive absorption with one's body. Thoughts may include the terrifying belief that each pain or symptom is life-threatening, that *this time* it is serious. There may be a vague sense that "something is wrong with my body," even in the absence of specific complaints. This preoccupation can have a paranoid-like intensity and is associated with a deep reluctance to relinquish physical symptoms or divert attention to other aspects of life. Many explanations have been suggested for this, including that the symptoms represent a way of taking care of conscious or unconscious feelings of guilt; that they are ways of dealing with early, hostile caregivers who have been internalized and equated with the ill body organs; and that they justify the patient's being cared for. Insight level varies widely across patients suffering from this disorder, with some cases of almost delusional beliefs about having severe illness.

Somatic States

Somatic states are central to the diagnosis itself. In illness anxiety disorder a patient is characteristically preoccupied with his or her body, sometimes to the exclusion of all else. Symptoms of increased arousal are quite frequent.

Relationship Patterns

Others may be perceived as powerful, healthy, and indifferent. The persistence of symptoms is often felt as evidence of a physician's ineffectiveness. Hostility to physicians and other health care professionals may be conscious or unconscious.

The Subjective Experience of the Therapist

The subjective experience of health care professionals encountering these patients, and of the therapists involved, may include similar feelings of hostility, as well as feelings of being useless to such patients or bothered by them.

S53 Factitious Disorders

In DSM-IV and -IV-TR, factitious disorders had their own category. DSM-5 has incorporated them into the category of somatic symptom and related disorders. They remain in ICD-10's "miscellaneous" category as "intentional production or feigning of symptoms or disabilities, either physical or psychological." Sometimes called "Munchausen's syndrome," factitious disorders are conditions in which a patient intentionally produces or feigns physical or psychological symptoms. Unlike in malingering, there is no obvious secondary gain. Little is known about the etiology, family patterns, or predisposing factors, except that individuals with factitious disorders typically have a prior history of early (and possibly traumatizing) medical treatment. Psychoanalytic experience suggests that, not infrequently, factitious phenomena may be understood as variants of PTSD, in which patients reenact painful illnesses or surgeries in an effort to feel that *this* time, they are in control of what in childhood was inflicted on them; that is, a form of repetition compulsion motivated by the desire for mastery. They may also have defined their sense of self in terms of their physical suffering. Individuals with factitious disorders are famously difficult to treat medically and are highly refractory to psychotherapy.

DSM-5's factitious disorder imposed on another, also called "Munchausen's syndrome by proxy," applies to individuals (usually parents, but sometimes nurses or other caregivers) who repeatedly cause illness or physical harm to their children or to persons in their care. Perpetrators of these acts deny their role in the damage—sometimes even in the face of video-recorded evidence of their destructive activity—and present themselves to medical personnel in states of great distress over the health crises of the persons they have harmed.

The Subjective Experience of Factitious Disorders

Affective States

Individuals with factitious disorders may exhibit a wide range of affective states, from anxiety over alleged physical symptoms to dysphoria and hostile expectations that medical professionals do not believe them. The overriding affective tone, however, is one of superficiality rather than emotional depth. A manipulative, opportunistic quality is often present. Despite such a patient's seemingly sincere insistence on the seriousness of a physical or psychological ailment, it may be difficult for a clinician to feel empathy or concern.

Cognitive Patterns

Cognitive patterns involve the physical or psychological complaints of the moment, coupled with ruminations about how to get medical professionals to take the complaints seriously. Patients with factitious disorders may be chronically preoccupied cognitively with persuading themselves as well as others of the reality of their suffering. They may be more or less obsessed with their connections to physicians and others on whom they feel medically dependent.

Somatic States

Somatic states may include chronic tension when desired care is not forthcoming. Some with factitious disorders, in their quest for attention from doctors or hospital personnel, inflict serious injury upon themselves. Others have persuaded previous physicians to do unnecessary surgeries; in such instances, their bodies may be permanently harmed. In Munchausen's syndrome by proxy, patients deliberately damage the bodies of others, usually their children—evidently out of an unconscious wish to enact a personal drama and to reinforce the strength of relationships with medical professionals who figure in their fantasy lives.

Relationship Patterns

Relationship patterns tend to be needy and dependent, with a great deal of negativism and dissatisfaction underlying an initial overt compliance. In their effort to get their complaints taken seriously, patients may exaggerate their symptom descriptions, thereby eliciting irritation from others. It is common for others to experience individuals with these disorders as unreliable, manipulative, self-dramatizing, and difficult.

The Subjective Experience of the Therapist

The most specific, and difficult, countertransference experience is anger, which is likely to affect all clinicians involved: physicians, psychiatrists, therapists, nurses, and others. Clinicians are devoted to curing real illness, not fake illness. It is tempting to dismiss patients with factitious disorders as a waste of time and resources. Frustration is also common to the extent that such patients are resistant to recognizing what they do and to entering into therapy.

Clinical Illustration

A 42-year-old woman with a history of multiple surgeries for congenital abnormalities was convinced she needed gall bladder surgery "because I have pain in my stomach all the time." Multiple medical evaluations, including full gastrointestinal workups, were negative. During psychotherapy, she accessed feelings of anger, fear, and helplessness about her childhood surgeries, complaining poignantly about her parents' "handling me like a fragile piece of glass." She gradually explored her potential for assertiveness. Eventually she confessed, "I ate spicy foods that gave me pain because I felt like my stomach pain was a friend."

S6 Specific Symptom Disorders

The large S6 grouping is borrowed from ICD-10 (all from its F50s and F60s), and explains the contiguity of a number of DSM-5 diagnostic groups and their ICD-10 codes, according to Table 3.2 (pp. 245–250).

S61 Feeding and Eating Disorders

Anorexia nervosa and bulimia nervosa (hereinafter shortened to anorexia and bulimia) appear to be more prevalent in industrialized societies, where there is an abundance of food and where conceptions of attractiveness involve being thin.

Through mass media and websites, images of physical perfection have spread globally, leading to eating disorders in societies where they had not been present before. Even in cultures with food shortages, people may aspire to cultural patterns of contemporary Western societies. Eating disorders have become common in immigrants from countries where eating disorders are rare (e.g., in university students who move from one country to another).

Women and girls make up 90% of reported cases, but there is some evidence that eating disorders are increasing among adolescent males. Populations especially at risk for these disorders include fashion models, athletes, and dancers. Anorexia usually begins in early adolescence, and bulimia in late adolescence or early adulthood. Course and outcome are variable: Some conditions are severe, compromising health and increasing the risk of mortality. There is often a switch or a lifetime co-occurrence between one disorder and the other. There is an elevated family history among first-degree relatives of anorexia and bulimia, along with mood disorders, suggesting some common genetic predisposition. Binge-eating disorder commonly overlaps with anxiety, mood, and impulse-control disorders, and with obesity.

Eating disorders may begin with a problem with food but extend to body discomfort and, in severe cases, a distorted body image. Disturbed affect regulation, low self-esteem, difficulties in mentalization, and impaired self-development are also common. Some eating disorders may arise from the spectrum of developmental trauma, beginning with conflictual family dynamics and proceeding through disordered attachment to more overt emotional and physical neglect, and to overt emotional, physical, and sexual abuse. Such severity generally accounts for the comorbidity that often complicates diagnosis and treatment. Thus, eating disorders are complex psychological phenomena with aspects that are often not obvious or discernible to the outside observer.

The Subjective Experience of Eating Disorders

Eating disorders appear in a heterogeneous group of people. Patients with a diagnosis of anorexia or bulimia differ in their average personality traits. Those with anorexia generally tend to be more obsessive–compulsive and narcissistic; they may refuse not only food, but any new experience, including relationships with people, or they may resist any psychological change, employing mental "no entry" mechanisms. Those with bulimia tend to be more emotionally dysregulated (with borderline functioning), with subjective feelings of emptiness and emotional hunger that they try to solve with food. As a result, they continue to feel empty, but disgusted in two senses: with anger and with self-loathing. Empirical data seem to suggest that it is possible to find high-functioning, perfectionistic personalities in some patients with eating disorders (particularly those with anorexia), both in adolescence and in adulthood, and that the presence of an emotionally dysregulated (borderline) personality worsens the clinical presentation of any eating disorder. Moreover, several patients with eating disorders may show overconstricted personality styles with relevant deficits in mentalization.

The onset of anorexia is often associated with a stressful life event, such as leaving home for college, a family disturbance, or the experience of loss. Bulimia frequently arises when a young person moves from early adolescence to late adolescence, with difficulties handling the progressive emergence of sexuality. Symptoms often arise during or following a diet. Anorexia and bulimia may range from minor to life-threatening, depending on both intrinsic severity and comorbidity. Minor transient anorexic episodes are common in middle adolescence, and may come to clinical attention only in passing when one is reviewing the past history of someone presenting with another condition, such as depression or anxiety, or a somatoform, dissociative, sexual, impulse-control, substance use, or personality disorder.

Comorbidity often complicates the clinical picture. Mood disorders and personality disorders are often comorbid, and so clinicians should be careful to ask about eating patterns when evaluating patients with these disorders. Patients will try to render their symptoms ego-syntonic by claiming them to be a "lifestyle." Paradoxically, patients with anorexia often feel better as their health worsens because at the same time they get closer to their thin ideal. Details about actual food consumption may be difficult to ascertain.

Affective States

Affective states may include symptoms of depression, anxiety, alexithymia, impulsivity, and shame. Depressive symptoms may include depressed mood, social withdrawal, and low self-esteem, and include both anaclitic and characterological depression. Anxiety symptoms commonly suffered include social phobic and obsessive–compulsive symptoms (only sometimes food-related). Alexithymia is not uncommon. Anorexic patients exhibit diminished interest in sex, while bulimic patients are more commonly involved in impulsive sexual behavior, increasing the risk of sexually transmitted diseases and pregnancy. In both conditions, it is common to eat alone, while feeling shame, anxiety, and sadness. Symptoms are generally kept hidden for long periods. Shame is common. Anorexic patients feel shame about the shape of their bodies, while bulimic patients feel shame about their lack of behavioral control, which often extends beyond food to self-harm and addiction. Parasuicidal gestures are frequent in this population, prompted by both depressed mood and by failure to attain one's ideal body figure.

The following emotional concerns are common in both anorexia and bulimia:

- Feelings of being starved for care and affection, and longing to be protected and cherished.
- Feelings of failure, weakness, guilt, and shame.
- Feelings of being unworthy and ineffective (e.g., "I would feel like I couldn't eat, and then if I did, I would feel guilty, like I did something I wasn't supposed to do or took in something I didn't deserve").
- Fear that others will abandon one or will withdraw their love.
- Anger and aggressiveness, which, because they are frightening, dangerous, and intolerable, are denied, muted, or hated (e.g., "I'm a bubbly person who never gets angry. It doesn't feel good to get angry, and nobody around me feels good when I get angry. They would get hurt, and you can't hurt the people you care about").
- Fear that emotional expression will lead to loss of control (e.g., an anorexic woman stated that if she were to talk freely about feelings, she would find herself "blowing in the wind").
- Feelings of emptiness or losing control.

Cognitive Patterns

Cognitive patterns include rigid thinking and perceptual distortions of patients' own bodies or body images. In minor or emerging symptoms, there may be dissatisfaction with the body or part of it. In more severe conditions, body image may be distorted to the point of compromised reality testing. Eating disorders span the spectrum from neurosis to psychosis, though most are more closely related to personality disorders.

Anorexic patients frequently manifest narcissistic issues, perfectionism, self-criticism, and asceticism. Omnipotence and idealization are common defenses. In severe cases, the defenses of splitting, withdrawal from external reality, and autistic fantasy may be present. Bulimic patients more commonly manifest dysregulated conditions, with identity diffusion, acting out, splitting of self- and object representations, devaluation, and idealization.

Cognitive patterns may include the following:

- Preoccupation with being devalued, inadequate, incompetent, or unloved, together with coping strategies and defenses to deal with these issues.
- A focus on being young, "little," childlike, and innocent, which implies the unconscious wish to avoid puberty and adulthood. For example, a young woman dresses herself as a girl; her starved body looks like a prepubertal girl's; she does not behave like a young woman; and her mother controls her life.
- Excessive interest in body image, and excessive dependence on viewing one's body in a mirror to track its shape and changes. Sometimes emotions distort body image, as in the case of a 15-year-old girl who constantly monitors her body: When bathing, after eating, after toileting, or when passing in front of any mirror, she stops and surveys certain areas. Before and after eating or

toileting, she inspects her belly and thighs, looking for changes in her body every time something goes in or out of it.

Somatic States

Somatic states involve the effect on the real body of mental conflict. Complaints are often nonspecific, and there may be difficulty differentiating between mental and somatic states. Hunger may express the subjective feelings of emptiness or desire for emotional bonds. Identity diffusion is common during binges or purges, again reflecting a difficulty in distinguishing between mental and somatic states. There may be confusion about sensations that ordinarily accompany eating and elimination, such as an inability to sense whether one is full. People with eating disorders are always at risk, and so general clinical attention is important (e.g., the complaint of a sensation of "plumpness" in the legs may be evidence of hypokalemia).

Somatic states may include the following:

- Feelings of physical emptiness in the stomach may be associated with the sense of an empty, depleted self (e.g., "I have a void that I can't seem to fill. It's a lonely existence").
- Confusion of mental and somatic states; (e.g., an adolescent woman related that when she ate, she felt totally confused, without a clear notion of herself, and she entered into "narcotic" states which she could leave only by expelling them through vomiting).

Relationship Patterns

These individuals may go to great lengths to keep their problems secret, making genuine emotional intimacy impossible. They may relate to others superficially and in ways that seem immature for their age. Relationships tend to be characterized by control and perfectionism in anorexic patients. They need to be admired, but from a distance that poses no threat. These patients may handle their wish to be lovable by compliance, politeness, and ingratiating behavior. They have difficulties accepting positive gestures from others. Bulimic patients are hungry for love, but their relationships tend to be unstable. In close relationships, they may suffer from frequent abandonment or engulfment anxieties. They may feel themselves unworthy or useless when they lose relationships, and may rage or act out against themselves.

The Subjective Experience of the Therapist

Clinical literature suggests that patients with eating disorders are often hard to treat because they are able to induce strong emotions in therapists, such as rage, hate, hopelessness, pity, sorrow, and love. This large spectrum of feelings tends to affect staff performance, treatment process, and outcome; several clinicians have suggested that moving the focus from patients' to therapists' emotional responses can become an important way to work with these patients. Countertransference issues often reflect a patient's level of personality functioning and comorbid personality disorders, with the prominent use of splitting and the resultant diffusion of identity, polarized and intense affective states, and the tendency to act out if the eating disorder is associated with a borderline personality organization.

Clinical Illustration

A 22-year-old woman, a former athlete and self-described "tomboy," was the youngest child and only girl in a family that was very strict about nutrition, exercise, and studies. After graduating from college, she became worried about "being thin enough to be a high-fashion model." She began a series of diets and then began feeling anxiety and nausea every time she went near food. She noted that "even when I force myself to eat, so I won't get sick, I can't tell if I'm hungry or not. I can never tell if I've eaten enough." Her worries about being too fat and her regimen of exercise, nutrition, and study became ever more severe. She thought she looked pregnant and justified her avoidance of dating by claiming, "I don't want to get pregnant." Eventually, her symptoms became severe enough to require treatment.

S62 Sleep–Wake Disorders

ICD-10 and DSM-5 classify sleep–wake disorders according to Table 3.2 (pp. 245–250).

Sleep–wake disorders considered "primary" include dyssomnias and parasomnias (although DSM-5 no longer uses the former term). Dyssomnias are problems in initiating or maintaining sleep (insomnia) or experiences of excessive sleepiness (hypersomnolence). The defining feature of insomnia disorder is trouble falling or staying asleep, sleep that is not restful, or a combination of these, lasting at least 3 nights per week for 3 months, and causing clinically significant difficulties in social, occupational, or other areas of functioning. Insomnia disorder has been found to be associated with physical or mental stimulation at nighttime in conjunction with negative conditioning for sleep. Significant preoccupation with the problem may exacerbate it: The more one tries to sleep, the more upset and angry one becomes, and the less likely one is to sleep. Chronic insomnia engenders deterioration of mood and motivation, lowered energy and attention, and increased exhaustion and sickness. Insomnia is more prevalent with age and in women.

Hypersomnolence disorder is defined by extreme sleepiness, extended sleep periods, or excessive napping for at least 3 months, causing clinically significant difficulty or impairment in social, occupational, or other areas of functioning. Individuals often carry out routine automatic behavior with little or no recall. True prevalence is unknown. Hypersomnolence disorder typically begins between ages 15 and 30, with gradual progression and a chronic and stable course.

The essential features of narcolepsy are repeated episodes of irresistible attacks of refreshing sleep, as well as episodes of cataplexy (sudden loss of muscle tone, usually following an outburst of intense emotion), hypocretin deficiency, and intrusion of rapid eye movement (REM) sleep. The sleepiness typically decreases after an attack, only to reappear later.

Breathing-related sleep disorders (sleep apneas) are sleep disruptions caused by ventilation abnormalities during sleep, leading to excessive sleepiness or insomnia. Symptoms may include nocturnal chest discomfort, a sense of choking or suffocation, intense anxiety, dryness of the mouth, extreme difficulty awakening, and inappropriate behavior. Breathing-related sleep disorders have an insidious onset, a gradual progression, and a chronic course.

Circadian rhythm sleep–wake disorder is an ongoing pattern of sleep difficulty resulting from a difference between a person's individual sleep–wake cycle and the demands of the outer world. Individuals with this disorder may experience wakefulness at regular points in each 24-hour period (e.g., at 11:00 P.M.) and excessive sleepiness at other points (e.g., at 11:00 A.M.). Without intervention, the symptoms may last for years or decades.

Parasomnias are characterized by abnormal behavioral or physiological events occurring in association with sleep, specific sleep stages, or sleep–wake transitions. These involve activation of the autonomic nervous system, motor system, and/or cognitive processes during sleep or sleep–wake transitions. They include nightmare disorder, non–rapid eye movement (NREM) sleep arousal disorders (sleep terror and sleepwalking types), and others. The essential feature of nightmare disorder is the repeated occurrence of frightening dreams from which the sleeper wakes, resulting in significant distress and/or social or occupational dysfunction. Dreams tend to involve severe anxiety about imminent physical danger.

The sleep terror type of NREM sleep arousal disorder (formerly known as sleep terror disorder or *pavor nocturnus*) involves abrupt awakenings, usually beginning with a panicky scream or cry, lasting about 10 minutes. It also includes intense anxiety and symptoms of autonomic arousal, such as sweating, rapid breathing, flushing of the skin, and pupil dilation. In children, the disorder usually begins between ages 4 and 12 and resolves spontaneously in adolescence. In adults it begins between ages 20 and 30, and tends to become chronic.

The sleepwalking type of NREM sleep arousal disorder (formerly known as sleepwalking disorder) is characterized by repeated episodes of complex motor behavior initiated during sleep (rising from bed and walking about). Episodes include a variety of behaviors, including sitting up; walking into closets, down stairs, or out of buildings; using the bathroom; eating; talking; and even operating machinery. Internal and external stimuli, psychosocial stressors, and alcohol or sedative use increase the likelihood of sleepwalking. Episodes occur between ages 4 and 8 and tend to peak at age 12. Most commonly, the pattern of sleepwalking includes repeated episodes occurring over a period of several years.

Many sleep–wake disorders are consequences of mood and anxiety disorders, including posttraumatic syndromes. The pathophysiological mechanisms responsible for these disorders also affect sleep–wake regulation. Their course generally follows that of the underlying mental disorder. Sleep disturbances resulting from intoxication or withdrawal of a substance are distinguished from other sleep–wake disorders by a consideration of their onset and course. Onset of a substance/medication-induced sleep disorder can occur up to 4 weeks after cessation of substance use.

The Subjective Experience of Sleep–Wake Disorders

Affective States

Affective states include feelings of helplessness, frustration, and anger about not being able to sleep: "I just lie there tossing and turning!" Sleep deprivation can cause depressed, demoralized, anxious, and irritable feelings: "I'm just so tired all day, it makes me annoyed and short-tempered with everyone around me."

Cognitive Patterns

Cognitive patterns include confusion, distractedness, and an inability to concentrate (e.g., "I can't concentrate, I can't think; I just feel horrible"). Individuals may feel overwhelmed by their inability to think clearly when sleep-deprived. Thoughts are disproportionately concerned with getting to sleep or staying asleep and may include theories about why sleep is so evasive.

Somatic States

Somatic states include fatigue, agitation, irritability, and hypo- or hypervigilance.

Relationsip Patterns

Relationship patterns may suffer from the patient's preoccupation with sleep and feelings of fatigue, anxiety, anger, and/or agitation.

Clinical Illustration

A 45-year-old woman who was about to receive a promotion began finding it hard to fall asleep; she was preoccupied with fears of being humiliated "when they find out I can't do the job." She pictured her military officer father laughing at her, and worried that she was upsetting her husband by being more successful. She was guiltily apprehensive that she would soon have even less time with her children. As she lay awake, she became anxious "that tomorrow I will be too tired even to think" and began being anxious about the insomnia itself.

S63 Sexual Dysfunctions

DSM-5 and ICD-10 now divide sexual disorders into sexual dysfunctions (F52) and paraphilic disorders (F65). A section on gender dysphoria (F64) can be found on pages 240–244 (see the Appendix: Psychological Experiences That May Require Clinical Attention) as gender incongruence. The current view is that gender incongruence ought to be interpreted, like homosexuality, as a nonpathological condition, rather than as a psychiatric disorder.

ICD-10 and DSM-5 classify sexual dysfunctions according to Table 3.2 (pp. 245–250).

Sexual dysfunctions had been subdivided in DSM-IV-TR, but DSM-5 has collapsed the subdivisions into a single list: delayed ejaculation, erectile disorder, female orgasmic disorder, female sexual interest arousal disorder, genito-pelvic pain/penetration disorder, male hypoactive sexual desire disorder, premature ejaculation, substance/medication-induced sexual dysfunction, and other specified/unspecified sexual dysfunction. For some reason, DSM-IV's sexual dysfunction due to a general medical condition has been omitted.

The Subjective Experience of Sexual Dysfunctions

Affective States

Affective states vary in relation to the wide range of sexual dysfunctions and, within the same diagnostic labels, across patients suffering from a specific dysfunction. Individuality is perhaps even more marked in sexual life than in other realms. However, some patterns are quite common (e.g., the tendency toward anxiety and/or depression, low self-esteem, lack of confidence, and worries about general adequacy).

Cognitive Patterns

Cognitive patterns may involve preoccupation with inadequacy or compensatory fantasies of power, or both.

Somatic States

Somatic states may include a sensory hyperreactivity in which certain types of touch feel irritating rather than comforting or arousing. This response may lead to additional feelings of anxiety and the sense that "something is wrong with my body." Other individuals may experience sensory hyporeactivity in which they feel a lack of physical reactions.

Relationship Patterns

Relationship patterns may be significantly influenced by the age at onset of the dysfunction. In general, they may be characterized by avoidance of mature emotional and sexual intimacy or by themes of domination and power.

Clinical Illustration

A 48-year-old single man with intermittent difficulties maintaining an erection during intercourse became increasingly anxious that he would not be able to "perform" with his next girlfriend. He became preoccupied with images of his father's "huge penis," in comparison to his "modest" organ. His anxiety grew to the point that whenever he was in the company of women about whom he would ordinarily have sexual fantasies, he would feel "my muscles tensing up, my stomach churning. I can hardly sit still," and had thoughts that "they know I can't perform." He became unable to sustain an erection "even with women I really like." He began avoiding social situations and limited himself more and more to work and his apartment.

S64 Paraphilic Disorders

ICD-10 and DSM-5 classify paraphilic disorders according to Table 3.2 (pp. 245–250).

Paraphilic disorders, also called "paraphilias" (Greek root) or "sexual perversions" (Latin root), are recurrent, intense sexual urges, fantasies, or behaviors that involve unusual objects, activities, or situations. To be classified as disorders, paraphilias must have the characteristic of being the most frequent fantasies or behaviors that induce sexual interest or pleasure, and may involve rigidly ritualized sexual encounters. These disorders cause clinically significant distress or impairment in social, occupational, or other important areas of functioning.

Atypical sexual interests have historically been classified as psychiatric disorders, most notably in Krafft-Ebing's 19th-century work *Psychopathia Sexualis*. Sexologist Friedrich Salomon Krauss is credited with coining the term "paraphilia" in 1903. Freud (1905) called them "perversions," defining them as *deviations from the sexual object and aim*. Some contemporary analysts still use the term for fantasies and activities, sexual or otherwise, characterized by rigidity, repetitiveness, and strong hostile and aggressive components.

Early editions of DSM and ICD referred to paraphilias as "sexual deviations." ICD-11 is likely to reclassify ICD-10's "disorders of sexual preference" as "paraphilic disorders." DSM-5 includes a diagnosis of transvestic disorder for persons aroused by cross-dressing. In contrast to DSM-IV and -IV-TR's transvestic fetishism, limited to heterosexual men sexually aroused by cross-dressing, in DSM-5 this diagnosis can be applied to anyone who cross-dresses. ICD-11, on the other hand, is likely to delete its similar category of fetishistic transvestitism and include the following diagnoses: exhibitionistic disorder, voyeuristic disorder, pedophilic disorder, coercive sexual sadism disorder, frotteuristic disorder, other paraphilic disorder involving non-consenting adults, and paraphilic disorder involving solitary behavior or consenting individuals. Paraphilic disorders are much more common in men than women. It is not unusual for a person with such a disorder to have more than one paraphilic interest.

Paraphilic diagnoses have been criticized for their highly subjective nature and their use of scientific and medical language to disguise moral opprobrium. They are often seen as an effort to control sexual behaviors, much as masturbation, oral sex, anal sex, and homosexuality were once considered mental disorders or symptoms of mental disorders. In response to these criticisms, DSM-5 considers it possible for an individual to engage in consensual atypical sexual behavior without being diagnosed with mental disorder. In contrast to previous editions, DSM-5 distinguishes individuals with atypical sexual fantasies, urges, and behaviors (paraphilias) from those with a diagnosable mental condition (paraphilic disorders). Diagnosing a DSM-5 paraphilic disorder requires a person who either (1) feels personal distress about his or her sexual interest, not just because of social disapproval or (2) has a sexual desire or behavior that involves another person's psychological distress, injury, or death, or a desire for sexual behaviors involving unwilling persons or persons unable to give legal consent.

Although the causes of paraphilias remain unknown, many have formulated psychodynamic explanations. While it is possible that therapeutic explorations may reduce paraphilic desires and behaviors in some cases, such outcomes are not easily obtained, perhaps because of the extremely reinforcing nature of behaviors that have become associated with orgasm.

The Subjective Experience of Paraphilic Disorders

The subjective experience of a paraphilic disorder may vary, depending on its specific nature (not all paraphilias are experienced equally), a patient's level of self-acceptance or rejection of paraphilic interests (due to factors such as religious beliefs, culture of origin, social class, etc.), the patient's degree of openness about them (which may range from being completely secretive, to sharing with one's spouse, to active membership in a community with similar interests, to shaming public arrest for illegal sexual activity), and the relative degree of social opprobrium attached to a particular paraphilic interest.

Affective States

Affective states vary. Some individuals regard their interests in a matter-of-fact and self-accepting way and express no conscious feelings about them. Other feelings may include pleasure when engaged in or thinking about the paraphilic interest; anxiety, depression, guilt, and self-loathing about the paraphilic interest; anxiety and fear of being discovered; or grandiose feelings of superiority to those who engage in conventional ("vanilla") sexual practices.

Cognitive Patterns

Cognitive patterns can include obsessing about (but not acting upon) a paraphilic interest or elaborately planning to act upon a specific desire. Some individuals immerse themselves, even compulsively, in sex research literature, acquiring technical knowledge about their paraphilia equal to or greater than that of recognized experts. Some rationalize their satisfying their own desires at another's expense. Others may seek to inhibit any open expressions of their paraphilic interests.

Somatic States

Somatic states may include high levels of arousal and vigilance when patients are engaged in sexual pursuits or behaviors and numbness and emptiness when they are not. Some individuals may use drugs or alcohol as a necessary prelude to engaging in a paraphilic activity.

Relationship Patterns

Relationship patterns also vary. Paraphilic interests may be dissociated from the rest of an individual's life, or the individual may belong to a community with similar interests. Some paraphilic disorders involve exploitation of nonconsenting individuals (or, in the case of pedophilic disorder, individuals who are not legally allowed to give consent). Some individuals with pedophilic disorder may enter into adult, heterosexual marriages while secretly acting on their paraphilic interests with children. On the other hand, so-called "virtuous pedophiles" have formed online communities to help prevent one another from acting upon their sexual interests.

The Subjective Experience of the Therapist

Subjective experiences of clinicians may include feelings of anxiety, concern, pity, judgment, revulsion, or voyeuristic curiosity about a paraphilic activity. Legal reporting requirements of pedophilic activity in particular may either tap into clinicians' authoritarian impulses to control or punish patient behavior or evoke antiauthoritarian responses to shield a patient (and the "sanctity" of the therapeutic encounter) from outside scrutiny.

Clinical Illustration

A 25-year-old man worked a midnight shift. On nights off, he would get drunk or high on cannabis and go to an area with some nightlife. There he would fall on the ground in a way that would "inadvertently" cause his pants to drop and expose his underwear to passing women. This evolved into making it appear as if his trousers were accidentally hooked on a fence, and torn as he tried to get free (he bought pants in large quantities at thrift shops). He would later masturbate to orgasm while thinking about the looks on the women's faces.

S65 Disruptive, Impulse-Control, and Conduct Disorders

ICD-10 and DSM-5 classify disruptive, impulse-control, and conduct disorders according to Table 3.2 (pp. 245–250).

In DSM-5, disruptive, impulse-control, and conduct disorders are now limited to pyromania and kleptomania for adults, with the curious addition of antisocial personality disorder, which is listed twice, both within this category and in the personality disorders section (the one other diagnosis listed twice in DSM-5 is schizotypal personality disorder; see Section S13, p. 144). For the PDM-2 discussion of antisocial personality disorder, see the section on psychopathic personalities in Chapter 1 on the P Axis (pp. 50–51). For child and adolescent disorders in this category (oppositional defiant disorder, intermittent explosive disorder, conduct disorder), see Chapters 6 and 9 on the SC and SA Axes, respectively. Other DSM-IV and –IV-TR impulse-control disorders have migrated: Pathological gambling is now among the substance-related and addictive disorders; trichotillomania is among the obsessive–compulsive and related disorders. The essential feature of impulse-control disorders is failure to resist the urge to perform an act that is harmful to oneself or others. For most of these disorders, a person feels an increasing sense of tension before committing the act; experiences pleasure, gratification, or relief at the time of committing it; and may feel regret, self-reproach, or guilt following the act.

Kleptomania is characterized by the recurrent failure to resist impulses to steal objects not needed for any personal or monetary value. Many individuals with kleptomania experience the impulse to steal as ego-dystonic and morally problematic. They fear being apprehended and may feel depressed or guilty about the thievery. Pyromania is characterized by a pattern of fire setting for pleasure or relief of tension, often with advance planning and preparation. Fire-setting incidents are episodic and may wax and wane in frequency.

Epidemiological studies suggest that subjects affected by these disorders are at a higher risk for comorbid alcohol and other substance abuse, OCD, anxiety disorders, and mood disorders. While kleptomania is more frequent in women, pyromania and other impulse-control disorders or behavioral addictions (see section S71.2, p. 228) are more common in men. There is limited information on the course of most of the impulse-control disorders.

The Subjective Experience of Impulse-Control Disorders

Affective States

As stated before, affective states in individuals with kleptomania or pyromania often include vacillation between feelings of emptiness or apathy, longing for the excitement or soothing that the behavior provides, and shame, fear, and depression. Often absent is a mature sense of regret that motivates change.

Cognitive Patterns

Cognitive patterns are more notable for absence of thought than for presence of problematic thoughts. The behaviors may have a pure ego-syntonic quality, also reflecting an impairment of thinking processes that involve the consideration of the short- and long-term effects of the behaviors. Early personal memories may be curiously vague or lacking. There also may be a sort of obsessive concern with getting opportunities to enact the impulsive behavior.

Somatic States

Somatic states that accompany these disorders may include hypo- and hyperarousal, as well as a wide variety of somatic symptoms (e.g., gastrointestinal symptoms and palpitations).

Relationship Patterns

Relationship patterns often suffer from the disorders themselves and the psychology that tends to accompany them. People living with someone who sets fires or steals are rarely tolerant and forgiving. Most individuals suffering from impulse-control disorders have disruptive relationships, on which their behavior takes a severe toll. Also, they tend to be reluctant patients; they are frequently seen by court order or when confronted with the legal consequences of their actions. Genuine therapeutic relationships are, as a result, difficult to make in the absence of strong internal motivation to change, and require patience with patients' reluctance to try to understand and control obviously problematic behaviors.

The Subjective Experience of the Therapist

The subjective experience of the therapist encountering or treating patients with impulse-control disorders may be characterized by the same reluctance to be engaged in treatment as the patients experience, as well as by difficulties in empathizing.

S7 Disorders Related to Addiction and to Other Medical Conditions

S71 Addictions

S71.1 *Substance-Related Disorders*

ICD-10 and DSM-5 classify substance-related and addictive disorders according to Table 3.2 (pp. 245–250).

Substance-related disorders affect millions of people around the world, with nicotine-related disorders being the most common type. The next most commonly misused substance is alcohol, followed by marijuana, cocaine, heroin, prescription pain relievers, and designer drugs such as methamphetamines. The primary psychodynamic view of addictive disorders is that the motivation to use and misuse drugs or to engage in an addictive behavior is born from unresolved conflicts and traumatic experiences that arouse intolerably dysphoric affects, which are then defended against with substance abuse or an addictive behavior.

The most prominent psychodynamic model of addiction interprets addiction as a form of self-medication against dysphoria or disordered mood. This formulation has also influenced cognitive-behavioral views of addiction. Consonant with the syndrome view, the self-medication hypothesis argues that there are common underlying biopsychosocial pathological processes underlying all addictions. Because an addiction serves a defensive function, it is very hard to stop. It ameliorates suffering, but because that relief is only temporary, the person needs to engage again in the defensive behavior of addiction once the relief wears off. This reflects the chronic, compulsive nature of addictive attitudes and disorders.

Addictive disorders affect all areas of a person's life, including emotional regulation, effective self-care, finding fulfilling relationships, and maintaining self-esteem. Although addictive disorders co-occur in approximately 50% of all people who present for mental health treatment, an addictive disorder may not be part of a patient's presenting complaint. Comorbidity between substance-related disorders and personality disorders varies widely across the different substances, with rates ranging from 10 to 100%, depending on the disorder. Highest correlations are between excessive substance use and psychopathic, emotionally dysregulated, and narcissistic personalities; temperamental factors such as impulsivity, sensation seeking, and novelty seeking may act as mediators between personality and the abuse of substances. In general, the presence of a personality disorder increases the severity of addiction and weakens cooperation in treatment. The prevalence of comorbid personality disorders seems higher in patients who misuse multiple substances—a clinical population that has been growing in recent years.

In intakes, especially with patients with personality disorders, it is therefore important to ask about addictions when these are not mentioned spontaneously by the patients. This should be done in a caring and nonjudgmental manner. Because denial of addiction is common, it is critical for a therapist to tolerate the fact that revealing an addiction may take time. This is perhaps inevitable, given the important defensive function that addictions play in a person's psychic life.

The Subjective Experience of Substance-Related Disorders

Affective States

Psychoactive drugs help people who misuse substances to tolerate intolerable feelings. The effects of drugs and alcohol are specific and temporary; the main emotions the person feels will generally determine which type of substance is preferred. Opiates help a person to feel "calm," "mellow," or "normal." Stimulants counter low energy, feelings of weakness, and feelings of being unloved; they may also be employed by high-energy individuals to augment a preferred hypomanic adaptation or to combat depression. Sedatives (e.g., alcohol, benzodiazepines, barbiturates), in low doses, can overcome feelings of isolation and allow feelings of closeness and warmth (e.g., "I can feel like one of the guys . . . I can join the human race"); in high doses, they drown out negative, unwelcome feelings and lead to social isolation.

The following are some ways in which addiction-prone individuals experience their emotional lives:

- Feelings of boredom and depression and of unworthiness alternating with demandingness.
- Intense feelings of rage or anger can fester or erupt. Such feelings may be associated with agitation or a sense of falling apart. Individuals dependent on opiates, for example, say that the drugs act to calm or contain their feelings or to make them feel normal.
- Chronic use causes physical addiction and the need not to be deprived of the substance. Patients report feeling awful without their substance of choice; they may feel panic if they cannot obtain the substance.
- As physical dependence develops, many of the feelings relieved by drugs are made more intense and intolerable when the drugs are abruptly withdrawn.

Cognitive Patterns

Cognitive patterns are notable for centering on rationalizations and denial that support addiction (e.g., "My drinking isn't as bad my father's. He was a *real* drunk"). The dangers of addiction are denied, via comments such as "I never thought about it." The fact of addiction is often disavowed via protests such as "I can stop at any time." When confronted with the realities of their condition, substance-misusing individuals tend to respond with comments prefaced by denial, such as "No, I'm not afraid when I shoot drugs."

Somatic States

In subjects with substance-related disorders we observe various somatic signs and symptoms. These somatic states may be a direct effect of the addictive substance (abuse or withdrawal) or the result of a lack of mentalization processes. In addition, there are cases in which the somatic complaint is the way patients seek help from a physician in order to get the prescription of the addictive substance (i.e., back pain, headache to obtain opiates).

Relationship Patterns

Relationship patterns may include intense feelings of neediness alternating with protests that one has no such needs. Life may feel unmanageable and unregulated to both substance-dependent persons and those close to them. Relationships may be described as shaky, untrustworthy, or disappointing. Partners who put pressure on the persons to get help are typically put off and devalued. We should note that many people who misuse substances experience themselves as helpless to control their worlds and lives, leading to a sense of rage. But internal prohibitions against expression of aggression lead to its displacement to addictive behaviors, which provide the persons with a sense of control and reduce the sense of helplessness and the dysphoric affects that arise because of the displaced aggression and rage.

Clinical Illustration

A 22-year-old patient first came to therapy after having started treatment in a methadone maintenance program. From early adolescence, he had heavily used sedatives and stimulants (amphetamines). "I was less afraid . . . I felt I could take on anyone when I was speeding." His long-standing shaky self-esteem and tenuous capacity to relate to others lent a self-effacing and reticent quality to his interpersonal dealings, including how he related in psychotherapy. Dating was difficult because he feared rejection, and he worried about how awkward he would appear if he showed his needs. His combination of charm and vulnerability made him highly appealing.

At the same time, a more brutal, violent, sadistic side was evident in the intensity of his boast that nobody could or would "screw me over." He could adopt a chilling veneer of self-sufficiency and disdain for other people's needs and feelings. He was not reluctant to tell the therapist how much he enjoyed stalking younger or weaker individuals "to beat on them and hurt them." He was keenly attracted to risky versions of athletics, martial arts, and high-performance motorcycles and automobiles, and was quick to dismiss the seriousness of injuries caused by such activities. If asked in therapy about a visible wound, he would say, "Nah, Doc, it doesn't bother me," even while wincing or moving in a guarded manner.

By the patient's late teens, uncontrolled violence and rage were interfering with his friendships, work, and life in general. He then discovered heroin and quickly became dependent on it. In contrast to the amphetamines and sedatives, narcotics immediately impressed him as calming and containing: "I felt calmer and more normal than I had ever felt in my life." In particular, once he got into the methadone maintenance program, he acknowledged a marked diminution in his rage, and he felt more organized, in control, and able to work.

Psychodynamic psychotherapy helps patients by helping to reduce their emotional suffering. It can be useful to tell patients early in treatment that as they feel better, they will likely become less interested in engaging in their addictions. This helps them realize that their emotional pain is the motivation for the substance misuse, and that the way to improve their substance-related problems is to heal their emotional pain. Psychodynamic therapy gives clinicians a wide range of supportive and expressive therapeutic techniques to use in treating people who are diagnosed with addictions, including psychodynamic treatments that are empirically supported, such as supportive–expressive therapy and dynamic deconstructive psychotherapy. Some therapists make treatment conditional on a patient's participation in a program such as Alcoholics Anonymous because of the risk that the person will never get the courage to try to stop or reduce the substance use. The addition of a community that supports sobriety can be important to treatment.

S71.2 *Behavioral Addictions (Gambling, Internet Addiction, Sex Addiction)*

Behavioral addictions belong to the same addiction syndrome as substance-related disorders and occur for the same psychological reasons. In all addictions, the brain's endogenous opioid systems are implicated and eventually affected. The aim of all behavioral addictions— pathological gambling, internet addiction, and sex addiction—is to relieve dysphoria. In pathological gambling, a person who wins and enjoys that feeling will continue to seek it out; losing money will not dissuade the person from doing so because the hope of winning again, and once again feeling that "high," fuels the motivation to relieve both the dysphoria that underlies the addiction and the new dysphoria that is created by the addiction.

Sexual addiction has clear psychopathological affinities with substance and gambling addictions. The closest ICD-10 designation would be excessive sexual drive, classified as a sexual dysfunction, but this rather misses the point of the condition: There is generally no sexual dysfunction per se; the behavior may occur in the context of elevated, normal, or even low-average sexual drive. It is not the drive that is problematic, but the addictive behavior.

The Subjective Experience of the Therapist

Negative countertransferences are common in work with patients diagnosed with either substance-related disorders or behavioral addictions, and these countertransferences can interfere with effective treatment. They are consistent with the negative attitudes that most people have toward those with addictive disorders. It is not unusual for therapists to cease trying to understand the mental lives of their patients when the patients' problems include addictions. Instead, they may berate them, may believe that all people with an addiction are liars, and/or may become frustrated with their slow progress. Supervision, consultation, and continued personal therapy are valuable. In addition, setting up a "therapeutic contract" stipulating that a patient undergo medical detoxification (as necessary for substance-related disorders) and rehabilitation before starting treatment may help the clinician and the patient to build a solid therapeutic frame and maintain the alliance.

S72 Mental Disorders Due to Another Medical Condition

ICD-10 keeps to the older terminology of "organic brain syndrome" in its category of organic, including symptomatic, mental disorders. DSM-III and -IV divided them into two categories: delirium, dementia, and amnestic and other cognitive disorders and mental disorders due to a general medical condition not elsewhere classified. DSM-5 has incorporated many of these disorders into their parent symptomatic groups, allowing for a more narrowly classified grouping of neurocognitive disorders, with a few residuals in the section on other mental disorders. Table 3.2 (pp. 245–250) presents the concordance of PDM-2 and ICD-10/DSM-5 classifications.

Although these classifications are lengthy, psychotherapeutic interventions are relatively limited and rare in most of these conditions, with the major exception of HIV-related neurocognitive disorder. Consequently, we begin with some general remarks about disorders related to another medical condition and then focus more narrowly on the HIV-related disorder. For descriptions of the clinical features and subjective experiences of other neurocognitive disorders, which are commonly observed in elderly persons, please refer to the discussion of these disorders in Chapter 14 on the SE Axis.

Mental disorders based on another medical condition cover a wide range from degenerative dementia of the Alzheimer's type to disorders produced by various patterns of substance misuse. The category also covers a wide range of reactions, from gradual changes in memory, mood, thinking, and behavior, to acute states of delirium. DSM-5 describes in detail each of these types, along with their associated symptoms. The following brief description of the subjective states that may accompany these disorders may encourage clinicians to try to capture the distinctive qualities of their patients' experiences with organic compromise.

The Subjective Experience of Mental Disorders Due to Another Medical Condition

Affective States

Affective states may include anxiety, fear, and/or depression. Depression or sadness often emerges with intimate awareness of lost capacities. Extreme feelings of helplessness and resignation can intensify depressive mood states and may also lead to secondary memory loss. Along with memory loss, there are often compromises in the individual's capacity to sequence actions and ideas, to follow directions, or to carry out novel problem-solving activities. These problems may further lead to feelings of helplessness, inadequacy, loss, and depression.

Not infrequently, individuals also experience significant fear and anxiety because of their difficulties in carrying out what in the past had been effortless daily activities. The anxieties range from fear of being alone and unprotected, to fear of injury, to fear of losing control and hurting others. These anxieties, sometimes reaching the point of panic attacks, can occur in especially challenging situations without adequate and familiar support. Acute states of delirium are often accompanied by catastrophic affective reactions involving intense fear, panic, and agitation. Affective states are often so intense and overwhelming that only the provision of supportive soothing structure, along with appropriate medical management, can alter them.

Cognitive Patterns

Cognitive patterns tend to parallel affective states, with the most common types of gradual-onset organicity involving memory loss. Thus depressive states, for example, may be attended by preoccupations with helplessness, further loss, and intermittent anger and suspiciousness in some individuals (sometimes secondary to compromised reality testing). Inability to accept or comprehend, and need to deny diminishing mental capacities, may also characterize thoughts (e.g., individuals may insist on the reality of their immediate perceptions, ignoring evidence that they have gotten something wrong). As memory loss progresses, individuals may live more and more in the affective states and mental content of the moment, sometimes showing immediate insight and cleverness without a sense of continuity to the recent past. During states of delirium, there are often rapidly shifting mental contents expressed in a fragmented manner.

Somatic States

Somatic states may mirror the affective states. They may include chest pain, palpitations, headaches, gastrointestinal symptoms, and sleeping and eating difficulties.

Relationship Patterns

Relationship patterns may range from needy and dependent to unrealistically independent and abusive. Supportive relationships that provide continuity, soothing guidance, and appropriate levels of challenge are often needed and appreciated (even if not acknowledged verbally).

S72.1 *HIV-Related Neurocognitive Disorder*

The HIV/AIDS epidemic remains a critical health issue worldwide, with 39 million people dead and 35 million more living with HIV. HIV impairs mental functioning directly but also indirectly: By weakening the immune system, it creates opportunities for brain infections that would otherwise likely be suppressed, such as cerebral toxoplasmosis, cryptococcal meningitis, progressive multifocal leukoencephalopathy, and cytomegalovirus encephalitis. A weakened immune system also facilitates other conditions, such as central nervous system (CNS) lymphoma, that impair mental functioning. When HIV is detected early and anti-retroviral medications are available to prevent these opportunistic infections, mental functioning is not indirectly impaired.

Thanks to improved medications, HIV can be a chronic, manageable condition in resource-rich settings; successfully treating HIV in the periphery, however, allows the virus to replicate into millions of copies per milliliter of blood in the CNS. HIV replicates in the CNS because nearly all anti-retroviral medications are unable to cross the blood–brain barrier. Unimpeded HIV replication in the CNS causes inflammation and other kinds of direct damage to mental functioning. Therefore, as more people are living with HIV over greater periods of time, more HIV-related neurocognitive impairment is developed and detected.

HIV-related neurocognitive disorder is the slowing of cognitive functioning indirectly and directly attributable to HIV infection. It affects approximately 0.002% of the world's population, but the prevalence is growing. While it can present in many ways, it is primarily a subcortical dementia creating problems with memory, mood, and movement. DSM-5 divides this condition, as it does other neurocognitive disorders, into major and mild neurocognitive disorder. HIV-related neurocognitive disorder is thus a spectrum disorder, but one name is used here to communicate patterns common to early and late stages.

Affective States

HIV-related neurocognitive disorder often creates apathy. While some people experience sad hopelessness and others no mood changes, most experience emotional indifference. It can be striking to clinicians delivering diagnoses of HIV-related neurocognitive disorder how few follow-up questions are asked and how little negative affect is displayed. In later states of the disorder, irritability and agitation are more frequent and intense.

Cognitive Patterns

As other subcortical dementias do, HIV-related neurocognitive disorder slows abilities to access and manipulate information. Affected persons may notice this slowing and may refer to "operating at half power" or "walking in molasses." When they notice gaps in memory, sufferers, even those who otherwise react in more mature ways, may adopt simple defensiveness such as frank denial or projective blaming. Sometimes memory lapses prompt the use of new mnemonic devices and increased support from others. The structures of daily routines are important mental contents, especially as the condition progresses.

Somatic States

HIV-related neurocognitive disorder decreases psychomotor speed and coordination. Dyskinesias that appear similar to either Parkinson's or Huntington's types of movement can develop. Apathy and depression can decrease self-care and create poor hygiene. Patients report increased experiences of physical pain, especially the tingling or burning sensations of HIV-related peripheral neuropathy.

Relationship Patterns

Dynamics of rescuing and distancing occur when people with HIV-related neurocognitive disorder turn to family members for support. Apathy and emotional isolation can create social isolation even from long-standing, close relationships. In later stages, regression challenges relationships in maintaining a previously achieved mature intimacy.

Clinical Illustration

A 62-year-old man living with HIV for over 20 years describes forgetting appointments and medications despite being previously conscientious. A high HIV load is found in his CNS. He reports not caring that he does not get as much pleasure from life, but "wanting to throw a tantrum" at his memory lapses or when his legs "don't work right."

SApp Appendix: Psychological Experiences That May Require Clinical Attention

This appendix to the S Axis addresses the clinically significant subjective experiences of important nonpathological populations that may require or seek help because of some distress.

A word on the SApp3 grouping in particular seems in order here. DSM-III, -IV, and -IV-TR clustered sexual dysfunction, paraphilic disorders, and gender identity disorder together under sexual and gender identity disorders. DSM-5 separates all three into their own categories, with sexual dysfunctions and gender dysphoria in sequence and paraphilic disorders relegated to the end of the manual's main listing of disorders. Gender identity disorder in DSM-III, -IV, and -IV-TR became DSM-5's gender dysphoria. We go a step further to depathologize gender incongruence completely, following the trajectory of homosexuality, which went from disorder to dysphoria before disappearing from the DSM. See section SApp3 (pp. 240–244) for further discussion.

SApp1 Demographic Minority Populations (Ethnic, Cultural, Linguistic, Religious, Political)

Boundaries between so-called "normality" and "illness," well-being and suffering, are not universal and vary across cultural settings. Culture provides interpretive, regulatory, and value contexts that shape attitudes and behavior, as well as subjective experiences and manifestations of signs and symptoms that become the diagnostic criteria of the different psychopathological pictures. Despite considerable efforts to provide a transcultural diagnostic *lingua franca*, the ICD and DSM configurations of mental disorders are strongly influenced by cultural patterns and by the medical approach of the Western societies from which they are derived.

Psychoanalytic theory has been criticized for decontextualizing individual development. Some early analysts such as Géza Róheim and Abraham Kardiner, however, and many analytic scholars over the last two decades in particular, have examined aspects of social context as they affect intrapsychic and interpersonal processes. Systematic inclusion of cultural sensitivity as a core area of emphasis in psychoanalytic psychotherapy is currently needed, along with specific approaches to cultural competence that extend existing psychodynamic theories about sociocultural context. These include attention to historical trauma, indigenous cultural narratives, context in language use and affect expression, effects of social oppression and stereotypes on therapeutic process and outcome, and the dynamic nature of cultural identifications.

Object relations and relational theories suggest that social location and racial positioning are reflected in and reproduced in the transference. When compared with other psychoanalytic traditions, the interpersonal, intersubjective, and relational approaches tend not to separate intrapsychic experience from social experience.

Although the study of race and racism in psychoanalysis has focused on racial tensions and dynamics between those of European and of African descent, recent scholarship has begun to explore racial dynamics across other cultural groups. For example, the concept of ethnocultural transference developed by Comas-Díaz and Jacobsen (1991) highlights how sociocultural histories and realities of client and therapist influence therapeutic dynamics. Comas-Díaz uses the term "postcolonization stress disorder" to describe the psychological experience of colonized people of color, including pervasive identity conflicts, alienation, self-denial, assimilation, and ambivalence resulting from experiences of racism and imperialism. Postcolonization stress disorder, in this integrative view, contrasts with PTSD, in that PTSD as a diagnosis does not reflect the repetitive and ethnic/political aspects of racism and imperialism (Tummala-Narra, 2015).

Other scholars have addressed the intersection of race and immigration and its relevance to the therapeutic relationship. For example, Eng and Han (2000) coined the term "racial melancholia" to describe an immigrant's wish to preserve a lost ideal of whiteness in the face of race hierarchies that impose the internalization of stereotypes, contributing to ambivalent identifications with the heritage culture and the new culture.

To obtain an accurate diagnostic assessment, the clinician must take into account the complex interactions among individual variables and norms, along with cultural, social, and family values, in relation to which mental disorders are shaped and defined. An accurate diagnostic assessment has to include: (1) a definition of the patient's cultural identity; (2) understanding of the individual's subjective experience—of the possible symptoms with which he or she may present, and of how they are mediated by the person's culture and language; (3) summary of relevant information about the patient's psychosocial environment; and (4) understanding of the patient's representation of the relationship with the clinician.

There follow some subjective experiences of demographic minority populations and of therapists encountering minority subjects. No pathology is implied.

SApp1.1 *Ethnic and Cultural Minorities*

Subjective Experiences of Ethnic and Cultural Minorities

Affective States

Affective states can vary widely with the personality of the particular individual and the specific situation. Persons in ethnic and cultural minorities may feel anxious or concerned with not being adequate. They may feel sad, isolated, and lonely. In challenging circumstances (e.g., at work or when starting new relationships), they may feel dysphoric and experience sudden mood swings.

Cognitive Patterns

Cognitive patterns vary, depending on the patient's background and on how authority is perceived within that person's culture. Individuals from hierarchical or autocratic/theocratic cultures may expect other people to be more active and directive and may become, by the standards of more egalitarian cultures, overcompliant and submissive to fulfill the role of "good patient." In the presence of societal power differences between self and others, such reactions are reasonable. To avoid their own ethnic prejudices or fears, people from minority backgrounds may become "color-blind" to their own ethnicity and deny ethnic/cultural differences between themselves and other people in their social context, including their therapists.

Somatic States

If somatic complaints are present, they are usually related to anxiety and hyperarousal. Individuals from some ethnic, cultural, and linguistic minorities may communicate their distress more via somatic complaints than via explicitly psychic symptoms (see section S51 on somatic symptom disorder, pp. 208–210).

Relationship Patterns

Relationship patterns can range from milder feelings of concern and wariness, to more mixed feelings of ambivalence (i.e., attachment coexists with suspicion), to more extreme feelings of mistrust and resentment toward others from different backgrounds (including the therapist). If a person sees his or her own background as of lower status than the therapist's current social environment and status, this power differential can invite projection of the wished-for omniscient parent, leading to primitive idealization of others. Conversely, individuals from ethnic backgrounds seen as more privileged may have difficulty trusting others, fearing they will get suboptimal care and defending against these prejudices by devaluing or idealizing their therapist.

The Subjective Experience of the Therapist

Therapists' internal experiences with patients from ethnic and cultural minorities may include feelings of doubt about being able to connect with and deeply understand these patients, which in effect can create estrangement: "We are miles apart from each other." Depending on therapists' preconscious prejudices and unconscious conflicts about their own ethnicity vis-à-vis certain ethnic minorities, powerful and deep feelings may be projected onto the patients.

Therapists who find it hard to empathize with certain ethnic/cultural minority patients may find themselves feeling angry, anxious, envious, or bored. Or they may feel guilty for belonging to an ethnicity that at some point (currently or historically) exploited or abused (in reality or fantasy) people like these patients. Therapists' ambivalence about their own ethnicity may also lead to ambivalence toward their patients. Both overidentification and reaction formation may lead therapists to pity and infantilize minority patients. A therapist may collude with a patient's maladaptive and pathological behavior, potentially compromising treatment and endangering aspects of the patient's life outside treatment.

Therapists may also have stereotypical beliefs that narrow and distort their perception of these patients. On the other hand, excessive curiosity about details of their patients' cultural nuances may strike the patients as voyeuristic and self-satisfying rather than therapeutically motivated.

Ethnic/cultural differences may lead to misinterpretations of nonverbal communications. Relative to the expected norm in a therapist's culture, higher or lower levels of verbal and emotional expressiveness can be interpreted respectively as a patient's being indiscreet and alarmingly histrionic or else withdrawn and inhibited.

SApp1.2 *Linguistic Minorities*

The Subjective Experience of Linguistic Minorities

Affective States

Affective states may include feelings of anxiety about being misunderstood and shame at making linguistic mistakes. Depressive mood swings may occur, with accompanying feelings of unacceptability to others. Language barriers may frustrate the person over real or fantasized difficulties in using appropriate words to convey needs and/or inner feelings and may make the person feel "regressed" to the situation of a child with inadequate words for complete self-expression. Fear and shame about mispronunciation may impede an otherwise fluid free association during psychoanalytic treatment. The resultant silence or affective dissonance may become a source for misunderstanding and misinterpretation on the part of the therapist.

Cognitive Patterns

Cognitive patterns may include "I don't think people can understand me." Preoccupation with perceived linguistic limitations may cause rumination about how to talk with others. Patients may rehearse wording and phrasing to ensure effective communication—a practice that can jeopardize the spontaneity needed for authentic communication.

Somatic States and Relationship Patterns

Both somatic states and relationship patterns largely overlap with those of persons from ethnic and cultural minorities (see above).

The Subjective Experience of the Therapist

Therapists may feel anxious apprehension that language will be a barrier to effective communication. If they feel a frequent need to ask patients to repeat certain words or phrases, they may find themselves irritated at having to intervene so often instead of maintaining their customary reserve. Alternatively, if they choose to remain relatively quiet and not interrupt, they may fail to take in much of the patients' material. A therapist may conclude, "Only a therapist who speaks the language could possibly treat this person," while a patient may be thinking, "What a relief that this therapist doesn't speak my language. They all know each other. And they all gossip. All my secrets would become public!" Thus the apparently rational and sympathetic wish to match the patient with an appropriate therapist may both distance therapist from patient and foster erroneous conclusions by both.

SApp1.3 *Religious Minorities*

Affective States

Affective states may include anxiety, anger, resentment, mistrust, and hostility. Given the potential divisive power of religious differences, patients may find it difficult or impossible to trust or like people in their neighborhoods or to have confidence in a therapist from a different religious background, especially a background with a history of conflict with theirs. Despite this, however, some patients seek a therapist of any religion other than their own, especially when hoping to escape trauma or pain that they attribute to the religion in question.

Cognitive Patterns

Cognitive patterns may include a sense of moral inferiority with attendant misperceptions arising from the projection of self-attacking mental states onto others, including the therapist. A patient may assume the therapist's religious convictions are either repressive and primitive or dangerously latitudinal; either assumption can undermine the working alliance.

Somatic States and Relationship Patterns

Somatic states can include a general state of tension and/or physical sensations of anxiety. Relationship patterns can range from virtual absence of any contacts with similar religious backgrounds in one's social circle (with consequent uncomfortable feelings of isolation) to the need to associate exclusively with others in the same religious minority.

The Subjective Experience of the Therapist

Internal experiences of therapists may include anxiety, anger, resentment, contempt, or frank hatred. Given a long history of interreligious misunderstandings and maltreatments, they might find it difficult to empathize with a patient of another religion; agnostic/atheistic/secular therapists may have trouble empathizing with any religious sensibility, leading to feelings of mistrust, hostility, or moral superiority. Conversely, via reaction formation to counteract their own biases, therapists may become overly gratifying and permissive. Finally, therapists unfamiliar with certain religious practices may inappropriately label them as pathological.

SApp1.4 *Political Minorities*

The Subjective Experience of Political Minorities

Affective States

Affective states may include mistrust and hostility, dysphoria, mood swings, and anxiety. Feelings of hostility may objectively correspond to the political reality of external circumstances, or may be projections of the patient's conflicts and prejudices, or may represent some combination of these.

Cognitive Patterns

Cognitive patterns may be dominated by suspicion or fear, motivating a person to avoid politics in his or her social network, thereby censoring sensitive political issues with others. The patient may assume that anyone from a different political background (including the therapist) would be menacing and could not possibly understand the patient's values and involvements.

Somatic States and Relationship Patterns

Somatic states and relationship patterns largely overlap with those of individuals from religious minorities (see above).

The Subjective Experience of the Therapist

Therapists' internal experiences with patients of contrasting political persuasions may include feelings of entitlement and righteousness: "What I believe is common sense." As with ethno-cultural minority patients, a therapist working with political minorities may project deep unconscious conflicts onto the patient. The patient may pick up the therapist's suppressed anger, leading to negative feelings that the therapist defensively interprets as originating in the patient. Unresolved aggression may engender defensive boredom and detachment rather than anger in a therapist. Therapist and patient may collude, consciously or unconsciously, in declining to address politics at all, or righteous countertransferences may tempt the therapist to misinterpret the patient's politics as intrapsychic phenomena.

SApp2 Lesbian, Gay, and Bisexual Populations

The understanding of lesbian, gay, and bisexual populations has matured rapidly, as has nosology for sexual orientations. The term "homosexuality" has been almost completely replaced with once offensive terms such as "gay" and "queer." "Gay," "lesbian," and "bisexual" have become both positive social identities and acceptable adjectives for sexual orientations. "Queer" is now an umbrella term for sexual orientations and gender expressions other than orientations and expressions that "match" one's biological sex. Sexual orientation should not be confused with gender expression, as many combinations are possible. For example, (1) a gay man might be "masculine" in gender expression, (2) a heterosexual man might be "feminine" in gender expression, (3) a lesbian might be "feminine" in gender expression, and (4) a heterosexual woman might be "masculine" in gender expression. The term "gay" can refer to all lesbians, gays, and bisexuals, but it is used here only in referencing gay men.

While historically a psychoanalytic understanding of lesbian, gay, and bisexual populations posited an intrapsychic pathological etiology for sexual orientation, such as unresolved oedipal issues, current psychoanalytic understanding is informed by science supporting a biologically based, nonpathological etiology. The range of scientific inquiry is exemplified by documentation of same-gender sexual behavior in over 1,500 nonhuman species. A preponderance of evidence suggests genetic factors and early uterine environment as significant for sexual orientation. The evidence does not exclude psychodynamic etiologies (which need not equate with pathology), but does focus more on "nature" than "nurture." Of course, this strict dichotomy is obsolete with the rise of epigenetics, where nurture may directly affect gene expression.

Lesbian, gay, and bisexual populations are as a group as psychologically robust as heterosexual populations; they do not report mental health problems in greater frequency than the population as a whole. Some evidence exists that when a lesbian, gay, or bisexual person reports a mental health problem, it may reflect the kinds of distress to which they are subjected as sexual minorities. Lesbian, gay, and bisexual populations do not have common affective states, typical mental content, or known accompanying somatic states. Instead, they mirror the heterosexual population in diversity and range along these continua. Their relationship patterns may involve "families of choice"—nonbiologically related groups that self-select and organize to celebrate holidays together, support one another in times of need, and otherwise play roles typical of a nuclear or extended biological family.

Lesbians, gay men, and bisexuals are subjected to minority stress. Unlike other minorities, they cannot always rely on the recognition and support of their families; in fact, family members may be an additional source of stress. It is not unusual for homonegative dynamics to occur in a sociocultural context that is indifferent or even collusive. Episodes of discrimination and violence can have a profound emotional impact transcending their direct effects; that is, they may affect not only direct victims, but also those who cannot avoid thinking that such disasters could happen to them, too.

Many studies of minority stress have confirmed its role in distress in lesbians and gay men. Meyer (1995, 2003), who developed and tested a minority stress model in a community sample of 741 gay men, described a minority stress continuum ranging from distal stressors—objective events and conditions—to proximal personal processes based on individual perceptions and appraisals. We can therefore construct a continuum extending from objective to subjective experiences on three dimensions: (1) actual experiences of discrimination and violence; (2) perceived stigma, or expectations of rejection and discrimination; and (3) internalized homonegative prejudice, or the directing of societal negative attitudes toward the self.

Some lesbian, gay, and bisexual individuals who present in clinical settings may show internalized homophobia and the sequelae of homophobia-related affective states, mental content, accompanying somatic states, and associated relational patterns. Internalized homophobia is the mental condition of believing same-sex sexual orientation to be wrong, sick, or inferior, while simultaneously experiencing oneself as having that orientation. Understanding internalized homophobia improves psychoanalytic treatment. Although we describe the phenomenon in general in what follows, a spectrum of experience exists between robust, joyous self-acceptance and thorny, miserable self-rejection.

The process by which lesbians, gays, and bisexuals acknowledge their sexual orientation and come to feel comfortable being open about it is widely referred to as "coming out." The phrase originated colloquially as "coming out of the closet"; the prior state of mind is referred to as "being in the closet" or "closetedness." Given the invisibility of sexual orientation, lesbians, gays, and bisexuals are constantly faced with the choice of revealing or concealing their sexual orientation. This reality has a psychological cost; sometimes the decision to reveal or not must be made quickly and requires disconfirming standard heteronormative communication.

The Subjective Experience of Internalized Homophobia

Affective Patterns

Internalized homophobia among lesbians, gays, and bisexuals generates feelings of guilt and shame. In severe cases, it involves self-hatred and, in extreme cases, nearly constant self-loathing. Denial of same-gender attraction can engender feelings of emptiness or recurrent dissociative states. Splitting off of one's experience of same-sex orientation from one's homophobic beliefs may manifest itself in externalizing paranoid fears and aggression toward lesbians, gays, and bisexuals, who are perceived as being seductive. At a higher level of ego development, splitting off one's sexual orientation from one's homophobia may be expressed as moralization against homosexuality that lends itself to feelings of righteous indignation and pious anger. Repression of such intrapsychic conflicts results in depression and anxiety. Compartmentalization leads to separate types of feeling states such as a daily "normal" asexual self-perception and an occasional "gay" hypersexual self-state, as clearly described in Freud's concept of splitting of the ego in the process of defense.

For example, a 30-year-old man feels ashamed of his attraction to a male colleague, tries to push these feelings out of his mind, and then acts them out homophobically. He writes on the walls of the office bathroom "Kill the faggot" and repeatedly asks colleagues, "Hey, are you a faggot?"

Cognitive Patterns

Lesbians, gays, and bisexuals with internalized homophobia experience intrusive sexual fantasies and images about same-sex partners and/or body parts. At lower levels of developmental organization, they report paranoid ideation such as "The world is dangerous," and may personalize societal stigma in thoughts such as "I'm not acceptable." At borderline levels, they may wish to be different, good, healthy, or noninferior with respect to their sexuality. In severe cases, they may have suicidal ideation. Particularly in novel social contexts, they scan the environment for signs of aggression and ask themselves, "Is it safe?" Even those at higher levels of development, with significant self-acceptance, may experience passing confusion and momentary self-doubt when confronted with negative societal messages.

For example, a 27-year-old woman worries that she is "broken" because of her love for a woman and wonders who can see her secret damage. At home, at work, and with friends, she pretends to be looking for a boyfriend and is careful to hide any behaviors considered "masculine."

Somatic States

Lesbians, gays, and bisexuals with internalized homophobia endure hypervigilance and hyperarousal. Compartmentalization and dissociated states can lead to risk-taking behavior. They may suffer poor long-term physical health outcomes, such as stress-related symptoms and the effects of substances used to manage internal conflicts.

For example, a 25-year-old gay man has specific abuse memories related to homophobic bullying episodes in the bathrooms at school, and these are encoded in a specific elimination disorder.

Relationship Patterns

Minority stress can complicate the relationships of gay, lesbian, and bisexual people, and obstruct their resolution. Mental health professionals in general can receive relevant help from an understanding of the role played by minority stress in psychological and relational development in these populations. In many places, marriage is still denied to same-sex couples; the lack of civil rights may lead to feelings of delegitimization and inadequacy, as well as concrete difficulties. Splitting off one's experience of same-sex sexual orientation from one's homophobic beliefs can be manifested in sexual or aggressive acting out or in unconscious moralizing punitiveness. Moreover, discrepancies in the outness–closetedeness dimension between two partners may be a source of stress. For example, one partner may want to express affection in public (e.g., by holding hands), and the other may prefer to avoid the behaviors that make "visible" their sexual orientation. Some bisexuals may be challenged with the relational difficulty inherent in "passing," meaning pairing themselves with opposite-sex partners and thereby obscuring their sexual orientation. It should be noted that bisexuality also exists on a continuum of being more attracted to one sex relative to the other.

The Subjective Experience of the Therapist

Clinicians' prejudices—or simply lacking of knowledge about sexual minorities—can heavily obstruct their understanding and bias their clinical listening to lesbian, gay, and bisexual clients. In these cases, it could be useful to consult a supervisor. Conversely, respectful listening, awareness of one's own prejudices, and adequate knowledge are important in creating a nonharmful and effective mental health practice. The following vignette exemplifies such issues.

Clinical Illustration

Antonio is a 32-year-old Italian bank clerk who is a nonpracticing Catholic. He consults a psychiatrist at the public mental health services for a growing difficulty in handling a sensation of anxiety and irritability. When the psychiatrist asks for more details about the origin of his anxiety, Antonio reluctantly says it has probably to do with his "private life." At this point, the psychiatrist awkwardly hazards a guess: "Problems with your wife?" Antonio, becoming more and more anxious and irritated, turns his eyes away. "I have a boyfriend," Antonio mutters. The psychiatrist realizes how inappropriate his question was and tries to restart: "Oh . . . I see. Well, that is not a problem. Go ahead." This new start is even more awkward, as it reveals the doctor's uneasiness with gay or lesbian clients. In a way, his problem is more about knowledge and experience than about prejudice and hostility; he hardly thinks about homosexuality as something that could be connected with relational or family problems, although he does think that homosexuality is related to sexual promiscuity, solitude, and shame. In a flash, the many things he *does not* know about the lives of gay people pass through his mind. He feels professionally inadequate, but at the same time, challenged. Accordingly, he asks for help from a supervisor, who helps him to understand how prejudices can bias clinical listening.

SApp3 Gender Incongruence

DSM-5 includes a new diagnosis of gender dysphoria (F64) in adolescents and adults, which replaces gender identity disorder in adolescents and adults. ICD-10 also has a gender identity disorder category (F64), which is likely to be replaced in ICD-11 by gender incongruence of adolescence and adulthood. ICD's gender incongruence will not be classified among mental disorders and is likely be situated in a new group of disorders, "conditions related to sexual health." In this spirit, PDM-2, as in the case of homosexuality and bisexuality, does not treat gender incongruence as a mental disorder.

Western psychiatric and medical theorizing about transsexualism and transgender phenomena began in the 19th century. Until the middle of the 20th century, with rare exceptions, transgender presentations were classified as psychopathological. Early psychoanalytic theories conflated gender identity with sexual orientation, which is why Freud, for example, attributed some cases of homosexuality to identifications with the parent of the other gender. Modern sex researchers separate the desires of homosexuality (to have partners of the same sex) from those of transsexualism (to live as the other sex). Usually, one's gender identity provides little or no information about one's sexual orientation.

The placement of gender diagnoses shifted in various iterations of both ICD and DSM. The diagnosis "transsexualism" first appeared in ICD-9 (1975), where it was classified as a "sexual deviation." ICD-10's (1992) new disorder grouping of gender identity disorders (F64) included five diagnoses: transsexualism (F64.0), dual-role transvestism (F64.1), gender identity disorder of childhood (F64.2), other gender identity disorders (F64.3), and gender identity disorder, unspecified (F64.4).

Neither DSM-I (1952) nor DSM-II (1968) had gender diagnoses. DSM-III (1980) added gender identity disorder of childhood and transsexualism. DSM-IV (1994) and DSM-IV-TR (2000) combined these two diagnoses into one overarching diagnosis, gender identity disorder, with transsexualism renamed as gender identity disorder in adolescents or adults. The diagnoses changed categories over time: psychosexual disorders (DSM-III); disorders usually first evident in infancy, childhood, or adolescence (DSM-III-R); sexual and gender identity disorders (DSM-IV, DSM-IV-TR); and finally gender dysphoria (DSM-5).

Gender diagnoses are controversial. Some argue that gender variance is not a symptom of a mental disorder, and that these diagnoses, like the old diagnosis of homosexuality, should be expunged. Others argue that removing diagnoses leads to loss of health care coverage for necessary medical and surgical treatment. A growing number of studies posit physical rather than mental causes of transgenderism; in any event, its causes are unknown. Nevertheless, many countries use psychiatrists and other mental health professionals as gatekeepers to whom patients must prove they are the "right" kind of transsexuals to qualify for transition services (e.g., therapists are asked to rule out the possibility that patients' conviction that they are of the gender that does not conform with their morphology is a temporary psychotic belief rather than a lifelong internal sense). However, individuals seeking transition, who do not otherwise have any mental symptoms or desire for mental health treatment, experience the gatekeeping function as unnecessarily burdensome.

Clinical presentations of gender incongruence first presenting in childhood (early onset) differ from those that first appear in adolescence and adulthood (the subjective experience of children is discussed in Chapter 9 on the SC Axis). Most children with gender incongruence do not grow up to be transgender. They are called "desisters"; most of them become gay or bisexual and "cisgender" (non-transgender) adults. A few may become heterosexual and cisgender as adults. When childhood gender incongruence continues into adolescence ("persisters"), individuals may undergo puberty suppression and later seek cross-hormonal and surgical treatment. Gender incongruence first presenting in adolescence and adulthood (late onset) is highly unlikely to desist; therefore, gender reassignment is often the treatment of choice.

Prior to DSM-5, having a disorder of sexual development or intersex condition was an exclusionary criterion for making any diagnosis that was a forerunner of gender incongruence. DSM-5 recognizes that some intersex patients develop gender incongruence and adds a fifth-digit specifier for patients who both are dysphoric and have a disorder of sexual development.

In 2015, the American Psychological Association published a new resource: the "Guidelines for Psychological Practice with Transgender and Gender Nonconforming People." Also of value is the *Standards of Care* document from the World Professional

Association for Transgender Health (WPATH; formerly the Harry Benjamin International Gender Dysphoria Association), now in its seventh version and available in 10 languages (English, Chinese, Croatian, French, German, Japanese, Norwegian, Portuguese, Russian, and Spanish) (WPATH, 2011).

The Subjective Experience of Gender Incongruence

Gender incongruence is characterized by marked and persistent lack of alignment between an individual's *experienced* (subjective sense of) gender and the *birth-assigned (natal)* gender. This incongruence often leads to a desire to transition to live and be accepted as a person of the subjectively experienced gender. Although not all gender-incongruent individuals experience distress, many do when hormonal and/or surgical treatments are unavailable. Most individuals prefer being addressed and referred to with names that suit their experienced gender and with appropriately gendered pronouns.

Thanks to the internet, today's adolescents know about puberty suppression, hormone treatment, and gender reassignment surgery (often before their parents do) and may expect to be treated as persons of their experienced gender. Some adults may seek hormone treatment, others may choose surgery, and some may seek both. Where treatment is not readily accessible or covered by insurance, individuals may pay privately or seek out hormones on the black market. Inability to access care may lead to suicidal feelings and, in extreme cases, genital self-mutilation.

As noted earlier, one function of mental health gatekeeping is to make a differential diagnosis, which ought to include consideration of nonconformity (nonpsychopathological) to gender roles, transvestic disorder, body dysmorphic disorder, dissociative identity disorder, schizophrenia, and other psychotic disorders.

Affective States

Affective states include anxious and depressed moods, at times characterized by despair and suicidal ideation. Anxiety or depression may be of sufficient severity to warrant its own psychiatric diagnosis. Self-medication of anxiety with drugs and alcohol is not uncommon. Inability to express one's experienced gender may lead to rage directed at one's own body or at external factors or individuals who are seen as obstructing gender expression. In adolescence, panic may be induced by onset of menses or breast development in natal girls or by facial hair emergence and penis growth in natal boys. There may be a strong yearning for the primary and secondary sex characteristics of the other gender. Individuals report satisfaction and pleasure when permitted, either privately or publicly, to express their inner experienced gender.

Cognitive Patterns

Cognitive patterns include preoccupations with gender, bordering on the obsessional, in individuals who have not made a transition. This usually abates if and when transition services are available and provided. Autism spectrum disorder may be present in adolescents presenting with gender incongruence.

Somatic States

Somatic states in nontransitioned individuals are characterized by extreme discomfort with the natal body. In adolescents, this may involve negative responses to the anticipation of or actual body changes at puberty. Starting in adolescence, natal men may shave legs or bind genitals to make erections less visible. Natal women may bind breasts or disguise them with nonrevealing clothing. Efforts at body modification (e.g., cross-sex hormones, electrolysis) are common.

Relationship Patterns

Relationship patterns vary. Individuals with gender incongruence may be either "androphilic" (attracted to men) or "gynephilic" (attracted to women). Some are bisexual. Some live in ostensibly homosexual relationships before transition, others in heterosexual marriages with biological children. Some individuals may be socially isolated. It is not uncommon for a transitioning individual to lose many long-term relationships through lack of acceptance. There are some cases of heterosexually married couples staying married after a transition.

The Subjective Experience of the Therapist

Subjective experiences of clinicians who are cisgender may include anxiety, concern, revulsion, or voyeuristic curiosity. Responses may also range from lack of acceptance of a child's or adolescent's experienced or expressed gender (sometimes referred to as "transphobia") to uncritical acceptance of the stated gender preference without considering alternative explanations (or a differential diagnosis). Clinicians' attachment to their own cisgender identities may sometimes make it difficult to enter into the clinical subjectivity of those wishing to make a transition either socially or anatomically from one gender to the other.

Clinical Illustrations

Case 1

A 35-year-old previously lesbian-identified professional woman seeks transition services. Her wife accompanies her to the consultation. As a child, the woman was a tomboy who was more comfortable playing with boys than with girls. This was not a problem in her family or the community where she was raised. She always felt accepted, was a good student, and earned a graduate degree. She first was aware of being attracted to girls at puberty (age 12). She came out as a lesbian in high school at age 16 and had several long-term girlfriends before settling down, at age 28, with her wife. The couple has two children, each parent having conceived a child with the same anonymous donor. In the last 2 years, the patient has felt increasingly uncomfortable with her body—a feeling she connects with long-standing feelings of "being different" since adolescence. She now thinks of herself as transgender rather than lesbian. She has chosen a male name, but when asked about which pronouns the consultant should use, she seems comfortable being referred to with female pronouns. Her breasts feel "wrong," and she wants them removed. She would like to go on testosterone and wishes to grow a beard. Her wife is supportive of the transition; they have been seeing a family therapist, who is advising them on how to explain the transition process to young children. After seeing an endocrinologist for treatment with masculinizing hormones, the patient now prefers to go by his male name. His voice deepens, and he grows facial hair and develops male-pattern baldness. In the professional setting where he works, his transition is accepted by his employer and his fellow employees. He is referred to a surgeon for a double mastectomy. He is not interested in pelvic surgery; he is thinking he still might want to bear another child. He eventually gets a legal name change.

Case 2

A 20-year-old natal male, brought by parents for evaluation of gender incongruence, insists on being addressed by a female name and referred to with female pronouns. She has recently taken a leave of absence from college due to overwhelming anxiety and distress. She has had social difficulties since childhood and has been diagnosed with an autism spectrum disorder of low severity. She does not recall childhood memories of gender incongruence, although she admits to gender-atypical interests, including playing female "dressup" with an older sister at age 4. Although she insists she is a woman, she recently began thinking of herself as "trans." She began masturbating to orgasm at age 13 and has continued this up to the present; an ongoing source of sexual fantasy and excitement involves wearing articles of female clothing while masturbating. She occasionally cross-dresses in private, but not in public. She once sexually experimented with a male school friend, but has had no sexual experiences with women. She is made anxious by her sexual attraction to women (gynephilia), as she does not want to be a lesbian and believes she should be attracted to men. She occasionally desires to be rid of her penis and to have a vagina, although the thought of having surgery seems "disgusting." Nevertheless, she wishes to be treated as a woman. She wishes to be rid of her beard, to have a woman's smooth face, and to have no Adam's apple. Psychological testing shows no evidence of a thought disorder, but attests to an ongoing struggle with gender issues. After treatment of her anxiety and depression, the patient returns to school. Her gender incongruence persists, but she is not as desperate about an immediate transition (which her parents oppose). Instead, she chooses a gender-neutral name as a way to ease into transition and avoid being addressed with the male name she was given at birth. She starts to seek out other transgender individuals online and at school. She has gone out publicly with her nails done with colored polish. She plucks her beard and is thinking about getting electrolysis, but does not at the present time wish to take hormones or have surgery.

TABLE 3.2. Concordance of PDM-2 and ICD-10/DSM-5 Diagnostic Categories for Adults

PDM-2

S1 Predominantly psychotic disorders
 S11 Brief psychotic disorder (Hysterical psychosis, Bouffée Délirante Polymorphe Aigüe)
 S12 Delusional disorder (Pure paranoia)
 S13 Schizotypal disorder (Simple schizophrenia, Residual schizophrenia)
 S14 Schizophrenia and schizoaffective disorder

ICD-10	DSM-5
F20–29. Schizophrenia, schizotypal, and delusional disorders F20. Schizophrenia .0/.1/.2. Paranoid/hebephrenic/catatonic .4/.5/.6. Undifferentiated/residual/simple .8/.9. Other/unspecified schizophrenia F21. Schizotypal disorder F22. Persistent delusional disorder F23. Acute and transient psychotic disorder F24. Induced delusional disorder (*folie à deux*) F25. Schizoaffective disorder .0/.1/.2. Manic/depressed/mixed .8/.9. Other/unspecified schizoaffective disorder F28/29. Other/unspecified nonorganic psychoses	Schizophrenia spectrum and other psychotic disorders F21. Schizotypal (personality) disorder F22. Delusional disorder F23. Brief psychotic disorder F20.81. Schizophreniform disorder F20.9. Schizophrenia F25. Schizoaffective disorder .0/.1. Bipolar/depressive F06. Catatonia F28/29. Other specified/unspecified schizophrenia spectrum and other psychotic disorders

PDM-2

S2 Mood disorders
 S21 Persistent depressive disorder (dysthymia)
 S22 Major depressive disorder
 S23 Cyclothymic disorder
 S24 Bipolar disorders
 S25 Maternal affective disorders

ICD-10	DSM-5
F30–39. Mood (affective) disorders F30. Manic episode F31. Bipolar affective disorder .0. Current episode hypomanic .1/.2. Current episode manic without/with psychotic symptoms .3. Current episode mild/moderate depression .4/.5. Current episode severe depression without/ with psychotic symptoms .6. Current episode mixed .7. Currently in remission .8/.9. Other/unspecified bipolar affective disorder	Bipolar and related disorders F31. Bipolar I disorder Current or most recent episode manic .11/.12/.13. Mild/moderate/severe .2. With psychotic features .73/.74. In partial/full remission .0. Current or most recent episode hypomanic .73/.74. In partial/full remission Current or most recent episode depressed .31/.32. Mild/moderate .4. Severe .5. With psychotic features .75/.76. In partial/full remission F31.81. Bipolar II disorder F34.0. Cyclothymic disorder F31.89/.9. Other specified/unspecified bipolar and related disorder

(continued)

TABLE 3.2. *(continued)*

ICD-10	DSM-5
F32. Depressive episode .0/.1. Mild/moderate depressive episode .2/.3. Severe depressive episode without/with psychotic symptoms .8/.9. Other/unspecified depressive episode F33. Recurrent depressive disorder .0/.1. Current episode mild/moderate .2/.3. Current episode severe without/with psychotic symptoms .4. Currently in remission .8/.9. Other/unspecified recurrent depressive disorder F34. Persistent mood disorder .0. Cyclothymia .1. Dysthymia .8/.9. Other/unspecified F38/39. Other/unspecified mood disorders	Depressive disorders F32. Major depressive disorder (single episode) .0/.1/.2. Mild/moderate/severe .3. With psychotic features .4/.5. In partial/full remission F33. Major depressive disorder (recurrent episode) .0/.1/.2. Mild/moderate/severe .3. With psychotic features .41/.42. In partial/full remission F34.1 Persistent depressive disorder (dysthymia) N94.3. Premenstrual dysphoric disorder F32.8/.9. Other specified/unspecified depressive disorder *NB: For disruptive mood dysregulation disorder, see Tables 6.2 and 9.2 for the SA and SC Axes, Chapters 6 and 9.*

PDM-2

S3 Disorders related primarily to anxiety
- S31 Anxiety disorders
  - S31.1 Specific phobias
  - S31.2 Social phobia
  - S31.3 Agoraphobia and panic disorder
  - S31.4 Generalized anxiety disorder
- S32 Obsessive–compulsive and related disorders
  - S32.1 Obsessive–compulsive disorder
  - S32.2 Body dysmorphic disorder (Dysmorphophobia)
  - S32.3 Hoarding disorder
  - S32.4 Trichotillomania and excoriation disorder

ICD-10	DSM-5
F40–48. Neurotic, stress-related, and somatoform disorders	
F40. Phobic anxiety disorders .0. Agoraphobia (with and without panic) .1. Social phobias .2. Specific (isolated) phobias F41. Other anxiety disorders .0. Panic disorder [episodic paroxysmal anxiety] .1. Generalized anxiety disorder .2. Mixed anxiety and depressive disorder	Anxiety disorders F40.2x. Specific phobias F40.1. Social anxiety disorder (social phobia) F41.0. Panic disorder F40.00. Agoraphobia F41.1. Generalized anxiety disorder
.3. Other mixed anxiety disorder F42. Obsessive–compulsive disorder .0. Predominantly obsessional thoughts .1. Predominantly compulsive acts .2. Mixed obsessional thoughts and acts F63. Habit and impulse disorders .3. Trichotillomania	Obsessive–compulsive and related disorders F42. Obsessive–compulsive disorder F45.22. Body dysmorphic disorder F42. Hoarding disorder F63.3. Trichotillomania and Excoriation (skin-picking) disorder

(continued)

TABLE 3.2. *(continued)*

PDM-2
S4 Event- and stressor-related disorders S41 Trauma- and stressor-related disorders S41.1 Adjustment disorders S41.2 Acute and posttraumatic stress disorders S41.3 Complex posttraumatic stress disorder S42 Dissociative disorders S42.1 Depersonalization/derealization disorder S42.2 Dissociative amnesia ± fugue S42.3 Dissociative identity disorder and other specified dissociative disorder–1 S43 Conversion disorder

ICD-10	DSM-5
F40–48. Neurotic, stress-related, and somatoform disorders	
F43. Reaction to severe stress, and adjustment disorders .0. Acute stress reaction .1. Posttraumatic stress disorder .2. Adjustment disorders .20. Brief depressive reaction .21. Prolonged depressive reaction .22. Mixed anxiety and depressive reaction .23. With predominant disturbance of other emotions .24. With mixed disturbance of emotions and conduct	Trauma- and stressor-related disorders F43.10. Posttraumatic stress disorder F43.0. Acute stress disorder F43.2. Adjustment disorders .21. With depressed mood .22. With anxiety .23. With mixed anxiety and depressed mood .24. With disturbance of conduct .25. With mixed disturbance of emotions and conduct
Dissociative (conversion) disorders F44.0. Dissociative amnesia F44.1. Dissociative fugue F44.3. Trance and possession disorders F44.7. Mixed dissociative (conversion) disorders F44.8. Other dissociative (conversion) disorders .80. Ganser's syndrome .81. Multiple personality disorder .88. Other specified dissociative (conversion) disorders .89. Other specified dissociative disorder F44.9. Dissociative (conversion) disorder, unspecified F48. Other neurotic disorders F48.1. Depersonalization–derealization syndrome .2. Dissociative stupor .4. Dissociative motor disorders .5. Dissociative convulsions	Dissociative disorders F44.81. Dissociative identity disorder F44.0. Dissociative amnesia. *Specify if:* F44.1. With dissociative fugue F48.1. Depersonalization/derealization disorder F44.88. Other specified dissociative disorder F44.81. Chronic and recurrent syndromes of mixed dissociative symptoms F44.88. Identity disturbance due to prolonged and intense coercive persuasion F44.88. Acute dissociative reactions to stressful events F44.3. Dissociative trance F44.9. Unspecified dissociative disorder
	Somatic symptom and related disorders F44. Conversion disorder .4. With weakness or paralysis .4. With abnormal movement .4. With swallowing symptoms .4. With speech symptoms .5. With attacks or seizures .6. With anesthesia or sensory loss .6. With special sensory symptom .7. With mixed symptoms

(continued)

TABLE 3.2. *(continued)*

PDM-2
S5 Somatic symptom and related disorders
S51 Somatic symptom disorder
S52 Illness anxiety disorder (Hypochondriasis)
S53 Factitious disorders

ICD-10	DSM-5
F45. Somatoform disorders	Somatic symptom and related disorders
.0. Somatization disorder	F45.1. Somatic symptom disorder
.1. Undifferentiated somatoform disorder	F45.21. Illness anxiety disorder
.2. Hypochondriacal disorder	F68.10. Factitious disorder
.3. Somatoform autonomic dysfunction	F45.8/.9. Other specified/unspecified somatic symptom and related disorder
.4. Persistent somatoform pain disorder	
.8/.9. Other specified/unspecified	
F68. Other disorders of adult personality and behavior	
.1. Intentional production or feigning of symptoms or disabilities, either physical or psychological (factitious disorder)	

PDM-2
S6 Specific symptom disorders
S61 Feeding and eating disorders
S62 Sleep–wake disorders
S63 Sexual dysfunctions
S64 Paraphilic disorders
S65 Disruptive, impulse-control, and conduct disorders

ICD-10	DSM-5
F50–59. Behavioral syndromes associated with physiological disturbances and physical factors	
F50. Eating disorders	Feeding and eating disorders
.0. Anorexia nervosa	F50.01. Anorexia nervosa, restricting type
.2. Bulimia nervosa	F50.02. Anorexia nervosa, binge-eating/purging type
.8/.9. Other/unspecified	F50.2. Bulimia nervosa
	F50.8. Binge-eating disorder
	F50.8/.9. Other specified/unspecified feeding or eating disorder
F51. Nonorganic sleep disorders	Sleep–wake disorders
F51.0. Nonorganic insomnia	G47.00. Insomnia disorder
F51.1. Nonorganic hypersomnia	G47.10. Hypersomnolence disorder
F51.2. Nonorganic disorder of the sleep–wake schedule	G47.4x. Narcolepsy
	Breathing-related sleep disorders
F51.3. Sleepwalking (somnambulism)	G47.3x. Obstructive sleep apnea hypopnea, central sleep apnea, sleep-related hypoventilation
F51.4. Sleep terrors	
F51.5. Nightmares	G47.2x. Circadian rhythm sleep–wake disorders
F51.8/.9. Other/unspecified sleep disorders	Parasomnias
NB: G codes for DSM-5 disorders at right indicate that these are not considered psychiatric by ICD-10, and are listed elsewhere in ICD-10.	F51.3. Non-REM sleep arousal disorder, sleepwalking type
	F51.4. Non-REM sleep arousal disorder, sleep terror type
	F51.5. Nightmare disorder
	G47.52. REM sleep behavior disorder
	G47.8/.9. Other specified/unspecified sleep–wake disorder

(continued)

TABLE 3.2. *(continued)*

ICD-10	DSM-5
F52. Sexual dysfunction, not caused by organic disorder or disease .0. Male hypoactive sexual desire disorder .1. Sexual aversion and lack of sexual enjoyment .2. Failure of genital response .3. Orgasmic dysfunction .4. Premature ejaculation .5. Nonorganic vaginismus .6. Nonorganic dyspareunia .7. Excessive sexual drive .8/9. Other/unspecified	Sexual dysfunctions F52.32. Delayed ejaculation F52.21. Erectile disorder F52.31. Female orgasmic disorder F52.22. Female sexual interest/arousal disorder F52.6. Genito-pelvic pain/penetration disorder F52.0. Male hypoactive sexual desire disorder F52.4. Premature ejaculation F52.8/.9. Other specified/unspecified sexual dysfunction
F65. Disorders of sexual preference .0. Fetishism .1. Fetishistic transvestism .2. Exhibitionism .3. Voyeurism .4. Paedophilia .5. Sadomasochism .6. Multiple disorders of sexual preference .8/.9. Other/unspecified	Paraphilic disorders F65.3. Voyeuristic disorder F65.2. Exhibitionistic disorder F65.81. Frotteuristic disorder F65.51. Sexual masochism disorder F65.52. Sexual sadism disorder F65.4. Pedophilic disorder F65.0. Fetishistic disorder F65.1. Transvestic disorder F65.8. Other specified paraphilic disorder F65.9. Unspecified paraphilic disorder
F63. Impulse disorders .0. Pathological Gambling .1. Pyromania .2. Kleptomania .3. Trichotillomania .8. Other Impluse Disorders .9. Impulse Disorder, unspecified	*NB: Disruptive, impulse-control, and conduct disorders in DSM 5 are limited to Pyromania and Kleptomania for adults (see Chapter 3, text).*

PDM-2

S7 Disorders related to addiction and to other medical conditions
- S71 Addictions
  - S71.1 Substance-related disorders
  - S71.2 Behavioral addictions (Gambling, Internet addiction, Sex addiction)
- S72 Mental disorders due to another medical condition
  - S72.1 HIV-related neurocognitive disorder

ICD-10		DSM-5
F10–19. Mental and behavioral disorders due to psychoactive substance use Mental and behavioral disorder due to use of:		Substance-related and addictive disorders
F10. Alcohol	To specify clinical condition:	Substance-related disorders
F11. Opioids F12. Cannabinoids	x.0. Acute intoxication x.1. Harmful use	*NB: See abridged ICD-10 listing at left. For full listing, see pp. 483–585 of DSM-5.*
F13. Sedatives or hypnotics	x.2. Dependence syndrome x.3. Withdrawal state	Non-substance-related disorders F63.0. Gambling disorder
F14. Cocaine F15. Other stimulants (incl. caffeine) F16. Hallucinogens	x.4. Withdrawal state with delirium x.5. Psychotic disorder x.6. Amnesic syndrome	*NB: In ICD-10, gambling is in F60–69. Disorders of adult personality and behavior; F63. Habit and impulse disorders; F63.0. Pathological gambling.*

(continued)

TABLE 3.2. *(continued)*

ICD-10	DSM-5
F17. Tobacco F18. Volatile solvents F19. Multiple drug use and use of other psychoactive substances x.7. Residual and late-onset psychotic disorder x.8./9. Other/unspecified mental and behavioral disorders	
F52. Sexual dysfunction, not caused by organic disorder or disease Excessive sexual drive	*NB: Sexual addiction per se is not listed in either ICD-10 or DSM-5.*
F00–09. Organic, including symptomatic, mental disorders F00. Dementia in Alzheimer's disease F01. Vascular dementia F02. Dementia in other diseases classified elsewhere F03. Unspecified dementia F04. Organic amnesic syndrome (not substance-induced) F05. Delirium (not substance-induced) F06. Other mental disorders due to brain damage and dysfunction and to physical disease .0. Organic hallucinosis .1. Organic catatonic disorder .2. Organic delusional disorder .3. Organic mood disorder .4. Organic anxiety disorder .5. Organic dissociative disorder .6. Organic emotionally labile disorder .7. Mild cognitive disorder .8/.9. Other specified/unspecified F07. Personality and behavioral disorders due to brain disease, damage, and dysfunction F09. Unspecified organic or symptomatic mental disorder	F06. Mental disorders due to another medical condition (AMC) (each one in its respective diagnostic grouping): .2. Psychotic delusional disorder due to AMC .0. Psychotic hallucinatory disorder due to AMC .1. Catatonia associated with/due to AMC .3x. Depressive or bipolar and related disorder due to AMC .4. Anxiety disorder due to AMC .8. Obsessive–compulsive and related disorder due to AMC Neurocognitive disorders Delirium: Substance intoxication Substance withdrawal Medication-induced Due to AMC Major or mild neurocognitive disorder (numerous types, each with its own subtypes): Due to Alzheimer's disease; involving frontotemporal lobes; with Lewy bodies; of vascular origin; due to traumatic brain injury; due to a substance/medication; due to HIV infection; due to prion disease; due to Parkinson's disease; due to Huntington's disease; due to AMC; due to multiple etiologies *NB: For full listing, see pp. 591–643 of DSM-5.*

PDM-2

SApp Appendix: Psychological experiences that may require clinical attention
- SApp1 Demographic minority populations
  - SApp1.1 Ethnic and Cultural Minorities
  - SApp1.2 Linguistic Minorities
  - SApp1.3 Religious Minorities
  - SApp1.4 Political Minorities
- SApp2 Lesbian, gay, and bisexual populations
- SApp3 Gender incongruence

ICD-10	DSM-5
F64. Gender identity disorders F64.0. Transsexualism F64.1. Dual-role transvestism F64.8. Other gender identity disorders F64.9. Gender identity disorder, unspecified	F64. Gender dysphoria F64.1. Gender dysphoria in adolescents and adults

BIBLIOGRAPHY

General Bibliography

American Psychiatric Association. (1968). *Diagnostic and statistical manual of mental disorders* (2nd ed.). Washington, DC: Author.

American Psychiatric Association. (1980). *Diagnostic and statistical manual of mental disorders* (3rd ed.). Washington, DC: Author.

American Psychiatric Association. (1994). *Diagnostic and statistical manual of mental disorders* (4th ed.). Washington, DC: Author.

American Psychiatric Association. (2000). *Diagnostic and statistical manual of mental disorders* (4th ed., text rev.). Washington, DC: Author.

American Psychiatric Association. (2013). *Diagnostic and statistical manual of mental disorders* (5th ed.). Arlington, VA: Author.

Greenspan, S. I. (1997). *Developmentally based psychotherapy*. Madison, CT: International Universities Press.

PDM Task Force. (2006). *Psychodynamic diagnostic manual*. Silver Spring, MD: Alliance of Psychoanalytic Organizations.

World Health Organization. (1992). *The ICD-10 classification of mental and behavioural disorders*. Geneva: Author.

World Professional Association for Transgender Health (WPATH). (2011). *Standards of care for the health of transsexual, transgender and gender non-conforming people, Version 7*. Minneapolis, MN: Author. Retrieved from *www.wpath.org/site_page.cfm?pk_association_webpage_menu=1351&pk_association_webpage=3926*.

S1 Predominantly Psychotic Disorders

Andreasen, N. C., Liu, D., Ziebell, S., Vora, A., & Ho, B. C. (2013). Relapse duration, treatment intensity, and brain tissue loss in schizophrenia: A prospective longitudinal MRI study. *American Journal of Psychiatry, 170*, 609–615.

Arieti, S. (1974). *Interpretation of schizophrenia* (2nd ed.). New York: Basic Books.

Beck, A. T., Rector, N., Stolar, N., & Grant, P. M. (2009). *Schizophrenia: Cognitive theory, research, and therapy*. New York: Guilford Press.

Bion, W. R. (1962). *Learning from experience*. London: Tavistock.

Ciompi, L. (1980). Catamnestic long-term study on the course of life and aging of schizophrenics. *Schizophrenia Bulletin, 6*, 606–618.

Farkas, M. (2007). The vision of recovery today: What it is and what it means for services. *World Psychiatry, 6*, 1–7.

Garrett, M., & Turkington, D. (2011). CBT for psychosis in a psychoanalytic frame. *Psychosis, 3*, 2–13.

Ho, B. C., Andreasen, N. C., Ziebell, S., Pierson, R., & Magnotta, V. (2011). Long-term antipsychotic treatment and brain volumes: A longitudinal study of first-episode schizophrenia. *Archives of General Psychiatry, 68*, 128–137.

Karon, B. P., & VandenBos, G. R. (2004). *Psychotherapy of schizophrenia: The treatment of choice*. Lanham, MD: Rowman & Littlefield. (Original work published 1981)

Klerman, G. (1990). The contemporary American scene: Diagnosis and classification of mental disorders, alcoholism and drug abuse. In N. Sartorius, A. Jablensky, D. Regier, J. Burke, & R. Hirshfeld (Eds.), *Sources and traditions of classification in psychiatry*. Toronto, ON, Canada: Hogrefe & Huber.

Perris, C. (1974). A study of cycloid psychoses. *Acta Psychiatrica Scandinavica, 50*(Suppl. 253), 7–79.

Pichot, P. (1981). Les limites de la schizophrénie. In P. Pichot (Ed.), *Actualités de la schizophrénie*. Paris: PUF.

Pichot, P. (1990). The diagnosis and classifications of mental disorders in the French-speaking countries: Background, current values and comparison with other classifications. In N. Sartorius, A. Jablensky, D. Regier, J. Burke, & R. Hirshfeld (Eds.), *Sources and traditions of classification in psychiatry*. Toronto, ON, Canada: Hogrefe & Huber.

Read, J., Fosse, R., Moskowitz, A., & Perry, B. D. (2014). The traumagenic neurodevelopmental model of psychosis revisited. *Neuropsychiatry, 4*, 656–679.

Read, J., Van Os, J., Morrison, A. P., & Ross, C. A. (2005). Childhood trauma, psychosis and schizophrenia: A literature review with theoretical and clinical implications. *Acta Psychiatrica Scandinavica, 112*, 330–350.

Sullivan, H. S. (1962). *Schizophrenia as a human process*. New York: Norton.

Tienari, P., Wynne, L. C., Sorri, A., Lahti, I., Läksy, K., Moring, J., . . . Miettunen, J. (2002). Genotype–environment interaction in the Finnish Adoptive Family Study: Interplay between genes and environment? In H. Hafner (Ed.), *Risk and protective factors in schizophrenia*. Darmstadt, Germany: Springer-Verlag.

Turner, D. T., van der Gaag, M., Karyotaki, E., & Cuijpers, P. (2014). Psychological interventions for psychosis: A meta-analysis of comparative outcome studies. *American Journal of Psychiatry, 171*, 523–538.

Wallerstein, R. S. (1967). Reconstruction and mastery in the transference psychosis. *Journal of the*

American Psychoanalytic Association, 15, 551–583.

Wykes, T., Steel, C., Everitt, B., & Tarrier, N. (2008). Cognitive behavior therapy for schizophrenia: Effect sizes, clinical models, and methodological rigor. *Schizophrenia Bulletin, 34*, 523–537.

Zubin, J., & Spring, B. (1977). Vulnerability: A new view of schizophrenia. *Journal of Abnormal Psychology, 86*, 103–126.

S2 Mood Disorders

Akiskal, H. S., Benazzi, F., Perugi, G., & Rihmer, Z. (2005). Agitated "unipolar" depression reconceptualized as a depressive mixed state: Implications for the antidepressant–suicide controversy. *Journal of Affective Disorders, 85*, 245–258.

Barlow, A., Mullany, B., Neault, N., Goklish, N., Billy, T., Hastings, R., . . . Walkup, J. T. (2014). Paraprofessional-delivered home-visiting intervention for American Indian Teen mothers and children: 3-year outcomes from a randomized controlled trial. *American Journal of Psychiatry, 172*, 154–162.

Blatt, S. J. (1995). The destructiveness of perfectionism: Implications for the treatment of depression. *American Psychologist, 50*, 1003–1020.

Blatt, S. J. (2004). *Experiences of depression: Theoretical, clinical and research perspectives.* Washington, DC: American Psychological Association.

Blatt, S. J. (2008). *Polarities of experiences.* Washington, DC: American Psychological Association.

Bleichmar, H. B. (1986). *La depresión: Un estudio psicoanalítico.* Buenos Aires: Ediciones Nueva Visión.

Bowlby, J. (1980). *Attachment and loss: Vol. 3. Loss: Sadness and depression.* London: Hogarth Press.

Brockington, I. (1996). *Motherhood and mental health.* New York: Oxford University Press.

Brokington, I. (1993). The case for "pure postpartum psychosis." *Neurology, Psychiatry and Brain Research, 2*, 7–13.

Campos, R. C., Besser, A., & Blatt, S. J. (2013). Recollections of parental rejection, self-criticism and depression in suicidality. *Archives of Suicide Research, 17*, 58–74.

Chang, E. C. (2001). Life stress and depressed mood among adolescents: Examining a cognitive-affective mediation model. *Journal of Social and Clinical Psychology, 20*, 416–429.

Chaudrom, L. H. (2003). Postpartum depression: What pediatricians need to know. *Pediatrics in Review, 24*, 154–160.

Cochran, S. V., & Rabinowitz, F. E. (2003). *Men and depression: Clinical and empirical perspectives.* San Diego, CA: Academic Press.

Deutsch, H. (1945). *The psychology of women: A psychoanalytic interpretation: Vol. 2. Motherhood.* Oxford, UK: Grune & Stratton.

Erikson, E. H. (1959). *Identity and the life cycle: Psychological issues.* New York: International Universities Press.

Etzersdorfer, E., & Schell, G. (2006). Suicidality in bipolar disorders: Psychoanalytic contribution. *Archives of Suicide Research, 10*, 283–294.

Fonagy, P., Gergely, G., Jurist, E., & Target, M. (2004). *Affect regulation, mentalization, and the development of self.* London: Karnac.

Frosch, J. (1990). Pregnancy, childbirth and postpartum reactions. In J. Frosh (Ed.), *Psychodynamic psychiatry: Theory and practice* (Vol. 2). Madison, CT: International Universities Press.

George, E. L., Milkowitz, D. J., Richards, J. A., Simoneau, T. L., & Taylor, D. O. (2003). The comorbidity of bipolar disorder and Axis II personality disorders: Prevalence and clinical correlates. *Bipolar Disorders, 5*, 115–122.

Green, A. (1980). *Narcissisme de vie, narcissisme de mort.* Paris: Editions de Minuit.

Horney, K. (1945). *Our inner conflicts.* New York: Norton.

Jackson, M. (2001). *Weathering the storms: Psychotherapy for psychosis.* London: Karnac.

Kennerly, H., & Gath, D. (1989). Maternity blues I: Detection and measurement by questionnaire. *British Journal of Psychiatry, 155*, 356–362.

Kohut, H. (1972). Thoughts on narcissism and narcissistic rage. *Psychoanalytic Study of the Child, 27*, 360–400.

Kramer, E. U., de Roten, Y., Perry, C., & Despland, J.-N. (2009). Specificities of defense mechanisms in bipolar affective disorder. *Journal of Nervous and Mental Disease, 197*, 675–681.

Langer, M. (1964). *Maternidad y sexo: Estudio psicoanalítico y psicosomático.* Buenos Aires: Paidos.

Loeb, F. F., & Loeb, L. R. (1987). Psychoanalytic observations on the effect of lithium on manic attacks. *Journal of the American Psychoanalytic Association, 35*, 877–902.

Luby, J. L. (2010). Preschool depression: The importance of identification of depression early in development. *Current Directions in Psychological Science, 19*, 91–95.

Luyten, P., & Blatt, S. J. (2013). Interpersonal relatedness and self-definition in normal and disrupted personality development. *American Psychologist, 68*, 172–183.

McCullough, J. P., Jr., Klein D. N., Keller, M. B., Holzer, C. E., Davis, S. M., Kornstein, S. G., . . . Harrison, W. M. (2000). Comparison of DSM-III-R chronic major depression and major depression superimposed on dysthymia (double depression): Validity of the distinction. *Journal of Abnormal Psychology, 109*, 419–427.

National Institute for Health Care Management (NIHCM) Foundation. (2010). *Identifying and treating maternal depression: Strategies and considerations for health plans* (Issue Brief). Washington, DC: Author. Retrieved from *www.nihcm.org/pdf/FINAL_MaternalDepression6-7.pdf.*

O'Hara, M. W. (1997). The nature of postpartum depressive disorders. In L. Murray & P. J. Cooper (Eds.), *Postpartum depression and child development.* New York: Guilford Press.

O'Hara, M. W., Schlechte, J. A., Lewis, D. A., & Varner, M. W. (1991). A controlled prospective study of postpartum mood disorders: Psychological, environmental and hormonal variables. *Journal of Abnormal Psychology, 100*, 63–73.

Ogden, T. H. (1992). *Projective identification and psychotherapeutic technique.* London: Karnac.

Pitt, B. (1973). Maternity blues. *British Journal of Psychiatry, 122*, 431–433.

Priotto Wenzel, M., & Mardini, V. (2013). Gestação, parto e puerpério. In C. L. Eizirik & A. M. Siqueira Bassols (Eds.), *O ciclo da vida humana.* Porto Alegre, Brazil: Artmed.

Quitkin, F. M. (2002). Depression with atypical features: Diagnostic validity, prevalence, and treatment. *The Primary Care Companion to the Journal of Clinical Psychiatry, 4*, 94–99.

Rado, S. (1927). The problem of melancholia. *International Journal of Psycho-Analysis, 9*, 297–313.

Rey, H. (1994). *Manic–depressive psychosis: Universals of psychoanalysis in the treatment of psychotic and borderline states.* London: Free Association Books.

Roberts, J. E., & Monroe, S. E. (1998). Vulnerable self-esteem and social processes in depression: Toward an interpersonal model of self-esteem regulation. In T. E. Joiner, Jr. & J. C. Coyne (Eds.), *The interactional nature of depression.* Washington, DC: American Psychological Association.

Rojtemberg, S. (2006). *Depresiones: Bases clínicas, dinámicas, neurocientíficas y terapéuticas.* Buenos Aires: Editorial Polemos.

Rosenfeld, H. (1963). *Psychotic states.* London: Hogarth Press.

Rosenthal, N. E., Sack, D. A., Gillin, J. C., Lewy, A. J., Goodwin, F. K., Davenport, Y., . . . Wehr, T. A. (1984). Seasonal affective disorder: A description of the syndrome and preliminary findings with light therapy. *Archives of General Psychiatry, 41*, 72–80.

Røssberg, J. I., Hoffart, A., & Friis, S. (2003). Psychiatric staff members' emotional reactions toward patients: A psychometric evaluation of an extended version of the Feeling Word Checklist (FWC-58). *Nordic Journal of Psychiatry, 57*, 45–53.

Rothschild, A. J., Winer, J., Flint, A. J., Mulsant, B. H., Whyte, E. M., Heo, M., Fratoni, S., . . . Meyers, B. S. (2008). Missed diagnosis of psychotic depression at four academic medical centers. *Journal of Clinical Psychiatry, 69*, 1293–1296.

Shahar, G. (2001). Personality, shame, and the breakdown of social ties: The voice of quantitative depression research. *Psychiatry: Interpersonal and Biological Processes, 64*, 229–238.

Shahar, G., Ann-Scotti, M., Joiner, T. E., Jr., & Rudd, M. D. (2008). Hypomanic symptoms predict an increase in narcissistic and histrionic personality disorder features in suicidal young adults. *Depression and Anxiety, 25*, 892–898.

Shahar, G., Blatt, S. J., Zuroff, D. C., Krupnick, J., & Sotsky, S. M. (2004). Perfectionism impedes social relations and response to brief treatment for depression. *Journal of Social and Clinical Psychology, 23*, 140–154.

Shahar, G., & Henrich, C. C. (2010). Do depressive symptoms erode self-esteem in early adolescence? *Self and Identity, 9*, 403–415.

Soifer, R. (1971). *Psicología del embarazo, parto y puerperio.* Buenos Aires: Ediciones Kargieman.

Stern, D. N. (1995). *The motherhood constellation: A unified view of parent–infant psychotherapy.* New York: Basic Books.

Stowe, Z. N., Hostetter, A. L., & Newport, D. J. (2005). The onset of postpartum depression: Implication for clinical screening in obstetrical and primary care. *American Journal of Obstetrics and Gynecology, 192*, 522–526.

Warren, L. W. (1983). Male intolerance of depression: A review with implications for psychotherapy. *Clinical Psychology Review, 3*, 147–156.

Weissman, M. M., Feder, A., Pilowsky, D. J., Olfson, M. F., Blanco, C., Lantigua, R., . . . Shea, S. (2004). Depressed mothers coming to primary care: Maternal reports of problems with their children. *Journal of Affective Disorders, 78*. 93–100.

Winnicott, D. W. (1957). *Mother and child: A primer of first relationships.* New York: Basic Books.

Zetzel, E. R. (1965). Depression and the incapacity to bear it. In M. Schur (Ed.), *Drives, affect and behavior* (Vol. 2). New York: International Universities Press.

S3 Disorders Related Primarily to Anxiety

Beidel, D. C., & Turner, S. M. (1998). *Shy children, phobic adults: Nature and treatment of social phobia.* Washington, DC: American Psychological Association.

Feuser, J. D., Yaryura-Tobias, J., & Saxena, S. (2008). The pathophysiology of body dysmorphic disorder. *Body Image, 5*, 3–12.

Frances, A. (2013). *Essentials of psychiatric diagnosis: Responding to the challenge of DSM-5* (rev. ed.). New York: Guilford Press.

Freud, S. (1909a). Analysis of a phobia in a five-year-old boy. *Standard Edition, 10*, 5–147.

Freud, S. (1909b). Notes upon a case of obsessional neurosis. *Standard Edition, 10*, 151–318.

Gabbard, G. O. (1992). Psychodynamics of panic disorder and social phobia. *Bulletin of the Menninger Clinic, 56*, 3–13.

Horowitz, K., Gorfinkle, K., Lewis, O., & Phillips, K. A. (2002). Body dysmorphic disorder in an adolescent girl. *Journal of the American Academy of Child and Adolescent Psychiatry, 4*(1), 1503–1509.

Hurvich, M. (2000). Fears of being overwhelmed and psychoanalytic theories of anxiety. *Psychoanalytic Review, 87*, 615–649.

Hurvich, M. (2003). The place of annihilation anxieties in psychoanalytic theory. *Journal of the American Psychoanalytic Association, 51*, 579–616.

Hurvich, M. (2011). New developments in the theory and clinical application of the annihilation anxiety concept. In A. B. Druck, C. Ellman, N. Freedman, & A. Thaler (Eds.), *A new Freudian synthesis*. London: Karnac.

Lemma, A. (2009). Being seen or being watched?: A psychoanalytic perspective on body dysmorphia. *International Journal of Psychoanalysis, 90*, 753–771.

McHugh, P. (2005). Striving for coherence: Psychiatry's efforts over classification. *Journal of the American Medical Association, 293*, 2526–2528.

Røssberg, J. I., Hoffart, A., & Friis, S. (2003). Psychiatric staff members' emotional reactions toward patients: A psychometric evaluation of an extended version of the Feeling Word Checklist (FWC-58). *Nordic Journal of Psychiatry, 57*, 45–53.

Stern, M. (1951). Anxiety, trauma and shock. *Psychoanalytic Quarterly, 20*, 179–203.

Veale, D., Ennis, M., & Lambrou, C. (2002). Possible association of body dysmorphic disorder with an occupation or education in art and design. *American Journal of Psychiatry, 159*(10), 1788–1790.

Weiss, E. (1964). *Agoraphobia in the light of ego psychology*. New York: Grune & Stratton.

S4 Event- and Stressor-Related Disorders

Barach, P. M. M. (1991). Multiple personality disorder as an attachment disorder. *Dissociation, 4*, 117–123.

Bellak, L., Hurvich, M., & Gediman, H. K. (1973). *Ego functions in schizophrenics, neurotics, and normals: A systematic study of conceptual, diagnostic, and therapeutic aspects*. New York: Wiley.

Brenner, I. (2001). *Dissociation of trauma: Theory, phenomenology, and technique*. Madison, CT: International Universities Press.

Brenner, I. (2004). *Psychic trauma: Dynamics, symptoms and treatment*. Lanham, MD: Aronson.

Breuer, J., & Freud, S. (1895). Studies on hysteria. *Standard Edition, 2*, 1–305.

Bromberg, P. M. (1998). *Standing in the spaces: Essays on clinical process, trauma, and dissociation*. Hillsdale, NJ: Analytic Press.

Bromberg, P. M. (2009). Multiple self states, the relational mind, and dissociation: A psychoanalytic perspective. In P. F. Dell & J. A. O'Neil (Eds.), *Dissociation and the dissociative disorders: DSM-V and beyond* (pp. 637–652). New York: Routledge.

Chefetz, R. (2015). *Intensive psychotherapy for persistent dissociative processes: The fear of feeling real*. New York: Norton.

Courtois, C. A. (2010). *Healing the incest wound: Adult survivors in therapy* (2nd ed.). New York: Norton.

Courtois, C. A., & Ford, J. D. (2013). *Treatment of complex trauma: A sequenced, relationship-based approach*. New York: Guilford Press.

Courtois, C. A., & Gold, S. N. (2009). The need for inclusion of psychological trauma in the professional curriculum: A call to action. *Psychological Trauma: Theory, Research, Practice, and Policy, 1*(1), 3–23.

Dalenberg, C. (1991). *Countertransference and the treatment of trauma*. Washington, DC: American Psychological Association.

Danieli, Y., Brom, D., & Sills, J. (Eds.). (2005). *The trauma of terrorism: Sharing knowledge and shared care: An international handbook*. New York: Haworth Press.

Davies, J. M., & Frawley, M. G. (1994). *Treating the adult survivor of childhood sexual abuse: A psychoanalytic perspective*. New York: Basic Books.

Dell, P. F. (2009). Understanding dissociation. In P. F. Dell & J. A. O'Neil (Eds.), *Dissociation and the dissociative disorders: DSM-V and beyond* (pp. 709–825). New York: Routledge.

Elliott, D. E., Bjelajac, P., Fallot, R. D., Markoff, L. S., & Reed, B. G. (2005). Trauma-informed or trauma-denied: Principles and implementation of trauma-informed services for women. *Journal of Community Psychology, 33*(4), 461–477.

Fairbairn, W. R. D. (1944). Endopsychic structure considered in terms of object-relationships. *International Journal of Psycho-Analysis, 25*, 70–92.

Fairbairn, W. R. D. (1952). *Psychoanalytic studies of the personality*. London: Tavistock.

Federn, P. (1952). *Ego psychology and the psychoses*. New York: Basic Books.

Felitti, V. J., Anda, R. F., Nordenberg, D., Williamson, D. F., Spitz, A. M., Edwards, V., . . . Marks, J. S. (1998). Relationship of childhood abuse and household dysfunction to many of the leading casues of death in adults: The Adverse Childhood Experiences (ACE) Study. *American Journal of Preventive Medicine, 14*, 245–258.

Fenichel, O. (1945). *The psychoanalytic theory of neurosis*. New York: Norton.

Ferenczi, S. (1949). Confusion of tongues between the adult and the child. *International Journal of Psycho-Analysis, 30*, 225–231.

Finkelhor, D. (2008). *Childhood victimization: Violence, crime, and abuse in the lives of young people: Violence, crime, and abuse in the lives of young people*. New York: Oxford University Press.

Fraser, G. A. (2003). Fraser's "dissociative table technique" revisited, revised: A strategy for working with ego states in dissociative disorders and ego-state therapy. *Journal of Trauma and Dissociation, 4*(4), 5–28.

Freud, S. (1894). The neuro-psychoses of defence. *Standard Edition, 3*, 43–61.

Freud, S. (1904). Splitting of the ego in the process of defence. *Standard Edition, 23*, 271–278.

Freud, S. (1914). Remembering, repeating and working through. *Standard Edition, 12*, 145–156.

Freud, S. (1925). Some character-types met with in psychoanalytic work: I. The "exceptions." *Standard Edition, 14*, 311–315.

Gartner, R. B. (2014). Trauma and countertrauma, resilience and counterresilience. *Contemporary Psychoanalysis, 50*, 609–626.

Herman, J. L. (1992). *Trauma and recovery: The aftermath of violence from domestic to political terror*. New York: Basic Books.

Horowitz, M. J. (1997). *Stress response syndromes: PTSD, grief and adjustment disorders* (3rd ed.). Lanham, MD: Aronson.

Howell, E. (2005). *The dissociative mind*. Hillsdale, NJ: Analytic Press.

International Society for the Study of Trauma and Dissociation. (2011). Guidelines for treating dissociative identity disorder in adults, third revision: Summary version. *Journal of Trauma and Dissociation, 12*(2), 188–212.

Jacobson, E. (1959). Depersonalization. *Journal of the American Psychoanalytic Association, 7*, 581–610.

Janet, P. (1889). *L'automatisme psychologique*. Paris: Alcan.

Janoff-Bulman, R. (1992). *Shattered assumptions: Towards a new psychology of trauma*. New York: Free Press.

Jung, C. (1963). *Memories, dreams, reflections* (A. Jaffé, Ed.; R. Winston & C. Winston, Trans.) New York: Vintage Books.

Karpman, S. (1968). Fairy tales and script drama analysis. *Transactional Analysis Bulletin, 26*(7), 39–43.

Kira, I. A. (2010). Etiology and treatment of post-cumulative traumatic stress disorders in different cultures. *Traumatology. 16*, 128–141.

Kluft, R. P. (1987). First-rank symptoms as a diagnostic clue to multiple personality disorder. *American Journal of Psychiatry, 144*, 293–298.

Kluft, R. P. (1992). Discussion: A specialist's perspective on multiple personality disorder. *Psychoanalytic Inquiry, 12*, 139–171.

Kluft, R. P. (2000). The psychoanalytic psychotherapy of dissociative identity disorder in the context of trauma therapy. *Psychoanalytic Inquiry, 20*, 259–286.

Kluft, R. P. (2009). A clinician's understanding of dissociation: Fragments of an acquaintance. In P. F. Dell & J. A. O'Neil (Eds.), *Dissociation and the dissociative disorders: DSM-V and beyond* (pp. 599–624). New York: Routledge.

Kohut, H. (1984). *How does psychoanalysis cure?* Chicago: University of Chicago Press.

Krystal, H. (Ed.). (1968). *Massive psychic trauma*. Boston: Little, Brown.

Krystal, H., & Krystal, J. H. (1988). *Integration and self-healing: Affect, trauma, alexithymia*. Hillsdale, NJ: Analytic Press.

Liotti, G. (2009). Attachment and dissociation. In P. F. Dell & J. A. O'Neil (Eds.), *Dissociation and the dissociative disorders: DSM-V and beyond* (pp. 53–65). New York: Routledge.

Loewenstein, R. J. (1991). An office mental status examination for complex chronic dissociative symptoms and multiple personality disorder. *Psychiatric Clinics of North America, 14*, 567–604.

Loewenstein, R. J., & Ross, D. R. (1992). Multiple personality and psychoanalysis: An introduction. *Psychoanalytic Inquiry, 12*, 3–48.

Nijenhuis, E. R. S., & Den Boer, J. A. (2009). Psychobiology of traumatization and trauma-related structural dissociation of the personality. In P. F. Dell & J. A. O'Neil (Eds.), *Dissociation and the dissociative disorders: DSM-V and beyond* (pp. 337–366). New York: Routledge.

O'Neil, J. A. (2009). Dissociative multiplicity and psychoanalysis. In P. F. Dell & J. A. O'Neil (Eds.), *Dissociation and the dissociative disorders: DSM-V and beyond* (pp. 287–325). New York: Routledge.

Pearlman, L. A., & Saakvitne, K. W. (1995). *Trauma and the therapist: Countertransference and vicarious traumatization in psychotherapy with incest survivors*. New York: Norton.

Putnam, F. W. (1989). *Diagnosis and treatment of multiple personality disorder*. New York: Guilford Press.

Putnam, F. W. (1997). *Dissociation in children and adolescents*. New York: Guilford Press.

Schilder, P. (1935). *The image and appearance of the human body*. Oxford, UK: Kegan Paul.

Schilder, P., & Rapaport, D. (1953). *Medical*

psychology. New York: International Universities Press.

Schnurr, P., & Green, B. L. (2004). *Trauma and health: Physical health consequences of exposure to extreme stress*. Washington, DC: American Psychological Association.

Schore, A. N. (2009). Attachment trauma and the developing right brain: Origins of pathological dissociation. In P. F. Dell & J. A. O'Neil (Eds.), *Dissociation and the dissociative disorders: DSM-V and beyond* (pp. 107–141). New York: Routledge.

Shengold, L. (1989). *Soul murder: The effects of childhood abuse and deprivation*. New Haven, CT: Yale University Press.

Sierra, M., & Berrios, G. E. (2000). The Cambridge Depersonalization Scale: A new instrument for the measurement of depersonalization. *Psychiatry Research, 93*, 153–164.

Simeon, D., & Abugel, J. (2006). *Feeling unreal: Depersonalization disorder and the loss of the self*. New York: Oxford University Press.

Smith, C. P., & Freyd, J. (2014). Institutional betrayal. *American Psychologist, 69*, 575–587.

Steele, K. S., Van der Hart, O., & Nijenhuis, E. R. S. (2009). The theory of trauma-related structural dissociation of the personality. In P. F. Dell & J. A. O'Neil (Eds.), *Dissociation and the dissociative disorders: DSM-V and beyond* (pp. 239–258). New York: Routledge.

Tarnopolsky, A. (2003). The concept of dissociation in early psychoanalytic writers. *Journal of Trauma and Dissociation, 4*, 7–25.

Terr, L. (1990). *Too scared to cry: Psychic trauma in childhood*. New York: Basic Books.

Terr, L. (1995). *Unchained memories: True stories of traumatic memories lost and found*. New York: Basic Books.

Tschöke, S., Uhlmann, C., & Steinert, T. (2011) Schizophrenia or trauma-related psychosis?: Schneiderian first rank symptoms as a challenge for differential diagnosis. *Neuropsychiatry, 1*(4), 349–360.

Ulman, R. B., & Brothers, D. (1988). *The shattered self*. Hillsdale, NJ: Analytic Press.

van der Hart, O., Nijenhuis, E. R. S., & Steele, K. (2006). *The haunted self: Structural dissociation and the treatment of chronic traumatization*. New York: Norton.

van der Kolk, B. A., McFarlane, A. C., & Weisaeth, L. (Eds.). (1996). *Traumatic stress: The effects of overwhelming experience on mind, body and society*. New York: Guilford Press.

Varvin, S., & Rosenbaum, B. (2003). Extreme traumatisation: Strategies for mental survival. *International Forum of Psychoanalysis, 12*, 5–16.

Watkins, J. G., & Watkins, H. H. (1997). *Ego states: Theory and therapy*. New York: Norton.

Wilson, J. P., & Raphael, B. (1993). *International handbook of traumatic stress syndromes*. New York: Plenum Press.

Wolff, P. H. (1987). *The development of behavioral states and the expression of emotions in early infancy*. Chicago: University of Chicago Press.

Wurmser, L. (1981). *The mask of shame*. Baltimore: Johns Hopkins University Press.

Yehuda, R., & McFarlane, A. C. (1995). Conflict between current knowledge about posttraumatic stress disorder and its original conceptual basis. *American Journal of Psychiatry, 152*, 1705–1713.

S5 Somatic Symptom and Related Disorders

Deutsch, F. (1939). The associative anamnesis. *Psychoanalytic Quarterly, 8*, 354.

Fenichel, O. (1945). *The psychoanalytic theory of neurosis*. New York: Norton.

Marty, P., & de M'Uzan, M. (1963). La pensée opératoire. *Revue Français, 27*(Suppl.), 345–356.

Sifneos, P. E. (1973). The prevalence of "alexithymic" characteristics in psychosomatic patients. *Psychotherapy and Psychosomatics, 22*, 255–262.

S6 Specific Symptom Disorders

Bemporad, J. R., Beresin, E., Ratey, J. J., O'Driscoll, G., Lindem, K., & Herzog, D. B. (1992a). A psychoanalytic study of eating disorders: I. A developmental profile of 67 cases. *Journal of the American Academy of Psychoanalysis, 20*, 509–531.

Bemporad, J. R., O'Driscoll, G., Beresin, E., Ratey, J. J., Lindem, K., & Herzog, D. B. (1992b). A psychoanalytic study of eating disorders: II. Intergroup and intragroup comparisons. *Journal of the American Academy of Psychoanalysis, 20*, 533–541.

Birsted-Breen, D. (1989). Working with an anorexic patient. *International Journal of Psychoanalysis, 70*, 29–40.

Blatt, S. (1974). Levels of object representation in anaclitic and introjective depression. *Psychoanalytic Study of the Child, 29*, 107–157.

Blatt, S. (2004). *Experiencies of depression: Theoretical, clinical, and research perspectives*. Washington, DC: American Psychological Association.

Bradley, S. J. (2000). *Affect regulation and the development of psychopathology*. New York: Guilford Press.

Bromberg, P. M. (2001). Treating patients with symptoms and symptoms with patience: Reflections on shame, dissociation and eating disorders. *Psychoanalytic Dialogues, 11*, 891–912.

Bruch, H. (1973). *Eating disorders: Obesity, anorexia nervosa and the person within.* New York: Basic Books.

Brusset, B. (1998). *Psychopathologie de l'anorexie mentale.* Paris: Dunod.

Colli, A., & Ferri, M. (2015). Patient personality and therapist countertransference. *Current Opinion in Psychiatry, 2*, 46–56.

Di Nicola, V. F. (1990). Anorexia multiforme: Self-starvation in historical and cultural context. *Transcultural Psychiatric Research Review, 27*, 165–196.

Fischer, N. (1989). Anorexia nervosa and unresolved rapprochement conflicts: A case study. *International Journal of Psychoanalysis, 70*, 41–54.

Freud, S. (1905). Three essays on the theory of sexuality. *Standard Edition, 7*, 125–143.

Fonagy, P., Gergely, G., Jurist, E., & Target, M. (2004). *Affect regulation, mentalization, and the development of the self.* London: Karnac.

Fonagy, P., & Target, M. (1996). Playing with reality: I. Theory of mind and the normal development of psychic reality. *International Journal of Psychoanalysis, 77*, 217–233.

Gazzillo, F., Lingiardi, V., Peloso, A., Giordani, S., Vesco, S., Zanna, V., . . . Vicari, S. (2013). Personality subtypes in adolescents with eating disorders. *Comprehensive Psychiatry, 54*(6), 702–712.

Green, A. (1980). *Narcissisme de vie, narcissisme de mort.* Paris: Éditions de Minuit.

Jeammet, P. (1984). L'anorexie mentale. *Encyclopédie Médico-Chirurgicale: Psychiatrie, 37350*, A10–A15.

Jeammet, P. (1991). Dysrégulations narcissiques et objectales dans la boulimie. In B. Brusset, C. Couvreur, & A. Fine (Eds.), *Boulimie, monographie de la Revue Française de Psychanalyse* (pp. 81–104). Paris: PUF.

Kächele, H., Kordy, H., Richard, M., & Research Group TR-EAT. (2001). Therapy amount and outcome of inpatient psychodynamic treatment of eating disorders in Germany: Data from a multicenter study. *Psychotherapy Research, 11*(3), 239–257.

Karasic, D., & Drescher, J. (Eds.). (2005). *Sexual and gender diagnoses of the* Diagnostic and Statistical Manual *(DSM): A reevaluation.* New York: Routledge. [Simultaneously published as *Journal of Psychology and Human Sexuality, 17*(3–4).]

Keating, L., Tasca, G. A., & Hill, R. (2013). Structural relationships among attachment insecurity, alexithymia and body esteem in women with eating disorders. *Eating Behaviors, 14*(3), 366–373.

Kernberg, O. F. (1984). *Severe personality disorders: Psychotherapeutic strategies.* New Haven, CT: Yale University Press.

Kernberg, O. F. (1992). *Aggression in personality disorders and perversion.* New Haven, CT: Yale University Press.

Kernberg, P. F. (1987). Mother–child interaction and mirror behavior. *Infant Mental Health Journal, 8*(4), 329–339.

Laufer, M., & Laufer, E. (1984). *Adolescence and developmental breakdown: A psychoanalytic view.* London: Karnac.

Lowenkopf, E. L., & Wallach, J. D. (1985). Bulimia: Theoretical conceptualizations and therapies. *Journal of the American Academy of Psychoanalysis, 13*, 489–503.

Moser, C., & Kleinplatz, P. J. (2005). *DSM-IV-TR* and the paraphilias: An argument for removal. *Journal of Psychology and Human Sexuality, 17*(3–4), 91–109.

Persano, H. L. (2005). Abordagem psicodinâmica do paciente com trastornos alimentares. In C. L. Eizirik, R. W. Aguiar, & S. S. Schestatsky (Eds.), *Psicoterapia de orientação analítica: Fundamentos teóricos e clínicos* (Cap. 49, pp. 674–688). Porto Alegre, Brazil: Artmed Editora.

Persano, H. L. (2006). Contratransferência em pacientes com transtornos alimentares. In J. Zaslavsky, & M. J. Pires dos Santos (Eds.), *Contratransferência: Teoria e prática clínica* (Cap. 10, pp. 150–166). Porto Alegre, Brazil: Artmed Editora.

Persano, H. L. (2014). El hospital de día para sujetos con trastornos de la conducta alimentaria: Abordaje interdisciplinario en comunidad terapéutica con enfoque psicodinámico. In *Programa de actualización en psiquiatría III*(10) (pp. 129–168). Buenos Aires: Editorial Médica Panamericana.

Rozen, D. L. (1993). Projective identification and bulimia. *Psychoanalytic Psychology, 10*, 261–273.

Schwartz, H. J. (1986). Bulimia: Psychoanalytic perspectives. *Journal of the American Psychoanalytic Association, 34*, 439–462.

Stein, R. (2005). Why perversion?: False love and the perverse pact. *International Journal of Psychoanalysis, 86*(3), 775–799.

Thompson-Brenner, H., Satir, D. A., Franko, D. F., & Herzog, D. B. (2012). Clinician reactions to patients with eating disorders: A review. *Psychiatric Services, 63*, 73–78.

Williams, G. (1997a). Reflections on some dynamics of eating disorders: "No entry" defences and foreign bodies. *International Journal of Psychoanalysis, 78*, 927–941.

Williams, G. (1997b). *Internal landscapes and foreign bodies: Eating disorders and other pathologies.* London: Karnac.

Zukerfeld, R. (1996). *Acto bulímico, cuerpo y tercera tópica.* Buenos Aires: Edicion Paidos.

S7 Disorders Related to Addiction and to Other Medical Conditions

Gottdiener, W. H. (2013). Understanding, treating, and preventing substance use disorders: A psychodynamic perspective. In N. E. Suchman, M. Pajulo, & L. C. Mayes (Eds.), *Parenting and substance abuse: Developmental approaches to intervention* (pp. 87–99). New York: Oxford University Press.

Khantzian, E. J., & Albanese, M. J. (2008). *Understanding addiction as self-medication: Finding hope behind the pain.* Lanham, MD: Rowman & Littlefield.

Shaffer, H. J., LaPlante, D. A., LaBrie, R. A., Kidman, R. C., Donato, A. N., & Stanton, M. V. (2004). Toward a syndrome model of addiction: Multiple expressions, common etiology. *Harvard Review of Psychiatry, 12*, 367–374.

Treisman, G., & Angelino, A. (2004). *The psychiatry of AIDS: A guide to diagnosis and treatment.* Baltimore: Johns Hopkins University Press.

U.S. Department of Health and Human Services. (2015). Global HIV statistics. Retrieved March 20, 2015, from *www.aids.gov/hiv-aids-basics/hiv-aids-101/global-statistics.*

SApp Psychological Experiences That May Require Clinical Attention

SApp1 *Demographic Minority Populations*

Comas-Diaz, L. (2007). Ethnopolitical psychology: Healing and transformation. In E. Aldarondo (Ed.), *Advancing social justice through clinical practice.* New York: Routledge.

Comas-Diaz, L., & Jacobsen, F. M. (1991). Ethnocultural transference and countertransference in the therapeutic dyad. *American Journal of Orthopsychiatry, 61*, 392–402.

Eng, E. L., & Han, S. (2000). A dialogue on racial melancholia. *Psychoanalytic Dialogues, 10*(4), 667–700.

Tummala-Narra, P. (2007). Skin color and the therapeutic relationship. *Psychoanalytic Psychology, 24*(2), 255–270.

Tummala-Narra, P. (2015). Cultural competence as a core emphasis of psychoanalytic psychotherapy. *Psychoanalytic Psychology, 32*(2), 275–292.

SApp2 *Lesbian, Gay, and Bisexual Populations*

Bagemihl, B. (1999). *Biological exuberance: Animal homosexuality and natural diversity.* New York: St. Martin's Press.

Blum, A., Danson, M., & Schneider, S. (1997). Problems of sexual expression in adult gay men: A psychoanalytic reconsideration. *Psychoanalytic Psychology, 14*(1), 1–11.

Cohen, K. M., & Savin-Williams, R. C. (2012). Coming out to self and others: Developmental milestones. In P. Levounis, J. Drescher, & M. E. Barber (Eds.), *The LGBT casebook* (pp. 17–33). Arlington, VA: American Psychiatric Publishing.

Dimen, M., & Goldner, V. (2002). *Gender in psychoanalytic space: Between clinic and culture.* New York: Other Press.

Dimen, M., & Goldner, V. (2012). Gender and sexuality. In G. O. Gabbard, B. E. Litowitz, & P. Williams (Eds.), *Textbook of psychoanalysis* (2nd ed., pp. 133–154). Arlington, VA: American Psychiatric Publishing.

Drescher, J. (1998). *Psychoanalytic therapy and the gay man.* Hillsdale, NJ: Analytic Press.

Drescher, J. (2012). What's in your closet? In P. Levounis, J. Drescher, & M. E. Barber (Eds.), *The LGBT casebook* (pp. 3–16). Arlington, VA: American Psychiatric Publishing.

Hatzenbuehler, M. L. (2009). How does sexual minority stigma "get under the skin"?: A psychological mediation framework. *Psychological Bulletin, 135*(5), 707–730.

Isay, R. A. (1989). *Being homosexual: Gay men and their development.* New York: Farrar, Straus, & Giroux.

Isay, R. A. (1996). Psychoanalytic therapy with gay men: Developmental considerations. In R. P. Cabaj, T. S. Stein, R. P. Cabaj, & T. S. Stein (Eds.), *Textbook of homosexuality and mental health* (pp. 451–469). Washington, DC: American Psychiatric Association.

LeVay, S. (2011). *Gay, straight, and the reason why: The science of sexual orientation.* New York: Oxford University Press.

Lingiardi, V. (2015). No maps for uncharted lands: What does gender expression have to do with sexual orientation? In A. Lemma & P. Lynch (Eds.), *Sexualities: Contemporary psychoanalytic perspectives* (pp. 101–120). London: Routledge.

Lingiardi, V., & Nardelli, N. (2012). Partner relational problem: Listening beyond homo-ignorance and homo-prejudice. In P. Levounis, J. Drescher, & M. E. Barber (Eds.), *The LGBT casebook* (pp. 223–230). Arlington, VA: American Psychiatric Publishing.

Lingiardi, V., Nardelli, N., & Drescher, J. (2015). New Italian lesbian, gay, and bisexuals psychotherapy guidelines: A review. *International Review of Psychiatry, 27*(5), 405–415.

Meyer, I. H. (1995). Minority stress and mental health in gay men. *Journal of Health and Social Behavior, 36*, 38–56.

Meyer, I. H. (2003). Prejudice, social stress, and mental health in lesbian, gay, and bisexual populations: Conceptual issues and research evidence. *Psychological Bulletin, 129*, 674–697.

Meyer, I. H., & Northridge, M. E. (2007). *The health of sexual minorities: Public health perspectives on lesbian, gay, bisexual, and transgender populations*. New York: Springer.

Mitchell, S. A. (1978). Psychodynamics, homosexuality, and the question of pathology. *Psychiatry: Journal for the Study of Interpersonal Processes, 41*, 254–263.

SApp3 Gender Incongruence

American Psychological Association. (2015). Guidelines for psychological practice with transgender and gender nonconforming people. *American Psychologist, 70*(9), 832–864.

Cohen-Kettenis, P. T., & Pfäfflin, F. (2010). The DSM diagnostic criteria for gender identity disorder in adolescents and adults. *Archives of Sexual Behavior, 39*(2), 499–513.

Drescher, J. (2010). Queer diagnoses: Parallels and contrasts in the history of homosexuality, gender variance, and the *Diagnostic and Statistical Manual* (DSM). *Archives of Sexual Behavior, 39*, 427–460.

Drescher, J. (2014). Controversies in gender diagnoses. *LGBT Health, 1*(1), 9–15.

Drescher, J., & Byne, W. (2013). *Treating transgender children and adolescents: An interdisciplinary discussion*. New York: Routledge.

Drescher, J., Cohen-Kettenis, P., & Winter, S. (2012). Minding the body: Situating gender diagnoses in the ICD-11. *International Review of Psychiatry, 24*(6), 568–577.

Meyer-Bahlburg, H. F. (2010). From mental disorder to iatrogenic hypogonadism: Dilemmas in conceptualizing gender identity variants as psychiatric conditions. *Archives of Sexual Behavior, 39*, 461–476.

Money, J., Hampson, J. G., & Hampson, J. L. (1955). Hermaphroditism: Recommendations concerning assignment of sex, change of sex, and psychological management. *Bulletin of the Johns Hopkins Hospital, 97*, 284–300.

Stoller, R. J. (1964). A contribution to the study of gender identity. *International Journal of Psycho-Analysis, 45*, 220–226.

Zucker, K. J. (2010). The DSM diagnostic criteria for gender identity disorder in children. *Archives of Sexual Behavior, 39*, 477–498.

Zucker, K. J., Cohen-Kettenis, P. T., Drescher, J., Meyer-Bahlburg, H. F. L., Pfäfflin, F., & Womack, W. M. (2013). Memo outlining evidence for change for gender identity disorder in the DSM-5. *Archives of Sexual Behavior, 42*, 901–914.

PART II

Adolescence

CHAPTER 4

Profile of Mental Functioning for Adolescents

MA Axis

CHAPTER EDITORS

Mario Speranza, MD, PhD **Nick Midgley, PhD**

CONSULTANTS

Mark Carter, MA, MSc
Martin Debbané, PhD
George Halasz, MS, MRCPsych
Annette Streeck-Fischer, MD, PhD

Introduction

The assessment of mental functioning is essential for diagnostic formulation, treatment planning, and implementation. Because it must include the developmental progression of mental functions, assessment of mental functioning in adolescents is a more complex process than assessment with adults. This chapter describes categories of basic mental functions for adolescents ages 12–19, with the goal of providing clinicians with the tools necessary to offer a clear clinical description of each adolescent's presentation and to place it within the proper developmental context.

Adolescence is a time of great change for young people at the physical, cognitive, social-emotional, and interpersonal levels. Although it is true that each teenager is an individual with a unique personality, there are also numerous developmental issues that everyone faces during the early, middle, and late adolescent years. These can be categorized into four broad areas: cognitive changes, moving toward independence, forming of identity (with morality), and sexuality. In chronological terms, adolescence can be separated into three stages: early adolescence (approximately 12–14 years), middle adolescence (approximately 15–16 years), and late adolescence (approximately 17–19 years; issues of late adolescence may extend into the early 20s). Whenever possible, descriptions of mental functioning in this chapter refer to these developmental issues and these broad age periods.

The MA-Axis domains are built on diverse psychodynamic, cognitive, and developmental models. As in the M Axis for adults, adolescents' mental functioning is organized into 12 distinct capacities referencing different levels of psychological adaptation, ranging from more compromised to more functional. Although conceptually distinct, these capacities are not completely separate; mental functioning should be conceptualized as a unified, integrated set of processes. According to a transactional model, personality and mental functioning are determined by the integration of constitutional features (temperament, genetic predispositions) with aspects of the relational environment (learning, experience, attachment style, cultural and social context). Individuals develop at different rates within a genetically influenced developmental continuum.

The MA Axis covers a variety of areas. Each section is accompanied by a general description of the capacity, with reference to the principal developmental task. For each capacity, we provide an annotated list of relevant assessment tools. We have also introduced an assessment procedure (see Table 4.1, pp. 306–307) whereby clinicians can indicate on a 5-point scale the level of each mental function in a specific patient (descriptors for key characteristics of levels of functioning 5, 3, and 1 are provided for *each* mental function). Finally, to provide a better understanding of the underlying constructions of the capacities, each section presents the most pertinent clinical and empirical literature.

Because adolescence has continuities and discontinuities with childhood and adulthood, we suggest referring to the corresponding sections of PDM-2. Although no profile can hope to capture the full panoply of mental life, the categories summarized for adults in the M Axis (see Chapter 2, pp. 76–77) highlight a number of critical areas illuminating the complexity and individuality of a person's mental functioning. We elaborate on those categories below, with an emphasis on adolescence.

Empirically Grounded Assessment of MA-Axis Capacities

The assessment of adolescents' mental functioning presents some special issues. Like that of children, the assessment of adolescents must integrate multiple sources, as each source provides unique information about adolescents' functioning. This includes adolescents' and parents' interview-based assessments, adolescents' performance-based measures, parents' and teachers' reports, and adolescents' self-rated scales. If adolescents are in a better position to describe their internal experience, parents and teachers may be more at ease in identifying symptoms that express themselves externally.

Information gathered should focus on an adolescent's present level of functioning, developmental history, and family mental health background. Finally, clinical observations should be made across diverse contexts such as school, home, and activities, and completed with informal reports from other adults in regular contact with the adolescent. The aim is to bring together all pieces of the puzzle to create a psychodynamic diagnostic profile of the adolescent.

In the following sections, the adolescent's mental functioning capacities are described in detail. For each capacity, we provide a list of well-validated clinical tools that can aid in assessment. For a broader array of assessment instruments, along with strategies for integrating information derived from them, please refer to Chapter 15 on assessment tools. In addition, specific PDM-2-referenced measures such as the Psychodiagnostic Chart–2 (PDC-2) and its adolescent counterpart (the PDC-A) are provided in the Appendix to this manual.

1. Capacity for Regulation, Attention, and Learning

For a broader definition of the first capacity, see Chapter 2 (p. 77).

In adolescence, the functions included in this capacity can be integrated under the broad concept of "self-regulation." Self-regulation refers to internal and/or transactional processes that manage emotion, cognition, and behavior. It encompasses the capacity to restrain behavior, detect errors, and engage in planning; it includes the ability to manage attention and to initiate (activational control) and inhibit (inhibitory control) behavior to adapt to contextual demands. Self-regulation plays a crucial role in the development of various aspects of functioning. It is associated with increased social competence, superior coping abilities, and academic success. Poorer regulatory capacities, on the other hand, are thought to underlie various forms of psychopathology (both externalizing and internalizing types). During development, the evolution of self-regulation depends on cognitive resources and the adjustment of scaffolding or regulation by adults or peers. Adolescence is characterized by significant improvements in self-regulatory abilities. Performances on tasks of cognitive and emotional control have been found to improve through adolescence and early adulthood, and to parallel the maturation of higher-order association cortices within the prefrontal brain regions.

Self-regulating abilities vary with individual factors (genetic predisposition, temperament, developmental hazards) and are strongly influenced by environmental factors (beginning in the early child–caregiver interactions) and situational contexts (with associated emotions), resulting in variations in performances across situations and settings. The assessment of this capacity should consequently integrate several sources of information: direct clinical and neuropsychological assessment, self-reports, and reports from knowledgeable informants.

Rating Scale

For this and each of the other MA-Axis capacities, a 5-point rating scale, in which each mental function can be assessed from 5 to 1, is provided in Table 4.1 (pp. 306–307). Descriptions of the anchor points for levels 5, 3, and 1 are provided for each capacity in the text.

5. At this level, adolescents are focused, well organized, and able to adapt and learn from experience, even under stress. They can express thoughts, affects, and other inner experiences verbally and nonverbally. Memory, attention, and executive function are at high levels and are well integrated.

3. These adolescents can be focused, organized, and able to adapt and learn when motivated. When not fully engaged, they may show moderate decline. Even when functioning optimally, individuals at this level can attend and focus only for relatively short periods and to a limited degree. Learning capacities are highly reliant

on external support, with significant difficulty protecting attentional processes from emotional interference. Under stress, there may be significant decline, with emergence of problems in language, information processing, and/or executive function.

1. These adolescents have fleeting attention and find it hard to stay focused, organized, and attentive. They may have difficulty adapting to the environment and learning from experience, and may be self-absorbed, lethargic, or passive. Learning capacity is severely limited because of one or more processing difficulties. Their verbal expressions may be compromised, impoverished, or peculiar.

Most Relevant Assessment Tools

Numerous tools are available to assess adolescents' regulation, attention, and learning. Self-questionnaires and informant-based checklists give critical information about this capacity. Assessment of complex cognitive processes, however, may require neuropsychological tests. In these situations, the clinician should refer the adolescent to an appropriately trained neuropsychologist. In the following section we list measures that may be useful in assessing intelligence, attention, executive functions, and learning. Those that specifically assess emotional and cognitive regulation are presented in other sections of this chapter, especially in the "Capacity for Affective Range, Communication, and Understanding" section.

Wechsler Intelligence Scale for Children

The Wechsler Intelligence Scale for Children—Fourth Edition (WISC-IV; Wechsler, 2005), the most widely used intelligence test for children, was normed on children between 6 years, 0 months and 16 years, 11 months of age. It is available in many languages. Administration requires 60–90 minutes and generates a full scale IQ (FSIQ), a comprehensive measure of the child's overall intellectual ability, and four composite scores that identify abilities in discrete domains: a verbal comprehension index (VCI), perceptual reasoning index (PRI), processing speed index (PSI), and working memory index (WMI). There are 10 core subtests, given equal weighting toward the FSIQ. Crawford, Anderson, Rankin, and MacDonald (2010) have developed a short form for use when circumstances preclude administering the full-length WISC-IV, by selecting the subtests with the highest loadings on composite scores: vocabulary and similarities for the VCI, block design and matrix reasoning for the PRI, digit span for the WMI, and coding and symbol search for the PSI. The short-form indexes have high reliability and criterion validity (Crawford et al., 2010; Hrabok, Brooks, Fay-McClymont, & Sherman, 2014).

A fifth edition of the WISC (WISC-V; Wechsler, 2014) has been recently released. The main innovations are new measures of visual–spatial ability, fluid reasoning, and visual working memory, and several composite scores of cognitive abilities relevant to assessment and identification of learning problems. The normative sample has been updated, and a new interactive digital format has been introduced with a computerized method for coding and summarizing results. For adolescents over age 16, the Wechsler Adult Intelligence Scale—Fourth Edition (WAIS-IV; Wechsler, 2008) is more appropriate.

Leiter International Performance Scale—Revised

The Leiter International Performance Scale—Revised (Leiter-R; Roid & Miller, 1997) is a nonverbal intelligence assessment for children ages 2–18. This "gold standard" assessment tool for children and adolescents with hearing and speech problems addresses a range of cognitive functions similar to those found on more traditional measures, including visual scanning/discrimination, visual synthesis, and visual abstract reasoning. A distinctive quality is the preferential use of nonverbal and pantomime instructions, eliminating the need for verbal instructions throughout administration. This feature supports the test's validity as an impartial measure of nonverbal cognitive assessment in youngsters with varying levels of hearing loss. The Leiter-R has high reliability and validity, with internal consistency reliability coefficients of .75–.90 within the visualization and reasoning subtests, and .67–.85 within the attention and memory subtests (Roid & Miller, 1997). The battery is norm-referenced with a normative sample of 1,719 subjects (Roid & Miller, 1997).

Comprehensive Executive Function Inventory

The Comprehensive Executive Function Inventory (CEFI; Naglieri & Goldstein, 2013) is a rating scale that evaluates goal-directed behaviors controlled by executive functions in youth ages 5–18. It determines an individual's profile of strengths and weaknesses in executive functioning by comparing individual scores to a nationally representative group. It can be used to guide assessment, diagnosis, and treatment planning and to evaluate intervention programs. In addition to a full-scale score calculated by adding responses to 90 of the items, it uses nine rationally derived scales to pinpoint targets for intervention: attention, emotion regulation, flexibility, inhibitory control, initiation, organization, planning, self-monitoring, and working memory. Reliability and validity data are strong. The CEFI offers parent, teacher, and self-report (for ages 12–18 years) forms, allowing for a multiple-rater perspective.

Behavioural Assessment of the Dysexecutive Syndrome in Children

The Behavioural Assessment of the Dysexecutive Syndrome in Children (BADS-C; Emslie, Wilson, Burden, Nimmo-Smith, & Wilson, 2003) is a battery developed to measure ecologically valid executive functioning in children 8–16 years old. It consists of six tests: rule shift cards, action program, key search, temporal judgment, zoo map, and modified six elements. For each, a summary profile score is obtained (range = 0–4), summed for a total score (maximum = 24). Normative data were obtained on 265 healthy children and on 114 with developmental/neurological disorders in the United Kingdom. Construct validity was demonstrated by providing a different age-related profile on a sample of 208 children ages 8–15 years, divided into three age groups (8 years to 9 years, 11 months; 10 years to 11 years, 11 months; 12 to 15 years) (Engel-Yeger, Josman, & Rosenblum, 2009).

Behavior Rating Inventory of Executive Function

The Behavior Rating Inventory of Executive Function (BRIEF; Gioia, Isquith, Guy, & Kenworthy, 2000) assesses executive functioning at home and school for children and adolescents ages 5–18. The 86-item questionnaire, with forms for parents and teachers, takes 10–15 minutes to administer and 15–20 minutes to score. A self-report version for adolescents 11–18 (BRIEF-SR) is also available. Eight subscales are used to calculate two index scores: a behavioral regulation index (BRI), based on three subscales (inhibit, shift, and emotional control), and a metacognition index (MI), based on five subscales (initiate, working memory, plan/organize, organization of materials, and monitor). Because the BRIEF is not disorder specific, it may be used to assess executive functioning in children and adolescents with a wide range of difficulties, such as those related to learning, attention, brain injuries, developmental disorders, various psychiatric conditions, and medical issues. It was normed on data from 1,419 parents and 720 teachers from a representative socioeconomic distribution. It has good reliability, with high test–retest reliability (*r*'s = .88 for teachers, .82 for parents), internal consistency (Cronbach's alphas = .80–.98), and moderate correlations between parent and teacher ratings (*r*'s = .32–.34). Convergent and divergent validity have been found with other measures of emotional and behavioral functioning; the BRIEF is also useful in differentiating children and adolescents with attention-deficit/hyperactivity disorder (ADHD) and reading disorder (McCandless & O'Laughlin, 2007).

Brown Attention-Deficit Disorder Scale for Adolescents

The Brown Attention-Deficit Disorder Scale for Adolescents (BADDS-A; Brown, 2001) is a 40-item self-report scale to help assess executive function impairments associated with attentional problems. Items are rated from 0 (never) to 3 (almost daily) and grouped into six clusters, each representing an underlying aspect of ADD/ADHD: (1) organizing, prioritizing, and activating to work; (2) focusing, sustaining, and shifting attention to tasks; (3) regulating alertness, sustaining effort, and processing speed; (4) managing frustration and modulating emotions; (5) utilizing working memory and accessing recall; and (6) monitoring and self-regulating action. These groupings organize observations about an adolescent's functioning that can be clinically useful. Total scores can range from 0 to 120, with higher scores indicating more severe impairment. A score of 50 is the clinical cutoff in adolescents. The BADDS-A shows good sensitivity and specificity, with 4% false negatives and 6% false positives.

Conners–Wells Adolescent Self-Report Scale

The Conners–Wells Adolescent Self-Report Scale (CASS; Conners et al., 1997), the adolescent form of the Conners Rating Scales—Revised (Conners, 1997), is a self-report measure, available in two forms, that assesses behavioral difficulties in adolescents ages 12 through 17. The Long Form (CASS:L, 87 items) takes about 20 minutes to complete; the Short Form (CASS:S, 27 items) takes approximately 5 minutes. Both have been validated (Conners et al., 1997; Steer, Kumar, & Beck, 2001). The CASS can be used for screening, for treatment monitoring, as a research instrument, and as a clinical diagnostic aid.

Multidimensional Adolescent Functioning Scale

The Multidimensional Adolescent Functioning Scale (MAFS; Wardenaar et al., 2013) is a 23-item self-report questionnaire containing three subscales: general functioning, family-related functioning, and peer-related functioning. It was developed by clinical consensus and validated in a general population sample of 842 adolescents (mean age of 15.0 ± 0.4 years). A confirmatory factor analysis showed a good fit with the hypothesized three-factor structure. All scales showed adequate internal consistency (greatest lower bound: .75–.91) and sufficient discriminative ability (scale intercorrelations: rho = .15–.52). The general functioning subscale was the most strongly correlated with the General Health Questionnaire. The MAFS seems to be an easy-to-use instrument with good psychometric characteristics; it appears suitable for a broad range of future research applications, especially when a multidimensional and unbiased indication of normal adolescent functioning is required.

2. Capacity for Affective Range, Communication, and Understanding

The second capacity refers to an adolescent's ability to experience and regulate emotions, a key component of self-regulation. Emotion regulation is a complex process responsible for monitoring, evaluating, and modifying emotional reactions to respond to the ongoing demands of experience in a way that is appropriate for a particular situation and consistent with the expectations and norms of the cultural milieu. It may involve regulation of subjective experience (feelings), cognitive responses (thoughts), emotion-related physiological responses (e.g., heart rate or hormonal activity), or emotion-related behaviors (bodily actions or expressions). Emotion regulation includes the regulation of one's own feelings, as well as the regulation of responses to other people's feelings.

During adolescence, teens must learn how to cope with a much greater range of unfamiliar situations at a time when they are experiencing increasing demands on their physical, mental, and emotional resources. This challenge may lead to rapidly fluctuating emotions. At the same time, they show a marked increase in their capacities to regulate emotions, and decision making about emotion regulation becomes more complex, depending on multiple factors. The significance of interpersonal and social context increases for adolescents. For instance, they tend to display more emotions if they expect a sympathetic response from peers. Adolescents' focus on peer relationships creates a heightened sensitivity to the evaluation of others, which may increase the intensity of self-conscious emotions such as pride and shame. They also learn to manage emotions internally, taking ownership of their feelings and understanding that emotions do not reflect objective facts.

Clinical and research studies have shown that adolescents differ in the time course of emotional responses to stimuli. This temporal dynamic, also known as "affective chronometry," is partly genetically determined but is also influenced by social-emotional support provided by family, peers, or teachers. The ability to regulate emotions and manage emotional expression is important to establishing and maintaining positive social relationships, whether with peers or with potential romantic partners. Therefore, adolescents' ability to recognize, label, and regulate their own emotions, to identify emotions of others accurately, and to anticipate responses to emotional displays becomes key to successful development in this period and is an important preparation for transition into adulthood.

Rating Scale

5. Adolescents at this level can use, express, and understand a wide range of subtle emotions effectively. They can decipher and respond to most emotional signals flexibly and accurately, even when under stress (e.g., they comprehend safety vs. danger, approval vs. disapproval, acceptance vs. rejection, respect vs. disdain). Affective communication seems appropriate in quality and intensity to the situation experienced in the moment.
3. At this level, adolescents experience and communicate a constricted range of emotional states, and/or show some difficulty experiencing specific affects (e.g., anger). They decipher others' emotional states with difficulty, and may respond to emotional signals in a dysregulated and asynchronous way, especially when challenged or stressed. They may express and communicate emotions in a poor or inappropriate way out of proportion to the situation and social expectations.
1. These adolescents show mostly fragmented, chaotic emotional expressions, or communicate little emotion at all (they may be unable to display appropriate facial expression, modulate voice tone appropriately, or maintain body posture appropriate to the situation). They often distort the emotional signals of others (therefore feeling suspicious, mistreated, unloved, angry, etc.), and have difficulty identifying feelings and distinguishing them from bodily sensations of emotions. Affective responses may therefore be perceived by others as odd, inappropriate, or incongruous.

Most Relevant Assessment Tools

Where indicated below, measures (or their adult versions) are discussed in the "Most Relevant Assessment Tools" section for capacity 2 in Chapter 2 (pp. 85–88).

Thematic Apperception Test

The Thematic Apperception Test (TAT; Murray, 1943) is a performance-based measure intended to evaluate a person's patterns of thought, attitudes, observational capacities, and emotional responses to ambiguous test materials. Subjects are given a set of cards showing human figures in a variety of settings and situations and asked to tell the examiner a story about each that includes the event shown in the picture; what has led up to it; what the characters are feeling and thinking; and what will be the outcome. Although developed for adults, the TAT has been used extensively with adolescents (Archer, Maruish, Imhof, & Piotrowski 1991; Kroon, Goudena, & Rispens, 1998). Among numerous scoring methods, the Social Cognition and Object Relations Scales (SCORS) developed by Westen (1991) is among the best validated in adolescent samples, with good interrater reliabilities and discriminant validity (Westen, Ludolph, Block, Wixom, & Wiss, 1990).

Shedler–Westen Assessment Procedure for Adolescents, Version II

In the Shedler–Westen Assessment Procedure for Adolescents, Version II (SWAP-II-A; Westen, DeFife, Malone, & DiLallo, 2014), the capacity for affective experience, expression, and communication is covered by several items, which correspond to the

SWAP-200 items discussed for this capacity in adults in Chapter 2 (see that discussion for details).

Emotion Regulation Checklist

The Emotion Regulation Checklist (ERC; Shields & Cicchetti, 1997) is a survey measuring affective behaviors in school-age children. Two subscales are useful in assessing emotional competence: lability/negativity and emotion regulation. The lability/negativity subscale examines mood swings, angry reactivity, affective intensity, and dysregulated positive emotions. The emotion regulation subscale captures emotional understanding, empathy, and equanimity. Internal consistency for these subscales was .96 for lability/negativity and .83 for emotion regulation. The Emotion Regulation Q-Sort is related to the ERC; both measure emotion regulation. The Q-Sort measures reactivity, empathy, and socially appropriate expressions. Though somewhat cumbersome to administer, it is suitable for a wide age range and is useful for longitudinal research.

Behavioral and Emotional Rating Scale

The Behavioral and Emotional Rating Scale (BERS; Epstein & Sharma, 1998) is a standardized, norm-based measure that assesses emotional and behavioral strengths of adolescents. It is composed of 52 items that assess five areas of adolescents' strengths: interpersonal strength, family involvement, intrapersonal strength, school functioning, and affective strengths. It may be completed by any adult familiar with an adolescent. Adults are asked to rate each item on a 4-point scale (0 = not at all like the child; 1 = not like the child; 2 = like the child; 3 = very much like the child). Several studies document the BERS's strong psychometric properties, including internal consistency values around .95 (Epstein & Sharma, 1998), test–retest reliability values ranging from .87 to .93, discriminant validity ranging from .60 to .80, and convergent validity ranging from .55 to .80 (Epstein, Mooney, Ryser, & Pierce, 2004).

Multifactor Emotional Intelligence Scale, Adolescent Version

The Multifactor Emotional Intelligence Scale, Adolescent Version (MEIS-AV; Mayer, Salovey, & Caruso, 1997) is a competence-based measure assessing aspects of emotional intelligence in adolescents and young adults. The adolescent version consists of seven separate subtests that measure four areas: (1) identifying emotions, (2) using emotions, (3) understanding emotions, and (4) managing emotions. The validity and reliability of this self-report instrument have been positively assessed in several studies (Trinidad, Unger, Chou, Azen, & Johnson, 2004; Woitaszewski & Aalsma, 2004).

Bar-On Emotional Quotient Inventory, Youth Version

The Bar-On Emotional Quotient Inventory, Youth Version (EQ-i:YV; Bar-On & Parker, 2000), derived from the Bar-On model of the Emotional Quotient (EQ; Bar-On & Parker, 2000; Pfeffier, 2001), is a self-report inventory measuring emotional intelligence in adolescents and young adults. It yields scores on five primary dimensions (intrapersonal, interpersonal, adaptability, stress management, and general mood), as well as a total EQ score indicating the child's global emotional and social intelligence. It consists of 60 self-report questions rated on a 4-point Likert-type scale.

The EQ-i:YV was normed on a North American sample of 9,172 children and adolescents from 7 to 18 years old. It showed good internal consistency (Cronbach's alpha = .84) and good retest validity. Factorial structure closely matched major EQ scales. Construct validity was supported by the expected pattern of correlations with scales of the NEO Five-Factor Inventory in a sample of 102 adolescents and with several scales of internalizing and externalizing problem behavior (Bar-On & Parker, 2000). A short version of 30 items for time-limited situations is available.

Affect Intensity and Reactivity Scale for Youth

The Affect Intensity and Reactivity Scale for Youth (AIR-Y; Jones, Leen-Feldner, Olatunji, Reardon, & Hawks, 2009) is a 27-item self-report questionnaire measuring affect intensity according to Bryant, Yarnold, and Grimm's (1996) three-factorial conceptualization of affect intensity: positive affectivity (15 items; e.g., "When I feel happy it is a strong type of feeling"), negative intensity (6 items; e.g., "When I am nervous I get shaky all over"), and negative reactivity (6 items; e.g., "The sight of someone who is hurt badly affects me strongly"). It appears to be a psychometrically sound measure for assessing affect intensity in youths (Jones et al., 2009; Tsang, Wong, & Lo, 2012).

Affect Intensity Measure

The Affect Intensity Measure (AIM; Larsen & Diener, 1987) is a 40-item self-report measure (a 20-item short form is available) of how intensely a person tends to experience positive and negative affects. "Affect intensity" is defined as stable individual differences in the strength with which individuals experience their emotions, irrespective of their valence (Larsen, 2009). Each item inquires about an individual's typical emotional reaction to everyday life events. Six-point items are used to measure affect intensity, anchored by "never" and "always." Larsen and Diener (1987) presented evidence concerning internal consistency, test–retest reliability, and validity of the AIM.

Emotional Intensity Scale

The Emotional Intensity Scale (EIS; Bachorowski & Braaten, 1994) is a 12-item self-report questionnaire that assesses emotional intensity of positive and negative emotional states. It asks about emotional responses to relatively detailed or noncontextualized scenarios. Respondents endorse one of five choices for each item. A total score and subtest scores for positive and negative emotions is generated. The EIS focuses exclusively on intensity of emotions and not on emotional reactivity and duration.

Emotional Reactivity Scale

The Emotional Reactivity Scale (ERS; Nock, Wedig, Holmberg, & Hooley, 2008) is a 21-item self-report measure assessing three aspects of emotion reactivity in adolescents: sensitivity (8 items; e.g., "I tend to get emotional very easily"), arousal/intensity (10 items; e.g., "When I experience emotions, I feel them very strongly/intensely"), and persistence (3 items; e.g., "When I am angry/upset, it takes me much longer than most people to calm down"). Each is rated on a 0–4 scale (0 = not at all like me, 4 = completely like me). The ERS factors correspond to Linehan's (1993) dimensions of activation, intensity, and duration. Adolescents with mood, anxiety, or eating disorders report significantly higher reactivity than controls or those with substance use problems, suggesting that emotional reactivity is associated with specific forms of psychological disorders (Nock et al., 2008). The authors' factor analysis yielded only one factor, and the measure showed good internal reliability (Cronbach's alpha = .94). The sensitivity, arousal/intensity, and persistence subscales demonstrated strong internal consistency, suggesting that both the total ERS score and the subscales are reliable indicators of emotional reactivity. The ERS showed good correlations with compatible and unlike constructs, respectively. Although a useful global measure of emotional reactivity, the ERS is limited by not considering the valence of emotional stimuli; all items have a negative valence.

Levels of Emotional Awareness Scale

The Levels of Emotional Awareness Scale (LEAS; Lane, Quinlan, Schwartz, & Walker, 1990) is available in several languages and has been widely used in adolescent samples (Nandrino et al., 2013). See Chapter 2 for further discussion.

Positive and Negative Affect Scale—Expanded Version

The Positive and Negative Affect Scale—Expanded Version (PANAS-X; Watson & Clark, 1994) has been used with adolescents and young adults and has demonstrated acceptable psychometric properties and reliability (i.e., Cronbach's alphas > .80) for all subscale scores (Sheeber et al., 2009). Again, see Chapter 2 for further discussion.

Emotion Regulation Questionnaire for Children and Adolescents

The Emotion Regulation Questionnaire for Children and Adolescents (ERQ-CA; Gullone & Taffe, 2012), a modified version of the adult ERQ (Gross & John, 2003), is a 10-item self-report measure of habitual expressive suppression (4 items) and reappraisal (6 items) of emotion regulation strategies. Revisions included simplification of item wording (e.g., "I control my emotions by not expressing them" was reworded to "I control my feelings by not showing them"), and reduction of response scale length to 5 points (1 = strongly disagree to 5 = strongly agree). Range of scores for each scale was 6–30 for reappraisal and 4–20 for expressive suppression. It was evaluated with a sample of 827 participants between ages 10 and 18 years. Results indicated sound internal consistency and stability over a 12-month period. Sound construct and convergent validity were also demonstrated (Gullone & Taffe, 2012). The ERQ-CA appears a valid, age-appropriate measure for investigating two strategies of emotion regulation during childhood and adolescence.

Cognitive Emotion Regulation Questionnaire

The Cognitive Emotion Regulation Questionnaire (CERQ; Garnefski, Kraaij, & Spinhoven, 2001, 2002) is a 36-item questionnaire constructed to identify the cognitive coping strategies used after negative events or situations. In contrast to coping questionnaires that do not separate thoughts and actions, the CERQ refers exclusively to an individual's thoughts. It consists of nine conceptually distinct subscales of four items, each referring to what someone thinks after experiencing threatening or stressful life events: self-blame, other-blame, rumination, catastrophizing, putting into perspective, positive refocusing, positive reappraisal, acceptance, and planning. Individual cognitive emotion regulation strategies are measured on a 5-point Likert scale from 1 (almost never) to 5 (almost always); subscale scores are obtained by summing scores on items belonging to that subscale (ranging from 4 to 20). The CERQ has been used in several adolescent studies exploring relationships between cognitive emotion regulation strategies and maladjustment. Its psychometric properties were found to be good in adolescent samples: Principal component analyses provided empirical support to the allocation of items to subscales; internal consistencies ranged from .68 to .83, with most Cronbach's alphas exceeding .80. Test–retest correlations ranged between .40 and.60, reflecting moderately stable styles (D'Acremont & Van der Linden, 2007; Garnefski et al., 2001).

Difficulties in Emotion Regulation Scale

Psychometric properties of the Difficulties in Emotion Regulation Scale (DERS; Gratz & Roemer, 2004) were examined in a community sample of 428 adolescents ages 13–17 years (Weinberg & Klonsky, 2009). Exploratory factor analysis supported a six-factor structure consistent with the six subscales. Internal consistencies for subscales were good to excellent (Cronbach's alphas ranged from .76 to .89). Robust correlations were shown with psychological problems of emotion dysregulation, specifically depression, anxiety, suicidal ideation, eating disorders, and alcohol and drug use. General reliability and validity of the DERS as a measure of emotion dysregulation in adolescents is thus good (Neumann, van Lier, Gratz, & Koot, 2010). For a fuller discussion of this measure, see Chapter 2.

3. Capacity for Mentalization and Reflective Functioning

For a broader definition of the third capacity, see Chapter 2 (p. 77).

Although mentalizing capacities change across the lifespan, theoretical and empirical studies have focused on the early foundation of mentalizing in childhood and later assessment of mentalizing in adulthood; as a result, little is known about adolescent mentalization. Because of changes in cognitive development during this period, when adolescents are beginning to integrate mental state knowledge and are able to make explicit references using mental state language, adolescents are hypersensitive both to their own mental states and to those of persons around them. When this integration becomes too demanding, impairments in mentalizing can become apparent. This difficulty in integration may derive from the increased complexity of cognitions related to the mental states of self and others, underscored by insufficient language capacity that may be necessary for explicit mentalization. Adolescence is also marked by the earlier maturation of the limbic affective system, with the cognitive prefrontal cortex (the regions implicated in social cognition and mentalization) maturing later, well into the teens and early 20s. Therefore, cortical regions important to explicit mentalization are likely to be underdeveloped during adolescence, furthering the potential for difficulties in integrating mental state knowledge and language. Because impairments in this capacity may lay the foundation for present and future psychopathology, knowing more about the development of mentalization is important beyond a normative understanding.

Rating Scale

5. Adolescents at this level can reflect on their internal mental states (emotions, thoughts, desires, needs), and understand internal experiences behind others' behaviors, even when challenged or stressed. They are highly capable of distinguishing inner from outer reality, have insight into their own motives and behaviors, and can think about self and others in subtle and sophisticated ways. Emotions are experienced and represented in complex and nuanced ways, in the context of social-emotional relationships and behavior patterns. These internal representations are used to modulate and inhibit impulses and also allow the adaptive expression of impulses when appropriate.

3. Adolescents at this level are generally able to understand and reflect on their own behavior and reactions in terms of mental states, to infer others' internal experiences from behavioral and contextual cues, and to construct and use internal representations to experience a cohesive sense of self and others. Except in situations of conflict or emotional intensity, however, there may be a notable decline from usual levels of awareness and understanding of their own and others' mental states, with difficulties in perceiving and representing emotions as they are being experienced. There may be limited ability to elaborate on a feeling in its own right and a tendency toward external justifications; wishes and feelings may be expressed via acting out or somatization.

1. These adolescents are unable to infer, understand, reflect upon, and symbolize either others' mental states or their own affective experiences. They have severe difficulties distinguishing between internal and external reality and between mental and emotional processes and real-world interactions; it seems that what exists in the mind must exist "out there," and vice versa. They may misunderstand, misinterpret, or be confused by others' actions and generally cannot represent emotions as they are being experienced. They remain embedded in the emotion itself, unable to express it in words. Behaviors and responses are largely unmediated by understanding or language, resulting in an inability to regulate affective states effectively. When this capacity is extremely low, especially under stress, there is no sense of connection between internal experiences and self-observation; the self may be experienced as incoherent, depleted, or altogether absent.

Most Relevant Assessment Tools

Existing measures to assess mentalization in adolescents include, among others, advanced theory-of-mind measures, self-reports, vignette-based measures, and scales derived from projective assessments. In an effort to approximate the demands of everyday life on social cognition, advanced tests using video footage have been developed. Examples of each type are given below.

Reflective Function Questionnaire for Youths

The Reflective Function Questionnaire for Youths (RFQY; Sharp et al., 2009), a 46-item self-report measure, follows the principles of the Reflective Functioning Scale (RFS; Fonagy, Target, Steele, & Steele, 1998) of the Adult Attachment Interview (AAI). Originally developed for adults, it was adapted for adolescents by simplifying items to be more developmentally appropriate. Responses are scored on a 6-point Likert scale from "strongly disagree" to "strongly agree." It contains both polar items (e.g., "I'm often curious about the meaning behind others' actions") and central items, which elicit a balanced mentalizing perspective (e.g., "I can tell how someone is feeling by looking in their eyes"). A total score is derived by summing scores of all items, with higher scores indicating higher reflective function. The maximum optimal reflective function score is 12. The psychometric properties of the RFQY have been explored in a sample of 146 inpatient adolescents between ages 12 and 17 (Ha, Sharp, Ensink, Fonagy, & Cirino, 2013). Results show good internal consistency (Cronbach's alpha = .71) and convergent validity with other assessments of mentalization. Construct validity was supported by the high correlations between levels of borderline features and low reflective function. These findings support the reliability and construct validity of the RFQY as an adapted measure of social cognition (mentalization) for adolescents and as a useful tool for clinicians to assess mentalization in inpatient adolescents.

Reflective Functioning Questionnaire, Short Version

The Reflective Functioning Questionnaire (RFQ), short version (Badoud, Luyten, Fonagy, Eliez, & Debbané, 2015; Luyten, Fonagy, Lowyck, & Vermote, 2012) is a measure of reflective functioning, defined as the capacity to understand one's own and others' actions in terms of cognitive and affective mental states. Eight items are rated on a 7-point scale, from which three scores are derived. The two subscale scores measure how confident versus doubtful one is that actions are intrinsically intentional (i.e., driven by mental states); the total is a difference score that brings the two certainty and uncertainty polarities back to one continuum. Thus the total score is distributed between two polarities: Negative scores identify individuals with poor recognition that actions of self and other are driven by mind states; positive scores designate people who are strongly convinced that behaviors originate from intentions. Based on the factorial structure provided by its authors (Luyten et al., 2012), four raw data items need to be rescored beforehand in two ways—namely, either (1 = 0) (2 = 0) (3 = 0) (4 = 0) (5 = 1) (6 = 2), or (1 = 2) (2 = 1) (3 = 0) (4 = 0) (5 = 0) (6 = 0). The French version of the RFQ has shown good psychometric properties in French-speaking adolescents and young adults. Groups of 123 adolescents (61 females, M_{age} = 15.72 years, SD_{age} = 1.74) and 253 adults (168 females, M_{age} = 23.10, SD_{age} = 2.56) from a general population completed a battery assessing both clinical (alexithymia, borderline traits, internalizing–externalizing symptoms) and psychological (empathy, mindfulness, attachment) variables. Data showed measurement invariance of the original two-factor structure and satisfactory construct validity and reliability of the two subscales, supporting the RFQ as a useful tool for clinicians to assess mentalization in community adolescents and young adults.

Social Cognition and Object Relations Scale

The Social Cognition and Object Relations Scale (SCORS; Westen, Lohr, Silk, & Kerber, 1985, 1990) is a performance-based measure developed to analyze TAT narratives in terms of mentalization. It requires respondents to make up a story based on their personal response to a series of line drawings. Two subscales have been used to measure mentalization (Rothschild-Yakar, Levy-Schiff, Fridman-Balaban, Gur, & Stein,

2010): complexity of representations, measuring the degree of differentiation between perspectives of self and others and integration of positive and negative attributes of self and others; and understanding social causality, measuring the degree to which attributions to actions performed by people in the narrative are logical, accurate, and psychologically minded.

Mentalization Stories for Adolescents

Mentalization Stories for Adolescents, version 2 (MSA-v.2; Rutherford et al., 2012; Vrouva & Fonagy, 2009), a multiple-choice questionnaire derived from an initial open-ended version that was cumbersome and too dependent on written communication, was recently developed to measure mentalizing abilities across ages 12–18. It is a scenario-based test consisting of 21 items showing everyday situations of adolescence. Each involves a protagonist in a negative interaction or verbal exchange with another character. They are intended to suggest feelings of sadness, guilt, jealousy, disappointment, or shame in the protagonist, who then does or says something as a result. Participants must select from three responses the one best reflecting their own opinion of the reasons for the protagonist's choice. Reponses are scored according to level of mentalizing: accurate, excessive, or distorted attributions. Response values were selected with reference to the median score of a group of clinicians and researchers with expertise in mentalization, who independently rated answers on a 0–9 scale. A composite score is calculated by summing a participant's scores for each item, ranging from a possible minimum of 24.5 to a possible maximum of 136.5. There are no normalized scores available, but composite scores above the median of 81 may be considered in the upper range of mentalizing ability, while those below 81 may be considered in the low range. The MSA-v.2 was administered to groups of adolescents (N = 116) and young adults (N = 58). In both, females scored on average higher than males—a finding in agreement with studies suggesting a female advantage in social cognition. Older female adolescents did better. The group score of young adults was higher than that of the adolescents. Psychometric properties were robust and were replicated in a study of 49 predominantly disadvantaged, inner-city North American adolescents (Rutherford et al., 2012).

Adolescent Levels of Emotional Awareness Scale

The Adolescent Levels of Emotional Awareness Scale (ALEAS; Pratt, 2006), a scenario-based measure examining aspects of mentalization, assesses participants' ability to provide differentiated and complex descriptions of emotional experiences of self and others. In each situation, constructed to elicit emotional responses, examinees are asked to write how they would feel and how they think the other person would feel, which can be expressed with varying levels of complexity.

Movie for Assessment of Social Cognition

The Movie for Assessment of Social Cognition (MASC; Dziobek et al., 2006) uses short video-recorded scenes to assess implicit mentalizing in typical peer and romantic relationships. It uses classical social cognition concepts such as false belief, *faux pas*, metaphor, and sarcasm to display a broad range of mental states both verbally and nonverbally. The storyline involves four characters getting together, preparing dinner, and playing a board game. Adolescents are presented with 46 video clips, and at the end of each scene are asked to imagine what the characters thought or felt. Answers are presented in a multiple-choice format with four response options. Each is coded as hypermentalizing (e.g., "Angry, her friend forgot she doesn't like sardines"), undermentalizing (e.g., "Surprised, she didn't expect sardines"), no mentalizing (e.g., "Sardines are salty and slippery"), or accurate mentalizing (e.g., "Repelled, she doesn't like sardines"). A total mentalizing score is derived from summing the total correct responses. Additionally, three separate scales are computed for the degree of incorrect mentalization, including hypermentalizing, undermentalizing, and no mentalizing, by summing total responses for each subscale. Psychometric properties have been found to be adequate (Dziobek et al., 2006); the MASC is sensitive in discriminating patients with borderline personality disorder (BPD) from individuals without BPD (Preißler, Dziobek, Ritter, Heekeren, & Roepke, 2010; Sharp et al., 2011).

Basic Empathy Scale

The Basic Empathy Scale (BES; Jolliffe & Farrington, 2006), a 20-item self-report measure assessing multidimensional aspects of empathic responsiveness in adolescence, has two subscales: affective empathy (11 items), measuring congruence with another person's emotions, and cognitive empathy (9 items), measuring ability to understand another's emotions. Each item asks for degree of agreement on a 5-point, Likert-type scale from 1 (strongly disagree) to 5 (strongly agree). Validation was conducted on a sample of 720 British 15-year-olds (Jolliffe & Farrington, 2006). The BES showed sufficient construct validity (significant differences in expected direction and magnitude between males and females) and good convergent and divergent validity. It can be considered a valid tool for measuring empathic responsiveness in adolescents.

Meta-Cognitions Questionnaire—Adolescent

The Meta-Cognitions Questionnaire—Adolescent (MCQ-A; Cartwright-Hatton et al., 2004) is a 30-item scale measuring metacognitive beliefs in adolescents, adapted from the MCQ for adults (Cartwright-Hatton & Wells, 1997). "Metacognition" refers to beliefs about thinking and worry processes. The MCQ-A items are rated on a 4-point Likert scale from "do not agree" to "agree very much." Five categories of meta-cognition are evaluated via five subscales: (1) positive beliefs about worry (e.g., "I need to worry in order to work well"); (2) beliefs about uncontrollability of thoughts and its dangers (e.g., "When I start worrying, I cannot stop"); (3) cognitive confidence (e.g., "I have a poor memory"); (4) beliefs about superstition, punishment, and responsibility (e.g., "I will be punished for not controlling certain thoughts"); and (5) cognitive self-consciousness (e.g., "I monitor my thoughts"). Item content and scoring are very close to those of the adult version, albeit the language was sometimes slightly modified for use with younger individuals. The MCQ-A was validated in a sample of 177 schoolchildren ages 13 through 17, together with other self-report measures of emotional well-being. Factor analysis supports a five-factor solution, as in the adult version. Internal consistency and validity indices are good, suggesting that the MCQ-A is a reliable and valid instrument for measuring metacognitive beliefs in adolescents.

4. Capacity for Differentiation and Integration (Identity)

For a broader definition of the fourth capacity, see Chapter 2 (p. 77).

A core task of adolescence is to develop a coherent and stable sense of identity. The term "identity" can refer to many phenomena, including people's goals, values, beliefs, group memberships, and roles in society. In psychological terms, however, identity comprises self-image, self-esteem, and individuality, as well as self-reflection and awareness of self. It implies both continuity ("subjective self") and coherence of personal experience ("definitory self"). The construction of identity is a process that involves the ego's ability to synthesize and integrate earlier identifications into a new form, uniquely one's own, that progressively coalesces into a realistic, essentially positive, and increasingly integrated self-definition. This process is supported by the advent of formal operational thought and abstract thinking, permitting adolescents to imagine what the future could be and allowing them to consider future "possible identities" that they might wish to become (or to avoid becoming). Assessing this feeling of agency is an important aspect of assessing identity in adolescence.

A paradox of identity is that it occurs via identifications with significant others (primarily with parents and other individuals during one's biographical experiences and also with "groups" as they are perceived). Identification with social roles, such as those in intimate relationships, can be considered as a driving force behind personality maturation and identity formation. Observing an adolescent's relational capacities gives important information on his or her identity status.

Adolescents with high levels of this capacity show a stability of identity-giving goals, talents, commitments, roles, and relationships, and have good and stable access to emotions. They show a clear self-definition as a result of self-reflective awareness, accompanied by consistency in self-images, autonomy/ego strength, and differentiated mental representations. In contrast, adolescents with low levels of this capacity lack a clear self-related perspective, and they experience no feelings of belonging and affiliation. They lack access to emotional levels of reality and mistrust the durability of positive emotions. They have poor access to cognitions and motives, accompanied by superficial and diffuse mental representations. They may experience distress, may have difficulties in maintaining healthy relationships with others, and may engage in self-destructive behaviors.

The following is a developmental guideline, based on James Marcia's (1966) theory of ego identity status, to age-expected attainments for adolescents and young adults in the capacity for identity formation.

(text resumes on page 281)

Developmental Guideline: Capacity for Identity Formation in Adolescence/Young Adulthood

Status	Description
	Early adolescence (ages 12–14)
Identity diffusion	The adolescent has not yet made a commitment to a specific developmental task and may or may not have explored alternatives in this domain. Adolescents at this stage show low levels of autonomy, self-esteem, and identity. They have a low sense of personal integration and difficulties adapting to new situations. They appear to be most influenced by peer pressure toward conformity and are generally self-focused. Cognitively, they rely on intuitive or dependent styles of decision making or show an absence of systematic approaches to solving problems. They demonstrate low levels of moral reasoning. They have no close relationships or have relationships focused on superficial issues.
	Middle adolescence (ages 15–16)
Foreclosure	The adolescent has not yet engaged in identity experimentation and has established an identity based on the choices or values of others. Adolescents at this stage show high levels of conformity, and their aspirations change rapidly. They rely on dependent strategies for decision making and are not generally open to new experiences. They have an external locus of control and are especially oriented toward the more distant future. Cognitively, adolescents at this stage have difficulties integrating ideas and thinking analytically. They may make errors in judgment because of reduced attention. They tend to show a preconventional or conventional level of moral reasoning. They can be oriented toward others' needs only in their ability to care. Interpersonally, they are most likely to be stereotyped in their styles of intimacy (more concerned with superficial features of a relationship) with friends sharing this similar ego identity status.
	Late adolescence (ages 17–19)
Moratorium	Adolescents at this stage are exploring various choices, but have not yet made a clear commitment to any. Their active exploration thus may be anxiety-filled. They may use denial, projection, and identification to keep general anxieties at bay. The more self-exploration they have engaged in, the more prepared they are to undertake tasks in a self-directed manner, without looking to others for reassurance and emotional support. They may regress adaptively. Cognitively, they show an analytic style and are able to integrate and analyze information from several perspectives. Interpersonally, they are most frequently in a pre-intimate state. They establish close friendship relationships characterized by respect for others' integrity, openness, and nondefensiveness, but they do not yet commit to a partner.
	Young adulthood (ages 20+)
Identity achievement	Adolescents and youth at this stage have attained a coherent and committed identity based on personal decisions and prior commitments. They show high levels of achievement motivation and self-esteem, low use of immature defense mechanisms, and internal locus of control. In terms of cognitive processes, they can function well under stress and use planned, rational, and logical decision-making strategies. They demonstrate a high level of moral reasoning about issues of both justice and care. Interpersonally, they demonstrate high levels of intimacy. They are able to develop mutual interpersonal relationships with both close friends and a partner, and they are genuinely interested in others.

Rating Scale

5. Adolescents at this level can appreciate the separateness and relatedness of different affect states, motives, and wishes of self and others, even when they are nuanced and ambiguous. They can organize varieties of experience and social-emotional demands over time and across contexts with contrasting role demands. They have reliable access to emotions and trust the stability of their affects. They show clear self-definition in terms of goals, commitments, and roles, accompanied by consistency in self-images, autonomy, and self-agency. They can engage in intimate relationships and interact spontaneously and flexibly with an increasingly complex and demanding environment.
3. Adolescents at this level can differentiate and integrate experience, but with some constriction and oversimplification, especially under stress. Intense emotions can lead to temporary fragmentation or polarization (all-or-nothing extremes) of internal experience. At this level, capacities for differentiation and integration are limited to a few realms (e.g., superficial relationships). Challenges outside these areas often lead to diminished functioning and impaired coping.
1. Internal experience is fragmented or rigidly compartmentalized and oversimplified most of the time; in extreme cases, internal experience may be detached from external context, and representations of self and other may be confused. Adolescents at this level lack a self-related perspective and a sense of belonging and affiliation. They lack access to emotional levels of reality and mistrust the durability of positive emotions. They have little ability to move through a range of emotional states either autonomously or with others without intense anxiety (often expressed as guilt or shame), acting out, or reliance on maladaptive defenses (self-soothing strategies), with concomitant impairment in reality testing (e.g., severe splitting and dissociation).

Most Relevant Assessment Tools

Where indicated below, measures (or their adult versions) are discussed in the "Most Relevant Assessment Tools" section for capacity 4 in Chapter 2 (pp. 92–94).

Assessment of Identity Development in Adolescence

The Assessment of Identity Development in Adolescence (AIDA; Goth, Foelsch, Schlüter-Müller, & Schmeck, 2012b), a self-report questionnaire assessing pathological identity development in adolescents ages 12–18, integrates identity constructs from psychodynamic and social-cognitive theories. The model distinguishes two fundamental dimensions, continuity and coherence. The AIDA was developed by a Swiss–German–U.S. research group, with special attention to culture-independent formulations and generic application of constructs (Goth et al., 2012b). It consists of 58 five-step format items that give a total score ranging from identity integration to identity diffusion, as well as two subscales, discontinuity and incoherence. Psychometric properties were explored in a mixed sample of 305 students, 52 adolescent psychiatric inpatients, and 52 adolescent outpatients with personality or other mental disorders (Goth et al., 2012a). There was excellent internal consistency for the total score (Cronbach's alpha = .94) and two scales (discontinuity = .86; incoherence

= .92). High levels of discontinuity and incoherence were associated with low levels of self-directedness, indicating maladaptive personality functioning. Both scales differentiated significantly between patients with personality disorders and controls, with remarkable effect sizes (*d*) of 2.17 and 1.94 standard deviations. An unrestricted exploratory factor analysis on the item level showed a joint higher-order factor, identity integration, explaining 24.3% of the variance and thus supporting test construction. Although it requires further validation, the AIDA seems a reliable and valid instrument that may provide insight into relevant aspects of adolescent identity development (Jung, Pick, Schlüter-Müller, Schmeck, & Goth, 2013; Kassin, De Castro, Arango, & Goth, 2013).

Social Cognition and Object Relations Scale—Global Rating Method

The Social Cognition and Object Relations Scale—Global Rating Method (SCORS-G; Stein, Hilsenroth, Slavin-Mulford, & Pinsker, 2011; Westen, 1985) is discussed more fully in Chapter 2. Two subscales (identity and coherence of self and complexity of representation of people) are useful for evaluating the capacity for differentiation and integration (identity). The SCORS-G reliably differentiates personality-disordered adolescents from normal adolescents (DeFife, Goldberg, & Westen, 2015) and incrementally improves prediction of therapy engagement and global functioning for adolescents beyond what Global Assessment of Functioning scores account for (Haggerty et al., 2015).

Identity Disturbance Questionnaire for Adolescents

The Identity Disturbance Questionnaire for Adolescents (IDQ-A; Westen, Betan, & DeFife, 2011), a 35-item adaptation of the IDQ for adults (Wilkinson-Ryan & Westen, 2000), assesses a range of potential manifestations of identity disturbance among adolescents on a 7-point scale (1 = not true at all, 4 = somewhat true, 7 = very true). The adolescent and adult forms are similar, but several items were revised to reflect age-appropriate identity issues for adolescents. Items in both versions were based on an extensive review of the clinical, theoretical, and empirical literatures on identity. For example, based on Erikson's (1968) concept of a negative identity, there are items assessing the extent to which an adolescent defines him- or herself in terms of a stigmatized group, negative label, or identity as "bad." Multiple items capture commitment to roles, affiliations, values, goals, and aspirations. Items representing subjective feelings and thoughts about identity disturbance were based on clinical literature and observation (e.g., "Tends to feel like a 'false self,' whose social persona does not match his/her inner experience," "Subjectively feels as [if] s/he is a different person depending on who s/he is with"). The IDQ-A addresses phenomena more readily observed by a clinically trained observer (e.g., "Holds beliefs that are grossly inconsistent with one another and seems unconcerned by contradictions," "Patient has trouble telling life story; narrative accounts have large gaps or inconsistencies"). Questions are written in straightforward language with minimal jargon. The IDQ-A was validated by asking a national random sample of 139 experienced psychiatrists and clinical psychologists to complete a battery of instruments on a randomly selected adolescent patient in their care. Of the 35 IDQ-A items, 33 significantly discriminated patients with or without a DSM-IV identity disturbance criterion according to clinicians' ratings. Factor analysis yielded four clinically and conceptually coherent factors that resembled dimensions previously identified in adults: lack of normative commitment, role absorption, painful incoherence, and lack of consistency.

Depressive Experiences Questionnaire—Adolescent Version

The Depressive Experiences Questionnaire—Adolescent Version (DEQ-A; Blatt, D'Afflitti, & Quinlan, 1976; Blatt, Schaffer, Bers, & Quinlan, 1992), a 66-item self-report scale, assesses the introjective and anaclitic personality dimensions hypothesized by Blatt and Zuroff (1992), who posit that the development of individual personality is structured around two fundamental and mutually interacting tasks: the establishment of satisfying interpersonal relationships and the achievement of a positive and cohesive sense of self. The specific configurations of these axes have important implications for self- and other-representations, for how individuals cope with external events, and for vulnerabilities to specific types of psychopathology. Derived from the adult version, items of the DEQ-A were rephrased for younger individuals (Blatt et al., 1992). Initial factor analyses have identified two principal factors: internally directed items, reflecting concerns about self-identity (self-criticism); and externally directed items, pointing to disturbances in interpersonal relationships (dependency). Scales derived from these factors have shown high internal consistency and substantial test–retest reliability in adolescents (Blatt et al., 1992). Subsequent theoretical developments and factor analyses have suggested that different levels can be identified, each following a trajectory from immature to more mature forms of relatedness and self-definition. The DEQ-A appears to measure adaptive and maladaptive dimensions of interpersonal relatedness (McBride, Zuroff, Bacchiochi, & Bagby, 2006), as well as adaptive and maladaptive dimensions of self-definition (Blatt, 2004). Fichman, Koestner, and Zuroff (1994) shortened the original DEQ-A by selecting eight statements with the highest loading on the dependency and self-criticism factors. Shahar and Priel (2003) found adequate reliability for both scales (.70, .82) of this short form of the DEQ-A.

Shedler–Westen Assessment Procedure for Adolescents, Version II

In the SWAP-II-A (Westen, DeFife, Malone, & DiLallo, 2014), identity is covered by several items, which correspond to the SWAP-200 items discussed for this capacity in adults in Chapter 2 (see that discussion for details).

5. Capacity for Relationships and Intimacy

For a broader definition of the fifth capacity, see Chapter 2 (p. 78).

The capacity to engage in stable, mutually satisfying relationships is dependent on the quality of attachment patterns and on coherence of the internal working models elaborated during development. An organized attachment pattern fosters healthy interpersonal relatedness and allows accepting support from and providing support to others. Adolescents with high levels of this capacity experience relationships as a support of their emerging identity. Individuation and relatedness are not mutually exclusive but are two complementary dimensions in adolescent development.

This capacity reflects an adolescent's ability to adjust interpersonal distance and closeness in response to specific relationships. An adolescent who is functioning well in this capacity can flexibly adjust interpersonal behaviors and attitudes (closeness, intimacy), depending on interpersonal and intrapersonal demands and circumstances (family relationships, friendships, romantic relationships). This may include the adolescent's emerging sexuality. The integration of sexuality is a specific developmental task of adolescence. A positive capacity for relationships and intimacy allows the adolescent's exploration of sexuality and the blend of sexuality with emotional intimacy.

The following is a developmental guideline to age-expected attainments for adolescents in the capacity for relationships and intimacy.

Developmental Guideline: Capacity for Relationships and Intimacy in Adolescence

Description
Early adolescence (ages 12–14)
At this stage, adolescents show a greater interest in privacy. Relational emotions are frequent; shyness, blushing, and modesty are common. Relationships are mainly superficial, but girls tend to be ahead of boys in more intimate connections. Experimentation with the body (including masturbation) appears, along with worries about being normal.
Middle adolescence (ages 15–16)
At this stage, adolescents show feelings of both tenderness and fear toward their sexual objects. They have concerns about sexual attractiveness and frequently change relationships. Heterosexual adolescents may be anxious about possible homosexuality; homosexual adolescents may feel marginalized and estranged. At these ages, adolescents begin to show feelings of love and passion, but tend to be stereotyped in their styles of intimacy (they may be more concerned with superficial features of a relationship).
Late adolescence (ages 17–19)
At this stage, adolescents are concerned with serious relationships. They begin to show a clear sexual identity and are open to tender and sensual love. They are able to develop mutual interpersonal relationships with close friends and partners, and they are genuinely interested in others.

Rating Scale

5. Adolescents at this level show an age-appropriate capacity for intimacy, caring, and empathy, even when feelings are strong or under stress, in a variety of expectable contexts (in family settings, with peers, with objects of romantic interest). They show the desire and capacity to seek closeness in relationships and can flexibly adjust to changing social-emotional demands, both interpersonally and intrapersonally. Sexuality is associated with emotional intimacy. An adolescent may provide support to others and accept support from others on the basis of situational needs.

3. At this level, adolescents show an age-appropriate capacity for intimacy, caring, and empathy, but the capacity is disrupted by strong emotions such as anger, shame, or separation anxiety. In such situations, they may withdraw or act out; conversely, they may become overly needy, clingy, and dependent. Sexuality may be dissociated from emotional intimacy. They find it difficult to adjust to situational demands and have some deficits in either the ability to accept support from others or the ability to provide others with support.

1. These adolescents show a superficial, need-oriented capacity for intimacy and caring; relationships lack mutuality and empathy. They are indifferent to the needs of others and appear withdrawn, socially isolated, and detached. Interactions tend to be one-way, lacking in mutuality, and characterized by marked deficits in the ability to support others or to accept support from others.

Most Relevant Assessment Tools

Where indicated below, measures (or their adult versions) are discussed in the "Most Relevant Assessment Tools" section for capacity 5 in Chapter 2 (pp. 96–98).

Network of Relationships Inventory

The Network of Relationships Inventory (NRI; Furman & Buhrmester, 1985), a widely used measure for assessing dyadic relationships with parents, siblings, teachers, or friends, explores how frequently different relationships are used to fulfill the functions of three behavioral systems—attachment, caregiving, and affiliation. It has several three-item subscales assessing relationship characteristics, rated on a 5-point Likert scale (1 = a little or not at all; 5 = more is not possible). Two overall scores can be calculated: social support (companionship, instrumental aid, intimacy, nurturance, affection, admiration, satisfaction, support, reliable alliance) and negative interchanges (conflict, antagonism, criticism, dominance, punishment). Psychometric analyses reported by the authors (Furman & Buhrmester, 1985) and by others (Spilt, Van Lier, Branje, Meeus, & Koot, 2014) show satisfactory internal consistency coefficients of the scale scores (Cronbach's alpha = .80).

Experiences in Close Relationships—Revised

The Experiences in Close Relationships—Revised (ECR-R) inventory (Fraley, Waller, & Brennan, 2000; see the discussion of the ECR in Chapter 2) has shown good psychometric properties in adolescent samples (Feddern Donbaek & Elklit, 2014). Wilkinson (2011) provided a shortened, modified version of the instrument (ECR-R-GSF) to assess general relationship attachment anxiety and avoidance in adolescents. Ten items from the anxiety scale and 10 items from the avoidance scale were selected as suitable for adolescents and amenable to word alteration to suit a general rather than romantic partner attachment. Validation of the ECR-R-GSF was explored on a sample of 1,187 individuals between ages 11 and 22. Both anxiety and avoidance items produced reliable scales (Cronbach's alpha = .88 for both) and were weakly correlated (r = .39), thus supporting the application of the ECR-R-GSF to assessing relationship-specific adolescent attachment structures.

Inventory of Interpersonal Problems—Circumplex—Short Form

The Inventory of Interpersonal Problems—Circumplex—Short Form (IIP-C-SF; Soldz, Budman, Demby, & Merry, 1995), a 32-item self-report measure of problematic aspects of relational functioning, is a shorter version of the original 64-item inventory (IIP-C; Horowitz, Alden, Wiggins, & Pincus, 2000; see discussion in Chapter 2). Like the original, the IIP-C-SF provides eight subscales (domineering, vindictive, cold, socially avoidant, nonassertive, exploitable, overly nurturant, intrusive), with items rated from 0 (not at all) to 4 (extremely). Psychometric properties have been validated in two samples of college students (mean age of 18), suggesting that the IIP-C-SF can be effectively used with adolescents and young adults.

Interview of Personality Organization Processes in Adolescence

The Interview of Personality Organization Processes in Adolescence (IPOP-A; Ammaniti, Fontana, Kernberg, Clarkin, & Clarkin, 2011) is a semistructured interview assessing personality organization as defined in Kernberg's theory of personality development and disorder (Kernberg, 1998; Kernberg, Weiner, & Bardenstein, 2000). It was created to help clinicians address emerging personality patterns, taking into account adolescents' difficulties and resources (Ammaniti, Fontana, & Nicolais, 2015). The IPOP-A is a reliable, validated 1-hour interview for adolescents ages 13–21 that assesses key dimensions of identity formation, quality of object relations, affect regulation, and risky behaviors (Ammaniti et al., 2012). The current version has 41 items and is available in several languages. It may be used for both clinical assessment and research. Accordingly, the scoring system is divided into research and clinical forms. The research system is a detailed, item-per-item coding procedure, while the clinical system guides therapists in scoring each domain. The validation process evidences high interrater reliability; convergent validity with self-report questionnaires such as the Millon Adolescent Clinical Inventory (Millon, Millon, & Davies, 1993) and the DERS (Gratz & Roemer, 2004); and construct validity, as the exploratory factor analysis shows five factors coherent with the underlying model: (1) quality of object relation inside the family, (2) identity, (3) commitment, (4) quality of object relation with peers and romantic mates, and (5) affect regulation.

Shedler–Westen Assessment Procedure for Adolescents, Version II

In the SWAP-II-A (Westen, DeFife, Malone, & DiLallo, 2014), relationships and intimacy are covered by several items (see the discussion of the SWAP-200 in Chapter 2 for details).

Social Cognition and Object Relations Scale—Global Rating Method

In the SCORS-G (Stein, Hilsenroth, Slavin-Mulford, & Pinsker, 2011; Westen, 1985), the scale for affective quality of representations is particularly pertinent to adolescents. It can be used to code affective elements of respondent narratives related to affective communication. It may also be useful in providing insights about affective experiences and expression. See Chapter 2 for further discussion.

6. Capacity for Self-Esteem Regulation and Quality of Internal Experience

The sixth capacity involves the degree to which an adolescent has a sense of internal control, self-efficacy, and agency. Self-esteem reflects the adolescent's overall emotional evaluation of his or her own worth. It is a judgment of self as well as an attitude toward the self. It includes evaluation of one's actual self in comparison to one's desired self and is closely associated with self-consciousness.

Adolescents have varying levels of self-esteem, influenced by factors such as gender, ethnicity, and socioeconomic status. While their self-esteem can fluctuate, studies have found that self-esteem stabilizes or even increases during middle and late adolescence and into early adulthood. Individuals with high self-esteem in childhood are likely to be adolescents with high self-esteem. Level of self-esteem is related to quality of primary relationships with attuned caregivers who convey to infants that they are worthwhile people, that their lives are meaningful, and that they will be valued by others. Positive self-esteem allows an adolescent to deal with a diversity of tasks and challenges, including novel situations. Low self-esteem may diminish adaptation and resilience and is associated with problems including depression, anorexia nervosa, delinquency, self-harm, and even suicide. Although causal direction is unclear, self-esteem is related to school performance and delinquency.

Rating Scale

5. At this level, adolescents show an appropriate capacity to maintain a stable sense of well-being, confidence, and realistic self-esteem in varying contexts and even under stress. Self-esteem is balanced with and appropriate to internal and external situations, and adolescents have an adequate level of confidence in their capacity to deal with multiple tasks and challenges, including novel situations. These characteristics positively influence the way in which an adolescent thinks, feels, and relates to others and the larger world.
3. Adolescents' sense of well-being, confidence, vitality, and self-esteem is generally adequate at this level, but may be easily disrupted by strong emotions and stressful situations. Feelings of vulnerability and inadequacy may result in diminished confidence in their capacity to deal with certain tasks (school or leisure activities), to achieve desired ends, or to act effectively in the world.
1. These adolescents have feelings of emptiness, incompleteness, or excessive self-preoccupation. Self-esteem is unstable and may fluctuate rapidly between extremes. There may be a discrepancy between internal experience and external behavior (e.g., there may be overcompensation for underlying feelings of vulnerability) and a discrepancy between implicit and explicit self-esteem; both discrepancies are associated with diminished adaptation and resilience.

Most Relevant Assessment Tools

Where indicated below, measures (or their adult versions) are discussed in the "Most Relevant Assessment Tools" section for capacity 6 in Chapter 2 (pp. 99–100).

Shedler–Westen Assessment Procedure for Adolescents, Version II

In the SWAP-II-A (Westen, Shedler, Durrett, Glass, & Martens, 2003), the capacity for self-esteem regulation and quality of internal experience is covered by several items (see the discussion of the SWAP-200 in Chapter 2 for details).

Rosenberg Self-Esteem Scale

The Rosenberg Self-Esteem Scale (RSES; Rosenberg, 1965) has demonstrated good reliability and validity across various healthy and nonhealthy adolescent samples (Isomaa, Väänänen, Fröjd, Kaltiala-Heino, & Marttunen, 2013). See Chapter 2 for further discussion of the RSES.

Scales of Psychological Capacities

Greenfield and colleagues (2013) have recently adapted the Scales of Psychological Capacities (SPC; Huber, Brandl, & Klug, 2004; see Chapter 2 for discussion) to use in adolescence (Ad-SPC) by rewording the questions for adolescents and adding two potentially critical capacities: (1) tolerance of ambivalence and (2) pursuit of self-interest. Given the high valence of sexuality in adolescence, the sequence on regulation of sexual experience was moved to the end to minimize the adverse impact of questions on the alliance. High interrater reliability was achieved for individual scale items. Construct validity was determined by using Pearson's correlations between multiple items and coadministered validated measures of psychopathology. These preliminary psychometric properties support the Ad-SPC's applicability in adolescent psychotherapy.

Self-Perception Profile for Adolescents

The Self-Perception Profile for Adolescents (SPPA; Harter, 1988), one of the better-known self-concept questionnaires, is one of only a few specific to adolescents. Constructed primarily for research purposes, it also has applications to educational and clinical areas. This self-report scale taps how adolescents assess their "competence" or "adequacy" in different areas and how they evaluate their overall self-worth. It contains 45 items, eight domain-specific subscales, and one self-esteem subscale providing measures of global and specific self-esteem and generating individual profiles. The original SPPA had an idiosyncratic and time-consuming item format describing two adolescents with opposite characteristics on each item. Wichstrøm (1995) revised the original for a large national representative sample of 11,315 Norwegian adolescents, using only one description on each item. This version has substantially better for reliability, convergent validity, and factorial validity than the original, with similar discriminant validity and social desirability. This revised version is thus well suited for assessing self-esteem in adolescents (Rudasill & Callahan, 2008).

Self-Description Questionnaire–II

The Self-Description Questionnaire–II (SDQ-II; Marsh, 1992; Marsh, Ellis, Parada, Richards, & Heubeck, 2005) is a self-report instrument based on the Shavelson, Hubner, and Stanton (1976) multidimensional self-concept model, measuring areas of self-concept in adolescence. It can be used across clinical and research settings to describe the structure of the self in adolescents ages 12–18. It focuses on three components of academic self-concept (math, verbal, and general school), seven components of nonacademic self-concepts (physical abilities, physical appearance, parent relations, opposite-sex relations, same-sex relations, honesty–trustworthiness, and emotional stability), and a global component (general self). Each scale is based on responses to 4–5 items (a total of 51 items); items are simple declarative sentences to which participants respond on a 6-point Likert scale from 1 (false) to 6 (true). Since its development in Australia (Marsh, 1992), reliability evidence (based on internal consistency coefficients) and validity evidence (based on internal structure) have been examined in different languages, including American English (Marsh, Plucker, & Stocking, 2001), Chinese (Marsh, Hau, & Kong, 2002), French (Guerin, Marsh, & Famose, 2003), Japanese (Nishikawa, Norlander, Fransson, & Sundbom, 2007), and Swedish (Nishikawa et al., 2007). The SDQ-II generalizes well to special populations (e.g., gifted and talented; Marsh et al., 2001). In a recent study of a sample of 903 French-speaking adolescents (mean age = 12.6 years), correlations between the 11 SDQ-II factors and the 7 mental health problems of the Youth Self-Report (YSR) showed a highly differentiated multivariate pattern of relations (from .11 to –.83; mean r = –.35), thus supporting a multidimensional perspective of self-concept in adolescence (Marsh, Parada, & Ayotte, 2004).

Multidimensional Self-Esteem Inventory

The Multidimensional Self-Esteem Inventory (MSEI; O'Brien & Epstein, 1998) is a 116-item self-report measure of individuals' perception of their overall social value. Respondents rate items on a 5-point scale according to the degree or frequency with which they feel each item applies to them. There are 10 subscales and a validity scale measuring the tendency to make oneself look better through socially desirable answers. Internal consistency reliability has been examined for each subscale, with Cronbach's alphas from .80 to .90. The stability of subscales has also been examined by test–retest correlations over a 1-month interval. Studies have supported convergent and discriminant validity by comparing MSEI subscale scores with other personality tests, measures of academic achievement, and other indices. The MSEI offers *T* scores based on a community sample of adolescents.

Multidimensional Self-Esteem Questionnaire

The Multidimensional Self-Esteem Questionnaire (SEQ; DuBois, Felner, Brand, Phillips, & Lease, 1996) is a 42-item self-report instrument assessing the multiple dimensions of adolescents' self-esteem, defined as the evaluation of one's actual self in comparison to one's desired self or the degree of liking for and satisfaction with the self. Each item asks about the extent of satisfaction or dissatisfaction with a described aspect of self (e.g., "I do as well on tests in school as I want to," "I like my body just the way it is"). Items are rated on a 4-point scale from "strongly disagree" to "strongly agree." The measure yields scores of self-evaluation pertaining to five separate life domains: peer relations, school achievement, family, body image, and sports/athletics. A separate, 8-item global self-esteem scale measures overall perceptions of self-worth (e.g., "I am happy with myself as a person"). The SEQ was developed and validated with a large (N = 1,800) and demographically diverse sample of physically healthy youth. It has demonstrated strong internal consistencies and test–retest reliabilities of subscales, plus factorial validity of the underlying multidimensional, hierarchical structure (DuBois et al., 1996; DuBois, Tevendale, Burk-Braxton, Swenson, & Hardesty, 2000).

7. Capacity for Impulse Control and Regulation

For a broader definition of the seventh capacity, see Chapter 2 (p. 78).

Accumulating evidence attests to a decrease in impulsivity and increase in self-regulation from childhood into adulthood, with a significant change during adolescence. Neuroimaging data suggest that this trend is associated with maturation of brain regions underscoring inhibitory control (mainly the orbitofrontal cortex and the anterior cingulate cortex in the right hemisphere). Evidence also points, however, to an increase in risk-taking behaviors that peaks in adolescence and then decreases during young adulthood. This pattern may be explained by dissociation between the relatively slow, linear development of top-down control systems during adolescence and the nonlinear development of the reward system, which is often hyperresponsive to rewards in adolescence. This combination of disproportionately activated reward circuitry and an underdeveloped and overtaxed neural control system may explain why adolescents appear to place emphasis on the potentially rewarding aspects of risk taking while showing a reduced capacity for regulatory control. It also implies that decision making in adolescence may be particularly modulated by emotional and social factors (e.g., when adolescents are with peers or in other affectively charged contexts).

Emotional and cognitive regulation is directly related to primary relationships during childhood, which help build a child's capacity for self-regulation. Traumatic experiences, neglect, or unstable infant–caregiver relationships may negatively influence the development of this capacity in adolescence, resulting in an excessive dependence on external supports. When rating the capacity for impulse control and regulation, a clinician should attend to an adolescent's overall developmental level (early, middle, or late adolescence) and the distal and proximal social-emotional factors that may influence this capacity (environmental factors, peer influence, stress situations, powerful emotional rewards).

Rating Scale

5. Adolescents at this level can express impulses in a manner appropriate to the situation at hand and to their cultural milieu. Impulse control is flexible and effective, so that urges and affects are expressed in a modulated and adaptive manner and in ways that strengthen interpersonal ties.

3. These adolescents are somewhat able to control and regulate impulses, but may have difficulties in certain affect- and conflict-laden situations (e.g., with a romantic partner, with a teacher, with peers, or when faced with frustration). Adolescents at this level may show a characteristic pattern of overcontrol (rigidity) or undercontrol (dysregulation) that carries across many situations.

1. Adolescents at this level are unable to control or regulate impulses appropriately, leading to profound difficulties in familial, social, and sexual relationships. Impulse control may be so weak that they are incapable of modulating anger and other negative affects; alternatively, impulse control may be so rigid that impulses remain almost completely unexpressed.

Most Relevant Assessment Tools

Where indicated below, measures (or their adult versions) are discussed in the "Most Relevant Assessment Tools" section for capacity 7 in Chapter 2 (pp. 101–103).

Barratt Impulsiveness Scale—Version 11—Adolescent

The Barratt Impulsiveness Scale—Version 11—Adolescent (BIS-11-A; Fossati, Barratt, Acquarini, & Di Ceglie, 2002) is a 30-item self-report questionnaire measuring impulsiveness in adolescents. Items are rated on a 4-point Likert scale (1 = rarely/never to 4 = almost always/always) and summed; the higher the total score, the higher the impulsiveness. The BIS-11-A is an adaptation of the adult BIS-11 (Patton, Stanford, & Barratt, 1995; see Chapter 2 for discussion), with 15 of the 30 original items reworded to correspond with adolescents' experiences. The adult version had three subfactors (motor impulsiveness, nonplanning impulsiveness, and attentional impulsiveness), but because of high intercorrelations among the subfactors for adolescents, total scores are the best index of impulsivity for this age group. Past research has found good internal consistency in adolescent samples (Fossati et al., 2002; Hartmann, Rief, & Hilbert, 2011; von Diemen, Szobot, Kessler, & Pechansky, 2007). Construct validity is evident from the relationship between BIS-11-A scores and other measures of impulse-related disorders (e.g., attention-deficit/hyperactivity disorder, aggression, drug consumption; Fossati et al., 2002). It has been translated into several languages, requires a third- to fourth-grade reading level, and can be considered a reliable tool to investigate impulsiveness in adolescents (Panwar et al., 2014; Reynolds, Penfold, & Patak, 2008).

Sensitivity to Punishment and Sensitivity to Reward Questionnaire

The Sensitivity to Punishment and Sensitivity to Reward Questionnaire (SPSRQ; Franken & Muris, 2006; Torrubia, Avila, Molto, & Caseras, 2001) is a self-report measure of sensitivity to cues signaling reward and punishment, in line with Gray's concepts of the behavioral activation system and behavioral inhibition system. The original SPSRQ had 48 items in a yes–no format rating for two scales, sensitivity to punishment and sensitivity to reward; both demonstrated acceptable Cronbach's alphas of internal consistency and test–retest reliability, as well as convergent and discriminant validity (Torrubia et al., 2001). Principal components analysis confirmed this two-factor structure. Further analyses have been conducted with shorter, more reliable versions (Aluja & Blanch, 2011; Caci, Deschaux, & Bayle, 2007; Cooper & Gomez, 2008; O'Connor, Colder, & Hawk, 2004), with specific adaptations for children (Luman, van Meel, Oosterlan, & Geurts, 2012) and adolescents (Matton, Goossens, Braet, & Vervaet, 2013), making the SPSRQ a suitable instrument for exploring sensivity to reward and punishment across development.

Urgency, Premeditation, Perseverance, and Sensation-Seeking Impulsive Behavior Scale

The Urgency, Premeditation, Perseverance, and Sensation-Seeking (UPPS) Impulsive Behavior Scale (Whiteside & Lynam, 2001) is discussed in Chapter 2. The four-factor model of the UPPS was replicated in a sample of teenagers (314 girls and 314 boys), using exploratory and confirmatory factor analyses. Girls had a higher score for urgency, and boys a higher score for sensation seeking. All four subscales had good to very good internal reliability (Van der Linden et al., 2006), suggesting that the UPPS is a promising tool for studying impulsivity in adolescence (D'Acremont & Van der Linden, 2005; Urben, Suter, Pihet, Straccia, & Stéphan, 2014).

Brief Self-Control Scale

The Brief Self-Control Scale (BSCS; Tangney, Baumeister, & Boone, 2004), also discussed in Chapter 2, is face-valid for adolescents and has been used in several adolescent samples, with results showing internal consistency, test–retest reliability, and convergent and discriminant validity (Duckworth, Kim, & Tsukayama, 2012; Farley & Kim-Spoon, 2014).

Behavioral Inhibition System and Behavioral Activation System Scales

The Behavioral Inhibition System and Behavioral Activation System (BIS/BAS) Scales (Carver & White, 1994), a 20-item questionnaire with two 4-point scales (1 = strongly disagree to 4 = strongly agree), measure dispositional sensitivity to the behavioral inhibition system and three types of reactivity to the behavioral activation system: reward responsiveness, drive, and fun seeking. Validity has been found sufficient in both adolescent (Gruber et al., 2013; Yu, Branje, Keijsers, & Meeus, 2011) and young adult (Franken, Muris, & Rassin, 2005; Heubeck, Wilkinson, & Cologon, 1998) samples.

8. Capacity for Defensive Functioning

For a broader definition of the eighth capacity, see Chapter 2 (p. 78).

Defensive functioning should be looked at developmentally, as different defenses emerge at different periods of development, with more mature and complex defenses appearing in late adolescence and young adulthood. There is a decrease from early to late adolescence in the use of immature and neurotic defenses, such as disavowal, denial, projection, and repression, and an increase in the use of mature defenses, such as identification, intellectualization, and sublimation. These age-related effects parallel cognitive changes (the consolidation of formal operational thinking and abstract reasoning), progress in individuation, and increase in mentalizing capacities. These changes lead older teenagers to be more independent and simultaneously more empathetic and involved with others. This shift to more mature defenses is progressive through late maturity.

Defensive functioning should be looked at from an adaptive perspective as well, although defenses may differ with respect to overall level of adaptiveness. Adolescents tend to use the same defense mechanisms in similar situations. They differ in degree of insight into their defense styles. Better insight into one's personal style is correlated with adaptation and well-being.

The following is a developmental guideline to age-expected attainments for adolescents in the capacity for defensive functioning.

Developmental Guideline: Capacity for Defensive Functioning in Adolescence

Description
Early adolescence (ages 12–14)
Early adolescence is characterized by a quantum leap in cognitive thinking (development of formal operational thinking and abstract reasoning), which fosters a softening of the psychic structure. However, pressures related to hormonal, pubertal, social, and physical changes make early adolescents vulnerable to shifting and volatile states of mind and to a sense of self-fragmentation. Use of immature defenses such as disavowal, denial, projection, and splitting is still common at this age. These upheavals cause early adolescents to be self-centered and sensitive to the external supports on which they rely.
Middle to late adolescence (ages 15–19)
In middle to late adolescence, an integration of self occurs. The consolidation of formal operational thinking, along with a relative calmness and a greater sense of stability, allows high-functioning older adolescents to rely more on internal supports. This greater sense of a firm foundation allows them to use more mature and sophisticated defenses such as sublimation, humor, affiliation, self-assertion, and intellectualization. High-functioning older teenagers are more empathic and involved with others, particularly with their families. They are much more in control of their feelings and actions.

Rating Scale

5. At this level, adaptive and developmentally appropriate defenses predominate. The use of mature defenses allows adolescents to experience a broad range of affects, and to be aware of and to manage thoughts and feelings in ways that promote continued growth and exploration in relationships and the world at large. Neurotic-level defenses (isolation, intellectualization, repression) may be used in some situations, but they do not significantly impair functioning, as these adolescents typically revert to more adaptive defenses (sublimation, humor) when anxiety, conflict, and stress diminish.

3. Adolescents at this level often respond to internal or external sources of stress by viewing problems as external, minimizing or ignoring internal causes. Hence, in situations of threat or anxiety, there may be modest distortions of reality. Adolescents may appear defensive and may disavow aspects of their own experience through denial and projection. Or they may mask negative self-states (e.g., shame, powerlessness, disappointment) by devaluing or idealizing self or others or by maintaining an illusion of omnipotence. Overall, defensive strategies may be unpredictable and fluctuating, with immature defenses (splitting, projection, acting out) appearing at times of greatest stress.

1. These adolescents are overwhelmed by anxiety, fear of dissolution/annihilation of the self, and/or physical harm or death. These fears come from the adolescents' difficulties in dealing with internal conflicts or external demands. External reality may be grossly distorted, anxiety poorly contained, and adaptation highly impaired. Lower-level defenses such as splitting, distortion, fragmentation, delusional projection, and psychotic denial are predominant in these adolescents. Their capacity to function in the context of relationships or on their own is severely restricted and impaired.

Most Relevant Assessment Tools

Where indicated below, measures (or their adult versions) are discussed in the "Most Relevant Assessment Tools" section for capacity 8 in Chapter 2 (pp. 104–107).

Shedler–Westen Assessment Procedure for Adolescents, Version II

In the SWAP-II-A (Westen, Shedler, Durrett, Glass, & Martens, 2003), the capacity for defensive functioning is covered by several items (see Chapter 2, page 85, for discussion of corresponding items in the SWAP-200).

Defense Style Questionnaire

The Defense Style Questionnaire (DSQ; Andrews, Singh, & Bond, 1983) is discussed in Chapter 2. The shorter version (DSQ-40), with 40 items (Andrews et al., 1993) measuring 20 defenses, is considered best suited for adolescents (Muris, Winands, & Horselenberg, 2003). Its psychometric properties have been investigated in normal and clinical samples of adolescents, with results showing good internal consistency and good discriminant and concurrent validity (Ruuttu et al., 2006). It appears to be a reliable and valid instrument for measuring defense style in adolescents.

Defense Mechanism Rating Scales and Defense Mechanism Rating Scales Q-Sort

The Defense Mechanism Rating Scales (DMRS; Perry, 1990) and the DMRS Q-Sort (Di Giuseppe, Perry, Petraglia, Janzen, & Lingiardi, 2014) are also discussed in Chapter 2 (pp. 104 and 105).

Response Evaluation Measure–71

The Response Evaluation Measure–71 (REM-71; Araujo, Ryst, & Steiner, 1999; Steiner, Araujo, & Koopman. 2001), likewise discussed in Chapter 2, can be considered a good screening instrument for assessing defenses in normal and clinical populations of adolescents (Plattner et al., 2003).

Comprehensive Assessment of Defense Style

The Comprehensive Assessment of Defense Style (CADS; Laor, Wolmer, & Cicchetti, 2001) assesses defensive behavior in children and adolescents based on observer reports. The CADS asks parents to answer 26 Likert-type questions about their child's behavioral tendencies. It was validated on a sample of 124 children and adolescents in a mental health clinic and 104 nontreated children. A factor analysis of 28 defenses yielded one mature factor, one immature factor of defenses expressed in relation to the environment (other-oriented), and one immature factor expressed in relation to the self (self-oriented). The CADS significantly discriminated between patients and nonpatients, with patients using more immature and fewer mature defenses than controls and adolescents using more mature and fewer other-oriented defenses than children (Wolmer, Laor, & Cicchetti, 2001). Preliminary reliability and validity data for the CADS are encouraging, suggesting areas of implementation such as longitudinal examination of defenses, psychopathology screening, and therapeutic improvement.

Defense Mechanisms Inventory

The Defense Mechanisms Inventory (DMI; Gleser & Ihilevich, 1969; Ihilevich & Gleser, 1986) is a paper-and-pencil test of the relative intensity of five major groups of defenses: turning against the object, principalization, turning against the self, reversal, and protection. Participants are asked to describe their reaction to 10 hypothetical dilemmas. Via a forced-choice method, each response represents one of the five defense clusters. Initially developed for adults, the DMI has been adapted for adolescents and used in several studies with suicidal and psychiatric inpatient adolescents (Noam & Recklitis, 1990; Recklitis, Noam, & Borst, 1992). Reliability, validity, and normative studies support its use at this age. There is also a six-story short form. Correlations between the short and long forms ranged from .90 to .95 on the five scales. The short form is thus an acceptable substitute for the lengthier inventory and is more usable in clinical and research settings (Recklitis, Yap, & Noam, 1995).

9. Capacity for Adaptation, Resiliency, and Strength

For a broader definition of the ninth capacity, see Chapter 2 (p. 78).

"Adaptation" in this capacity implies a critical, nonconformist adaptation to specific contexts that does not result in a restriction of psychic functioning. It enables an adolescent to transcend obstacles and turn setbacks into opportunities for growth and positive change. "Resiliency" reflects a complex process of personal, interpersonal, and contextual protective mechanisms, resulting in an anomalous, positive outcome in the face of adversity. At a personal level, the construct implies the adolescent's ability to self-regulate dynamically and appropriately (at behavioral and emotional levels) to contexts of abuse, neglect, violence, chronic illness, discrimination, or poverty and to adapt more quickly to changing circumstances. Resiliency is a dynamic process, consistent with a biopsychosocial, person-in-environment model of development. There is a growing recognition that risk and protective factors for resiliency may operate differently at different points and trajectories across the life course. In adolescence, resiliency implies a growing capacity for assertiveness, self-protection, and adequate perspective taking, as well as the use of creative ways of dealing with challenge and threat.

Rating Scale

5. At this level, adolescents can respond flexibly and age-appropriately to unexpected stress in ways that do not significantly compromise overall functioning and ongoing maturation. They can ask for support and help when necessary. They show a flexible repertoire of responses when confronted with stressful situations and seem implicitly aware of their strengths and vulnerabilities. They can manage shifts in emotional states without compromising their personal and interpersonal functioning.

3. These adolescents can respond flexibly and age-appropriately to most unexpected and stressful situations. They can generally use their strengths in the service of their functioning. When in more complex social-emotional contexts, however, they may use less adaptive strategies that can interfere temporarily with behavior regulation, and they may show mild symptomatology. These experiences do not significantly restrict their growth and overall functioning over time.

1. These adolescents are extremely vulnerable and dependent on the external world to maintain their emotional and behavioral equilibrium. Regulatory mechanisms are severely lacking, leading to maladaptive patterns of response and a strong tendency to regress to early modes of functioning (avoidance, overcontrol, dissociation) when faced with unpredictable or stressful situations. They cannot manage complex social-emotional situations, show more severe forms of symptomatology, and suffer more lasting compromise to their personal and interpersonal functioning.

Most Relevant Assessment Tools

Where indicated below, measures (or their adult versions) are discussed in the "Most Relevant Assessment Tools" section for capacity 9 in Chapter 2 (pp. 108–110).

Resilience Scale for Adolescents

The Resilience Scale for Adolescents (READ; Hjemdal, Friborg, Stiles, Martinussen, & Rosenvinge, 2006), a derivation of the Resilience Scale for Adults (RSA; Hjemdal, Friborg, Martinussen, & Rosenving, 2001), is a 28-item test with items rated on a 5-point Likert-type scale. The response set for the READ was changed to a Likert-type scale, as the semantic differential used in the RSA proved difficult for teens. It was validated on 425 Norwegian adolescents between 13 and 15 years of age (Hjemdal et al., 2006). It contains five factors: (1) personal competence, (2) social competence, (3) structured style, (4) family cohesion, and (5) social resources. The scale shows good discriminant validity with the Short Mood and Feeling Questionnaire and Social Phobia Anxiety Index for Children and good predictive validity of depressive symptoms (Hjemdal, Aune, Reinfjell, Stiles, & Friborg, 2007). Cronbach's alphas for the five factors ranged from .85 to .69. Gender differences were found, with girls reporting higher levels of social resources and boys reporting higher scores on personal competence. The READ appears both reliable and valid. A parent/significant adult version of the scale (READ-P) is also available. A Norwegian validation of a shorter, 23-item version of the scale has been reported as yielding acceptable psychometric properties (von Soest, Mossige, Stefansen, & Hjemdal, 2010).

Resiliency Scale for Children and Adolescents

The Resiliency Scale for Children and Adolescents (RSCA; Prince-Embury, 2008) was developed for use in preventive screening for psychological vulnerability. It consists of three scales that assess for resilience in children and adolescents: sense of mastery, sense of relatedness, and emotional reactivity (Prince-Embury & Courville, 2008a). Sense of mastery, a 20-item scale rated on a 5-point Likert scale, consists of three content areas: optimism, self-efficacy, and adaptability. Sense of relatedness consists of 24 items encompassing comfort and trust in others, perceived access to support by others, and capacity to tolerate differences in others. The emotional reactivity scale has 20 items consisting of sensitivity/threshold for and intensity of reaction, length of recovery time, and impairment while upset. Validation of the RSCA included normative samples of 226 children ages 9–11, 224 adolescents ages 12–14, and 200 adolescents ages 15–18 (Prince-Embury & Courville, 2008b), as well as a clinical sample of 169 adolescents ages 15–18 (Prince-Embury, 2008). All three measures exhibited strong internal consistency and construct validity.

Adolescent Resilience Scale

The Adolescent Resilience Scale (ARS; Oshio, Kaneko, Nagamine, & Nakaya, 2003) for college-age youth is a 21-item scale with three factors: novelty seeking, emotional regulation, and positive future orientation. Construct validation involved a Japanese population of 207 young adults between the ages of 19 and 23 (Oshio et al., 2003). It differentiated among vulnerable (high stressors, high psychopathology), resilient (high stressors, low psychopathology), and well-adjusted (low stressors, low psychopathology) groups. The initial validation study (Oshio, Nakaya, Kaneko, & Nagamine, 2002) found acceptable internal reliability. Cronbach's alphas for the total scale (.85) and three factors were all acceptable (novelty seeking = .79; emotional regulation = .77; positive future orientation = .81). Correlations averaged .75 among the resilience total and subscales. It has shown good convergent and discriminant validity with the Big Five Personality Inventory (Nakaya, Oshio, & Kaneko, 2006).

Resilience Skills and Abilities Scale

The Resilience Skills and Abilities Scale (RSAS), originally the Adolescent Resiliency Belief System Scale (Jew, 1997), consists of 35 items rated on a 5-point Likert scale (Jew, Green, & Kroger, 1999). It draws on Mrazek and Mrazek's (1987) cognitive appraisal theory, operationalizing resiliency by using characteristics of individuals in stressful contexts. Validation involved four studies of 408 high school students ages 14–15. The current version has three subscales: active skill acquisition, future orientation, and independence/risk taking. It appears both reliable and valid, with acceptable intraclass correlations indicating test–retest reliability (.36–.70) and internal consistency (Cronbach's alphas = .68–.95).

Ego Resiliency Scale–89—Revised

The Ego Resiliency Scale–89—Revised (ER89-R; Alessandri, Vecchio, Steca, Caprara, & Caprara, 2008; Vecchione, Alessandri, Barbaranelli, & Gerbino, 2010) is a brief inventory of 10 items on a 4-point Likert scale, drawn from the original 14 items included in the ER89 scale of Block and colleagues (Letzring, Block, & Funder, 2005). It has been used to assess the development of ego resiliency from late adolescence to emerging adulthood, focusing on different ways to define continuity and change. Psychometric properties have been confirmed in both cross-cultural and longitudinal research (Alessandri et al., 2014; Vecchione et al., 2010). The scale predicts externalizing and internalizing problems, both concurrently and 2 and 4 years later. Findings suggest that it is a valid and reliable instrument that can be fruitfully used for studying ego resiliency through various developmental stages (Vecchione et al., 2010).

Multidimensional Adolescent Functioning Scale

The MAFS (Wardenaar et al., 2013), described earlier in this chapter as an assessment tool for capacity 1, is a 23-item self-report questionnaire developed by clinical consensus to assess normal adolescent functioning. It comprises three subscales: general functioning, family-related functioning, and peer-related functioning. See the earlier description for further details.

Strengths and Difficulties Questionnaire

The Strengths and Difficulties Questionnaire (SDQ; Goodman, 1997) is a brief screening tool for 3- to 16-year-olds. It exists in several versions and several languages to meet the needs of researchers, clinicians, and educators. Each version includes between one and three of the following: (1) 25 items on psychological attributes; (2) an impact statement asking whether the informant thinks the young person has a problem; and (3) follow-up questions containing the 25 items modified to read "within the last month," plus 2 additional follow-up questions about effect of interventions. All versions ask about 25 attributes, some positive and others negative. Items are divided into five scales (five items each): (1) emotional problems, (2) conduct problems, (3) hyperactivity/inattention, (4) peer social relationships, and (5) prosocial behavior. Scales 2, 3, and 4 are summed to generate a "total difficulties" score; 10 items deal with strengths. The same items are included in questionnaires for parents and teachers of 4- to 16-year-olds (Goodman, 1997). Self-report versions are available for children ages 11–16, depending on level of understanding and literacy (Goodman, Meltzer, & Bailey, 1998). The measure has been used extensively in studies around the world and has good psychometric properties, comparing favorably with the Achenbach and other, longer problem-related scales. Its advantages are its brevity, coverage across the age spectrum, and ease of use by professionals who are not psychometricians. While primarily problem-focused, it includes strengths related to resiliency.

Behavioral and Emotional Rating Scale–2

The Behavioral and Emotional Rating Scale–2 (BERS-2; Epstein, 2004), a later version of the BERS described as an assessment tool for capacity 2, is designed to aid in strength-based assessment. Consisting of 52 Likert-type items, it provides an overall strength index and five-factor analytically derived subscales assessing key areas of functioning: (1) interpersonal strength, (2) family involvement, (3) intrapersonal strength, (4) school functioning, and (5) affective strength. Scores are calculated for each dimension and then combined in an overall strength index. Higher scores reflect greater perceived strengths. Investigations suggest that the BERS-2 is a psychometrically sound instrument (Duppong Hurley, Lambert, Epstein, & Stevens, 2014; Epstein, Mooney, Ryser, & Pierce, 2004). Technical adequacy has been addressed with respect to content validity, convergent validity, discriminant validity, interrater reliability, and short- and long-term test–retest reliability.

10. Self-Observing Capacities (Psychological Mindedness)

For a broader definition of this set of capacities, see Chapter 2 (p. 78).

Self-observing capacities (psychological mindedness) play a key role in organizing an adolescent's emotional experiences and evaluating internal affective shifts by reflecting on them coherently. Psychological mindedness develops in childhood and adolescence as a complex cognitive capacity involving the child's increasing capacity for abstraction and comprehension of the motives, attitudes, and characteristics of the self and others. This capacity is built on both cognitive and emotional skills acquired during development.

Social perspective taking is a core feature in the developmental progression of psychological mindedness. It begins with a simple egocentric judgment (i.e., the self's own viewpoint is the same as that of others) between the ages of 3 and 5. This gives way to a self-reflective level between 6 and 8, when the individual recognizes the self as a possible focus of others' perspectives. Between 9 and 15 years of age, there is a mutual perspective, characterized by the ability to recognize the perspectives of the self and others even when not in relationship. During adolescence, individuals further develop the ability to perceive others' points of view and to analyze their own and others' behaviors and emotions. These skills provide a basis for the capacity for self-observation. Finally, as a person moves into young adulthood, there is an understanding of a network of perspectives binding individuals into a social system.

A low level of psychological mindedness in adolescence may be related to alexithymia (again, see the discussion of psychological mindedness in Chapter 2 for more details).

Rating Scale

5. At this level, adolescents seem highly motivated and able to observe and understand the self in relation to others, showing an ability to reflect on a full range of their own and others' feelings and experiences. They can reflect on both the present and the past and have a long-term view of the self, values, and goals. They can reflect on multiple relationships between feelings and experiences, across the full range of age-expected experiences in the context of new challenges.

3. These adolescents seem somewhat motivated and able to recognize and reflect on meanings that underlie overt words and actions. They have some insight into their own and others' motives, and can link past and present experience. Under stress, their self-awareness, self-reflection, and self-examination may fluctuate or deteriorate, along with their awareness of others' subjective experience. In these situations, they may be only partly able to use such information effectively.

1. These adolescents seem poorly motivated or unable to reflect genuinely on feelings, thoughts, and behaviors in either the present or the past. They seem not to value psychological constructs. Self-awareness is typically limited to polarized affect states or simple emotional reactions. They have deficient awareness of others' subjectivity, and often tend toward fragmentation. They cannot reflect on specific emotional experiences or affect states and may resort to primitive defenses, acting out impulsively or dissociating in the face of intense affect.

Most Relevant Assessment Tools

Where indicated below, measures (or their adult versions) are discussed in the "Most Relevant Assessment Tools" section for capacity 10 in Chapter 2 (pp. 111–113).

Adolescent Version of the Psychological Mindedness Scale

The Adolescent Version of the Psychological Mindedness Scale (PMS-A; Boylan, 2006) is an adaptation of the PMS originally developed by Conte and colleagues to assess self-understanding and interest in the motivation and behavior of others and to explore suitability for psychodynamic psychotherapy (Conte, Ratto, & Karusa, 1996;

Shill & Lumley, 2002; see Chapter 2 for discussion). Several studies have used the PMS in adolescent populations (Cecero, Beitel, & Prout, 2008; Roxas & Glenwick, 2014). The PMS was adapted in a sample of 107 normal-intelligence adolescents between ages 13 and 18, with 12 items deleted based on lack of relevance to adolescents. The reduced version yields a score from 33 to 132. A component factor analysis found that four of Conte and colleagues' (1996) five factors accounted for 43% of the variance: (1) interest in the meaning of one's behavior and that of others, (2) access to feelings, (3) willingness to try to understand oneself and others, and (4) openness to new ideas and capacity for change. There was good internal consistency at baseline (Cronbach's alpha = .84) and at postmeasurement (Cronbach's alpha = .81), and moderate to high alphas for individual factors: interest (.78), access (.67), willingness (.80), and openness (.64). The adolescent adaptation seems easy to understand, making it suitable for adolescents (Parker, Eastabrook, Keefer, & Wood, 2010).

Toronto Alexithymia Scale–20

The Toronto Alexithymia Scale–20 (TAS-20; Bagby, Parker, & Taylor, 1994; see Chapter 2 for discussion) is being increasingly used with adolescent respondents, although psychometric properties have been shown to be less reliable with adolescents (Rieffe, Oosterveld, & Meerum Terwogt, 2006). Parker and colleagues (2010) examined measurement invariance of factor structure, internal reliability, and mean levels of responses in younger adolescents (ages 13–14), middle adolescents (15–16), and older adolescents (17–18), and in a comparison group of young adults (19–21). A formal readability analysis was also conducted. Results revealed systematic age differences in factor structure and psychometric properties, with quality of measurement progressively deteriorating with younger age. Much of this effect may be attributable to the reading difficulty of the scale. The authors concluded that use of the TAS-20 with young teenage respondents is not recommended without appropriate adaptation.

Shedler–Westen Assessment Procedure for Adolescents, Version II

In the SWAP-II-A (Westen, DeFife, Malone, & DiLallo, 2014), self-observing capacities are covered by several items (see the discussion of the SWAP-200 in Chapter 2, page 85, for details).

11. Capacity to Construct and Use Internal Standards and Ideals

The 11th capacity indexes an adolescent's personal sense of morality. Internal standards and ideals (related to the construct of superego) are internalized early in life through interactions with parents and other caregivers, and are then elaborated and refined in adolescence in subsequent interactions with peers and models (e.g., teachers, mentors). As moral values are learned within social contexts, maturation of moral development in adolescence implies the capacity to manage interpersonal relations and to protect oneself from negative peer influence. This capacity is an outgrowth of other mental functions and integrates a number of them. Empathy and perspective taking play an essential role in moral development and in ethical decision-making processes in adolescence.

The following is a developmental guideline of age-expected attainments for adolescents in the capacity to construct and use internal standards and ideals.

Developmental Guideline: Capacity to Construct and Use Internal Standards and Ideals in Adolescence

Description
Early adolescence (ages 12–14)
Although young adolescents develop the capacity for abstract reasoning, they are still at a preconventional level of moral reasoning. The morality of an action is judged by its consequences, and rules and limits are tested. Young adolescents focus on the direct consequences of their actions for themselves (reward vs. punishment), and only later does the right behavior become defined by whatever is in an individual's best interest (self-interest).
Middle adolescence (ages 15–16)
Interest in moral reasoning appears in middle adolescence with the development of ideals and the selection of role models. Adolescents at around 15 years show more consistent evidence of self-conscience and a greater capacity for goal setting. Morality is characterized by an acceptance of society's conventions about right and wrong. Adolescents begin to be receptive to approval or disapproval from others as it reflects concordance with perceived roles (driven by interpersonal accord and conformity). In a later stage, they will integrate the principle of obeying laws because of their importance in maintaining a functioning society (authority and social order obedience). At this point, however, morality is predominantly dictated by outside forces.
Late adolescence (ages 17–19)
With the development of more mature introspection, a sense of personal dignity and self-esteem, and ability to set goals and follow through, late adolescents become capable of accepting social institutions and cultural traditions. By age 20, adolescents and young adults reach a postconventional level of moral development, in which one's own perspective may take precedence over society's view. People with postconventional morality view rules as useful but changeable. First, laws are regarded as social contracts. Later, moral reasoning becomes based on abstract reasoning using universal ethical principles. Laws are valid only insofar as they are grounded in justice, and a commitment to justice carries an obligation to disobey unjust laws.

Rating Scale

5. Adolescents at this level have internal standards that seem flexible and integrated with a realistic sense of their capacities, values, and ideals, and with social contexts. Internal standards provide opportunities for meaningful striving and feelings of authenticity and self-esteem. Feelings of guilt are used as a signal for reappraising one's own behavior. Others are also viewed with a balance of compassion, empathy, and objective criticism.

3. At this level, internal standards and ideals tend to be either moderately rigid and inflexible, or inconsistent across contexts, driven more by needs, desires, and feelings than by a coherent set of moral guidelines. They are integrated neither with a realistic sense of one's own capacities, values, and ideals nor with social contexts. Self-esteem is overly dependent on peer influence. Guilt feelings are experienced more as self-criticism than as signals for reappraising one's behavior.

1. Internal standards and ideals are rigid and inflexible; based on harsh and punitive expectations; poorly integrated with a realistic sense of one's capacities, values, and

ideals; and inconsistent with the social and cultural context. Feelings of guilt are denied and associated with internalizing and externalizing behaviors. The moral sense seems to have either a tyrannical or an insignificant role in organizing self-experience and in interpreting behavior of self and others. Guilt feelings are not balanced with compassion and objective criticism; self and others are often viewed as "totally bad" or "totally good." Internal standards, ideals, and a sense of morality are for the most part absent.

Most Relevant Assessment Tools

Where indicated below, measures (or their adult versions) are discussed in the "Most Relevant Assessment Tools" section for capacity 11 in Chapter 2 (pp. 114–116).

Shedler–Westen Assessment Procedure for Adolescents, Version II

In the SWAP-II-A (Westen, DeFife, Malone, & DiLallo, 2014), the capacity to construct and use internal standards and ideals is covered by several items (see the discussion of the SWAP-200 in Chapter 2 for details).

Prosocial Reasoning Objective Measure

The Prosocial Reasoning Objective Measure (PROM; Carlo, Eisenberg, & Knight, 1992) is discussed in Chapter 2. Psychometric properties have been reported in studies with students from middle childhood to early adulthood (Carlo et al., 1992; Roskam & Marchal, 2003).

Defining Issues Test, Version 2

Version 2 of the Defining Issues Test (DIT2; Rest, Narvaez, Bebeau, & Thoma, 1999) is a measure of moral judgment based on Kohlberg's (1984) theory of moral development, defined as a universal, continual cognitive process that develops in stages. It consists of five dilemma stories, each followed by 12 issue statements. The subject reads a story and ranks corresponding statements in terms of their moral importance, resulting in scores of the degree to which a subject uses the personal interest (stages 2 and 3), maintaining norms (stage 4), or postconventional (stages 5 and 6) schema of Kohlberg's model. The DIT2 has been widely used to measure moral judgment and has been shown to be a reliable and valid measure of characteristics of moral judgment in youth (Thoma & Dond, 2014).

Psychopathy Checklist: Youth Version

The Psychopathy Checklist: Youth Version (PCL:YV; Forth, Kosson, & Hare, 2003), an adapted version of Hare's Psychopathy Checklist—Revised (PCL-R; Hare, 2003; see Chapter 2), is a 20-item clinician-rated assessment of psychopathic characteristics in young people. The authors suggest a 60- to 90-minute semistructured interview to assess a youth's interpersonal style, to get information on history and current functioning, and to assess credibility of statements. Items are scored on a 3-point scale (0 = not present, 1 = somewhat present, and 2 = definitely present). As in adults, factor analyses on community and incarcerated adolescent samples identify four factors:

deceitful and manipulative (interpersonal factor); emotional detachment (affective factor); reckless, impulsive, and irresponsible (lifestyle factor); and propensity to violate social norms (antisocial factor) (Jones, Cauffman, Miller, & Mulvey, 2006; Vitacco, Neumann, Caldwell, Leistico, & Van Rybroek, 2006). Studies using an item response theory model have shown that items that were most discriminating (or most sensitive to changes) of the posited latent trait of psychopathy among adolescents included "glibness/superficial charm," "lack of remorse," and "need for stimulation" (Tsang, Piquero, & Cauffman, 2014). The PCL:YV has shown good reliability and validity and is widely used to assess psychopathic personality traits in adolescents and young adults (Sevecke, Pukrop, Kosson, & Krischer, 2009).

12. Capacity for Meaning and Purpose

For a broader definition of the final capacity, see Chapter 2 (p. 79).

This capacity is strongly related to identity construction and moral development in adolescence, and to a realistic acknowledgment of personal potentials and limitations. It is also influenced by the development of mentalizing capacities, which allow an adolescent to be sensitive to the attitudes, values, thoughts, and feelings of others and to experience a feeling of sharing and participation. This capacity allows for creativity and affiliation as well. A delayed maturation of this capacity may be related to inhibition, self-sabotage, or uncritical adhesion to ideologies via parental or peer influence.

Rating Scale

5. Adolescents at this level show a clear, unwavering sense of purpose and meaning, along with an intrinsic sense of agency and self-direction and the ability to look outside the self and transcend immediate situational concerns. Subjectivity and intersubjectivity play a major role in the life of these adolescents, who are able to have a critical involvement in personal and general projects.
3. Adolescents at this level show some sense of purpose and meaning, along with periods of uncertainty and doubt. They are able to look outside the self with effort, and have some sense of connectedness with other people and the world. They can grasp the broader implications of attitudes and beliefs, and accept alternative perspectives only in certain conflict-free domains.
1. These adolescents show a lack of direction, aimlessness, and little or no sense of purpose; when asked, they appear unable to articulate a cohesive personal philosophy or set of life goals. Subjectivity and intersubjectivity have little or no importance. They may be unaware of this lack of direction, and may experience and express a pervasive sense of isolation and meaninglessness, while being uncritically involved in projects and ideologies.

Most Relevant Assessment Tools

Where indicated below, measures (or their adult versions) are discussed in the "Most Relevant Assessment Tools" section for capacity 12 in Chapter 2 (pp. 116–118).

Shedler–Westen Assessment Procedure for Adolescents, Version II

In the SWAP-II-A (Westen, DeFife, Malone, & DiLallo, 2014), the capacity for meaning and purpose is covered by several items (see the Chapter 2 discussion of the SWAP-200 for details).

Dispositional Flow Scale–2

The Dispositional Flow Scale–2 (DFS-2; Jackson & Ecklund, 2002; see Chapter 2 for discussion) has been used in several studies with adolescent samples and was found to have acceptable reliability and convergent validity (Moreno Murcia, Cervellò Gimeno, & Gonzàlez-Cutre Coll, 2008). Confirmatory factor analyses showed good reliability and validity for the nine first-order factors and for higher-order flow (Wang, Liu, & Khoo, 2009). In adolescents, flow is correlated with beneficial outcomes, such as increased concentration, enjoyment, happiness, strength, motivation, self-esteem, optimism, and future-mindedness (Hektner & Asakawa, 2000). It is also associated with intrinsic motivation and enjoyment in adolescents (Hektner & Csikszentmihalyi, 1996).

Future Orientation Scale

The Future Orientation Scale (FOS; Steinberg et al., 2009) is a relatively new 15-item self-report measure to explore future orientation in adolescents and young adults. Items were generated by developmental psychologists with expertise in adolescent psychosocial development. Respondents are given 10 pairs of statements separated by the word "BUT," are asked to choose the better descriptor, and then are asked whether the description is "really true" or "sort of true." Responses are coded on a 4-point scale from "really true" for one descriptor to "really true" for the other, and averaged. Higher scores indicate greater future orientation. Items are grouped into three five-item subscales: time perspective (e.g., "Some people would rather be happy today than take their chances on what might happen in the future BUT Other people will give up their happiness now so that they can get what they want in the future"); anticipation of future consequences (e.g., "Some people like to think about all of the possible good and bad things that can happen before making a decision BUT Other people don't think it's necessary to think about every little possibility before making a decision"); and planning ahead (e.g., "Some people think that planning things out in advance is a waste of time BUT Other people think that things work out better if they are planned out in advance"). Intercorrelations among subscales suggest that these aspects of future orientation are related but not identical. Confirmatory factor analysis has shown that a three-factor model provides a satisfactory and better fit to data than a one-factor model. The FOS is also correlated with other self-report instruments. Discriminant validity is suggested by its weak correlation with IQ and with other executive function measures (Steinberg et al., 2009).

Junior Temperament and Character Inventory

The Junior Temperament and Character Inventory (JTCI; Luby, Svrakic, McCallum, Przybeck, & Cloninger, 1999), an adaptation of Cloninger's TCI (Cloninger, Przybeck, Svrakic, & Wetzel, 1994) for children and adolescents, is a self-report measure of temperament and emerging personality characteristics (see Chapter 2, page 117, for a description of the TCI-R). Items were modified to capture underlying temperamental or personality features using examples appropriate for children and adolescents. Psychometric properties were tested in a sample of 322 nonreferred children (mean age = 12.0 years, *SD* = 1.3). Both fit and internal consistency emerged as satisfactory. Schmeck and Poustka (2001) investigated psychometric properties in a sample of older German adolescents (188 psychiatrically referred and 706 nonreferred adolescents ages 12–18) and found good support for Cloninger's model. Goodness-of-fit indices were remarkably high for both temperament and character dimensions, with a better fit for adolescents than for children ages 9–13 years (Luby et al., 1999), indicating that structure of personality is further developed and stabler in the older group and more comparable to the personality structure of adults. The JTCI has been translated into several languages (Korean: Lyoo et al., 2004; French: Asch et al., 2009; Swedish: Kerekes et al., 2010; Italian: Andriola et al., 2012) and is a widely validated instrument for use in child and adolescent populations (Kim et al., 2006).

Qualitative and Structural Dimensions of Self-Descriptions

The Qualitative and Structural Dimensions of Self-Descriptions (QSDSD; Blatt, Bers, & Schaffer, 1993) is described in Chapter 2. Using open-ended descriptions of the self, Blatt and colleagues' scoring system enables clinicians to generate ratings of self-attributions and complexity of self-representation and to track changes in these areas over time (e.g., during psychotherapy; see Bers, Blatt, Sayward, & Johnston, 1993; Blatt, Auerbach, & Levy, 1997). The QSDSD can also be used by a clinician as a prompt for discussing an adolescent's goals, aspirations, and feelings regarding past, present, and future events.

Adolescent Life Goal Profile Scale

The Adolescent Life Goal Profile Scale (ALGPS; Gabrielsen, Ulleberg, & Watten, 2012), a 16-item self-questionnaire scored on a 5-point Likert scale, measures perceived importance and perceived attainability of four life goal categories: relations, generativity, religion, and achievements. It can be useful for general adolescent research and for individual mental health care. Exploratory factor analyses found a two-dimensional structure with life goals and attainability ratings. Data support the reliability and convergent validity of the ALGPS (Gabrielsen, Watten, & Ulleberg, 2013).

Summary of Basic Mental Functioning

Following the same approach introduced in Chapter 2 on the M Axis, we recommend that clinicians summarize basic mental functioning for adolescents quantitatively (see Table 4.1).

TABLE 4.1. Summary of Basic Mental Functioning: MA Axis

To obtain a rating of an adolescent patient's overall mental functioning, a clinician should add up the 1–5 point ratings assigned to each capacity (Table 4.1a), yielding a single numerical index of overall functioning ranging from 12 to 60. This index permits provisionally assigning a patient to one of the categories outlined in Table 4.1b, which provides short qualitative descriptions of seven levels of mental functioning. Schematically, *healthy* mental functioning corresponds to MA1; *neurotic* to MA2 and MA3; *borderline* to MA4, MA5, and MA6 (from high to low, from moderate impairments to significant defects); and *psychotic* to MA7.

TABLE 4.1a. MA-Axis Functioning: Total Score

MA-Axis capacities	Rating scale				
1. Capacity for regulation, attention, and learning	5	4	3	2	1
2. Capacity for affective range, communication, and understanding	5	4	3	2	1
3. Capacity for mentalization and reflective functioning	5	4	3	2	1
4. Capacity for differentiation and integration (identity)	5	4	3	2	1
5. Capacity for relationships and intimacy	5	4	3	2	1
6. Capacity for self-esteem regulation and quality of internal experience	5	4	3	2	1
7. Capacity for impulse control and regulation	5	4	3	2	1
8. Capacity for defensive functioning	5	4	3	2	1
9. Capacity for adaptation, resiliency, and strength	5	4	3	2	1
10. Self-observing capacities (psychological mindedness)	5	4	3	2	1
11. Capacity to construct and use internal standards and ideals	5	4	3	2	1
12. Capacity for meaning and purpose	5	4	3	2	1
	Total score = __				

TABLE 4.1b. Levels of Mental Functioning

Level; range	Heading	Description
		Healthy
MA1; 54–60	Healthy/optimal mental functioning	The adolescent shows optimal or very good functioning in all or most mental capacities, with modest, expectable variations in flexibility and adaptation across life contexts.
		Neurotic
MA2; 47–53	Good/appropriate mental functioning with some areas of difficulty	The adolescent shows an appropriate level of mental functioning, with some specific areas of difficulty (e.g., in three or four mental capacities) that reflect conflicts or challenges related to specific life situations or events.
MA3; 40–46	Mild impairments in mental functioning	The adolescent shows mild constrictions and areas of inflexibility in some domains of mental functioning, implying impairments in areas such as self-esteem regulation, impulse and affect regulation, defensive functioning, and self-observing capacity.

(continued)

TABLE 4.1b. *(continued)*

Level; range	Heading	Description
		Borderline
MA4; 33–39	Moderate impairments in mental functioning	The adolescent shows moderate constrictions and inflexibility in most or almost all domains of mental functioning, affecting quality and stability of relationships, sense of identity, and range of affects tolerated. Functioning at this level reflects the significantly impaired adaptations denoted as "borderline-level" in many psychoanalytic writings.
MA5; 26–32	Major impairments in mental functioning	The adolescent shows major constrictions and alterations in almost all domains of mental functioning (e.g., tendencies toward fragmentation and difficulties in self–object differentiation), along with limited experience of feelings and/or thoughts in major life areas (i.e., love, work, play).
MA6; 19–25	Significant defects in basic mental functions	The adolescent shows significant defects in most domains of mental functioning, along with problems in the organization and/or integration–differentiation of self and others.
		Psychotic
MA7; 12–18	Major/severe defects in basic mental functions	The adolescent shows major and severe defects in almost all domains of mental functioning, with impairment in reality testing, fragmentation, or self–object differentiation; disturbances in perception, integration, and regulation of affect and thought; and severe defects in one or more basic mental functions (perception, integration, motor, memory, regulation, judgment, etc.)

BIBLIOGRAPHY

General Bibliography

Adams, G. R., & Berzonsky, M. D. (2003). *Blackwell handbook of adolescence.* Malden, MA: Blackwell.

Ammaniti, M., Fontana, A., Clarkin, A., Clarkin, J. F., Nicolais, G., & Kernberg, O. F. (2012). Assessment of adolescent personality disorders through the Interview of Personality Organization Processes in Adolescence (IPOP-A): Clinical and theoretical implications. *Adolescent Psychiatry, 2*(1), 36–45.

Amsel, E., & Smetana, J. G. (2011). *Adolescent vulnerabilities and opportunities: Developmental and constructivist perspectives.* New York: Cambridge University Press.

Atzil-Slonim, D., Tishby, O., & Shefler, G. (2015). Internal representations of the therapeutic relationship among adolescents in psychodynamic psychotherapy. *Clinical Psychology and Psychotherapy, 22*(6), 502–512.

Atzil-Slonim, D., Wiseman, H., & Tishby, O. (2016). Relationship representations and change in adolescents and emerging adults during psychodynamic psychotherapy. *Psychotherapy Research, 26*(3), 279–296.

Bychkova, T., Hillman, S., Midgley, N., & Schneider, C. (2011). The psychotherapy process with adolescents: A first pilot study and preliminary comparisons between different therapeutic modalities using the Adolescent Psychotherapy Q-Set. *Journal of Child Psychotherapy, 37*(3), 327–348.

Haggerty, G., Zodan, J., Mehra, A., Zubair, A., Ghosh, K., Siefert, C. J., . . . DeFife, J. (2016). Reliability and validity of prototype diagnosis for adolescent psychopathology. *Journal of Nervous and Mental Disease, 204*(4), 287–290.

Lanyado, M., & Horne, A. (Eds.). (2009). *The handbook of child and adolescent psychotherapy: Psychoanalytic approaches* (2nd ed.). New York: Routledge.

Lerner, R. M., & Steinberg, L. (Vol. Eds.). (2009). *Handbook of adolescent psychology: Vol 1. Individual bases of adolescent development* (3rd ed.). Hoboken, NJ: Wiley.

Midgley, N., & Kennedy, E. (2011). Psychodynamic psychotherapy for children and adolescents: A critical review of the evidence base. *Journal of Child Psychotherapy, 37,* 232–260.

Nakashi-Eisikovits, O., Dutra, L., & Westen, D. (2002). Relationship between attachment patterns and personality pathology in adolescents. *Journal of the American Academy of Child and Adolescent Psychiatry, 41*(9), 1111–1123.

Porcerelli, J. H., Cogan, R., & Bambery, M. (2011). The Mental Functioning axis of the *Psychodynamic Diagnostic Manual*: An adolescent case study. *Journal of Personality Assessment, 93*(2), 177–184.

Schwartz, S. J., Donnellan, M. B., Ravert, R. D., Luyckx, K., & Zamboanga, B. L. (2013). Identity development, personality, and well-being in adolescence and emerging adulthood: Theory, research, and recent advances. In I. B. Weiner (Series Ed.) & R. M. Lerner, M. A. Easterbrooks, & J. Mistry (Vol. Eds.), *Handbook of psychology: Vol. 6. Developmental psychology* (2nd ed., pp. 339–364). Hoboken, NJ: Wiley.

Tibon Czopp, S. (2012). Invited commentary: Applying psychodynamic developmental assessment to explore mental functioning in adolescents. *Journal of Youth and Adolescence, 41*(10), 1259–1266.

Westen, D., DeFife, J. A., Malone, J. C., & DiLallo, J. (2014). An empirically derived classification of adolescent personality disorders. *Journal of the American Academy of Child and Adolescent Psychiatry, 53*, 528–549.

1. Capacity for Regulation, Attention, and Learning

Beaver, K. M., Ratchford, M., & Ferguson, C. J. (2009). Evidence of genetic and environmental effects on the development of low self-control. *Criminal Justice and Behavior, 36*, 1158–1172.

Blakemore, S. J., & Choudhury, S. (2006). Development of the adolescent brain: Implications for executive function and social cognition. *Journal of Child Psychology and Psychiatry, 47*(3–4), 296–312.

Boelema, S. R., Harakeh, Z., Ormel, J., Hartman, C. A., Vollebergh, W. A., & van Zandvoort, M. J. (2014). Executive functioning shows differential maturation from early to late adolescence: Longitudinal findings from a TRAILS study. *Neuropsychology, 28*(2), 177–187.

Brown, T. E. (2001). *Brown Attention-Deficit Disorder Scales for Children and Adolescents: Manual.* San Antonio, TX: Psychological Corporation.

Brydges, C. R., Anderson, M., Reid, C. L., & Fox, A. M. (2013). Maturation of cognitive control: Delineating response inhibition and interference suppression. *PLoS ONE, 8*(7), e69826.

Carver, C. S., & Scheier, M. F. (1998). *On the self-regulation of behavior.* New York: Cambridge University Press.

Casey, B. J., Getz, S., & Galvan, A. (2008) The adolescent brain. *Developmental Review, 28*(1), 62–77.

Clarebout, G., Horz, H., & Schnotz, W. (2010). The relations between self-regulation and the embedding of support in learning environments. *Educational Technology Research and Development, 58*(5), 573–587.

Conners, C. K. (1997). *Conners Rating Scales—Revised: Technical manual.* North Tonawanda, NY: Multi-Health Systems.

Conners, C. K., Wells, K. C., Parker, J. D., Sitarenios, G., Diamond, J. M., & Powell, J. W. (1997). A new self-report scale for assessment of adolescent psychopathology: Factor structure, reliability, validity, and diagnostic sensitivity. *Journal of Abnormal Child Psychology, 25*(6), 487–497.

Crawford, J. R., Anderson, V., Rankin, P. M., & MacDonald J. (2010). An index-based short-form of the WISC-IV with accompanying analysis of the reliability and abnormality of differences. *British Journal of Clinical Psychology, 49*, 235–58.

DeThorne, L. S., & Schaefer, B. A. (2004). A guide to child nonverbal IQ measures. *American Journal of Speech–Language Pathology, 13*(4), 275–290.

Emslie, H., Wilson, F., Burden, V., Nimmo-Smith, I., & Wilson, B. A. (2003). *Behavioural Assessment of the Dysexecutive Syndrome for Children (BADSC).* London: Harcourt Assessment/Psychological Corporation.

Engel-Yeger, B., Josman, N., & Rosenblum, S. (2009). Behavioural assessment of the Dysexecutive Syndrome for Children (BADS-C): An examination of construct validity. *Neuropsychological Rehabilitation, 19*(5), 662–676.

Fan, J., McCandliss, B. D., Fossella, J., Flombaum, J. I., & Posner, M. I. (2005). The activation of attentional networks. *NeuroImage, 26*, 471–479.

Farley, J. P., & Kim-Spoon, J. (2014). The development of adolescent self-regulation: Reviewing the role of parent, peer, friend, and romantic relationships. *Journal of Adolescence, 37*(4), 433–440.

Gioia, G., Isquith, P. K., Guy, S. C., & Kenworthy, L. (2000). Test review: Behavior Rating Inventory of Executive Function. *Child Neuropsychology, 6*(3), 235–238.

Hrabok, M., Brooks, B. L., Fay-McClymont, T. B., & Sherman, E. M. (2014). Wechsler Intelligence Scale for Children—Fourth Edition (WISC-IV) short-form validity: A comparison study in pediatric epilepsy. *Child Neuropsychology, 20*(1), 49–59.

Luna, B. (2009). Developmental changes in cognitive control through adolescence. *Advances in Child Development and Behavior, 37*, 233–278.

McCandless, S., & O' Laughlin, L. (2007). The clinical utility of the Behavior Rating Inventory of Executive Function (BRIEF) in the diagnosis of ADHD. *Journal of Attention Disorders 10*(4), 381–389.

Montalvo, F. T., & Torres, M. C. (2008). Self-regulated

learning: Current and future directions. *Electronic Journal of Research in Educational Psychology, 2*(1), 1–34.

Naglieri, J. A., & Goldstein, S. (2013). *Comprehensive Executive Function Inventory.* Toronto, ON, Canada: Multi-Health Systems.

Roid, G., & Miller, L. (1997). *Leiter International Performance Scale—Revised.* Wood Dale, IL: Stoelting.

Sawyer, S. M., Afifi, R. A., Bearinger L. H., Blakemore, S. J., Dick, B., Ezeh, A. C., & Patton, G. C. (2012). Adolescence: A foundation for future health. *Lancet, 379*(9826), 1630–1640.

Steer, R. A., Kumar, G., & Beck, A. T. (2001). Use of the Conners–Wells' Adolescent Self-Report Scale: Short Form with psychiatric outpatients. *Journal of Psychopathology and Behavioral Assessment, 23*(4), 231–239.

Vijayakumar, N., Whittle, S., Dennison, M., Yücel, M., Simmons, J., & Allen, N. B. (2014). Development of temperamental effortful control mediates the relationship between maturation of the prefrontal cortex and psychopathology during adolescence: A 4-year longitudinal study. *Developmental Cognitive Neuroscience, 9*, 30–43.

Vohs, K. D., & Baumeister, R. F. (Eds.). (2016). *Handbook of self-regulation: Research, theory, and applications* (3rd ed.). New York: Guilford Press.

Wardenaar, K. J., Wigman, J. T., Lin, A., Killackey, E., Collip, D., Wood, S. J., . . . Yung, A. R. (2013). Development and validation of a new measure of everyday adolescent functioning: The Multidimensional Adolescent Functioning Scale. *Journal of Adolescent Health, 52*(2), 195–200.

Wechsler, D. (2005). *Wechsler Intelligence Scale for Children—Fourth Édition: Canadian (WISC-IV).* Toronto ON, Canada: Psychological Corporation.

Wechsler, D. (2008). *Wechsler Adult Intelligence Scale—Fourth Edition: Technical and interpretive manual.* San Antonio, TX: Pearson.

Wechsler, D. (2014). *Wechsler Intelligence Scale for Children—Fifth Édition (WISC-V).* San Antonio, TX: Pearson.

2. Capacity for Affective Range, Communication, and Understanding

Adrian, M., Zeman, J., & Veits, G. (2011). Methodological implications of the affect revolution: A 35-year review of emotion regulation assessment in children. *Journal of Experimental Child Psychology, 110*(2), 171–197.

Archer, R. P., Maruish, M., Imhof, E. A., & Piotrowski, C. (1991). Psychological test usage with adolescent clients: 1990 survey findings. *Professional Psychology: Research and Practice, 22*, 247–252.

Bachorowski, J., & Braaten, E. B. (1994). Emotional intensity: Measurement and theoretical implications. *Personality and Individual Differences, 17*(2), 191–199.

Bar-On, R., & Parker, J. (2000). *The Emotional Quotient Inventory: Youth Version: Technical manual.* Toronto, ON, Canada: Multi-Health Systems.

Barchard, K. A., Bajgar, J., Leaf, D. E., & Lane, R. D. (2010). Computer scoring of the Levels of Emotional Awareness Scale. *Behavior Research Methods, 42*(2), 586–595.

Bryant, F. B., Yarnold, P. R., & Grimm, L. G. (1996). Toward a measurement model of the Affect Intensity Measure: A three-factor structure. *Journal of Research in Personality, 30*, 223–247.

D'Acremont, M., & Van der Linden, M. (2007). How is impulsivity related to depression in adolescence?: Evidence from a French validation of the Cognitive Emotion Regulation Questionnaire. *Journal of Adolescence, 30*(2), 271–282.

Davidson, R. J., Jackson, D. C., & Kalin, N. H. (2000). Emotion, plasticity, context, and regulation: Perspectives from affective neuroscience. *Psychological Bulletin, 126*(6), 890–909.

Epstein, M. H., Mooney, P., Ryser, G., & Pierce, C. D. (2004). Validity and Reliability of the Behavioral and Emotional Rating Scale (2nd Edition): Youth Rating Scale. *Research on Social Work Practice, 14*(5), 358–367.

Epstein, M. H., & Sharma, H. M. (1998). *Behavioral and Emotional Rating Scale: A strength-based approach to assessment.* Austin, TX: PRO-ED.

Farley, J. P., & Kim-Spoon, J. (2014). The development of adolescent self-regulation: Reviewing the role of parent, peer, friend, and romantic relationships. *Journal of Adolescence, 37*(4), 433–440.

Fonagy, P., Gergely, G., Jurist, E. L., & Target, M. (2004). *Affect regulation, mentalization and the development of the self.* London: Karnac.

Garnefski, N., Kraaij, V., & Spinhoven, P. (2001). Negative life events, cognitive emotion regulation and depression. *Personality and Individual Differences, 30*, 1311–1327.

Garnefski, N., Kraaij, V., & Spinhoven, P. (2002). *Manual for the use of the Cognitive Emotion Regulation Questionnaire.* Leiderdorp, The Netherlands: DATEC.

Gratz, K. L., & Roemer, L. (2004). Multidimensional assessment of emotion regulation and dysregulation: Development, factor structure, and initial validation of the Difficulties in Emotion Regulation Scale. *Journal of Psychopathology and Behavioral Assessment, 36*, 41–54.

Gross, J. J., & John, O. P. (2003). Individual differences in two emotion regulation processes:

Implications for affect, relationships, and well-being. *Journal of Personality and Social Psychology, 85*, 348–362.

Gullone, E., & Taffe, J. (2012). The Emotion Regulation Questionnaire for Children and Adolescents (ERQ-CA): A psychometric evaluation. *Psychological Assessment, 24*(2), 409–417.

Hussong, A. M., & Hicks, R. E. (2003). Affect and peer context interactively impact adolescent substance use. *Journal of Abnormal Child Psychology, 31*, 413–426.

Jones, R. E., Leen-Feldner, E. W., Olatunji, B. O., Reardon, L. E., & Hawks, E. (2009). Psychometric properties of the Affect Intensity and Reactivity Measure adapted for Youth (AIR-Y). *Psychological Assessment, 21*(2), 162–175.

Kroon, N., Goudena, P. P., & Rispens, J. (1998). Thematic apperception tests for child and adolescent assessment: A practitioner's consumer guide. *Journal of Psychoeducational Assessment, 16*(2), 99–117.

Lane, R. D., & Garfield, D. A. S. (2005). Becoming aware of feelings: Integration of cognitive-developmental, neuroscientific, and psychoanalytic perspectives. *Neuro-Psychoanalysis, 7*, 5–30.

Lane, R. D., Quinlan, D. M., Schwartz, G. E., & Walker, P. A. (1990). The Levels of Emotional Awareness Scale: A cognitive-developmental measure of emotion. *Journal of Personality Assessment, 55*(1–2), 124–134.

Lane, R. D., & Schwartz, G. E. (1987). Levels of emotional awareness: A cognitive-developmental theory and its application to psychopathology. *American Journal of Psychiatry, 144*(2), 133–143.

Larsen, R. J. (2009). Affect intensity. In M. R. Leary & R. H. Hoyle (Eds.), *Handbook of individual differences in social behavior* (pp. 241–254). New York: Guilford Press.

Larsen, R. J., & Diener, E. (1987). Affect intensity as an individual difference characteristic: A review. *Journal of Research in Personality, 21*, 1–39.

Linehan, M. M. (1993). *Cognitive-behavioral treatment of borderline personality disorder.* New York: Guilford Press.

Mayer, J. D., Salovey, P., & Caruso, D. R. (1997). *Multifactor Emotional Intelligence Scale, Student Version*. Unpublished manuscript, Durham, NH.

Murray, H. A. (1943). *Thematic Apperception Test: Manual.* Cambridge, MA: Harvard University Press.

Nandrino, J. L., Baracca, M., Antoine, P., Paget, V., Bydlowski, S., & Carton, S. (2013). Level of emotional awareness in the general French population: Effects of gender, age, and education level. *International Journal of Psychology, 48*(6), 1072–1079.

Neumann, A., van Lier, P. A. C., Gratz, K. L., & Koot, H. M. (2010). Multidimensional assessment of emotion regulation difficulties in adolescents using the Difficulties in Emotion Regulation Scale. *Assessment, 17*(1), 138–149.

Nock, M. K., Wedig, M. M., Holmberg, E. B., & Hooley, J. M. (2008). The Emotion Reactivity Scale: Development, evaluation, and relation to self-injurious thoughts and behaviors. *Behavior Therapy, 39*(2), 107–116.

Pfeffier, S. I. (2001). Emotional intelligence: Popular but elusive construct. *Roeper Review, 23*(3), 138–149.

Schore, A. N. (2003). *Affect dysregulation and disorders of the self.* New York: Norton.

Sheeber, L. B., Allen, N. B., Leve, C., Davis, B., Shortt, J. W., & Katz, L. F. (2009). Dynamics of affective experience and behavior in depressed adolescents. *Journal of Child Psychology and Psychiatry, 50*(11), 1419–1427.

Shields, A. M., & Cicchetti, D. (1997). Emotion regulation and autonomy: The development and validation of two new criterion Q-sort scales. *Developmental Psychology, 33*, 906–916.

Subic-Wrana, C., Beutel, M. E., Brähler, E., Stöbel-Richter, Y., Knebel, A., Lane, R. D., & Wiltink, J. (2014). How is emotional awareness related to emotion regulation strategies and self-reported negative affect in the general population? *PLoS ONE, 9*(3), e91846.

Trinidad, D. R., Unger, J. B., Chou, C. P., Azen, S. P., & Johnson, C. A. (2004). Emotional intelligence and smoking risk factors in adolescents: Interactions on smoking intentions. *Journal of Adolescent Health, 34*(1), 46–55.

Tsang, K. L., Wong, P. Y., & Lo, S. K. (2012). Assessing psychosocial well-being of adolescents: A systematic review of measuring instruments. *Child: Care, Health and Development, 38*(5), 629–646.

Watson, D., & Clark, L. A. (1994). *The PANAS-X: Manual for the Positive and Negative Affect Schedule—Expanded Form.* Iowa City: University of Iowa.

Weinberg, A., & Klonsky, E. D. (2009). Measurement of emotion dysregulation in adolescents. *Psychological Assessment, 21*(4), 616–621.

Westen, D. (1991). Social cognition and object relations. *Psychological Bulletin, 109*, 429–455.

Westen, D., Ludolph, P., Block, J., Wixom, J., & Wiss, C. (1990). Developmental history and object relations in psychiatrically disturbed adolescent girls. *American Journal of Psychiatry, 147*, 1061–1068.

Woitaszewski, S. A., & Aalsma, M. C. (2004). The contribution of emotional intelligence to the social and academic success of gifted adolescents as measured by the Multifactor Emotional Intelligence Scale—Adolescent Version. *Roeper Review, 27*, 25–30.

Yurgelun-Todd, D. (2007). Emotional and cognitive changes during adolescence. *Current Opinion in Neurobiology, 17*(2), 251–257.

Zeman, J., Cassano, M., Perry-Parrish, C., & Stegall, S. (2006). Emotion regulation in children and adolescents. *Journal of Developmental and Behavioral Pediatrics, 27*(2), 155–168.

3. Capacity for Mentalization and Reflective Functioning

Allen, J. G., Fonagy, P., & Bateman, A. W. (2008). *Mentalizing in clinical practice.* Washington, DC: American Psychiatric Publishing.

Badoud, D., Luyten, P., Fonagy, P., Eliez, S., & Debbané, M. (2015). The French version of the Reflective Functioning Questionnaire: Validity data for adolescents and adults and its association with non-suicidal self-injury. *PLoS ONE, 10*(12), e0145892.

Barchard, K. A., Bajgar, J., Leaf, D. E., & Lane, R. D. (2010). Computer scoring of the Levels of Emotional Awareness Scale. *Behavior Research Methods, 42*(2), 586–595.

Bateman, A. W., & Fonagy, P. (2012). *Handbook of mentalizing in mental health practice.* Arlington, VA: American Psychiatric Publishing.

Blakemore, S. J. (2012). Development of the social brain in adolescence. *Journal of the Royal Society of Medicine, 105*(3), 111–116.

Carlson, S. M., Moses, L. J., & Brenton, C. (2002). How specific is the relationship between executive functioning and theory of mind?: Contributions of inhibitory control and working memory. *Infant and Child Development, 11,* 73–92.

Cartwright-Hatton, S., Mather, A., Illingworth, C., Brocki, J., Harrington, R., & Wells, A. (2004). Development and preliminary validation of the Meta-Cognitions Questionnaire—Adolescent Version. *Journal of Anxiety Disorders, 18,* 411–422.

Cartwright-Hatton, S., & Wells, A. (1997). Beliefs about worry and intrusions: The Meta-Cognitions Questionnaire and its correlates. *Journal of Anxiety Disorders, 11*(3), 279–296.

Casey, B. J., Getz, S., & Galvan, A. (2008). The adolescent brain. *Developmental Review, 28*(1), 62–77.

Dziobek, I., Fleck, S., Kalbe, E., Rogers, K., Hassenstab, J., Brand, M., . . . Convit, A. (2006). Introducing MASC: A movie for the assessment of social cognition. *Journal of Autism and Developmental Disorders, 36,* 623–636.

Fonagy, P., & Target, M. (2006). The mentalization-focused approach to self-pathology. *Journal of Personality Disorders, 20*(6), 544–76.

Fonagy, P., Target, M., Steele, H., & Steele, M. (1998). *Reflective Functioning Scale manual.* Unpublished manuscript.

Ha, C., Sharp, C., Ensink, K., Fonagy, P., & Cirino, P. (2013). The measurement of reflective function in adolescents with and without borderline traits. *Journal of Adolescence, 36*(6), 1215–1223.

Jolliffe, D., & Farrington, D. P. (2006). Development and validation of the Basic Empathy Scale. *Journal of Adolescence, 29*(4), 589–611.

Lane, R. D., Quinlan, D. M., Schwartz, G. E., Walker, P. A., & Zeilin, S. B. (1990). The Levels of Emotional Awareness Scale: A cognitive-developmental measure of emotion. *Journal of Personality Assessment, 55,* 124–134.

Lane, R. D., & Schwartz, G. E. (1987). Levels of emotional awareness: A cognitive-developmental theory and its application to psychopathology. *American Journal of Psychiatry, 144,* 113–143.

Luyten, P., Fonagy, P., Lowyck, B., & Vermote, R. (2012). Assessment of mentalization. In A. W. Bateman & P. Fonagy (Eds.), *Handbook of mentalizing in mental health practice* (pp. 43–66). Washington, DC: American Psychiatric Press.

Nandrino, J. L., Baracca, M., Antoine, P., Paget, V., Bydlowski, S., & Carton, S. (2013). Level of emotional awareness in the general French population: Effects of gender, age, and education level. *International Journal of Psychology, 48*(6), 1072–1079.

Parling, T., Mortazavi, M., & Ghaderi, A. (2010). Alexithymia and emotional awareness in anorexia nervosa: Time for a shift in the measurement of the concept? *Eating Behaviors, 11*(4), 205–120.

Pratt, B. M. (2006). *Emotional intelligence and the emotional brain: A battery of tests of ability applied with high school students and adolescents with high-functioning autistic spectrum disorders.* Unpublished doctoral dissertation, University of Sydney, Sydney, Australia.

Preißler, S., Dziobek, I., Ritter, K., Heekeren, H. R., & Roepke, S. (2010). Social cognition in borderline personality disorder: Evidence for disturbed recognition of the emotions, thoughts, and intentions of others. *Frontiers in Behavioral Neuroscience, 4,* 1–8.

Rothschild-Yakar, L., Levy-Shiff, R., Fridman-Balaban, R., Gur, E., & Stein, D. (2010). Mentalization and relationships with parents as predictors of eating disordered behavior. *Journal of Nervous and Mental Disease, 198*(7), 501–507.

Rutherford, H. J., Wareham, J. D., Vrouva, I., Mayes, L. C., Fonagy, P., & Potenza, M. N. (2012). Sex differences moderate the relationship between adolescent language and mentalization. *Personality Disorders, 3*(4), 393–405.

Sharp, C., Pane, H., Ha, C., Venta, A., Patel, B., Sturek, J., & Fonagy, P. (2011). Theory of mind and emotion regulation difficulties in adolescents with borderline traits. *Journal of the American Academy of Child and Adolescent Psychiatry, 50,* 563–573.

Sharp, C., Williams, L., Ha, C., Baumgardner, J., Michonski, J., Seals, R., . . . Fonagy, P. (2009). The development of a mentalization-based outcomes and research protocol for an adolescent in-patient unit. *Bulletin of the Menninger Clinic, 73*, 311–338.

Siegel, D. J. (2012). *The developing mind: How relationships and the brain interact to shape who we are* (2nd ed.). New York: Guilford Press.

Sterck, E., & Begeer, S. (2010). Theory of mind: Specialized capacity or emergent property? *European Journal of Developmental Psychology, 7*, 1–16.

Subic-Wrana, C., Beutel, M. E., Brähler, E., Stöbel-Richter, Y., Knebel, A., Lane, R. D., & Wiltink, J. (2014). How is emotional awareness related to emotion regulation strategies and self-reported negative affect in the general population? *PLoS ONE, 9*(3), e91846.

Vrouva, I., & Fonagy, P. (2009). Development of the Mentalizing Stories for Adolescents (MSA). *Journal of the American Psychoanalytic Association, 57*(5), 1174–1179.

Vrouvra, I., Target, M., & Ensink, K. (2012) Measuring mentalization in children and young people. In N. Midgley & I. Vrouvra (Eds.), *Minding the child: Mentalization-based interventions with children, young people and their families* (pp. 54–76). London: Routledge.

Westen, D., Lohr, N., Silk, K. R., & Kerber, K. (1985). *Measuring object relations and social cognition using the TAT: Scoring manual.* Unpublished manuscript, University of Michigan, Ann Arbor, MI.

Westen, D., Lohr, N., Silk, K. R., & Kerber, K. (1990). Object relations and social cognition in borderlines, major depressives, and normals: A Thematic Apperception Test analysis. *Psychological Assessment, 2*(4), 355–364.

4. Capacity for Differentiation and Integration

Blatt, S. J. (2004). *Experiences of depression: Theoretical, clinical, and research perspectives.* Washington, DC: American Psychological Association.

Blatt, S. J., & Blass, R. B. (1996). Relatedness and self-definition: A dialectic model of personality development. In G. G. Noam & K. W. Fischer (Eds.), *Development and vulnerabilities in close relationships* (pp. 309–338). Hillsdale, NJ: Erlbaum.

Blatt, S. J., D'Afflitti, J. P., & Quinlan, D. M. (1976). *Depressive Experiences Questionnaire.* New Haven, CT: Yale University Press.

Blatt, S. J., Schaffer, C. E., Bers, S. A., & Quinlan, D. M. (1992). Psychometric properties of the Depressive Experiences Questionnaire for Adolescents. *Journal of Personality Assessment, 59*(1), 82–98.

Blatt, S. J., Zohar, A. H., Quinlan, D. M., Zuroff, D. C., & Mongrain, M. (1995). Subscales within the dependency factor of the Depressive Experiences Questionnaire. *Journal of Personality Assessment, 64*, 319–339.

Blatt, S. J., & Zuroff, D. C. (1992). Interpersonal relatedness and self-definition: Two prototypes for depression. *Clinical Psychology Review, 12*, 527–562.

DeFife, J. A., Goldberg, M., & Westen D. (2015). Dimensional assessment of self- and interpersonal functioning in adolescents: Implications for DSM-5's general definition of personality disorder. *Journal of Personality Disorders, 29*(2), 248–260.

Erikson, E. H. (1968). *Identity: Youth and crisis.* New York: Norton.

Eudell-Simmons, E. M., Stein, M. B., DeFife, J. A., & Hilsenroth, M. J. (2005). Reliability and validity of the Social Cognition and Object Relations Scale (SCORS) in the assessment of dream narratives. *Journal of Personality Assessment, 85*(3), 325–333.

Fichman, L., Koestner, R., & Zuroff, D. C. (1994). Depressive styles in adolescence: Assessment, relation to social functioning, and developmental trends. *Journal of Youth and Adolescence, 23*, 315–330.

Goth, K., Foelsch, P., Schlüter-Müller, S., Birkhölzer, M., Jung, E., Pick, O., & Schmeck, K. (2012a). Assessment of identity development and identity diffusion in adolescence—Theoretical basis and psychometric properties of the self-report questionnaire AIDA. *Child and Adolescent Psychiatry and Mental Health, 6*(1), 27.

Goth, K., Foelsch, P., Schlüter-Müller, S., & Schmeck, K. (2012b). *AIDA: A self report questionnaire for measuring identity in adolescence—Short manual.* Basel, Switzerland: Child and Adolescent Psychiatric Hospital, Psychiatric University Hospitals Basel.

Haggerty, G., Blanchard, M., Baity, M. R., DeFife, J. A., Stein, M. B., Siefert, C. J., . . . Zodan, J. (2015). Clinical validity of a dimensional assessment of self- and interpersonal functioning in adolescent inpatients. *Journal of Personality Assessment, 97*(1), 3–12.

Jung, E., Pick, O., Schlüter-Müller, S., Schmeck, K., & Goth, K. (2013). Identity development in adolescents with mental problems. *Child and Adolescent Psychiatry and Mental Health, 7*, 26.

Kassin, M., De Castro, F., Arango, I., & Goth, K. (2013). Psychometric properties of a culture-adapted Spanish version of AIDA (Assessment of Identity Development in Adolescence) in Mexico. *Child and Adolescent Psychiatry and Mental Health, 7*, 25.

Klimstra, T. A., Luyckx, K., Branje, S., Teppers, E., Goossens, L., & Meeus, W. H. (2013). Personality traits, interpersonal identity, and relationship stability: Longitudinal linkages in late adolescence and young adulthood. *Journal of Youth and Adolescence, 42*(11), 1661–1673.

Kroger, J. (2004). *Identity in adolescence: The balance between self and other.* London: Psychology Press.

Kroger, J., Martinussen, M., & Marcia, J. E. (2010). Identity status change during adolescence and young adulthood: A meta-analysis. *Journal of Adolescence, 33*, 683–698.

Leary, M. R., & Tangney, J. P. (Eds.). (2012). *Handbook of self and identity* (2nd ed.). New York: Guilford Press.

Marcia, J. E., (1966). Development and validation of ego identity status, *Journal of Personality and Social Psychology, 3*, 551–558.

McBride, C., Zuroff, D., Bacchiochi, J., & Bagby, M. R. (2006). Depressive Experiences Questionnaire: Does it measure maladaptive and adaptive forms of dependency? *Social Behavior and Personality, 34*(1), 1–16.

Meeus, W., van de Schoot, R., Keijsers, L., Schwartz, S. J., & Branje, S. (2010). On the progression and stability of adolescent identity formation: A five-wave longitudinal study in early-to-middle and middle-to-late adolescence. *Child Development, 81*(5), 1565–1581.

Shahar, G., & Priel, B. (2003). Active vulnerability, adolescent distress, and the mediating–suppressing role of life events. *Personality and Individual Differences, 35*, 199–218.

Stein, M., Hilsenroth, M., Slavin-Mulford, J., & Pinsker, J. (2011). *Social Cognition and Object Relations Scale: Global Rating Method (SCORS-G)* (4th ed.). Unpublished manuscript, Massachusetts General Hospital and Harvard Medical School, Boston, MA.

Westen, D. (1985). *Social Cognition and Object Relations Scale: Original manual to use for training.* Ann Arbor: Department of Psychology, University of Michigan.

Westen, D., Betan, E., & DeFife, J. A. (2011). Identity disturbance in adolescence: Associations with borderline personality disorder. *Development and Psychopathology, 23*(1), 305–313.

Wilkinson-Ryan, T., & Westen, D. (2000). Identity disturbance in borderline personality disorder: An empirical investigation. *American Journal of Psychiatry, 157*, 528–541.

Zuroff, D. C., Quinland, D. M., & Blatt, S. J. (1990). Psychometric properties of the Depressive Experience Questionnaire in a college population. *Journal of Personality Assessment, 55*, 65–72.

5. Capacity for Relationships and Intimacy

Ammaniti, M., Fontana, A., Kernberg, O., Clarkin, A., & Clarkin, J. (2011). *Interview of Personality Organization Processes in Adolescence (IPOP-A).* Unpublished manuscript, Sapienza University of Rome and Weill Medical College of Cornell University, New York.

Ammaniti, M., Fontana, A., & Nicolais, G. (2015). Borderline personality disorder in adolescence through the lens of the Interview of Personality Organization Processes in Adolescence (IPOP-A): Clinical use and implications. *Journal of Infant, Child, and Adolescent Psychotherapy, 14*, 1–15.

Brenning, K., Soenens, B., Braet, C., & Bosmans, G. (2011). An adaptation of the Experiences in Close Relationships Scale—Revised for use with children and adolescents. *Journal of Social and Personal Relationships, 28*(8), 1048–1072.

Chen, X., & Graham, S. (2012). Close relationships and attributions for peer victimization among late adolescents. *Journal of Adolescence, 35*(6), 1547–1556.

Cozolino, L. (2006). *The neuroscience of human relationships: Attachment and the developing social brain.* New York: Norton.

Feddern Donbaek, D., & Elklit, A. (2014). A validation of the Experiences in Close Relationships—Relationship Structures scale (ECR-RS) in adolescents. *Attachment and Human Development, 16*(1), 58–76.

Fraley, R. C., Waller, N. G., & Brennan, K. A. (2000). An item-response theory analysis of self-report measures of adult attachment. *Journal of Personality and Social Psychology, 78*, 350–365.

Furman, W., & Buhrmester, D. (1985). Children's perceptions of the personal relationships in their social networks. *Developmental Psychology, 21*, 1016–1024.

Gratz, K., & Roemer, L. (2004). Multidimensional assessment of emotion regulation and dysregulation: Development, factor structure, and initial validation of the Difficulties in Emotion Regulation Scale. *Journal of Psychopathology and Behavioral Assessment, 26*, 41–54.

Hopwood, C. J., Pincus, A. L., DeMoor, R. M., & Koonce, E. A. (2008). Psychometric characteristics of Inventory Problems—Short Circumplex (IIP-SC) with college students. *Journal of Personality Assessment, 90*(6), 615–618.

Horowitz, L. M., Alden, L. E., Wiggins, J. S., & Pincus, A. L. (2000). *Inventory of Interpersonal Problems.* London: Psychological Corporation.

Hutman, H., Konieczna, K. A., Kerner, E., Armstrong, C. R., & Fitzpatrick, M. (2012). Indicators of relatedness in adolescent male groups: Toward a qualitative description. *The Qualitative Report, 17*(30), 1–23.

Imamoglu, E. O. (2003). Individuation and relatedness: Not opposing but distinct and complementary. *Genetic, Social, and General Psychology Monographs, 129*(4), 367–402.

Kernberg, O. F. (1998). The diagnosis of narcissistic and antisocial pathology in adolescence. *Annals of the American Society of Adolescent Psychiatry, 22*, 169–186.

Kernberg, P., Weiner, A., & Bardenstein, K. (2000). *Personality disorders in children and adolescence.* New York: Basic Books.

Millon, T., Millon, C., & Davis, R. (1993). *Millon Adolescent Clinical Inventory (MACI) manual.* Minneapolis, MN: National Computer Systems.

Oudekerk, B. A., Allen, J. P., Hessel, E. T., & Molloy, L. E. (2015). The cascading development of autonomy and relatedness from adolescence to adulthood. *Child Development, 86*(2), 472–485.

Sibley, C. G., Fischer, R., & Liu, J. H. (2005). Reliability and validity of the Revised Experiences in Close Relationships (ECR-R) self-report measure of adult romantic attachment. *Personality and Social Psychology Bulletin, 31*(11), 1524–1536.

Soldz, S., Budman, S., Demby, A., & Merry, J. (1995). A short form of the Inventory of Interpersonal Problems Circumplex scales. *Assessment, 2*, 53–63.

Spilt, J. L., Van Lier, P. A., Branje, S. J., Meeus, W., & Koot, H. M. (2015). Discrepancies in perceptions of close relationships of young adolescents: A risk for psychopathology? *Journal of Youth and Adolescence, 44*(4), 910–921.

Stein, M., Hilsenroth, M., Slavin-Mulford, J., & Pinsker, J. (2011). *Social Cognition and Object Relations Scale: Global Rating Method (SCORS-G)* (4th ed.). Unpublished manuscript, Massachusetts General Hospital and Harvard Medical School, Boston, MA.

Westen, D. (1985). *Social Cognition and Object Relations Scale: Original manual to use for training.* Ann Arbor: Department of Psychology, University of Michigan.

Wilkinson, R. B. (2011). Measuring attachment dimensions in adolescents: Development and validation of the Experiences In Close Relationships—Revised—General Short Form. *Journal of Relationships Research, 2*, 53–62.

6. Capacity for Self-Esteem Regulation and Quality of Internal Experience

Aasland, A., & Diseth, T. H. (1999). Can the Self-Perception Profile for Adolescents (SPPA) be used as an indicator of psychosocial outcome in adolescents with chronic physical disorders? *European Child and Adolescent Psychiatry, 8*(2), 78–85.

DuBois, D. L., Felner, R. D., Brand, S., Phillips, R. S. C., & Lease, A. M. (1996). Early adolescent self-esteem: A developmental-ecological framework and assessment strategy. *Journal of Research on Adolescence, 6*, 543–579.

DuBois, D. L., Tevendale, H. D., Burk-Braxton, C., Swenson, L. P., & Hardesty, J. L. (2000). Self-system influences during early adolescence: Investigation of an integrative model. *Journal of Early Adolescence, 20*, 12–43.

Finzi-Dottan, R., & Karu, T. (2006). From emotional abuse in childhood to psychopathology in adulthood: A path mediated by immature defense mechanisms and self-esteem. *Journal of Nervous and Mental Disease, 194*(8), 616–621.

Greenfield, B., Filip, C., Schiffrin, A., Bond, M., Amsel, R., & Zhang, X. (2013). The Scales of Psychological Capacities: Adaptation to an adolescent population. *Psychotherapy Research, 23*(2), 232–246.

Guerin, F., Marsh, H. W., & Famose, J. P. (2003). Construct validation of the Self-Description Questionnaire II with a French sample. *European Journal of Psychological Assessment, 19*, 142–150.

Harter, S. (1988). *Manual for the Self-Perception Profile for Adolescents.* Denver, CO: University of Denver.

Horvath, S., & Morf, C. C. (2010). To be grandiose or not to be worthless: Different routes to self-enhancement for narcissism and self-esteem. *Journal of Research in Personality, 44*(5), 585–592.

Huber, D., Brandl, T., & Klug, G. (2004). The Scales of Psychological Capacities: Measuring beyond symptoms. *Psychotherapy Research, 14*(1), 89–106.

Huber, D., Henrich, G., & Klug, G. (2005). The Scales of Psychological Capacities: Measuring change in psychic structure. *Psychotherapy Research, 15*(4), 445–456.

Hughes, A., Galbraith, D., & White, D. (2011). Perceived competence: A common core for self-efficacy and self-concept? *Journal of Personality Assessment, 93*(3), 278–289.

Isomaa, R., Väänänen, J. M., Fröjd, S., Kaltiala-Heino, R., & Marttunen, M. (2013). How low is low?: Low self-esteem as an indicator of internalizing psychopathology in adolescence. *Health Education and Behavior, 40*(4), 392–399.

Marsh, H. W., Ellis, L. A., Parada, R. H., Richards, G., & Heubeck, B. G. (2005). A short version of the Self Description Questionnaire II: Operationalizing criteria for short-form evaluation with new applications of confirmatory factor analyses. *Psychological Assessment, 17*(1), 81–102.

Marsh, H. W., Hau, K. T., & Kong, C. K. (2002). Multilevel causal ordering of academic self-concept and achievement: Influence of language of instruction (English compared with Chinese) for Hong Kong students. *American Educational Research Journal, 39*(3), 727–763.

Marsh, H. W., Parada, R. H., & Ayotte, V. (2004). A multidimensional perspective of relations between self-concept (Self Description Questionnaire II) and adolescent mental health (Youth Self-Report). *Psychological Assessment, 16*, 27–41.

Marsh, H. W., Plucker, J. A., & Stocking, V. B. (2001). The Self-Description Questionnaire II and gifted students: Another look at Plucker, Taylor, Callahan, and Tomchin's (1997) "Mirror, mirror on the wall." *Educational and Psychological Measurement, 61*, 976–996.

Marsh, H. W. (1992). *SDQ II: Manual.* Sydney, Australia: Self Research Centre, University of Western Sydney.

Molloy, L. E., Ram, N., & Gest, S. D. (2011). The storm and stress (or calm) of early adolescent self-concepts: Within- and between-subjects variability. *Developmental Psychology, 47*(6), 1589–1607.

Nishikawa, S., Norlander, T., Fransson, P., & Sundbom, E. (2007). A cross-cultural validation of adolescent self-concept in two cultures: Japan and Sweden. *Social Behavior and Personality, 35*, 269–286.

O'Brien, E. J., & Epstein, S. (1998). *MSEI: The Multidimensional Self-Esteem Inventory professional manual.* Odessa, FL: Psychological Assessment Resources.

Rosenberg, M. (1965). *Society and the adolescent self-image.* Princeton, NJ: Princeton University Press.

Rudasill, K. M., & Callahan, C. M. (2008). Psychometric characteristics of the Harter Self-Perception Profiles for Adolescents and Children for use with gifted populations. *Gifted Child Quarterly, 52*(1), 70–86.

Shavelson, R. J., Hubner, J. J., & Stanton, G. C. (1976). Self-concept: Validation of construct interpretations. *Review of Educational Research, 46*(3), 407–441.

Short, J. L., Sandler, I. N., & Roosa, M. W. (1996). Adolescents' perceptions of social support: The role of esteem enhancing and esteem threatening relationships. *Journal of Social and Clinical Psychology, 15*(4), 397–341.

Siegel, D. J. (2012). *The developing mind: How relationships and the brain interact to shape who we are* (2nd ed.). New York: Guilford Press.

Tafarodi, R. W., & Milne, A. B. (2002). Decomposing global self-esteem. *Journal of Personality, 70*(4), 443–483.

Wichstrøm, L. (1995). Harter's Self-Perception Profile for Adolescents: Reliability, validity, and evaluation of the question format. *Journal of Personality Assessment, 65*(1), 100–116.

7. Capacity for Impulse Control and Regulation

Aluja, A., & Blanch, A. (2011). Neuropsychological Behavioral Inhibition System (BIS) and Behavioral Approach System (BAS) assessment: A shortened Sensitivity to Punishment and Sensitivity to Reward Questionnaire version (SPSRQ-20). *Journal of Personality Assessment, 93*(6), 628–636.

Blakemore, S. J. (2012). Imaging brain development: The adolescent brain. *NeuroImage, 61*, 397–406.

Blakemore, S. J., & Choudhury, S. (2006). Development of the adolescent brain: Implications for executive function and social cognition. *Journal of Child Psychology and Psychiatry, 47*, 296–312.

Blakemore, S. J., & Robbins, T. W. (2012). Decision-making in the adolescent brain. *Nature Neuroscience, 15*(9), 1184–1191.

Burrus, C. (2013). Developmental trajectories of abuse: An hypothesis for the effects of early childhood maltreatment on dorsolateral prefrontal cortical development. *Medical Hypotheses, 81*, 826–829.

Caci, H., Deschaux, O., & Bayle, F. J. (2007). Psychometric properties of the French versions of the BIS/BAS scales and the SPSRQ. *Personality and Individual Differences, 42*, 987–998.

Carver, C. S., & White, T. L. (1994). Behavioral inhibition, behavioral activation, and affective responses to impending reward and punishment: The BIS/BAS scales. *Journal of Personality and Social Psychology, 67*, 319–333.

Cooper, A., & Gomez, R. (2008). The development of a short form of the Sensitivity to Punishment and Sensitivity to Reward Questionnaire. *Journal of Individual Differences, 29*(2), 90–104.

D'Acremont, M., & Van der Linden, M. (2005). Adolescent impulsivity: Findings from a community sample. *Journal of Youth and Adolescence. 34*(5), 427–435.

Dalley, J. W., Everitt, B. J., & Robbins, T. W. (2011). Impulsivity, compulsivity, and top-down cognitive control. *Neuron, 69*, 680–694.

Duckworth, A. L., Kim, B., & Tsukayama. E. (2012). Life stress impairs self-control in early adolescence. *Frontiers in Psychology, 3*, 608.

Farley, J. P., & Kim-Spoon, J. (2014). The development of adolescent self-regulation: Reviewing the role of parent, peer, friend, and romantic relationships. *Journal of Adolescence, 37*(4), 433–440.

Fonagy, P., Gergely, G., Jurist, E. L., & Target, M. (2002). *Affect regulation, mentalization, and the development of the self.* New York: Other Press.

Fossati, A., Barratt, E. S., Acquarini, E., & Di Ceglie, A. (2002). Psychometric properties of an adolescent version of the Barratt Impulsiveness Scale–11 for a sample of Italian high school students. *Perceptual and Motor Skills, 95*(2), 621–635.

Franken, I. H. A., & Muris, P. (2006). BIS/BAS personality characteristics and college students' substance use. *Personality and Individual Differences, 40*, 1497–1503.

Franken, I. H. A., Muris, P., & Rassin, E. (2005). Psychometric properties of the Dutch BIS/BAS Scales. *Journal of Psychopathology and Behavioral Assessment, 27*(1), 25–30.

Galván, A. (2014). Insights about adolescent behavior, plasticity, and policy from neuroscience research. *Neuron, 83*(2), 262–265.

Giedd, J. N. (2008). The teen brain: Insights from neuroimaging. *Journal of Adolescent Health, 42*, 335–343.

Gruber, J., Gilbert, K. E., Youngstrom, E., Youngstrom, J. K., Feeny, N. C., & Findling, R. L. (2013). Reward dysregulation and mood symptoms in an adolescent outpatient sample. *Journal of Abnormal Child Psychology, 41*(7), 1053–1065.

Hartmann, A. S., Rief, W., & Hilbert, A. (2011). Psychometric properties of the German version of the Barratt Impulsiveness Scale, Version 11 (BIS-11) for adolescents. *Perceptual and Motor Skills, 112*(2), 353–368.

Heubeck, B. G., Wilkinson, R. B., & Cologon, J. (1998). A second look at Carver and White's (1994) BIS/BAS scales. *Personality and Individual Differences, 2*(5), 785–800.

Luman, M., van Meel, C. S., Oosterlaan, J., & Geurts, H. M. (2012). Reward and punishment sensitivity in children with ADHD: Validating the Sensitivity to Punishment and Sensitivity to Reward Questionnaire for children (SPSRQ-C). *Journal of Abnormal Child Psychology, 40*(1), 145–157.

Matton, A., Goossens, L., Braet, C., & Vervaet, M. (2013). Punishment and reward sensitivity: Are naturally occurring clusters in these traits related to eating and weight problems in adolescents? *European Eating Disorders Review, 21*(3), 184–194.

O'Connor, R. M., Colder, C. R., & Hawk, L. W. (2004). Confirmatory factor analysis of the Sensitivity to Punishment and Sensitivity to Reward Questionnaire. *Personality and Individual Differences, 37*, 985–1002.

Ordaz, S. J., Foran, W., Velanova, K., & Luna, B. (2013). Longitudinal growth curves of brain function underlying inhibitory control through adolescence. *Journal of Neuroscience, 33*(46), 18109–18124.

Panwar, K., Rutherford, H. J., Mencl, W. E., Lacadie, C. M., Potenza, M. N., & Mayes L. C. (2014). Differential associations between impulsivity and risk-taking and brain activations underlying working memory in adolescents. *Addictive Behaviors, 39*(11), 1606–1621.

Patton, J. H., Stanford, M. S., & Barratt, E. S. (1995). Factor structure of the Barratt Impulsiveness Scale. *Journal of Clinical Psychology, 51*, 768–774.

Reynolds, B., Penfold, R. B., & Patak, M. (2008). Dimensions of impulsive behavior in adolescents: Laboratory behavioral assessments. *Experimental and Clinical Psychopharmacology, 16*(2), 124–131.

Richards, J. M., Plate, R. C., & Ernst, M. (2012). Neural systems underlying motivated behavior in adolescence: Implications for preventive medicine. *Preventive Medicine, 55*(Suppl.), S7–S16.

Schore, A. N. (2003). *Affect dysregulation and disorders of the self.* New York: Norton.

Steinberg, L. (2007). Risk taking in adolescence: New perspectives from brain and behavioral science. *Current Directions in Psychological Science, 15*(2), 55–59.

Steinberg, L. (2014). *Age of opportunity: Lessons from the new science of adolescence.* New York: Houghton Mifflin Harcourt.

Tangney, J. P., Baumeister, R. F., & Boone, A. L. (2004). High self-control predicts good adjustment, less pathology, better grades, and interpersonal success. *Journal of Personality, 72*(2), 271–324.

Torrubia, R., Avila, C., Molto, J., & Caseras, X. (2001). The Sensitivity to Punishment and Sensitivity to Reward Questionnaire (SPSRQ) as a measure of Gray's anxiety and impulsivity dimensions. *Personality and Individual Differences, 3*, 837–862.

Urben, S., Suter, M., Pihet, S., Straccia, C., & Stéphan, P. (2014). Constructive thinking skills and impulsivity dimensions in conduct and substance use disorders: Differences and relationships in an adolescents' sample. *Psychiatric Quarterly, 86*(2), 207–218.

Van der Linden, M., d'Acremont, M., Zermatten, A., Jermann, F., Larøi, F., Willems, S., . . . Bechara, A. (2006). A French adaptation of the UPPS Impulsive Behavior Scale: Confirmatory factor analysis in a sample of undergraduate students. *European Journal of Psychological Assessment, 22*(1), 38–42.

von Diemen, L., Szobot, C. M., Kessler, F., & Pechansky, F. (2007). Adaptation and construct validation of the Barratt Impulsiveness Scale (BIS 11) to Brazilian Portuguese for use in adolescents. *Revista Brasileira de Psiquiatria, 29*(2), 153–156.

White, A. M. (2009). Understanding adolescent brain development and its implications for the clinician. *Adolescent Medicine: State of the Art Reviews, 20*, 73–90.

Whiteside, S. P., & Lynam, D. R. (2001). The five factor model and impulsivity: Using a structural model of personality to understand impulsivity. *Personality and Individual Differences, 30*(4), 669–689.

Whiteside, S. P., Lynam, D. R., Miller, J. D., & Reynolds, S. K. (2005). Validation of the UPPS Impulsive Behaviour Scale: A four-factor model of impulsivity. *European Journal of Personality, 19*, 559–574.

Yu, R., Branje, S. J., Keijsers, L., & Meeus, W. H. (2011). Psychometric characteristics of Carver and White's BIS/BAS scales in Dutch adolescents and their mothers. *Journal of Personality Assessment, 93*(5), 500–507.

8. Capacity for Defensive Functioning

Andrews, G., Singh, M., & Bond, M. (1993). The Defense Style Questionnaire. *Journal of Nervous and Mental Disease, 181*(4), 246–256.

Araujo, K., Ryst, E., & Steiner, H. (1999). Adolescent defense style and life stressors. *Child Psychiatry and Human Development, 30*(1), 19–28.

Cramer, P. (1987). The development of defense mechanisms. *Journal of Personality, 55*, 597–614.

Cramer, P. (2007). Longitudinal study of defense mechanisms: Late childhood to late adolescence. *Journal of Personality, 75*(1), 1–24.

Di Giuseppe, M. G., Perry, J. C., Petraglia, J., Janzen, J., & Lingiardi, V. (2014). Development of a Q-sort version of the Defense Mechanism Rating Scales (DMRS-Q) for clinical use. *Journal of Clinical Psychology, 70*, 452–465.

Erickson, S., Feldman, S., & Steiner, H. (1997). Defense reactions and coping strategies in normal adolescents. *Child Psychiatry and Human Development, 28*(1), 45–56.

Evans, D. W., & Seaman, J. L. (2000). Developmental aspects of psychological defenses: Their relation to self-complexity, self-perception and symptomatology in adolescents. *Child Psychiatry and Human Development, 30*, 237–254.

Feldman, S., Araujo, K., & Steiner, H. (1996). Defense mechanisms in adolescents as a function of age, sex, and mental health status. *Journal of the American Academy of Child and Adolescent Psychiatry, 35*, 1344–1354.

Gleser, G. C., & Ihilevich, D. (1969). An objective instrument for measuring defense mechanisms. *Journal of Consulting and Clinical Psychology, 33*(1), 51–60.

Ihilevich, D., & Gleser, G. C. (1986). *Defense mechanisms.* Owosso, MI: DMI Associates.

Laor, N., Wolmer, L., & Cicchetti, D. V. (2001). The comprehensive assessment of defense style: Measuring defense mechanisms in children and adolescents. *Journal of Nervous and Mental Disease, 189*(6), 360–368.

Muris, P., Winands, D., & Horselenberg, R. (2003). Defense styles, personality traits, and psychopathological symptoms in nonclinical adolescents. *Journal of Nervous and Mental Disease, 191*(12), 771–780.

Noam, G. G., & Recklitis, C. J. (1990). The relationship between defenses and sympoms in adolescent psychopathology. *Journal of Personality Assessment, 54*, 311–327.

Perry, J. C. (1990). *The Defense Mechanism Rating Scale manual* (5th ed.). Cambridge, MA: Author.

Plattner, B., Silvermann, M. A., Redlich, A. D., Carrion, V. G., Feucht M, . . . Steiner, H. (2003). Pathways to dissociation: Intrafamilial versus extrafamilial trauma in juvenile delinquents. *Journal of Nervous and Mental Disease, 191*, 781–788.

Prunas, A., Preti, E., Huemer, J., Shaw, R. J., & Steiner, H. (2014). Defensive functioning and psychopathology: A study with the REM-71. *Comprehensive Psychiatry, 55*(7), 1696–1702.

Recklitis, C. J., Noam, G. G., & Borst, S. R. (1992). Adolescent suicide and defensive style. *Suicide and Life-Threatening Behavior, 22*(3), 374–387.

Recklitis, C. J., Yap, L., & Noam, G. G. (1995). Development of a short form of the adolescent version of the Defense Mechanisms Inventory. *Journal of Personality Assessment, 64*(2), 360–370.

Ruuttu, T., Pelkonen, M., Holi, M., Karlsson, L., Kiviruusu, O., Heilä, H., . . . Marttunen, M. (2006). Psychometric properties of the Defense Style Questionnaire (DSQ-40) in adolescents. *Journal of Nervous and Mental Disease, 194*(2), 98–105.

Schave, D., & Schave, B. (1989). *Early adolescence and the search for self: A developmental perspective.* New York: Praeger.

Steiner, H., Araujo, K., & Koopman, C. K. (2001). The Response Evaluation Measure (REM-71): A new instrument for the measurement of defenses in adults and adolescents. *American Journal of Psychiatry, 158*, 467–473.

Tuulio-Henriksson, A., Poikolainen, K., Aalto-Setala, T., & Lonnqvist, J. (1997). Psychological defense styles in late adolescence and young adulthood: A follow-up study. *Journal of the American Academy of Child and Adolescent Psychiatry, 36*(8), 1148–1153.

Wolmer, L., Laor, N., & Cicchetti, D. V. (2001). Validation of the Comprehensive Assessment of Defense Style (CADS): Mothers' and children's responses to the stresses of missile attacks. *Journal of Nervous and Mental Disease, 189*(6), 369–376.

9. Capacity for Adaptation, Resiliency, and Strength

Ahern, N. R., Kiehl, E. M., Sole, M. L., & Byers, J. (2006). A review of instruments measuring resilience. *Comprehensive Child and Adolescent Nursing, 29*(2), 103–125.

Alessandri, G., Luengo Kanacri, B. P., Eisenberg, N., Zuffianò, A., Milioni, M., Vecchione, M., & Caprara, G. V. (2014). Prosociality during the transition from late adolescence to young adulthood: The role of effortful control and ego-resiliency. *Personality and Social Psychology Bulletin, 40*(11), 1451–1465.

Alessandri, G., Vecchio, G., Steca, P., Caprara, M. G., & Caprara, G. V. (2008). A revised version of Kremen and Block's ego-resiliency scale in an Italian sample. *Testing, Psychometrics, Methodology in Applied Psychology, 14*, 1–19.

Charney, D. S. (2004). Psychobiological mechanisms of resilience and vulnerability: Implication for successful adaptation to extreme stress. *American Journal of Psychiatry, 161*, 195–216.

Deighton, J., Croudace, T., Fonagy, P., Brown, J., Patalay, P., & Wolpert, M. (2014). Measuring mental health and wellbeing outcomes for children and adolescents to inform practice and policy: A review of child self-report measures. *Child and Adolescent Psychiatry and Mental Health, 29*, 8–14.

Denckla, C. A., & Mancini, A. D. (2014). Multimethod assessment of resilience. In C. J. Hopwood & R. F. Bornstein (Eds.), *Multimethod clinical assessment* (pp. 254–282). New York: Guilford Press.

Duppong Hurley, K., Lambert, M. C., Epstein, M. H., & Stevens, A. (2014). Convergent validity of the Strength-Based Behavioral and Emotional Rating Scale with youth in a residential setting. *Journal of Behavioral Health Services and Research, 42*(3), 346–354.

Egeland, B., Carlson, E., & Sroufe, L. A. (1993). Resilience as a process. *Development and Psychology, 5*, 517–528.

Epstein, M. H., Mooney, P., Ryser, G., & Pierce, C. D. (2004). Validity and Reliability of the Behavioral and Emotional Rating Scale (2nd Edition): Youth Rating Scale. *Research on Social Work Practice, 14*(5), 358–367.

Epstein, M. (1999). The development and validation of a scale to assess the emotional and behavioral strengths of children and adolescents. *Remedial and Special Education, 20*(5), 258–262.

Epstein, M. H. (2004). *Behavioral and Emotional Rating Scale—Second Edition.* Austin, TX: PRO-ED.

Fraser, M., & Galinsky, M. (1997). *Toward a resilience-based model of practice.* Washington, DC: NASW Press.

Goodman, R. (1997). The Strengths and Difficulties Questionnaire: A research note. *Journal of Child Psychology and Psychiatry, 38*, 581–586.

Goodman, R., Meltzer, H., & Bailey, V. (1998). The Strengths and Difficulties Questionnaire: A pilot study on the validity of the self-report version. *European Child and Adolescent Psychiatry, 7*, 125–130.

Hennighausen, K. H., Hauser, S. T., Billings, R. L., Schultz, L. H., & Allen, J. P. (2004). Adolescent ego-development trajectories and young adult relationship outcomes. *Journal of Early Adolescence, 24*(1), 29–44.

Hjemdal, O., Aune, T., Reinfjell, T., Stiles, T. C., & Friborg, O. (2007). Resilience as a predictor of depressive symptoms: A correlational study with young adolescents. *Clinical Child Psychology and Psychiatry, 12*, 91–104.

Hjemdal, O., Friborg, O., Martinussen, M., & Rosenvinge, J. H. (2001). Preliminary results from the development and validation of a Norwegian scale for measuring adult resilience. *Journal of the Norwegian Psychological Association, 38*, 310–317.

Hjemdal, O., Friborg, O., Stiles, T. C., Martinussen, M., & Rosenvinge, J. H. (2006). A new scale for adolescent resilience: Grasping the protective resources behind healthy development. *Measuring and Evaluation in Counseling and Development, 39*, 84–96.

Jew, C. L. (1997). *Adolescent Resiliency Belief System Scale.* Thousand Oaks, CA: California Lutheran University.

Jew, C. L., Green, K. E., & Kroger, J. (1999). Development and validation of a resiliency measure. *Measurement and Validation in Counseling and Development, 2*, 75–90.

Letzring, T. D., Block, J., & Funder, D. C. (2005). Ego-control and ego-resiliency: Generalization of self-report scales based on personality descriptions from self, acquaintances, and clinicians. *Journal of Research in Personality, 39*, 395–422.

Luthar, S. S. (2006). Resilience in development: A synthesis of research across five decades. In D. Cicchetti & D. J. Cohen (Eds.), *Developmental psychopathology: Vol. 3. Risk, disorder, and adaptation* (pp. 739–795). Hoboken, NJ: Wiley.

Mrazek, P. J., & Mrazek, D. (1987). Resilience in child maltreatment victims: A conceptual exploration. *Child Abuse and Neglect, 11*, 357–365.

Nakaya, M., Oshio, A., & Kaneko, H. (2006). Correlations for Adolescent Resilience Scale with Big Five personality traits. *Psychological Reports, 98*(3), 927–930.

Oshio, A., Kaneko, H., Nagamine, S., & Nakaya, M. (2003). Construct validity of the Adolescent Resilience Scale. *Psychological Reports, 93*, 1217–1222.

Oshio, A., Nakaya, M., Kaneko, H., & Nagamine, S. (2002). Development and validation of an Adolescent Resilience Scale. *Japanese Journal of Counseling Science, 35*, 57–65.

Prince-Embury, S. (2008). The Resiliency Scale for Children and Adolescents, psychological symptoms, and clinical status in adolescents. *Canadian Journal of School Psychology, 23*, 41–56.

Prince-Embury, S., & Courville, T. (2008a). Comparison of one-, two-, and three-factor models of personal resiliency using the Resiliency Scales for Children and Adolescents. *Canadian Journal of School Psychology, 23*, 11–25.

Prince-Embury, S., & Courville, T. (2008b). Measurement invariance of the Resiliency Scales for Children and Adolescents with respect to sex and age cohorts. *Canadian Journal of School Psychology, 23*, 26–44.

Rutter, M. (2012). Resilience as a dynamic concept. *Development and Psychopathology, 24*, 335–344.

Smith-Osborne, A., & Whitehill Bolton, K. (2013). Assessing resilience: A review of measures across the life course. *Journal of Evidence-Based Social Work, 10*, 111–126.

Southwick, S. M., Litz, B. T., Charney, D., & Friedman, M. J. (Eds.). (2011) *Resilience and mental health: Challenges across the lifespan*. New York: Cambridge University Press.

Vecchione, M., Alessandri, G., Barbaranelli, C., & Gerbino, M. (2010). Stability and change of ego resiliency from late adolescence to young adulthood: A multiperspective study using the ER89-R Scale. *Journal of Personality Assessment, 92*(3), 212–221.

von Soest, T., Mossige, S., Stefansen, K., & Hjemdal, O. (2010). A validation study of the Resilience Scale for Adolescents (READ). *Journal of Psychopathology and Behavioural Assessment, 32*, 215–225.

Waaktaar, T., & Torgersen, S. (2009). How resilient are resilience scales?: The Big Five scales outperform resilience scales in predicting adjustment in adolescents. *Scandinavian Journal of Psychology, 51*(2), 157–163.

Wagnild, G. M., & Young, H. M. (1993). Development and psychometric evaluation of the Resilience Scale. *Journal of Nursing Measurement, 1*, 165–178.

Wardenaar, K. J., Wigman, J. T., Lin, A., Killackey, E., Collip, D., Wood, S. J., . . . Yung, A. R. (2013). Development and validation of a new measure of everyday adolescent functioning: The Multidimensional Adolescent Functioning Scale. *Journal of Adolescent Health, 52*(2), 195–200.

Werner, E., & Smith, R. (1992). *Overcoming the odds: High risk children from birth to adulthood.* Ithaca, NY: Cornell University Press.

10. Self-Observing Capacities (Psychological Mindedness)

Bagby, R. M., Parker, J. D. A., & Taylor, G. J. (1994). The twenty-item Toronto Alexithymia Scale: I. Item selection and cross validation of the factor structure. *Journal of Psychosomatic Research, 38*, 23–32.

Beitel, M., Ferrer, E., & Cecero, J. J. (2005). Psychological mindedness and awareness of self and others. *Journal of Clinical Psychology, 61*, 739–750.

Boylan, M. B. (2006). Psychological mindedness as a predictor of treatment outcome with depressed adolescents. *Dissertation Abstracts International: Section B Sciences and Engineering, 67*(6), 3479.

Cecero, J. J., Beitel, M., & Prout, T. (2008). Exploring the relationships among early maladaptive schemas, psychological mindedness and self-reported college adjustment. *Psychology and Psychotherapy, 81*(1), 105–118.

Cicchetti, D., Ackerman, B. P., & Izard, C. E. (1995). Emotions and emotion regulation in developmental psychopathology. *Development and Psychopathology. 7*, 1–10.

Conte, H. R., Ratto, R., & Karusa, T. B. (1996). The Psychological Mindedness Scale: Factor structure and relationship to outcome of psychotherapy. *Journal of Psychotherapy Practice and Research, 5*(3), 250–259.

Eastabrook, J. M., Flynn, J. J., & Hollenstein, T. (2013). Internalizing symptoms in female adolescents: Associations with emotional awareness and emotion regulation. *Journal of Child and Family Studies, 23*(3), 487–496.

Fonagy, P., Gergely, G., Jurist, E. L., & Target, M. (2002). *Affect regulation, mentalization, and the development of the self.* New York: Other Press.

Hatcher, R. L., & Hatcher, S. L. (1997). Assessing the psychological mindedness of children and adolescents. In M. McCallum & W. E. Piper (Eds.), *Psychological mindedness: A contemporary understanding* (pp. 59–75). Mahwah, NJ: Erlbaum.

Karukivi, M., Vahlberg, T., Pölönen, T., Filppu, T., & Saarijärvi, S. (2014). Does alexithymia expose to mental disorder symptoms in late adolescence?: A 4-year follow-up study. *General Hospital Psychiatry, 36*(6), 748–752.

Lane, R. D., Quinlan, D. M., Schwartz, G. E., Walker, P. A., & Zeitlin, S. B. (1990). The Levels of Emotional Awareness Scale: A cognitive-developmental measure of emotion. *Journal of Personality Assessment, 55*, 124–134.

McCallum, M., & Piper, W. E. (Eds.). (1997). *Psychological mindedness: A contemporary understanding.* Mahwah, NJ: Erlbaum.

Parker, J. D., Eastabrook, J. M., Keefer, K. V., & Wood, L. M. (2010). Can alexithymia be assessed in adolescents?: Psychometric properties of the 20-Item Toronto Alexithymia Scale in younger, middle, and older adolescents. *Psychological Assessment, 22*(4), 798–808.

Rieffe, C., Oosterveld, P., & Meerum Terwogt, M. (2006). An alexithymia questionnaire for children: Factorial and concurrent validation results. *Personality and Individual Differences, 40*(1), 123–133.

Roxas, A. S., & Glenwick, D. S. (2014). The relationship of psychological mindedness and general coping to psychological adjustment and distress in high-school adolescents. *Individual Differences Research, 12*(2), 38–49.

Shill, M. A., & Lumley, M. A. (2002). The Psychological Mindedness Scale: Factor structure, convergent validity and gender in a non-psychiatric sample. *Psychology and Psychotherapy, 75*, 131–150.

Speranza, M., Loas, G., Guilbaud, O., & Corcos, M. (2011). Are treatment options related to

alexithymia in eating disorders?: Results from a three-year naturalistic longitudinal study. *Biomedicine and Pharmacotherapy, 65*(8), 585–589.
Taylor, G. J., & Taylor, H. S. (1997). Alexithymia. In M. McCallum & W. E. Piper (Eds.), *Psychological mindedness: A contemporary understanding* (pp. 77–104). Mahwah, NJ: Erlbaum.

11. Capacity to Construct and Use Internal Standards and Ideals

Burnett, S., & Blakemore, S. J. (2009). The development of adolescent social cognition. *Annals of the New York Academy of Sciences, 1167*, 51–56.
Caravita, S. C., Sijtsema, J. J., Rambaran, J. A., & Gini, G. (2014). Peer influences on moral disengagement in late childhood and early adolescence. *Journal of Youth and Adolescence, 43*(2), 193–207.
Carlo, G., Eisenberg, N., & Knight, G. P. (1992). An objective measure of adolescents' prosocial moral reasoning. *Journal of Research on Adolescence, 2*(4), 331–349.
Daniel, E., Dys, S. P., Buchmann, M., & Malti, T. (2014). Developmental relations between sympathy, moral emotion attributions, moral reasoning, and social justice values from childhood to early adolescence. *Journal of Adolescence, 37*(7), 1201–1214.
De Caroli, M. E., Falanga, R., & Sagone, E. (2014). Prosocial behavior and moral reasoning in Italian adolescents and young adults. *Research in Psychology and Behavioral Sciences, 2*(2), 48–53.
Decety, J., & Howard, L. H. (2014). Emotion, morality, and the developing brain. In M. Mikulincer & P. R. Shaver (Eds.), *Mechanisms of social connection: From brain to group* (pp. 105–122). Washington, DC: American Psychological Association.
Eisenberg, N., Carlo, G., Murphy, B., & Van Court, P. (1995). Prosocial development in late adolescence: A longitudinal study. *Child Development, 66*(4), 1179–1197.
Eisenberg-Berg, N., & Mussen, P. (1978). Empathy and moral development in adolescence. *Developmental Psychology, 14*(2), 185–186.
Eisenberg, N., Cumberland, A., Guthrie, I. K., Murphy, B. C., & Shepard, S. A. (2005). Age changes in prosocial responding and moral reasoning in adolescence and early adulthood. *Journal of Research on Adolescence, 15*(3), 235–260.
Forth, A., Kosson, D., & Hare, R. (2003). *The Hare Psychopathy Checklist: Youth Version, Technical Manual.* North Tonawanda, NY: Multi-Health Systems.
Gfellner, B. M. (1986a). Changes in ego and moral development in adolescents: A longitudinal study. *Journal of Adolescence, 9*(4), 281–302.
Gfellner, B. M. (1986b). Ego development and moral development in relation to age and grade level during adolescence. *Journal of Youth and Adolescence, 15*(2), 147–163.
Hardy, S. A., Walker, L. J., Olsen, J. A., Woodbury, R. D., & Hickman, J. R. (2014). Moral identity as moral ideal self: Links to adolescent outcomes. *Developmental Psychology, 50*(1), 45–57.
Hare, R. D. (2003). *Manual for the Revised Psychopathy Checklist* (2nd ed.). Toronto, ON, Canada: Multi-Health Systems.
Hart, D., & Carlo, G. (2005). Moral development in adolescence. *Journal of Research on Adolescence, 15*(3), 223–233.
Jesperson, K., Kroger, J., & Martinussen, M. (2013). Identity status and moral reasoning: A meta-analysis. *Identity, 13*, 266–280.
Jones, S., Cauffman, E., Miller, J., & Mulvey, E. (2006). Investigating different factor structures of the Psychopathy Checklist—Youth Version: Confirmatory factor analytic findings. *Psychological Assessment, 18*, 33–48.
Kohlberg, L. (1984). *Essays on moral development: Vol. 2. The psychology of moral development.* San Francisco: Harper & Row.
Krettenauer, T., Colasante, T., Buchmann, M., & Malti, T. (2014). The development of moral emotions and decision-making from adolescence to early adulthood: A 6-year longitudinal study. *Journal of Youth and Adolescence. 43*(4), 583–596.
Lai, F. H., Siu, A. M., Chan, C. C., & Shek, D. T. (2012). Measurement of prosocial reasoning among Chinese adolescents. *Scientific World Journal, 2012*, 174845.
Rest, J., Narvaez, D., Bebeau, M., & Thoma, S. (1999). DIT-2: Devising and testing a new instrument of moral judgment. *Journal of Educational Psychology, 91*(4), 644–659.
Roskam, I., & Marchal, J. (2003). An objective measure of French-speaking adolescents' prosocial moral reasoning. *Archives de Psychologie, 70*, 227–240.
Sevecke, K., Pukrop, R., Kosson, D. S., & Krischer, M. K. (2009). Factor structure of the Hare Psychopathy Checklist: Youth Version in German female and male detainees and community adolescents. *Psychological Assessment, 21*(1), 45–56.
Thoma, S. J., & Dond, Y. (2014). The defining issues test of moral judgment development. *Behavioral Development Bulletin, 19*(3), 55–61.
Tsang, S., Piquero, A. R., & Cauffman E. (2014). An examination of the Psychopathy Checklist: Youth Version (PCL:YV) among male adolescent offenders: An item response theory analysis. *Psychological Assessment, 26*(4), 1333–1346.
Van der Graaff, J., Branje, S., De Wied, M., Hawk, S.,

Van Lier, P., & Meeus, W. (2014). Perspective taking and empathic concern in adolescence: Gender differences in developmental changes. *Developmental Psychology, 50*(3), 881–888.

Vitacco, M. J., Neumann, C. S., Caldwell, M. F., Leistico, A. M., & Van Rybroek, G. J. (2006). Testing factor models of the Psychopathy Checklist: Youth Version and their association with instrumental aggression. *Journal of Personality Assessment, 87*(1), 74–83.

12. Capacity for Meaning and Purpose

Andriola, E., Donfrancesco, R., Zaninotto, S., Di Trani, M., Cruciani, A. C., Innocenzi, M., . . . Cloninger, C. R. (2012). The Junior Temperament and Character Inventory: Italian validation of a questionnaire for the measurement of personality from ages 6 to 16 years. *Comprehensive Psychiatry, 53*(6), 884–892.

Asch, M., Cortese, S., Perez Diaz, F., Pelissolo, A., Aubron, V., Orejarena, S., . . . Purper-Ouakil, D. (2009). Psychometric properties of a French version of the Junior Temperament and Character Inventory. *European Child and Adolescent Psychiatry, 18*(3), 144–153.

Blatt, S. J., Auerbach, J. S., & Levy, K. N. (1997). Mental representations in personality development, psychopathology, and the therapeutic process. *Review of General Psychology, 1*, 351–374.

Blatt, S. J., Bers, S. A., & Schaffer, C. E. (1993). *The assessment of self descriptions.* Unpublished manuscript, Yale University.

Bers, S. A., Blatt, S. J., Sayward, H. K., & Johnston, R. S. (1993). Normal and pathological aspects of self-descriptions and their change over long-term treatment. *Psychoanalytic Psychology, 10*, 17–37.

Bronk, K. C. (2011). The role of purpose in life in healthy identity formation: A grounded model. *New Directions for Youth Development, 132*, 31–44.

Cloninger, C. R., Przybeck, T. R., Svrakic, D. M., & Wetzel, R. D. (1994). *The Temperament and Character Inventory (TCI): A guide to its development and use.* St. Louis, MO: Center for Psychobiology of Personality, Washington University.

Csikszentmihalyi, M. (1990). *Flow: The psychology of optimal experience.* New York: Harper & Row.

Damon, W., Menon, J., & Bronk, K. C. (2003). The development of purpose during adolescence. *Applied Developmental Science, 7*(3), 119–128.

Gabrielsen, L. E., Ulleberg, P., & Watten, R. G. (2012). The Adolescent Life Goal Profile Scale: Development of a new scale for measurements of life goals among young people. *Journal of Happiness Studies, 13*(6), 1053–1072.

Gabrielsen, L. E., Watten, R. G., & Ulleberg, P. (2013). Differences on Adolescent Life Goal Profile Scale between a clinical and non-clinical adolescent sample. *International Journal of Psychiatry in Clinical Practice, 17*(4), 244–252.

Habermas, T., & Bluck, S. (2000). Getting a life: The emergence of the life story in adolescence. *Psychological Bulletin, 126*, 748–769.

Hektner, J. M., & Asakawa, K. (2000). Learning to like challenges. In M. Csikszentmihalyi & B. Schneider (Eds.), *Becoming adult: How teenagers prepare for the world of work* (pp. 95–112). New York: Basic Books.

Hektner, J. M., & Csikszentmihalyi, M. (1996). *A longitudinal exploration of flow an intrinsic motivation in adolescents.* Paper presented at the annual meeting of the American Education Research Association, Alfred Sloan Foundation, New York.

Jackson, S. A., & Eklund, R. C. (2002). Assessing flow in physical activity: The Flow State Scale–2 and Dispositional Flow Scale–2. *Journal of Sport and Exercise Psychology, 24*, 133–150.

Kerekes, N., Brändström, S., Ståhlberg, O., Larson, T., Carlström, E., Lichtenstein, P., . . . Nilsson, T. (2010). The Swedish version of the parent-rated Junior Temperament and Character Inventory (J-TCI). *Psychological Reports, 107*(3), 715–725.

Kim, S. J., Lee, S. J., Yune, S. K., Sung, Y. H., Bae, S. C., Chung, A., . . . Lyoo, I. K. (2006). The relationship between the biogenetic temperament and character and psychopathology in adolescents. *Psychopathology, 39*(2), 80–86.

Luby, J. L., Svrakic, D. M., McCallum, K., Przybeck, T. R., & Cloninger, C. R. (1999). The Junior Temperament and Character Inventory: Preliminary validation of a child self-report measure. *Psychological Reports, 84*(3), 1127–1138.

Lyoo, I. K., Han, C. H., Lee, S. J., Yune, S. K., Ha, J. H., Chung, S. J., . . . Hong, K. E. (2004). The reliability and validity of the Junior Temperament and Character Inventory. *Comprehensive Psychiatry, 45*(2), 121–128.

Mariano, J. M., & Going, J. (2011). Youth purpose and positive youth development. *Advances in Child Development and Behavior, 41*, 39–68.

McAdams, D. P. (2013). The psychological self as actor, agent, and author. *Perspectives on Psychological Science, 8*, 272–295.

McAdams, D. P., & Olson, B. D. (2010). Personality development: Continuity and change over the life course. *Annual Review of Psychology, 61*, 517–542.

Moreno Murcia, J. A., Cervelló Gimeno, E., & González-Cutre Coll, D. (2008). Relationships among goal orientations, motivational climate and flow in adolescent athletes: Differences by gender. *Spanish Journal of Psychology, 11*(1), 181–191.

Pitzer, M., Esser, G., Schmidt, M. H., & Laucht, M. (2007). Temperament in the developmental course: A longitudinal comparison of New York Longitudinal Study-derived dimensions with the Junior Temperament and Character Inventory. *Comprehensive Psychiatry, 48*(6), 572–582.

Poustka, L., Parzer, P., Brunner, R., & Resch, F. (2007). Basic symptoms, temperament and character in adolescent psychiatric disorders. *Psychopathology, 40*(5), 321–328.

Schmeck, K., & Poustka, F. (2001). Temperament and disruptive behavior disorders. *Psychopathology, 34*(3), 159–163.

Steinberg, L., Graham, S., O'Brien, L., Woolard, J., Cauffman, E., & Banich M. (2009). Age differences in future orientation and delay discounting. *Child Development, 80*(1), 28–44.

Wang, C. K. J., Liu, W. C., & Khoo, A. (2009). The psychometric properties of Dispositional Flow Scale–2 in internet gaming. *Current Psychology, 28*, 194–201.

CHAPTER 5

Emerging Personality Patterns and Syndromes in Adolescence

PA Axis

CHAPTER EDITORS

Johanna C. Malone, PhD **Norka Malberg, PsyD**

CONSULTANTS

Line Brotnow, MSc
Antonello Colli, PhD
Nakia Hamlett, PhD
Eirini Lympinaki, MSc
Larry Rosenberg, PhD
Matthew Steinfeld, PhD
Danijela Stojanac, MD

Introduction

Personality patterns form during childhood and continue to develop over the course of life. By adolescence, most individuals will have a relatively stable emerging personality style that serves as a framework for their thoughts, feelings, behaviors, and ways of being in the world. The emerging personality includes strengths and weaknesses that respond to an individual's contextual world. In trying to conceptualize adolescent personality, one can consider three domains: (1) wishes, fears, values, and conflicts; (2) psychological or adaptive resources; and (3) aspects of relatedness (i.e., the experiences of the self and other). See, for example, Westen and Chang (2001) for a review. Thinking historically in psychoanalytic terms, Westen and Chang link the first domain to classical perspectives of conflict, compromise formations, and motivations; the second domain to an ego-psychological perspective, including mechanisms of defense; and the third domain to object relations, self-psychological, and relational frameworks. Yet these domains are also tied to research areas beyond psychoanalytic theories. Moreover, depending on a number of factors—including biological dispositions, cognitive capacities, age and developmental stage, the nature of the family and broader cultural influences, and life events—personality may change or stabilize.

Readers of this chapter on the PDM-2 PA Axis should note that many issues related to personality development and etiological factors are discussed at greater length in Chapter 8 on the child personality axis (the PC Axis). Similarly, theoretical and conceptual issues related to adult personality pathology overlap greatly with those of adolescent personality, and for more in-depth background, readers should refer to Chapter 1 on the adult personality axis (the P Axis). In this chapter, we focus on the issues specifically related to adolescent personality.

To characterize adolescent mental health and mental health disorders, it is important to describe both emerging and relatively formed personality patterns. Personality syndromes are not fully fixed at a specific age; they imply a sufficiently formed personality structure, which may become apparent toward adolescence. As for the adult P Axis, the major organizing principles for the PA Axis are (1) level of personality organization and (2) personality style. Level of personality organization is a severity index that describes any of the personality styles, which themselves do not directly convey health or pathology but rather characteristic ways of being in the world.

We first provide a brief overview of recent research, which increasingly demonstrates the importance of assessing adolescent personality. Next, we discuss the unique aspects of the developmental stage and clinical issues that clinicians and researchers should consider when assessing adolescent personality. We then provide an overview of current adolescent-focused assessment instruments that clinicians and researchers might utilize. Next, we detail an approach to diagnosing the level of personality organization and emerging personality style with adolescent populations. We also provide three brief clinical illustrations that demonstrate how a clinician might apply the PA Axis to understanding adolescent patients.

Adolescents and Emerging Personality: Background and Significance

A growing body of evidence suggests that emerging patterns of personality pathology in adolescence are both highly prevalent and persistent (Grilo & McGlashan, 1998; Kongerslev, Chanen, & Simonsen, 2015; Levy, 2005; Nock & Kessler, 2006; Westen, Dutra, & Shedler, 2005). Yet the *Diagnostic and Statistical Manual of Mental Disorders* (most recently DSM-IV-TR and DSM-5; American Psychiatric Association, 2000, 2013) and the *International Classification of Diseases* (currently ICD-10; World Health Organization, 1992) caution against diagnosing adolescent personality disorders, in part because there needs to be evidence that such a disorder is longstanding and enduring, which is difficult to establish at a young age. ICD-10 suggests that a personality disorder diagnosis will be unlikely before age 16 or 17; DSM-5 states that for those under 18, the diagnosis is unlikely, and traits will need to be present for at least a year. These recommendations likely arose less from empirical evidence and more from efforts both to differentiate characteristics normative to a developmental stage characterized by "storm and stress" from persistent pathology (Casey, Jones, & Levita, 2010), and to protect youth from social stigma (Catthoor, Feenstra, Hutsebaut, Schrijvers, & Sabbe, 2015; Chanen, Jovev, & Mcgorry, 2008; Laurensenn, Hutsebaut, Feenstra, Van Busschbach, & Luyten, 2013). However, clinical evidence and empirical research indicate that adolescent personality pathology is distinct from both normal development and abnormal psychopathology. This finding has critical importance for shaping how clinicians might develop treatments when working with adolescent patients.

Parsing out the distinction between developmental stage and pathology, Kernberg (1998) differentiates adolescents who face an identity crisis from those who face identity diffusion (see also Erikson, 1956). Whereas identity crisis is a normal part of adolescence, reflecting issues of identity relating to individuation from the family and managing conflicting feelings about sexual urges, identity diffusion—as evidenced by the lack of integration of representations of both the self and others—is indicative of personality pathology (Chen, Cohen, Johnson, Kasen, & Crawford, 2004; Johnson, Chen, & Cohen, 2004; Wiley & Berman, 2013). In other words, adolescents with identity diffusion lack a sense of who they are and have trouble understanding and relating to other people without disruptive distortions. The distinction between adolescent personality pathology and attributes of the developmental stage is further supported by longitudinal studies of personality development showing that personality pathology co-occurs with other forms of impairment, and that it predicts not only adult personality pathology but also a range of other interpersonal functioning and pathological outcomes in the years following adolescence (Daley, Copeland, Wright, Roalfe, & Wales, 2006; Feenstra, Van Busschbach, Verheul, & Hutsebaut, 2011; Kasen et al., 2007).

Attending to personality pathology in adolescents is important for a number of reasons. First, by assessing adolescent personality pathology, clinicians may more effectively shape their treatments of psychiatric disorders. Personality dynamics influence the presentation and severity of internalizing, externalizing, and eating pathology (Freeman & Reinecke, 2007; Johnson et al., 2000). Comorbid patterns of psychiatric psychopathology can also be tied to common personality features (Allertz & van Voorst, 2007; Chen, Cohen, Kasen, & Johnson, 2006; Lavan & Johnson, 2002). Next, there is increasing evidence that personality pathology begins even prior to adolescence and may at times be stable into adulthood (Chanen et al., 2004; Cohen, Crawford, Johnson, & Kasen, 2005). For example, childhood diagnoses of disruptive behavior disorders with callous–unemotional characteristics are now thought to persist as a form of psychopathy or adult antisocial personality disorder (Cohen et al., 2005; Rey, Morris-Yates, Singh, Andrews, & Stewart, 1995). These characteristics are not only stable but are also comorbid with disorders such as substance use disorders, which are diagnosable in adolescence (Biederman et al., 2008; Chanen et al., 2004; Cohen et al., 2005; DiLallo, Jones, & Westen, 2009; Frick, Stickle, Dandreaux, Farrell, & Kimonis, 2005; Jones & Westen, 2010; Rey et al., 1995). Such research highlights the need for earlier interventions that specifically target emerging personality pathology while young people are still in structured environments with more sources of support. At the same time, developmental pathways are not linear or deterministic; concepts from a developmental psychopathology framework such as "equifinality" and "multifinality" suggest that outcomes of personality pathology may have diverse contributing factors, and that risk factors for personality pathology do not always result in outcomes of personality disorder diagnoses.

Diagnosing emergent personality pathology in adolescents is often more difficult than in adults. In addition, research shows that therapists are often hesitant to diagnose such pathology because of concerns that they will label the adolescents with stigmatizing disorders and because DSM warns clinicians against diagnosing personality disorders in adolescents (Johnson et al., 2005; Kasen et al., 2007; Laurensenn et al., 2013). Yet adolescents do have personalities, and these personalities can be characterized by both adaptive and maladaptive qualities. Clinicians working with adolescents should take into account their patients' ages and developmental stages (e.g., a 13-year-old is quite different from an 18-year-old). In addition, clinicians should consider the sensitivity of adolescents to family and environmental factors and think about how these factors might contribute to the personality traits seen in adolescence. Ultimately, the decision as to whether an adolescent's personality patterns are sufficiently rigid and maladaptive to constitute personality pathology depends on a clinician's consideration of all the factors outlined. Without compelling evidence that a personality pattern is significantly compromising the 12 mental capacities listed later in this chapter, the clinician may characterize a relatively stable personality pattern as the adolescent's unique personal signature of strengths and vulnerabilities (as would be done with an adult).

When considering the development and presentation of adolescent personality, a clinician must consider characteristics that emerge from ongoing interactions among a number of factors. Some of these causal mechanisms are discussed in greater depth in Chapter 8 on the PC Axis, and what follows is a brief review.

- An individual is born with certain biological dispositions, such as activity level and ability to be soothed (i.e., temperament). The infant's unique neuropsychological state develops over time in response to interactions with the environment.
- Within the activities of daily life, unique caregiver–infant patterns develop that ideally allow the child to master, modulate, and regulate affective responses. With maturation, the field of core relationships widens. By adolescence, there may be a tendency to repeat early patterns of interaction (i.e., attachment styles).
- There is a gradual development of a pattern of inner experience and behavior that continues to affect and be affected by interactions with the people in the adolescent's interpersonally expanding environment—an environment that the young person has increasing power to shape. The adolescent's self-esteem develops as a result of the conscious and unconscious meanings attached to these experiences.
- During development, a variety of adaptive and defensive operations emerge as ways of mastering both unusual or traumatic experiences and the normal frustrations of growing up. Adolescents with high levels of aggression and irritability are often in chronic conflict with parents, teachers, and peers. In contrast, adolescents with more internalizing patterns and with behavioral inhibition may elicit overprotective responses or be overlooked, resulting in increased inhibition and consequent feelings of inferiority.

Developmental Aspects of Adolescent Emerging Personality Patterns

Puberty ushers in a period of expansion and potential inner turmoil. Although most adolescents manage to navigate it successfully (i.e., without undue storminess), some may show temporary difficulties that will not develop into disorders during adulthood, and others may experience persistent pathological functioning.

Over the course of adolescence, a young person has to accomplish three major tasks: (1) adapting to hormonal and other changes in the body (i.e., neurophysiology);

(2) beginning the process of transferring attachment from the family of origin to other love objects; and (3) constructing a more nuanced and competent capacity to compare and evaluate experiences realistically in the context of an emerging, increasingly complex sense of self.

Early Adolescence

Early adolescence (approximately 12–14 years) is characterized by important physical changes (growth in body hair, gains in height and weight), among which the most important is the sexual maturation of girls (onset of menstruation) and boys (growth in testicles and penis). Body issues may arise, ranging from mild to extreme as adolescents integrate the physical changes. According to the most common gender stereotypes, for example, some girls either hide themselves in baggy clothes or wear overly revealing outfits. Some boys may either become overly focused on evidencing masculinity or withdraw into a more cerebral stance. Ways of coping with physical changes vary enormously. Many adolescents may also struggle with their sense of identity, feel awkward about their selves and their bodies, and worry intensely about being "normal."

With hormonal changes and more sexual feelings, it is normative for both boys and girls to engage in masturbation, which may include eroticized fantasy. They may become more aware of sexual preferences as such fantasies develop (Adelson, 2012). Gender identity may become more articulated with the onset of secondary sex characteristics. While most children and adolescents may have some gender-nonconforming behaviors, some adolescents begin to express discordance between gender and phenotypic sex characteristics. Cognitively, young adolescents show a growing capacity for abstract thinking and self-reflection, but their attention is generally focused on the present rather than the future. Some show moodiness and—when stressed—a tendency to return to childlike behaviors. There may be an increased inclination toward the testing of rules and limits.

Middle Adolescence

During middle adolescence (approximately 15–16 years), physical growth slows for girls and continues for boys. Self-reflection increases, permitting adolescents to explore and reflect about inner experience with an interest in moral reasoning and thinking about the meaning of life. There is an increase in conflicts with parents and an increased focus on peer interactions. During this period, adolescents are especially vulnerable to peer pressure; because of the absence of a clear sense of self, they look to peers for guidance. In moving away from family members as the principal objects of affection and in diminishing identifications with parents, adolescents may show a variety of patterns: identifications with (and imitation of) a range of peers and other adults; sexual experimentation and/or a hypermoralistic stance; obsessive involvement with idealistic or intellectual pursuits; and/or egocentric hedonism. The adolescent may deny vulnerability and mortality with counterphobic, impulsive acts or may withdraw from action in the world. Empirical studies show that risk taking, novelty seeking, and hunger for stimulation increase during adolescence and are present in about the 50% of adolescents (Irwin, 1989; Kelley, Schochet, & Landry, 2004). Generally speaking, dismissive youth may seek to distance themselves from parents as soon as possible, whereas preoccupied youth may be unwilling or unable to embrace parental demands for greater autonomy. Although families may experience an increase in conflict and a decline in warmth, this may represent a new wave of insecurity more than an overall worsening of relationships.

As adolescents become more aware of sexual desires and more sexually experienced, they will usually develop increased certainty about aspects of sexual identity and orientation. Development of sexual identity in adolescents will be influenced by a range of demographic factors (e.g., age, culture), as well as by sexual experience (D'Augelli & Patterson, 2001; Mustanski, Kuper, & Greene, 2014). Gender identity may also become increasingly clearly developed; some transgender youth may wish to find ways to have more conformity between their gender identity and their biological sex. Like other minority groups, gender and sexual minorities may be more vulnerable to bullying and exclusion in certain social and cultural contexts (for lesbian, gay, bisexual, and transgender issues, see also Chapter 6 on the SA Axis, pp. 442–444).

Family relationships and dynamics play a critical role in adolescent personality development: Parent–child relationships require realignment during adolescence, and midlife reevaluation may compromise parents' abilities to meet their adolescents' needs to negotiate increasing autonomy. Parental socialization behaviors may influence adolescents' development of cognitive attributions and emotion regulation and generally affect how adolescents face the developmental tasks of this period. Given the importance of both family and peer relationships, parent training, school services, and peer programs all have great therapeutic and preventive value during adolescence.

Late Adolescence

In late adolescence (approximately 17–19 years; issues may extend into the early 20s), young women are generally fully developed, while young men continue to gain weight and height. In this last phase of emerging adulthood, adolescents show an increasing capacity for delayed gratification and insight, accompanied by a firmer sense of identity, increased emotional stability, and continued interest in moral reasoning. In late adolescence, youth ideally continue to develop a more nuanced view of their sexualities and gender identities.

Significant Contextual Factors in the Treatment of Adolescents

In addition to considering the developmental sequence of adolescence, clinicians must pay attention to a complicated array of contextual factors. A brief overview follows.

Family Relationships

Given the vast evidence for the role of family stress in the emergence of personality, clinicians should evaluate how family relationships contribute to the emergence and/or maintenance of personality symptomatology. Risk factors such as negative parenting behaviors (e.g., abuse, neglect, low parental affection or nurturing) (Keinänen, Johnson, Richards, & Courtney, 2012); parental conflict; parental psychiatric disorders (Cohen et al., 2005); early separation from parents, particularly before the age of 5 (Lahti, Pesonen, Räikkönen, & Erikson, 2012); parental suicide attempts or completion; parental incarceration history; and domestic violence (Afifi et al., 2011) should be taken into consideration during the assessment process.

Personality problems such as interpersonal oversensitivity, emotional dysregulation, and self-harm in adolescents are empirically correlated with negative parenting (higher levels of conflict, negative affect, lack of support for managing emotions, and invalidating emotion socialization practices), while caregivers' positive affective behaviors are associated with a faster rate of decline in borderline personality severity scores across time (Adrian, Zeman, Erdley, Lisa, & Sim, 2011; Crowell, Beauchaine, & Lenzenweger, 2008; Keenan et al., 2010; Yap et al., 2011; Zalewski et al., 2014). When the family environment fails to helps children manage negative emotions—that is, when parents create an insensitive, punitive, chaotic, or hostile environment—children's negative emotionality tends to increase over time (Bates, Schermerhorn, & Petersen, 2014; Lengua & Wachs, 2012). High levels and increasing levels of family conflict from early to late adolescence are associated with higher levels of antisocial behavior (Hofer et al., 2013; Lansford et al., 2009)

Parenting styles may affect adolescents' development of emotion regulation in different ways. Authoritarian parenting, characterized by high levels of parental control and demandingness and low levels of warmth and acceptance, may inhibit the development of self-regulation by leading children to be emotionally overaroused and to suppress negative emotions (Sroufe, 1996). With permissive/indulgent parenting, marked by high levels of warmth and acceptance and very low levels of behavioral control (Baumrind, 1991), teens are unable to learn how or when to self-regulate and are more likely to engage in impulsive, dysregulated behaviors.

To facilitate diagnostic and therapeutic processes, a clinician should involve an adolescent patient's parents in treatment. This practice helps in constructing a more complex and in-depth picture of the young person's emerging personality and helps parents to understand how family dynamics contribute to the patient's personality development and to the perseverance of personality symptoms. Working with parents may increase their own capacity to respond in a supportive and positive way to their child, especially during times of conflict and stress. This is particularly crucial for adolescents at risk for developing borderline functioning, given the link between the formation of a cohesive sense of identity and feelings of positive interpersonal contact and connectedness (Stanley & Siever, 2009). Involving parents may help them shift from coercive, nonmentalizing cycles of engagement to mentalizing discussions that promote trust, security, attachment, and effective communication (Bleiberg, 2004). A clinician is thus not only assessing the young person, but also the capacity of the caregiving system to engage in and support the therapeutic process.

Peer Relationships

As adolescents recognize that their parents are not infallible, they increasingly question and resist the parents' attempts to influence and guide them. A relational vacuum can result, which tends to be filled by peers. Although parental influence does not disappear over the adolescent years, it may decline relative to that of peers. Peer influence may be protective. For example, preadolescents who have friends and attain friendships of higher quality show fewer depressive symptoms, have higher self-esteem, and experience less internalized problems than adolescents whose friendships are of lower quality (Rubin et al., 2004; Updegraff & Obeidallah, 1999). Positive relationships with peers can moderate the association between negative parenting and externalizing behavior problems (Lansford, Criss, Pettit, Dodge, & Bates, 2003); buffer children from the negative effects of chronic maltreatment in the family on their self-esteem (Bolger, Patterson, & Kupersmidt, 1998); and, in economically disadvantaged families, protect adolescents from the negative effects of economic stress on their life satisfaction (Raboteg-Šarić, Šakić, & Brajša-Žganec, 2009). Similarly, the school environment can affect the emergence and continuation of personality problems; in schools with a strong focus on learning, students show declines in borderline, narcissistic, antisocial, and histrionic personality features (Kasen et al., 2007).

But peer relationships can also put adolescents at risk for maladaptive personality development. Risky behaviors tend to occur within a peer context (Wolfe, Jaffe, & Crooks, 2006); within their peer groups, teens experience a host of interactions that shape their attitudes about such behaviors (Dishion, Spracklen, Andrews, & Patterson, 1996; Patterson, Dishion, & Yoerger, 2000). Peer group members tend to develop similar attitudes and behaviors over time in the areas of substance use (Urberg, Değirmencioğlu, & Pilgrim, 1997), general delinquency (Kiesner, Cadinu, Poulin, & Bucci, 2002), dropping out of school (Cairns, Cairns, & Neckerman, 1989), and unsafe sexual practices (Henry, Schoeny, Deptula, & Slavick, 2007). Peer pressure has been identified as a risk factor for substance use and deviant behavior (e.g., Claesen, Brown, & Eicher, 1986; Santor, Messervey, & Kusumakar, 2000). During the evaluation process, clinicians should take adolescents' social climates into account; those characterized by high conflict and shallow interpersonal relationships predict the emergence of personality problems (Kasen, Cohen, Chen, Johnson, & Crawford, 2009).

Socioeconomic and Cultural Factors

Low familial socioeconomic status (SES) has been identified as a factor in several types of personality syndromes, even after researchers have controlled for the effects of trauma, stressful life events, IQ, parenting, and comorbid symptoms (Cohen et al., 2005; Johnson, Cohen, Dohrenwend, Link, & Brook, 1999). Neighborhood characteristics may influence personality problems as well (Hart & Marmorstein, 2009). There is also evidence of cultural influences on the prevalence and presentation of personality patterns; the prominence of various symptoms within a given diagnostic category may vary by cultural background (Newhill, Eack, & Conner, 2009). Cultural factors may account for the fact that antisocial and borderline personalities are more common in Western cultures (Mulder, 2012). Clinicians need to be aware of how cultural values and beliefs may influence what is seen as normative adolescent behavior within a specific cultural group, especially while gathering parental reports and exploring issues such as separation–individuation. Clinicians should approach cultural issues from a mentalizing stance of genuine curiosity and inquisitiveness, fostering the atmosphere of respect, trust, and safety that will facilitate exploration of how cultural dynamics might be affecting young persons and their families (see also Chapter 6 on the SA Axis).

Clinical Issues Arising in the Treatment of Adolescents

The physical, emotional, and cognitive developmental changes outlined above make working with adolescent patients different from working with either children or adults. See Loughran (2004) for a review of working psychodynamically with adolescent patients. Fonagy, Gergely, Jurist, and Target (2002) emphasize two critical developmental challenges to keep in mind: first, the adolescent patient's recent development of formal operations, which leads to the intensification of interpersonal understanding—a potentially overwhelming process in which the adolescent can be flooded by new affective experiences of self and other; second, the separation from both the external caregiver and the internal representation of the caregiver. In this individuation process, some adolescents have difficulties resulting from early caregiving issues that were largely concealed until this stage.

Unlike in work with adults, current attachment relationships should be more directly addressed with adolescents. This may mean considering with an adolescent and family whether, in addition to individual sessions, there should be family meetings, consultations with teachers, and separate communication or meetings with parents without the adolescent. When caregivers are involved, an additional focus should be on helping them become more reflective and consistent in how they think about their child and the child's personality. When deciding which family member(s) to meet with first, rather than having predetermined rules, a clinician should consider the nature of the presenting problem and how the meeting may influence the family system and treatment alliance. Issues surrounding confidentiality are particularly important in this age group. The clinician should discuss with the adolescent and the family the limits of confidentiality and consider how to handle communications about sex, drug/alcohol use, and other risky behaviors.

In listening to an adolescent and achieving an understanding of his or her personality, a clinician should consider all modes of communication. This includes paying close attention to nonverbal cues of affect, body language, and clothing/physical appearance. There should be an emphasis on thinking about how the adolescent patient is adapting to his or her cultural surroundings at many levels (home, school, friend groups, neighborhood, culture of origin, religious background, etc.). It may be useful to think about ways that the adolescent is perceiving self and others in each of these settings, and to notice when things feel either congruent or in conflict. For example, are there different expectations about identity and relationships that exist across settings? If so, how does the adolescent make sense of those disparities and navigate this challenge? It is essential for the clinician to consider actively the strengths of the adolescent patient, the family, and the community to facilitate growth.

An engaged affirming stance is necessary for forming a treatment alliance and helps the adolescent become more curious about him- or herself. A clinician's treatment approach should be guided by an assessment of the adolescent's personality organization and personality style. For example, the interventions and transference–countertransference dynamics with a patient who has a depressive personality style and a neurotic level of organization may differ dramatically from those with an adolescent who has an antisocial personality style and a psychotic level of personality organization. This difference is clearly important, regardless of whether both patients qualify for a DSM-5 diagnosis of major depressive disorder.

When a clinician is evaluating an adolescent's personality and planning for effective treatment, it is essential to take into consideration *personality strengths* as well as *protective factors* in the family and wider social systems. Important general protective factors that may differentiate adolescents who go through a tumultuous period but do not develop a personality disorder from adolescents who then develop a personality disorder are "mentalizing capacities." Clinicians should consider three key protective factors: (1) "reflective function," or the capacity and willingness to recognize, experience, and reflect on one's thoughts, feelings and motivations; (2) "agency," or a sense of oneself as being effective and responsible for one's actions; and (3) "relatedness," or a valuing of relationship that takes the form of openness to others' perspectives and of efforts to engage with others (Bleiberg, 2004; Hauser, Allen, & Golden, 2006). Mentalizing may enable adolescents to perceive and label emotions stemming from difficult life experiences, and engaging in a reflective process about these experiences may then reduce the negative impact of such experiences (Fonagy et al., 2002). Moreover, mentalizing capacities appear to protect against the development of psychopathology in individuals who have experienced early abuse and neglect, and such capacities moderate the link between psychopathy and aggressive behavior in male adolescents (Taubner, White, Zimmermann, Fonagy, & Nolte, 2012). For a more detailed description of this aspect of development, see Chapter 4 on the MA Axis.

Other contextual and intrapersonal factors may provide additional information during the process of assessment, clinical formulation, and treatment planning. For instance, higher IQ, talents, and positive self-perceptions are associated with good developmental outcomes among children who have overcome diverse disadvantages and adversities (Sapienza & Masten, 2011). Contextual factors that have been identified as promoting resilience in youth include positive parenting, effective schools, and connections to prosocial organizations such as places of worship (Masten, 2007). Competent functioning in any of the important life tasks of adolescence (school and peer relationships) may be yet another source of resilience (Skodol et al., 2007). Considering these aspects is essential for developing a diagnostic profile, planning treatment, and making clinical recommendations.

Personality Assessment in Adolescence

Generally speaking, clinical tests should provide data to inform and guide decisions regarding diagnosis/main problems and treatment planning, as well as to document change across treatment. A number of issues pertaining to the clinical use of standardized assessments should be considered, not the least of which is the choice of informants. Indeed, research on the interrater reliability of clinical assessments in childhood and adolescence has consistently shown low to moderate correlations among informants (e.g., De Los Reyes & Kazdin, 2005), and factors such as child age, setting, and type of child problem influence agreement. In adolescence, agreement among youth, parents, and other informants (usually teachers) is lower than in childhood (see Smith, 2007, for a clinically based review). In part, this trend can be understood as a function of adolescents' relatively greater understanding of social desirability and possibly unwanted consequences of truthfully representing the extent of their suffering. In terms of understanding parents' and teachers' inaccuracies, the increased autonomy of adolescents can cause authority figures to become less likely confidants and can also cause informants' observations to reflect highly context-specific youth behavior/self-expression. In support of the latter point, informants with similar roles in the life of an adolescent (such as two parents) demonstrate higher interrater reliability than do informants exposed to the youth in different settings (e.g., parents and teachers) (Shiner & Allen, 2013). The specific biases and unique contributions of different informants (and assessment methods) highlight the importance of collecting information about the adolescent patient from multiple sources. Clinically speaking, the level of agreement among youth, parents, and other reporters can inform the clinical formulation and become an independent target and measure of treatment outcome.

Self-Report Measures of Personality Functioning in Adolescence

Personality Assessment Inventory—Adolescent

The Personality Assessment Inventory—Adolescent (PAI-A) is a 264-item self-administered, multidimensional measure of personality functioning and psychopathology. Adolescents evaluate how true each statement is for them on a 4-point Likert scale, and the measure can be given to youth ages 12–18 (Morey, 2007). Substantially shortened and worded at a fourth-grade reading-level, the PAI-A retains the basic structure of the well-validated adult PAI. Initial empirical analyses suggest adequate psychometric properties (Morey, 2007; Rios & Morey, 2013). Like the PAI for adults, the PAI-A includes multiple, nonoverlapping scales: 4 test validity scales (identifying tendencies to over- or underreport symptoms, defensiveness, inattention), 11 clinical scales, 5 treatment consideration scales (including suicidality, aggressiveness, and treatment rejection), and 2 interpersonal scales (dominance and warmth). The nonoverlapping nature of the scales provides the PAI-A with good discriminant validity, which is a concern with other assessment tools.

Minnesota Multiphasic Personality Inventory—Adolescent

The Minnesota Multiphasic Personality Inventory—Adolescent (MMPI-A) is normed on a sample of ethnically diverse 14- to 18-year-olds and is among the most frequently used personality and psychopathology assessments for this age group (Butcher et al., 1992; Sellbom & Jarrett, 2014). Like the MMPI-2, it has been the target of extensive empirical testing and has been translated into a number of languages. The MMPI-A includes 478 true–false items making up 3 validity scales and 10 empirically derived clinical scales. In terms of clinical practice and treatment planning, research studies have consistently found good concurrent and predictive validity, namely with regard to diagnostic severity (e.g., Archer, 2004). Although it is somewhat shorter and has undergone substantial changes with regard to item contents, the reading level required to fill out the questionnaire adequately is higher than for similar scales (seventh to ninth grade), and the length of administration places considerable demands on attention capacities.

Big Five Inventory—Adolescent

The Big Five Inventory—Adolescent (BFI-A) is a 5-minute 44-item scale constructed to assess the prototype definitions of neuroticism, extraversion, openness, agreeableness, and conscientiousness in the "Big Five" model of personality (John, Donahue, & Kentle, 1991). This theoretical approach has proven to be a useful framework for characterizing personality in adolescence (John, Caspi, Robins, Moffit, & Stouthamer-Loeber, 1994; Lynam et al., 2005) and to be predictive of personality functioning and psychopathology across cultures (Vazsonyi, Ksinan, Mikuška, & Jiskrova, 2015). Importantly, the inclusion of measures in this personality assessment battery that capture adaptive elements of functioning is an important part of the clinical formulation (Cicchetti, 1993; Rashid & Ostermann, 2009; Rawana & Brownlee, 2009; Shiner, 2009; Tedeschi & Kilmer, 2005; Westen & Shedler, 2007), which in turn can inform treatment planning. The BFI-A consists of easily worded statements (sixth-grade reading comprehension) evaluated by adolescents on a 5-point Likert scale indexing the extent to which they feel that the item captures an essential feature of their functioning. The psychometric qualities of the BFI-A have been found to be adequate (Hahn, Gottschling, & Spinath, 2012), and the scale has been validated for use with Hispanic populations (Benet-Martinez & John, 1998). It does not contain any scales to evaluate validity.

Millon Adolescent Clinical Inventory

The Millon Adolescent Clinical Inventory (MACI) is a 165-item 31-scale self-report inventory designed to assess a broad range of clinical syndromes and dimensions of personality pathology in adolescence (Millon & Davis, 1993; Millon, Millon, Davis, & Grossman, 2006). Based on Millon's theory of personality, the MACI was developed and normed on clinical samples and has proven to be predictive of severity and functioning across clinical settings (McCann, 1999). It is among the most frequently used adolescent personality measures in clinical practice, and it has received robust empirical validation (Murrie & Cornell, 2002; Romm, Bockian, & Harvey, 1999). The MACI scales were not designed to be orthogonal (mutually exclusive), and recent factor analyses suggest that they can be used to distinguish three principal underlying personality factors ("prototypes"): demoralization (lack of core sense of self, borderline tendencies); acting out (manipulation, domination, callous–unemotional tendencies); and detachment (low self-esteem, fear of rejection, inhibited tendencies) (Adkisson, Burdsal, Dorr, & Morgan, 2012). Recent studies also suggest that the scales are predictive of specific defense mechanisms (Rachão & Campos, 2015). In addition to the clinical scales, the MACI includes validity scales to detect attitudes to self-disclosure, desirability, and debasement. The MACI takes 20–30 minutes to administer, and items are worded at a sixth-grade reading level.

Interview-Based or Clinician-Reported Measures of Adolescent Personality Functioning

Adolescent to Adult Personality Functioning Assessment

The Adolescent to Adult Personality Functioning Assessment (AD-APFA) is a clinician-administered interview asking an adolescent about functioning over periods of between 2 and 5 years (Naughton, Oppenheim, & Hill, 1996). Six domains are covered: education/work; love relationships (cohabiting and noncohabiting sexual relationships); friendships; nonspecific social contacts (social exchanges with strangers or acquaintances); negotiations (assertive interactions in order to achieve a goal); and coping with practical, day-to-day matters. The interviewer uses nonfixed questions to obtain adequate information; ratings are made on the basis of youth's descriptions of behavior, and do not take account of their own evaluation of functioning. The scale can only be used with adolescents age 18 and over, covering the periods 16–20 and 21–25 years of age. As the adult parent version of this scale does, the AD-APFA has good interrater reliability (Naughton et al., 1996).

Shedler–Westen Assessment Procedure–II—Adolescent

The Shedler–Westen Assessment Procedure–II—Adolescent (SWAP-II-A[1]) is a clinician-reported personality pathology measure for adolescents ages 14–18 (Westen, Shedler, Durrett, Glass, & Martens, 2003; Westen, DeFife, Malone, & DiLallo, 2014). It includes 200 statements regarding diverse aspects of adolescent personality, worded in jargon-free language common to clinicians across theoretical orientations. Each statement is sorted by the clinician into a number of categories based on their applicability to the patient (i.e., Q-sort methodology). The sorting takes place *following* in-depth clinical interviewing or longitudinal knowledge of the patient, and previous literature has found that experienced clinicians need 6 contact hours to produce adequate ratings (Shedler & Westen, 2007). In an attempt to increase clinical relevance, the items were drawn from multiple sources (including DSM-IV-TR) and have been revised multiple times based on clinician feedback (Shedler & Westen, 2007). The score profiles scale provides (1) dimensional scores for DSM-IV-TR and DSM-5 personality disorder diagnoses, (2) dimensional scores for an alternative set of personality syndromes identified empirically through SWAP research, and (3) dimensional trait scores derived via factor analysis of the SWAP item set. These dimensional scores are accompanied as well by suggested cutoffs to yield DSM-compatible diagnostic categories, and top-rated items can be grouped to form the basis of a narrative case formulation, using the descriptions on the sorting cards to create the outline of a written evaluation (Shedler & Westen, 2007). The SWAP-II-A also generates a Psychological Health Index (PHI), which measures adaptive psychological resources and capacities, or ego strengths. The RADIO Index uses the item content of the SWAP-200 to categorize personality functioning into five domains: reality testing and thought process; affect regulation and tolerance; defensive organization; identity integration; and object relations (Waldron et al., 2011, p. 363). Initial empirical studies support the validity of both the adult (Blagov, Bi, Shedler, & Westen, 2012) and adolescent (DeFife, Malone, DiLallo, & Westen, 2013; Westen et al., 2005) versions of the SWAP. Additional information can be found in Chapters 4 and 15 of this manual.

Structured Interview of Personality Organization—Adolescent Version

The Structured Interview of Personality Organization—Adolescent Version (STIPO-A) is used to make dimensional assessments of core concepts of Kernberg's theory of personality organization, including identity consolidation, quality of object relations, use of primitive defenses, quality of aggression, adaptive coping versus character rigidity, and moral values. Compared with the STIPO for adults, the STIPO-A represents a simplification of item wording and reorganization of the scoring scheme (Ammaniti et al., 2012). Initial empirical testing suggests adequate reliability and validity (Fontana & Ammaniti, 2010; Stern et al., 2010). The considerable length of administration (over 2 hours) causes this measure to be out of reach for patients with limited attention capacities, however. The STIPO blends self-report and performance-based/clinician-rating methodology, as the interviewer or rater makes scoring judgments based on the content and process of the interview (Bram & Yalof, 2015).

---

[1]Unlike the SWAP for adults, whose electronic version on CD is available in different translations, the SWAP-II (adults) and the SWAP-II-A (adolescents) are not currently available.

Interview of Personality Organization Processes in Adolescence

The Interview of Personality Organization Processes in Adolescence (IPOP-A) is a semistructured 41-item clinical interview for youth ages 13–21 years (Ammaniti, Fontana, Kernberg, Clarkin, & Clarkin, 2011). The scale was constructed on the model of the STIPO-A but takes only an hour to administer. The IPOP-A emphasizes developmental processes of personality rather than its purported structure and takes into consideration gender as well as stage of adolescent development. Rather than using direct questioning, the instrument elicits adolescents' responses to scenes from daily life to inquire about affective experiences. The assessment yields scores in three domains: identity formation (differentiating between normal identity crisis and identity diffusion), object relations (quality of interpersonal functioning), and affect regulation (insight into and ability to modulate affect) (Ammaniti et al., 2012).

Identity Disturbance Questionnaire

The Identity Disturbance Questionnaire for Adolescents (IDQ-A) is a brief 35-item instrument; each item is rated by the clinician on a 7-point scale to capture its applicability to the patient (Wilkinson-Ryan & Westen, 2000). The evaluation can follow a clinical interview or can be part of an ongoing clinical observation. The IDQ yields a score on four identity disorder factors (role absorption, painful incoherence, inconsistency, and lack of normative commitment) and has been found to be particularly predictive of borderline functioning in adult and adolescent samples (Westen, Betan, & DeFife, 2011).

Performance-Based Methods of Measuring Personality Functioning in Adolescence

The assumption underlying projective tests is that, when confronted with ambiguous or amorphous material, an individual's desires and conflicts can be gleaned from his or her attempts to restructure or impose meaning on the image (Obrzut & Boliek, 2003).

Rorschach Inkblot Test

The Rorschach Inkblot Test includes 10 intentionally amorphous images to be described freely by the respondent. The Rorschach has been used with adolescents since soon after its initial publication (see, e.g., Gorlow, Zimet, & Fine, 1952), and it can be scored and interpreted by using either Exner's Comprehensive System (Exner, 2003) or the Rorschach Performance Assessment System (Meyer, Viglione, Mihura, Erard, & Erdberg, 2011). The Comprehensive System makes use of different cutoff scores for some variables for which the normative data demonstrate significant developmental changes (i.e., Egocentricity Index, WSUM6, Affective Ratio), and it does not employ the Suicide Constellation (SCON) below the age of 16. The Rorschach has been found to have acceptable reliability, and meta-analytic studies have demonstrated validity effect sizes within the range of self-report measures such as the MMPI-A (e.g., Hiller, Rosenthal, Bornstein, Berry, & Brunell-Neuleib 1999; Mihura, Meyer, Dumitrascu, & Bombel, 2013) with both adolescent and adult populations.

Rorschach research has identified constellations of variables that assess difficulties with reality testing and thinking, hypervigilance, difficulties with self-image or relationships, high experienced levels of affective distress, difficulties with controls and stress tolerance, and difficulties with affect regulation. Validity studies based on these configurations have established that elements contained within those constellations related to thinking and reality testing (i.e., SCZI and PTI) are able to differentiate children (Stokes & Pogge, 2001) and adolescents (Hilsenroth, Eudell-Simmons, DeFife, & Charnas, 2007) with psychotic disorders from youth without such disorders. The Ego Impairment Index (EII) is a broad measure of impaired adjustment that weights elements such as those related to reality testing, thinking problems, object relations, and occurrence of critical thought content to provide an overall index of impaired functioning. This index, in particular, seems to be a measure of personality structure apart from symptom status and has been found to be predictive of poor long-term outcome in psychiatric inpatients across a range of psychopathology, including thinking problems. Administration of the Rorschach requires at least 1 hour, and scoring and interpretation require approximately 2 additional hours. Its administration, scoring, and interpretation are complex and require considerable formal training and experience.

Storytelling Techniques

Thematic Apperception Test

The Thematic Apperception Test (TAT) contains 31 cards depicting people involved in implied actions and interactions (Bellak, 1993; Murray, 1943, 1971) created to elicit responses revealing the patient's dominant emotions, drives, traits, and conflicts. Generally, 10 cards are selected by the clinician as a function of the patient's age to elicit meaningful responses. With adolescents, cards 1, 2, 5, 7GF, 12F, 12M, 15, 17BM, 18BM, and 18GF may be of particular interest. In spite of over 50 years of clinical applications, the TAT does not have well-developed normative data, and critics have additionally raised concerns with respect to the lack of appropriate representation of figures from diverse cultures. This absence can in part be understood in light of the multiple, vastly different scoring schemes applied to the TAT. Of particular interest, Cramer and Blatt (1990) developed a scoring system for TAT defenses (denial, projection, identification); proposed a developmental theory of defenses; and found that children exposed to trauma who demonstrated the greatest use of defenses, and especially age-appropriate defenses, showed least emotional impairment (Dollinger & Cramer, 1990). Kelly (1997) and others recommend using the Social Cognition and Object Relations Scale (SCORS; Westen, Lohr, Silk, Gold, & Kerber, 1985) to facilitate the interpretation of the TAT results of children and adolescents (see Bram, 2014; Kelly, 2007).

Tell-Me-A-Story

The Tell-Me-A-Story (TEMAS) was designed to be a multiculturally sensitive instrument for youth under the age of 18 (Costantino, Malgady, & Rogler, 1988). It consists of 23 cards (with parallel sets for minorities and nonminority youth) from which a child or adolescent will narrate a description. A quantitative system was developed that evaluates 18 cognitive functions, 9 personality functions (interpersonal relationships, aggression, anxiety/depression, achievement motivation, delay of gratification, self-concept, sexual identity, moral judgment, and reality testing), and 7 affective functions (happy, sad, angry, fearful, neutral, ambivalent, and inappropriate affect).

Roberts Apperception Test for Children–2

The Roberts Apperception Test for Children–2 (Roberts-2) was developed with a standardization sample ranging in age from 6 to 18, whose demographic features roughly matched 2004 U.S. Census figures (Roberts, 2005). Constructed to assess youth's interpretation of interpersonal situations, the Roberts-2 includes 27 stimulus cards with parallel sets for minority and nonminority populations, 11 of which have parallel male and female versions. This instrument is one of the few thematic procedures with an explicit and standardized scoring system, and interrater reliability has generally been in the good to excellent range across the scales provided. These scales have included the following: theme overview; available resources; problem identification (five levels); problem resolution (five levels); emotions (anxiety, aggression, depression, and rejection); outcome scales (unresolved, nonadaptive, maladaptive, or unrealistic); and unusual or atypical responses (nine categories). Validity was established by examining the instrument's ability to document developmental differences and to distinguish between nonreferred and referred samples. Although all variables showed a statistically significant ability to differentiate respondents by age and clinical group, there are as yet limited findings pertaining to whether variables distinguish among various clinical samples.

Social Cognition and Object Relations Scale

The Social Cognition and Object Relations Scale (SCORS) comprises multiple scales on which cognitive and affective dimensions of object relations are rated based on narrative data (Stein, Hilsenroth, Slavin-Mulford, & Pinsker, 2011; Westen et al., 1985). The SCORS Global Rating Method (SCORS-G; Stein et al., 2011) is the most recent format and yields eight scales: complexity of representation of people; affective quality of representation; emotional investment in relationships; emotional investment in values and moral standards; understanding of social causality; self-esteem; identity and coherence of self; and experience and management of aggressive impulses. The SCORS-G is well validated for both adults and adolescents (Haggerty et al., 2015; see Stein et al., 2011, for a review).

The PA-Axis Diagnostic Approach

Below, we outline a two-step process of first considering severity through *level of personality organization* and then assessing *emerging personality style.*

Level of Personality Organization

Level of personality organization exists on a continuum from relatively healthy to compromised. This continuum can also be described as including healthy, neurotic, borderline, and psychotic levels. Consistent with the evaluation of child personality in the PC Axis, the severity of personality problems in adolescents may be evaluated alongside the MA Axis in relation to the 12 capacities of mental functioning included on that axis. These capacities are as follows:

- Cognitive and affective processes
  1. Capacity for regulation, attention, and learning
  2. Capacity for affective range, communication, and understanding
  3. Capacity for mentalization and reflective functioning
- Identity and relationships
  4. Capacity for differentiation and integration (identity)
  5. Capacity for relationships and intimacy
  6. Capacity for self-esteem regulation and quality of internal experience
- Defense and coping
  7. Capacity for impulse control and regulation
  8. Capacity for defensive functioning
  9. Capacity for adaptation, resiliency, and strength
- Self-awareness and self-direction
  10. Self-observing capacities (psychological mindedness)
  11. Capacity to construct and use internal standards and ideals
  12. Capacity for meaning and purpose

At the healthy end of the personality continuum all of these capacities are working together in a healthy, flexible, age-expected manner, and the adolescent employs one or a number of personality traits or patterns to support healthy functioning. For example, an adolescent may become a bit more compulsive when challenged by a difficult school assignment in order to master it. At the same time, the adolescent may be able to relax and be silly with his or her friends or romantic interest.

At the other end of the continuum are adolescents who evidence personality patterns characterized by rigid or limited capacities for relationships, emotional range, imagination, and so forth. Such patterns are often viewed as emerging personality disorders. A teenager who is chronically involved in antisocial behavior and has little awareness or concern about the feelings of others, relating to them largely as things rather than people, may show considerable limitations in all the mental functioning capacities in the MA Axis and may legitimately be considered to have psychopathic or antisocial personality pathology.

Below are described four common patterns of personality organization. These can be thought of as general patterns of engaging the world, arranged from healthiest to most maladaptive.

"Normal" Emerging Personality Patterns (Healthy)

Adolescents with healthy patterns demonstrate cohesive personality organizations in which their biological endowments, including their temperamental vulnerabilities, are managed adaptively within developmentally appropriate relationships with families, peers, and others. In relation to their stage of adolescent development, they have an increasingly organized sense of self, including age-appropriate coping skills and empathic, conscientious ways of dealing with feelings about self and others. Barring unforeseen, unmanageable adversities, such adolescents are likely to grow into the rich array of healthy characters.

Mildly Dysfunctional Emerging Personality Patterns (Neurotic)

Adolescents with neurotic patterns demonstrate less cohesive personality organizations in which their biological endowments, including their temperamental vulnerabilities, are managed less adaptively. Early in life, their primary caregivers may have had trouble helping them manage these constitutional dispositions. Thus their relationships with families, peers, and others are more fraught with problems. Such adolescents do not navigate the various developmental levels described earlier as successfully as those with less problematic endowments and/or more responsive caregivers. However, their sense of self and their sense of reality are pretty solid. As development proceeds, their adaptive mechanisms may be apparent in moderately rigid defensive patterns, and their reactions to adversities may be somewhat dysfunctional.

Dysfunctional Emerging Personality Patterns (Borderline)

Adolescents with borderline emerging personality patterns demonstrate vulnerabilities in reality testing and sense of self. Such problems may be manifested by maladaptive ways of dealing with feelings about themselves and others. Their defensive operations may distort reality (e.g., their own feelings may be perceived in others, rather than in themselves; the intentions of others may be misperceived; etc.).

Severely Dysfunctional Emerging Personality Patterns (Psychotic)

Adolescents with psychotic emerging personality patterns demonstrate significant deficits in their capacity for reality testing and forming a sense of self, manifested by consistently maladaptive ways of dealing with feelings about themselves and others. Their defensive operations interfere with their basic capacities to relate to others and to separate their own feelings and wishes from those of others.

Emerging Adolescent Personality Styles

In addition to considering level of organization, clinicians need to consider their adolescent patients' emerging personality styles. Rather than thinking of these styles as categorical diagnoses, it is more useful for clinicians to think of the relative degree to which each patient might be considered a match for a particular clinical description or prototype (see DeFife et al., 2015b; Haggerty et al., 2016; Westen, Shedler, & Bradley, 2006; Westen, Shedler, Bradley, & DeFife, 2012).

Consistent with the P and PC Axes of PDM-2, the PA-Axis classification system is derived from clinical expertise in theory and observation as well as empirical research. As discussed in Chapter 1 on the P Axis, personality styles can be organized under empirically identified superordinate categories or spectra, "internalizing" and "externalizing" (Markon, Krueger, & Watson, 2005; Westen et al., 2012). However, recent initial research utilizing adolescent samples has broadened these spectra in adolescent samples to consider "internalizing," "externalizing," and "borderline–dysregulated" spectra, and "obsessional" character style, based on outcomes from empirical research (Westen, DeFife, Malone, & DiLallo, 2014). See Figure 5.1. An overarching framework of spectra/character styles may have clinical utility in helping clinicians create formulations and develop treatments.

Below, an overview of the personality styles tied to each spectrum is provided, based on clinical observations, theory, and research. These styles were recently identified in a study of adolescent personality by Westen and colleagues (2014) and are also quite consistent with those found across other samples of adults and adolescents (see, e.g., Westen et al., 2003, 2012) and those outlined in the first PDM (PDM Task Force, 2006). Future research will need to validate these specific styles further, but we present them here as a framework for clinicians to work from, rather than as a final understanding of personality diagnostic categories.

In addition to a brief overview of extant theory and research tied to each style, we provide a prototype based on the summary of the SWAP-II-A items associated with each style, to create an empirical description of what patients with these personality styles might look like (for specific SWAP-II-A items and item scale correlations, clinicians may refer to Westen et al., 2014). To help guide clinicians' thinking, we also provide a "Match to Description" scale for each prototype, so that clinicians can match the extent to which they feel each adolescent patient matches that particular prototype (see DeFife, Goldberg, & Westen, 2015a; Westen et al., 2006, 2012).

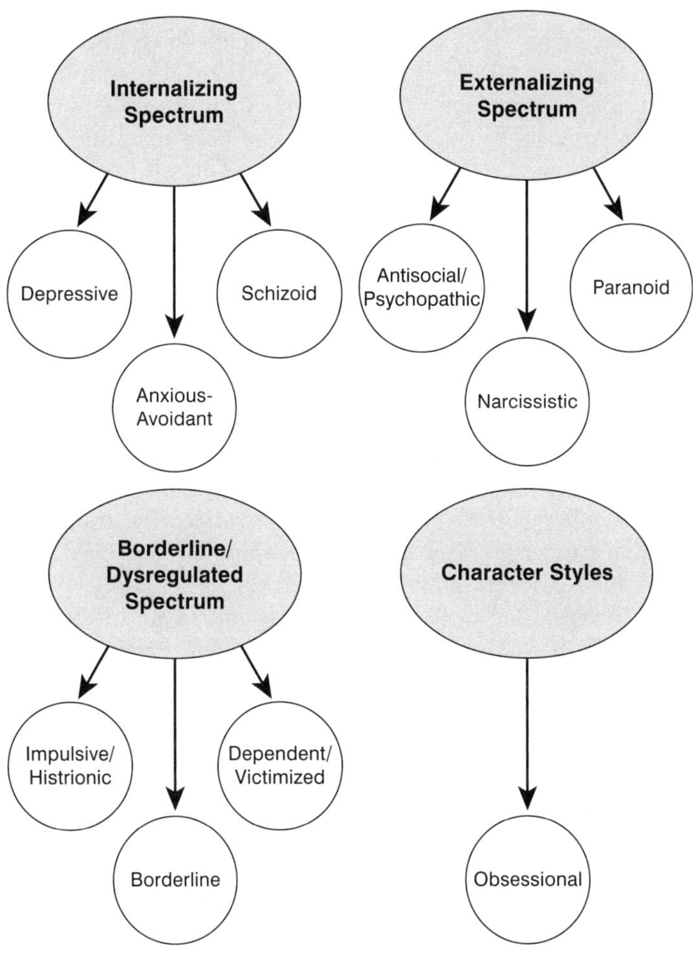

FIGURE 5.1. Empirically derived personality spectra and styles in adolescents. From Westen, DeFife, Malone, and DiLallo (2014). Copyright © 2014 Elsevier. Reprinted by permission.

PA-Axis Personality Syndromes[2]

Internalizing Spectrum

Depressive Personalities

When adolescents with depressive personality pathology present for treatment, they are likely to have unique treatment needs. Whereas adolescents with clinical depression present with physiological, behavioral, and vegetative symptoms (e.g., low appetite, fatigue, chronic pain, anhedonia), youth with depressive personalities may or may not exhibit these symptoms; they are nonetheless plagued by less concrete but more pervasive difficulties. Fortunately, several important theoretical frames offer perspective as well as an organizing framework for understanding variations of depressive personality. Blatt's (2004) model is perhaps the most widely referenced, having delineated two major forms of depressive characterology: the "introjective" and the "anaclitic." Introjective depression involves a focus on internal defectiveness, low self-worth, and self-critical tendencies, as well as a pervasive sense of internal "badness," "evil," or irreversible damage. Anaclitic depression has a more overt outward focus on interpersonal relationships, emphasizing themes related to dependency issues, abandonment fears, feelings of emptiness, loneliness, and helplessness. Blatt's early work spanned several decades and provided robust evidence that these subtypes respond differently to therapist and therapy factors and that they differ with regard to the role of early attachment relationships. Further distinctions have determined that the introjective type of depression is a better descriptor for those classified as having a depressive personality, whereas the anaclitic dynamics may also fit the diagnoses of narcissistic or dependent personality disorder (PDM Task Force, 2006). Blatt's seminal framework has clear implications for understanding the development of depressive personality characteristics in children and adolescents.

Empirical Description

Adolescents with depressive personality characteristics are often unhappy, depressed, or despondent. They regularly feel inadequate, inferior, worthless, or like "failures." They tend to be self-critical, setting unrealistically high standards for themselves, and also experience high levels of guilt. In contrast, it may be difficult for them to acknowledge or express anger toward others. They may regularly feel fatigued or lacking in energy. These adolescents may be prone to feeling "empty," believing that life has no meaning, and finding little satisfaction or enjoyment in their activities. They may be conflicted about pleasurable emotions and achievement and at times will deny or squelch realistic dreams in order to protect themselves from disappointment. In some cases, these adolescents will have a deep sense of "inner badness" and may appear that they want to punish the self or deny themselves pleasure. They also may be preoccupied with thoughts of death and dying. In relationships, they may experience fears of being rejected or abandoned.

Match to Description				
5	4	3	2	1
Very good match	Good match	Significant match (features)	Slight match	Little or no match

[2]PA axis, as PC axis, do not have codes for each personality syndrome. Because the adolescent and child personality are emerging patterns, we preferred not to reify in a code.

KEY FEATURES

Contributing constitutional–maturational patterns: Possible genetic predisposition to depression; depressive personality traits coalescing and consolidating through complex interactions between the environment (including family/parenting, trauma, school/community), temperament, attachment style, and growth in developmental stages across domains (i.e., social, biological, psychosexual, cognitive); also viewed in terms of deviations from the normative "storm and stress" of adolescent emotional and social growth.

Central tension/preoccupation: Goodness/badness (with accompanying attacks on the self); aloneness/relatedness (and accompanying experience of loss).

Central affects: Sadness, guilt, shame, negative self-evaluations, repressed anger/rage.

Characteristic pathogenic beliefs about self: "There is something essentially bad or inadequate about me," "Someone or something necessary for well-being has been irretrievably lost."

Characteristic pathogenic belief about others: "People who really get to know me will reject me."

Central ways of defending: Introjection, reversal, idealization of others, devaluation of self, denial, repression.

Countertransference and Transference Reactions

COUNTERTRANSFERENCE

Clinicians may get drawn into enactments that could confirm patients' pathogenic beliefs about the self; clinicians may feel compelled to "rescue" patients by attempts to "convince" the patients of their positive aspects, rather than helping the patients more fully explore pathogenic self-beliefs; clinicians may experience detachment or irritation toward the patients for rigid, inflexible "clinging" to pathogenic self-beliefs and negative beliefs about the social world, despite the clinicians' efforts to help the patients develop a more nuanced, balanced image of self and other; painful feelings may also occur in the context of managing suicidality occurring in the context of severe depression superimposed on a depressive personality style.

TRANSFERENCE

Patients may become increasingly dependent on clinicians for ego strength, due to overwhelming feelings of helplessness and low self-efficacy; patients may idealize clinicians, particularly in comparison to their own negative self-evaluations; patients may become increasingly paranoid, angry, or mistrusting of the therapists for refuting or otherwise challenging strongly held negative self-beliefs or may view clinicians' unconditional positive regard as "fake" or an indication that the clinicians cannot be trusted as intelligent professionals (e.g., "How can Dr. Smith be so kind to me when I'm so terrible? It must be false, not genuine," or "Dr. Smith may not be skilled enough to see how defective I am").

The following illustration is offered with the purpose of guiding clinicians in their thinking regarding the clinical picture emerging from the diagnostic process, as well as demonstrating the importance of an initial clinical formulation in the process of treatment planning, intervention, and ongoing assessment.

Clinical Illustration

Doris, an attractive 17-year-old, was referred for psychological evaluation and psychotherapy by her family doctor 1 year after the loss of her mother to cancer. Doris seemed to be having trouble working through grief; she cried constantly, had abandoned her goal of entering university, and had problems staying at home alone. She also found no pleasure in beach volleyball, which used to be her favorite hobby, and wanted to quit her team. Her father described Doris as being a quiet and undemanding child, who did not engage in close friendships but was always very likable. She had reached her developmental milestones within the expected time frame and had been an easygoing baby and toddler, but tired easily and was often sick with colds and ear infections. During her school years, Doris didn't seem to feel confident in her school performance and was hesitant to participate actively in class, although she performed very well on tests. She rarely expressed anger toward her parents or her peers. She easily showed compassion and blamed herself, feeling sad and ashamed, when she interfered in a conflict. Although she was a "smiley" child, her father said she often had a melancholic look in her eyes, and sometimes she shared with her parents her doubt about her self-value and sought their support. Doris had a sister 5 years her senior, who had always been a very dynamic child and left Doris somewhat in the shadows. However, Doris didn't complain or compete with her sister; indeed, she seemed happy to be around her and often asked for her advice and support.

Doris's mother had been a career woman who worked a lot and had not wanted children. It was Doris's father who insisted on having a second child, with the promise that the paternal grandmother and aunt would help in Doris's upbringing. Doris only saw her mother for a few hours daily, but (as she mentioned in her therapy sessions) she felt that her mother was full of energy and always emotionally available for her and that this compensated for her absence. Doris's father was her primary caregiver but he felt that he couldn't emotionally approach his daughter as well as his wife had. Doris herself confirmed his impression, stating that it was always easier for her to talk to her mother about her problems. The parents had had a warm and loving relationship.

The mother first fell ill when Doris was 13½ years old. Both parents and children were shocked, and the family's life changed dramatically. Doris tried to avoid thinking about it at first and soothed herself by thinking that her mother would be fine. However, a sudden metastasis after 2 years of treatment forced reality violently into Doris's life, and her mother passed away within a few months. During her mother's sickness, Doris became more depressed. She would not stay at home and clung to her boyfriend and friends, meeting them every day after school until late at night. During therapy, she confessed feeling enormous guilt over not being able to stay at home with her mother, as her father had asked her to. Similarly, she acknowledged feeling devastated and powerless in the face of her grief and sadness. After her mother's death, life in Doris's house changed, with both her sister and her father preoccupied with keeping her mother's business going. Doris's sister expected her to help by working some hours per week, but Doris felt too weak. She blamed herself for this feeling of weakness, maintaining that she should have been stronger in order to help her family more. Some months after her mother's death, Doris's boyfriend, to whom she felt very close and who had been her main source of emotional support, left her for another girl. Doris explained in tears that she felt shattered and terribly lonely. Her boyfriend asked to get together again after 2 months, and she forgave him, since she loved him so much and could acknowledge and feel gratitude, after his supporting her for such a long time. However, she was afraid that he remained somehow ambivalent about this reunion, and she felt very jealous of the girl he used to be with. She described these thoughts of jealousy as being dominant in her mind, and she strongly feared that her boyfriend would abandon her again for this girl (although she could understand that this was an irrational thought, since he had left this girl to return to her). Doris's constant feelings of sadness had been stressful for her friends and boyfriend, and she tried to restrain herself from expressing her grief and crying in front of them. In the last 2 months before referral, Doris had felt increasingly that she was not good at anything and wanted to abandon beach volleyball and her dream to study nutrition. She was very concerned about having upset her father with her problems and felt guilty about it. Although she had thought of getting help from a mental health professional, she was reluctant to ask her father for help, fearing she would cause him further troubles. Therefore, she felt great relief when her father suggested it himself.

During her therapy sessions, Doris made an immediate emotional connection with her therapist and communicated openly and accurately about her emotional experiences. She was keenly interested in investigating her internal world, although she sometimes expressed her fear that she was too weak to endure the pain that was unraveled through the therapeutic process. The therapist felt sympathy for Doris and found it easy to establish a warm attachment and a good therapeutic alliance with her.

Evaluating the Case

In evaluating the case of Doris, we first characterize the level of mental functioning by drawing upon clinical observations for each MA-Axis capacity. We then identify the primary emerging personality style.

COGNITIVE AND AFFECTIVE PROCESSES

1. *Capacity for regulation, attention, and learning*: Good gross and fine motor skills; good ability to concentrate and learn when not under stress.
2. *Capacity for affective range, communication, and understanding*: Wide range of emotions, but little reference to feelings of anger. Rich capacity for emotional expression and communication.
3. *Capacity for mentalization and reflective functioning:* Strong capacity for reflective functioning and empathy.

IDENTITY AND RELATIONSHIPS

4. *Capacity for differentiation and integration (identity):* Good capacity for mental representations of self and others and for differentiation of these representations. Confusion under stress between wish-fulfilling fantasies and reality, as in the case of her mother's illness (belief that the mother would be fine).
5. *Capacity for relationships and intimacy:* Close relationship with her parents and sister (especially her deceased mother). Close relationship with peers, by whom she

feels supported and valued. Fear of abandonment in romantic relationship under stressful circumstances, starting with her mother's death.

6. *Capacity for self-esteem regulation and quality of internal experience:* Frequent breakdowns in self-esteem regulation, accompanied by doubts about her value and feelings of weakness. Seeks help with self-esteem regulation from her environment.

DEFENSE AND COPING

7. *Capacity for impulse control and regulation:* Imposes strict controls on her affects, particularly aggressive impulses. Feelings of sadness and despair challenge her capacity for regulation.
8. *Capacity for defensive functioning:* Turning anger inward, repression, avoidance, idealization of others. Reality testing is slightly challenged in extremely stressful circumstances (such as the mother's illness).
9. *Capacity for adaptation, resiliency, and strength:* Although Doris has a good capacity for reflective function and secure internal representations, she frequently feels powerless and insufficiently able to face stressful situations.

SELF-AWARENESS AND SELF-DIRECTION

10. *Self-observing capacities (psychological mindedness):* Curiosity about her external and internal world. Good capacity to reflect on her own and others' emotions, as well as on interpersonal relationships.
11. *Capacity to construct and use internal standards and ideals*: Imposes strict demands on herself and displays intolerance for perceived weakness and need. Easily feels inadequate and guilty.
12. *Capacity for meaning and purpose:* Has a developed sense of meaning and purpose, which has faced some disruption by her depressive experience and loss.

Level of functioning: Neurotic.
Primary emerging personality style: Depressive.

Anxious–Avoidant Personalities

The roots of anxious–avoidant personality organization are intimately linked to important aspects of the early caregiving environment and individual differences in temperament. In particular, temperamental characteristics such as shyness, fearfulness, exaggerated or pronounced startle response, tearfulness, and social withdrawal are early precursors to a personality style described as avoidant or anxious. Not surprisingly, these personality characteristics often develop in a context where one or both parents exhibit a similar constellation of anxious–avoidant personality traits. Thus a child who might be classified by Thomas, Chess, and Birch (1968) as "slow to warm up" may be more likely to live in a familial environment structured, at least in part, by efforts (1) to contain and manage interpersonal anxiety and inhibitions shared by infant and caregiver, (2) to create social distance from persons who are not family members, (3) to limit exposure to social awkwardness or fear-inducing interactions, and (4) to manage concerns about separation and individuation. In this familial environment, the child begins to develop and internalize working models or representations of self and others (Bowlby, 1969, 1988) or "internalized relationships" (Loewald, 1962) that not only will determine the child's growing sense of self and the world, but will also influence the developmental trajectory across various dimensions. Specifically, these internal working models will predict the degree (1) of emotional distance or closeness to other that is tolerable or unacceptable, (2) to which others are experienced as overwhelming and frightening versus safe and calming, (3) of internalized sense of deficiency or incompetence, and (4) to which the individual avoids social interactions or situations due to fear of embarrassment. Internal working models also have an impact on how the individual is perceived by others and often the degree to which the person misperceives being the subject of persecution or ridicule. The overwhelming characterological anxiety associated with feeling impotent, intensely afraid, socially isolated, and utterly ineffective can lead to the development and use of primitive defensive strategies geared toward keeping the severe anxiety from becoming completely overwhelming. Unfortunately, these defenses are often ineffective, leading to the experience of "free-floating anxiety" that forms the core of this personality structure.

Fears of annihilation, cues signaling interpersonal danger, and separation anxiety (i.e., the terror associated with losing an interpersonal object), as well as the fear of disintegrating or fragmenting, dominate the developing personality. Moreover, most children and adolescents with anxious–avoidant traits have often been reared by parents who, unable to manage their own anxiety and terrors, have inadequately contained their children's emotions or provided a secure base for development. As such, individuals with anxious–avoidant personality features typically suffer from a severe lack of coping capacities, resulting in severe affective regulation difficulties and other associated somatic and physiological complaints. As early as preschool, these characteristics may lead to school refusal, neglect by peers, social isolation, hypersensitivity to environmental stimuli, social avoidance, and noticeable inhibition. Over the course of development, as the core of this temperamental predisposition becomes consolidated, the individual may become increasingly avoidant of people and social situations until the person is essentially isolated in an interpersonal world of his or her own creation. Furthermore, a vicious cycle ensues: The socially avoidant behaviors become negatively reinforcing, ensuring more avoidance and fewer opportunities to form new object relationships and representations. Because a child with a developing personality organization of this kind has little opportunity to disconfirm the growing sense of self as incompetent and fragile and the world as dangerous and unsafe, social terror and anxiety become the organizing components of the stabilizing character structure.

Avoidant children may interact and express themselves quite well in a safe, comfortable, well-known milieu, such as their own home or that of relatives. At the adaptive end of the continuum, adolescents with this pattern may be very sensitive, sweet, empathetic, thoughtful, and creative, with a few close friends and a capacity to pursue interests in depth. At the maladaptive end of the continuum, children may limit themselves emotionally and intellectually to a degree where they avoid or retreat from many age-expected peer and school activities.

Empirical Description

Adolescents with an anxious–avoidant personality style experience high levels of anxiety and tend to be shy and self-conscious in social situations. Consequently, fears of humiliation and embarrassment frequently cause them to avoid social situations, and they are more focused on avoiding fears or harm than on pursuing their desires. Some may fairly rigidly adhere to a routine to avoid anxiety, and separations from their parents or caregivers may be particularly challenging. Interpersonally, they tend to be passive, unassertive, and overly compliant with authority. They may lack social skills, appearing at times awkward or inappropriate. These adolescents may be inhibited and constricted in expressing their wishes or impulses. They may have trouble making decisions, ruminate, and have recurrent obsessional thoughts. Some adolescents matching this profile may experience panic attacks, experience somatic symptoms in response to stress, or have exaggerated fears on contracting medical illnesses. Finally, some of these adolescents may be unduly frightened by sexuality and associate it with danger.

Match to Description				
5	**4**	**3**	**2**	**1**
Very good match	Good match	Significant match (features)	Slight match	Little or no match

KEY FEATURES

Contributing constitutional–maturational patterns: Possible anxious or timid disposition/temperament (i.e., slowness to warm up); genetic liability for anxiety or timid disposition.

Central tension/preoccupation: Safety/danger.

Central affects: Fear, anxiety, shame, embarrassment, guilt, confusion.

Characteristic pathogenic beliefs about self: "I am in constant danger that I must somehow elude," "Something catastrophic could happen at any moment," "I must not be separated from my caregiver."

Characteristic pathogenic beliefs about others: "Others are sources of either unimagined dangers or magical protection," "Others may create situations that would cause me humiliation, shame, or embarrassment."

Central ways of defending: Symbolization, displacement, avoidance, rationalization; general anxieties that may hide more upsetting specific anxieties (i.e., anxieties may serve a defensive function).

Countertransference and Transference Reactions

COUNTERTRANSFERENCE

Clinicians may inadvertently attempt to rescue patients by trying to convince them that the extent of their fear and anxiety is disproportional to actual life events; therapists may also try to counter the patients' distorted thought processes; due to patients' expectations, paranoid fears, and anxiety, therapists may inadvertently get pulled into enactments that result in the patients' actually becoming (or perceiving themselves to become) more embarrassed, more ashamed, more worried, and so on; clinicians may then begin to feel increasingly responsible for patients and unconsciously act in an effort to avoid worsening or being the cause of the patients' anxiety.

TRANSFERENCE

Clinicians may be idealized and viewed as "saviors" or sources of safety. Dependency issues may begin to present prominently in treatment; conversely, paranoid fears may be projected onto clinicians, resulting in patients' mistrusting the clinicians and becoming more inhibited or resistant; patients may be expecting to and waiting to feel embarrassed, ashamed, or otherwise uncomfortable due to the social nature of interactions with therapists; due to separation anxieties, patients may have anxiety associated with separations from therapists (at the end of sessions, during vacations, etc.).

Schizoid Personalities

Although they may also crave relationships, schizoid adolescents have a pervasive pattern of detachment from social relationships and have a very restricted range of expression of emotions in interpersonal settings. They seem to avoid social interactions very actively and are seen by others as "loners." In contrast to avoidant and constricted children, who may be likable and popular, they have few or no friends. Because of either severe inhibition or lack of social skills, schizoid children cannot spontaneously interact appropriately with others. When asked about their withdrawals, they may assert that others do a variety of ills to them. Clinical experience suggests that they may have learned to fear the negative consequences of their need for love.

More than other personality organizations, the schizoid pattern constitutes a continuum that ranges from mild or neurotic impairment to severe psychotic disorders. Temperamentally distinct as being easily overstimulated and hyperreactive (McWilliams, 2011), children and adolescents with this personality style understand early that they are in some way distinct or "different" from others and may subsequently increasingly isolate or separate themselves from others. At the mild end of the continuum, individuals appear indifferent to others, detached, and largely uninterested in building and maintaining relationships. At the extreme end, their detachment from the social world is due less to indifference and due more to their active fantasy lives, loss of touch with reality, and subsequent odd behaviors and perceptions. This latter group tends to lack the defensive capacities to maintain internal integrity and cohesion, almost as if there is no barrier between themselves and others, leaving them unable to keep themselves from becoming dysregulated by external stimuli. These individuals, diffuse as they are, become even more disorganized when in close contact with others, as fears of engulfment, annihilation, and other forms of vulnerability pervade their being. At either end of the spectrum, aloneness is valued as a primary defensive strategy that allows a person to project outward the unbearable sensations of "object hunger" or "love made hungry" (Fairbairn, 1952; McWilliams, 2011) onto others "out there." The schizoid individual withdraws, becoming lost in fantasies, in staunch rejection of and contrast to the outer world. Given that individuals with this personality style tend to prefer solitary status and seem uninterested in relationships with others, there have been long-held perceptions that they lack the typical human desire and need for close attachments. However, contemporary literature suggests that some schizoid people long for intimacy and social connection as much as most individuals do (Shedler & Westen, 2004).

In addition to being physically isolated from others, these individuals are isolated by the uniqueness of their thoughts, ideas, and perceptions of the world. Highly sensitive and reactive to social stimuli, they tend to react to social triggers by withdrawing into themselves and creating their own worlds. There is literature to suggest that both a low-warmth, unemotional, detached parenting style and an overbearing, smothering parenting style are linked to the development of schizoid personality traits. Importantly, there is equifinality, in that either parenting style leads to the overwhelming internal need to distance oneself from others as much as absolutely possible. In contrast, the goals of schizoid individuals with differing early parenting experiences may be distinct. Whereas a child of an overbearing caregiver is consumed by fears of engulfment or being controlled, a child of a detached mother is most concerned with avoiding psychic contact with his or her own overwhelming desire and longing for nurturing and intimacy. Moreover, this latter type's intense rejection of unmet dependency needs leads to the use of defensive strategies such as projection and denial, which allow these intense feelings to be placed outside the self. As a primary strategy, when such persons feel afraid or overwhelmed, they hide—whether they do so in reclusive settings or only by virtue of their imaginations (McWilliams, 2011). It is important to note also that, particularly in childhood, schizoid personality traits can be difficult to distinguish from autism spectrum disorder. Given that both pathologies are characterized by social differences, odd behaviors, isolation, and apparent lack of interest in interpersonal relationships, from this perspective children and adolescents with schizoid personality traits may not behave and "look" drastically different from those who might be considered as having "high-functioning" autism.

Empirical Description

Adolescents with a schizoid personality style lack social skills and tend to be socially awkward. They lack close friendships and tend to be ignored or avoided by peers. Their appearance or manner might seem odd or peculiar (e.g., grooming, eye contact). They may appear to have a limited range of emotions and to be emotionally detached from or indifferent with other people. They often feel like outcasts or outsiders and may be bullied or teased. Such adolescents may seem childish for their age and think in overly concrete terms. Their descriptions of important people in their life may seem two-dimensional, and they may have difficulty making sense of other people's behavior. Some of these adolescents may use reasoning processes that seem odd or idiosyncratic (e.g., arbitrary inferences), and they may also elicit boredom in others (e.g., by talking incessantly, without feeling, or about inconsequential matters).

Match to Description				
5	4	3	2	1
Very good match	Good match	Significant match (features)	Slight match	Little or no match

KEY FEATURES

Contributing constitutional–maturational patterns: Highly sensitive, shy, easily overstimulated, prone to odd thinking and strange behaviors, potential risk for psychosis.

Central tension/preoccupation: Fear of closeness/longing for closeness.

Central affects: General emotional pain when overstimulated; overwhelming affects and annihilation fears that must be suppressed.

Characteristic pathogenic belief about the self: "Dependency and love are dangerous."

Characteristic pathogenic beliefs about others: "The social world is dangerous and impinging on my boundaries," "The social world is dangerously engulfing."

Central ways of defending: Withdrawal, both physically and into fantasy and idiosyncratic preoccupations.

Countertransference and Transference Reactions

COUNTERTRANSFERENCE

Clinicians may become parental toward patients in an effort to "protect" them and attempt to assuage their severe anxieties and limit the impact of their social impairments on their daily lives; clinicians may struggle to establish an appropriate amount of closeness and distance in therapy that will allow for a relationship to develop and trust to build, but that will also avoid triggering or worsening patients' fears of engulfment or intrusion; clinicians may feel tempted to get patients to "open up" and let the clinicians into their intrapsychic worlds before the patients are ready; due to patients' character structure, clinicians may unconsciously begin to view the patients as members of an "interesting species" (McWilliams, 2011, p. 207), rather than simply as other human beings.

TRANSFERENCE

Patients may struggle to make sense of clinicians' behaviors as well as their own; they may not know how to relate to clinicians in a meaningful way in therapy; patients may "test" clinicians to see whether the clinicians will react to the patients' strange or provocative communications and behaviors in the same ways that others in the patients' lives have; they are hoping against hope that the clinicians will still be interested and attempt to help, despite their odd, unpredictable, and unusual ways of being and interacting; patients may take an inordinately long time to "learn" how to speak to clinicians because they feel afraid, lost, empty, and disconnected during the early stages of therapy (McWilliams, 2011).

Externalizing Spectrum

Psychopathic–Antisocial Personalities

Adolescents with significant sociopathic or psychopathic tendencies show some degree of disregard for, and violation of, the rights of others, and are notable for deceitfulness and lack of remorse. There is a belief that temperaments characterized by excessive aggression in infancy and early childhood predispose individuals to antisocial or psychopathic personality tendencies. People with antisocial tendencies or psychopathy also tend to have a higher threshold for thrill-seeking and sensory stimulation than others do, and have often been exposed to deprivation, neglect, or abuse throughout childhood. Similarly to children who develop narcissistic personalities (and there is significant overlap), those with psychopathic tendencies were often overindulged as children, frequently given material goods and deprived of emotional care (McWilliams, 2011).

Because a sense of omnipotent control serves as a primary defensive strategy for individuals with psychopathy (McWilliams, 2011), such individuals tend to feel most powerful and masterful when devising and implementing strategies that seek to gain control and advantage over others. These behaviors are evident as early as elementary school, with the challenge being a determination of the extent to which there is a pervasive lack of empathy and personal regard for others. There is an inherently diminished capacity for attachment and self–other relatedness and perspective.

Like most other personality patterns, psychopathy exists on a continuum, with lower-functioning individuals displaying problems with thinking, poor reality testing, less internal integration, and a greater likelihood for displaying serious, dangerous, and aggressive behaviors (including armed robbery, rape, murder, or other acts that violate the rights and feelings of others). At the higher-functioning end of the spectrum, persons with psychopathic traits may tend to hide their cruel, coercive intentions better than others, often behind a cool veneer of narcissistic aloofness, while using their intelligence to outwit and manipulate others. Frequently, higher-functioning persons with psychopathy can build "friendships" and achieve great success in academic, social, and occupational or economic domains.

Historically, there has been a widespread clinical belief that persons with psychopathy are untreatable––but, more recently, there is increasing evidence that some treatment approaches can alter the relatedness problems, empathic sensibilities, and behavioral patterns of persons exhibiting psychopathy. Bateman and Fonagy (2004, 2008, 2013) and their colleagues have begun to investigate the effectiveness of mentalization-based therapy in the treatment of antisocial personality. This model presumes that these persons lack the capacity to understand their own internal worlds; they also struggle to place themselves "in someone else's shoes," and thus lack the capacity to understand the internal states of others or to read or perceive certain emotions in others (most disturbingly, fear). Alternatively, these persons may be able to understand others' emotional states on a cognitive (but not emotional) level and often use this knowledge to coerce, manipulate, or otherwise control others. As such, mentalization-based treatment for antisocial personality focuses on increasing mentalizing capacities, including building empathy and accurate perspective taking. Additionally, because people with psychopathy seem to experience singular emotional sensations (either "manic exhilaration or blind rage"; McWilliams, 2011, p. 160), mentalization-based therapy may focus on helping identify and articulate a wider range of emotional states in individuals with psychopathy.

Empirical Description

Adolescents who match this prototype tend to demonstrate a reckless disregard for the rights, property, or safety of others. They show little remorse when they cause harm or injury and they may routinely take advantage of others. These adolescents tend to be rebellious and defiant toward authority figures. They can be deceitful, manipulative, with little empathy, seeming unable or unwilling to respond to others' feelings. They may be impervious to consequences, with a tendency to act impulsively, be unreliable, and blame others for their shortcomings or circumstances. They tend to be thrill seeking, to engage in criminal or delinquent behavior, and to abuse alcohol and drugs. Some of these adolescents may be prone to violence or gain pleasure from being aggressive and from being seen as "bad" or "tough." They may dominate and intimidate their significant others. They may repeatedly try to convince others that they are committed to change, but then revert to maladaptive behavior.

Match to Description				
5	4	3	2	1
Very good match	Good match	Significant match (features)	Slight match	Little or no match

KEY FEATURES

Contributing constitutional–maturational patterns: Genetic vulnerability, possible congenital aggressiveness, early exposure to violence and trauma, high threshold for emotional stimulation.

Central tension/preoccupation: Instrumental relational and physical aggression, fear of being controlled.

Central affects: Rage, envy.

Characteristic pathogenic belief about self: "I can do whatever I want."

Characteristic pathogenic beliefs about others: "No one can be trusted," "Everyone is selfish, manipulative, dishonorable, and/or weak."

Central ways of defending: Reaching for omnipotent control.

Countertransference and Transference Reactions

COUNTERTRANSFERENCE

Clinicians may respond positively to (and be seduced by) patients' charming manner and may get drawn into enactments characterized by "bending the rules" for the patients, advocating for the patients in atypical ways, or exhibiting blurred boundaries; when the clinicians realize the patients' agendas and strategies, they may feel powerless, afraid, or resistant to the differing dynamics in the relationship; contempt, moralistic outrage, hate, and hostility are common reactions once clinicians realize the degree to which the patients lack sincerity, emotion, and empathy (McWilliams, 2011); clinicians may develop negative feelings toward patients that are, counterintuitively, reflections of the patients' inability to care for (and feel empathic toward) the therapist; clinicians may feel disarmed, controlled, and frightened by patients due to the nature and impact of their character pathology (i.e., cold, callous, unemotional traits).

TRANSFERENCE

Patients may project predation tendencies onto their therapists, such that the therapists are viewed as being involved for personal gain or other selfish reasons; patients may be exceedingly charming with clinicians for secondary gains that may or may not be apparent to the clinicians; patients, having no experiences with emotion and love, may struggle to figure out clinicians' "angles" and make meaning of the clinicians' perspective and behaviors (e.g., kindness, unconditional positive regard).

The following illustration is offered with the purpose of guiding clinicians in their thinking regarding the clinical picture emerging from the diagnostic process, as well as demonstrating the importance of an initial clinical formulation in the process of treatment planning, intervention, and ongoing assessment.

Clinical Illustration

Tom was 13 years old when his mother and stepfather referred him for diagnosis and treatment following several incidents of delinquency, as well as poor school performance over the previous 2 years. At the age of 12, Tom began hanging around with older adolescents who were engaged in drug dealing and arms possession. At the time of referral, Tom was participating in acts of school vandalism and smoking. In addition, he had repeatedly stolen money from his stepfather, his mother, and his older sister. After he was caught stealing, he always spoke of his regret and apologized; however, both his mother and stepfather believed that he apologized to avoid their anger and punishment, not out of true remorse. He exhibited no guilt about the stealing and repeated it as soon as he wanted to have something he could not afford with his pocket money. He didn't seem to care about the consequences of his acts and showed little compassion, even when his sister or mother was crying after he stole from one of them. When his mother scolded him, he responded by telling her he feared no punishment and exhibiting an emotionally flat, tough attitude. On occasion, however, he displayed a tender and giving side of himself by trying to help his stepfather fix his boat (this was his stepfather's main hobby) and sometimes cleaning the house to surprise his mother when she would get back from work. On family outings, Tom always wanted to be neat and well dressed and behaved politely to people who were not family members. He clearly identified with his stepfather's upper-class status. These two contradicting sides of his personality puzzled the rest of the family members in their efforts to understand who he was and how they should relate to him.

Tom's childhood years were very traumatic. His mother, a young, immature woman who already felt stressed after the birth of her daughter (3 years older than Tom), did not want another child. Tom's father, who worked for the government, was described as a man with a difficult temperament and a tendency toward addictions (alcohol and gambling). In addition, he was not keen on caring for the children. The parental couple was already experiencing difficulties before the added strain of Tom's birth. Following his birth, the parents' relationship deteriorated further, and they were constantly engaging in arguments. Tom was described by his mother as a very quiet and easygoing baby who asked for nothing. In contrast, she was demanding toward him, coaxing him to walk from an early age and toilet-training him at 15 months. Convinced that she had to help her children be independent and tough, she avoided cuddling them when they cried. When Tom was 20 months old, his maternal grandmother died suddenly. Tom's mother entered a long period of grief in which she was emotionally unavailable to her children. Similarly, Tom's father started spending days away from home; some months later, when Tom was 2½ years old, he abandoned his family. He remained disconnected from his children. While grieving, Tom's mother found out that her husband had used her credit cards to withdraw large amounts of money for gambling and that she was left with substantial debts. The family had to face extreme poverty, deprived of food and a stable place to live. Thus Tom's mother decided to take on two jobs, leaving her children alone for several hours with only the inadequate care of their disabled maternal grandfather. Tom experienced great emotional deprivation from the age of 2½ until he was 9 years old, with his mother being absent and his sister (who mainly took care of him) enjoying terrifying him after dark. Tom himself reported in his therapy sessions—while laughing—that he had spent several hours when he was little under the sheets, feeling terrified, until his mother returned home. In later years, he tried to overcome his fears on his own and "toughen up" by rewatching movies that had scared him in the past, like *Saw*.

Things changed for the family when Tom was about 9 years old: His mother remarried, and they moved to her new, well-off husband's house. The family experienced no more financial deprivation, and Tom's mother stopped working a lot and started spending time with Tom and his sister. Tom changed schools, but his classmates bullied him at his new school. Some months later, his behavior at school changed from being shy and quiet to causing trouble during lessons and getting involved in fights with his classmates. He also started to compete with older kids by engaging in risky behaviors with bicycles and engaging in truancy. After the stealing incidents, his mother started to believe that Tom was just like his father; Tom seemed irritated, but also somehow proud, when hearing his mother's comments.

Tom attended the diagnostic sessions unwillingly, complaining that he had promised to "be good" and that he expected his parents to withdraw their punishment of sending him to mental health specialists. He had a blank, expressionless face and showed no interest in emotional contact, although he cooperated well in testing; he talked about himself and his family in a mainly emotionally flat and superficial manner. Psychological testing revealed fears of deprivation, loss, and loneliness and experiences of sadness and pain, against which he defended himself through avoidance, detachment, projection, and acting out. It seemed that Tom's need to feel adequate and strong had alienated him from his painful internal world, and thus reinforced his feelings of deprivation and internal emptiness. Prior evaluation by a school psychologist had revealed average intelligence and no specific learning difficulties. However, he displayed difficulties in focusing his attention for long periods, especially when required to participate in problem solving; he abandoned his tasks easily since he lost his motivation when faced with something difficult that required effort.

In his therapy sessions, Tom talked about his need to be popular in school by being the "tough one" that everyone respected or feared. His relationships with his peers seemed to have been superficial, focusing on impressing others with tricks and toughness. He also disliked discussing school lessons or problems of any kind with his classmates since he stated he felt these were "boring" topics. He talked to his therapist a lot about the experiences of financial deprivation when he was young and his current impulsive needs to buy things he wished for.

In therapy, Tom's attitude changed rapidly from one session to the next. Sometimes he was happy to be with his therapist, and tried to charm her either by talking about his physical abilities in sports and bicycle tricks or by showing his strength or lack of respect for punishment or danger. He also expressed wanting to be something special that would make himself and his parents proud, although he didn't have a clear picture of how to achieve this. At these times, the therapist felt in emotional contact with Tom, who responded by allowing some of his painful feelings to come to the fore while describing incidents of the past (e.g., terrifying dreams he had or movies that frightened him). At other times—especially after fights with his mother—he came across as being cold and emotionally detached, demanding to stop therapy, since he felt very good about himself and needed nothing to change. In those moments, Tom seemed to be unreachable; the therapist felt as if they had "hit a brick wall," and experienced countertransference feelings of disappointment and sadness.

Evaluating the Case

In evaluating the case of Tom, we first characterize the level of mental functioning by drawing upon clinical observations for each MA-Axis capacity. We then identify the primary emerging personality style.

COGNITIVE AND AFFECTIVE PROCESSES

1. *Capacity for regulation, attention, and learning:* Good fine and gross motor skills, good verbal abilities, poor behavior regulation; impulsive actions and limited motivation to focus attention on learning activities.
2. *Capacity for affective range, communication, and understanding:* Restricted range of emotions; can talk about his fears and understand them, but is not in touch with his feelings in order to communicate them. Emotions can escalate rapidly and lead to outbursts and acting out.
3. *Capacity for mentalization and reflective functioning:* Failure to understand the emotional functioning consequences of his actions for others. Poor capacity for empathy.

IDENTITY AND RELATIONSHIPS

4. *Capacity for differentiation and integration (identity):* Incoherent sense of self; exhibits contradictory sides of himself without consciously experiencing the conflict. Cannot differentiate his internal wishes from external world and feels he can satisfy his wishes regardless of others' will.
5. *Capacity for relationships and intimacy:* Wishes to have friends, but his relationships are superficial. Mother's early behavior seems to have fostered an avoidant attachment pattern. Attachment trauma of abandonment from father and lack of adequate parental care through most of his childhood. Current conflicts with his sister, mother, and stepfather.
6. *Capacity for self-esteem regulation and quality of internal experience:* Self-esteem seems unstable and is based on others' acceptance. Self-image oscillates between images of a kind, well-off young man and a tough, rebellious, and fearless individual.

DEFENSE AND COPING

7. *Capacity for impulse control and regulation:* Poor emotion and behavior regulation. Impulsivity in actions and limited frustration tolerance. Frequent aggression outbursts, mainly toward his mother and peers.

8. *Capacity for defensive functioning*: Emotional detachment and avoidance, identification with the aggressor, projection, and acting out.
9. *Capacity for adaptation, resiliency, and strength:* Regardless of all the relational adversity he has experienced, some brief moments of meeting with the therapist, indicating perhaps a desire to connect with another.

SELF-AWARENESS AND SELF-DIRECTION

10. *Self-observing capacities (psychological mindedness):* Restricted curiosity about the world and limited capacity for self-reflection. Very confused about his wishes and values.
11. *Capacity to construct and use internal standards and ideals:* Lack of capacity for remorse, disregard for the consequences of his actions, and general belief that anything is permissible so long as he is careful not to get caught.
12. *Capacity for meaning and purpose:* Lacks an age-appropriate sense of meaning that helps organize his personal choices. Has trouble seeing beyond the present moment.

Level of functioning: Borderline.
Primary emerging personality style: Psychopathic–antisocial.

Narcissistic Personalities

There is a full range of narcissistic patterns in adolescents. At the healthier end of the narcissistic spectrum, adolescents are highly focused on realistic pride in accomplishment. Toward the more dysfunctional end, narcissistically motivated adolescents may show pervasive patterns of grandiose fantasy and/or behavior. They may exhibit arrogance, entitlement, need for admiration, and lack of empathy for others. Or they may seem depressed, irritated, and full of complaints behind which are frustrated grandiose aspirations. Although some narcissistic adolescents seem "spoiled" and entitled, most are clearly defending against feelings of low self-esteem and are trying to avoid shame and humiliation.

People with narcissistic personalities are driven by an insatiable need for adoration, admiration, and adulation from others. Having at the core an unyielding sense of being fraudulent and unlovable (McWilliams, 2011), such people operate between the polarities of devaluation and idealization. The roots of narcissism begin in childhood with a natural and necessary sense of omnipotence and grandiosity that good parenting supports and mirrors. According to Kohut (1968), it is also from this early inflated sense of the self—of existing at the center of the universe as the master of one's realm—that the roots of healthy personality structure are born. More precisely, the development of the self begins with mirroring by an empathic, loving parent; this mirroring reflects the essence of the individual until this sense of being is internalized. In this context, one first feels grandiose, special, and superior, eventually developing a more balanced and nuanced perspective on the self and others. Alternatively, in the context of cold and unresponsive parenting, a developmental arrest can occur such that an individual becomes stuck and a "disorder of the self" develops (Kohut & Wolf, 1978).

Contemporary theorists suggest that disorders of the self can occur as many subtypes within a range of varying predominant personality traits. At the core, all individuals with narcissistic personalities have a terrifying, intolerably painful sense of being deficient and broken. Often, as children, these people have been narcissistic extensions of self-involved parents who value the children only in relation to themselves. In this confusing, enmeshed familial environment, the grandiosity of childhood becomes a facade or defense against the painful reality of having never been seen, recognized, or valued as a separate self. As Winnicott (1960) notes, from this experience, the "false sense" develops—an identity not based on any sense of one's true self but rather formed on the basis of what is acceptable. At the other extreme, a child who is mirrored to such an extent as never to experience frustration or to come into contact with any true sense of personal limitation is also at risk for the development of narcissistic personality. As McWilliams (2011) points out, the experience of being constantly judged, even if positively, leads to equal measures of self-doubt and insecurity. Feeling much like a fraud, the overidealized child also becomes a self-caricature, feeling both entitled (by virtue of being constantly indulged) but also secretly concerned that he or she is wholly undeserving of such indiscriminate latitude and adulation. In either instance (i.e., when a child is either over- or undervalued, in an atmosphere typified by constant scrutiny and evaluation), concerns with perfectionism, social status, and the opinions of others form the core of the person's identity.

The resulting psychological fragility of this early developmental experience engenders a self-preoccupation that only values others as a means to an end. Vacillating between devaluing and idealizing themselves or others, individuals with narcissistic personalities can only locate their self-esteem in others, by viewing themselves as either superior or inferior by comparison. This external barometer replaces an inner core of identity and self-esteem, such that when this "narcissistic supply" is limited or unavailable, there is an overwhelming sense of internal emptiness and utter depletion. The fragile veneer of the individual with narcissistic traits, the screen of narcissistic perfection, and the projection of deficiency and inferiority onto others are also intimately linked with powerful emotions such as envy, rage, and intense shame. These emotions rise to the surface when the person experiences emotional injury in the form of ridicule, insult, or other forms of embarrassing public "undressing." The emotional vulnerability and pain experienced by individuals with narcissistic traits are, in ways, unparalleled. With few internal mechanisms for maintaining coherence and esteem, they perceive themselves as victims of their circumstances; they are entirely dependent on an unpredictable, external social world to maintain internal equilibrium and organization.

Empirical Description

Adolescents with an emerging narcissistic personality style appear to feel privileged and expect preferential treatment. They have an exaggerated sense of self-importance and tend to be dismissive, arrogant, and controlling. These adolescents seek to be the center of attention and seem to treat others as an audience to witness their own importance. They believe that they should be appreciated and associated with people perceived to be of higher status or superior. In their interactions they tend to be critical, manipulative, and lacking in empathy. They are competitive and envious of others, but also may expect themselves to be "perfect" and have an underlying sense of being inadequate or inferior. At the same time, they may be invested in portraying themselves as emotionally strong and untroubled.

Match to Description				
5	4	3	2	1
Very good match	Good match	Significant match (features)	Slight match	Little or no match

KEY FEATURES

Contributing constitutional–maturational patterns: No clear data (see Kohut, 1968, for some suggestions).

Central tension/preoccupation: Inflation–deflation of self-esteem.

Central affects: Shame, humiliation, contempt, envy.

Characteristic pathogenic beliefs about self: "I need to be perfect to feel OK," "I need to feel that I am superior to others to feel OK."

Characteristic pathogenic belief about others: "Others enjoy riches, beauty, power, and fame; the more I have of these things, the better I feel; others envy me."

Central ways of defending: Idealization, devaluation, denial.

Countertransference and Transference Reactions

COUNTERTRANSFERENCE

Clinicians may respond positively to (and be seduced by) patients' idealizations; clinicians may experience negative countertransference reactions (e.g., rage, hate, boredom) toward the patients when the clinicians feel devalued or when interacting with aspects of a patient's false self (e.g., grandiosity, conceit, severe devaluation of others); clinicians may also feel bored, annoyed, or sleepy during sessions, as the sense that "nothing 'real' is going on" predominates; clinicians may be surprised or "thrown off" by patients' lack of interest in exploring the therapeutic relationship; clinicians may have a sense of "being invisible" or being obliterated by the patients and not viewed as real persons (McWilliams, 2011)

TRANSFERENCE

Clinicians may be alternatingly idealized and devalued; patients project parts of themselves onto therapists (i.e., the devalued or idealized parts), so that transference to the clinicians is as self-objects rather than as real, separate persons; clinicians are used as "containers" for split-off parts of the patients as a strategy for maintaining self-esteem (McWilliams, 2011); various self-object transferences may occur, including mirroring, twinship, and alter-ego patterns during the course of therapy (Kohut, 1968).

Paranoid Personalities

A pervasive pattern of distrustfulness and suspiciousness is relatively rare in childhood. In adolescence it is less rare, but is often part of another emerging personality pattern, such as an antisocial pattern or multidimensionally impaired (borderline) clinical picture. These adolescents have mild to moderate to pervasive distrust and suspiciousness of others, whose motives they interpret as malevolent. Shame and humiliation are important predeterminants to this emerging personality pattern. In interactions with peers and adults, such children expect shame and humiliation to occur. They therefore project, avoid, and attack in a preemptive fashion, in words and/or in actions.

The period of development as adolescents make the transition into early adulthood is one of great uncertainty. Their perspective and positionality regarding their bodies, familial relationships, and friendships are frequently in flux, and thus they may experience increased anxiety amidst a shifting social landscape. Research has found that humans, under conditions of prolonged uncertainty, heightened anxiety, and fear, may develop beliefs that assume inequity in relationships, uncertainty about how the world works, and the potential for imminent risk to oneself if not careful. Adolescents who grew up in family systems, or social conditions, in which these beliefs were accurate descriptions of daily life may psychologically organize around these relational contingencies in such ways that even when they later find relationships and social settings in which there is no present basis to assume threat and risk, or to experience fear, they may continue to perceive and experience them nonetheless.

For example, imagine a child growing up in a home in which a parent has magical beliefs outside the cultural norm, labile and unpredictable mood, and impaired reality testing, and is emotionally intrusive into the child's psychological privacy. The parent habitually barges into the child's room speaking loudly in the middle of the night, about things that don't make total sense and that may not have a basis in consensual reality. It would be reasonable to assume that such a child might feel fear or confusion and might need to find a way to conceptually organize interactions that are difficult to hold in mind in any coherent way. Over time, the child might accommodate to the parent's interpersonal style (due in no small part to the fact that no matter how impaired the parent may be, the child needs the parent to survive), bending his or her perceptual reality to make the parent's mode of interaction make sense. By doing so, the child would be able to maintain connection with, and proximity to, the parent, but in the process would configure him- or herself in a way necessitating suspicion and guardedness against the ever-present possibility and fear of mistreatment and exploitation by the closest of relations. This self-configuration would set in motion the belief that all relationships, no matter how close, carry the potential for threat and manipulation, at times that are not predictable.

It should be noted that while paranoid personality patterns may be observable and understood from a characterological perspective in adolescence, this is also a period of development during which early symptomatic expressions of psychotic spectrum illnesses may first become evident. For individuals with genetic loading for schizophrenia, schizoaffective disorders, and mood disorders with psychotic features, treating clinicians will have to pay close attention to the fine-grained distinctions that may disambiguate paranoia (whose etiology is in large part attributable to character pathology) from paranoia in the context of the onset or prodromal phase of a psychotic spectrum illness. Differentiating between the two may be done in part by assessing the extent to which paranoid thinking is porous, or believed in 100%, and thus constituting delusional thinking.

Empirical Description

Adolescents with a paranoid personality style may be prone to intense anger disproportionate to the situation at hand. They tend to blame their own failures and shortcomings on others, hold grudges, and have extreme reactions to slights and criticism. They are often hostile and suspicious, assuming that others will harm, deceive, or betray them. These adolescents generally lack close friendships and feel misunderstood, disliked, and/or ignored by others. They tend to see their own unacceptable feelings and impulses in others rather than themselves; relatedly, they often manage to elicit in others feeling similar to their own. When upset, they tend to have difficulty seeing positive and negative qualities in the same person at the same time. Strong emotions may also lead them to be more irrational than is customary, and sometimes their perception of reality may seem impaired. These adolescents often lack psychological insight and have difficulty making sense of their own behavior and that of others. They may ruminate, dwell on problems, and sometimes be preoccupied by aggressive ideas/fantasies.

Match to Description				
5	4	3	2	1
Very good match	Good match	Significant match (features)	Slight match	Little or no match

KEY FEATURES

Contributing constitutional–maturational patterns: Being subjected to irritating/aggressive interactions over the course of development; being subjected to unexplained, bizarre experiences over the course of development; possible higher fear sensitivity.

Central tension/preoccupation: Attacking or being attacked by humiliating others.

Central affects: Fear, rage, shame, contempt.

Characteristic pathogenic belief about self: "I am in constant danger."

Characteristic pathogenic belief about others: "The world is full of potential dangers and people who may cause me harm."

Central ways of defending: Projection, projective identification, denial, reaction formation.

Countertransference and Transference Reactions

COUNTERTRANSFERENCE

Clinicians may find themselves wanting to make logical appeals regarding everything being OK, as well as feeling a strong pull to "lend their ego functioning" and organize patients' thought processes. Feelings of frustration and impatience over the persistent and compulsive nature of patients' irrational thoughts are common.

TRANSFERENCE

Feelings of fear, suspicion, anger, and hostility are often projected onto clinicians. As a result, establishing a therapeutic alliance based on trust and genuine connection is extremely difficult with these patients. In the transference, clinicians are often suspected of manipulative agendas, hidden desires, and unpredictable responses. This often creates an extremely challenging therapeutic environment filled with helplessness and frustration for both clinicians and patients.

Borderline–Dysregulated Spectrum

Impulsive–Histrionic Personalities

Impulsive–histrionic adolescents demonstrate a pattern of self-dramatizing, attention-seeking, provocative behavior, which is often both sexual and aggressive. Adolescence is a period of time in which prefrontal inhibitory control is a work in progress. Impulse control, temporal discounting, distress tolerance, and learning how to share are all developmental tasks that begin in childhood, but they frequently require more practice during this phase of growth—albeit in settings and relationships that often involve greater complexity and consequence. This period of time is also one in which adolescents may be experimenting with different facets of their identity, as well as engaging in performative acts to try other facets on for size. This is all part of the intricate dance of negotiating adolescent peer groups and social circles associated with school and locale, which pulls for certain valued behaviors (while disincentives others). Attention seeking in the form of dress and speech may enable adolescents to distinguish themselves, as well as to garner social capital, enhance a felt sense of positive self-regard, and practice acts of agency. For adolescents coming from family systems in which they do not feel (or are not in actuality) seen, histrionic and impulsive acts may be aimed at attracting the attention that they are looking for from primary caregivers, but that seems unattainable in any other way. Additionally, some adolescents may be temperamentally predisposed to be sensation seekers, and thus seek out dangerous acts for the thrill of the risk involved.

However, while all of the aforementioned personality attributes may be considered normative forms of experimentation and/or performative acts to locate boundaries of consensual social norms, adolescents who routinely transgress these boundaries (experiencing negative social, occupational, interpersonal, medical, and legal consequences as a result) may be evidencing histrionic and impulsive personality traits that are more rigid than fluid—more diagnostic of developmental thresholds initially not met as opposed to core aspects of one's emerging "self." These individuals may use histrionic traits as "work-arounds" for attention and self-esteem, making impulsive decisions to evoke highly charged interactions with others. Risk taking here may serve to demonstrate to others that an adolescent is "fearless," "carefree," and "cool," but may paradoxically evoke from within the very emotional states that the adolescent is attempting to compensate for.

Empirical Description

Adolescents with an emerging impulsive–histrionic personality style may find themselves in relationships that tend to be unstable, chaotic, and rapidly changing. They may be sexually promiscuous for persons of their age and show a tendency toward being sexually seductive or provocative. Their sexual or romantic partners may seem "inappropriate" in terms of age and/or status. They may get drawn into extrafamilial relationships in which they are emotionally or physically abused or in which they needlessly put themselves in dangerous situations. These adolescents may act impulsively, seek thrills or high levels of stimulation, and be prone to drug or alcohol abuse. In relationships, they may become attached quickly or intensely to people who may or may not be available; develop feelings and expectations that are not warranted by the history or context of the relationship; or at times get drawn into romantic or sexual "triangles." Some may fantasize about ideal or perfect love. Their emotions change rapidly and unpredictably, are often exaggerated or theatrical, and tend to spiral out of control. They may try to override feelings of fear or anxiety by rushing headlong into feared situations. These adolescents may surround themselves with peers who are delinquent or alienated or may draw peers into scenarios that feel alien or unfamiliar (e.g., being uncharacteristically insensitive or cruel, feeling like the only person in the world who can help). They lack a clear sense of who they are and seem untroubled by the inconsistency of contradicting feelings or beliefs.

Match to Description				
5	**4**	**3**	**2**	**1**
Very good match	Good match	Significant match (features)	Slight match	Little or no match

KEY FEATURES

Contributing constitutional–maturational patterns: Possible sensitivity, sociophilia.

Central tension/preoccupation: Power over others.

Central affects: Fear, shame, guilt (over competition).

Characteristic pathogenic belief about self: "There is something problematic/lacking about me that needs to be overcompensated for."

Characteristic pathogenic belief about others: "Others will not like me/will reject me unless I quickly do something to attract their attention."

Central ways of defending: Repression, regression, sexualizing, acting out; overcompensation.

Countertransference and Transference Reactions

COUNTERTRANSFERENCE

Clinicians may find themselves wanting to please, feeling flattered, and often feeling under pressure to act in response to these patients. However, as the treatment progresses, clinicians find themselves feeling disconnected and somewhat tired of the high levels of engagement required by the patients and often feel pressured to "keep up" with the high intensity of the interaction.

TRANSFERENCE

Clinicians often become the target of patients' attention seeking and impulsive behaviors. In the transference, clinicians are often seen as potential gratifying figures, providers of attention and love. When these attempts are not reciprocated according to their expectations, these patients respond with diverse strategies, ranging from passive–aggressive maneuvers to quite theatrical ways of expressing emotions, but setting the clinicians up for failure one way or another. Both idealization and denigration are prevalent ways of relating in these patients in the context of the transference.

Borderline Personalities

The strength and tempo of contingencies that govern the regulation of distress between infants and caregivers are believed to directly affect the formation of personality, with different early attachment patterns predicting distinct kinds of personality organization that later emerges. A disorganized early attachment pattern between a caregiver and infant is generally believed to be the seed that later grows into borderline personality style (Fonagy, Target, Gergely, Allen, & Bateman, 2003; Liotti, 2004). Unlike secure, avoidant, and anxious early attachment patterns (which, from the perspective of an infant, allow the infant to assess the reliability of receiving a soothing behavior vs. an unpleasant one from a caregiver in relation to the baby's own distress), disorganized early attachment does not provide an opportunity for the infant to experience stable, reliable, or predictable interpersonal interactions due to the caregiver's disorganized mode of engagement. This results in the infant's having no reliable reference point with which to locate his or her own contours and no opportunity at the developmentally appropriate time to realize that the regulation of distress is possible in a relationship (let alone that self-regulation—its one-person counterpart—is possible). As a result, the adult develops a borderline personality organization, in the absence of any opportunity for the sense of self to cohere (Fineberg, Steinfeld, Brewer, & Corlett, 2014).

In the absence of being able to self-regulate easily, individuals with a borderline personality organization are left in the labor-intensive position of having to deploy interpersonal "work-arounds" in order to change their internal states. For example, if they feel sad and do not know how to change that internal feeling of sadness, they will have to induce in another person the desire to assuage that feeling or risk "drowning" in it. Whereas those with a flexible repertoire of self-regulatory skills might go for a run, watch a comedy movie, talk to a friend, or engage in any other pleasurable activity, people with borderline organization have great difficulty with this. Instead of being able to self-regulate, they have to regulate others to get their needs met; this is frequently accomplished via projective identification (Klein, 1946; Ogden, 1979; Spillius & O'Shaughnessy, 2013).

In adolescence, it may be normal for young people to make demands and test the boundaries of close adults in their lives as they learn the unspoken norms that govern adult social relationships. This is distinct, however, from borderline personality pathology in which there is a pervasive and unchanging mode of interpersonal engagement, which is felt as disorganizing by the young adult's interlocutor. In addition to projective identification, and in the absence of self-regulatory skills, adolescents with an emerging borderline organization may use self-harming behaviors such as cutting, substance misuse, and relationships of all kinds as means of changing their internal states.

Empirical Description

Adolescents with an emerging borderline personality style tend to experience emotions that spiral out of control and change rapidly and unpredictably. They are prone to painful feelings of emptiness and are unable to soothe or comfort themselves without the help of another person. When strong emotions are stirred up, they may become irrational. These individuals tend to make repeated suicidal threats or gestures, either as "cries for help" or as efforts to manipulate others, and they may also engage in self-mutilating behavior. In some cases, they may struggle with genuine wishes to kill themselves. Relationships for these adolescents tend to be unstable and chaotic. They have a tendency to become attached quickly, but when they become upset, they have trouble simultaneously seeing the positive and negative qualities in the same person. They can be simultaneously needy and rejecting of others, with fears of being alone, rejected, or abandoned. These adolescents may lack a stable sense of who they are and may have a deep sense of inner "badness." They tend to feel unhappy, depressed, and misunderstood, and may believe that life has no meaning. When they are distressed, their sense of reality may become impaired, and they may enter altered or dissociative states.

Match to Description				
5	4	3	2	1
Very good match	Good match	Significant match (features)	Slight match	Little or no match

KEY FEATURES

Contributing constitutional–maturational patterns: Disorganized early attachment relationships; prolonged periods of physical, emotional, and/or sexual abuse during early development.

Central tension/preoccupation: Difficulty with self-regulation; diffuse sense of self; the use of other people in attempts to regulate self in the absence of being able to do this oneself.

Central affects: Emptiness, confusion, loss, desperation, betrayal, paranoid thinking.

Characteristic pathogenic beliefs about self: "I am unlovable," "I am helpless when left alone," "People will pay attention only when I act in extreme ways."

Characteristic pathogenic belief about others: "Other people are either all good or all bad."

Central ways of defending: Splitting, projective identification, acting out.

Countertransference and Transference Reactions

COUNTERTRANSFERENCE

Clinicians may experience feelings of having wronged someone, alongside heightened emotional intensity and loss of metacognitive awareness. Affective shifts between strong positive and negative feelings, as well as feelings of being "pushed" and "pulled" and feeling manipulated, are often experienced when treating patients in this category.

TRANSFERENCE

In the transference, patients' perceptions of the clinician are distorted by primitive defense mechanisms, such as projective identification and splitting. In response to those perceptions of the clinician, patients tend to manifest quick shifts between extreme affects, rapid shifts between idealization and devaluation, and suicidal gestures.

The following illustration is offered with the purpose of guiding clinicians in their thinking regarding the clinical picture emerging from the diagnostic process, as well as demonstrating the importance of an initial clinical formulation in the process of treatment planning, intervention, and ongoing assessment.

Clinical Illustration

Linda, a 15-year-old, appeared shy and hesitant. Her parents requested a psychological assessment due to her serious behavior problems, especially during the last 2 years. She cried for no apparent reason, was prone to sudden outbursts of verbal rage toward her parents, and sometimes physically attacked her sister (3 years her junior). She had started smoking at the age of 14 and occasionally smoked marijuana with her friends. Linda experienced many difficulties in her relationships with her peers and she had to change schools to avoid bullying and constant fights with her older classmates. She was also prone to risky behavior when out with her friends, ignoring danger and unintended consequences. In the last year before her referral, her school performance had declined considerably, and her mother had recently discovered that Linda was repeatedly engaging in self-mutilating behavior (cutting).

Linda's mother was a very beautiful woman who had suffered anxiety attacks and depression during extended periods of her life. Linda's father was a successful businessman; he was very handsome, seemed to have invested a lot in his looks, and exhibited many narcissistic personality traits. The parents had had a stormy relationship after Linda's birth, with constant fights and periods of separation, during which Linda's father left home for months and dated other women. They officially divorced 2 years ago, although Linda's mother had not worked through her grief and hoped for a reunion.

Linda had a troublesome upbringing. She was born with a serious heart disease, and after 20 months of repeated examinations and changes in medication, her doctors had decided she needed surgery. Linda's health issue shocked her parents. They seemed to have experienced it as a narcissistic wound, which still caused them pain, although her health problem had been fully remedied. Her father reacted with aggression, repeatedly accusing his wife of not taking good enough care of the baby. Her mother was very anxious and often felt unable to soothe her baby when she was upset. During her health examinations and surgery, Linda, who was just a toddler, openly expressed her fears and asked her parents not to leave her side. After the birth of her younger sister, Linda became deeply jealous and often attacked her sister's nanny physically. Due to Linda's health problems, her parents seemed to have been reluctant in placing firm limits on her behavior. When she was first enrolled in day care (at age 3½), she suffered from separation anxiety for almost a year, making her adaptation difficult. During her first school years, she had always been unreliable with her homework but otherwise performed well academically until the year before referral, when she was almost held back a grade.

During her diagnostic sessions and subsequent five preparative sessions—before she was referred for psychotherapy in a specialized therapeutic unit for adolescents and their families—Linda was very ambivalent about attending her appointments and cooperating with the clinician. Her mood and attitude toward the therapist oscillated between extremes from one session to the next. Sometimes she was warm and would open up; in the next session, she would be aggressive, sabotaging every attempt of the therapist to establish emotional contact and claiming furiously that she needed no help from her.

Linda spoke with emotional flatness about her earlier school years when she was bullied by her peers. She said that she didn't care about it and that her classmates' reaction was "racist," due to the music she preferred. She claimed she had no friends there, only boyfriends. It seemed that Linda had accepted all romantic proposals with the aim of making friends, but she admitted that nothing good came out of this. She was happy to change schools and claimed she had very close friends there already, having established a strong bond with these new friends from the first day they met. They accepted her style of clothes and music, and one friend even told her almost daily that he admired her for all the things she had done in her life. Linda said that she revealed things about herself slowly, so as to maintain suspense and not allow people to get bored with her. In later sessions, however, she mentioned her great disappointment with some of these friends. She maintained that they didn't really care about how she felt, and that they only pretended to empathize with her for a moment before she would see them laughing and being in a good mood. She felt that they were "cheating" on her, and when challenged by the therapist, she failed to think of any other perspective that would explain their behavior.

When asked about her self-harming behavior, Linda said that at first she did it after a fight with her best friend in order to punish herself. She initially felt enormous physical pain, which subsided, giving way to excitement—"a real thrill!" Linda admitted cutting herself every time she felt sad. Whenever she had an urge to cry, she crouched and felt her body grow cold. Then she cut herself, and the sensation of the warm blood on her skin made her feel alive again. She usually carved song lyrics on her wrists; she felt that doing so would cause the words to enter into her soul and make her feel stronger. Linda felt that self-cutting was nothing to worry about and said that it was something she wouldn't like to stop doing. The same was true of her other risky behaviors (such as running in the street half naked for fun, or jumping from high junk piles into strangers' houses): She felt that these things were keeping her alive and made life worth living.

Linda displayed a rather childish and artistic idea about death. When she was 8, a classmate of hers had died, and the whole class went to the funeral. There she saw her classmate lying in the casket, and she thought he was sleeping. From then on, she had associated death with an eternal sleep, and she claimed she had felt no fear of death ever since.

Linda's relationship with her parents was shaky. She felt that they had no capacity to think like her, and so they had never really understood her. Thus she had always felt lonely even in their presence. She concealed her self-mutilating behavior from her father since she felt he would be very disappointed. The psychological assessment revealed a depressive disorder and elements of borderline personality disorder. The therapist felt at times great sympathy for Linda, who tried with all means to defend herself against painful emotions of low self-esteem, loneliness, and fear of death. At other times, though, when she experienced Linda's aggression, the therapist felt surprised at being targeted without any obvious reason. This feeling was accompanied by heightened emotional intensity later in such sessions, reducing the therapist's ability to think clearly.

Evaluating the Case

In evaluating the case of Linda, we first characterize the level of mental functioning by drawing upon clinical observations for each MA-Axis capacity. We then identify the primary emerging personality style.

COGNITIVE AND AFFECTIVE PROCESSES

1. *Capacity for regulation, attention, and learning:* Good motor and verbal skills. Capacity for learning disrupted during periods of affect dysregulation.
2. *Capacity for affective range, communication, and understanding:* Restricted range of affective communication. Emotional outbursts. Frequent use of the body as a means to regulate. Extreme shifts in affect.
3. *Capacity for mentalization and reflective functioning:* Failure to mentalize about her own and others' internal states. Limited ability to think of alternative perspectives, representing her own beliefs as facts.

IDENTITY AND RELATIONSHIPS

4. *Capacity for differentiation and integration (identity):* Great difficulty in differentiating internal states from external events and experiences. Reacts with rigidity in interpersonal relationships when affect regulation is challenged.
5. *Capacity for relationships and intimacy:* Relationships are unstable and oscillate between extremes: sudden overinvestment in relationships, accompanied by the fantasy of a strong emotional bond, suddenly followed by the feeling that the other persons are "cheating." A strong need for closeness and intimacy but inability to tolerate the frustration caused by the difference between others' and her own mental states. Thus relationships are often superficial.
6. *Capacity for self-esteem regulation and quality of internal experience:* Precarious sense of self-esteem. Efforts to devaluate others in order to keep her self-esteem intact. Need for admiration. Engaging in self-mutilating or dangerous actions in order to feel internally alive.

DEFENSE AND COPING

7. *Capacity for impulse control and regulation:* Easy dysregulation and oscillation between extremes. Poor capacity for behavior control. Frequent outbursts and acting out.
8. *Capacity for defensive functioning:* Projection, rationalization, flight into fantasy, acting out, turning anger toward the self, devaluation of others. Sometimes poor reality testing.
9. *Capacity for adaptation, resiliency, and strength:* Very poor capacity to cope in stressful or painful situations. Easy dysregulation in the face of any environmental challenge.

SELF-AWARENESS AND SELF-DIRECTION

10. *Self-observing capacities (psychological mindedness):* Limited capacity to explore her internal world, and restricted interpersonal curiosity aimed at understanding others' mental states and perspectives.
11. *Capacity to construct and use internal standards and ideals:* Very loose moral values. Superego oscillates between extremes: sometimes severe physical punishments (self-cutting) and at other times no restrictions on attacks upon family members (no conscious guilt).
12. *Capacity for meaning and purpose:* Trouble thinking beyond the current moment, and a limited sense of the meaning and purpose of her attitudes, actions, and beliefs.

Level of functioning: Borderline.
Primary emerging personality style: Borderline.

Dependent–Victimized Personalities

Adolescents with excessively dependent personalities experience a compelling need to be taken care of. They fear separation, either recurrently or pervasively, and typically engage in submissive and clinging behavior. They are often anxious in new situations and shrink from taking risks or new steps. Adolescence is also a period in which, as teenagers become young adults, they frequently venture out of their family systems and are confronted with different kinds of rules that govern social relationships. This can be especially challenging for young adults who grow up in two particular familial settings:

1. In family systems in which there is a high degree of other-orientation (vs. self-orientation) and in which each member looks out for the others, adolescents may be used to attending to other people's needs and expecting somebody else to do the same for them. However, when entering social settings where this is not the case, adolescents may look to others for the same support and care they offer, and may be disappointed not to receive it in turn.
2. For adolescents who grow up either having all of their needs met and not having had to reflect on this, or, conversely, being depended on by caregivers who could not take care of themselves, this too may lead to dependent personality styles in which the young adults may look to proximal others with disappointment and confusion at unmet interpersonal expectations.

Adolescents who experience real or perceived traumas and/or slights may also harbor unarticulated anger and criticism about others' attitudes and actions toward them—reactions that are resistant to a change in perspective. The feelings of victimization, which may have roots in real lived experiences, may also in this age range stem from feelings of social alienation, teasing, adolescent social pressures, loneliness, poor school performance, bullying, and other forms of negative experience or abuse. Compensatory behaviors may involve desperately seeking social acceptance, participating in risky forms of behavior to accumulate the social currency valued by one's peers, and finding one's mood dependent on the validation and praise of others.

Empirical Description

Adolescents with a dependent–victimized personality style may have trouble acknowledging or expressing anger toward others and instead may become depressed, self-critical, and self-punitive. Anger may be expressed in passive and indirect ways. These adolescents tend to be ingratiating or submissive with peers. They tend to be passive and unassertive, needy, or dependent, with fears they will be rejected or abandoned. They may fear being alone. They tend to be suggestible or easily influenced and are insufficiently concerned with meeting their own needs. They may feel that they are not their "true self" with others and have the tendency to seek out or create interpersonal relationships in which they are in the role of caring for, rescuing, or protecting the other people. They are prone to idealizing others and may fantasize about ideal or perfect love. Yet they tend to become attached to or interested in people who are unavailable, or to choose sexual or romantic partners who seem inappropriate (in terms of age, status, etc.). They are vulnerable to getting drawn into relationships outside the family in which they are emotionally or physically abused or to put themselves needlessly in dangerous situations. They may tend to feel helpless, powerless, or at the mercy of forces outside their control.

Match to Description				
5	**4**	**3**	**2**	**1**
Very good match	Good match	Significant match (features)	Slight match	Little or no match

KEY FEATURES

Contributing constitutional–maturational patterns: Real or perceived losses, particularly involving close relationships, early in development.

Central tension/preoccupation: Abandonment: Feeling a pervasive need for another person to confirm safety and care; relying on others for one's own emotional stability; minimizing interpersonal conflict to avoid the feared consequences of interpersonal rupture.

Central affects: Depression and self-criticism.

Characteristic pathogenic belief about self: "If I voice discontent or voice my needs, others will leave me."

Characteristic pathogenic belief about others: "People will abandon me if I do something wrong."

Central ways of defending: Sublimating fear and anger; maintaining continuity and proximity of relationships, despite not meeting one's own needs, to avoid negative affect.

Countertransference and Transference Reactions

COUNTERTRANSFERENCE

Early in treatment, clinicians may experience a range of affects, including positive emotions resulting from identifications with patients' projections of being omniscient authorities, pressure to collude to avoid negative affect, and impulses toward crossing boundaries to provide help. Later in treatment, these feelings may change to those of irritation and disengagement and/or a sense of being burdened and constrained.

TRANSFERENCE

Patients may experience feelings of abandonment and rage in response to what they perceived as the clinicians' rejection of their expressed dependency needs. In the transference, patients tend to perceive clinicians as not sensitive and attuned enough and often as yet other rejecting attachment figures.

Character Style

Obsessive–Compulsive Personalities

Adolescents with obsessive–compulsive personalities are preoccupied with orderliness, perfectionism, and mental and interpersonal control, at the expense of flexibility, openness, and efficiency. They may be countering unconscious or preconscious aggression. On the more disturbed end of the spectrum, they may be defending against overwhelming anxiety, wishes to regress, loss of reality testing, or loss of impulse control. On the healthy end of the obsessive–compulsive spectrum, they may be obedient, follow rules readily, and be very conscientious about such duties as schoolwork and house chores. At the most maladaptive end are adolescents whose need for control has a stubborn quality that oppresses their family members and their environment.

Adolescence is a time in which numerous pressures are placed on emerging adults in the form of life plans, academic achievement, clarity of future career paths, and expectations from others (family members, the school system, peers, etc.). In the aggregate, or in specific instances to an extreme, these pressures can create very intense existential anxiety that requires defense. Some adolescents respond to these affective states with the development of a highly organized and perfectionist self-stance—constantly judging themselves for perceived weaknesses, imperfections, and mistakes, and striving to present the opposite image to the outside world. Others may experience pervasive rumination and resentment toward others they perceive as more "perfect" than themselves. It is not uncommon to see students in the middle school to high school years working furiously to attain good grades, maintain social standing, and other people's affections, only to feel that no matter how hard they try, it is never enough to secure these goals in the eyes of others. In attempting to exert control over what are felt to be uncertain and anxiety-inducing circumstances (in which "failure" signals severe negative consequences), these individuals paradoxically contribute to increasing the anxiety and misperception that there are high-stakes outcomes riding on even the most mundane activities.

These obsessions, which are largely cognitive and affective events in the body, may sometimes reach a magnitude requiring behavioral regulation. Actions such as bingeing and purging, exercising, nail biting, self-cutting, or other repetitive and compulsive behaviors may all serve to reduce obsessional ideation. These compensatory behaviors in adolescence are frequently hidden from caregivers, teachers, and peers to preserve a patina of "normality." Treating clinicians thus need to be willing to probe further than one exchange when assessing the presence of these symptoms.

Empirical Description

Adolescents with an obsessive–compulsive personality style expect themselves to be "perfect" and tend to be overly concerned with rules, procedures, order, and organization. They generally adhere rigidly to daily routines and are excessively devoted to school, work, or productivity, to the detriment of fun, pleasure, or friendships. They may see themselves as logical, rational, and uninfluenced by emotion, and tend to think in abstract, intellectualized terms. Yet they are also constricted and inhibited, with a limited range of emotions. These adolescents tend to become absorbed in details to the point of missing what is significant. They may be self-critical and self-righteous, with unrealistically high standards. They tend to deny or disavow a need for nurturance, caring, or comfort, and are invested in seeing themselves as emotionally strong and untroubled. In their relationships, they may be competitive, controlling, stingy, or withholding.

Match to Description				
5	4	3	2	1
Very good match	Good match	Significant match (features)	Slight match	Little or no match

KEY FEATURES

Contributing constitutional–maturational patterns: Fear of losing control; conflict over aggression; limited experiences of autonomy during development.

Central tension/preoccupation: Wish to be in control of one's emotions and impulses.

Central affects: Anger and anxiety.

Characteristic pathogenic belief about self: "I must be perfect, or bad things will happen."

Characteristic pathogenic beliefs about others: "Others are judging me and trying to control me," "Others are better than I am."

Central ways of defending: Obsessive thinking to manage anxiety; intellectualization; isolation of affect; reaction formation; overvaluing of thought versus feeling.

Countertransference and Transference Reactions

COUNTERTRANSFERENCE

Clinicians experience feelings of frustration and of being controlled. These often result in retaliatory fantasies toward patients, as well as a sense of boredom, distance, and futility.

TRANSFERENCE

Clinicians are often perceived as controlling. Anger and hostility often manifest themselves in response to anxiety about being controlled and a constant struggle for freedom and autonomy.

BIBLIOGRAPHY

Adelson, S. L. (2012). Practice parameter on gay, lesbian, or bisexual sexual orientation, gender nonconformity, and gender discordance in children and adolescents. *Journal of the American Academy of Child and Adolescent Psychiatry, 51*, 957–974.

Adkisson, R., Burdsal, C., Dorr, D., & Morgan, C. (2012). Factor structure of the Millon Adolescent Clinical Inventory scales in psychiatric inpatients. *Personality and Individual Differences, 53*(4), 501–506.

Adrian, M., Zeman, J., Erdley, C., Lisa, L., & Sim, L. (2011). Emotional dysregulation and interpersonal difficulties as risk factors for nonsuicidal self-injury in adolescent girls. *Journal of Child Psychology and Psychiatry, 39*(3), 389–400.

Aelterman, N., Decuyper, M., & De Fruyt, F. (2010). Understanding obsessive–compulsive personality disorder in adolescence: A dimensional personality perspective. *Journal of Psychopathology and Behavioral Assessment, 32*(4), 467–478.

Afifi, T. O., Mather, A., Boman, J., Fleisher, W., Enns, M. W., Macmillan, H., & Sareen J. (2011). Childhood adversity and personality disorders: Results from a nationally representative population-based study. *Journal of Psychiatric Research, 45*(6), 814–822.

Ahktar, S. (1990). Paranoid personality disorder: A synthesis of developmental, dynamic and descriptive features. *American Journal of Psychotherapy, 44*, 5–25.

Alden, L. E., Laposa, J. M., Taylor, C. T., & Ryder, A. G. (2002). Avoidant personality disorder: Current status and future directions. *Journal of Personality Disorders, 16*, 1–29.

Allertz, A., & van Voorst, G. (2007). Personality disorders from the perspective of child and adolescent psychiatry. In B. van Luyn, S. Akhtar, & W. J. Livesley (Eds.), *Severe personality disorders: Everyday issues in clinical practice* (pp. 79–92). New York: Cambridge University Press.

American Psychiatric Association. (2000). *Diagnostic and statistical manual of mental disorders* (4th ed., text rev.). Washington, DC: Author.

American Psychiatric Association. (2013). *Diagnostic and statistical manual of mental disorders* (5th ed.). Arlington, VA: Author.

Ammaniti, M., Fontana, A., Clarkin, A. F., Clarkin, J., Nicolais, G. F., & Kernberg, O. (2012). Assessment of adolescent personality disorders through the Interview of Personality Organization Processes in Adolescence (IPOP-A): Clinical and theoretical implications. *Adolescent Psychiatry, 2*(1), 36–45.

Ammaniti, M., Fontana, A., Kernberg, O., Clarkin, J., & Clarkin, A. (2011). *Interview of Personality Organization Processes in Adolescence (IPOP-A)*. Unpublished manuscript, Sapienza University of Rome and Weill Medical College of Cornell University, New York.

Ammaniti, M., Fontana, A., & Nicolais, G. (2015). Borderline personality disorder in adolescence through the lens of the Interview of Personality Organization Processes in Adolescence (IPOP-A): Clinical use and implications. *Journal of Infant, Child, and Adolescent Psychotherapy, 14*, 82–97.

Anastasopoulos, D. (2007). The narcissism of depression or the depression of narcissism and adolescence. *Journal of Child Psychotherapy, 33*(3), 345–362.

Archer, R. P. (2004). Overview and update on the Minnesota Multiphasic Personality Inventory—Adolescent. In M. E. Marushin (Ed.), *The use of psychological testing for treatment planning and outcomes assessment: Vol. 2. Instruments for children and adolescents* (pp. 81–122). London: Routledge.

Bagby, R. M., & Farvolden, P. (2004). The Personality Diagnostic Questionnaire, PDQ-4. In M. Hersen (Ed.), *Comprehensive handbook of psychological assessment: Vol. 2. Personality assessment* (pp. 122–133). Hoboken, NJ: Wiley.

Barry, C. T., & Kauten, R. L. (2014). Nonpathological and pathological narcissism: Which self-reported characteristics are most problematic in adolescents? *Journal of Personality Assessment, 96*(2), 212–219.

Bateman, A. W., & Fonagy, P. (2004). *Psychotherapy of borderline personality disorder: Mentalisation based treatment*. New York: Oxford University Press.

Bateman, A., & Fonagy, P. (2008). Comorbid antisocial and borderline personality disorders: Mentalization-based treatment. *Journal of Clinical Psychology, 64*(2), 181–194.

Bateman, A., & Fonagy, P. (2013). Mentalization-based treatment. *Psychoanalytic Inquiry, 33*(6), 595–613.

Bates, J. E., Schermerhorn, A. C., & Petersen, I. T. (2014). Temperament concepts in developmental psychopathology. In K. Rudolph & M. Lewis (Eds.), *Handbook of developmental psychopathology* (3rd ed., pp. 311–329). New York: Springer.

Baumrind, D. (1991). The influence of parenting style on adolescent competence and substance use. *Journal of Early Adolescence, 11*(1), 56–95.

Bellak, L. (1993). *The T.A.T., C.A.T., and S.A.T. in clinical use* (5th ed.). Boston: Allyn & Bacon.

Bemporad, J. R., Smith, H. F., Hanson, G., & Cicchetti, D. (1982). Borderline syndromes in childhood: Criteria for diagnosis. *American Journal of Psychiatry, 139*, 596–602.

Bene, A. (1979). The question of narcissistic personality disorders: Self pathology in children. *Bulletin of the Hampstead Clinic, 2*, 209–218.

Benet-Martinez, V., & John, O. P. (1998). Los Cinco Grandes across cultures and ethnic groups: Multitrait multimethod analyses of the Big Five in Spanish and English. *Journal of Personality and Social Psychology, 75*, 729–750.

Biederman, J., Ball, S. W., Monuteaux, M. C., Mick, E., Spencer, T. J., McCreary, M., . . . Faraone, S. V. (2008). New insights into the co-morbidity between ADHD and major depression in adolescent and young adult females. *Journal of the American Academy of Child and Adolescent Psychiatry, 47*, 426–434.

Blagov, P. S., Bi, W., Shedler, J., & Westen, D. (2012). The Shedler–Westen Assessment Procedure (SWAP): Evaluating psychometric questions about its reliability, validity, and impact of its fixed score distribution. *Assessment, 19*(3), 270–282.

Blagov, P. S., & Westen, D. (2008). Questioning the coherence of histrionic personality disorder: Borderline and hysterical personality subtypes in adults and adolescents. *Journal of Nervous and Mental Disease, 196*, 785–797.

Blair, R. J., Budhani, S., Colledge, E., & Scott, S. (2005). Deafness to fear in boys with psychopathic tendencies. *Journal of Child Psychology and Psychiatry, 46*, 327–336.

Blatt, S. (2004). *Experiences of depression: Theoretical, clinical, and research perspectives*. Washington, DC: American Psychological Association.

Bleiberg, E. (1984). Narcissistic disorders in children. *Bulletin of the Menninger Clinic, 48*, 501–517.

Bleiberg, E. (2000). Borderline personality disorder in children and adolescents. In T. Lubbe (Ed.), *The borderline psychotic child: A selective integration* (pp. 39–68). London: Routledge.

Bleiberg, E. (2004). Treatment of dramatic personality disorders in children and adolescents. In J. J. Magnavita (Ed.), *Handbook of personality disorders: Theory and practice* (pp. 467–497). New York: Wiley.

Bleiberg, E., & Markowitz, J. C. (2012). IPT for borderline personality disorder. In J. C. Markowitz & M. M. Weissman (Eds.), *Casebook of interpersonal psychotherapy*. New York: Oxford University Press.

Blos, P. (1979). *The adolescent passage: Developmental issues*. New York: International Universities Press.

Blum, H. P. (1974). The borderline childhood of the Wolf Man. *Journal of the American Psychoanalytic Association, 22*, 721–742.

Bolger, K. E., Patterson, C. J., & Kupersmidt, J. B. (1998). Peer relationships and self-esteem among children who have been maltreated. *Child Development, 69*, 1171–1197.

Bornstein, R. F. (1996). Beyond orality: Toward an object relations/interactionist reconceptualization of the etiology and dynamics of dependency. *Psychoanalytic Psychology, 13*, 177–203.

Bornstein, R. F. (2005). *Dependent patient: A practitioner's guide*. Washington, DC: American Psychological Association.

Bornstein, R. F. (2012). From dysfunction to adaptation: An interactionist model of dependency. *Annual Review of Clinical Psychology, 8*, 291–316.

Bowlby, J. (1969). *Attachment and loss: Vol. 1: Attachment*. London: Hogarth Press.

Bowlby, J. (1988). *A secure base*. London: Routledge.

Bram, A. D. (2014). Object relations, interpersonal functioning, and health in a nonclinical sample: Construct validation and norms for the TAT SCORS-G. *Psychoanalytic Psychology, 31*(3), 314–342.

Bram, A. D., & Yalof, J. (2015). Quantifying complexity: Personality assessment and its relationship with psychoanalysis. *Psychoanalytic Inquiry, 35*, 74–97.

Bullard, D. M. (1960). Psychotherapy of paranoid patients. *Archives of General Psychiatry, 2*, 137.

Butcher, J. N., Williams, C. L., Graham, J. R., Archer, R. P., Tellegen, A., Ben-Porath, Y. S., & Kaemmer, B. (1992). *Minnesota Multiphasic Personality Inventory—Adolescent (MMPI-A): Manual for administration, scoring, and interpretation*. Minneapolis: University of Minnesota Press.

Cairns, R. B., Cairns, B. D., & Neckerman, H. J. (1989). Early school dropout: Configurations and determinants. *Child Development, 60*, 1437–1452.

Calvo, N., Gutiérrez, F., Andión, O., Caseras, X., Torrubia, R., & Casas, M. (2012). Psychometric properties of the Spanish version of the self-report Personality Diagnostic Questionnaire–4+ (PDQ-4+) in psychiatric outpatients. *Psicothema, 24*, 156–160.

Campos, R. C. (2013). Conceptualization and preliminary validation of a depressive personality concept. *Psychoanalytic Psychology, 30*, 601–620.

Carroll, A. (2009). Are you looking at me?: Understanding and managing paranoid personality disorder. *Advances in Psychiatric Treatment, 15*, 40–48.

Carstairs, K. (1992). Paranoid–schizoid or symbiotic? *International Journal of Psychoanalysis, 73*, 71–85.

Casey, B. J., Jones, R. M., & Levita, L. (2010). The storm and stress of adolescence: Insights from human imaging and mouse genetics. *Developmental Psychobiology, 52*(3), 225–235.

Catthoor, K., Feenstra, D. J., Hutsebaut, J., Schrijvers, D., & Sabbe, B. (2015). Adolescents with personality disorders suffer from severe psychiatric stigma: Evidence from a sample of 131 patients. *Adolescent Health, Medicine and Therapeutics, 6*, 81–89.

Chanen, A. M., Jackson, H. J., McGorry, P. D., Allot, K. A., Clarkson, V., & Yuen, H. P. (2004). Two-year stability of personality disorder in older adolescent outpatients. *Journal of Personality Disorders, 18*(6), 526–541.

Chanen, A. M., Jovev, M., & Mcgorry, P. D. (2008). Borderline personality disorder in young people and the prospects for prevention and early intervention. *Current Psychiatry Reviews, 4*(1), 48–57.

Chen, H., Cohen, P., Johnson, J. G., Kasen, S., & Crawford, T. N. (2004). Adolescent personality disorders and conflict with romantic partners during the transition to adulthood. *Journal of Personality Disorders, 18*(6), 507–525.

Chen, H., Cohen, P., Kasen, S., & Johnson, J. G. (2006). Adolescent Axis I and personality disorders predict quality of life during young adulthood. *Journal of Adolescent Health, 39*(1), 14–19.

Chess, S., & Thomas, A. (1977). Temperamental individuality: From childhood to adolescence. *Journal of the American Academy of Child Psychiatry, 16*, 218–226.

Chess, S., & Thomas, A. (1986). *Temperament in clinical practice*. New York: Guilford Press.

Chused, J. (1999). Obsessional manifestations in children. *Psychoanalytic Study of the Child, 54*, 219–232.

Cicchetti, D. (1993). Developmental psychopathology: Reactions, reflections, projections. *Developmental Review, 13*, 471–502.

Claesen, D. R., Brown, B. B., & Eicher, S. A. (1986). Perceptions of peer pressure, peer conformity dispositions, and self-reported behavior among adolescents. *Developmental Psychology, 22*(4), 521–530.

Clark, D., & Bolton, D. (1985). Obsessive–compulsive adolescents and their parents: A psychometric study. *Journal of Child Psychology and Psychiatry, 26*, 267–276.

Cohen, P., Crawford, T. N., Johnson, J. G., & Kasen, S. (2005). The children in the community: Study of developmental course of personality disorder. *Journal of Personality Disorders, 19*(5), 466–486.

Coker, L. A., & Widiger, T. A. (2005). Personality disorders. In J. E. Maddux & B. A. Winstead (Eds.), *Psychopathology: Foundations for a contemporary understanding* (pp. 201–228). Mahwah, NJ: Erlbaum.

Conklin, C. Z., & Westen, D. (2005). Borderline personality disorder in clinical practice. *American Journal of Psychiatry, 162*, 867–875.

Costantino, G., Malgady, R. G., & Rogler, I. H. (1988). *TEMAS (Tell-Me-A-Story) manual*. Los Angeles: Western Psychological Services.

Cramer, P. (1982). *Defense mechanism manual*. Unpublished manuscript, Williams College.

Cramer, P., & Blatt, S. J. (1990). Use of the TAT to measure change in defense mechanisms following intensive psychotherapy. *Journal of Personality Assessment, 54*, 236–251.

Crowell, S. E., Beauchaine, T. P., & Lenzenweger, M. F. (2008). The development of borderline personality and self-injurious behavior. In T. P. Beauchaine & S. P. Hinshaw (Eds.), *Child and adolescent psychopathology* (pp. 510–539). Hoboken, NJ: Wiley.

Dahl, E. K. (1995). Daughters and mothers: Aspects of the representation world during adolescence. *Psychoanalytic Study of the Child, 50*, 187–204.

Daley, A. J., Copeland, R. J., Wright, N. P., Roalfe, A., & Wales, J. K. (2006). Exercise therapy as a treatment for psychopathologic conditions in obese and morbidly obese adolescents: A randomized, controlled trial. *Pediatrics, 118*, 2126–2134.

da Silva, D. R., Rijo, D., & Salekin, R. T. (2013). Child and adolescent psychopathy: Assessment issues and treatment needs. *Aggression and Violent Behavior, 18*, 71–78.

D'Augelli, A. R., & Patterson, C. J. (Eds.). (2001). *Lesbian, gay, and bisexual identities and youth: Psychological perspectives*. New York: Oxford University Press.

DeFife, J. A., Goldberg, M., & Westen, D. (2015a). Dimensional assessment of self-and interpersonal functioning in adolescents: Implications for DSM-5's general definition of personality disorder. *Journal of Personality Disorders, 29*(2), 248–260.

DeFife, J. A., Haggerty, G., Smith, S. W., Betancourt, L., Ahmed, Z., & Ditkowsky, K. (2015b). Clinical validity of prototype personality disorder ratings in adolescents. *Journal of Personality Assessment, 97*(3), 271–277.

DeFife, J. A., Malone, J. C., DiLallo, J., & Westen, J. (2013). Assessing adolescent personality disorders with the Shedler–Westen Assessment Procedure for Adolescents. *Clinical Psychology: Science and Practice, 20*(4), 393–407.

De Los Reyes, A., & Kazdin, A. E. (2005). Informant discrepancies in the assessment of childhood psychopathology: A critical review, theoretical framework, and recommendations for further study. *Psychological Bulletin, 131*(4), 483–509.

de Reus, R. J., & Emmelkamp, P. M. (2012). Obsessive–compulsive personality disorder: A review of current empirical findings. *Personality and Mental Health, 6*, 1–21.

DiLallo, J. J., Jones, M., & Westen, D. (2009). Personality subtypes in disruptive adolescent males. *Journal of Nervous and Mental Disease, 197*(1), 15–23.

Dishion, T. J., Spracklen, K. M., Andrews, D. W., & Patterson, G. R. (1996). Deviancy training in male adolescent friendships. *Behavior Therapy, 27*, 373–390.

Disney, K. L. (2013). Dependent personality disorder: A critical review. *Clinical Psychology Review, 33*, 1184–1196.

Dollinger, S., & Cramer, P. (1990). Children's defensive responses and emotional upset following a disaster: A projective assessment. *Journal of Personality Assessment, 54*, 55–62.

Dowling, S. (1989). The significance of infant observations for psychoanalysis in later states of life: A discussion. In S. Dowling & A. Rothstein (Eds.), *The significance of infant observational research for clinical work with children, adolescents and adults* (pp. 213–226). Madison, CT: International Universities Press.

Edens, J. F., Marcus, D. K., & Morey, L. C. (2009). Paranoid personality has a dimensional latent structure: Taxometric analyses of community and clinical samples. *Journal of Abnormal Psychology, 118*, 545–553.

Egan, J., & Kernberg, P. F. (1984). Pathological narcissism in childhood. *Journal of the American Psychoanalytic Association, 32*, 39–62.

Eggum, N. D., Eisenberg, N., Spinrad, T. L., Valiente, C., Edwards, A., Kupfer, A. S., & Reiser, M. (2009). Predictors of withdrawal: Possible precursors of avoidant personality disorder. *Development and Psychopathology, 21*, 815–838.

Ensink, K., Biberdzic, M., Normandin, L., & Clarkin, J. (2015). A developmental psychopathology and neurobiological model of borderline personality disorder in adolescence. *Journal of Infant, Child, and Adolescent Psychotherapy, 14*, 46–69.

Erikson, E. H. (1956). The problem of ego identity. *Journal of the American Psychoanalytic Association, 4*, 56–121.

Erikson, E. H. (1959). *Identity and the life cycle: Selected papers*. New York: International Universities Press.

Esterberg, M. L., Goulding, S. M., & Walker, E. F. (2010). Cluster A personality disorders: Schizotypal, schizoid and paranoid personality disorders in childhood and adolescence. *Journal of Psychopathology and Behavioral Assessment, 32*, 515–528.

Evans, M. (2011). Pinned against the ropes: Understanding anti-social personality-disordered patients through use of the counter-transference. *Psychoanalytic Psychotherapy, 25*(2), 143–156.

Exner, J. E. (2003). *The Rorschach: A comprehensive system: Vol. 1. Basic foundations and principles of interpretation* (4th ed.). New York: Wiley.

Fairbairn, W. R. D. (1952). *An object-relations theory of the personality*. New York: Basic Books.

Feenstra, D. J., Van Busschbach, J. J., Verheul, R., & Hutsebaut, J. (2011). Prevalence and comorbidity of Axis I and Axis II disorders among treatment refractory adolescents admitted for specialized psychotherapy. *Journal of Personality Disorders, 25*(6), 842–850.

Fineberg, S., Steinfeld, M., Brewer, J., & Corlett, P. (2014). A computational account of borderline personality disorder: Impaired predictive learning about self and others through bodily simulation. *Frontiers in Psychiatry, 5*, 111.

Fischer, N., & Fischer, R. (1991). Adolescence, sex, and neurogenesis: A clinical perspective. In S. Akhtar & H. Parens (Eds.), *Beyond the symbiotic orbit: Advances in separation-individuation theory: Essays in honor of Selma Kramer, M.D.* (pp. 209–226). Hillsdale, NJ: Analytic Press.

Flament, M. F., Koby, E., Rapoport, J. L., Berg, C. J., Zahn, T., Cox, C., . . . Lenane, M. (1990). Childhood obsessive–compulsive disorder: A prospective follow-up study. *Journal of Child Psychology and Psychiatry, 31*, 363–380.

Flynn, D., & Skogstad, H. (2006). Facing towards or turning away from destructive narcissism. *Journal of Child Psychotherapy, 32*, 35–48.

Fonagy, P., & Bateman, A. (2008). The development of borderline personality disorder-a mentalizing model. *Journal of Personality Disorders, 22*, 4–21.

Fonagy, P., Gergely, G., Jurist, E. L., & Target, M. (2002). *Affect regulation, mentalization, and the development of the self*. New York: Other Press.

Fonagy, P., Target, M., Gergely, G., Allen, J. G., & Bateman, A. W. (2003). The developmental roots of borderline personality disorder in early attachment relationships: A theory and some evidence. *Psychoanalytic Inquiry, 23*, 412–459.

Fonseca-Pedrero, E., Paino, M., & Lemos-Giráldez, S. (2013). Maladaptive personality traits in adolescence: Psychometric properties of the Personality Diagnostic Questionnaire–4+. *International Journal of Clinical and Health Psychology, 13*(3), 207–215.

Fontana, A., & Ammaniti, M. (2010). *Adolescent STIPO: Psychometric properties, convergent validity and comparison with normal adolescents.* White Plains, NY: Weill Medical College of Cornell University.

Fournier, J. C., DeRubeis, R. J., & Beck, A. T. (2012). Dysfunctional cognitions in personality pathology: The structure and validity of the Personality Belief Questionnaire. *Psychological Medicine, 42,* 795–805.

Francis, G., & D'Elia, F. (1994). Avoidant disorder. In M. C. Roberts (Series Ed.) & T. H. Ollendick, N. J. King, & W. Yules (Vol. Eds.), *Issues in clinical child psychology: International handbook of phobic and anxiety disorders in children and adolescents* (pp. 131–143). New York: Plenum Press.

Francis, G., & Gragg, R. A. (1996). *Developmental clinical psychology and psychiatry: Vol. 35. Childhood obsessive compulsive disorder.* Thousand Oaks, CA: SAGE.

Francis, G., Last, C., & Strauss, C. (1992). Avoidant disorder and social phobia in children and adolescents. *Journal of the American Academy of Child and Adolescent Psychiatry, 31,* 1086–1089.

Freeman, A., & Reinecke, M. A. (Eds.). (2007). *Personality disorders in childhood and adolescence.* Hoboken, NJ: Wiley.

Freud, A. (1963). The concept of developmental lines. *Psychoanalytic Study of the Child, 18,* 245–265.

Freud, A. (1965). *Normality and pathology in childhood: Assessments of development.* New York: International Universities Press.

Freud, A. (1981). The concept of developmental lines: Their diagnostic significance. *Psychoanalytic Study of the Child, 36,* 129–136.

Friborg, O., Martinussen, M., Kaiser, S., Øvergård, K. T., & Rosenvinge, J. H. (2013). Comorbidity of personality disorders in anxiety disorders: A meta-analysis of 30 years of research. *Journal of Affective Disorders, 145,* 143–155.

Frick, P. J., Stickle, T. R., Dandreaux, D. M., Farrell, J. M., & Kimonis, E. R. (2005). Callous-unemotional traits in predicting the severity and stability of conduct problems and delinquency. *Journal of Abnormal Child Psychology, 33*(4), 471–487.

Gabbard, G. O. (2005). Mind, brain, and personality disorders. *American Journal of Psychiatry, 162,* 648–655.

Gabbard, G. O., Gunderson, J. G., & Fonagy, P. (2002). The place of psychoanalytic treatments within psychiatry. *Archives of General Psychiatry, 59*(6), 505–510.

Gibson, P. R. (2004). Histrionic personality. In P. G. Caplan & L. Cosgrove (Eds.), *Bias in psychiatric diagnosis* (pp. 201–206). Northvale, NJ: Aronson.

Gorlow, L., Zimet, C. N., & Fine, H. J. (1952). The validity of anxiety and hostility Rorschach content scores among adolescents. *Journal of Consulting Psychology, 16*(1), 73–75.

Greenman, D. A., Gunderson, J. G., Cane, M., & Saltzman, P. R. (1986). An examination of the borderline diagnosis in children. *American Journal of Psychiatry, 143,* 998–1003.

Greenspan, S. I. (1989a). The development of the ego: Biological and environmental specificity in the psychopathological developmental process and the selection and construction of ego defenses. *Journal of the American Psychoanalytic Association, 37,* 605–638.

Greenspan, S. I. (1989b). *The development of the ego: Implications for personality theory, psychopathology, and the psychotherapeutic process.* Madison, CT: International Universities Press.

Greenspan, S. I., & Pollock, G. H. (Eds.). (1991). *The course of life: Vol. 4. Adolescence.* Madison, CT: International Universities Press.

Grilo, C. M., & McGlashan, T. H. (1998). Frequency of personality disorders in two age cohorts of psychiatric inpatients. *American Journal of Psychiatry, 155*(1), 140–142.

Grigsby, J., & Stevens, D. (2000). *Neurodynamics of personality.* New York: Guilford Press.

Haggerty, G., Blanchard, M., Baity, M. R., Defife, J. A., Stein, M. B., Siefert, C. J., . . . & Zodan, J. (2015). Clinical validity of a dimensional assessment of self-and interpersonal functioning in adolescent inpatients. *Journal of Personality Assessment, 97*(1), 3–12.

Haggerty, G., Zodan, J., Mehra, A., Zubair, A., Ghosh, K., Siefert, C. J., . . . DeFife, J. (2016). Reliability and validity of prototype diagnosis for adolescent psychopathology. *Journal of Nervous and Mental Disease, 204*(4), 287–290.

Hahn, E., Gottschling, J., & Spinath, F. M. (2012). Short measurements of personality: Validity and reliability of the GSOEP Big Five Inventory (BFI-S). *Journal of Research in Personality, 46*(3), 355–359.

Hart, D., & Marmorstein, N. R. (2009). Neighborhoods and genes and everything in between: Understanding adolescent aggression in social and biological contexts. *Development and Psychopathology, 21,* 961–973.

Hauser, S. T., Allen, J. P., & Golden, E. (2006). *Out of the woods: Tales of resilient teens.* Cambridge, MA: Harvard University Press.

Henry, D. B., Schoeny, M. E., Deptula, D. P., & Slavick, J. T. (2007). Peer selection and socialization effects on adolescent intercourse without a condom and attitudes about the costs of sex. *Child Development, 78,* 825–838.

Hiller, J. B., Rosenthal, R., Bornstein, R. F., Berry, D. T., & Brunell-Neuleib, S. (1999). Comparative meta-analysis of Rorschach and MMPI validity. *Psychological Assessment, 11*(3), 278–296.

Hilsenroth, M. J., Eudell-Simmons, E. M., DeFife, J. A., & Charnas, J. W. (2007). The Rorschach Perceptual and Thinking Index (PTI): An examination of reliability, validity and diagnostic efficiency. *International Journal of Testing, 7*(3), 269–291.

Hofer, C., Eisenberg, N., Spinrad, T. L., Morris, A. S., Gershoff, E., Valiente, C., . . . Eggum, N. D. (2013). Mother–adolescent conflict: Stability, change, and relations with externalizing and internalizing behavior problems. *Social Development, 22*(2), 259–279.

Horowitz, K., Gorfinkle, K., Lewis, O., & Phillips, K. (2002). Body dysmorphic disorder in an adolescent girl. *Journal of the American Academy of Child and Adolescent Psychiatry, 14*, 1503–1509.

Horowitz, L. M. (2004). *Interpersonal foundations of psychopathology*. Washington, DC: American Psychological Association.

Horvath, S., & Morf, C. C. (2009). Narcissistic defensiveness: Hypervigilance and avoidance of worthlessness. *Journal of Experimental Social Psychology, 45*(6), 1252–1258.

Houghton, S., West, J., & Tan, C. (2005). The nature and prevalence of psychopathic tendencies among mainstream school children and adolescents: Traditional and latent-trait approaches. In R. F. Waugh (Ed.), *Frontiers in educational psychology* (pp. 259–280). Hauppague, NY: Nova Science.

Huprich, S., Rosen, A., & Kiss, A. (2013). Manifestations of interpersonal dependency and depressive subtypes in outpatient psychotherapy patients. *Personality and Mental Health, 7*, 223–232.

Huprich, S. K., & Frisch, M. B. (2004). The Depressive Personality Disorder Inventory and its relationship to quality of life, hopefulness, and optimism. *Journal of Personality Assessment, 83*, 22–28.

Hyler, S. E. (1994). *Personality Diagnostic Questionnaire, PDQ-4+*. New York: New York State Psychiatric Institute.

Irwin, C. E., Jr. (1989). Risk-taking behavior in the adolescent patient: Are they impulsive? *Pediatric Annals, 18*, 122–134.

John, O. P., Caspi, A., Robins, R. W., Moffitt, T. E., & Stouthamer-Loeber, M. (1994). The "Little Five": Exploring the nomological network of the five factor model of personality in adolescent boys. *Child Development, 65*(1), 160–178.

John, O. P., Donahue, E. M., & Kentle, R. L. (1991). *The Big Five Inventory, Versions 4a and 54*. Berkeley: University of California, Institute of Personality and Social Research.

Johnson, J. G., Chen, H., & Cohen, P. (2004). Personality disorder traits during adolescence and relationships with family members during the transition to adulthood. *Journal of Consulting and Clinical Psychology, 72*, 923–932.

Johnson, J. G., Cohen, P., Dohrenwend, B. P., Link, B. G., & Brook, J. S. (2009). A longitudinal investigation of social causation and social selection processes involved in the association between socioeconomic status and psychiatric disorders. *Journal of Abnormal Child Psychology, 108*, 490–499.

Johnson, J. G., Cohen, P., Smailes, E., Kasen, S., Oldham, J., & Brook, J. S. (2000). Adolescent personality disorders associated with violence and criminal behavior during adolescence and early adulthood. *American Journal of Psychiatry, 157*, 1406–1412.

Johnson, J. G., First, M. B., Cohen, P., Skodol, A. E., Kasen, S., & Brooks, J. S. (2005). Adverse outcomes associated with personality disorder not otherwise specified in a community sample. *American Journal of Psychiatry, 162*(10), 1926–1932.

Jones, M., & Westen, D. (2010). Diagnosis and subtypes of adolescent antisocial personality disorder. *Journal of Personality Disorders, 24*(2), 217–243.

Juni, S. (1979). Theoretical foundations of projection as a defence mechanism. *International Review of Psychoanalysis, 6*, 115–121.

Kasen, S., Cohen, P., Chen, H., Johnson, J. G., & Crawford, T. N. (2009). School climate and continuity of adolescent personality disorder symptoms. *Journal of Child Psychology and Psychiatry, 50*(12), 1504–1512.

Kasen, S., Cohen, P., Skodol, A. E., First, M. B., Johnson, J. G., Brook, J. S., & Oldham, J. M. (2007). Comorbid personality disorder and treatment use in a community sample of youths: A 20-year follow up. *Acta Psychiatrica Scandinavica, 115*, 56–65.

Kaser-Boyd, N. (2006). Rorschach assessment of paranoid personality disorder. In S. K. Huprich (Ed.), *Rorschach assessment of personality disorder* (pp. 57–84). Mahwah, NJ: Erlbaum.

Keenan, K., Hipwell, A. E., Chung, T., Stepp, S., Loeber, R., Stouthamer-Loeber, M., . . . McTigue, K. (2010). The Pittsburgh Girls Study: Overview and initial findings. *Journal of Clinical Child and Adolescent Psychology, 39*(4), 506–521.

Keinänen, M. T., Johnson, J. G., Richards, E. S., & Courtney, E. A. (2012). A systematic review of the evidence-based psychosocial risk factors for understanding of borderline personality disorder. *Psychoanalytic Psychotherapy, 26*, 65–91.

Kelley, A. E., Schochet, T., & Landry, C. F. (2004). Risk taking and novelty seeking in adolescence: Introduction to Part I. *Annals of the New York Academy of Sciences, 1021*, 27–32.

Kelly, F. D. (1997). *The assessment of object relations phenomena in adolescents: TAT and Rorschach Measures*. Mahwah, NJ: Erlbaum.

Kelly, F. D. (2007). The clinical application of the

social cognition and object relations scale with children and adolescents. In S. Smith & L. Handler (Eds.), *The clinical assessment of children and adolescents: A practitioner's handbook*. Mahwah, NJ: Erlbaum.

Kendler, K. S. (1993). Twin studies of psychiatric illness: Current status and future directions. *Archives of General Psychiatry, 50*, 905–915.

Kendler, K. S., & Eaves, L. J. (1986). Models for the joint effect of genotype and environment on liability to psychiatric illness. *American Journal of Psychiatry, 143*, 279–289.

Kernberg, O. F. (1987). Projection and projective identification: Developmental and clinical aspects. *Journal of the American Psychoanalytic Association, 35*, 795–819.

Kernberg, O. F. (1998). The diagnosis of narcissistic and antisocial pathology in adolescence. In A. H. Esman (Ed.), *Adolescent psychiatry: Developmental and clinical studies* (Vol. 22, pp. 169–186). Hillsdale, NJ: Analytic Press.

Kernberg, O. F. (1999). A severe sexual inhibition in the course of the psychoanalytic treatment of a patient with a narcissistic personality disorder. *International Journal of Psychoanalysis, 80*, 899–908.

Kernberg, O. F. (2010). Narcissistic personality disorder. In J. Clarkin, P. Fonagy, & G. Gabbard (Eds.), *Psychodynamic psychotherapy for personality disorders: A clinical handbook*. (pp. 257–287). Arlington, VA: American Psychiatric Publishing.

Kernberg, P. F. (1983). Borderline conditions: Childhood and adolescent aspects. In K. S. Robson (Ed.), *The borderline child: Etiology, diagnosis, and treatment* (pp. 101–119). New York: McGraw-Hill.

Kernberg, P. F. (1988). Children with borderline personality organization. In C. J. Kestenbaum & D. T. Williams (Eds.), *Handbook of clinical assessment of children and adolescents* (pp. 604–625). New York: New York University Press.

Kernberg, P. F. (1989). Narcissistic personality disorder in childhood. *Psychiatric Clinics of North America, 112*, 671–693.

Kernberg, P. F., & Chazan, S. E. (1998). The Children's Play Therapy Instrument (CPTI): Description, development, and reliability studies. *Journal of Psychotherapy Practice and Research, 7*(3), 196–207.

Kernberg, P. F., Weiner, A. S., & Bardenstein, K. K. (2000). *Personality disorders in children and adolescents*. New York: Basic Books.

Kiesner, J., Cadinu, M., Poulin, F., & Bucci, M. (2002). Group identification in early adolescence: Its relation with peer adjustment and its moderator effect on peer influence. *Child Development, 73*(1), 196–208.

Klein, D. N., Kotov, R., & Bufferd, S. J. (2011). Personality and depression: Explanatory models and review of the evidence. *Annual Review of Clinical Psychology, 7*, 269–295.

Klein, D. N., Schatzberg, A. F., McCullough, J. P., Dowling, F., Goodman, D., Howland, R. H., . . . Keller, M. B. (1999). Age of onset in chronic major depression: Relation to demographic and clinical variables, family history, and treatment response. *Journal of Affective Disorders, 55*, 149–157.

Klein, M. (1946). Some notes on schizoid mechanisms. *International Journal of Psychoanalysis, 27*, 99–110.

Kohut, H. (1968). The psychoanalytic treatment of narcissistic personality disorders: Outline of a systematic approach. *Psychoanalytic Study of the Child, 23*, 86–113.

Kohut, H., & Wolf, E. (1978). The disorders of the self and their treatment: An outline. *International Journal of Psycho-Analysis, 59*, 413–425.

Kongerslev, M. T., Chanen, A. M., & Simonsen, E. (2015). Personality disorder in childhood and adolescence comes of age: A review of the current evidence and prospects for future research. *Scandinavian Journal of Child and Adolescent Psychiatry and Psychology, 3*(1), 31–48.

Lahey, B. B., Loeber, R., Burke, J. D., & Applegate, B. (2005). Predicting future antisocial personality disorder in males from a clinical assessment in childhood. *Journal of Consulting and Clinical Psychology, 73*, 389–399.

Lahti, M., Pesonen, A. K., Räikkönen, K., & Erikson, J. G. (2012). Temporary separation from parents in early childhood and serious personality disorders in adult life. *Journal of Personality Disorders, 26*(5), 751–762.

Lansford, J. E., Criss, M. M., Dodge, K. A., Shaw, D. S., Pettit, G. S., & Bates, J. E. (2009). Trajectories of physical discipline: Early antecedents and developmental outcomes. *Child Development, 80*(5), 1385–1402.

Lansford, J. E., Criss, M. M., Pettit, G. S., Dodge, K. A., & Bates, J. E. (2003). Friendship quality, peer group affiliation, and peer antisocial behavior as moderators of the link between negative parenting and adolescent externalizing behavior. *Journal of Research on Adolescence, 13*, 161–184.

Laurenssen, E. M. P., Hutsebaut, J., Feenstra, D. J., Van Busschbach, J. J., & Luyten, P. (2013). Diagnosis of personality disorders in adolescents: A study among psychologists. *Child and Adolescent Psychiatry and Mental Health, 7*(1), 3.

Lavan, H., & Johnson, J. G. (2002). The association between Axis I and Axis II psychiatric symptoms and high-risk sexual behavior during adolescence. *Journal of Personality Disorders, 16*, 73–94.

Leckman, J. F., & Mayes, L. C. (1998). Understanding developmental psychopathology: How useful are evolutionary accounts? *Journal of the American*

Academy of Child and Adolescent Psychiatry, 37, 1011–1021.

Lengua, L. J., & Wachs, T. D. (2012). Temperament and risk: Resilient and vulnerable responses to adversity. In M. Zentner & R. L. Shiner (Eds.), *Handbook of temperament* (pp. 519–540). New York: Guilford Press.

Lenzenweger, M. F. (2010). A source, a cascade, a schizoid: A heuristic proposal from the Longitudinal Study of Personality Disorders. *Development and Psychopathology, 22*, 867–881.

Levy, K. N. (2005). The implications of attachment theory and research for understanding borderline personality disorder. *Development and Psychopathology, 4*, 959–986.

Liotti, G. (2004). Trauma, dissociation, and disorganized attachment: Three strands of a single braid. *Psychotherapy: Theory, Research, Practice, Training, 41*, 472–487.

Loas, G., Baelde, O., & Verrier, A. (2015). Relationship between alexithymia and dependent personality disorder: A dimensional analysis. *Psychiatry Research, 225*, 484–488.

Loeber, R., & Schmaling, K. B. (1985). The utility of differentiating between mixed and pure forms of antisocial child behavior. *Journal of Abnormal Child Psychology, 73*, 315–335.

Loewald, H. W. (1962). Internalization, separation, mourning, and the super-ego. *Psychoanalytic Quarterly, 31*(4), 483–504.

Loughran, M. J. (2004). Psychodynamic therapy with adolescents. In H. Steiner (Ed.), *Handbook of mental health interventions in children and adolescents: An integrated developmental perspective* (pp. 586–620). San Francisco: Jossey-Bass.

Lubbe, T. (2000). The borderline concept in childhood: Common origins and developments in clinical theory and practice in the USA and the UK. In T. Lubbe (Ed.), *The borderline psychotic child: A selective integration* (pp. 3–38). London: Routledge.

Lubbe, T. (2003). Diagnosing a male hysteric: Don Juan-type. *International Journal of Psychoanalysis, 84*, 1043–1059.

Lynam, D. R., Caspi, A., Moffitt, T. E., Raine, A., Loeber, R., & Stouthamer-Loeber, M. (2005). Adolescent psychopathy and the Big Five: Results from two samples. *Journal of Abnormal Child Psychology, 33*(4), 431–443.

Mahler, M. S. (1971). A study of the separation–individuation process and its possible application to borderline phenomena in the psychoanalytic situation. *Psychoanalytic Study of the Child, 26*, 403–424.

Mahler, M. S., & Kaplan, L. (1977). Developmental aspects in the assessment of narcissistic and so-called borderline personalities. In P. Hartocollis (Ed.), *Borderline personality disorders: The concept, the syndrome, the patient* (pp. 71–89). New York: International Universities Press.

Mancebo, M. C., Eisen, J. L., Grant, J. E., & Rasmussen, S. A. (2005). Obsessive compulsive personality disorder and obsessive compulsive disorder: Clinical characteristics, diagnostic difficulties, and treatment. *Annals of Clinical Psychiatry, 17*, 197–204.

March, J. S., & Leonard, H. L. (1996). Obsessive–compulsive disorder in children and adolescents: A review of the past 10 years. *Journal of the American Academy of Child and Adolescent Psychiatry, 34*, 1265–1273.

Markon, K. E., Krueger, R. F., & Watson, D. (2005). Delineating the structure of normal and abnormal personality: An integrative hierarchical approach. *Journal of Personality And Social Psychology, 88*(1), 139–157.

Markowitz, J. C., Skodol, A. E., Petkova, E., Xie, H., Cheng, J., Hellerstein, D. J., . . . McGlashan, T. H. (2005). Longitudinal comparison of depressive personality disorder and dysthymic disorder. *Comprehensive Psychiatry, 46*, 239–245.

Masten, A. S. (2007). Resilience in developing systems: Progress and promise as the fourth wave rises. *Development and Psychopathology, 19*(3), 921–930.

Masterson, J. F. (1980). *From borderline adolescent to functioning adult*. New York: Brunner/Mazel.

Masterson, J. F. (2013). *Treatment of the borderline adolescent: A developmental approach*. London: Routledge.

McCann, J. T. (1999). *Assessing adolescents with the MACI: Using the Millon Adolescent Clinical Inventory*. New York: Wiley.

McLean, P. D., & McLean, C. P. (2004). Family therapy of avoidant personality disorder. In M. M. MacFarlane (Ed.), *Family treatment of personality disorders: Advances in clinical practice* (pp. 273–303). Binghamton, NY: Haworth Clinical Practice Press.

McWilliams, N. (1994). *Psychoanalytic diagnosis*. New York: Guilford Press.

McWilliams, N. (2006). Some thoughts about schizoid dynamics. *Psychoanalytic Review, 93*, 1–24.

McWilliams, N. (2011). *Psychoanalytic diagnosis: Understanding personality structure in the clinical process* (2nd ed.). New York: Guilford Press.

Meyer, G. J., Viglione, D. J., Mihura, J. L., Erard, R. E., & Erdberg, P. (2011). *Rorschach Performance Assessment System: Administration coding, interpretation and technical manual*. Toledo, OH: Rorschach Performance Assessment System.

Mihura, J. L., Meyer, G. J., Dumitrascu, N., & Bombel, G. (2013). The validity of the individual Rorschach variables: Systematic reviews and meta-analyses of the comprehensive system. *Psychological Bulletin, 136*, 548–605.

Millon, T., & Davis, R. D. (1993). The Millon Adolescent Personality Inventory and the Millon Adolescent Clinical Inventory. *Journal of Counseling and Development, 71*(5), 570–574.

Millon, T., Millon, C., Davis, R., & Grossman, S. (2006). *Millon Adolescent Clinical Inventory manual* (2nd ed.). Minneapolis, MN: National Computer Systems.

Minne, C. (2011). The secluded minds of violent patients. *Psychoanalytic Psychotherapy, 25*, 38–51.

Moffitt, T. E. (1993). Adolescence-limited and life course-persistent antisocial behavior: A developmental view. *Psychological Review, 100*, 674–701.

Moffitt, T., Caspi, A., Dickson, N., Silva, P., & Stanton, W. (1996). Childhood-onset versus adolescent-onset antisocial conduct problems in males: Natural history from ages 3 to 18 years. *Development and Psychopathology, 8*, 399–425.

Moffitt, T. E., Caspi, A., Harrington, H., & Milne, B. J. (2002). Males on the life-course-persistent and adolescence-limited antisocial pathways: Follow-up at age 26 years. *Development and Psychopathology, 14*(1), 179–207.

Morey, L. (2007). *Personality Assessment Inventory—Adolescent professional manual.* Lutz, FL: Psychological Assessment Resources.

Morgan, T. A., & Clark, L. A. (2010). Passive-submissive and active-emotional trait dependency: Evidence for a two-factor model. *Journal of Personality, 78*, 1325–1352.

Mulder, R. T. (2012). Cultural aspects of personality disorder. In T. Widiger (Ed.), *The Oxford handbook of personality disorders* (pp. 260–274). New York: Oxford University Press.

Murray, H. A. (1943). *Thematic Apperception Test: Manual.* Cambridge, MA: Harvard University Press.

Murray, H. A. (1971). *Thematic Apperception Test: Manual* (rev. ed.). Cambridge, MA: Harvard University Press.

Murrie, D. C., & Cornell, D. G. (2002). Psychopathy screening of incarcerated juveniles: A comparison of measures. *Psychological Assessment, 14*, 390–396.

Mustanski, B., Kuper, L., & Greene, G. J. (2014). Development of sexual orientation and identity. In D. L. Tolman, L. M. Diamond, J. A. Bauermeister, W. H. George, J. G. Pfaus, L. M. Ward, . . . L. M. Ward (Eds.), *APA handbook of sexuality and psychology: Vol. 1. Person-based approaches* (pp. 597–628). Washington, DC: American Psychological Association.

Naughton, M., Oppenheim, A., & Hill, J. (1996). Assessment of personality functioning in the transition from adolescent to adult life: Preliminary findings. *British Journal of Psychiatry, 168*, 33–37.

Newhill, C. E., Eack, S. M., & Conner, K. O. (2009). Racial differences between African and White Americans in the presentation of borderline personality disorder. *Race and Social Problems, 1*, 87–96.

Nock, M. K., & Kessler, R. C. (2006). Prevalence of and risk factors for suicide attempts versus suicide gestures: Analysis of the National Comorbidity Survey. *Journal of Abnormal Psychology, 115*, 616–623.

Normandin, L., Ensink, K., & Kernberg, O. F. (2015). Transference-focused psychotherapy for borderline adolescents: A neurobiologically informed psychodynamic psychotherapy. *Journal of Infant, Child, and Adolescent Psychotherapy, 14*, 98–110.

Obrzut, J. E., & Boliek. C. A. (2003). Thematic approaches to personality assessment with children and adolescents. In H. M. Knoff (Ed.), *The assessment of child and adolescent personality* (pp. 173–198). New York: Guilford Press.

Offer, D., Ostrow, E., & Howard, K. I. (1981). *The adolescent: A psychological self-portrait.* New York: Basic Books.

Ogden, T. H. (1979). On projective identification. *International Journal of Psycho-Analysis, 60*(2), 357–373.

Ørstavik, R. E., Kendler, K. S., Czajkowski, N., Tambs, K., & Reichborn-Kjennerud, T. (2007). The relationship between depressive personality disorder and major depressive disorder: A population-based twin study. *American Journal of Psychiatry, 164*, 1866–1872.

Pajer, K. A. (1998). What happens to "bad" girls?: A review of the adult outcome of antisocial adolescent girls. *American Journal of Psychiatry, 155*, 862–870.

Palombo, J. (1982). Critical review of the concept of the borderline child. *Clinical Social Work Journal, 10*, 246–264.

Palombo, J. (1983). Borderline conditions: A perspective from self psychology. *Clinical Social Work Journal, 11*, 323–338.

Palombo, J. (1985). The treatment of borderline neurocognitively impaired children: A perspective from self psychology. *Clinical Social Work Journal, 13*, 117–128.

Palombo, J. (1987). Self-object transferences in the treatment of borderline neurocognitively impaired children. In J. S. Grotstein, M. F. Solomon, & J. A. Lang (Eds.), *The borderline patient: Emerging concepts in diagnosis, psychodynamics, and treatment* (Vol. 2, pp. 317–345). Hillsdale, NJ: Analytic Press.

Palombo, J. (1988). Adolescent development: A view from self psychology. *Child and Adolescent Social Work Journal, 5*, 171–186.

Palombo, J. (1990). The cohesive self, the nuclear self, and development in late adolescence. *Adolescent Psychiatry, 17*, 338–359.

Patalay, P., Fonagy, P., Deighton, J., Belsky, J., Vostanis, P., & Wolpert, M. (2015). A general psychopathology factor in early adolescence. *British Journal of Psychiatry, 207*, 15–22.

Patterson, G. R., Dishion, T. J., & Yoerger, K. (2000). Adolescent growth in new forms of problem behavior: Macro- and micro-peer dynamics. *Prevention Science, 1*, 3–13.

Paul, R., Cohen, D. J., Klin, A., & Volkmar, E. (1999). Multiplex developmental disorders: The role of communication in the construction of a self. *Child and Adolescent Psychiatric Clinics of North America, 8*, 189–202.

Petti, T. A., & Vela, R. M. (1990). Borderline disorders in childhood: An overview. *Journal of the American Academy of Child and Adolescent Psychiatry, 29*, 327–337.

Pine, F. (1974). On the concept "borderline" in children: A clinical essay. *Psychoanalytic Study of the Child, 29*, 341–368.

PDM Task Force. (2006). *Psychodynamic diagnostic manual.* Silver Spring, MD: Alliance of Psychoanalytic Organizations.

Raboteg-Šarić, Z., Šakić, M., & Brajša-Žganec, A. (2009). Quality of school life in primary schools: Relations with academic achievement, motivation and students' behavior. *Društvena Istraživanja, 18*(4–5), 697–716.

Rachão, I., & Campos, R. C. (2015). Personality styles and defense mechanisms in a community sample of adolescents: An exploratory study. *Bulletin of the Menninger Clinic, 79*(1), 14–40.

Rashid, T., & Ostermann, R. F. (2009). Strength-based assessment in clinical practice. *Journal of Clinical Psychology, 65*(5), 488–498.

Rawana, E. P., & Brownlee, K. (2009). Making the possible probable: A strength-based assessment and intervention framework for clinical work with parents, children and adolescents. *Families in Society: Journal of Contemporary Social Services, 90*, 255–260.

Rettew, D. C., Zanarini, M. C., Yen, S., Grilo, C. M., Skodol, A. E., Shea, M. T., . . . Gunderson, J. G. (2003). Childhood antecedents of avoidant personality disorder: A retrospective study. *Journal of the American Academy of Child and Adolescent Psychiatry, 42*, 1122–1130.

Reus, R., Berg, J. F., & Emmelkamp, P. M. (2013). Personality Diagnostic Questionnaire 4+ is not useful as a screener in clinical practice. *Clinical Psychology and Psychotherapy, 20*(1), 49–54.

Rey, J. M., Morris-Yates, A., Singh, M., Andrews, G., & Stewart, G. W. (1995). Continuities between psychiatric disorders in adolescents and personality disorders in young adults. *American Journal of Psychiatry, 152*(6), 895–900.

Rinsley, D. B. (1980). Diagnosis and treatment of borderline and narcissistic children and adolescents. *Bulletin of the Menninger Clinic, 44*, 147–170.

Rios, J., & Morey, L. C. (2013). Detecting feigned ADHD in later adolescence: An examination of three PAI-A negative distortion indicators. *Journal of Personality Assessment, 95*(6), 594–599.

Robbins, M. (1982). Narcissistic personality as a symbiotic character disorder. *International Journal of Psycho-Analysis, 63*, 457–473.

Roberts, G. E. (2005). *Roberts-2 manual.* Los Angeles: Western Psychological Services.

Robson, K. S. (Ed.). (1983). *The borderline child: Etiology, diagnosis, and treatment.* New York: McGraw-Hill.

Romm, S., Bockian, N., & Harvey, M. M. (1999). Factor-based prototypes of the Millon Adolescent Clinical Inventory in adolescents referred for residential treatment. *Journal of Personality Assessment, 72*, 125–143.

Rossouw, T. I. (2015). The use of mentalization-based treatment for adolescents (MBT-A) with a young woman with mixed personality disorder and tendencies to self-harm. *Journal of Clinical Psychology, 71*, 178–187.

Rubin, K. H., Dwyer, K. M., Booth-LaForce, C., Kim, A. H., Burgess, K. B., & Rose-Krasnor, L. (2004). Attachment, friendship, and psychosocial functioning in early adolescence. *Journal of Early Adolescence, 24*(4), 326–356.

Russ, E., Shedler, J., Bradley, R., & Westen, D. (2008). Refining the construct of narcissistic personality disorder: Diagnostic criteria and subtypes. *American Journal of Psychiatry, 165*, 1473–1481.

Rygaard, N. P. (1998). Psychopathic children: Indicators of organic dysfunction. In T. Millon, E. Simonsen, M. Birket-Smith, & R. D. Davis (Eds.), *Psychopathy: Antisocial, criminal, and violent behavior* (pp. 247–259). New York: Guilford Press.

Salekin, R. T., & Frick, P. J. (2005). Psychopathy in children and adolescents: The need for a developmental perspective. *Journal of Abnormal Child Psychology, 33*(4), 403–409.

Salihovic, S., Kerr, M., & Stattin, H. (2014). Under the surface of adolescent psychopathic traits: High-anxious and low-anxious subgroups in a community sample of youths. *Journal of Adolescence, 37*(5), 681–689.

Sander, L. W. (1985). Toward a logic of organization in psychobiological development. In H. Klar & L. Siever (Eds.), *Biologic response styles: Clinical implications* (pp. 20–36). Washington, DC: American Psychiatric Association.

Sander, L. W. (1987). A 25-year follow-up: Some reflections on personality development over the long term. *Infant Mental Health Journal, 8*(3), 210–220.

Sandler, J. (1972). The role of affects in psychoanalytic theory. *Ciba Foundation Symposium, 8*, 31–46.

Sanislow, C. A., da Cruz, K., Gianoli, M. O., & Reagan, E. R. (2012). Avoidant personality disorder, traits, and type. In T. A. Widiger (Ed.), *The Oxford handbook of personality disorders* (pp. 549–565). New York: Oxford University Press.

Santor, D. A., Messervey, D., & Kusumakar, V. (2000). Measuring peer pressure, popularity, and conformity in adolescent boys and girls: Predicting school performance, sexual attitudes, and substance abuse. *Journal of Youth and Adolescence, 29*(2), 163–182.

Sapienza, J. K., & Masten, A. S. (2011). Understanding and promoting resilience in children and youth. *Current Opinion in Psychiatry, 24*(4), 267–273.

Sellbom, M., & Jarrett, M. A. (2014). Conceptualizing youth BPD within an MMPI-A framework. In C. Sharp & J. L. Tackett (Eds.), *Handbook of borderline personality disorder in children and adolescents* (pp. 65–79). New York: Springer.

Sharp, C., & Fonagy, P. (2015). Practitioner review: Borderline personality disorder in adolescence: Recent conceptualization, intervention, and implications for clinical practice. *Journal of Child Psychology and Psychiatry, 56*(12), 1266–1288.

Sharp, C., & Vanwoerden, S. (2015). Hypermentalizing in borderline personality disorder: A model and data. *Journal of Infant, Child, and Adolescent Psychotherapy, 14*, 33–45.

Shedler, J., & Westen, D. (2004). Dimensions of personality pathology: An alternative to the five-factor model. *American Journal of Psychiatry, 161*(10), 1743–1754.

Shedler, J., & Westen, D. (2007). The Shedler–Westen Assessment Procedure (SWAP): Making personality diagnosis clinically meaningful. *Journal of Personality Assessment, 89*(1), 41–55.

Sheets, E. S., & Craighead, W. E. (2007). Toward an empirically based classification of personality pathology. *Clinical Psychology: Science and Practice, 14*, 77–93.

Shiner, R. L. (2009). The development of personality disorders: Perspectives from normal personality development in childhood and adolescence. *Development and Psychopathology, 21*(3), 715–734.

Shiner, R. L., & Allen, T. A. (2013). Assessing personality disorders in adolescents: Seven guiding principles. *Clinical Psychology: Science and Practice, 20*(4), 361–377.

Shiner, R. L., & Tackett, J. L. (2014). Personality disorders in children and adolescents. In E. J. Mash & R. A. Barkley (Eds.), *Child psychopathology* (3rd ed., pp. 848–896). New York: Guilford Press.

Sigmund, D., Barnett, E., & Mundt, C. (1998). The hysterical personality disorder: A phenomenological approach. *Psychopathology, 31*, 318–330.

Skodol, A. E., Bender, D. S., Pagano, M. E., Shea, M. T., Yen, S., Sanislow, C. A., . . . Gunderson, J. G. (2007). Positive childhood experiences: Resilience and recovery from personality disorder in early adulthood. *Journal of Clinical Psychiatry, 68*(7), 1102–1108.

Smith, S. R. (2007). Making sense of multiple informants in child and adolescent psychopathology: A guide for clinicians. *Journal of Psychoeducational Assessment, 25*(2), 139–149.

Spillius, E., & O'Shaughnessy, E. (2013). *Projective identification: The fate of a concept.* London: Routledge.

Sroufe, L. A. (1996). *Emotional development: The organization of emotional life in the early years.* New York: Cambridge University Press.

Stanley, B., & Siever, L. J. (2009). The interpersonal dimension of borderline personality disorder: Toward a neuropeptide model. *American Journal of Psychiatry, 167*(1), 24–39.

Stein, M., Hilsenroth, M., Slavin-Mulford, J., & Pinsker, J. (2011). *Social Cognition and Object Relations Scale: Global Rating Method (SCORS-G).* Unpublished manuscript, Massachusetts General Hospital and Harvard Medical School.

Stern, B. L., Caligor, E., Clarkin, J. F., Critchfield, K. L., Hörz, S., MacCornack, V., . . . Kernberg, O. (2010). Structured Interview of Personality Organization (STIPO): Preliminary psychometrics in a clinical sample. *Journal of Personality Assessment, 92*(1), 35–44.

Stokes, J. M., & Pogge, D. L. (2001). The relationship of the Rorschach SCZI to psychotic features in a child psychiatric sample. *Journal of Personality Assessment, 76*(2), 209–228.

Syed, M., & Seiffge-Krenke, I. (2013). Personality development from adolescence to emerging adulthood: Linking trajectories of ego development to the family context and identity formation. *Journal of Personality and Social Psychology, 104*(2), 371–384.

Taubner, S., White, L. O., Zimmermann, J., Fonagy, P., & Nolte, T. (2013). Attachment-related mentalization moderates the relationship between psychopathic traits and proactive aggression in adolescence. *Journal of Abnormal Child Psychology, 41*, 929–938.

Taylor, C. T., Laposa, J. M., & Alden, E. (2004). Is avoidant personality disorder more than just social avoidance? *Journal of Personality Disorders, 18*, 571–594.

Tedeschi, R., & Kilmer, R. (2005). Assessing strengths, resilience, and growth to guide clinical interventions. *Professional Psychology: Research and Practice, 36*(3), 230–237.

Thomas, A., Chess, S., & Birch, H. (1968). *Temperament and behavior disorders in children.* New York: New York University Press.

Tillfors, M., Furmark, T., Ekselius, L., & Fredrikson, M. (2004). Social phobia and avoidant personality disorder: One spectrum disorder? *Nordic Journal of Psychiatry, 58*, 147–152.

Tuvblad, C., Wang, P., Bezdjian, S., Raine, A., & Baker, L. A. (2016). Psychopathic personality development from ages 9 to 18: Genes and environment. *Development and Psychopathology, 28*(1), 27–44.

Tyson, P., & Tyson, R. L. (1990). *Psychoanalytic theories of development: An integration.* New Haven, CT: Yale University Press.

Updegraff, K., & Obeidallah, D. A. (1999). Young adolescents' patterns of involvement with siblings and friends. *Social Development, 8*, 52–69.

Urberg, K. A., Değirmencioğlu, S. M., & Pilgrim, C. (1997). Close friend and group influence on adolescent cigarette smoking and alcohol use. *Developmental Psychology, 33*(5), 834.

Vazsonyi, A. T., Ksinan, A., Mikuška, J., & Jiskrova, G. (2015). The Big Five and adolescent adjustment: An empirical test across six cultures. *Personality and Individual Differences, 83*, 234–244.

Waldron, S., Moscovitz, S., Lundin, J., Helm, F., Jemerin, J., & Gorman, B. (2011). Evaluating the outcomes of psychotherapies: The Personality Health Index. *Psychoanalytic Psychology, 28*, 363–388.

Weise, K. L., & Tuber, S. (2004). The self and object representations of narcissistically disturbed children: An empirical investigation. *Psychoanalytic Psychology, 21*, 244–258.

Westen, D. (1990). The relations among narcissism, egocentrism, self-concept, and self-esteem: Experimental, clinical, and theoretical considerations. *Psychoanalysis and Contemporary Thought, 13*(2),183–239.

Westen, D., Betan, E., & DeFife, J. A. (2011). Identity disturbance in adolescence: Associations with borderline personality disorder. *Development and Psychopathology, 23*(1), 305–313.

Westen, D., & Chang, C. (2001). Personality pathology in adolescence: A review. *Adolescent Psychiatry, 25*, 61–100.

Westen, D., DeFife, J. A., Malone, J. C., & DiLallo, J. (2014). An empirically derived classification of adolescent personality disorders. *Journal of the American Academy of Child and Adolescent Psychiatry, 53*(5), 528–549.

Westen, D., Dutra, L., & Shedler, J. (2005). Assessing adolescent personality pathology. *British Journal of Psychiatry, 186*, 227–238.

Westen, D., Lohr, N., Silk, K., Gold, L., & Kerber, K. (1985). Object relations and social cognition in borderline personality disorder and depression: A TAT analysis. *Psychological Assessment, 2*, 355–364.

Westen, D., & Shedler, J. (2007). Personality diagnosis with the Shedler–Westen Assessment Procedure (SWAP): Integrating clinical and statistical measurement and prediction. *Journal of Abnormal Psychology, 116*, 810–822.

Westen, D., Shedler, J., & Bradley, R. (2006). A prototype approach to personality disorder diagnosis. *American Journal of Psychiatry, 163*(5), 846–856.

Westen, D., Shedler, J., Bradley, B., & DeFife, J. A. (2012). An empirically derived taxonomy for personality diagnosis: Bridging science and practice in conceptualizing personality. *American Journal of Psychiatry, 169*(3), 273–284.

Westen, D., Shedler, J., Durrett, C., Glass, S., & Martens, A. (2003). Personality diagnoses in adolescence: DSM-IV Axis II diagnoses and an empirically derived alternative. *American Journal of Psychiatry, 160*, 952–966.

Wheeler, Z. (2013). *Treatment of schizoid personality: An analytic psychotherapy handbook.* Unpublished doctoral dissertation, Pepperdine University.

Widiger, T. A., & Bornstein, R. F. (2001). Histrionics, dependent, and narcissistic personality disorders. In P. B. Sutker & H. E. Adams (Eds.), *Comprehensive handbook of psychopathology* (3rd ed., pp. 509–531). New York: Plenum Press.

Wiley, R. E., & Berman, S. L. (2013). Adolescent identity development and distress in a clinical sample. *Journal of Clinical Psychology, 69*(12), 1299–1304.

Wilkinson-Ryan, T., & Westen, D. (2000). Identity disturbance in borderline personality disorder: An empirical investigation. *American Journal of Psychiatry, 157*(4), 528–541.

Willock, B. (1987). The devalued (unloved, repugnant) self: A second facet of narcissistic vulnerability in the aggressive, conduct-disordered child. *Psychoanalytic Psychology, 3*, 219–240.

Winarick, D. J., & Bornstein, R. F. (2015). Toward resolution of a longstanding controversy in personality disorder diagnosis: Contrasting correlates of schizoid and avoidant traits. *Personality and Individual Differences, 79*, 25–29.

Winnicott, D. W. (1953). Transitional objects and transitional phenomena: A study of the firstnot-me possession. *International Journal of Psycho-Analysis, 34*, 89–97.

Winnicott, D. W. (1960). Ego distortion in terms of true and false self. In D. W. Winnicott (Ed.), *The maturational processes and the facilitating environment* (pp. 140–152). New York: International Universities Press.

Winnicott, D. W. (1965). *The maturational processes and the facilitating environment: Studies in the theory of emotional development* (J. D. Sutherland, Ed.). New York: International Universities Press.

Wolfe, D. A., Jaffe, P. G., & Crooks, C. V. (2006). *Adolescent risk behaviors: Why teens experiment and strategies to keep them safe.* New Haven, CT: Yale University Press.

Wolff, S. (1991). "Schizoid" personality in childhood and adult life: III. The childhood picture. *British Journal of Psychiatry, 159*, 629–635.

Wolff, S., & Barlow, A. (1979). Schizoid personality in childhood: A comparative study of schizoid, autistic and normal children. *Journal of Child Psychology and Psychiatry, 20*, 29–46.

Wolff, S., Townshend, R., McGuire, R. J., & Weeks, D. J. (1991). "Schizoid" personality in childhood and adult life: II. Adult adjustment and the continuity with schizotypal personality disorder. *British Journal of Psychiatry, 159*, 620–629.

World Health Organization. (1992). *The ICD-10 classification of mental and behavioural disorders: Clinical descriptions and diagnostic guidelines.* Geneva: Author.

Yap, M. B. H., Allen, N. B., O'Shea, M., di Parsia, P., Simmons, J. G., & Sheeber, L. (2011). Early adolescents' temperament, emotion regulation during mother–child interactions, and depressive symptomatology. *Development and Psychopathology, 23*(1), 267–282.

Zalewski, M., Stepp, S. D., Scott, L. N., Whalen, D. J., Beeney, J. E., & Hipwell, A. E. (2014). Maternal borderline personality disorder symptoms and parenting of adolescent daughters. *Journal of Personality Disorders, 28*(4), 541–554.

Zanarini, M. C., Gunderson, J. G., Marino, M. F., Schwartz, E. O., & Frankenberg, E. R. (1989). Childhood experiences of borderline patients. *Comprehensive Psychiatry, 30*, 18–25.

CHAPTER 6

Adolescent Symptom Patterns: The Subjective Experience

SA Axis

CHAPTER EDITOR

Mario Speranza, MD, PhD

CONSULTANTS

Corinne Blanchet-Collet, MD
Jacques Dayan, MD, PhD
Martin Debbané, PhD
George Halasz, MS, MRCPsych
Jonathan Lachal, MD, PhD
Nick Midgley, PhD
Massimiliano Orri, PhD

Introduction

This chapter focuses on adolescents' subjective experience of symptom patterns as described by international classifications of mental disorders, such as the *Diagnostic and Statistical Manual of Mental Disorders*, fifth edition (DSM-5; American Psychiatric Association, 2013) and the *International Classification of Diseases*, 10th revision (ICD-10; World Health Organization, 1992). Adolescents falling into the same diagnostic category may vary widely in their subjective experience of symptom patterns (Fonagy & Target, 2002). We emphasize that exploring adolescents' subjective experience is an essential aspect of the diagnostic process. Because response to treatments is powerfully predicted by subjective experience (Blatt, Quinlan, Pilkonis, & Shea, 1995; McCallum, Piper, Ogrodniczuk, & Joyce, 2003), the PDM-2 person-centered approach to mental suffering has important therapeutic consequences.

Symptom patterns in adolescents are best viewed in a developmental, dynamic context that includes environmental determinants. Clinicians who work with adolescents are continually reminded of the many factors that contribute to different symptom patterns, as well as the unique developmental pathways leading to them. This period presents multiple challenges that test adolescents' capacities for adaptation and overall emotional and behavioral flexibility (school environment, autonomy, peer relationships, sexuality, social roles, etc.). In addition, adolescents develop rapidly and therefore experience relatively sudden changes in their behaviors, feelings, thoughts, fantasies, and symptom patterns.

The meaning of a symptom may be quite different at different developmental stages. It is important to consider the specific maturation of adolescents' mental capacities that may influence symptom expression—especially in the areas of identity and relational capacities, mentalization, regulation of self-esteem, and defensive functioning. Special attention to variations in these capacities should be given to adolescents with histories of neurodevelopmental disorders, who may experience and express symptoms patterns differently from adolescents with more typical development. In general, clinicians must be aware of the unstable expression of symptom patterns in adolescence and favor observations over extended periods before considering any specific diagnosis at this age.

In this chapter, we limit our presentation to features observed in the most common symptom patterns in adolescence. For comprehensive descriptions, clinicians are invited to read the corresponding adult and child chapters of PDM-2 (Chapters 3 and 9), and in some cases to refer to the symptom descriptions of DSM-5 (American Psychiatric Association, 2013). At the end of the chapter, we include a table (Table 6.2) showing the concordance between the PDM-2 system and the DSM-5 and ICD-10 systems in the area of symptom patterns.

The subjective experience of the therapist treating an adolescent may vary widely, ranging from loving protectiveness to exasperated rage. Although the emotional response of clinicians in relation to adolescent symptoms is in large part mediated by patient personality characteristics (see Chapter 5 on the PA Axis), it is possible to trace some clinician responses that occur specifically in relation to adolescents' symptoms. We discuss some characteristics of therapists' experience in treating adolescents, referring to Chapter 3 on the S Axis for more detailed descriptions of specific symptoms. In comparison to work with adults, interactions with adolescents and their families can evoke particularly complex and confusing feelings, which, if unrecognized, can significantly affect clinical judgment and behavior.

A therapist should be aware that countertransferences with adolescents can stem from three domains: the adolescent; the parents, other caregivers, and the family system in general; and the therapist. Adolescents with histories of neglect and abuse may incite particularly strong emotional responses in their therapists, triggering hostile feelings toward neglecting and/or maltreating parents and evoking "overparental" and overprotective responses toward the adolescents. Unrecognized, these responses can put clinicians at odds with family members and lead to a failure to recognize the parents' own underlying feelings of guilt and shame (Rasic, 2010). Work with an adolescent can also arouse a clinician's own adolescent conflicts, facilitating identification or counteridentification and thus leading to distortion in the perception and interpretation of the patient's dynamics.

Table 6.1 provides an overview of the SA Axis, listing the sections and subsections of the various conditions we address.

TABLE 6.1. Adolescent Symptom Patterns: The Subjective Experience—SA Axis

SA0	**Healthy responses**		
	SA01	Developmental and situational crises	
SA1	**Predominantly psychotic disorders**		
	SA11	Brief psychotic disorder	
	SA14	Schizophrenia and schizoaffective disorder	
SA2	**Mood disorders**		
	SA22	Depressive disorders	
	SA24	Bipolar disorders	
	SA26	Disruptive mood dysregulation disorder	
	SA27	Suicidality	
	SA28	Nonsuicidal self-injury	
SA3	**Disorders related primarily to anxiety**		
	SA31	Anxiety disorders	
		SA31.1	Specific phobias
		SA31.2	Social phobia
		SA31.3	Agoraphobia and panic disorder
		SA31.4	Generalized anxiety disorder
	SA32	Obsessive–compulsive and related disorders	
		SA32.1	Obsessive–compulsive disorder
		SA32.2	Body dysmorphic disorder (dysmorphophobia)
SA4	**Event- and stressor-related disorders**		
	SA41	Trauma- and stressor-related disorders	
		SA41.1	Adjustment disorders
		SA41.2	Acute and posttraumatic stress disorders
		SA41.3	Complex posttraumatic stress disorder
	SA42	Dissociative disorders	
	SA43	Conversion disorder	
SA5	**Somatic symptom and related disorders**		
	SA51	Somatic symptom disorder	
	SA52	Illness anxiety disorder (hypochondriasis)	
	SA53	Factitious disorders	
SA8	**Psychophysiological disorders**		
	SA81	Feeding and eating disorders	
SA9	**Disruptive behavior disorders**		
	SA91	Conduct disorder	
	SA92	Oppositional defiant disorder	
	SA93	Substance-related disorders	
	SA94	Internet addiction disorder	

(continued)

TABLE 6.1. *(continued)*

SA10	**Patterns in adolescence of infancy/childhood-onset disorders**	
	SA101	Autism spectrum disorder
	SA102	Attention-deficit/hyperactivity disorder
	SA103	Specific learning disorders
SAApp	**Appendix: Psychological experiences that may require clinical attention**	
	SAApp1	Demographic minority populations (ethnic, cultural, linguistic, religious, political)
	SAApp2	Lesbian, gay, and bisexual populations
	SAApp3	Gender incongruence

SA0 Healthy Responses

SA01 Developmental and Situational Crises

Adolescence is a challenging period characterized by major changes at the physical, cognitive, and social-emotional levels. In cultures in which teenagers are pushed toward autonomy and independence, they are forced to build their own identities and find their places in society. Because these goals are not always achieved without difficulty, adolescents may show seemingly contradictory progressive and regressive attitudes simultaneously. Friends and relatives of the adolescents can feel confused and pressured by these ambivalent behaviors.

Aggression in maturing adolescents is a natural part of their development as they test the limits of their emerging personalities (Winnicott, 1969). Consequently, crises are inherent to adolescent development. A crisis can be considered a temporary moment of disequilibrium, a destabilizing of the familiar organization in the life of an individual. It may be developmentally driven (when an adolescent is confronted with autonomy, with new cognitive demands, or with new types of emotional relationships) or may result from an outside factor that shatters the adolescent's internal equilibrium (grief, trauma, educational conflicts).

A crisis is not a disorder. Certain crises that characterize adolescence are healthy processes, necessary for identity construction. Sometimes, in fact, the *absence* of a crisis can be pathological. A crisis can have a favorable or unfavorable outcome, depending on internal as well as external factors. A favorable solution may allow an adolescent to access new functioning with new potentialities. An unfavorable solution may create a breakdown in development characterized by regressive behaviors. The issue does not depend solely on the adolescent's ability to develop a stable defensive organization; it also depends on the resources that the relational environment is able to mobilize. This double-sided potential of a crisis is well captured in the Chinese pictogram that simultaneously represents the dimension of danger and the opportunity of change.

When a system can adapt to evolving changes in an adolescent's development, anxiety is contained. When it fails to find new solutions and employs rigid mechanisms to control the situation, the acute onset of a symptom or pathological behavior in the adolescent may ensue. The adolescent acts as the designated victim of the dysfunction of the whole system. The crisis becomes an emergency. But the behavior that leads to the emergency is not a disorder in itself; it is only the tip of the much larger iceberg, the entire familial and social system. This perspective does not exclude the existence of true psychopathology in the adolescent; it simply emphasizes the role played by the environment in initiating or maintaining symptom expression.

There are two main vectors of a crisis. The first is an emergency, such as a brief psychotic episode, manic–depressive disorder, temper outburst, anxiety attack, or suicide attempt. The second consists of reactions to challenges encountered with the family and/or social environment. These two vectors often intersect and may give rise to a dangerous intolerance of the adolescent within the social environment (family, peers, educators). Almost all psychopathology in adolescence challenges the containing and reassuring capacities of involved adults. When they fail, anxiety progressively invades the psychic functioning of the adolescent and those involved with him or her. Anxiety, regardless of its basis (whether it is about fragmentation, depersonalization, or loss and separation), is the common element of every emergency situation in adolescence. Acting out can sometimes be the only way for adolescents to express intense feelings and evacuate unbearable anguish about their mental integrity. Acting out takes the place of a mental representation. It can thus provide a transforming moment, insofar as it inscribes into reality something that cannot be registered at the psychic level.

For the therapist of an adolescent, giving adequate responses to this anxiety and to the acting out is an essential step. The family and other involved individuals usually ask for fast relief of their anguish, which can take the form of attributing a psychiatric diagnosis to the adolescent. A professional should avoid a reductionist solution and leave the situation open to several perspectives. The therapist's contribution must also go beyond relieving anxiety and containing the psychic outbursts and instead move toward the opening of a space that the crisis and the acting out bring. The aftermath of the acting out may paradoxically include a special time to restore less pathological communication and raise questions about the individual and relational dynamics that have led to the situation. An adequate answer to these crises in adolescence requires working with those in relationship to the adolescent and more generally adopting a systemic approach to the situation. Family involvement is fundamental to a good prognosis (Tompson, Boger, & Asarnow, 2012).

SA1 Predominantly Psychotic Disorders

Psychotic disorders are also discussed in Chapter 3 on the S Axis (see pp. 139–141).

Psychosis is defined as a severe disruption of thought and behavior, resulting in the loss of reality testing. The diagnosis of psychosis is based on overt changes in a person's behavior and functioning, with evidence of disrupted thinking. Although psychotic symptoms are characteristic of schizophrenia, they may present as aspects of other illnesses, including mood disorders, neurological conditions, and acute intoxication. Psychosis should thus be regarded more as a symptom than as a diagnosis.

Despite the lack of precise epidemiological data, it is generally agreed that the prevalence of psychotic disorders increases markedly during adolescence, with an estimated prevalence of 7.5% among adolescents ages 13–18 years (Kelleher et al., 2012). Generally, the symptoms of a psychotic disorder begin between the ages of 18 and 24, but the onset of less severe symptoms usually begins during the early teen years. Five percent of adults with schizophrenia report onset of psychosis before the age of 15. Once the full disorder is present, the clinical picture of adolescent psychoses is very similar to what is observed in adults. Psychotic disorders severely disrupt an adolescent's ability to function normally in daily activities and are often quite debilitating and disabling.

There is increasing evidence that the early recognition and treatment of psychotic disorders can lead to substantial improvements in recovery and overall functioning (Thompson et al., 2015). As a consequence, there is now a growing drive to identify psychotic disorders at their earliest possible stages and to identify young people who appear to be at high risk of developing a psychotic disorder. By assisting adolescents who appear to be at increased risk, we may be able to prevent the illness from occurring or at least to reduce its impact on these adolescents' lives.

As the clinical pictures of the different psychotic disorders are well described in the section of Chapter 3 on these disorders, we focus in this chapter on two questions: the clinical outcomes of brief psychotic disorder and the prodromal phase of adolescent-onset schizophrenia.

SA11 Brief Psychotic Disorder

As in adults, the essential feature of a diagnosed brief psychotic disorder in adolescence is the sudden onset of positive symptomatology characterized by delusions, hallucinations, formal thought disorders, and grossly disorganized behavior, including catatonia. In adolescents, these psychotic symptoms are frequently associated with phenomena of depersonalization and/or derealization, extreme mood lability, and a dream state of consciousness without proper confusion. The constant presence of somatic signs (insomnia, motor agitation) makes this disorder a true emergency situation needing a protective setting. The clinical picture, which resembles the description of Valentin Magnan's (1893) *bouffée délirante polymorphe aigüe*, has an acute, rich, polymorphous presentation and a relatively brief and self-limited clinical course. The change from a nonpsychotic to a clearly psychotic state occurs within a very short time period (less than 2 weeks, but sometimes within hours), usually without a prodromal period. Psychosocial stressors may precipitate the onset of the episode. These symptoms are transient by definition. An episode of the disturbance usually lasts less than 1 month, with a full return to the premorbid level of functioning. When the symptoms persist beyond a month, a different diagnosis should be given. This convention recalls the perspective contained in the diagnosis of *bouffée délirante polymorphe aigüe*, which was supposed to be a provisional diagnosis that left completely open the long-term outcome after the episode.

Adolescents' psychiatrists have since moderated this optimistic perspective on the basis of epidemiological studies showing that brief psychotic episodes in adolescence do not have a consistently positive outcome and do have negative consequences on personality development (Lachman, 2014). A brief psychotic disorder as diagnosed in DSM-5 may eventually become a diagnosable bipolar disorder with psychotic features, schizophrenia, or the short psychotic episodes that may occur in personality disorders. Schizophrenia and bipolar disorders are the most common outcomes. Fewer than one-third of adolescents diagnosed with brief psychotic disorder develop no long-term psychiatric problem. Known prognostic factors for a schizophrenic outcome compared to other outcomes (including bipolar disorders) include longer onset, longer duration of recovery, only partial recovery, problematic premorbid personality, and catatonic symptoms (Cohen et al., 2005).

Brief psychotic disorder seems to be more frequent in adolescents and young adults with a fragile personality organization, such as those Chapters 1 and 5 consider as at the psychotic level on the P and PA Axes. The presence of traumatic stressors may include positive emotional experiences, such as falling in love or being touched by an aesthetic experience (as has been described for the "Stendhal syndrome," recalling the psychotic-like experience of the romantic French writer during his initial journey in Italy). Adolescents with heightened sensibilities and fragile personalities characterized by strong dependent features can experience the loss of ego boundaries when faced with such intense emotions. This is also what probably happens in adolescents with emerging borderline personality disorder when they are faced with stressful relational situations. The quality of the psychotic experience in these situations may have a predominantly persecutory tone, related to the attributional bias frequently elicited by the activation of disorganized attachment patterns. But beyond possible psychiatric outcomes, the major consequences of a brief psychotic disorder in adolescence may include the secondary reorganization of the adolescent personality toward the avoidance of intimate relationships of any kind, as well as the development of a constrained personality and a diminished sense of self.

Clinical Illustration

Paul is a 15-year-old boy with no known psychiatric history. His parents, who are alarmed about his recent behavior, bring him to the emergency service. For a few days, he has mentioned weird ideas; for instance, he thinks a stranger who offered him some food 2 days earlier has drugged him. These ideas have appeared suddenly after a short period of excitement and endless existential questioning. In recent weeks, he has smoked a lot of hashish with his band of "marginal" friends. In the weeks preceding this episode, Paul has had several moments of anxiety accompanied by concerns about his sexual orientation (fear of being homosexual). He has had moderate insomnia and has lost 11 pounds in a month.

In the consultation, Paul appears perplexed, confused, and incoherent. He acknowledges feeling "weird," and he describes ideas of persecution. Although he does not report hallucinations, he looks very anxious. His mood changes quickly, switching from an excited state to a state of prostration. Paul is afraid his parents will be killed in a political plot related to his participation in a student demonstration the day before. By the time of the consultation, he seems very preoccupied. He can stop suddenly in the middle of a sentence, fixing his gaze on the wall and whispering things like "Life is beautiful."

SA14 Schizophrenia and Schizoaffective Disorder

"Early-onset schizophrenia" (EOS) is defined as onset before 18 years of age. Onset before 13 years is often described as "childhood-onset schizophrenia" (COS). EOS and COS are considered more severe forms of schizophrenia, with a high genetic loading. The diagnosis in children and adolescents uses the same criteria as in adults and is characterized by positive and negative symptoms. Positive symptoms include hallucinations, delusions, and thought disorders. Negative symptoms include deficits such as social withdrawal, blunted affectivity, and paucity of speech or thought. Disorganized behavior may represent an independent third domain, including disorganized speech, bizarre behavior, and poor attention (McClellan, Stock, & American Academy of

Child and Adolescent Psychiatry Committee on Quality Issues, 2013). One important adaptation of the criteria compared to those used in adults is that a failure to achieve age-appropriate interpersonal, academic, or occupational progress can substitute for significant deterioration in functioning below premorbid levels.

Hallucinations, thought disorder, and flattened affect have been consistently found in EOS, whereas systematic delusions and catatonic symptoms occur less frequently. Developmental variation in language and cognition may affect the range and quality of symptom presentation. Most youth who develop schizophrenia show a large array of premorbid abnormalities. Common premorbid difficulties include social withdrawal and isolation, disruptive behaviors, attentional deficits, speech and language problems, cognitive delays, and symptoms on the autism spectrum. The gradual development of psychotic symptoms in children with neurodevelopmental disorders can be difficult to recognize. The onset is insidious, the negative symptoms are more prominent, and the course of the illness is relatively poor compared to more acute onsets. In these insidious onsets, an adolescent may experience his or her symptoms as ego-syntonic and may thus expresses incoherent, imaginative, or delusional ideas without being conscious of the impact they may have on others. Schizophrenia with an acute early onset is relatively easy to diagnose and generally has a more favorable course. Atypical clinical presentations (such as visual hallucinations, confusion, catatonic symptoms, symptom fluctuations, and paradoxical reactions to classical antipsychotic treatments) should alert the clinician to the possible expression of a treatable organic disease that presents with a schizophrenia-like symptomatology (Sedel et al., 2007).

The Prodromal Phase of Schizophrenia

The period of functional decline and gradual emergence of attenuated positive symptoms preceding the first psychotic episode—the "psychosis prodrome"—can last from a few months to several years. The prodromal syndrome usually becomes apparent in adolescence; it is characterized by subclinical manifestations of positive and negative symptoms, as well as nonspecific symptoms, associated with a decline in interpersonal and academic functioning (Yung & McGorry, 2007).

Adolescents in the prodromal phase may experience an array of nonspecific psychotic symptoms, such as odd beliefs (unusual/extraordinarily intense new ideas, strange new feelings); troubles in concentrating or thinking clearly; mistrust of others; and unusual perceptual experiences (increased sensitivity to sounds or sights, mistaking noises for voices). Depersonalization and derealization are frequently reported during these periods and may create a flickering sense of reality in an adolescent. These progressive changes in the subjective experiences of the self, the world, and relationships are frequently associated with a negative emotionality (such as dysphoric mood and inappropriate affects) and with behavioral changes such as odd behaviors, social withdrawal, a dramatic drop in academic performance, or a marked decline in personal hygiene or self-care.

Many view the prodromal phase as affording a critical opportunity for preventive intervention (Compton, McGlashan, & McGorry, 2007); consequently, it has become the focus of intense research. Whether certain constellations of experiences represent the prodromal phase of a severe psychotic disorder is difficult to answer prospectively. If frank psychosis develops in up to 40% of affected patients within 12 months of symptom onset, the concept of the prodromal syndrome is in fact a retrospective one. The progression from prodromes to disease is not linear. In some cases, the "prodromal" phase may decrease in intensity and may not lead to overt psychosis. Some German authors (e.g., Huber, Gross, Schuttler, & Linz, 1980) have accordingly considered the prodrome as a syndrome that confers an increased vulnerability to psychosis but does not inevitably lead to it. Thus the prodrome is a risk factor for psychosis and not a precursor. In fact, because it implies that psychosis is inevitable, the use of this term could be considered misleading. For this reason, Yung and McGorry (1996) have introduced the term "at-risk mental state" (ARMS) for adolescents exhibiting subthreshold psychotic symptoms and the term "ultra-high-risk" (UHR) for those who experience clear-cut psychotic symptoms that resolve spontaneously, without antipsychotic medication, within 7 days.

ARMS and UHR are thus prospective concepts introduced to identify adolescents and young adults for whom intervention at an early stage, before the onset of frank psychosis, may be justified in order to prevent further deterioration and suffering. Transition rates to psychosis for adolescents and young adults who are positive for UHR criteria are about 30–35% within 1–2 years of follow-up (Cannon, Cornblatt, & McGorry, 2007). This is substantially higher than the incidence rate of psychosis among transition-age youth in the general population. However, many attenuated symptoms are quite stable and do not lead to more severe illness—as in individuals with schizotypal personality disorder, who rarely become psychotic, or in the nearly 10% of normal individuals who have attenuated psychotic-like symptoms such as mild hallucinations and/or delusions.

For the moment, there are no clear treatments for this prodromal syndrome. Attempts to institute early antipsychotic treatments have shown no clear long-lasting effects. On the contrary, data seem to indicate that for this population, an integrated model of treatment—including assertive community treatment, social skills training, and psychoeducation in multiple-family groups—allows a 15% reduction of the rate of conversion to full-blown psychosis (Nordentoft, Rasmussen, Melau, Hjorthøj, & Thorup, 2006). These interventions should be weighed against the negative impact that a premature diagnosis may have on the expectations and acceptance of others in the adolescent's social environment.

The Subjective Experience of Schizophrenia in Adolescence

Affective States

A mix of anxiety and depressive symptoms frequently characterizes the emotional experience of adolescents with schizophrenia. This mix may vary according to the main features manifested during the course of the illness. Intense feelings of anxiety or even terror, with psychomotor agitation, may be associated with hallucinations and delusions and with a sense of being controlled by external forces. Depersonalization and derealization phenomena may be very disturbing.

Depression is common in adolescents with schizophrenia at every phase of the illness. It may take the form of blunted or inappropriate affect or of an inability to feel pleasure (anhedonia). Depressive symptoms may also appear once positive symptoms are reduced by medication. They are frequently associated with progressive insight into the illness. These periods put an adolescent at great risk for self-harm and suicide attempts. The association of schizophrenic and affective symptoms (with an identifiable cycle) is frequent in adolescence and may lead to a diagnosis of schizoaffective disorder. Adolescents with this diagnosis show bizarre and persecutory delusions, mood-incongruent hallucinations with lability of mood, and significant functional deterioration.

Cognitive Patterns

Data from the Early Onset of Schizophrenia study of the U.S. National Institute of Mental Health have shown that children and adolescents with schizophrenia report high rates of hallucinations across all sensory modalities. Nearly all patients described significant auditory hallucinations, but up to 80% also reported significant rates of visual hallucinations during their hospitalizations. High rates for tactile (60%) and olfactory (30%) hallucinations were also observed in this pediatric sample; they occurred exclusively in patients with auditory hallucinations. Auditory hallucinations are very real for the adolescents hearing them and can be deeply confusing for others to witness. The voices may be critical, threatening, or neutral, and are often unknown to the person hearing them. As in adults, hallucinations may lead to delusions (synesthesia may lead to delusions of infestations by foreign bodies; olfactory hallucinations may lead to delusions of body putrefaction). In adolescents with an acute onset, the most frequent delusional themes are similar to those observed in adults: persecution, control, ideas of reference, and somatic delusions. In adolescents with more insidious onset, delusional themes may be more difficult to identify, with unspecified and mood-incongruent themes.

Thought processes and behaviors may be impaired by hallucinations or delusions. Adolescents experiencing new-onset psychoses may have trouble organizing their thoughts, as they doubt their perceptions and feelings. The environment may suddenly be perceived as incomprehensible. Hallucinations can decrease an adolescent's ability to pay attention to external stimuli, memorize and process information, prioritize tasks, make decisions, and plan for the future. Some teens may experience intense anxiety or feelings of shame about these uncontrollable changes and may not want to report the symptoms to parents or professionals for fear of being seen as "crazy."

Somatic States

Adolescents with schizophrenia may report a variety of unusual body experiences that may be related to the presence of synesthesia or to delusional themes focused on the body (loss of control of the body, infestations by insects or worms, emitting a foul odor, delusion of body defects). These experiences can be terrifying and may be associated with ritualistic behaviors (endless verifications, gazing into the mirror) and self-injuring acts. Catatonic phenomena (body rigidity and unresponsiveness to outside stimuli) may also be observed in adolescence.

Changes in sleeping and eating patterns are common in adolescents with schizophrenia and may be amplified by medication. Although antipsychotic medications can have a positive effect on psychotic symptoms, these drugs have several negative effects. Adolescents frequently complain about emotional numbing that reduces their capacity to interact with others. Weight gain and the resultant transformation of self-image may pose major problems for adolescents taking medication and constitute a common reason for discontinuing treatment (Vandyk & Baker, 2012).

Relationship Patterns

Qualitative studies exploring the social adjustment of adolescents with schizophrenia have shown that they have great difficulties with interpersonal relationships and social adaptation (Byrne & Morrison, 2010). Difficulties in relationships are also an important part of the emotional burden of parents of adolescents with schizophrenia spectrum disorders (Knock, Kline, Schiffman, Maynard, & Reeves, 2011).

There are several possible reasons for the social withdrawal and reduced peer engagement of adolescents with schizophrenia: their blunted emotional expression and lack of interest in the outside world, their odd and suspicious behaviors, and their difficulties in self-care. Moreover, as in adults, specific deficits in mentalizing capacities and in the integration of contextual information may impair these adolescents' understanding of the social world. Such difficulties may directly contribute to the development and perpetuation of unusual psychological experiences and may increase their reluctance to communicate them to others. In addition, fear of stigma may lead to their concealing their difficulties and to delaying their seeking help (Byrne & Morrison, 2010). For adolescents with psychotic functioning, improvement of social understanding and communication (including the expression of their unusual experiences) may be key to improving their emotional well-being and recovering from the disorder.

SA2 Mood Disorders

In this section we describe the most common mood disorders found in adolescence along with two conditions that have been introduced in DSM-5 but deserve future research (suicidality and nonsuicidal self-injury). Although suicidality and nonsuicidal self-injury are transnosographic behaviors that can be found in almost every clinical context, they are frequently associated with mood disorders and are thus presented in this section. It is worthwhile to remind that in the clinical encounter with an adolescent, suicidality and nonsuicidal self-injury should be systematically explored, especially in the context of a depressive symptomatology.

SA22 Depressive Disorders

Both diagnosing depressive disorders and helping families in recognizing their symptoms during adolescence remain challenges for every clinician. Adolescents themselves tend to confound depression with sadness. Close family members or individuals in the school environment are usually the first to perceive the early behavioral manifestations of the inner suffering of depressive adolescents. The first report of the DSM-5 Childhood and Adolescent Disorders Work Group focused on the need to consider developmental extensions of DSM-IV syndromes (Pine, 2009). Unfortunately, except for irritability in children or adolescents and failure to make expected weight gains, the description of major depressive disorder remains more closely applicable to adults than applicable to adolescents.

If there is a shared phenomenology of depression through the lifespan, qualitative studies have highlighted some specific features of the lived experience of depressed adolescents. These studies support contributions from Blatt's conceptualization (Blatt

& Homann, 1992; Blatt & Zuroff, 1992) of different experiences of depression, as well as from interpersonal psychopathology (Lachal et al., 2012).

The Subjective Experience of Depression in Adolescence

Depressive dynamics remain hard to diagnose (and treat) in adolescence, mainly because of difficulties in recognizing what belongs to depressive disorders and what is part of a normal developmental process. The DSM Work Group (Pine, 2009) proposed some adolescent specifiers to the clinical picture of adult depression (mainly irritability, either replacing or in addition to depressive mood), but there is a clear overlap of symptoms between adults and adolescents.

Classical psychoanalytic theories of adult depression focused mainly on issues related to loss and a sense of responsibility for having attacked and damaged an ambivalently loved or lost object—sometimes described as "guilty depression." With increasing attention to the development of the self, there has been growing interest among psychoanalytic thinkers in issues of narcissistic vulnerability and "narcissistic depression." Research has given support for the idea that these two formulations may capture different subtypes of depression, each describing a group of depressed individuals with differing presentations and differing vulnerabilities, and with potentially differing responses to therapy (Blatt, 1998). The concerns of the first involve disruption in relationships with others (with feelings of loss, abandonment, and loneliness); those of the second center on problems of identity (associated with low self-esteem, feelings of failure, culpability, lack of self-confidence).

According to Blatt and Zuroff (1992), these two depressive experiences correspond to different personality configurations derived from distinct developmental lines, which are thought to be in synergistic interaction throughout development: the anaclitic (or dependent) line, which concerns the establishment of satisfying interpersonal relationships; and the introjective (self-critical) line, which concerns the achievement of a positive and cohesive sense of self.

Blatt and his colleagues (e.g., Blatt & Homann, 1992) have advocated for a view of depression as more than a clinical disorder, depicting it as an affective state that varies from normality to pathology—from mild, transient, appropriate dysphoric reactions to untoward life events to severe, disabling, persistent, and intense reactions that have little justification in current life circumstances. Therapists of adolescents have supported this dimensional view and emphasized the importance of understanding the dynamics of depression in adolescence, particularly of integrating the perspective of a developmental crisis with issues concerning the management of conflicted anger (Midgley, Cregeen, Hughes, & Rustin, 2013). In adolescence, the anaclitic subtype of depression focuses particularly on interpersonal issues related to dependency, as this period elicits questions about autonomy and the consolidation of personal identity. A fragile self (narcissistic vulnerability) remains more sensitive to breakdowns and grief.

"Metabolization" of anger is an issue specific to the introjective (or self-critical) subtype of depression in adolescence. Its clinical presentation involves frequent outbursts; depressed adolescents fear the loss of approval and acceptance from significant others too much to engage in angry tirades. Impulsive acts and internal fights against depressive affects can be misunderstood as other psychiatric conditions, including attention-deficit/hyperactivity disorder (ADHD), oppositional defiant disorder (ODD), and other impulse-control disorders or personality disorders (Blatt & Zuroff, 1992).

Affective States

The core symptoms described by depressed adolescents are persistent overwhelming sadness and despair and a sense of "spiralling down and within" (Dundon, 2006; see also Midgley et al., 2015). In the anaclitic subtype, feelings of shame, humiliation, and low self-esteem can lead to chronic feelings of insecurity and fears of being abandoned and left unprotected. In the introjective subtype, the feeling of failure and guilt dominates; these depressed adolescents strive for perfection. Frequently adolescents look for exterior events to explain their suffering. Such searches can be understood as attempts to give meaning to their internal experience; they give professionals access to the adolescents' cognitive distortions or difficulties in coping with normal life events. More severely depressed adolescents may explicitly express their inner experience of emotional emptiness (Lachal et al., 2012).

Cognitive Patterns

Depression in adolescents often leads to academic downslide, mostly due to mental slowing and decreased concentration. Self-scrutiny and criticism overcome the adolescents, leading to loss of the desire to live and sometimes to the determination to die, with a high risk of suicide in severe cases.

Somatic States

Qualitative studies depict a constant experience of "being weighed down." In the context of their sexually maturing bodies, fatigue and lack of self-care are often the first symptoms of depression that adolescents perceive and report. These symptoms are usually accompanied by a change in sleeping habits (insomnia more commonly than hypersomnia).

Relationship Patterns

Depressed adolescents' persistent "spiralling down and within" takes them away from school and relatives, especially if they commit impulsive acts and convey unrelenting anger toward parents, friends, or teachers. Qualitative studies highlight a decreased investment in nonschool activities, with marked distress and loss of motivation. Clinicians' experience and sensitivity to countertransference are invaluable for both establishing the diagnosis and having a therapeutic impact. Perception of irrepressible sadness and, in more severe cases, intense silent distress can be indicators of depression, especially during the first consultation when adolescents show more than tell about their inner pain.

Clinical Illustration

A 15-year-old girl came with her parents to consult a psychiatrist because her teachers noticed a progressive onset of frequent outbursts of anger and crying. This behavior started at home and then extended to school a few weeks later. Her only complaint was of sleep disturbances; her parents described a recent tendency toward isolation and mistrust. Their daughter had also dropped out of singing lessons and was convinced she would never be able to succeed in her preparation for the choir concert at the end of the year. She told the clinician that he was wasting his time talking to her because nobody could help her. The psychiatrist noted her sad tone and felt for the distress of his patient and her parents. He rapidly diagnosed an introjective depression and advised treatment with psychotherapy.

SA24 Bipolar Disorders

Bipolar disorders are described in more detail in Chapter 3 on the S Axis (pp. 158–160) and in Chapter 9 on the SC Axis (pp. 548–551).

Bipolar disorders are a group of mood disorders characterized by unusual shifts in a person's mood, energy, and ability to function that are different from the ordinary ups and downs everyone goes through. The most common form of bipolar disorder has long been known as manic–depressive illness, in which a person experiences cycles of manic episodes of abnormally elevated mood alternating with depressive episodes or symptoms.

Diagnosis of bipolar disorders in children and adolescence has been a controversial topic. In the United States, the prevalence of diagnosed bipolar disorders in children and adolescents has risen rapidly (from 0.42% in 1994 to 6.7% in 2003). The concomitantly increasing prescription of antipsychotic medication for children and adolescents has concerned both scientists and clinicians. Several researchers have noted that this trend is influenced by certain methodological assumptions, and especially by the criteria used to identify bipolar disorders in these populations. As Carlson and Klein (2014) have stated, the core of the disagreement is whether mania in adolescents should be diagnosed narrowly, with discrete episodes representing a clear departure from prior functioning and with symptoms equivalent to those of adults (the conservative or narrow viewpoint); or whether it should be diagnosed more broadly to include early childhood onset of chronic emotion dysregulation, usually superimposed on symptoms of ADHD and ODD with multiple other comorbidities. This broader phenotype includes severe irritability manifested by intense and protracted rage outbursts.

The DSM-5 Work Group on Bipolar Disorders eventually decided to limit the diagnosis of bipolar disorders in young people to the narrow phenotype resembling that of the adult. This choice was based on longitudinal studies showing that nonepisodic chronic irritability predicts unipolar depressive and anxiety disorders, but not bipolar disorders. They proposed a new diagnostic category, disruptive mood dysregulation disorder (DMDD), to explore the broader phenotype further (see the next section below).

Notwithstanding these clarifications, symptoms of bipolar disorders differ in young people compared to adults in several significant ways. Unlike adult-onset disease, where mania appears in elevated moods or euphoria, mania in adolescence is more likely indicated by heightened irritability, extreme sensitivity to negative reactions from others, destructive outbursts, and highly disruptive and/or aggressive behaviors, with significant difficulty in interpersonal relationships. This presentation may complicate the differential diagnosis between bipolar disorders and emerging borderline personality disorder. Moreover, adolescents are more likely than adults to experience mixed symptoms and symptoms that cycle more continually and more rapidly between depressive and manic states. In contrast, adults may have distinct periods of depression and mania that last for weeks or months. Delusional symptoms during manic episodes, which may be misdiagnosed as schizophreniform disorder, are also more frequent in adolescents than in adults.

Finally, as previously noted, adolescents with bipolar disorders have high rates of comorbid disorders (e.g., depression, ADHD, disruptive behavior problems, substance use disorders) that may complicate the differentiation of truly bipolar symptoms from those of other disorders. A comprehensive longitudinal history of the illness course, with a clear definition of episodes, may help disentangle bipolar disorders from other problems.

DSM-5 identifies several bipolar disorder diagnoses that can be applied to adolescents: bipolar I disorder, defined by manic or mixed episodes; bipolar II disorder, defined by a pattern of depressive episodes and hypomanic episodes without full-blown manic or mixed episodes; and cyclothymic disorder, a mild form of bipolar disorder. Yet many adolescents who experience bipolar-like phenomena with clinically significant distress and impairment do not meet the criteria for one of these disorders; these youth may receive a DSM-5 diagnosis of other specified or unspecified bipolar and related disorder.

The Subjective Experience of Bipolar Disorders in Adolescence

Affective States and Cognitive Patterns

The emotional states of young people with bipolar disorders are unusually intense and may change dramatically. Extreme highs and lows of mood are accompanied by extreme changes in energy, activity, sleep, and behavior. These shifts are usually unpredictable and uncontrollable, and most of the time adolescents experience mixed states. During manic episodes, they feel a great surge of energy, with intense pleasure and a decreased need for sleep. They may feel unrealistically self-confident and powerful and have grandiose fantasies of invincibility and exceptionality. This state can be associated with poor inhibition and risk-taking behaviors, such as misuse of alcohol and drugs, reckless driving, and sexual promiscuity. At the same time, bipolar adolescents may experience an intense irritability—a feeling of internal tension and hypersensitivity, especially to criticism, which may lead to extreme temper outbursts. Their thoughts are often confused and illogical, and they appear unable to concentrate on a specific topic. The overall internal experience is of being out of control, with an unstable sense of self that oscillates between feeling weak and strong, competent and incompetent.

Somatic States

The biological rhythms of bipolar adolescents are highly disrupted in all phases of the illness. Somatic states include increased energy, restlessness, and sleeplessness. But adolescents with bipolar conditions also experience states of hyperarousal, frequently associated with irritability and anxiety.

Relationship Patterns

Adolescents with bipolar disorders frequently show unpredictable, chaotic, and impulsive relationship patterns. They experience immense difficulty in psychosocial functioning. Family relationships are highly disturbed. The therapeutic relationship is also challenged by their mood swings. Bipolar adolescents are at serious risk for adverse outcomes, including suicide, substance misuse, risky sexual behaviors, and borderline personality disorder.

SA26 Disruptive Mood Dysregulation Disorder

DMDD is characterized by chronic, severe, persistent irritability. This irritability has two prominent manifestations: (1) severe, frequent temper outbursts that appear disproportionate to the situation and inconsistent with developmental level and (2) chronic, persistently irritable or angry mood between the temper outbursts. The clinical presentation of DMDD must be carefully distinguished from other, related conditions, especially pediatric bipolar disorders. This category was recently added to DSM-5 to address concerns about the appropriate classification and treatment of children with chronic, persistent irritability relative to children with classic (i.e., episodic) bipolar disorders.

Some symptoms associated with DMDD are also present in other child psychiatric disorders, such as depression, bipolar disorders, and ODD. Differentiating DSM-5 DMDD from other disorders relies primarily on careful characterization of irritable nonepisodic mood and the severity, high frequency, and long duration of the temper outbursts. Many adolescents who meet the criteria for this disorder also meet the criteria for ADHD and for anxiety disorders. In these cases, adolescents show more symptoms of hyperarousal.

The Subjective Experience of DMDD in Adolescence

Affective States

The affective experience of adolescents with DMDD is a chronic irritability with angry mood, expressed in frequent temper outbursts. This difficulty in regulating emotions may be associated with risky behaviors, suicide attempts, and severe aggression, which may lead to psychiatric hospitalizations.

Cognitive Patterns

The internal experience of these adolescents may include being out of control of their frequent temper outbursts. This subjective dyscontrol may be associated with a negative self-perception and with an unstable sense of self. These adolescents may have limited insight into their behaviors and experience the setting of limits as a painful injustice.

Somatic States

Although hyperarousal is not among the DSM-5 criteria for DMDD, adolescents with this clinical profile frequently present symptoms of hyperarousal, such as insomnia, distractibility, or intrusiveness.

Relationship Patterns

The chronic, severe irritability of DMDD is associated with marked disruption in a child's family and peer relationships as well as in school performance. Because of their extremely low frustration tolerance, such children generally have difficulty succeeding in school; they are often unable to participate in the activities typically enjoyed by healthy children; their family lives are severely disrupted by their outbursts and irritability; and they have trouble initiating or sustaining friendships. Levels of dysfunction in children with bipolar disorders and DMDD are generally comparable.

SA27 Suicidality

The essential manifestation of suicidal behavior disorder is a suicide attempt, defined as a behavior that the individual has undertaken with at least some intent to die. According to the manual, the behavior may or may not lead to injury or serious medical consequences because several factors can influence the outcome of the suicide attempt (including poor planning, lack of knowledge about the lethality of the method chosen, low intentionality or ambivalence, or chance intervention by others after the behavior has been initiated). Moreover, determining the degree of intent can be challenging because individuals may not clearly acknowledge their intent.

Risk markers for suicidal behavior disorder include degree of planning, including selection of a time and place to minimize rescue or interruption, and the individual's mental state at the time of the behavior. Suicidal behavior is seen in the context of a variety of mental disorders, most commonly bipolar disorders, major depressive disorder, schizophrenia, schizoaffective disorder, anxiety disorders (particularly panic disorder associated with catastrophic content), posttraumatic stress disorder (PTSD), substance use disorders (especially alcohol use disorders), borderline personality disorder, antisocial personality disorder, eating disorders, and adjustment disorders.

DSM-5 specifies that the act must not meet the criteria for nonsuicidal self-injury (NSSI); that is, it does not involve self-injury directed to the surface of the body, undertaken to induce relief from a negative feeling or cognitive state or to achieve a positive mood state. NSSI (see section SA28, pp. 404–406) is another new diagnostic category on which future research is also encouraged. A current diagnosis of suicidal behavior disorder is given if the attempt has occured in the last 12 months. A diagnosis of early remission is given if 12–24 months have passed since the last attempt.

The Subjective Experience of Suicidality in Adolescence

Adolescent suicide is a major public health concern in all Western countries, and it is the second leading cause of death worldwide among persons under age 29. Attempted suicide is a more statistically widespread phenomenon, with prevalences of 8–10% worldwide. The highest reported attempted suicide rate is among those ages 15–24; their attempted-to-completed suicide ratio is estimated as between 50:1 and 100:1. The prevention of suicidal behavior is therefore a primary concern worldwide. Studies conducted from multiple perspectives (psychological, psychiatric, and sociological) find that a critical risk factor for attempted suicide is a prior attempt, thus justifying a separate diagnostic category.

Adolescents and young adults' suicidal attempts are frequently seen in the context of different mental disorders. But they are also observed in youth with no discernible pathology, particularly in some cultural contexts (e.g., India, China). A feature found in almost all who attempt suicide is an intense psychic suffering associated with a feeling of being at a central life impasse. Exploration of adolescents' feelings before and after suicide attempts, along with the expectations and meanings that they connect to this action, is thus essential to develop adequate preventive and therapeutic strategies.

Phenomenological analysis of the narratives of adolescents and young adults involved in suicidal acts has identified several themes that can be organized into three major domains: individual experience, relational experience, and the sociocultural experience.

Affective States and Cognitive Patterns

Three significant aspects frequently emerge in the narratives of suicidal adolescents: sadness, negative emotions toward the self, and the need for some control over one's own life (Lachal et al., 2015). Adolescents and young adults describe sadness, sorrow, mental pain, despair, detachment, anger, and irritability. They depict a devalued self characterized by the experience of failure: decreased self-esteem, with feelings of uselessness, incompetence, and worthlessness. They sometimes mention self-hatred. Many have the impression that they have lost control of their existence, that they can no longer take part in decisions that concern them. Dealing with problems seems impossible. They no longer understand themselves. Life becomes hopeless and senseless. The inner experience is of loss of life's meaning and the feeling of being trapped in a suffering present, with no possible better future. The suicidal act appears as an escape from an overwhelming, unmanageable life situation and is therefore associated with positive emotions. Suicide attempts seem to give devastated adolescents a feeling of mastery over their bodies and the lives they feel they have lost. Self-injuries, frequently associated with suicidal attempts, can express the same effort to regain control. Failure of the suicidal act may be experienced as yet another demonstration of ineptitude and thus may reinforce an adolescent's negative perception of the self.

Somatic States

Suicidal adolescents often experience high levels of anxiety, frequently expressed in somatic forms. Anxiety can be a proximal risk factor for the suicidal act and should be monitored attentively in at-risk adolescents.

Relationship Patterns

Adolescents frequently describe communication problems and impasses in their interactions with family members that seem to parallel, at the relational level, the negative emotions described at the individual level. Family dynamics are perceived as rigid and overwhelming, without acceptance or trust. The family situation is experienced as unbearable. Relational difficulties, separations, or feelings of insecurity engender suicidal ideation. Conflicts, separations, losses, and absences can all explain the decision to act. Alternative relationships with friends or lovers, frequently characterized by a dependent quality, fail to compensate for the family difficulties, thus increasing feelings of loneliness and not being understood. The experience of feeling unheard is central to the suicidal process: before the suicide attempt, in its precipitating factors, and while an adolescent is in care.

Another invasive feeling is that of being different and rejected. Suicidal adolescents find themselves marginalized, isolated, and rejected, based on elements of reality (school, sexuality, religion, origins, etc.). The fear of being judged by others amplifies feelings of painful solitude.

In adolescents' suicide attempts, communication issues are fundamental. The suicidal act seems primarily an interpersonal act concerning not only the self, but also the environment of significant others. It may be seen as the only choice, once every other communicative possibility has failed. Then suicide attempts can serve to express distress to others, or to take vengeance on one or more family members or friends. This consideration highlights the importance of attentively considering the resolution of the suicidal crisis. Adolescents who successfully emerge from their suicidal crises are those who describe a progressive opening of the lines of communication with others—a process that establishes a basis for a change in family relationships. The rapprochement with their families, the reconnection, the improvement of relationships, and better communication are simultaneously conditions for, and consequences of, getting better. Getting better requires that those around these adolescents, including empathetic professionals, express their understanding.

This need for empathic relationship is often a problem in the care of suicidal teens. Adolescents who are at the greatest risk of repeated attempts have the feeling that dialogue and communication remain as impossible after a suicide attempt as before. The message in the attempt is still unanswered, with the effect of reinforcing the feelings that led to it. The relational dimension of a suicidal attempt may include aggressive feelings such as revenge, addressed to significant others, with the intent of making these others feel both guilty and at last aware of an adolescent's suffering (Orri et al., 2014).

Finally, the experience of suicide by adolescents is affected by the ways in which the peer group and society respond to their distress. Suicidal adolescents describe how difficult it is to belong to a peer group, a cultural group, or, more broadly, the social group. Self-esteem is based on standards and values inculcated by family, religious, and cultural souces (e.g., hard work, school success, integrity, beauty, and other ideals). Inability to meet these standards brings shame and the sense of stigma, guilt, or anger at others. Religious beliefs function as both protective and precipitating factors of suicide attempts. Adolescents also report the impact of the mass media. The way a society understands suicidal acts or stigmatizes the suicidal person has an impact on attempts.

Adolescents involved in suicidal behavior seem to feel stuck in an individual and relational impasse from which there is no exit. They continually try to link their individual state of distress, helplessness, and loneliness to the presence of others, seeking to connect. Suicidal behavior represents a means of establishing, through the act itself, a connection between personal distress and other people. Failure to make that link appears to be a major factor responsible for keeping an adolescent in the state of mind that led to the initial act and thus keeping him or her at risk for repeating it.

SA28 Nonsuicidal Self-Injury

In nonsuicidal self-injury (NSSI), an adolescent repeatedly inflicts shallow yet painful injuries on the surface of his or her body. These behaviors should be differentiated from suicidal behaviors, which may sometimes coexist in the same person. Most commonly, the aim of self-harming behaviors is to reduce negative emotions, such as tension, anxiety, and self-reproach, and/or to resolve an interpersonal difficulty. In some cases, the injury is conceived as self-punishment. Self-injuring adolescents often report an immediate sensation of relief. Frequent self-harm may be associated with a sense of urgency and craving, such that the resultant behavioral pattern resembles an addiction.

Until recently, NSSI was primarily associated with developmental disabilities, eating disorders, and borderline personality disorder. A sizable percentage of adolescents and young adults who engage in self-harming acts, however, may not meet the criteria for depressive, anxiety, eating, substance use, or other major psychiatric disorders. In fact, nonsuicidal self-harm appears to be a common, nonspecific psychiatric symptom found in a variety of disorders, and also in adolescents without a specific psychiatric diagnosis. It seems more useful to understand such behaviors in functional terms than as a distinct diagnosis. Recent community studies have found that one-third of adolescents in the United States have engaged in some type of NSSI, with an onset typically around age 13 or 14 and a clear female predominance.

The Subjective Experience of NSSI in Adolescence

Affective States

Self-harming behaviors serve both intrapersonal and interpersonal functions. Their major purposes appear to be affect regulation and management of distressing thoughts. Experimental data support the regulating aspect of diagnosed NSSI (Zetterqvist, Lundh, Dahlström, & Svedin, 2013). Most commonly, NSSI functions temporarily to alleviate overwhelming negative emotions such as anxiety, depression, anger, frustration, guilt, shame, or even a sense of deadness. Intense negative emotions precede these acts, and their performance results in reduced negative emotions as well as feelings of calm and relief. They may also help adolescents to gain a sense of control, change their distressing or suicidal thoughts, or stop dissociative experiences. Some report that they self-injure as a form of self-directed anger or self-punishment. NSSI can serve multiple other functions, such as the desire to influence others, obtain attention, or produce a physical sign of emotional distress, but each of these is relevant only to a minority of adolescents who self-injure.

Cognitive Patterns

Adolescents experience a range of negative emotions and thoughts in the period immediately preceding a self-injurious act. They are frequently self-critical. Prior to the act, they experience a period of preoccupation with the intended behavior that is difficult to control. Thinking about self-injury occurs frequently, even when the impulse is not acted upon. Suicidal thoughts may also be present in some adolescents who self-injure. Some adolescents report hurting themselves specifically to stop suicidal ideation or to stop themselves from actually attempting suicide. Self-injury is generally not inflicted with suicidal intent, however. Nonsuicidal and suicidal behaviors serve distinctly different purposes. NSSI has been conceptualized as "a morbid form of self-help."

Somatic States

Adolescents who self-injure demonstrate high levels of emotional reactivity, emotional intensity, and physiological arousal, especially under stress. They also experience other somatic symptoms of anxiety. Self-harming behaviors help the adolescent in reducing this physiological and emotional arousal and may induce a state of psychic numbing.

Relationship Patterns

Self-harm may serve interpersonal functions for adolescents. Their behaviors may elicit positive reinforcement in the form of attention from others, although many who injure themselves do so in private and do not tell others. Self-injury might also help a teen to avoid difficult relational situations. The threat of self-harm might cause adults or peers to decrease interpersonal pressure or to stop attempting to get the teenager to complete homework, chores, or other tasks.

Such interpersonal functions can challenge the therapeutic alliance. Clinicians can feel a range of negative reactions to adolescents who injure themselves. They may perceive them as playing a game, being manipulative, or seeking attention. It is helpful to remember that impulsive self-harm in adolescents generally stems from emotional pain, not malevolent intentions, and that the teenager needs more effective skills to replace self-injury. Understanding NSSI requires clinicians to consider both intrapersonal and interpersonal functions. A therapist should adopt an attitude of respectful curiosity to gain an adolescent's trust and to establish a spirit of collaboration. Assessment should focus on the history of self-injury, its current manifestations, and especially its functions.

Several strategies have been suggested to reduce self-injurious behaviors, including mindfulness skills, deep breathing exercises, use of ice on the wrist to produce a physical distraction, talking to a friend about feelings, and exercise. Helping adolescents to improve their affective language and other communication skills is essential to reduce these behaviors. Since self-harming adolescents often have poor problem-solving abilities, it is important to improve these skills as well. Involving the family in the support and treatment of such an adolescent is critical, given that poor communication with family members has been associated with both NSSI and suicidal behavior in adolescents. Improving the family's understanding of the adolescent's self-harm can be useful in decreasing conflicts. It can be helpful for the family to learn deescalation strategies and to expand listening and communication skills.

SA3 Disorders Related Primarily to Anxiety

Disorders characterized by high anxiety are described in more detail in Chapter 3 on the S Axis (pp. 164–177) and Chapter 9 on the SC Axis (pp. 557–563).

DSM-5 identifies several patterns of anxiety and several specific anxiety disorders, such as specific phobia, social anxiety disorder (social phobia), panic disorder, agoraphobia, and generalized anxiety disorder (GAD). Obsessive–compulsive disorder (OCD) and body dysmorphic disorder (BDD or dysmorphophobia) now have their own category in DSM-5 (obsessive–compulsive and related disorders). The limits of all these disorders are less clear than in adulthood, and symptom patterns often overlap. There is also considerable heterogeneity in the onset of these disorders, with GAD, agoraphobia, panic disorder, OCD, and BDD mostly emerging in adolescence.

Epidemiological data show that anxiety disorders are the most frequent psychiatric disorders in children and adolescents. Overall, anxiety disorders are more prevalent in girls than in boys. Gender differences accentuate with development, with prevalence ratios reaching 2–3:1 by adolescence.

SA31 Anxiety Disorders

Manifestations of anxiety in adolescence may include feelings of overwhelming fear, panic states accompanied by somatic symptoms, school refusal, and acute anxiety states. While there are expectable transient anxieties that accompany new experiences (e.g., going to school, becoming part of a peer group, separating from parents), an anxiety disorder is characterized by continuing anxiety that may interfere with full mastery of age-expected experiences. Anxiety is the affective signal of danger. The content of what is dangerous may be conscious or unconscious, real or unreal. In adolescence it is often associated with basic safety and relationship issues (e.g., fear of illness, injury, loss of/damage to a caregiver or other love object, or even the imagined consequences of success).

Although anxiety appears in earliest childhood, the ability to regulate and metabolize it increases and changes with psychological development. Normally, as children grow, they are increasingly able to manage greater amounts of anxiety. The course of an anxiety disorder is highly variable, depending on the adolescent and the family. In some instances it is transient and episodic, while in others it is so intense that it interferes with an adolescent's functioning. Family patterns, peer relationships, the school environment, and the adolescent's internal stability can play significant roles in its course. The signs of anxiety may vary with the adolescent's age and stage of development.

The Subjective Experience of Anxiety Disorders in Adolescence

Affective States and Cognitive Patterns

The subjective experience of anxiety includes a sense of danger, a pervasive fear, and a heightened state of alertness. In its extreme form, there is a dread of impending doom. In its less extreme form, adolescents describe a vague sense of worry and nervousness. When the experience is more chronic, adolescents will sometimes use the words "stress" and "tension." These states may be handled with defense mechanisms ranging from denial to sublimation. When defensive functioning is not sufficient to contain the anxiety, there may be a repetitive, even compulsive, replaying of anxiety-producing situations or events until the anxiety is neutralized and the adolescent feels a sense of mastery over the imagined threat. Mild to moderate anxiety may stimulate cognitive activity, whereas moderate to severe anxiety can disrupt cognitive processes and thinking in general.

Excessive anxiety may lead adolescents not to communicate. They may see their anxiety as evidence of weakness or as a personal failing and may be unwilling to share what they are feeling because of shame, expectations of being misunderstood, or fear of being judged. Anxiety may also damage adolescents' confidence, concentration, and feelings about the future. Finally, it can interfere with sleep, eating, learning, normal activities, and peer relations, and affect the adolescent's ability to cope. Performance anxiety, for example, can range from mild apprehension about giving a book report to stage fright so extreme as to be paralyzing. In addition to these general signs, there are several specific symptom patterns, such as panic attacks, specific phobias, and social anxiety. Social anxiety is particularly frequent in adolescents with poor social skills or low self-esteem, who feel exaggerated fears of embarrassment, criticism, or rejection by peers.

Somatic States

Anxiety has a number of physical manifestations. Somatic states may include decreased or increased motor activity and changes in posture. Physiological responses may include increased heart rate, increased or decreased respiration, dilated pupils, increased muscle tension, and increases in galvanic skin responses. Chronic states of anxiety contribute to a variety of physical problems, including most notably eczema and neurodermatitis. Unmanaged anxiety may also be manifested as disorders of skin, muscles, or joints, and may affect gastrointestinal functioning and evacuation. There can also be physiological responses such as palpitations and sweating. Gross motor activity may increase in an effort to discharge anxiety, but this discharge usually provides only temporary relief and does not contribute significantly to mastery. Nightmares, eating and sleeping difficulties, and regressive behaviors are common in highly anxious children.

Relationship Patterns

Relationships may be interrupted, burdened, or compromised by anxiety disorders. Social and learning activities may suffer. When an adolescent has little or no capacity to cope with fears realistically, the result can be a complete breakdown in psychological functioning. In a vicious cycle of anxiety and failed efforts to master it, this breakdown leaves the anxiety unchecked, leading to an escalation of the breakdown and further escalation of anxiety. Relationships in this situation become disrupted by the adolescent's inability to attend to anything but the anxiety and the efforts to reduce it.

The clinical interview is the most important diagnostic tool in the assessment of anxiety. Multiple sources are ideal: Parents may provide the most reliable information about how their child is functioning at home and at school, but a teenager is likely to have the best sense of his or her own internal experience. Self-report questionnaires are useful in assessing anxiety because teenagers may endorse a symptom on a rating scale that they have denied or downplayed during the interview. Adolescents who are suspected of having an anxiety disorder should be assessed for core symptoms from other psychiatric categories. In particular, the adolescent should be asked about depressed mood, current or past thoughts of suicide, and NSSI.

Clinical Illustration

A 13-year-old girl was brought for assessment for recent severe panic attacks. A psychopharmacologist had prescribed an antidepressant and an anxiolytic and recommended attention to the dynamics of the anxiety. This girl was a straight-A student, popular among peers, and active in sports. It appeared that the onset of the anxiety was related to her concern about weight gain and attractiveness to boys. Although she clearly did not have a weight problem, she had made several unsuccessful attempts at dieting. Her mother was concerned about her worries, but her father teased her for being "fat." She felt enraged at her father and alienated from her mother, who did not protect her from the teasing. At first the parents did not take the attacks seriously, even though their daugher was extremely distressed. In time, the attacks escalated in intensity, at which point her parents became overly concerned, and the daughter felt vindicated in having convinced them of her distress. In therapy, she focused increasingly on the issues of independence and autonomy. When the attacks diminished in intensity and became more manageable, the girl was able to move on developmentally.

SA31.1 *Specific Phobias*

Specific phobias are described in more detail in Chapter 3 (pp. 168–169) and in Chapter 9 (pp. 560–561).

A phobia is an identifiable and persistent fear that is excessive or unreasonable and is triggered by the presence or anticipation of a specific object or situation. Adolescents with one or more phobias consistently experience anxiety when exposed to that object or situation. The fear, anxiety, or avoidance is almost always immediately induced by the phobic situation to a degree that is persistent and out of proportion to the actual risk posed. Common specific phobias include fear of animals, insects, blood, heights, closed spaces, and flying. In adolescents, the identified fear must last at least 6 months to be considered a specific phobia rather than a transient fear.

At this time, there is very limited scientific knowledge about how to prevent specific phobias in adolescents. However, early detection and intervention can reduce the severity of symptoms, enhance the adolescent's normal growth and development, and improve the quality of life experienced by adolescents with anxiety disorders.

SA31.2 *Social Phobia*

Social phobia (now called social anxiety disorder in DSM-5) is described in more detail in Chapter 3 (p. 169).

In social phobia, an adolescent is fearful about or avoidant of social interactions and situations that involve the possibility of being scrutinized. These include social interactions such as meeting unfamiliar people and situations in which the individual may be observed by others or may perform in front of others. Ideation involves being negatively evaluated by others by being embarrassed, humiliated, or rejected. Social anxiety disorder is a common condition among adolescents and young adults, with prevalence rates up to 28%, and is often associated with severe impairment in educational careers (Dell'Osso et al., 2014). Findings suggest that interpersonal stressors, including the particularly detrimental stressors of peer victimization and familial emotional maltreatment, may predict both depressive and social anxiety symptoms in adolescence (Hamilton et al., 2016).

SA31.3 *Agoraphobia and Panic Disorder*

Agoraphobia and panic disorder are also described in more detail in Chapter 3 (pp. 169–170).

The essential feature of agoraphobia is an excessive anxiety about being in (or anticipating) situations from which escape might be difficult or in which help may not be available in the event of having a panic attack (or panic-like symptoms). Agoraphobia is frequently associated with panic attacks, abrupt surges of intense fear, or intense discomfort, accompanied by physical and/or cognitive symptoms, in response to an unexpected or typically feared object or situation. Often in these situations, an individual may have the vague thought that something dreadful may happen.

Agoraphobia and panic disorder are extremely common in adolescence and are often associated with lifelong psychiatric disturbance (Creswell, Waite, & Cooper, 2014). In DSM-5, the agoraphobia core symptom criteria have been revised to require fear about multiple situations. This modification has been introduced to prevent the overdiagnosis of agoraphobia, based on the overestimation of danger or occasional fears. However, a recent study has shown that one-quarter of young people with symptom presentations consistent with the DSM-IV agoraphobia definition no longer met the criteria for DSM-5 agoraphobia, although they showed severity and impairment across most domains comparable to those of youth who did meet criteria for DSM-5 agoraphobia (Cornacchio, Chou, Sacks, Pincus, & Comer, 2015). Furthermore, these adolescents showed higher levels of anxiety sensitivity and internalizing psychopathology than youth with DSM-5 agoraphobia. Thus specific attention to anxiety sensitivity and to functional impairment related to anxiety should be given to adolescents and young people to increase the possibility that they will receive adequate psychotherapeutic and pharmacological treaments.

SA31.4 *Generalized Anxiety Disorder*

GAD is described in more detail in Chapter 3 (pp. 170–171).

The key features of GAD in adolescence are persistent and excessive anxiety over various domains that an adolescent finds difficult to control. Worries may include fears about poor school performance or a wide variety of other bad things' happening, such as failing to be on time, making mistakes, a loved one's becoming ill or dying, parents' divorcing, personal health crises, catastrophic world events, and natural disasters. The adolescent may experience physical symptoms, including restlessness or feeling keyed up or on edge; being easily fatigued; difficulty concentrating or mind going blank; irritability; muscle tension; and sleep disturbance. Adolescents suffering from GAD usually report hyper-arousal and constant exaggerated apprehension in dealing with most everyday activities.

Adolescent-onset anxiety disorders frequently persist into adulthood and place youth at risk for future psychiatric problems, including mood and substance use disorders. Existing studies support a number of pharmacological and psychotherapeutic treatments for childhood anxiety disorders. The strongest evidence supports separated and combined use of selective serotonin reuptake inhibitors (SSRIs) and cognitive-behavioral therapy (CBT). Early detection and treatment of childhood anxiety disorders can prevent substantial impairment over the course of a child's development and accumulation of functional disability (Mohatt, Bennett, & Walkup, 2014; Wehry, Beesdo-Baum, Hennelly, Connolly, & Strawn, 2015).

SA32 Obsessive–Compulsive and Related Disorders

SA32.1 *Obsessive–Compulsive Disorder*

OCD is described in more detail in Chapter 3 (pp. 173–174).

OCD in adolescence is an impairing condition with a specific set of distressing symptoms incorporating repetitive, intrusive thoughts (obsessions) and distressing, time-consuming rituals (compulsions). Symptoms can occur in children as young as 4 years of age, but more commonly they first appear between ages 6 and 9. Early adolescence and young adulthood are other common periods of new or recurrent onset, probably because these tend to be times of developmental stress. Once considered rare in youth, OCD has been found in epidemiological studies to have an estimated prevalence of 0.25–4% in children and adolescents. Symptoms in a young person are accompanied by anxiety that may be conveyed to, and sometimes magnified by, parents. Together, the parents and child are not able to quell the anxiety, which becomes acutely worse if the symptoms (ritual behaviors) are not allowed expression. OCD waxes and wanes in many adolescents, but it typically follows a chronic course, causing marked functional impairment across multiple domains (including home, school, and social settings). The etiology of pediatric OCD remains poorly understood. While genetic factors clearly influence its expression, little is known about the effects of environmental factors. Neuropsychological models propose that OCD arises from alterations in frontostriatal circuitry.

The Subjective Experience of OCD in Adolescence

Affective States

As with the other disorders in the SA3 section of PDM-2, the associated affective states involve pervasive anxiety. In OCD, its source is usually not clear. Both parent and adolescent tend to focus on the anxiety itself, rather than wishing to explore its origins. The characteristic patterns of symptom onset suggest that the sources of many obsessions and compulsions lie in developmental challenges. Anger and magical fears of loss of control may lie beneath the anxiety.

Cognitive Patterns

Thoughts and fantasies include a preoccupation with the obsessional ideation or ritual in the service of defending against underlying anxiety. Adolescents may have little insight into their obsessions and compulsions and may need age-appropriate education and motivation from clinicians.

Somatic States

An adolescent may also develop somatic symptoms similar to those described for both GAD and phobias. Obsessional thinking may make the adolescent's preoccupation with sensations such as stomachache and headache much greater than it is in other disorders related primarily to anxiety.

Relationship Patterns

The excessive preoccupation with the obsessional idea or compulsive ritual, along with the underlying anxiety, may interfere with relationships and with functioning in daily life. Even when obsessional anxiety is not interfering in routine activities, it may be present as a more generalized affective state. Adolescents with OCD are noted for their attempts to control situations and relationships as they try to keep their anxieties at manageable levels. Relationships may thus be characterized by a tendency toward rigidity, control, and dependency (often unacknowledged).

Clinical Illustration

A 17-year-old boy was exercising 4 hours a day, obsessively weighing and measuring everything he ate, and spending the rest of his day planning his eating and exercising. Although he had done well academically in previous years, he was ignoring schoolwork and doing poorly. Over 4 months, he lost 50 pounds. He had been mildly overweight as a child, labeled a "brainiac," and shunned by peers. His compulsive eating and exercising began in connection with an email liaison. He began psychoanalysis and after 4 months attempted suicide by purposely losing control of the family car at high speed. This attempt revealed his deep rage toward his parents, who he felt had prepared him poorly for the world; he was angry at his mother for holding on to him and at his father for seemingly abandoning him. With this insight, his preoccupation with his eating and exercise diminished; he began to make friends, to engage more fully in exploring his feelings, and to form healthier patterns of adaptation. Although this case illustrates difficulties with regulating eating, it demonstrates obsessive and compulsive patterns that can manifest themselves in a variety of symptoms.

SA32.2 *Body Dysmorphic Disorder (Dysmorphophobia)*

BDD is described in more detail in Chapter 3 (pp. 174–176).

BDD is a debilitating psychological condition characterized by preoccupations with perceived bodily flaws and physical appearance. Although flaws are often minimal, or nonexistent (Windheim, Veale, & Anson, 2011), adolescents diagnosed with BDD have a genuine, heartfelt belief in their physical ugliness, which provokes overwhelming anxieties about deformity, inadequacy, and judgments by others (Phillips, 2004). The central theme of the disorder is a delusional obsession centered on physical appearance. Adolescents with this obsession may describe themselves as unattractive and deformed. Although the face is frequently the primary source of concern, they may be worried about every bodily region (Windheim et al., 2011).

The delusional preoccupations in BDD appear to be relatively difficult to inhibit or control. Adolescents may spend several hours a day focusing on or attempting to modify their appearance. Although onset is typically in early adolescence, it can develop in middle to late childhood (Phillips, 2004). Symptoms tend to be consistent with several other psychological disorders and conditions, including those of depression, social phobia, OCD, eating disorders, and several personality disorders (Buhlmann & Winter, 2011). These similarities can often mask the recognition of BDD in adolescents, further complicating diagnosis.

The development and maintenance of BDD have major implications for social development, adjustment, and transitioning (Phillips, 2004). Unfortunately, the problem often goes unnoticed and unrecognized among teachers, friends, family, and health care professionals (Buhlmann & Winter, 2011). Studies from community samples suggest a general prevalence rate of 0.7–1.1%, while those in clinical samples are significantly more elevated, with reported rates between 2.2 and 6% (Grant, Won Kim, & Crow, 2001). The disorder negatively affects psychosocial functioning of all affected individuals, especially adolescents (Brewster, 2011). Although research remains relatively limited, the use of psychotropic drugs (antidepressants) and the integration of CBT appears to provide the best outcome for individuals with this diagnosis (Phillips, 2004). Given its adverse effects on adolescents, understanding the mechanisms of the disorder and promoting awareness of it are paramount in improving acceptance, decreasing stigma, and increasing access to care.

SA4 Event- and Stressor-Related Disorders

The event- and stressor-related disorders in PDM-2 include, first, trauma- and stressor-related disorders—that is, disorders in which exposure to a traumatic or stressful event is listed explicitly as a diagnostic criterion. These include adjustment disorders, acute stress disorder, PTSD, and complex PTSD (CPTSD). They also include dissociative disorders and conversion disorder. Previously, the trauma- and stressor-related disorders were considered anxiety disorders. However, they are now considered distinct because many patients do not have anxiety, but instead have symptoms of anhedonia or dysphoria, anger, aggression, or dissociation. For the whole SA4 group of disorders, we advise readers to refer also to the "Prefatory Comments" on the S4 grouping in Chapter 3 of this manual (p. 160).

SA41 Trauma- and Stressor-Related Disorders

SA41.1 *Adjustment Disorders*

In DSM-5, adjustment disorders are included in the new category of trauma- and stressor-related disorders. Their essential feature is that emotional or behavioral symptoms occur in response to an identifiable stressor. The individual's experience of distress seems out of proportion to the severity or intensity of the stressor, which produces significant impairments in several areas of functioning. Reaction to the stressor usually appears within 3 months of the experienced stress and may be characterized by anxiety, depressed mood, or disturbances of conduct in isolation or in combination.

The Subjective Experience of Adjustment Disorders in Adolescence

Reactions of adolescents to adverse events vary, from attempts to increase self-mastery to use of regressive defenses. These two responses may coexist; adjustment disorders may thus show different patterns from those in adults, and there are some gender differences as well. Adolescents show a greater tendency than adults to make decisions based on emotions, impulsive or not. They frequently misuse substances to escape from sad or anxious thoughts. Aggressive behavior, risk taking, suicidality, self-harm, and provocative behaviors are common ways for adolescents with adjustment disorders to express feelings. Such actions can hide the affects of depression and anxiety; the internal experience of loss, sadness, or anxiety may be hard for adolescents themselves to perceive.

The ordinary course of adolescence is usually characterized, at least in some periods, by changing behaviors accompanied by unstable mood changes, increased withdrawal, a tendency toward social isolation, and an insatiable and irrepressible gregariousness. Consequently, the diagnosis of adjustment disorders may be overestimated. Reciprocally, some reactions may be falsely attributed to the ordinary course of development. The point is that in adjustment disorders, reactions are triggered and sustained by notable events, such as family conflict, loss, harassment, interpersonal hostility, romantic deceit, or any potentially traumatic event. Family support appears critical to any sense of mastery in the wake of a painful occurrence. The experience of losing control of events, whether or not it is associated with self-reproaches and self-depreciation, is more common when multiple stressors are present. Heteroaggressive behaviors and restlessness, particularly in males, and self-attacking behavior in females, may be interpreted as specific ways to escape from passivity.

Clinical Illustration

A 14-year-old boy with no prior antisocial acts committed repeated robberies at school. His presentation was fierce and aggressive; he refused to speak to the psychiatrist assigned to him. The parents spoke of the declining health of his younger brother, with whom he had been highly competitive before his diagnosis of leukemia. The boy refused to speak about his brother. A week later, he was expelled from school for insulting a teacher. Suddenly, after a fourth consultation, he came into the office in tears, talking about a dream in which he saw his brother dying despite his own efforts to help him. His dream seemed to have lowered his sense of culpability and allowed him to speak about deep feelings of sadness and anxiety. After several therapeutic consultations (both with and without his parents), his depressed mood disappeared, and his aggressive and antisocial behaviors stopped.

SA41.2 Acute and Posttraumatic Stress Disorders

Acute stress disorder and PTSD are distinct disorders in DSM-5 that both show a common anxiety response reactivity to a traumatic event that includes some form of reexperiencing of or reactivity to the traumatic event. If acute stress disorder progresses to PTSD, it may also be a transient stress response that remits within 1 month of trauma exposure and does not result in PTSD. Approximately half of individuals who eventually develop PTSD initially present with acute stress disorder. Symptom worsening during the initial month can occur, often as a result of ongoing life stressors or further traumatic events.

In its treatment of the diagnosis of PTSD, DSM-5 has not emphasized adolescence. Current research, however, confirms the appropriate use of the adult criteria for adolescents. The potential effects of co-occurring exposures to extreme traumatic experiences (such as actual or threatened death, serious injury, sexual abuse, or the witnessing of domestic violence), and the significant interplay between trauma and loss, have been confirmed. Somatic reactions such as stomach pain, headaches, or episodes of tachycardia or tachypnea have also been observed in adolescent samples. A few developmental studies have established the presence of experimental memory and attentional biases that can be linked to clinical reactions. For adolescents, however, the clustering of PTSD symptoms in studies of unique or repeated traumas suggests that a three-symptom cluster model, including intrusion/active avoidance, arousal, and numbing/passive avoidance, may be a better fit than the DSM model.

The occurrence of PTSD is particularly high in late adolescence and young adulthood. This greater vulnerability may result both from developmental factors (such as a high level of risk taking) and from political and socioeconomic factors (such as an increased international involvement of youth in gangs or civil wars, both as perpetrators and as victims). In economically developed countries, the prevalence of the full syndrome of PTSD (particularly numbing and avoidance) in reaction to potentially traumatic events is lower before middle adolescence.

Freud (1895) described a particular feature of the adolescent period with the term *Nachträglichkeit*, translated into English as "deferred action." Initially, the term referred to a situation in which a sexual event, even one of low emotional intensity, creates a traumatic reaction during adolescence or young adulthood, as the resonant traumatic potentiality of some previous event or events is understood. This is particularly the case when sexual abuse during early childhood has been initially experienced as confusing rather than traumatizing, but then takes on new meaning and significance in the context of adolescent development. Contemporarily, this reaction is often interpreted as the result of biological patterns and/or of the exacerbation of the sexual drive: Development will contribute to the reinvestment of past traumatic events, sexual or nonsexual.

A third pattern during adolescence is the influence of trauma on the developing self that may be difficult to interpret in terms of psychopathology when dissociative responses appear, with or without depersonalization or derealization, particularly if the initial trauma is unknown or uncertain. These features may appear either as new symptoms accompanying a contemporary traumatic event or as the continuation of dissociative states triggered by the memory of a previous trauma. Childhood trauma may set the stage for various and severe dissociative states during adolescence and adulthood, most of them having being described with the outdated term hysteria. Recent findings suggest that prefrontal and limbic structures underlie these dissociative responses in PTSD.

The Subjective Experience of Acute Stress Disorder and PTSD in Adolescence

Affective States

Most affective states in adolescence are similar to those experienced during adulthood. Some are reinforced, however, by the conditions of adolescence—particularly feelings of existential despair, of life's having no value, and of being defective, or the feeling that no human beings (particularly parents or friends) are able to help. In the case of collective disasters, thoughts of revenge against the institutions that were supposed to protect adolescents have been shown to be particularly high in cases of PTSD symptoms of great intensity, especially when parents were involved as victims.

Suicidal ideation is frequent in adolescents' PTSD, particularly when the traumatic event has been associated with shame, as in the case of sexual abuse or sexual or psychological harassment. Feelings of body incompetence and body image dissatisfaction may be notable in these latter cases.

Cognitive Patterns

Mental content typically includes reexperiencing the traumatic event through flashbacks, ruminations, or nightmares that are particularly painful. These reexperiencings may be spontaneous or triggered by reminders of the trauma. Fantasies of revenge, of reparation, or of suicide may accompany such ideas. They are interpreted, even if inaccurate, as defenses against the unbearable passivity of being victimized. Dissociation or derealization may be present.

Cognitive patterns are characterized by vivid traumatic memories, disorganized in temporality, arising suddenly without any effort of recollection and even against efforts to forget. Conversely, other personal memories become overgeneralized. Autobiographical memories (information and personally relevant events acquired in a specific spatial–temporal context that enable a person to construct a sense of identity and continuity) may be impaired.

Memory and attentional biases for negative information may be responsible for errors or reduced speed of processing and may contribute to impaired judgment and lowered academic performance. These biases toward a pessimistic interpretation of the environment may explain some aspects of aggressive or depressive feelings. Amnesia for the trauma has not been found in most studies if the traumatic event happened after childhood.

Somatic States

Somatic states are similar to those that have been described in adults. Sleep disorders are common. Self-harm seems frequent in cases of sexual or psychological abuse, and an increased rate of suicidality has also been found in these latter cases (Scheeringa, Zeanah, & Cohen, 2011). Eating disorders and substance use may also be present. The few neuroimaging studies performed with adolescents show modifications comparable to those that have been described among adults (Jackowski, de Araújo, de Lacerda, Mari Jde, & Kaufman, 2009).

SA41.3 *Complex Posttraumatic Stress Disorder*

CPTSD is described in more detail in Chapter 3 (pp. 190–194).

Many traumatic events are time limited. In some cases, however, children and adolescents experience chronic trauma that continues or repeats for months or years. The current (DSM-5) PTSD diagnosis does not fully capture the severe psychological harm that occurs with prolonged trauma. The diagnosis of CPTSD has been proposed to capture this pattern of symptoms associated with a chronic neglect, abuse, and severe mistreatment over the course of childhood (National Center for PTSD, 2016). Such developmental trauma frequently compromises an adolescent's identity, self-worth, and personality, capacity to self-regulate, relations with others, and intimacy (van der Kolk, 2005). In the face of developmental trauma, dissociation may be a child's only survival strategy in the short term, even if this leads to depersonalization, derealization, and discontinuities of self and personal experience in the long term. Adolescence, with its growing need for sexuality and intimate relationships, may trigger dissociative episodes in children with developmental trauma.

Recovery from CPTSD requires restoration of control and power for the traumatized adolescent. Survivors can become empowered by healing relationships, which create safety, allow for remembrance and mourning, and promote reconnection with everyday life (Herman, 1997).

SA42 Dissociative Disorders

Dissociative disorders are described in more detail in Chapter 3 (p. 194).

According to DSM-5, dissociative disorders are a group of symptom patterns characterized by a disruption of and/or discontinuity in the normal integration of consciousness, memory, identity, emotion, perception, body representation, motor control, and behavior. Dissociative symptoms can potentially disrupt every area of psychological functioning.

Children and adolescents may describe a range of dissociative symptoms that reflect a lack of coherence in mental functioning (International Society for the Study of

Dissociation, 2004). These symptoms can be manifested as (1) inconsistent consciousness, which is reflected in symptoms of fluctuating attention and trance states; (2) autobiographical forgetfulness and fluctuations in access to knowledge, which reflect incoherence in developmental memory processes; (3) fluctuating moods and behavior, including rage episodes and regressions, which reflect difficulties in self-regulation; (4) beliefs in alternate selves or imaginary friends that control one's behavior, reflecting disorganization in the development of a cohesive self; and (5) depersonalization and derealization, which reflect a subjective sense of dissociation from normal body sensations and perceptions or from a sense of self.

Dissociation in children and adolescents may be seen as a malleable developmental phenomenon that may accompany a wide variety of childhood presentations. Symptoms of dissociation are seen in populations of children and adolescents with other disorders, including PTSD (Putnam, Hornstein, & Peterson, 1996), OCD (Stien & Waters, 1999), and reactive attachment disorders, as well as in general populations of traumatized and hospitalized adolescents (Atlas, Weissman, & Liebowitz, 1997) and delinquent adolescents (Carrion & Steiner, 2000).

Dissociative symptoms in adolescents have been found to correlate with traumatic histories of significant sexual and/or physical abuse (Macfie, Cicchetti, & Toth, 2001), and with neglectful, rejecting, and inconsistent parenting styles (Brunner, Parzer, Schuld, & Resch, 2000; Sanders & Giolas, 1991). Individual differences in adolescents' susceptibility to dissociative symptoms may be related to other inherited personality traits (Jang, Paris, Zweig-Frank, & Livesley, 1998). According to Siegel (2012), "interpersonal processes can facilitate integration by altering the restrictive ways in which the mind may have come to organize itself" (p. 376). Therapeutic intervention, therefore, can aim to provide those new interpersonal relationships that foster the integration and coherence of the self and improve adaptation.

The DSM-5 category of dissociative disorders includes depersonalization/derealization disorder (characterized by experiences of unreality or detachment from one's mind, self, or body and/or experiences of irreality in or detachment from one's surroundings), dissociative amnesia (characterized by an inability to recall autobiographical information), and dissociative identity disorder (characterized by the presence of two or more distinct personality states or an experience of possession and recurrent episodes of amnesia).

SA43 Conversion Disorder

Conversion disorder is described in more detail in Chapter 3 (pp. 206–207).

Conversion disorder is a condition in which symptoms and deficits in voluntary motor function suggest a neurological or other physical condition that is in fact not present. In most cases, symptoms date from a minor illness or injury (Leary, 2003). The prevalence of conversion disorders in youth is difficult to establish, but it is estimated to be about 1–3% of children and adolescents consulting for neurological problems. During childhood, conversion disorder occurs most commonly in the preadolescent years, roughly twice as often in girls as in boys. These cases place considerable demands on consulting time and diagnostic resources. Among predisposing factors, studies have identified rigid obsessional personality traits, states of anxiety and depression, and previous sexual abuse (Pehlivanturk & Unal, 2002). Environmental factors include domestic stress, feelings of parental rejection, poor intrafamilial communication, unresolved grief and unhappiness at school (Leary, 2003). The positive diagnosis of conversion disorder is frequently delayed by fear of misdiagnosis, which can lead to excessive medical investigations. In the great majority of cases, diagnosis can be achieved through a detailed physical examination and the identification of clinical incongruities. A delay in diagnosis can also be related to a refusal by parents or the adolescent to accept the absence of organic disease. Such refusal often goes with denial of any familial problems and with anger directed at medical personnel (Leary, 2003).

Intervention begins with an acknowledgment that the young person has a real illness that has seriously disrupted normal patterns of living. The presenting disability should be regarded as a symptom reflecting unconscious conflict. An effective therapeutic strategy is a graded physiotherapy program linked to a reward system and directed by an empathic physiotherapist (Brazier & Venning, 1997). This can be provided within the setting of children's hospital wards under the supervision of general pediatricians. Good results have also been achieved with behavior therapy (with both positive and negative reinforcement), psychotherapy, and hypnosis (Campo & Negrini, 2000).

SA5 Somatic Symptom and Related Disorders

Somatic symptom and related disorders are characterized by an intense focus (e.g., excessive and disproportionate thoughts, feelings and behaviors) on physical (somatic) phenomena, which cause significant distress and/or interfere with daily functioning. DSM-5 includes in this category somatic symptom disorder, illness anxiety disorder (hypochondriasis), and factitious disorders. Somatic symptom and related disorders are described in more detail in Chapter 3 (pp. 207–208).

SA51 Somatic Symptom Disorder

Somatic symptom disorder is characterized by bodily symptoms that cause significant distress or dysfunction and in which psychosocial factors are considered to play a role in initiating, deteriorating, or maintaining the symptoms. In DSM-5, the diagnosis is based on the presence of positive symptoms and signs (distressing somatic symptoms plus abnormal thoughts, feelings, and behaviors in response to them), rather than on the absence of a medical explanation for somatic symptoms. This is an important change from the DSM-IV criteria for somatization disorder, which overemphasized the centrality of medically unexplained symptoms. Such symptoms are present to various degrees, particularly in conversion disorder, but somatic symptom disorder can also accompany diagnosed medical disorders. In fact, a distinctive characteristic of many adolescents with somatic symptom disorder is not the somatic symptoms per se, but instead the way they present and interpret them.

Adolescents with somatic symptom disorder complain about a variety of physical problems: They may suffer stomachaches, headaches, nausea, urgency to urinate or defecate, and other similar problems. Although an adolescent usually does not associate the symptoms with particular stressors, they appear to be related to situations that evoke anxiety in the adolescent. Somatic symptom disorder tends to occur in families with difficulties integrating physical sensations, feelings, and thoughts. The symptoms, which are not produced intentionally, may begin spontaneously or after a minor illness. The adolescent is typically convinced that the ailment is purely physical. A pattern ensues in which the young patient progressively uses the symptoms in the service of avoidance. This pattern may become generalized to the point where the adolescent appears debilitated by the symptoms.

The Subjective Experience of Somatic Symptom Disorder in Adolescence

Affective States

An adolescent's affective state is often characterized by a high level of concerns about illnesses. The individual appears distressed and in pain. The distress may be compounded if the adolescent feels that caregivers question the reality of the illness. On feeling disbelieved, the adolescent is likely to protest loudly, to feel injured, and to become enraged.

Cognitive Patterns

The adolescent's thoughts often focus on the particular somatic symptoms, and there is often a narrowing of interests in age-expected domains. Some adolescents with this pattern also experience numerous fears characteristic of younger children. The patient's conviction of the gravity of the illness leads to concerns about dire physical consequences, which may be vague and ill defined or specific and elaborate. The adolescent may feel that he or she is seriously ill and in danger of dying.

Somatic States

It is important not to ignore the possibility of undiagnosed medical illness and to take into account any medical illness that may accompany the somatic symptom disorder. Whether or not such a condition can be found, taking the adolescent's pain and anxiety seriously may prevent an escalation of those complaints that are unconsciously designed to demonstrate just how bad the suffering is.

Relationship Patterns

Depending on the dynamics that trigger the somatic symptoms, relationships may be reasonably intact or may demonstrate severe regressive features. In the latter case, the adolescent may become excessively fearful of separating from caregivers or may become withdrawn and isolated. Relationships may be characterized by exaggerated dependency, and new relationships may be avoided.

Clinical Illustrations

A 12-year-old girl daughter of immigrants became unable to walk or move. Neurological tests failed to explain her paralysis. In therapy, she revealed an extreme conflict about whether to identify with her "new" culture (implying a move away from her parents) or to stay in the "old" culture with her parents (and avoid anxieties about new challenges). After 6 months in treatment, she began to move around the consultation room, and 2 years later she was back in school functioning normally.

In another case, a 14-year-old boy had trouble swallowing. He could not get his breakfast down or take medicine, but in the therapist's office he had no trouble downing a hamburger. He had ongoing conflicts with his mother, a strict disciplinarian, with whom he would provoke huge fights. In treatment, his symptom was seen as expressing difficulty "swallowing" what his mother was "feeding" him, and it remitted once he expressed his feelings about her harsh discipline.

SA52 Illness Anxiety Disorder (Hypochondriasis)

Illness anxiety disorder is described in more detail in Chapter 3 (pp. 210–211).

Illness anxiety disorder is preoccupation with and unrealistic fear of having or developing a serious disease in the absence of medical evidence of an illness. Illness anxiety disorder was previously called "hypochondriasis," a term that many now see as pejorative, but that persists. People with illness anxiety disorder are always thinking about their physical health. Fears may derive from misinterpreting nonpathological physical symptoms or normal bodily functions (e.g., abdominal bloating and crampy discomfort, awareness of heartbeat, sweating). Adolescents with illness anxiety disorder do not purposely create these symptoms and are unable to control them. They seek reassurance from family, friends, or health care providers repeatedly. They feel better for a short time and then begin to worry about the same symptoms or new symptoms. Symptoms may shift and change and are often vague. Some may recognize that their fear of having a serious disease is unreasonable or unfounded.

Transient hypochondriacal states frequently appear during periods of developmental changes; hence adolescence is a favorable period for the appearance of illness anxiety disorder. Adolescents need time and experience to integrate their body's changes into their total representation of the body. Those with illness anxiety disorder often believe with vivid imagery that something specific is wrong with their bodies, even if no medical abnormalities are found. In other cases, out of embarrassment, adolescents may hide somatic symptoms. This concealment can lead to further anxiety about the problem and to obsessive and compulsive behaviors. Treatment of illness anxiety disorder includes establishing a consistent, supportive physician–patient relationship; CBT has been found to be helpful (Sørensen, Birket-Smith, Wattar, Buemann, & Salkovskis, 2011; Wicksell, Melin, Lekander, & Olsson, 2009).

SA53 Factitious Disorders

Factitious disorders are described in more detail in Chapter 3 (pp. 211–213).

In the type of factitious disorder generally seen in adulthood (also called Munchausen's syndrome), a person intentionally produces or feigns physical or psychological symptoms. In childhood and adolescence, it is more common to see Munchausen's syndrome by proxy, in which an individual (usually a parent, but sometimes a nurse or other caregiver) repeatedly causes illness or physical harm to another person. The perpetrator denies playing any role and presents to medical personnel as in great distress over the health crisis of the person he or she has harmed. Unlike in malingering, there is no obvious secondary gain, though there may be some psychological reward in the attention received during medical dramas created by factitious crises. There are few studies of the etiology, family patterns, or predisposing factors, but parents with this diagnosis typically have a prior history of early (and possibly traumatizing) medical treatment.

SA8 Psychophysiological Disorders

SA81 Feeding and Eating Disorders

Feeding and eating disorders are also discussed in Chapter 3 (pp. 213–217).

DSM-5 has regrouped under feeding and eating disorders several conditions involving persistent disturbance of eating or eating-related behaviors that result in altered food consumption or absorption, producing significant impairment in health or psychosocial functioning. We focus on anorexia nervosa and bulimia nervosa, which have a frequent onset in adolescence, in this chapter. We include these disorders under the Psychophysiological Disorders category because they both imply a deep perturbation of the physiological process of eating.

The core diagnostic criteria for anorexia nervosa and bulimia nervosa are conceptually unchanged from DSM-IV, with one small exception: The requirement of amenorrhea in the diagnosis of anorexia nervosa has been eliminated. The only change in the DSM-IV criteria for bulimia nervosa is a reduction in the required minimum average frequency of binge eating and inappropriate compensatory behavior frequency (from twice to once weekly).

The frequent onset of eating disorders in adolescence is related to the physiological and psychological changes of adolescence. Puberty induces hormonal variations, body composition changes, and food intake regulation modifications. In this context, many transient and deviant food choices or eating disorders are encountered, including bingeing, craving, nibbling, and other temporary deviations from normal eating that are associated with adolescent empowerment and the individuation process. About 20% of adolescent girls experiment with restrictive or fasting behaviors but only a small minority will develop severe eating disorders. When these problems occur in the perimenarchal period, they may be a response to menstruation onset and accompanying anxiety about sexuality and maturation through puberty. Restrictive behaviors, weight loss, and dietary deficiencies retard the process of puberty and interfere with the development of secondary sexual features. Thus anorexia, bulimia, binge eating, and related behaviors may have dramatic somatic repercussions for puberty, fertility, and growth, along with an increased risk of osteoporosis (Roux, Blanchet, Stheneur, Chapelon, & Godart, 2013).

Anorexia nervosa is the most common eating disorder in clinical populations (70–80%) during the peripubertal period, with frequency peaks at about the ages of 12–13 and 17–19. Bulimia nervosa is more common in the older group. In Western populations, the prevalence of diagnosed anorexia nervosa has been stable over the last few decades: about 1% in girls and 0.03% in boys (Hoek, 2006). Epidemiological data in non-Western countries show increasing prevalence, particularly in eastern Asia. The disorders need to be approached from biological, psychological, familial, and sociocultural perspectives. Thus standard classifications use not only somatic criteria (e.g., weight changes or vomiting), but also psychological criteria (e.g., fear of being fat, disturbance in the experience of body weight or shape), and behavioral criteria (e.g., restriction of intake, binge eating, compulsive exercising, or laxative use). There are clear cross-cultural variations in the occurrence and presentation of these criteria.

Systemic psychotherapies and family-based treatments are essential in the care of adolescents with eating disorders (Findlay, Pinzon, Taddeo, & Katzman, 2010). The most recent studies and guidelines recommend a comprehensive approach and multidisciplinary care, including somatic, nutritional, and psychiatric regular and interactive interventions (American Psychiatric Association, 2006; Gowers & Bryant-Waugh, 2004; National Institute for Clinical Excellence, 2004).

Like adults, adolescents with eating disorders show different kinds of functioning, including obsessive–compulsive, narcissistic, and borderline features. It is also arguable that severely anorexic patients, who believe they must restrict eating even while at realistic risk of starvation, represent inherently a condition at the psychotic level of personality functioning (see Chapters 1 and 5 on the P and PA Axes). Bulimic patients and anorexic patients with purge symptoms tend to be at a borderline level of functioning.

All DSM-5 eating disorders have similar physiopathological bases, and frequent crossovers or categorical migrations occur between subtypes. In most adolescents (30–60%), there is a first stage of transient binge-eating episodes or bulimia nervosa; 80% of bulimic adults have experienced anorexic episodes (Milos, Spindler, & Schnyder, 2005). Adolescents with premorbid problems of being overweight, or with initial forms of the binge-eating/purging subtype of anorexia, are at greater risk of long-term bulimic disorders. Binge episodes usually occur in the first 3–5 years of anorexic episodes. Conversely, fewer than 5% of bulimic patients develop anorexia nervosa, a condition that seems much more resistant to change (symptomatic fixity = 50%). Yet Smink, van Hoeken, and Hoek (2013) found global favorable overcomes in more than 70% of cases of anorexia nervosa and in 55% of bulimia cases. Eating disorders thus overlap; although we cannot describe an anorexic or bulimic personality, temperament profiles can be considered as predisposing factors. Psychiatric comorbidity, familial factors, and anthropometric/symptomatic factors seem to predict crossover and eating symptomatology evolution.

There are some clinical features of eating disorders more specific to adolescence. Anorexia nervosa in boys often starts with premorbid obesity or being overweight. Somatic harm rapidly becomes severe, with much bingeing and purging. Difficulties in identity are central, often dominated by wishes to gain lean muscle mass. Anorexia sometimes follows a massive stress, such as sexual abuse, death in the family, attachment problems, or serious illness. Generally in such cases, adolescents report loss of appetite and sadness or other depressive symptoms rather than typically "anorexic" cognitions. Immigrant adolescents or the children of migrants may experience a clash of cultures that can interfere with identity construction. Anorexia nervosa, and eating disorders generally, may fulfill a positive acculturative function and be a culture-clash equivalent (Demarque et al., 2015). Finally, adolescents suffering from anorexia secondary to eating disorders during childhood may experience an exacerbation of the problem during puberty. In these cases, problems centering around identity building are often profound and severe.

The Subjective Experience of Eating Disorders in Adolescence

Affective States

As stated earlier, anorexic and bulimic adolescents share several features. They frequently lack an awareness of their emotional experiences; they are highly alexithymic, showing a chronic inability to recognize, identify, and label emotions. Emotions may be experienced as uncontrollable, rapidly oscillating, intense, painful, and threatening to a vulnerable self. Difficulty in coping with their own emotions is paradoxically associated with an oversensitivity to the emotions of others and with a constant preoccupation with others' responses. This state may lead to ingratiating or acquiescent behaviors. Self-depreciation, shame, and feelings of jealousy are frequently associated with this attitude.

Dependency and self-criticism are common in both anorexic and bulimic adolescents (Speranza et al., 2003). This is not surprising since one of the major problems of adolescents with eating disorders is a struggle for autonomy and self-definition that may reflect incomplete separation–individuation during earliest childhood. Anorexic adolescents show high dependency features. Self-critical depression seems a more specific feature of bulimic patients and may reflect the fragility of their identity and their difficulties regulating self-esteem. As Heatherton and Baumeister (1991) have emphasized, the motivation for binge eating may be an attempt to escape negative aspects of self-awareness and to control the dysphoric states associated with borderline-level personality organizations.

Cognitive Patterns

Low self-esteem and difficulties in self-affirmation are common experiences of adolescents with eating disorders. Pathological eating may be a way to cope with feelings of lack of control. Fears of leaving childhood for adulthood may create avoidance behaviors (e.g., maintaining a childlike physical appearance by reducing weight that affects endocrine stimulation, height, and development of secondary sex characteristics) or overinvestment in opposite behaviors (overfemininity or oversexuality with high-risk sexual behaviors). An adolescent may experience this paradox as having a split personality: a normal one that is rational and an anorexic/bulimic one that is completely irrational. The concretization of this split may take the form of inner voices guiding and controlling the adolescent's behavior. In contrast, some adolescents with eating disorders may perceive their condition as part of their identity and fear any modification of their situation as a threat to their core sense of self.

Eating disorders seem to provide a sense of safety and protection to adolescents at several levels, allowing them to regain self-control and power and to feel beautiful and special. Control over emotions and behaviors can take the form of obsessive symptoms that go beyond food themes and may be exerted in a tyrannical way that neglects basic bodily needs. Any failure in this idealized, draconian control may then be experienced with overwhelming shame and guilt.

Somatic States

Denial of physiological needs is an essential feature of eating disorders. Bruch (1973) considered weak interoceptive awareness (uncertainty between feelings and body sensations) as pathognomonic of anorexia nervosa. The alexithymic functioning of eating-disordered adolescents may also reduce their capacity to adapt to stress. Faced with the physiological arousal induced by emotional demands, alexithymic patients may resort to restricted patterns of repetitive and automated behaviors, such as the hyperactivity of anorexic individuals or the binge–purge cycles of bulimic patients, which temporarily relieve their feelings of discomfort and restore their inner equilibrium. Such practices may generate, in the long term, positive reinforcements of the eating disorder comparable to those observed in addictive disorders (Speranza et al., 2012).

Both types of eating disorders may be associated with somatic consequences in multiple organ systems. The risk of death is high in adolescents with anorexia nervosa.

A plethora of dermatological changes have been described, some (such as purpura, indicating a bleeding diathesis) signaling serious pathophysiology. There is a high risk of developing diabetic illness and gastrointestinal complications (gastric dilatation, Mallory–Weiss syndrome, and severe liver dysfunction), which may be serious. Acrocyanosis is common. Fatal arrhythmias are possible. Low-weight patients are at a high risk for osteopenia and osteoporosis. Nutritional abnormalities are also common, including sodium depletion, hypovolemia, hypophosphatemia, and hypomagnesemia (see Mitchell & Crow, 2006).

Relationship Patterns

Adolescents with eating disorders often find social contexts threatening—a reaction that may perpetuate avoidance and isolation. This social discomfort is the counterpart of overattachment to parents, particularly mothers. Current theories consider disordered eating behaviors as reflecting a developmental arrest in the separation–individuation process traceable to a caregiver's failure to provide essential functions during development. Symptoms may be attempts to cope with needs stemming from this incomplete self-development or from an interruption of the separation–individuation process. Relationships with parents are sometimes reversed; eating-disordered adolescents may feel the need to exert control over parents' lives, behaviors, or feelings. Relations with peers and love objects are characterized by a similar dependency and by emotional exclusivity. Separation experiences are hard to manage or avoided. Separations from an older brother or sister who leaves home, or separations secondary to parental separation or divorce, are frequently triggers of eating disorders.

Clinicians treating eating-disordered adolescents have countertransference reactions that may vary with the type of disorder. Anorexic adolescents are frequently alexithymic and controlling. Bulimic adolescents may be equally alexithymic, but are more impulsive and emotionally unstable. Rasting, Brosig, and Beutel (2005), who videotaped and evaluated facial affects in dyadic therapeutic interactions in a sample of psychosomatic and eating-disordered patients, observed that the predominant emotional reaction of therapists to alexithymic patients was contempt. Professionals should be aware of the potential impact of alexithymic features on therapeutic relationships and avoid misinterpreting their patients' emotional limitations as negative engagement in treatment.

Clinical Illustration

A 14-year-old girl with no history of childhood obesity had begun to lose weight after menarche. She was an excellent student, described by parents as a rigorous perfectionist. She had no best friend or boyfriend and shunned peers in favor of schoolwork and running competitions. Her beloved 19-year-old brother had left for college the preceding year. Restrictive eating behaviors had begun then, reportedly because she was feeling fat and was uncomfortable with pubertal body changes. Initially, she had avoided sugar, fat, and snacks and had to fight against hunger. She started controlling her food and trying to control her parents' eating behaviors and cooking habits. The parents suspected laxative abuse and noted some obsessive–compulsive symptoms. More recently, she was refusing family meals and insisting on eating alone with her mother, whom she called all day long. She told her physician she was doing well; she simply felt too fat. She was angry with him for prohibiting her physical exercise because of her dangerously low weight. Because of the severity of her weight loss, massive denial, anorexic cognitions, physical hyperactivity, purgative behaviors, obsessive–compulsive practices, and fused relationship with her mother, hospitalization was deemed necessary.

SA9 Disruptive Behavior Disorders

Disruptive behavior disorders are a group of conditions involving problems in control of one's emotions and behaviors, at a cost to others. DSM-5 has introduced a new category of disruptive, impulse-control, and conduct disorders, combining several disorders of emotional and behavioral self-control previously included among the disorders usually first diagnosed in infancy, childhood, or adolescence—notably oppositional defiant disorder (ODD) and conduct disorder (CD). The underlying causes of problems in controlling emotions and behaviors vary greatly across disorders and individuals with these diagnoses. Factors of temperament (including neurodevelopmental disorders such as ADHD) and environment both play a significant role in pathogenesis. Disruptive behavior disorders are heterogeneous, with different characteristics in terms of comorbid neuropsychiatric problems, neuropsychological profiles, and social–familial difficulties. They are best understood by taking account of the developmental trajectories of the youngsters diagnosed with them.

SA91 Conduct Disorder

CD is also discussed in Chapter 9 (pp. 571–573).

CD involves a repetitive, persistent pattern of behavior in which an adolescent violates the basic rights of others or violates age-appropriate societal norms or rules. DSM-5 groups such behaviors into aggressive conduct that causes or threatens physical harm to other people or animals; nonaggressive conduct causing property loss or damage; deceitfulness; and theft and serious rule violations. Conduct-disordered adolescents have major impairments in social, academic, and occupational functioning. Research has found two subtypes of antisocial behavior. The first emerges in early childhood and follows a persistent life course, whereas the second emerges in adolescence, reflects peer processes such as mimicry of antisocial peers, and remits in early adulthood. DSM-5 further postulates a subtype with limited prosocial emotions, displaying high callous–unemotional traits. These traits include flat affect and reduced empathy and remorse and are associated with more severe, varied, and persistent patterns of antisocial behavior and aggression.

Many children with CD have coexisting symptomatology, such as mood disorders, anxiety, posttraumatic syndromes, problems with attention and hyperactivity, learning problems, substance misuse, and thought disorders. Persisting CD in adolescence is a strong predictor of antisocial personality disorder, especially among boys from low-socioeconomic-status families of origin who show high callous–unemotional traits. Adolescents with CD are at high risk of negative outcomes that include substance use disorders, school dropout, unwanted pregnancies, conviction, and increased injuries and mortality.

Disruptive behavior disorders, including CD, are the most common reason for referral to child and adolescent mental health services. An estimated 6% of all children and adolescents have some form of CD, far more commonly in boys than in girls. Girls are more likely to develop adolescent-onset CD, whereas for boys onset is usually in childhood and involves more aggressiveness.

Many factors may contribute to the development of CD, including brain damage, child abuse, genetic vulnerability, school failure, inadequate relationships, and traumatic experiences. Oppositional behaviors and violence may reflect particular relational dynamics between a youngster and the social and family environment. Deviant behaviors are thus important signals to identify. They may occur in situations of mutual misunderstanding in which rigid attitudes provoke an escalation of aggression (e.g., in the absence of any mediation in situations of generational and cultural conflict, with a failure to find solutions other than direct confrontation). They may also be the youngster's reaction to familial or social rejection, real or perceived. Parental attitudes may play a role in the genesis of children's behavioral problems. Rigid or chaotic educational attitudes, emotional neglect, or harsh parental interactions characterized by insensitivity to a child's needs may be at the basis of insecure or disorganized attachment patterns between the child and the parents.

Research provides support for the hypothesis that life-course-persistent antisocial behavior is a neurodevelopmental disorder that emerges in the transactions between individual vulnerabilities and environmental adversity (Frick & Viding, 2009). Empirical findings also suggest that severe antisocial behaviors emerging in adolescence frequently have a negative prognosis and are rarely limited to the adolescent period (Fairchild, van Goozen, Calder, & Goodyer, 2013). Both forms of antisocial behavior are associated with emotion-processing deficits, changes in brain structure and function, alterations in cortisol secretion, and atypical personality traits (such as increased callous–unemotional traits).

The Subjective Experience of CD in Adolescence

Affective States

Adolescents with CD tend to be unaware of their own affective states and unresponsive to the feelings of others. This is particularly the case for those with callous–unemotional traits, who may lack remorse and appear unempathetic and opportunistic. Adolescents with this diagnosis show affect that is labile and not well regulated; they are usually unable to tolerate even small amounts of frustration or delay of gratification. They tend to express anger when they do not get their own way and to express satisfaction when they succeed. At times they acknowledge feelings of fear, and they may also admit to deeper feelings of pain and resentment at not being cared for and at being mistreated by others. They commonly express a defeated attitude of having given up on people.

Cognitive Patterns

Thoughts and fantasies often involve the conviction of being frequently wronged. Adolescents with CD may have a clearly defensive sense of invulnerability, and they tend to regard others with indifference. Their goals usually include material gain and power. Thoughts about any other aspects of interpersonal relationships are remarkably absent.

Somatic States

Somatic states most prominently seen in these individuals include arousal and hypervigilance. In addition, there may be somatic symptoms as a part of the core psychopathology or as a consequence of the frequent co-occurrence of substance use disorders.

Relationship Patterns

Relationship patterns may be characterized by impulsivity and indifference toward others. Because others tend to be seen as objects to manipulate in the service of power, excitement, or material benefits, it is not surprising that relationships tend to be poor and short-lived. Primary caregivers frequently describe living with an adolescent with CD as overwhelming, demanding, and unrelenting. Current treatment guidelines focus on parent training programs, but help in that context is frequently experienced as shaming, judgmental, and stigmatizing. When, by contrast, professionals are seen as nonjudgmental, normalizing, and sensitive to the wider family context, including the parents' own emotional needs, more positive outcomes are reported.

Clinical Illustration

A 16-year-old boy had failed eighth grade, had been stealing cars since age 12, and was acting intimidating toward peers. Eventually, he was arrested and sent to a detention center, where he was described as angry and entitled, with little regard for others. He tried to intimidate the staff—a significant problem, as he was a large, strong adolescent. An intuitive detention officer began talking sympathetically with him, often about his history of being treated unfairly, while also setting limits on his intimidation by giving him "time outs" in the county jail. After a year in this setting, he began to comply with its rules; within 2 years, he became one of its best students.

SA92 Oppositional Defiant Disorder

ODD is also discussed in Chapter 9 (see pp. 573–576).

ODD in adolescence is characterized by argumentativeness, negativity, hostility, and defiance toward authority. While all adolescents can be negative in the service of self-definition, openly provocative, uncooperative, and hostile behaviors become a serious concern when they take the form of a continuing pattern—markedly more frequent and consistent than the behaviors of other adolescents of the same age and developmental level and interfering with adaptive patterns in major areas of an adolescent's life. Symptoms such as temper tantrums, excessive arguing with adults, active defiance of requests and rules, deliberate attempts to annoy or upset people, blaming others, being touchy and easily annoyed by others, and expressing anger and resentment are frequent features of this problem. For children with ODD, adolescence can be even more complicated than it is for most youngsters, as these children may have more trouble than others with social interactions, academics, and control of their emotions.

In DSM-5, the symptoms of ODD fall into three groups: angry/irritable mood, argumentative/defiant behavior, and vindictiveness. The chronic irritability in these adolescents highlights links between oppositionality and mood disorders and reflects a deficit in emotion regulation behind a propensity toward explosive outbursts and disruptive, self-defeating behaviors.

Oppositional and defiant behaviors are among the most common reasons for referral to mental health services in childhood and adolescence. Symptoms are relatively stable during childhood and adolescence. They commonly occur alongside other disorders or conditions such as anxiety, depression, and ADHD, and they may ultimately develop into CD. Evidence indicates that diagnosed ODD not only acts as a precursor to CD and antisocial behaviors, but also predicts mood disorders and anxiety.

Adolescents with oppositional and defiant patterns often have low self-esteem and feel that they are not getting the attention they deserve. Behind the overt disruptiveness of oppositional adolescents are feelings of demoralization, resentment, self-doubt, and self-hatred. Such youngsters almost always feel poorly understood. A dramatic and persistent state of hyperalertness, oriented toward guarding their self-worth, characterizes their affective states. They are poised to feel put upon and righteously indignant. Their efforts to maintain their self-esteem may look more stimulating and euphoric than anxious. Problems with self-regulation are often present.

Although the causes of such behaviors are not fully known, the symptoms of ODD are frequently part of a pattern of problematic early interactions. However, it may be difficult to disentangle the relative contributions of the individual's characteristics from those of the problematic interactions of early family life. Fonagy (see Bateman & Fonagy, 2012) has proposed a bidevelopmental model of disruptive behavior disorders that takes into account the interplay between a child's temperamental difficulties and the parents' inability to attune to the child's needs because of their own difficulties. Insensitive behaviors by parents amplify the child's reactions and trigger a cycle of mutual misunderstanding. The environment does not contain the child's impulsiveness, hyperactivity, and irritability. These symptoms produce unsatisfactory relational exchanges that deprive the child of the positive emotional sharing experiences necessary for the development of a consistent self-representation and for confidence in others. Oppositional behaviors and aggressiveness may perform the function of protecting a fragile identity from feelings of dependence. The child develops compelling interactive strategies that later expand to other relational contexts.

Most adolescents with this diagnosis have weak insight into their problems. They typically do not regard themselves as angry, oppositional, or defiant. Instead, they justify their behavior as a response to unreasonable demands or circumstances and attribute the problem to others' demands for conformity. Their impulsivity leads to behaviors that evoke negative consequences, to which they seem oblivious. Although expressions of remorse or contrition may follow some defiant actions, oppositional adolescents more often feel justified in their behavior and see themselves as victims of injustice. Recurrent disapproval from others may erode their sense of self-cohesion, making oppositional adolescents more vulnerable to narcissistic injury and fragmentation. Their inability to demonstrate their competence leads them to feel especially vulnerable to criticism and to failure.

Social and family relationships are usually impaired because of these adolescents' disruptiveness, bossiness, and oppositionality. In a vicious cycle, the disapproval to which they are regularly subjected may lead oppositional adolescents to be more rebellious and defiant. These responses, along with their tendency to associate with similarly defiant peers, may drive them into delinquent patterns.

SA93 Substance-Related Disorders

Substance-related disorders are described in more detail in Chapter 3 (pp. 225–228) and Chapter 9 (p. 576). Although substance-related disorders is a specific group of conditions in adults, we included these disorders under adolescent disruptive behavior disorders because an increasing number of studies indicate that the deficits in emotional and behavioral self-control shown by these disorders strongly predict adolescent problems with substance use.

DSM-5 considers the essential feature of a substance use disorder to be a cluster of cognitive, behavioral, and physiological symptoms indicating that an individual continues using the substance despite significant substance-related problems. This diagnosis is based on four pathological patterns of behavior related to substance use: impaired control, social impairment, risky use, and pharmacological criteria (tolerance and withdrawal). It can apply to several classes of substances. Independently of the specific drug, all such disorders cause underlying changes in brain circuits that may persist beyond detoxification, particularly in individuals with severe disorders. The behavioral effects of these changes may include repeated relapses and intense craving upon exposure to drug-related stimuli.

Substance use during adolescence is common worldwide. Data from the 2014 Monitoring the Future Survey estimated that within the previous year, 60.2% of 12th graders had used alcohol, 35.1% had used marijuana, and 13.9% had used a prescription drug for nonmedical reasons (Johnston, Miech, O'Malley, Bachman, & Schulenberg, 2014). An estimated 11.4% of adolescents met DSM-IV criteria for a substance use disorder. Such use in adolescence often co-occurs with psychological distress and psychiatric illness. Adolescents with psychiatric disorders are at higher risk for developing a substance use disorder; conversely, high rates of psychiatric illness are seen in adolescents with substance use disorders. Co-occurring psychiatric illness and substance use disorders complicate adolescents' treatment course and prognosis.

An increasing number of studies indicate that childhood psychological dysregulation predicts adolescent substance use disorders, whether difficulties are of the externalizing (e.g., aggression) or internalizing (e.g., anxiety) type. Adolescents with externalizing behaviors seem to be most responsive to drug activation of the brain's reward cue system, while those who internalize appear to use drugs to control a hyperresponsive fear–anxiety system. Both types share a common deficit in psychological regulation with cognitive, behavioral, and emotional difficulties since childhood. The concept of psychological dysregulation comprises distinct but related components: executive cognitive dysfunction, behavioral impulsivity, and emotional lability.

Several environmental influences that affect the risk of accelerated and problematic use of alcohol and other drugs and the development of adolescent substance use disorders have been identified. These include child maltreatment and other traumatic events; parental influences, such as parenting practices and substance use by parents; and peer influences. Some of these also lead to manifestations of psychological dysregulation, such as CD, ADHD, anxiety-related disorders, and depressive disorders.

While it is developing, the brain is vulnerable to negative events. If a trauma occurs or an individual uses substances during adolescence, brain development can be disturbed, which can lead to reduced cognitive control over behavior and increased dominance of emotional responses. Substance misuse can increase adolescents' risk of trauma exposure and decrease their ability to cope adaptively with new distressing events. Adolescents with co-occurring psychiatric illness and substance use disorders need an integrated, multimodal treatment approach that includes psychotherapy, pharmacological interventions, family involvement, and collaboration with community supports.

The Subjective Experience of Substance-Related Disorders in Adolescence

Affective States

Social pressures and experimentation are the motives adolescents most frequently cite for initiating drug or alcohol use. They may start using to imitate peers and be accepted by them or to enhance social activities; they may also fear that if they refuse, their friends may exclude them. Many report curiosity as a motive for first use. Substance use may further serve as a coping strategy to deal with stress, forget unpleasant experiences, feel numb or indifferent to life challenges, and erase painful feelings (such as anxiety, emptiness, depression, embarrassment, humiliation, and rage). Reasons for initiating drug or alcohol use are likely distinct from those that contribute to the progression from initial use to regular use and ultimately to a diagnosis of a substance use disorder. The majority of adolescents using substances report that the drugs make them feel good, help them cope with difficulties, and enhance their sense of confidence and self-esteem.

Cognitive Patterns

Adolescents with problematic substance consumption frequently use rationalization and denial when confronted with their misuse. Cognitive patterns are often related to the main emotions that led to substance use. Once an adolescent regularly uses drugs, resultant cognitive patterns reflect the effect of the substance on the individual's brain: fragmented and paranoid thinking, fantasies of specialness and brilliance, wish-fulfilling convictions of desirability, potency, and invulnerability.

Somatic States

Somatic states accompany both the affects described above and the substances used. Teenagers can be creative and inventive in their efforts to maximize intoxication, which can put them at risk for complications in many organ systems, with both immediate and long-term consequences. Somatic states may vary from arousal and agitation to numbness and tranquility.

Relationship Patterns

Adolescents with substance-related disorders show a marked need for guidance and approval from others; they may perceive themselves as powerless and ineffective and may seek constant support and reassurance from others. Relationship patterns are frequently characterized by intense feelings of neediness, alternating with protests that the adolescents have no such needs. Relationships may be described as shaky, untrustworthy, or disappointing, and may range from active involvement in a social group where the substance misuse pattern is ritualized, to isolated, self-absorbed states of solitary withdrawal. Once a person is involved in regular substance misuse, relationships tend to be valued as a means of obtaining the desired substance and thus take on a manipulative quality.

Clinical Illustration

An 18-year-old male was brought for therapy by his mother for substance use interfering with his school performance. His father opposed the treatment. Parents had separated when the boy was 4 after his father, who was heavily involved in drugs, had overdosed, attempted suicide, been hospitalized, and lost his driver's license. At 14, the boy began using marijuana occasionally, escalating quickly to daily use. During a 4-year course of therapy that was only partially successful, it became apparent that his marijuana use constituted an effort to identify with his father. Escalation during high school also reflected a determination to distract himself from emerging homosexual feelings.

SA94 Internet Addiction Disorder

Internet addiction disorder (IAD; also referred to as "problematic internet use" or "compulsive internet use") reflects use of the internet to such an excessive extent that it interferes with daily life. IAD is often divided into subtypes by activity, such as gaming; online social networking; blogging; email checking; excessive, overwhelming, or inappropriate internet pornography use; or internet shopping (shopping addiction). These habits are troubling only to the extent that these activities interfere with normal life and show a cluster of cognitive and behavioral symptoms, including progressive loss of control, tolerance, and withdrawal symptoms, analogous to the symptoms of substance use disorders.

Notwithstanding these similarities, IAD has not been included in the DSM-5 chapter on substance-related disorders and addictive disorders because at this time there is insufficient peer-reviewed evidence to establish the specific diagnostic criteria and course descriptions needed to identify these behaviors as mental disorders. One internet problem that has been considered as a provisional diagnosis in DSM-5, however, is internet gaming disorder (IGD), which has been included in the section of the manual addressing conditions on which future research is encouraged.

The essential feature of IGD is persistent and recurrent participation in computer gaming, typically group games, for many hours (generally more than 8–10 hours per day). These games involve competition between groups of players, participating in complex structured activities that include a significant aspect of social interactions. As persons with substance use disorders do in regard to their substance use, individuals with IGD continue to sit at a computer and engage in gaming despite neglect of other activities. Attempts to direct them toward schoolwork, activities, or family obligations are strongly resisted. If prevented from using a computer and returning to the game, they become agitated and angry. An emerging consensus suggests that IGD is commonly defined by (1) withdrawal, (2) loss of control, and (3) conflict (King & Delfabbro, 2014b). Because money is not at risk, this condition is separate from gambling disorder involving the internet. When individuals are involved in internet games, certain brain pathways are triggered in the same direct and intense way that a drug affects an addicted brain. The gaming prompts a neurological response that influences feelings of pleasure and reward, and the result, in the extreme, is an addictive behavior.

The main reasons individuals give for excessive computer use include avoiding boredom rather than communicating or seeking information. King and Delfabbro (2014a) identified four underlying cognitive factors in IGD: beliefs about game reward value and tangibility; maladaptive and inflexible rules about gaming behaviors; overreliance on gaming to meet self-esteem needs; and gaming as a method of gaining social acceptance.

Much of the literature on diagnosed IGD comes from Asian countries and centers on young males, with a point prevalence of 8.4% and 4.5% for male and female adolescents between 15 and 19 years, respectively (Lam, 2014). A survey on a large European adolescent sample using the proposed DSM-5 criteria for IGD found that 1.6% of adolescents met the full criteria, with a further 5.1% at risk, meeting up to four criteria (Müller et al., 2015). IGD was closely associated with psychopathological symptoms, especially aggressive and rule-breaking behavior and social problems. In other studies, the problem has been associated with psychiatric diagnoses such as social anxiety, depressive disorders, ADHD, and OCD.

This growing literature demonstrates that IGD is common among adolescents and is related to psychosocial and psychiatric problems. Although classification of this phenomenon is still a matter of debate, there is a growing awareness of the risk of excessive use of online computer games, which can lead to functional impairment and intense distress in adolescents and young adults. There is an urgent need for more methodologically sound assessment procedures and youth-specific prevention and treatment programs (Petry et al., 2014).

SA10 Patterns in Adolescence of Infancy/Childhood-Onset Disorders

In this section, we present adolescents' common subjective experiences of the symptom patterns of three disorders that usually surface in infancy and/or childhood: autism spectrum disorder (ASD), attention-deficit/hyperactivity disorder (ADHD), and specific learning disorders. In DSM-5, all of these are classified as neurodevelopmental disorders—a group of conditions with early onset, characterized by developmental deficits that produce impairments of personal, social, academic, or occupational functioning. Developmental deficits range from specific limitations of learning or control of executive functions to global impairments of social skills or intelligence. Neurodevelopmental disorders often co-occur and have enduring patterns, with serious consequences that go well beyond childhood. We have chosen to describe these disorders in depth because of their high prevalence and because they involve specific challenges in adolescence.

Neurodevelopmental disorders are covered primarily in Chapter 9 of this manual on the SC Axis. For a complete description of each, please refer to the corresponding section of Chapter 9.

SA101 Autism Spectrum Disorder

ASD is a complex neurodevelopmental disorder characterized by qualitative impairment in social interaction, language, and communication, and by restricted interests and repetitive stereotyped behaviors. These symptoms are present from early childhood and cause severe limitation in several key areas of functioning. Manifestations vary greatly depending on the severity of cardinal symptoms, current language and intellectual ability, onset age and pattern, and concurrent genetic/medical or environmental/acquired conditions. DSM-5 explicitly recognizes the "spectrum" nature of autism—subsuming the DSM-IV pervasive developmental disorder categorical subgroups of autistic disorder, Asperger's disorder, Rett's disorder, pervasive developmental disorder not otherwise specified, and childhood disintegrative disorder, and placing them under the single umbrella term of ASD. DSM-5 has thus highlighted the dimensional nature of the cardinal behavioral domains of autistic psychologies and underlined their heterogeneity. The introduction of the notion of diagnostic specifiers speaks for the value of an individualized assessment of needs in designing therapeutic interventions.

The developmental trajectory for individuals with ASD is neither uniform nor linearly ascending. Adolescents on the spectrum display varying patterns of improvement into adolescence and early adulthood, although they continue to display behavioral characteristics of autism. Overall, such adolescents show improvements in communication and decreases in challenges related to stereotyped movements and patterns of behaviors. Impairments in social communication tend to persist into adolescence. Developmental trajectories depend on the severity of the disorder, language and intellectual levels, and the history of treatment interventions.

The Subjective Experience of ASD in Adolescence

Children with ASD are confronted with difficult challenges as they enter adolescence. Separation from the family, construction of a personal identity, opening to social relationships, and access to sexuality are particularly challenging to them.

Affective States

Adolescents with ASD may experience a range of anxious symptoms, including physiological arousal, separation anxiety, panic, and social anxiety. Anxiety is thought to increase during adolescence as teens on the spectrum, especially those without intellectual disabilities, become more aware of their differences from peers. Because adolescents with autistic patterns may not be able to recognize and describe how they feel, anxiety can be difficult to diagnose. Parents and care providers need to recognize diverse signs of anxiety, including changes in behaviors such as sleep patterns and eating habits, worry or rumination, withdrawal from normal daily activities, and increases in repetitive or destructive behaviors. Once an anxiety response is triggered, individuals with ASD can have difficulty controlling it. Anxiety can be debilitating, affecting individuals across environmental contexts. Relationships between social skill deficits and social anxiety can be reciprocal: Adolescents with poor social skills are likely to experience negative peer interactions, which may then lead to fear and distress about subsequent social interactions, resulting in avoidance and withdrawal. This behavior then limits opportunities to acquire social skills through exposure to social situations, thereby leading to social skill deficits.

Depression is also common among adolescents diagnosed with ASD. Studies of parent reports of depressed mood show a rate as high as 50% (Schall & McDonough, 2010). Emerging research finds an increased risk for suicidal thoughts and tendencies among teens with diagnosed ASD. As with anxiety, recognizing depression in autistic adolescents can be challenging, as some characteristics of ASD (e.g., decreased interactions with peers and reduced emotional expression) resemble signs of depression. Depression may appear as increased moodiness (including anger, irritability, and sadness), reduction of interest in prior favorite activities, and changes in eating and sleep habits.

Cognitive States

Adolescents with ASD, even those whose functioning is relatively good, have a deficit in the domain of social cognitions. They frequently fail to understand the subtleties of interpersonal relationships and are unable to take the point of view of others. They may struggle to understand irony, sarcasm, implicit messages, and other forms of nonliteral language. They are also unable to make inferences about information that is not directly presented. They are unable to use nonverbal means to understand or convey a message. These cognitive problems may hamper the development of social relations and increase their tendency to restrict their interests.

Somatic States

These adolescents may show different somatic signs of anxiety, including trembling hands, breathing difficulties, or stomachaches, especially when confronted with social demands. Sleep problems are common. Adolescents with ASD may be unable to recognize and describe their physiological needs or may express them in unusual ways—especially those with intellectual disabilities, who sometimes fail to react to pain or who express such reactions in behavior. They may ignore their physiological needs when captured by personal interests such as video games or internet surfing.

Relationship Patterns

Impairment in reciprocal social communication is an essential feature of ASD. Longitudinal studies report some improvements in communication but persisting impairments in social interaction in adolescence (Smith, Maenner, & Seltzer, 2012). It is in adolescence that most children with ASD start realizing they are not quite like others—a painful process not only for the adolescents themselves, but also for those who love them. Separation from their families is complicated by the social difficulties they encounter. For those who show an interest in peers, the quality of social interactions will depend on their level of insight. If they are unaware of their shortcomings in reading social cues, they may come across as rude, insulting, or boring. Lacking the ability to judge the depth or sincerity of others, they may become victims of teasing or targets of unscrupulous people wanting to take advantage of them. Adolescents with ASD can become attached to others but have great difficulty forming mature, empathic, reciprocal relationships. They are often oblivious to others' needs and interests and are exceedingly focused on their own. Autistic adolescents may find some true friends among people with common interests and may find their identity in autism via their special skills and knowledge.

In contrast with their slower social development, adolescents with ASD develop physiologically and sexually at the same pace as their peers. They tend, however, to be naive, immature, and inexperienced in sexual matters. The lack of reciprocity sets up a barrier at the first stages of intimacy. If parents and care providers feel uncomfortable talking about sex in general, it is critical that clinicians discuss these topics with these adolescents. Such conversations may involve talking about desires and worries, explaining how to initiate friendships that can lead to socially acceptable sexual relationships, talking about normal behaviors, and setting clear limits on inappropriate behaviors.

Clinical Illustration

A 15-year-old adolescent in the high-functioning range of the autism spectrum was brought by his mother for help with intense social anxiety, complaining of stomach pain in the morning and refusing to go to school. His mother had discovered that at school, some students had started to tease him for his "weird" behaviors, such as talking to himself or collecting tree leaves. His psychiatrist prescribed an antianxiety medication and a social skills group. An intervention in school was organized to explain Steven's difficulties to his peers. He was soon able to return and to function better there.

SA102 Attention-Deficit/Hyperactivity Disorder

ADHD is a neurodevelopmental disorder defined by impairing levels of inattention, disorganization, and/or hyperactivity–impulsivity. In DSM-5, ADHD is included in the chapter on neurodevelopmental disorders, although there are equally strong arguments (such as shared risk factors and high comorbidity) for placing it in the chapter on disruptive, impulse-control, and conduct disorders.

The core symptoms required for a diagnosis of ADHD are the same in adolescence as in childhood, but the pattern of symptoms and difficulties may change somewhat (see also the discussion of ADHD in Chapter 9, pp. 586–588). In most individuals with ADHD, symptoms of motor hyperactivity become less obvious in adolescence, but restlessness, inattention, poor planning, and impulsivity persist. Moreover, the difficulties that teens experience as a result of ADHD symptoms, such as poor school performance, may intensify in response to increased demands and expectations for independent functioning. These considerations led the DSM-5 Work Group on ADHD and Disruptive Behavior Disorders to raise the age requirement for the presence of significant symptoms to "prior to age 12 years." ADHD symptoms may in fact become problematic when increasing demands for autonomy, responsibility, and academic performance exceed an adolescent's adaptive capacities.

Some of the more pronounced symptoms in teens with ADHD (e.g., poor time management, procrastination, poor motivation, and difficulties sustaining attention) relate to deficits in executive functioning (Snyder, Miyake, & Hankin, 2015). Executive functioning allows individuals to foresee long-term consequences for actions, plan accordingly, evaluate progress, and shift plans as necessary. The development of executive function is related to the maturation of the frontal network that peaks during adolescence and young adulthood. Neuroimaging studies have shown that adolescents with ADHD have a delayed maturation of frontal networks that parallel their deficits on executive tasks.

In addition to such difficulties, adolescents with ADHD may exhibit lower frustration tolerance, more excessive emotional responses, or less emotional maturity than their peers. The disorder is relatively stable through early adolescence, but some individuals have a declining course, with the development of antisocial behaviors and substance misuse. In many children with ADHD, symptoms persist through adolescence, with resulting impairments of personal, social, academic, and occupational functioning.

The Subjective Experience of ADHD in Adolescence

Affective States and Cognitive Patterns

In adolescents with ADHD, the sense of self is frequently distorted by the cumulative effects of the symptoms and the negative responses they have elicited over the years. Studies of the personal narratives of these adolescents note their tendency to define themselves in terms of their ADHD traits and symptoms—a phenomenon that Krueger and Kendall (2001) labeled the "ADHD-defined self." That is, they seem to develop an identity that incorporates many of the stigmatizing beliefs and negative attributes of ADHD. Their ability to maintain a cohesive self often dissolves into anger and aggression as pressures from others increase. Their self-descriptions are frequently centered on feelings of disappointment and dissatisfaction with disruptive situations. Teenage girls with ADHD report feelings of inadequacy and self-deprecation, whereas boys may show increased anger and frustration.

Teens with ADHD may also experience stigma or embarrassment related to their diagnosis. They may feel different from their peers, and they may wish to believe that their symptoms have faded or disappeared with age. Such wishful beliefs can lead to their interrupting medications or dismissing psychoeducational interventions. Lack of confidence and low self-esteem may also leave teenagers with ADHD more vulnerable to peer pressures toward drug use and other high-risk behaviors. Such adolescents are consequently at higher risk than other adolescents in regulating their impulses, even when they know that their behaviors are self-destructive.

Somatic States

Somatic states experienced by adolescents with ADHD vary, largely depending on whether they are or are not on medication. Independent of medication, they are not always aware of their somatic states and their difficulties in regulating excitation. They frequently rely on comments from others to regulate their behaviors. When they grow up, they progressively improve their capacity to identify their somatic states. They can then better describe their excess of energy or their difficulties with control: "I can't control the way my brain works." Although hyperactivity tends to decline during adolescence, teens may perceive an inner feeling of jitteriness, restlessness, or impatience. Sleep patterns may be chaotic, with delayed sleep onset and difficulties in waking. A pattern of sleeping late may be the consequence of bad habits such as late-night internet use, but adolescents with ADHD may seek this rhythm because at night there is less stimulation that distracts from their preferred activities.

Adolescents in treatment may vary greatly in how they experience the positive and negative effects of medication. Many report that medication fosters improvements in their academic performance and social interactions, with "secondary" benefits such as building their confidence. But they also frequently report unwanted side effects, including difficulty sleeping, low appetite, mood swings, stomachaches, and headaches. Asking specific questions about side effects of the medication is invaluable to establish optimal dosages.

A central concern of some adolescents is the change in their subjective experience when they are on ADHD medications. They may feel less sociable or outgoing and less creative, as if the drugs have reduced the exuberance that is part of their identity. This experience can lead them to stop taking their medication, despite its positive effects on several aspects of their life. Adolescents in general, and those with ADHD in particular, are striving for independence and are present-oriented. Helping them become independent in managing medications, and teaching them effective self-management strategies, can increase their sense of agency.

Relationship Patterns

The relationships of adolescents with ADHD are often inconsistent, and interactions that are mutual and continuous may be hard to maintain. These young people are frequently self-centered and focused primarily on their own gratification. They may lack reciprocity with others. Their insight may be weak, with a tendency to attribute responsibility to others. Their difficulty in attending to social cues and organizing their behavior accordingly results in negative interactions at home and in school. Family relationships may be conflictful. Peer relationships are often disrupted by peer rejection, neglect, or teasing. Psychotherapy may be critical in helping adolescents with ADHD to stabilize their sense of self and to develop a sense of personal responsibility and an increased capacity for empathy.

Clinical Illustration

A 15-year-old boy was brought for consultation by his parents because he could no longer keep up with his class. He was unable to focus on assignments, was falling behind in homework, and was beginning to have learning gaps. He appeared tired and irritable. In fourth grade, he had been diagnosed with ADHD and had taken a stimulant medication for 3 years. He had earned grades slightly above average without any special services. He described himself as slow to write; he found it hard to take notes while listening to the teacher, and so he often missed parts of lessons. At home, he had problems in homework organization and time management. He was feeling exhausted and thinking of giving up on school.

SA103 Specific Learning Disorders

Specific learning disorders are also discussed in Chapter 9 (see pp. 591–597).

In DSM-5, specific learning disorder is a diagnostic category characterized by particular deficits in the basic cognitive mecanisms related to understanding or using written and/or spoken language or mathematics. As a result of these deficits, individuals have persistent and significant difficulty learning foundational academic skills, including listening, written expression, basic reading skills, mathematical calculation, and mathematical reasoning. Performance of the affected academic skills is well below average, or acceptable performance levels are achieved only with extraordinary effort. The learning difficulties are considered "specific" because they are not attributable to intellectual disabilities, to sensory or neurological problems, to psychosocial adversity, or to inadequate educational instruction.

Specific learning disorders are believed to arise from the interaction of genetic, epigenetic, and environmental factors that affect the brain's ability to perceive or process information efficiently and accurately. There are no known biological markers of these disorders. Neurocognitive, neuroimaging, or genetic testing is not useful for the diagnosis, which is instead based on performance tests. Generally, the learning difficulties are readily apparent in the early school years. In some children, however, they may not fully manifest themselves until the later school years, by which time learning demands have increased and exceed the person's limited capacities. For all individuals, specific learning disorders can produce lifelong impairments in activities dependent on the skills that are problematic and can interfere with later occupational performance.

Adolescents with specific learning disorders may perform daily activities in unconventional ways; thus they may not fully conform with ordinary classroom environments. They frequently encounter difficulties during their years in school and report lower self-esteem, less emotional support, and more problems with academic and emotional adjustment than peers without these disorders. They may also feel profound social isolation. Longitudinal studies have shown that emotional and behavioral disorders appear 2–3 years after the emergence of specific learning disorders, suggesting a possible causal link between learning disorders and emotional problems (Ingesson, 2007). This link is probably mediated by the quality of the self-image that an adolescent develops over time.

The Subjective Experience of Specific Learning Disorders in Adolescence

Affective States and Cognitive Patterns

According to Harter's (1999) model of self-development, an essential feature of the learning process is the feeling of mastery. The cognitive jubilation that a child experiences when experiencing success, and the narcissistic rewards that go with such experiences, are fundamental features of the motivation to learn. The perception of one's own competence deeply affects one's interest in an activity and one's subsequent efforts to attain competence in it. As a consequence of their repetitive failures, adolescents with specific learning disorders develop a negative evaluation of their competence. Avoidance of learning activities, for fear of failing and of criticisms from others, limits training opportunities and reduces the potential for improving one's competence. This may have strong effects on self-development, beyond the specific domain of competence.

Adolescents with specific learning disorders are characterized by inefficiencies in their learning procedures that oblige them to exert constant vigilance, for which they pay a high price in terms of fatigue. When there are additional attentional difficulties, performance further deteriorates, with a negative perception of the learning activity and a possible general refusal of all knowledge. But adolescents react differently to specific learning disorders. There are two basic response groups among adolescents: those who comply with the unwritten school "contract" and those who reject it.

In the first case, suffering is intense. These adolescents maintain the goal of academic success and value knowledge, but they realize the impact of their disability. The feeling of responsibility for their failures dominates their inner lives. An internal logic captures those who identify themselves with failure and, in conformance with the model of learned helplessness, anticipate future failures. The devaluation and demoralization often result in anxious and depressive suffering, a sense of paralysis, or a general inability to engage in learning activities. This may take the form of inhibition or passivity.

For adolescents who refuse the school contract, the suffering is less evident and experienced more by the environment. These individuals can adopt passive oppositional strategies, among which slowness is one of the most glaring. They can sometimes adopt a more provocative attitude as a reaction to feelings of incomprehension and rejection—an attitude that may be amplified by conflicts around school activities. In other cases, the oppositional/provocative attitudes are more severe, with outright refusal of the overall educational system and the appearance of CD. In the first type of response, the emotional and behavioral disorders are linked to the progressive school failure and to the low self-esteem associated with the learning disorders. In the second type of response, disruptive behaviors, which frequently follow early problems with attention and impulsivity, interfere with the subsequent acquisition of learning skills (Trzesniewski, Moffitt, Caspi, Taylor, & Maughan, 2006).

There are some key periods for the development of a child's "learning identity" (i.e., self-perception as an agent of the process of learning academic skills). Self-esteem is especially fragile in the first years of school in children with specific learning disorders, especially before the diagnosis, when feelings of inadequacy and helplessness are paramount. Self-esteem shows a general trend of improvement in adolescence, probably related to better understanding and acceptance of the disorder, adoption of more functional strategies (such as proactive attitudes and compartmentalization of the disabilities), and more adaptive school and professional choices (Ingesson, 2007). Adolescents in an informed, supportive environment (at school or at home) show a more positive self-image (Al-Yagon, 2007; Humphrey, 2002). Several factors have been associated with better outcome: self-awareness/understanding of disorders, self-advocacy/proactive attitudes, and presence and utilization of support systems (peer support and mentorship) (Raskind, Goldberg, Higgins, & Herman, 1999).

Somatic States

Adolescents with specific learning disorders have high levels of anxiety, expressed in performance anxiety, school refusal, or somatic complaints (chronic fatigue and sleep difficulties).

Relationship Patterns

Adolescents with specific learning disorders frequently struggle with dependency issues. As children, they may have had parents who were very involved in supporting them to achieve. With the push toward autonomy, they can become intolerant of parents' and teachers' help, although they may continue to need supervision. They may seek alternative support among peers. The choice of peers, along with the positive or negative role they eventually play, depends on an adolescent's self-confidence and personal resources. In some cases, an adolescent with a learning disorder may develop a strong intimate relationship with a partner that mimics past close experiences with parents.

Clinical Illustration

A 15-year-old boy was admitted after a suicide attempt that followed an argument with his mother. Conflicts between him and his parents about school had been increasing, and he had a highly symbiotic relationship with a girlfriend, about which he was very defensive. He had a history of severe developmental dyslexia. He devalued himself and the school environment, and had growing difficulties with paying attention. He could easily talk about his sadness, anger, and exhaustion concerning his learning disorder. He smoked cannabis to relax from school pressure.

SAApp Appendix: Psychological Experiences That May Require Clinical Attention

SAApp1 Demographic Minority Populations (Ethnic, Cultural, Linguistic, Religious, Political)

The intricate and complex task of understanding a person's inner functioning implies the integration of both individual and cultural dimensions, as long-standing systems are continuously involved in human beings' developmental processes. von Bertalanffy (1968, 1969) construes culture and the self as systems, conceived as "a complex of interacting elements" or a "set of elements standing in interrelation." Culture includes interrelated patterns of behavior reflecting values and beliefs related to individual and social functioning. This view focuses on investigating how selves and cultures affect each other's systemic functioning as they engage in ongoing dynamic interaction.

Human development has many facets, including physical, intellectual, economic, artistic, spiritual, emotional, social, and moral dimensions. Changes that take place in adolescence provide windows of opportunity for the expression and development of different individual attributes. During this long process, adolescents receive multiple cultural messages about what is expected from them (often with gendered formulations). The empirical and clinical literatures typically focus on individual (e.g., temperament), interactional (e.g., parenting behaviors), and relational (e.g., attachment, friendship) levels of analysis. Often forgotten is the role played by cultural beliefs and norms in the interpretation of the acceptability of individual characteristics and the types and ranges of interactions and relationships that are likely or permissible. Social categories such as culture, subculture, and ethnic and religious issues influence children's and parents' functioning by shaping the other ecological systems according to their unique, developmentally relevant characteristics.

Matsumoto (1997) defines culture as the "attitudes, values, beliefs, and behaviors shared by a group of people, communicated from one generation to the next" (p. 5). Cultural systems include predominant values and beliefs, economic and social resources, and available opportunities for personal growth. Rubin (1998) describes the significance of culture with respect to behavioral inhibition. Parents are generally concerned (Mills & Rubin, 1990; Schneider, Attili, Vermigli, & Younger, 1997), and peers often "mark" a child for rejection (Rubin, Chen, & Hymel, 1993), if he or she seems wary of social influence. During late childhood and early adolescence, socially wary children may develop a weak self-image and feel they have poor social skills and peer relationships (Boivin, Hymel, & Bukowski, 1995); two potential "outcomes" for such children are loneliness and depression (Boivin et al., 1995; Rubin, Chen, McDougall, Bowker, & McKinnon, 1995).

In China, however, these findings could not be replicated. In individualistic cultures, such as those in North America and Western Europe, assertive and competitive behaviors are explicity endorsed. Within the more collectivistic Chinese culture, shyness (*hai xiu* in Mandarin) is not regarded as maladaptive (e.g., Chen, Rubin, & Li, 1995). In fact, shy, inhibited behavior appears to be encouraged because group functioning requires restraint, obedience, and submission (e.g., Chen, Rubin, & Li, 1997; Ho & Kang, 1984). Thus parents and teachers describe reticent, quiet children as well behaved (Ho & Kang, 1984). Unlike their Western counterparts, these children think well of themselves and their social relationships. In some cultures, the response to an aggressive act may be to explain to the child why the behavior is unacceptable; in others, physical discipline may be the norm; in yet others, aggression may be ignored or even reinforced (see Segall, Dasen, Berry, & Poortinga, 1990).

Cultural awareness offers not just a way of viewing behavioral and emotional expression, but also a perspective on key concepts of the main theories in Western developmental literature. Fuligni (1998) conducted research with a large group of American adolescents from immigrant and native-born families with Mexican, Chinese, Filipino, and European backgrounds, examining whether parent–child conflict and cohesion during adolescence vary among families with different cultural traditions of parental authority and individual autonomy. Although the results are quite dated today, they showed that adolescents from Mexican, Chinese, and Filipino backgrounds held beliefs and expectations consistent with greater respect for parental authority and lower emphasis on autonomy than those of their European American peers.

Raeff (2004) has explored how developmental psychologists have conceptualized autonomy and connectedness as dichotomous dimensions. Characterizing cultures in such unidimensional terms, she argues, obscures the complexities of both cultural processes and self-development. The clinical and empirical literatures are slowly replacing the dichotomy between autonomy and connectedness with conceptions of autonomy and connectedness as co-occurring, positively coexisting dimensions of self, shaped by cultural values (Grotevant & Cooper, 1998; Guisinger & Blatt, 1994; Turiel, 1996).

Clinicians should consider all cultural systems in which an adolescent is involved: family (with its cultural and spiritual beliefs and practices), community (the nature of neighborhood in terms of resources and culture, as well as safety and other specific conditions), and peer relationships (predominant activities with peers, formal and informal; the nature of peer culture). Encouragement of cultural competence and multicultural training in psychotherapy training programs should increase the effectiveness of psychotherapy, as competence in managing the intersection of race and immigration has been found to be relevant to the therapeutic relationship (Hayes, Owen, & Bieschke, 2015; Tummala-Narra, 2015).

Thus clinicians should do the following:

- Recognize that specific racial and cultural factors influence the treatment process.
- Try to understand and respect each adolescent's cultural surround; be committed to a multilevel understanding of the person, encompassing family, community, helping systems, and culture.
- Consider symptoms from a cultural as well as a clinical perspective.
- Consider that an adolescent may be caught between two cultures—the values of the family versus those of the surrounding society. This may be of special relevance in identity formation, as the adolescent tries to integrate both cultural traditions.

- Incorporate relevant cultural, racial, and economic factors into treatment planning.
- Appreciate that an adolescent's "family" may be different from the Western nuclear family; in many cultures, it includes several generations and extended family relationships.

Clinicians should avoid:

- Failing to recognize the cultural dimension or minimizing its relevance; believing that "one developmental theory fits all," and that "everybody is the same."
- Considering single dimensions as separate from others (biological, emotional, familial, community, cultural).
- Devaluing spirituality and family belief systems. Spirituality may be a foundational support for adolescents in minority populations; statements that devalue spirituality or other pivotal cultural beliefs may alienate adolescents, provoking them to withdraw from treatment.

Ecklund (2012) suggests applying intersectionality theory to patients with multiple cultural group identities. "Intersectionality of identity" refers to how an individual embodies multiple cultural, ethnic, and group identities; a child may possess multiple intersecting identities, and the child's family members may each represent intersectionality of identity within the family unit (Mahalingam, Balan, & Haritatos, 2008). Such a perspective allows a therapist to understand simultaneous and multiple influences of the diverse cultural group values, norms, and expectations that contribute to a complex individual identity (Narváez, Meyer, Kertzner, Ouellette, & Gordon, 2009; Shih & Sanchez, 2009).

Enhanced cultural competence in clinicians is linked also with social justice issues, including access to mental health services (Sue, 2001). Ethnic differences influence the rates of retention and engagement in mental health services, and disparities may partly stem from the inability of services to fulfill the needs and expectations of ethnic minority populations (Polo, Alegrìa, & Sirkin, 2012).

Clinical Illustration

A 16-year-old Pakistani Muslim was advised to see a psychologist because of frequent school absences. He said he did not want to leave home anymore because he felt apathetic; specifically, he did not want to attend school ever again. Some boys had begun at lunch to tease him because his religion prohibited his eating certain foods. Although he had support from close friends, he felt in conflict between his religious values and the school context. The therapist tried to help him feel safe to express feelings, fears, needs, desires, and conflicts about the process of reaching an integrated identity.

SAApp2 Lesbian, Gay, and Bisexual Populations

As noted in the corresponding section of Chapter 3 (see pp. 237–240), lesbians, gay men, and bisexual individuals who live in stigmatizing environments are more routinely subject to "minority stress," including internalized homophobia, that can undermine psychological and relational well-being. Among youth, minority stress can affect the development of sexual identity because of its impact on the coming-out process. Lesbian, gay, and bisexual adolescents are often subjected to stigmatization, victimization, bullying, and cyberbullying. Their early attractions may be associated with beliefs that they are "sick"; feelings of being different from peers; and fear of disappointing the expectations of parents, teachers, or friends. In some cases, antipathy toward one's own same-sex feelings may be externalized by committing violence against peers perceived as gay. Some teenagers *question* their sexual identity, but do not identify themselves either as heterosexual or as lesbian, gay, or bisexual, even when they begin to become aware of their first same-sex attractions.

Given the pervasiveness of heteronormativity and sexism, development in children who grow up to be lesbian, gay, or bisexual is often characterized by "gender confusion" and "gender stress" (Drescher, 1998). In gender confusion, individuals interpret their first same-sex attractions by using gender stereotypes. For example, a girl may think, "Since I'm attracted to women, then I'm a man," or a boy may think, "Since I'm attracted to men, then I'm a woman." Self-stigmatizing responses such "I am depraved," "I will be alone," or "I am a sinner" may also be present. Gender stress can occur over a protracted period, as early same-sex attractions and feelings get linked to other gender-nonconforming interests, and as individuals come to realize they are failing to meet the cultural and social expectations of their assigned gender. Lesbian, gay, and bisexual adults, whether gender-conforming or nonconforming as children, recall gender stress in their attempts to integrate their early homoerotic feelings into their gender identity.

"Homonegativity" is pervasive in a variety of contexts; most youths are exposed to its effects. In school environments, homonegative bullying ranges from ridicule of gay people to disapproval and even violent attacks. In contrast to other types of bullying, homophobic bullying has several unique presentations, primarily because gender and sexuality are essential parts of identity (Lingiardi & Nardelli, 2014; Rivers, 2011). Moreover, sexual minority youths are subject to an increased risk of being bullied, compared with their heterosexual peers (Evans & Chapman, 2014). The internet and social media bring a higher risk of cyberbullying, which is often more insidious and more difficult to control, as it often relies on anonymity and has a far wider reach among bystanders (Cooper & Blumenfeld, 2012).

Sometimes an adolescent's family may be an additional source of discomfort and stress. Family rejection can interfere with developmental pathways and lead to negative health outcomes, including suicidal behaviors (Ryan, Huebner, Diaz, & Sanchez, 2009). In worst-case scenarios, some parents have thrown their children out of their homes when they learn of the children's sexual identity.

As noted in Chapter 3, coming out to family may be followed by a stage of crisis and then by a "new homeostasis." In such cases, communication and family and social relationships may become more authentic and promote the exchange of new and more empathetic feelings. Practitioners should evaluate as fully as possible the costs and benefits, as well as risk and protective factors, when helping adolescents decide how and when to disclose their sexual orientation. Some studies show that having a best friend offers the opportunity to share experiences related to a lesbian, gay, or bisexual identity and constitutes a protective factor against adverse family reactions and, more generally, against minority stress (Baiocco, Laghi, Di Pomponio, & Nigito, 2012). One should monitor any possible obstacle (e.g., family and social) to the evolving processes of self-discovery (Adelson & American Academy of Child and Adolescent Psychiatry Committee on Quality Issues, 2012; Lingiardi, Nardelli, & Drescher, 2015). We should note that although teenagers today have the ability to retrieve information from the internet about issues of sexual minorities, as well as information about HIV and other sexually transmitted diseases, they can also use the internet to engage more easily in multiple, anonymous sexual encounters.

Several frameworks purport to explain the development of lesbian, gay, and bisexual identities. They include stages of development from an initial confusion about sexual identity, to increasing integration, through stages of exploration and acceptance. These models have been criticized for being too rigid, linear, and simplistic, however, and for not taking into account differences between the various sexual minority identities and individual difficulties in integrating the many facets of identity (ethnicity, gender, religion, etc.). But such models may be useful in their generalizations about four typical but not universal age ranges in the development of sexual minority identities in adolescents: (1) initial awareness of same-sex sexual attraction (7–12 years); (2) initiation of same-sex sexual activity (13–18 years); (3) self-identification as gay, lesbian, or bisexual (14–18 years); and (4) disclosure to a significant other that one is gay, lesbian, or bisexual (15–19 years) (Mustanski, Kuper, & Greene, 2014).

A clinician should obtain an adolescent's history without presuming heterosexuality—asking, for example, "Is there someone special in your life?" rather than "Do you have a boyfriend/girlfriend?"

Clinical Illustration

A 16-year-old boy told his therapist:

> "I never questioned my heterosexuality until I felt turned on by another guy at my new school. I thought, 'There's no way I'm gay. I still dig girls, and sissy boys disgust me.' But I can't stop thinking about that guy. I hate him. But I feel angry and confused. I remember my parents making fun of a gay couple who lived in our neighborhood. I feel their disapproval aimed at me now."

SAApp3 Gender Incongruence

As noted in Chapter 3 (pp. 240–244), gender incongruence is characterized by marked and persistent lack of conformity between an individual's *experienced* (subjective sense of) gender and the *birth-assigned* (natal) gender.

Gender incongruence has been labeled in DSM-5 as gender dysphoria, replacing the previous diagnosis of gender identity disorder. This modification reflects a change in conceptualization of the disorder's defining features by emphasizing the phenomenon of gender incongruence rather than cross-gender identification per se. With this change in DSM, a cross-gender identity itself is no longer considered pathological. Instead, the focus is on the distress stemming from the incongruence between a person's inner perception of gender and an incongruous bodily reality and assigned gender. DSM-5 identifies two separate sets of criteria: one for children and one for adults and adolescents.

Several studies indicate that the more intense a child's gender incongruence is before puberty, the more likely it is to persist into adolescence; when gender incongruence intensifies in adolescence, the likelihood of long-term gender incongruence increases. In most children, however, gender incongruence does not persist into adolescence; in such cases, the youth are referred to as "desisters." The majority of those who desist before or during early adolescence grow up to be gay, lesbian, or bisexual rather than transgender; a smaller proportion grow up to be heterosexual. Adolescents with gender incongruence may be either "androphilic" (attracted to men) or "gynephilic" (attracted to women). Some are bisexual.

Because psychotherapeutic approaches have not proven successful in relieving gender incongruence, social, juridical, medical, and surgical gender reassignment is currently the treatment of choice. Gender reassignment with hormonal and/or surgical treatment has been reported to improve the social, psychological, and sexual well-being and functioning of gender-incongruent adolescents.

In contrast to the situation in the last century, today's transgender youth may have access to early medical intervention to alleviate gender incongruence. Progressive and accepting communities are increasingly creating safe spaces; positive transgender role models and networks of families with gender-variant children may be available (Institute of Medicine, 2011). Although many adolescents have a strong, persistent wish for gender reassignment, those seeking treatment for gender incongruence are a heterogeneous group. Some are ambivalent about reassignment; others may have concerns secondary to a coexisting gender condition (American Psychological Association, 2015; Cohen-Kettenis & Klink, 2015; de Vries, Cohen-Kettenis, & Delemarre-van de Waal, 2006; Drescher & Byne, 2012).

Often parents wish to know what a gender-variant child's eventual sexual and gender identity will be. It may be preferable to tell the youngster that it is too early to know which way development will unfold, rather than referring to gender-atypical behaviors and feelings as a "phase"—a response that may feel disapproving or minimizing. It may also be useful to explore what the child's gender-atypical presentation means (Adelson & American Academy of Child and Adolescent Psychiatry Committee on Quality Issues, 2012), and to educate youth and families about possibilities and limitations of different treatment approaches. Feeling accepted and free to talk can bring considerable relief to everyone. An interdisciplinary approach is strongly recommended. Mental health professionals should cooperate with a pediatric endocrinologist when reassignment treatment is needed (World Professional Association for Transgender Health [WPATH], 2011).

When childhood gender incongruence continues into adolescence, individuals may undergo puberty suppression and then later seek cross-hormonal and surgical treatment (such youth are referred to as "persisters"). In some cases, the incongruence desists only after puberty is suppressed; the treatment is stopped, and the child goes on to have a delayed puberty. As noted in the corresponding section of Chapter 9 (pp. 606–608), while there is no clinical consensus about the treatment of prepubertal children, the three clinical approaches outlined in that section all offer puberty suppression to children when clinically indicated—either to "buy time," in case the child desists after puberty or to prevent the development of secondary sex characteristics in those who persist. Gender incongruence first presenting in adolescence (late onset) usually does not come to clinical attention before puberty and is unlikely to desist, making gender reassignment often the treatment of choice.

The core features of gender incongruence in adolescents are the discrepancy between experienced gender and assigned gender and the subjective distress that this discrepancy produces. Adolescents with gender incongruence vary in how they experience and manage this discrepancy. Some have intense distress about the incongruence, and expect that clinicians will provide them with hormones and gender reassignment surgery as quickly as possible. Others feel only some unease or confusion about their gender identity and try to find ways to live with these feelings. There are also huge differences among adolescents in their ability to handle the complexities and adversities that often accompany gender variance. The ways the environment has responded to their gender-variant behavior can range from accepting and supporting to rejecting and stigmatizing.

In recent years, thanks mainly to the internet, many youth with gender incongruence have been coming to gender clinics with the clear aim of puberty suppression and gender reassignment (i.e., cross-sex hormone treatment and surgery). Many have a broad range of coexisting psychiatric problems, with anxiety and depressive disorders being the most common. As in adult gender clinics, nonclassic presentations are frequent, and there is an increasing need for detailed diagnoses and psychological treatments. As formalized in the Netherlands, decisions about gender reassignment in adolescence should be made only after a comprehensive medical and psychological evaluation (de Vries & Cohen-Kettenis, 2012).

The Subjective Experience of Gender Incongruence in Adolescence

Affective States

Affective states include anxious and depressed moods. Especially with the onset of secondary sexual characteristics, there may be feelings of hopelessness and suicidal thoughts. The discomfort may be relieved when an adolescent is permitted to express the experienced gender (e.g., wearing clothing associated with the experienced gender).

Cognitive Patterns

Cognitive patterns include preoccupations with gender, which usually disappear if and when transition services are available and provided. Change of first name and pronouns may be desired. ASD may be present and require a differential diagnosis because cross-gender identity may also be part of the rigid convictions that are typical for autism.

Somatic States

Somatic states may include extreme discomfort with one's own physical sexual characteristics. Actual and anticipated body characteristics may evoke dismay. Attempts to hide one's physical sexual characteristics are common: Natal girls may bind their breasts, and natal boys may bind their genitals to make erections less visible. If sexually active, they may exclude their primary sex characteristics from lovemaking.

Relationship Patterns

Relationship patterns vary. Adolescents may encounter social difficulties, often within school contexts, with gender-atypical interests leading to social isolation. They may also experience various kinds of discrimination (e.g., both transphobic and homophobic bullying). Sometimes their own families victimize them. Increasingly, progressive communities are creating safe spaces for them.

TABLE 6.2. Concordance of PDM-2 and DSM-5/ICD-10 Diagnostic Categories for Adolescents

PDM-2

SA0 Healthy responses
SA01 Developmental and situational crises

PDM-2

SA1 Predominantly psychotic disorders
SA11 Brief psychotic disorder
SA14 Schizophrenia and schizoaffective disorder

ICD-10	DSM-5
F20–29. Schizophrenia, schizotypal, and delusional disorders	Schizophrenia spectrum and other psychotic disorders
F23. Acute and transient psychotic disorders	F23. Brief psychotic disorder
F20. Schizophrenia	F20.81. Schizophreniform disorder
F25. Schizoaffective disorder	F20.9. Schizophrenia
	F25. Schizoaffective disorder

PDM-2

SA2 Mood disorders
SA22 Depressive disorders
SA24 Bipolar disorders
SA26 Disruptive mood dysregulation disorder
SA27 Suicidality
SA28 Nonsuicidal self-injury

ICD-10	DSM-5
F30–39. Mood (affective) disorders	Depressive disorders
F32. Depressive episode	F32. Major depressive disorder
F33. Recurrent depressive disorder	F34.8. Disruptive mood dysregulation disorder
F31. Bipolar affective disorder	Bipolar and related disorders
F92.0. Depressive conduct disorder	*Conditions for further study.* Suicidal behavior disorder
NB: Depressive conduct disorder is included in F90–98. Behavioral and emotional disorders with onset usually occurring in childhood and adolescence.	*Conditions for further study.* Nonsuicidal self-injury

PDM-2

SA3 Disorders related primarily to anxiety
SA31 Anxiety disorders
SA31.1 Specific phobias
SA31.2 Social phobia
SA31.3 Agoraphobia and panic disorder
SA31.4 Generalized anxiety disorder
SA32 Obsessive–compulsive and related disorders
SA32.1 Obsessive–compulsive disorder
SA32.2 Body dysmorphic disorder

ICD-10	DSM-5
F40. Phobic anxiety disorders	Anxiety disorders
F40.2. Specific (isolated) phobias	F40.2x. Specific phobias
F40.1. Social phobias	F40.10. Social anxiety disorder (social phobia)
F40.0. Agoraphobia	F40.00. Agoraphobia
F41. Other anxiety disorders	F41.0. Panic disorder

(continued)

TABLE 6.2. *(continued)*

ICD-10	DSM-5
F41.0. Panic disorder (episodic paroxysmal anxiety)	F41.1. Generalized anxiety disorder
F41.1. Generalized anxiety disorder	Obsessive–compulsive and related disorders
F42. Obsessive–compulsive disorder	F42. Obsessive–compulsive disorder
	F45.22. Body dysmorphic disorder

PDM-2

SA4 Event- and stressor-related disorders
- SA41 Trauma- and stressor-related disorders
  - SA41.1 Adjustment disorders
  - SA41.2 Acute and posttraumatic stress disorders
  - SA41.3 Complex posttraumatic stress disorder
- SA42 Dissociative disorders
- SA43 Conversion disorder

ICD-10	DSM-5
F43. Reaction to severe stress and adjustment disorders	Trauma- and stressor-related disorders
F43.2. Adjustment disorders	F43.2. Adjustment disorders
F43.0. Acute stress reaction	F43.0. Acute stress disorder
F43.1. Posttraumatic stress disorder	F43.10. Posttraumatic stress disorder
F44. Dissociative (conversion) disorders	Dissociative disorders
F44.0. Dissociative amnesia	F48.1. Depersonalization/derealization disorder
F44.8. Other dissociative (conversion) disorders	F44.0. Dissociative amnesia
F44.81. Multiple personality disorder	F44.81. Dissociative identity disorder
F44.4. Dissociative motor disorders	F44.4–.7. Conversion disorder
F44.5. Dissociative convulsions	*NB: Conversion disorder is included in F45 Somatic symptom and related disorders.*
F44.6. Dissociative anaesthesia and sensory loss	
F44.7. Mixed dissociative [conversion] disorders	
F48.1. Depersonalization–derealization syndrome	
NB: This syndrome is included in F48. Other neurotic disorders.	

PDM-2

SA5 Somatic symptom and related disorders
- SA51 Somatic symptom disorder
- SA52 Illness anxiety disorder (hypochondriasis)
- SA53 Factitious disorders

ICD-10	DSM-5
F45. Somatoform disorders	Somatic symptom and related disorders
F45.0. Somatization disorder	F45.1. Somatic symptom disorder
F45.2. Hypochondriacal disorder	F45.21. Illness anxiety disorder
F68.1. Intentional production or feigning of symptoms or disabilities, either physical or psychological (factitious disorder)	F68.10. Factitious disorders
NB: Factitious disorder is included in F68. Other disorders of adult personality and behaviour.	

(continued)

TABLE 6.2. *(continued)*

ICD-10	DSM-5
PDM-2	
SA8 Psychophysiological disorders SA81 Feeding and eating disorders	
F50. Eating disorders F50.0. Anorexia nervosa F50.2. Bulimia nervosa	Feeding and eating disorders F50.01–.02. Anorexia nervosa F50.2. Bulimia nervosa F50.8. Binge-eating disorder
PDM-2	
SA9 Disruptive behavior disorders SA91 Conduct disorder SA92 Oppositional defiant disorder SA93 Substance-related disorders SA94 Internet addiction disorder	
F90–98. Behavioural and emotional disorders with onset usually occurring in childhood and adolescence F91. Conduct disorders F91.3. Oppositional defiant disorder	Disruptive, impulse-control, and conduct disorders F91.2. Conduct disorder (adolescent-onset type) F91.3. Oppositional defiant disorder
F10–19. Mental and behavioural disorders due to psychoactive substance use	Substance-related and addictive disorders *Conditions for further study.* Internet gaming disorder
PDM-2	
SA10 Patterns in adolescence of infancy/childhood-onset disorders SA101 Autism spectrum disorder SA102 Attention-deficit/hyperactivity disorder SA103 Specific learning disorders	
F84. Pervasive developmental disorders F84.0. Childhood autism	Neurodevelopmental disorders F84.0. Autism spectrum disorder
NB: See Chapter 9 on the SC Axis. F81. Specific developmental disorders of scholastic skills F81.0. Specific reading disorder F81.2. Specific disorder of arithmetical skills F81.1. Specific spelling disorder F90.0. Disturbance of activity and attention	F81. Specific learning disorder F81.0. With impairment in reading F81.2. With impairment in mathematics F81.81. With impairment in written expression F90. Attention-deficit/hyperactivity disorder
PDM-2	
SAApp Appendix: Psychological experiences that may require clinical attention SAApp1 Demographic minority populations (ethnic, cultural, linguistic, religious, political) SAApp2 Lesbian, gay, and bisexual populations SAApp3 Gender incongruence	
F64. Gender identity disorders F64.0. Transsexualism F64.1. Dual-role transvestism F64.8. Other gender identity disorders	F64. Gender dysphoria F64.1. Gender dysphoria in adolescents and adults

The Subjective Experience of the Therapist

Subjective experiences of the clinician (countertransference) may range from lack of acceptance of gender incongruence and an adolescent's wish to make a gender transition to uncritical acceptance of the stated gender preference without considering alternative explanations (differential diagnosis).

Clinical Illustration

A 14-year-old natal girl has been a tomboy since age 6; s/he was always more comfortable playing with boys, though s/he was often socially isolated from both boys and girls. When s/he was a young child, the pediatrician advised her parents to discourage male behaviors. At present, s/he has only one friend. In the new school year, s/he started being harassed by peers. The parents are very concerned—especially since s/he has started to ask about surgical gender reassignment and asked to be called Alex. At the same time, s/he does not want to be addressed by masculine pronouns. The mother continues to try to discourage the cross-gender interests, while the father thinks they should try to better understand how to help by consulting a clinical psychologist specializing in gender incongruence.

BIBLIOGRAPHY

General Bibliography

American Psychiatric Association. (2013). *Diagnostic and statistical manual of mental disorders* (5th ed.). Arlington, VA: Author.

Blatt, S. J., Quinlan, D. M., Pilkonis, P. A., & Shea, M. T. (1995). Impact of perfectionism and need for approval on the brief treatment of depression: The National Institute of Mental Health Treatment of Depression Collaborative Research Program revisited. *Journal of Consulting and Clinical Psychology, 63*(1), 125–132.

Fonagy, P., & Target, M. (2002). The place of psychodynamic theory in developmental psychopathology. *Development and Psychopathology, 12*, 407–425.

McCallum, M., Piper, W. E., Ogrodniczuk, J. S., & Joyce, A. S. (2003). Relationships among psychological mindedness, alexithymia and outcome in four forms of short term psychotherapy. *Psychology and Psychotherapy: Theory, Research and Practice, 76*, 133–144.

Patalay, P., Fonagy, P., Deighton, J., Belsky, J., Vostanis, P., & Wolpert, M. (2015). A general psychopathology factor in early adolescence. *British Journal of Psychiatry, 207*(1), 15–22.

Rasic, D. (2010). Countertransference in child and adolescent psychiatry: A forgotten concept? *Journal of the Canadian Academy of Child and Adolescent Psychiatry, 19*(4), 249–254.

Tompson, M. C., Boger, K. D., & Asarnow, J. R. (2012). Enhancing the developmental appropriateness of treatment for depression in youth: Integrating the family in treatment. *Child and Adolescent Psychiatric Clinics of North America, 21*(3), 345–384.

Winnicott, D. W. (1969). The use of an object. *International Journal of Psycho-Analysis, 50*, 711–716.

World Health Organization. (1992). *The ICD-10 classification of mental and behavioural disorders: Clinical descriptions and diagnostic guidelines.* Geneva: Author.

SA1 Predominantly Psychotic Disorders

Abidi, S. (2013). Psychosis in children and youth: Focus on early-onset schizophrenia. *Pediatrics in Review, 34*(7), 296–305.

Byrne, R., & Morrison, A. P. (2010). Young people at risk of psychosis: A user-led exploration of interpersonal relationships and communication of psychological difficulties. *Early Intervention in Psychiatry, 4*(2), 162–168.

Cannon, T. D., Cornblatt, B., & McGorry, P. (2007). The empirical status of the ultra high-risk (prodromal) research paradigm. *Schizophrenia Bulletin, 33*(3), 661–664.

Cohen, D., Nicolas, J. D., Flament, M. F., Perisse, D., Dubos, P. F., Bonnot, O., . . . Mazet, P. (2005). Clinical relevance of chronic catatonic schizophrenia in children and adolescents: Evidence from a prospective naturalistic study. *Schizophrenia Research, 76*(2–3), 301–308.

Compton, M. T., McGlashan, T. H., & McGorry, P. D. (2007). Toward prevention approaches for schizophrenia: An overview of prodromal states, the duration of untreated psychosis, and early intervention paradigms. *Psychiatric Annals, 37*, 340–348.

David, C. N., Greenstein, D., Clasen, L., Gochman, P., Miller, R., Tossell, J. W., . . . Rapoport, J. L. (2011). Childhood onset schizophrenia: High rate of visual hallucinations. *Journal of the American Academy of Child and Adolescent Psychiatry, 50*, 681–686.

Huber, G., Gross, G., Schuttler, R., & Linz, M. (1980). Longitudinal studies of schizophrenic patients. *Schizophrenia Bulletin, 6*(4), 592–605.

Kelleher, I., Connor, D., Clarke, M. C., Devlin, N., Harley, M., & Cannon, M. (2012). Prevalence of psychotic symptoms in childhood and adolescence: A systematic review and meta-analysis of population-based studies. *Psychological Medicine, 42*(9), 1857–1863.

Knock, J., Kline, E., Schiffman, J., Maynard, A., & Reeves, G. (2011). Burdens and difficulties experienced by caregivers of children and adolescents with schizophrenia-spectrum disorders: A qualitative study. *Early Intervention in Psychiatry, 5*(4), 349–354.

Lachman, A. (2014). New developments in diagnosis and treatment update: Schizophrenia/first episode psychosis in children and adolescents. *Journal of Child and Adolescent Mental Health, 26*(2), 109–124.

Magnan, V. (1893). *Des signes physiques intellectuels et moraux de la folie héréditaire: Recherche sur les centres nerveux*. Paris: Masson.

McClellan, J., Stock, S., & American Academy of Child and Adolescent Psychiatry (AACAP) Committee on Quality Issues (CQI). (2013). Practice parameter for the assessment and treatment of children and adolescents with schizophrenia. *Journal of the American Academy of Child and Adolescent Psychiatry, 52*(9), 976–990.

Müller, H., Laier, S., & Bechdolf, A. (2014). Evidence-based psychotherapy for the prevention and treatment of first-episode psychosis. *European Archives of Psychiatry and Clinical Neuroscience, 264*(Suppl. 1), S17–S25.

Nordentoft, M., Rasmussen, J. O., Melau, M., Hjorthøj, C. R., & Thorup, A. A. (2014). How successful are first episode programs?: A review of the evidence for specialized assertive early intervention. *Current Opinion in Psychiatry, 27*(3), 167–172.

Rapado-Castro, M., McGorry, P. D., Yung, A., Calvo, A., & Nelson, B. (2015). Sources of clinical distress in young people at ultra high risk of psychosis. *Schizophrenia Research, 165*(1), 15–21.

Sedel, F., Baumann, N., Turpin, J. C., Lyon-Caen, O., Saudubray, J. M., & Cohen, D. (2007). Psychiatric manifestations revealing inborn errors of metabolism in adolescents and adults. *Journal of Inherited Metabolic Disease, 30*(5), 631–641.

Thompson, E., Millman, Z. B., Okuzawa, N., Mittal, V., DeVylder, J., Skadberg, T., . . . Schiffman, J. (2015). Evidence-based early interventions for individuals at clinical high risk for psychosis: A review of treatment components. *Journal of Nervous and Mental Disease, 203*(5), 342–351.

Trotman, H. D., Holtzman, C. W., Ryan, A. T., Shapiro, D. I., MacDonald, A. N., Goulding, S. M., . . . Walker, E. F. (2013). The development of psychotic disorders in adolescence: A potential role for hormones. *Hormones and Behavior, 64*(2), 411–419.

Vandyk, A. D., & Baker, C. (2012). Qualitative descriptive study exploring schizophrenia and the everyday effect of medication-induced weight gain. *International Journal of Mental Health Nursing, 21*(4), 349–357.

Yung, A. R., & McGorry, P. D. (1996). The initial prodrome in psychosis: Descriptive and qualitative aspects. *Australian and New Zealand Journal of Psychiatry, 30*, 587–599.

Yung, A. R., & McGorry, P. D. (2007). Prediction of psychosis: Setting the stage. *British Journal of Psychiatry, 51*, s1–s8.

Wong, M. M., Chen, E. Y., Lui, S. S., & Tso, S. (2011). Medication adherence and subjective weight perception in patients with first-episode psychotic disorder. *Clinical Schizophrenia and Related Psychoses, 5*(3), 135–141.

Zdanowicz, N., Mees, L., Jacques, D., Tordeurs, D., & Reynaert, C. (2014). Assessment and treatment of the risk of psychosis in adolescents: A review. *Psychiatria Danubina, 26*(2), 115–121.

SA2 Mood Disorders

SA22 *Depressive Disorders*

Blatt, S. (1998). Contribution of psychoanalysis to the understanding and treatment of depression. *Journal of the American Psychoanalytic Association, 46*, 722–752.

Blatt, S. J., & Homann, E. (1992). Parent–child interaction in the etiology of dependent and self-critical depression. *Clinical Psychology Review, 12*(1), 47–91.

Blatt, S. J., & Zuroff, D. C. (1992). Interpersonal relatedness and self-definition: Two prototypes for depression. *Clinical Psychology Review, 12*, 527–562.

Dundon, E. E. (2006). Adolescent depression: A metasynthesis. *Journal of Pediatric Health Care, 20*(6), 384–392.

Lachal, J., Speranza, M., Schmitt, A., Spodenkiewicz, M., Falissard, B., Moro, M. R., & Revah-Levy, A. (2012). Depression in adolescence: From qualitative research to measurement. *Adolescent Psychiatry, 2*, 296–308.

Midgley, N., Cregeen, S., Hughes, C., & Rustin, M. (2013). Psychodynamic psychotherapy as treatment for depression in adolescence. *Child and Adolescent Psychiatric Clinics of North America, 22*(1), 67–82.

Midgley, N., Parkinson, S., Holmes, J., Stapley, E., Eatough, V., & Target, M. (2015). Beyond a diagnosis: The experience of depression among clinically-referred adolescents. *Journal of Adolescence, 44*, 269–279.

Pine, D. (2009, April). Report of the DSM-5 Childhood and Adolescent Disorders Work Group. Retrieved from *www.dsm5.org/progressreports/pages/0904reportofthedsm-vchildhoodandadolescentdisordersworkgroup.aspx*.

SA24 *Bipolar Disorders*

Axelson, D., Birmaher, B., Strober, M., Gill, M. K., Valeri, S., Chiappetta, L., . . . Keller, M. (2006). Phenomenology of children and adolescents with bipolar spectrum disorders. *Archives of General Psychiatry, 63*, 1139–1148.

Birmaher, B., Axelson, D., Goldstein, B., Strober, M., Gill, M. K., Hunt, J., . . . Keller, M. (2009). Four-year longitudinal course of children and adolescents with bipolar spectrum disorders: The Course and Outcome of Bipolar Youth (COBY) study. *American Journal of Psychiatry, 166*, 795–804.

Carlson, G. A., & Klein, D. N. (2014). How to understand divergent views on bipolar disorder in youth. *Annual Review of Clinical Psychology, 10*, 529–551.

Carlson, G. A., & Meyer, S. E. (2006). Phenomenology and diagnosis of bipolar disorder in children, adolescents, and adults: Complexities and developmental issues. *Development and Psychopathology, 18*, 939–969.

DeFilippis, M. S., & Wagner, K. D. (2013). Bipolar depression in children and adolescents. *CNS Spectrums, 18*, 209–213.

Grimmer, Y., Hohmann, S., & Poustka, L. (2014). Is bipolar always bipolar?: Understanding the controversy on bipolar disorder in children. *F1000Prime Reports, 1*(6), 111.

SA26 *Disruptive Mood Dysregulation Disorder*

Brotman, M. A., Schmajuk, M., Rich, B. A., Dickstein, D. P., Guyer, A. E., Costello, E. J., . . . Leibenluft, E. (2006). Prevalence, clinical correlates, and longitudinal course of severe mood dysregulation in children. *Biological Psychiatry, 60*, 991–997.

Dougherty, L. R., Smith, V. C., Bufferd, S. J., Carlson, G. A., Stringaris, A., Leibenluft, E., & Klein, D. N. (2014). DSM-5 disruptive mood dysregulation disorder: Correlates and predictors in young children. *Psychological Medicine, 21*, 1–12.

Johnson, K., & McGuinness, T. M. (2014). Disruptive mood dysregulation disorder: A new diagnosis in the DSM-5. *Journal of Psychosocial Nursing and Mental Health Services, 52*(2), 17–20.

Krieger, F. V., & Stringaris, A. (2013). Bipolar disorder and disruptive mood dysregulation in children and adolescents: Assessment, diagnosis and treatment. *Evidence-Based Mental Health, 16*(4), 93–94.

Leibenluft, E. (2011). Severe mood dysregulation, irritability, and the diagnostic boundaries of bipolar disorder in youths. *American Journal of Psychiatry, 168*(2), 129–142.

Roy, A. K., Lopes, V., & Klein, R. G. (2014). Disruptive mood dysregulation disorder: A new diagnostic approach to chronic irritability in youth. *American Journal of Psychiatry, 171*(9), 918–924.

Stringaris, A., Cohen, P., Pine, D. S., & Leibenluft, E. (2009). Adult outcomes of youth irritability: A 20-year prospective community-based study. *American Journal of Psychiatry, 166*, 1048–1054.

SA27 *Suicidality*

Everall, R. D., Bostik, K. E., & Paulson, B. L. (2006). Being in the safety zone: Emotional experiences of suicidal adolescents and emerging adults. *Journal of Adolescent Research, 21*(4), 370–392.

Fazaa, N., & Page, S. (2003). Dependency and self-criticism as predictors of suicidal behavior. *Suicide and Life-Threatening Behavior, 33*(2), 172–185.

Jordan, J., McKenna, H. P., Keeney, S., Cutcliffe, J., Stevenson, C., Slater, P., & McGowan, I. (2012). Providing meaningful care: Learning from the experiences of suicidal young men. *Qualitative Health Research, 22*(9), 1207–1219.

Kaess, M., & Brunner, R. (2012). Prevalence of adolescents' suicide attempts and self-harm thoughts vary across Europe. *Evidence-Based Mental Health, 15*, 66.

Klomek, A. B., Orbach, I., Sher, L., Sommerfeld, E., Diller, R., Apter, A., . . . Zalsman, G. (2008). Quality of depression among suicidal inpatient youth. *Archives of Suicide Research, 12*(2), 133–140.

Lachal, J., Orri, M., Sibeoni, J., Moro, M. R., & Revah-Levy, A. (2015). Metasynthesis of youth suicidal behaviours: Perspectives of youth, parents, and health care professionals. *PLoS ONE, 10*(5), e0127359.

Orbach, I., Mikulincer, M., Blumenson, R., Mester, R., & Stein, D. (1999). The subjective experience of problem irresolvability and suicidal behavior: Dynamics and measurement. *Suicide and Life-Threatening Behavior*, 29(2), 150–164.

Orri, M., Paduanello, M., Lachal, J., Falissard, B. N., Sibeoni, J., & Revah-Levy, A. (2014). Qualitative approach to attempted suicide by adolescents and young adults: The (neglected) role of revenge. *PLoS ONE, 9*(5), e96716.

World Health Organization. (2014). *Preventing suicide: A global imperative.* Geneva: Author.

SA28 *Nonsuicidal Self-Injury*

Dickstein, D. P., Puzia, M. E., Cushman, G. K., Weissman, A. B., Wegbreit, E., Kim, K. L., . . . Spirito, A. (2015). Self-injurious implicit attitudes among adolescent suicide attempters versus those engaged in nonsuicidal self-injury. *Journal of Child Psychology and Psychiatry, 56*(10), 1127–1136.

Fischer, G., Brunner, R., Parzer, P., Resch, F., & Kaess, M. (2013). Short-term psychotherapeutic treatment in adolescents engaging in non-suicidal self-injury: A randomized controlled trial. *Trials, 13*(14), 294.

Glenn, C. R., & Klonsky, E. D. (2013). Nonsuicidal self-injury disorder: An empirical investigation in adolescent psychiatric patients. *Journal of Clinical Child and Adolescent Psychology, 42*(4), 496–507.

Hooley, J. M., & St Germain, S. A. (2013). Nonsuicidal self-injury, pain, and self-criticism: Does changing self-worth change pain endurance in people who engage in self-injury? *Clinical Psychological Science, 2*(3), 297–305.

Klineberg, E., Kelly, M. J., Stansfeld, S. A., & Bhui, K. S. (2013). How do adolescents talk about self-harm: A qualitative study of disclosure in an ethnically diverse urban population in England. *BMC Public Health, 13*, 572.

Klonsky, E. D., Victor, S. E., & Saffer, B. Y. (2014). Nonsuicidal self-injury: What we know, and what we need to know. *Canadian Journal of Psychiatry, 59*(11), 565–568.

Walsh, B. W. (2014). Clinical assessment of self-injury: A practical guide. *Journal of Clinical Psychology, 63*(11), 1057–1068.

Zetterqvist, M., Lundh, L. G., Dahlström, O., & Svedin, C. G. (2013). Prevalence and function of non-suicidal self-injury (NSSI) in a community sample of adolescents, using suggested DSM-5 criteria for a potential NSSI disorder. *Journal of Abnormal Child Psychology, 41*(5), 759–773.

SA3 Disorders Related Primarily to Anxiety

SA31 *Anxiety Disorders*

Bernstein, G. A., & Victor, A. M. (2011). Pediatric anxiety disorders. In K. Cheng & K. M. Myers (Eds.), *Child and adolescent psychiatry: The essentials* (2nd ed., pp. 103–120). Philadelphia: Lippincott Williams & Wilkins.

Cohen Kadosh, K., Haddad, A. D., Heathcote, L. C., Murphy, R. A., Pine, D. S., & Lau, J. Y. (2015). High trait anxiety during adolescence interferes with discriminatory context learning. *Neurobiology of Learning and Memory, 123*, 50–57.

Compton, S. N., Peris, T. S., Almirall, D., Birmaher, B., Sherrill, J., & Kendall, P. C. (2014). Predictors and moderators of treatment response in childhood anxiety disorders: Results from the CAMS trial. *Journal of Consulting and Clinical Psychology, 82*(2), 212–224.

Connolly, S. D., Bernstein, G. A., & Work Group on Quality Issues. (2007). Practice parameter for the assessment and treatment of children and adolescents with anxiety disorders. *Journal of the American Academy of Child and Adolescent Psychiatry, 46*(2), 267–283.

Mohatt, J., Bennett, S. M., & Walkup, J. T. (2014). Treatment of separation, generalized, and social anxiety disorders in youths. *American Journal of Psychiatry, 171*(7), 741–748.

Tassin, C., Reynaert, C., Jacques, D., & Zdanowicz, N. (2014). Anxiety disorders in adolescence. *Psychiatria Danubina, 26*(1), 27–30.

Wehry, A. M., Beesdo-Baum, K., Hennelly, M. M., Connolly, S. D., & Strawn, J. R. (2015). Assessment and treatment of anxiety disorders in children and adolescents. *Current Psychiatry Reports, 17*(7), 591.

SA31.1 *Specific Phobias*

Davis, T. E., Ollendick, T. H., & Öst, L. G. (2009). Intensive treatment of specific phobias in children and adolescents. *Cognitive and Behavioral Practice, 16*(3), 294–303.

SA31.2 *Social Phobia*

Dell'Osso, L., Abelli, M., Pini, S., Carlini, M., Carpita, B., Macchi, E., . . . Massimetti, G. (2014). Dimensional assessment of DSM-5 social anxiety symptoms among university students and its relationship with functional impairment. *Neuropsychiatric Disease and Treatment, 16*(10), 1325–1332.

Hamilton, J. L., Potter, C. M., Olino, T. M., Abramson, L. Y., Heimberg, R. G., & Alloy, L. B. (2016). The temporal sequence of social anxiety and depressive symptoms following interpersonal stressors during adolescence. *Journal of Abnormal Child Psychology, 44*(3), 495–509.

SA31.3 *Agoraphobia and Panic Disorder*

Cornacchio, D., Chou, T., Sacks, H., Pincus, D., & Comer, J. (2015). Clinical consequences of the revised DSM-5 definition of agoraphobia in treatment-seeking anxious youth. *Depression and Anxiety, 32*(7), 502–508.

Creswell, C., Waite, P., & Cooper, P. J. (2014). Assessment and management of anxiety disorders in children and adolescents. *Archives of Disease in Childhood, 99*(7), 674–678.

SA31.4 *Generalized Anxiety Disorder*

Mohatt, J., Bennett, S. M., & Walkup, J. T. (2014). Treatment of separation, generalized, and social anxiety disorders in youths. *American Journal of Psychiatry, 171*(7), 741–748.

Wehry, A. M., Beesdo-Baum, K., Hennelly, M. M., Connolly, S. D., & Strawn, J. R. (2015). Assessment and treatment of anxiety disorders in children and adolescents. *Current Psychiatry Reports, 17*(7), 52.

SA32 *Obsessive–Compulsive and Related Disorders*

SA32.1 *Obsessive–Compulsive Disorder*

Freeman, J., Garcia, A., Frank, H., Benito, K., Conelea, C., Walther, M., & Edmunds, J. (2014). Evidence base update for psychosocial treatments for pediatric obsessive–compulsive disorder. *Journal of Clinical Child and Adolescent Psychology, 43*(1), 7–26.

Krebs, G., & Heyman, I. (2015). Obsessive–compulsive disorder in children and adolescents. *Archives of Disease in Childhood, 100*(5), 495–499.

Rosa-Alcázar, A. I., Sánchez-Meca, J., Rosa-Alcázar, Á., Iniesta-Sepúlveda, M., Olivares-Rodríguez, J., & Parada-Navas, J. L. (2015). Psychological treatment of obsessive–compulsive disorder in children and adolescents: A meta-analysis. *Spanish Journal of Psychology, 18*, E20.

Wells, J. G. (2014). Obsessive–compulsive disorder in youth: Assessment and treatment. *Journal of Clinical Psychiatry, 75*(5), e13.

SA32.1 *Body Dysmorphic Disorder*

Brewster, K. (2011). Body dysmorphic disorder in adolescence: Imagined ugliness. *The School Psychologist*. Retrieved from *www.apadivisions.org/division-16/publications/newsletters/school-psychologist/2011/07/adolescent-dysmorphic-disorder.aspx.*

Buhlmann, U., & Winter, A. (2011). Perceived ugliness: An update on treatment-relevant aspects of body dysmorphic disorder. *Current Psyhiatry Report, 13*, 283–288.

Grant, J. E., Won Kim, S., & Crow, S. J. (2001). Prevalence and clinical features of body dysmorphic disorder in adolescent and adult psychiatric inpatients. *Journal of Clinical Psychiatry, 62*, 517–522.

Phillips, K. A. (2001). Body dysmorphic disorder. In K. A. Phillips (Ed.), *Somatoform and factitious disorders*. Washington, DC: American Psychiatric Publishing.

Phillips, K. A. (2004). Body dysmorphic disorder: Recognizing and treating imagined ugliness. *World Psychiatry, 3*(1), 12–17.

Windheim, K., Veale, D., & Anson, M. (2011). Mirror gazing in body dysmorphic disorder and health controls: Effects of duration of gazing. *Behaviour Research and Therapy, 14*(1), 1–10.

SA4 Event- and Stressor-Related Disorders

SA41 *Trauma- and Stressor-Related Disorders*

SA41.1 *Adjustment Disorders*

Casey, P., & Bailey, S. (2011). Adjustment disorders: The state of the art. *World Psychiatry, 10*(1), 11–18.

Casey, P., & Doherty, A. (2012). Adjustment disorder: Implications for ICD-11 and DSM-5. *British Journal of Psychiatry, 201*, 90–92.

Fernández, A., Mendive, J. M., Salvador-Carulla, L., Rubio-Valera, M., Luciano, J. V., Pinto-Meza, A., . . . Serrano-Blanco, A. (2012). Adjustment disorders in primary care: Prevalence, recognition and use of services. *British Journal of Psychiatry, 201*, 137–142.

Pelkonen, M., Marttunen, M., Henriksson, M., & Lonnqvist, J. (2005). Suicidality in adjustment disorder: Clinical characteristics of adolescent outpatients. *European Child and Adolescent Psychiatry, 14*, 174–180.

SA41.2 *Acute and Posttraumatic Stress Disorders*

Buchanan, N. T., Bluestein, B. M., Nappa, A. C., Woods, K. C., & Depatie, M. M. (2013). Exploring gender differences in body image, eating pathology, and sexual harassment. *Body Image, 10*(3), 352–360.

Freud, S. (1895). Project for a scientific psychology. *Standard Edition, 1*, 283–397.

Guillery-Girard, B., Clochon, P., Giffard, B., Viard, A., Egler, P. J., Baleyte, J. M., . . . Dayan, J. (2013). "Disorganized in time": Impact of bottom-up and top-down negative emotion generation on memory formation among healthy and traumatized adolescents. *Journal of Physiology (Paris), 107*(4), 247–254.

Jackowski, A. P., de Araújo, C. M., de Lacerda, A. L., Mari Jde, J., & Kaufman, J. (2009). Neurostructural imaging findings in children with post-traumatic stress disorder: Brief review. *Psychiatry and Clinical Neurosciences, 63*(1), 1–8.

Mazza, J. J., & Reynolds, W. M. (1999). Exposure to violence in young inner-city adolescents: Relationships with suicidal ideation, depression, and PTSD symptomatology. *Journal of Abnormal Child Psychology, 27*(3), 203–213.

Saul, A. L., Grant, K. E., & Smith Carter, J. (2008). Post-traumatic reactions in adolescents: How well do the DSM-IV PTSD criteria fit the real life experience of trauma exposed youth? *Journal of Abnormal Child Psychology, 36*(6), 915–925.

Scheeringa, M. S., Zeanah, C. H., & Cohen, J. A. (2011). PTSD in children and adolescents: Toward an empirically based algorithma. *Depression and Anxiety, 28*(9), 770–782.

SA41.3 *Complex Posttraumatic Stress Disorder*

Herman, J. (1997). *Trauma and recovery: The aftermath of violence from domestic abuse to political terror* (rev. ed.). New York: Basic Books.

National Center for PTSD. (2016, February 23). Complex PTSD. Retrieved from *www.ptsd.va.gov/professional/PTSD-overview/complex-ptsd.asp.*

Roth, S., Newman, E., Pelcovitz, D., van der Kolk, B., & Mandel, F. S. (1997). Complex PTSD in victims exposed to sexual and physical abuse: Results from the DSM-IV field trial for posttraumatic stress disorder. *Journal of Traumatic Stress, 10*, 539–555.

van der Kolk, B. (2005). Developmental trauma disorder. *Psychiatric Annals, 35*(5), 401–408.

SA42 *Dissociative Disorders*

Atlas, J., Weissman, K., & Liebowitz, S. (1997). Adolescent inpatients' history of abuse and dissociative identity disorder. *Psychological Reports, 80*(3, Pt. 2), 1086.

Brunner, R., Parzer, P., Schuld, V., & Resch, F. (2000). Dissociative symptomatology and traumatogenic factors in adolescent psychiatric patients. *Journal of Nervous and Mental Disease, 188*, 71–77.

Carrion, V. G., & Steiner, H. (2000). Trauma and dissociation in delinquent adolescents. *Journal of the American Academy of Child and Adolescent Psychiatry, 39*, 353–359.

International Society for the Study of Dissociation. (2004). Guidelines for the evaluation and treatment of dissociative symptoms in children and adolescents. *Journal of Trauma and Dissociation, 5*(3), 119–150.

Jang, K. L., Paris, J., Zweig-Frank, H., & Livesley, W. J. (1998). Twin study of dissociative experience. *Journal of Nervous and Mental Disease, 186*, 345–351.

Macfie, J., Cicchetti, D., & Toth, S. L. (2001). The development of dissociation in maltreated preschool-aged children. *Development and Psychopathology, 13*, 233–254.

Putnam, F. W., Hornstein, N. L., & Peterson, G. (1996). Clinical phenomenology of child and adolescent dissociative disorders: Gender and age effects. *Child and Adolescent Psychiatric Clinics of North America, 5*, 351–360.

Sanders, B., & Giolas, M. H. (1991). Dissociation and childhood trauma in psychologically disturbed adolescents. *American Journal of Psychiatry, 148*, 50–54.

Siegel, D. J. (2012). *The developing mind: How relationships and the brain interact to shape who we are* (2nd ed.). New York: Guilford Press.

Stien, P., & Waters, F. S. (1999). *Chronic traumatic stress in children as an etiological factor in the development of obsessive–compulsive disorder and attention-deficit/hyperactivity disorder.* Workshop presented at the 15th Annual Meeting of the International Society for Traumatic Stress, Miami, FL.

SA43 *Conversion Disorder*

Brazier, D. K., & Venning, H. E. (1997). Conversion disorders in adolescents: A practical approach to rehabilitation. *British Journal of Rheumatology, 36*(5), 594–598.

Campo, J. V., & Negrini, B. J. (2000). Case study: Negative reinforcement and behavioural management of conversion disorder. *Journal of the American Academy of Child and Adolescent Psychiatry, 39*, 787–790.

Leary, P. M. (2003). Conversion disorder in childhood—diagnosed too late, investigated too much? *Journal of the Royal Society of Medicine, 96*(9), 436–438.

Pehlivanturk, B., & Unal, F. (2002). Conversion disorder in children and adolescents: A four year follow up study. *Journal of Psychosomatic Research, 52*, 187–191.

SA5 Somatic Symptom and Related Disorders

Garralda, M. E. (1999). Practitioner review: Assessment and management of somatisation in childhood and adolescence: A practical perspective. *Journal of Child Psychology and Psychiatry, 140*, 1159–1167.

Klineberg, E., Rushworth, A., Bibby, H., Bennett, D., Steinbeck, K., & Towns, S. (2014). Adolescent chronic fatigue syndrome and somatoform disorders: A prospective clinical study. *Journal of Pediatrics and Child Health, 50*(10), 775–781.

Schulte, I. E., & Petermann, F. (2011). Somatoform disorders: 30 years of debate about criteria!: What about children and adolescents? *Journal of Psychosomatic Research*, 70(3), 218–228.

SA52 *Illness Anxiety Disorder (Hypochondriasis)*

Ehrlich, S., Pfeiffer, E., Salbach, H., Lenz, K., & Lehmkuhl, U. (2008). Factitious disorder in children and adolescents: A retrospective. *Psychosomatics, 49*(5), 392–398.

Morrell, B., & Tilley, D. S. (2012). The role of nonperpetrating fathers in Munchausen syndrome by proxy: A review of the literature. *Journal of Pediatric Nursing, 27*(4), 328–335.

Sørensen, P., Birket-Smith, M., Wattar, U., Buemann, I., & Salkovskis, P. (2011). A randomized clinical trial of cognitive behavioural therapy versus short-term psychodynamic psychotherapy versus no intervention for patients with hypochondriasis. *Psychological Medicine, 41*, 431–441.

Squires, J. E., & Squires, R. H. (2013). A review of Munchausen syndrome by proxy. *Pediatric Annals, 42*(4), 67–71.

Wicksell, R. K., Melin, L., Lekander, M., & Olsson, G. L. (2009). Evaluating the effectiveness of exposure and acceptance strategies to improve functioning and quality of life in longstanding pediatric pain: A randomized controlled trial. *Pain, 141*(3), 248–257.

SA8 Psychophysiological Disorders

SA81 *Feeding and Eating disorders*

American Psychiatric Association, Work Group on Eating Disorders. (2006). Practice guideline for the treatment of patients with eating disorders, third edition. *American Journal of Psychiatry, 163*(Suppl.), 1–54.

Bruch, H. (1973). *Eating disorders: Obesity, anorexia nervosa, and the person within.* New York: Basic Books.

Demarque, M., Guzman, G., Morrison, E., Ahovi, J., Moro, M. R., & Blanchet-Collet, C. (2015).

Anorexia nervosa in a girl of Chinese origin: Psychological, somatic and transcultural factors. *Clinical Child Psychology and Psychiatry, 20*(2), 276–288.

Findlay, S., Pinzon, J., Taddeo, D., & Katzman, D. K. (2010). Family-based treatment of children and adolescents with anorexia nervosa: Guidelines for the community physician. *Paediatrics and Child Health, 15*(1), 31–35.

Gazzillo, F., Lingiardi, V., Peloso, A., Giordani, S., Vesco, S., Zanna, V., . . . Vicari, S. (2013). Personality subtypes in adolescents with eating disorders. *Comprehensive Psychiatry, 54*(6), 702–712.

Gowers, S., & Bryant-Waugh, R. (2004). Management of child and adolescent eating disorders: The current evidence base and future directions. *Journal of Child Psychology and Psychiatry, 45*, 63–83.

Heatherton, T. F., & Baumeister, R. F. (1991). Binge eating as escape from self-awareness. *Psychological Bulletin, 110*(1), 86–108.

Hoek, H. W. (2006). Incidence, prevalence and mortality of anorexia nervosa and other eating disorders. *Current Opinion in Psychiatry, 19*(4), 389–394.

Milos, G., Spindler, A., & Schnyder, U. (2005). Instability of eating disorder diagnoses: Prospective study. *British Journal of Psychiatry, 187*, 574–578.

Mitchell, J. E., & Crow, S. (2006). Medical complications of anorexia nervosa and bulimia nervosa. *Current Opinion in Psychiatry, 19*(4), 438–443.

National Institute for Clinical Excellence. (2004). *Eating disorders: Core interventions in the treatment and management of anorexia nervosa, bulimia nervosa and related eating disorders* (NICE Clinical Guidelines, No. 9). Leicester, UK: British Psychological Society.

Rasting, M., Brosig, B., & Beutel, M. E. (2005). Alexithymic characteristics and patient therapist interaction: A video analysis of facial affect display. *Psychopathology, 38*, 105–111.

Roux, H., Blanchet, C., Stheneur, C., Chapelon, E., & Godart, N. (2013). Somatic outcome among patients hospitalised for anorexia nervosa in adolescence: Disorders reported and links with global outcome. *Eating and Weight Disorders, 18*(2), 175–182.

Smink, F. R., van Hoeken, D., & Hoek, H. W. (2013). Epidemiology, course, and outcome of eating disorders. *Current Opinion in Psychiatry, 26*(6), 543–548.

Speranza, M., Atger, F., Corcos, M., Loas, G., Guilbaud, O., Stéphan, P., . . . Jeammet, P. (2003). Depressive psychopathology and adverse childhood experiences in eating disorders. *European Psychiatry, 18*(8), 377–383.

Speranza, M., Loas, G., Guilbaud, O., & Corcos, M. (2011). Are treatment options related to alexithymia in eating disorders?: Results from a three-year naturalistic longitudinal study. *Biomedicine and Pharmacotherapy, 65*, 585–589.

Speranza, M., Revah-Levy, A., Gicquel, L., Loas, G., Venisse, J. L., Jeammet, P., & Corcos, M. (2012). An investigation of Goodman's addictive disorder criteria in eating disorders. *European Eating Disorders Review, 20*(3), 182–189.

SA9 Disruptive Behavior Disorders

SA91 *Conduct Disorder*

Baker, R. H., Clanton, R. L., Rogers, J. C., & De Brito, S. A. (2015). Neuroimaging findings in disruptive behavior disorders. *CNS Spectrums, 10*, 1–13.

Blair, R. J., Leibenluft, E., & Pine, D. S. (2015). Conduct disorder and callous–unemotional traits in youth. *New England Journal of Medicine, 371*(23), 2207–2216.

Fairchild, G., van Goozen, S. H., Calder, A. J., & Goodyer, I. M. (2013). Research review: Evaluating and reformulating the developmental taxonomic theory of antisocial behaviour. *Journal of Child Psychology and Psychiatry, 54*(9), 924–940.

Frick, P. J., & Viding, E. (2009). Antisocial behavior from a developmental psychopathology perspective. *Development and Psychopathology, 21*, 1111–1131.

Johnson, A. C. (2015). Developmental pathways to attention-deficit/hyperactivity disorder and disruptive behavior disorders: Investigating the impact of the stress response on executive functioning. *Clinical Psychology Review, 36*, 1–12.

Lewis, R. M., Petch, V., Wilson, N., Fox, S., & Craig, C. E. (2015). Understanding conduct disorder: The ways in which mothers attempt to make sense of their children's behaviour. *Clinical Child Psychology and Psychiatry, 20*(4), 570–584.

Lindsey, L. M. (2015). The challenges for primary caregivers of adolescents with disruptive behavior disorders. *Journal of Family Nursing, 21*(1), 1491–1467.

Polanczyk, G. V., Salum, G. A., Sugaya, L. S., Caye, A., & Rohde, L. A. (2015). Annual research review: A meta-analysis of the worldwide prevalence of mental disorders in children and adolescents. *Journal of Child Psychology and Psychiatry, 56*(3), 345–365.

SA92 *Oppositional Defiant Disorder*

Bateman, A. W., & Fonagy, P. (2012). Antisocial personality disorder. In A. W. Bateman & P. Fonagy (Eds.), *Handbook of mentalizing in mental health practice* (pp. 289–308). Washington, DC: American Psychiatric Publishing.

Keenan, K., & Wakschlag, L. S. (2004). Are oppositional defiant and conduct disorder symptoms normative behaviors in preschoolers?: A comparison of referred and nonreferred children. *American Journal of Psychiatry, 161*(2), 356–358.

Kelsberg, G. (2006). What are effective treatments for oppositional defiant behaviors in adolescents? *Journal of Family Practice, 55*, 10.

Kimonis, E. R., & Frick, P. J. (2010). Oppositional defiant disorder and conduct disorder grown-up. *Journal of Developmental and Behavioral Pediatrics, 31*(3), 244–254.

Lindhiem, O., Bennett, C. B., Hipwell, A. E., & Pardini, D. A. (2015). Beyond symptom counts for diagnosing oppositional defiant disorder and conduct disorder? *Journal of Abnormal Child Psychology, 43*(7), 1379–1387.

Maughan, B., Rowe, R., Messer, J., Goodman, R., & Meltzer, H. (2004). Conduct disorder and oppositional defiant disorder in a national sample: Developmental epidemiology. *Journal of Child Psychology and Psychiatry, 45*(3), 609–621.

Steinberg, E. A., & Drabick, D. A. (2015). A developmental psychopathology perspective on ADHD and comorbid conditions: The role of emotion regulation. *Child Psychiatry and Human Development, 46*(6), 951–966.

SA93 *Substance-Related Disorders*

Clark, D. B., Chung, T., Thatcher, D. L., Pajtek, S., & Long, E. C. (2012). Psychological dysregulation, white matter disorganization and substance use disorders in adolescence. *Addiction, 107*(1), 206–214.

Donovan, J. E (2004). Adolescent alcohol initiation: A review of psychosocial risk factors. *Journal of Adolescent Health, 35*, 529e7–529e18.

Grotstein, J. S. (1986). The psychology of powerlessness: Disorders of self-regulation and interactional regulation as a newer paradigm for psychopathology. *Psychoanalytic Inquiry, 6*, 93–118.

Hammond, C. J., Mayes, L. C., & Potenza, M. N. (2014). Neurobiology of adolescent substance use and addictive behaviors: Treatment implications. *Adolescent Medicine: State of the Art Reviews, 25*(1), 15–32.

Johnston, L. D., Miech, R. A., O'Malley, P. M., Bachman, J. G., & Schulenberg, J. E. (2014, December 16). Use of alcohol, cigarettes, and number of illicit drugs declines among U.S. teens. University of Michigan News Service. Retrieved from *www.monitoringthefuture.org.*

Merikangas, K. R., He, J. P., Burstein, M., Swanson, S. A., Avenevoli, S., Cui, L., . . . Swendsen, J. (2010). Lifetime prevalence of mental disorders in U.S. adolescents: Results from the National Comorbidity Survey Replication—Adolescent Supplement (NCS-A). *Journal of the American Academy of Child and Adolescent Psychiatry, 49*(10), 980–989.

Migliorini, R., Stewart, J. L., May, A. C., Tapert, S. F., & Paulus, M. P. (2013). What do you feel?: Adolescent drug and alcohol users show altered brain response to pleasant interoceptive stimuli. *Drug and Alcohol Dependence, 133*(2), 661–668.

Roberts, R. E., Roberts, C. R., & Xing, Y. (2007). Comorbidity of substance use disorders and other psychiatric disorders among adolescents: Evidence from an epidemiologic survey. *Drug and Alcohol Dependence, 88*(S1), S4–S13.

Tarter, R. E., Kirisci, L., Mezzich, A., Cornelius, J. R., Pajer, K., Vanyukov, M., . . . Clark, D. (2003). Neurobehavioral disinhibition in childhood predicts early age at onset of substance use disorder. *American Journal of Psychiatry, 160*(6), 1078–1085.

Thatcher, D. L., & Clark, D. B. (2008). Adolescents at risk for substance use disorders: Role of psychological dysregulation, endophenotypes, and environmental influences. *Alcohol Research and Health, 31*(2), 168–176.

Titus, J. C., Godley, S. H., & White, M. K. (2006). A post-treatment examination of adolescents' reasons for starting, quitting, and continuing the use of drugs and alcohol. *Journal of Child and Adolescent Substance Abuse, 16*(2), 31–49.

Wetherill, R., & Tapert, S. F. (2013). Adolescent brain development, substance use, and psychotherapeutic change. *Psychology of Addictive Behaviors, 27*(2), 393–402.

Yule, A. M., & Wilens, T. E. (2015). Substance use disorders in adolescents with psychiatric comorbidity: When to screen and how to treat: Consider pharmacotherapy, psychotherapy when treating substance use disorders. *Current Psychiatry, 14*(4), 37–51.

SA94 *Internet Addiction Disorder*

King, D. L., & Delfabbro, P. H. (2014a). The cognitive psychology of internet gaming disorder. *Clinical Psychology Review, 34*(4), 298–308.

King, D. L., & Delfabbro, P. H. (2014b). Internet gaming disorder treatment: A review of definitions of diagnosis and treatment outcome. *Journal of Clinical Psychology, 70*(10), 942–955.

King, D. L., Haagsma, M. C., Delfabbro, P. H.,

Gradisar, M., & Griffiths, M. D. (2013). Toward a consensus definition of pathological video-gaming: A systematic review of psychometric assessment tools. *Clinical Psychology Review, 33*(3), 331–342.

Lam, L. T. (2014). Risk factors of internet addiction and the health effect of internet addiction on adolescents: A systematic review of longitudinal and prospective studies. *Current Psychiatry Reports, 16*(11), 508.

Müller, K. W., Janikian, M., Dreier, M., Wölfling, K., Beutel, M. E., Tzavara, C., . . . Tsitsika, A. (2015). Regular gaming behavior and internet gaming disorder in European adolescents: Results from a cross-national representative survey of prevalence, predictors, and psychopathological correlates. *European Child and Adolescent Psychiatry, 24*(5), 565–574.

Petry, N. M., Rehbein, F., Gentile, D. A., Lemmens, J. S., Rumpf, H. J., Mößle, T., . . . O'Brien, C. P. (2014). An international consensus for assessing internet gaming disorder using the new DSM-5 approach. *Addiction, 109*(9), 1399–1406.

Tam, P., & Walter, G. (2013). Problematic internet use in childhood and youth: Evolution of a 21st century affliction. *Australasian Psychiatry, 21*(6), 533–536.

SA10 Patterns in Adolescence of Infancy/Childhood-Onset Disorders

SA101 *Autism Spectrum Disorder*

Bellini, S. (2004). Social skill deficits and anxiety in high functioning adolescents with autism spectrum disorders. *Focus on Autism and Other Developmental Disabilities, 19*(2), 78–86.

Hedges, S., White, T., & Smith, L. (2015, February). *Anxiety in adolescents with ASD.* Chapel Hill: University of North Carolina, Center on Secondary Education for Students with ASD (CSESA).

Lai, M. C., Lombardo, M. V., Chakrabarti, B., & Baron-Cohen, S. (2013). Subgrouping the autism "spectrum": Reflections on DSM-5. *PLoS Biology, 11*(4), e1001544.

Ozbayrak, R. K. (2016). Meeting the challenges of adolescence: A guide for parents. Retrieved from *www.aspergers.com/adolesc.html.*

Reaven, J., Blakeley-Smith, A., Leuthe, E., Moody, E., & Hepburn, S. (2012). Facing your fears in adolescence: Cognitive-behavioral therapy for high-functioning autism spectrum disorders and anxiety. *Autism Research and Treatment, 2012,* 423905.

Schall, C. M., & McDonough, J. T. (2010). Autism spectrum disorders in adolescence and early adulthood: Characteristics and issues. *Journal of Vocational Rehabilitation, 32,* 81–88.

Shattuck, P. T., Orsmond, G. I., Wagner, M., & Cooper, B. P. (2011). Participation in social activities among adolescents with an autism spectrum disorder. *PLoS ONE, 6*(11), e27176.

Smith, L. E., Maenner, M. J., & Seltzer, M. M. (2012). Developmental trajectories in adolescents and adults with autism: The case of daily living skills. *Journal of the American Academy of Child and Adolescent Psychiatry, 51*(6), 622–631.

SA102 *Attention-Deficit/Hyperactivity Disorder*

Brinkman, W. B., Sherman, S. N., Zmitrovich, A. R., Visscher, M. O., Crosby, L. E., Phelan, K. J., & Donovan, E. F. (2012). In their own words: Adolescent views on ADHD and their evolving role managing medication. *Academic Pediatrics, 12*(1), 53–61.

Bussing, R., Zima, B. T., Mason, D. M., Porter, P. C., & Garvan, C. W. (2011). Receiving treatment for attention-deficit hyperactivity disorder: Do the perspectives of adolescents matter? *Journal of Adolescent Health, 49*(1), 7–14.

Charach, A., Yeung, E., Volpe, T., Goodale, T., & Dosreis, S. (2014). Exploring stimulant treatment in ADHD: Narratives of young adolescents and their parents. *BMC Psychiatry, 14,* 110.

Krueger, M., & Kendall, J. (2001). Descriptions of self: An exploratory study of adolescents with ADHD. *Journal of Child and Adolescent Psychiatric Nursing, 14,* 61–72.

Meaux, J. B., Hester, C., Smith, B., & Shoptaw, A. (2006). Stimulant medications: A trade-off?: The lived experience of adolescents with ADHD. *Journal for Specialists in Pediatric Nursing, 11,* 214–226.

Snyder, H. R., Miyake, A., & Hankin, B. L. (2015). Advancing understanding of executive function impairments and psychopathology: Bridging the gap between clinical and cognitive approaches. *Frontiers in Psychology, 26*(6), 328.

SA103 *Specific Learning Disorders*

Al-Yagon, M. (2007). Socioemotional and behavioral adjustment among school-age children with learning disabilities: The moderating role of maternal personal resources. *Journal of Special Education, 40*(4), 205–217.

Harter, S. (1999). *The construction of the self: A*

developmental perspective. New York: Guilford Press.

Humphrey, N. (2002). Teacher and pupil ratings of self-esteem in developmental dyslexia. *British Journal of Special Education, 29*, 29–36.

Ingesson, S. G. (2007). Growing up with dyslexia. *School Psychology International, 28*(5), 574–591.

Raskind, M. H., Goldberg, R. J., Higgins, E. L., & Herman, K. L. (1999). Patterns of change and predictors of success in individuals with learning disabilities: Results from a twenty-year longitudinal study. *Learning Disabilities Research and Practice, 14*, 35–49.

Rosetti, C. W., & Henderson, S. J. (2013). Lived experiences of adolescents with learning disabilities. *The Qualitative Report, 18*(47), 1–17.

Trzesniewski, K. H., Moffitt, T. E., Caspi, A., Taylor, A., & Maughan, B. (2006). Revisiting the association between reading achievement and antisocial behavior: New evidence of an environmental explanation from a twin study. *Child Development, 77*(1), 72–88.

SAApp Appendix: Psychological Experiences That May Require Clinical Attention

SAApp1 *Demographic Minority Populations (Ethnic, Cultural, Linguistic, Religious, Political)*

Boivin, M., Hymel, S., & Bukowski, W. M. (1995). The roles of social withdrawal, peer rejection, and victimization by peers in predicting loneliness and depressed mood in childhood. *Development and Psychopathology, 7*, 765–785.

Chen, X., Rubin, K. H., & Li, B. (1995). Social and school adjustment of shy and aggressive children in China. *Developmental and Psychopathology, 7*, 337–349.

Chen, X., Rubin, K. H., & Li, B. (1997). Maternal acceptance and social and school adjustment: A four-year longitudinal study. *Merrill–Palmer Quarterly, 43*, 663–681.

Ecklund, K. (2102). Intersectionality of identity in children: A case study. *Professional Psychology: Research and Practice, 43*, 256–264.

Fuligni, A. J. (1998) Authority, autonomy, and parent–adolescent conflict and cohesion: A study of adolescents from Mexican, Chinese, Filipino, and European backgrounds. *Developmental Psychology, 34*, 782–792.

Grotevant, H. D., & Cooper, C. R. (1998). Individuality and connectedness in adolescent development: Review and prospects for research on identity, relationships, and context. In E. E. A. Skoe & A. L. van der Lippe (Eds.), *Personality development in adolescence*. London: Routledge.

Guisinger, S., & Blatt, S. J. (1994). Individuality and relatedness: Evolution of a fundamental dialectic. *American Psychologist, 49*, 104–111.

Hayes, J. A., Owen, J., & Bieschke, K. J. (2015), Therapist differences in symptom change with racial/ethnic minority clients. *Psychotherapy, 52*(3), 308–314.

Ho, D. Y. R., & Kang, T. K. (1984). Intergenerational comparisons of child-rearing attitudes and practices in Hong Kong. *Developmental Psychology, 20*, 1004–1016.

Mahalingam, R., Balan, S., & Haritatos, J. (2008). Engendering immigrant psychology: An intersectionality perspective. *Sex Roles, 59*, 326–336.

Matsumoto, D. (1997). *Culture and modern life*. Pacific Grove, CA: Brooks/Cole.

Mills, R. S. L., & Rubin, K. H. (1990). Parental beliefs about problematic social behaviors in early childhood. *Child Development, 61*, 138–151.

Narváez, R. F., Meyer, I., Kertzner, R., Ouellette, S., & Gordon, A. (2009). A qualitative approach to the intersection of sexual, ethnic, and gender identities. *Identity: International Journal of Theory and Research, 9*, 63–86.

Polo, A. J., Alegrìa, M., & Sirkin, J. T. (2012). Increasing the engagement of Latinos in services through community-derived programs: The Right Question Project–Mental Health. *Professional Psychology: Research and Practice, 43*, 208–216.

Raeff, C. (2004). Within-culture complexities: Multifaceted and interrelated autonomy and connectedness characteristics in late adolescent selves. *New Directions for Child and Adolescent Development, 104*, 61–78.

Rubin, K. H. (1998). Social and emotional development from a cultural perspective. *Developmental Psychology, 34*(4), 611–615.

Rubin, K. H., Chen, X., & Hymel, S. (1993). Socioemotional characteristics of aggressive and withdrawn children. *Merrill–Palmer Quarterly, 49*, 518–534.

Rubin, K. H., Chen, X., McDougall, P., Bowker, A., & McKinnon, J. (1995). The Waterloo Longitudinal Project: Predicting adolescent internalizing and externalizing problems from early and mid-childhood. *Development and Psychopathology, 7*, 751–764.

Schneider, B. H., Attili, G., Vermigli, P., & Younger, A. (1997). A comparison of middle-class English-Canadian and Italian mothers' beliefs about children's peer directed aggression and social withdrawal. *International Journal of Behavioral Development, 21*, 133–154.

Segall, M. H., Dasen, P. R., Berry, J. W., & Poortinga, Y. H. (1990). *Human behavior in global perspective*. New York: Pergamon Press.

Shih, M., & Sanchez, D. (2009). When race becomes even more complex: Toward understanding the landscape of multiracial identity and experiences. *Journal of Social Issues, 65*, 1–11.

Sue, D. W. (2001). Multidimensional facets of cultural

competence. *The Counseling Psychologist, 29*, 790–821.

Tummala-Narra, P. (2015). Cultural competence as a core emphasis of psychoanalytic psychotherapy. *Psychoanalytic Psychology, 32*(2), 275–292.

Turiel, E. (1996). Equality and hierarchy: Conflict in values. In E. S. Reed, E. Turiel, & T. Brown (Eds.), *Values and knowledge*. Mahwah, NJ: Erlbaum.

von Bertalanffy, L. (1968). *Organismic psychology and systems theory*. Barre, MA: Clark University Press, with Barre Publishers.

von Bertalanffy, L. (1969). *General System Theory*. New York: Braziller.

SAApp2 *Lesbian, Gay, and Bisexual Populations*

Adelson, S. L., & American Academy of Child and Adolescent Psychiatry (AACAP) Committee on Quality Issues (CQI). (2012). Practice parameter on gay, lesbian, or bisexual sexual orientation, gender nonconformity, and gender discordance in children and adolescents. *Journal of the American Academy of Child and Adolescent Psychiatry, 51*(9), 957–974.

Baiocco, R., Laghi, F., Di Pomponio, I., & Nigito, C. S. (2012). Self-disclosure to the best friend: Friendship quality and internalized sexual stigma in Italian lesbian and gay adolescents. *Journal of Adolescence, 35*(2), 381–387.

Cooper, R. M., & Blumenfeld, W. J. (2012). Responses to cyberbullying: A descriptive analysis of the frequency of and impact on LGBT and allied youth. *Journal of LGBT Youth, 9*(2), 153–177.

Drescher, J. (1998). *Psychoanalytic therapy and the gay man*. Hillsdale, NJ: Analytic Press.

Evans, C. R., & Chapman, M. V. (2014). Bullied youth: The impact of bullying through lesbian, gay, and bisexual name calling. *American Journal of Orthopsychiatry, 84*(6), 644–652.

Lingiardi, V., & Nardelli, N. (2014). Negative attitudes to lesbians and gay men: Persecutors and victims. In G. Corona, E. A. Jannini, M. Maggi, G. Corona, E. A. Jannini, & M. Maggi (Eds.), *Emotional, physical and sexual abuse: Impact in children and social minorities* (pp. 33–47). Cham, Switzerland: Springer International.

Lingiardi, V., Nardelli, N., & Drescher, J. (2015). New Italian lesbian, gay and bisexual psychotherapy guidelines: A review. *International Review of Psychiatry, 27*(5), 405–415.

Mustanski, B., Kuper, L., & Greene, G. J. (2014). Development of sexual orientation and identity. In D. L. Tolman & L. M. Diamond (Series Eds.) & J. A. Bauermeister, W. H. George, J. G. Pfaus, & L. M. Ward (Vol. Eds.), *APA handbook of sexuality and psychology: Vol. 1. Person-based approaches* (pp. 597–628). Washington, DC: American Psychological Association.

Rivers, I. (2011). *Homophobic bullying: Research and theoretical perspectives*. New York: Oxford University Press.

Ryan, C., Huebner, D., Diaz, R., & Sanchez, J. (2009). Family rejection as a predictor of negative health outcomes in white and Latino lesbian, gay, and bisexual young adults. *Pediatrics, 123*(1), 346–352.

SAApp3 *Gender Incongruence*

Adelson, S. L., & American Academy of Child and Adolescent Psychiatry (AACAP) Committee on Quality Issues (CQI). (2012). Practice parameter on gay, lesbian, or bisexual sexual orientation, gender nonconformity, and gender discordance in children and adolescents. *Journal of the American Academy of Child and Adolescent Psychiatry, 51*(9), 957–974.

American Psychological Association. (2015). Guidelines for psychological practice with transgender and gender nonconforming people. *American Psychologist, 70*(9), 832–864.

Cohen-Kettenis, P. T., & Klink, D. (2015). Adolescents with gender dysphoria. *Best Practice & Research. Clinical Endocrinology & Metabolism, 29*(3), 485–495.

de Vries, A. L., & Cohen-Kettenis, P. T. (2012). Clinical management of gender dysphoria in children and adolescents: The Dutch approach. *Journal of Homosexuality, 59*, 301–320.

de Vries, A. L., Cohen-Kettenis, P. T., & Delemarre-van de Waal, H. (2006). Clinical management of gender dysphoria in adolescents. *International Journal of Transgenderism, 9*(3–4), 83–94.

Drescher, J., & Byne, W. (2012). Gender dysphoric/gender variant (GD/GV) children and adolescents: Summarizing what we know and what we have yet to learn. *Journal of Homosexuality, 59*(3), 501–510.

Institute of Medicine. (2011). *The health of lesbian, gay, bisexual, and transgender people: Building a foundation for better understanding*. Washington, DC: National Academies Press.

World Professional Association for Transgender Health (WPATH). (2011). *Standards of care for the health of transsexual, transgender and gender-non-conforming people, Version 7*. Minneapolis, MN: Author. Retrieved from *www.wpath.org/site_page.cfm?pk_association_webpage_menu=1351&pk_association_webpage=3926*.

PART III
Childhood

CHAPTER 7

Profile of Mental Functioning for Children

MC Axis

CHAPTER EDITORS

Norka Malberg, PsyD **Larry Rosenberg, PhD**

CONSULTANTS

Karin Ensink, PhD
Melinda Kulish, PhD
Karin Lindqvist, PhD
Eirini Lympinaki, PhD
Janet A. Madigan, MD
Johanna C. Malone, PhD

Introduction

This chapter describes basic mental functions for children ages 4–11. Our goal is to provide a clinician with the tools necessary to offer a clear clinical description of a child's presentation and place it within the proper developmental context. To allow for greater appreciation of continuities and discontinuities during critical periods of development, the chapters on childhood and adolescence are presented separately in PDM-2. The MC Axis, described in this chapter, integrates psychodynamic, cognitive, and developmental models of growth. Each category of functioning described here is accompanied by a general description, followed by a guideline to expected developmental accomplishments in the area described. For some categories, we have further segregated age groups to illustrate the maturational changes that take place within specific age cohorts. The idea is to further distinguish the developmental expectations for the purpose of diagnostic profiling.

The overall framework guiding the descriptions is based on the idea that every individual develops at a different rate within the developmental continuum, as determined by the interaction between constitutional aspects of the child and his or her relational environment. Compared to the first edition, PDM-2 takes a stronger developmental psychopathology focus, using the same categories of mental functioning as those in the adolescence and adult chapters of the manual. This structure offers the possibility of retracing the developmental path of emerging pathological manifestations in the context of growth and maturation. The assessment of children's mental functioning is a fluid, dynamic, and complex process. In this chapter, we offer what we hope is a clinician-friendly guide to assessment and formulation of a child's overall mental functioning—one that takes into consideration the uniqueness of each child's developmental process.

As the other M Axes do, the MC Axis includes an assessment procedure (see Table 7.2 at the end of the chapter, pp. 493–494) whereby a clinician can indicate on a 5-point scale the level at which each mental function is articulated. In conjunction with the PC Axis, the MC Axis thus allows clinicians to construct an individual profile leading to formulations that integrate both the overall emerging personality of the child (PC Axis) and the specific aspects of mental functioning (MC Axis) influencing emerging patterns of personality and symptomatology.

Again, we subdivide descriptions of child functioning into age subgroups, in the hope that this will highlight for the reader the different capacities and developmental tasks associated with each developmental substage, and thus offer a baseline of normality in assessing a child's current mental functioning. Although no profile can hope to capture the full panoply of mental life, the categories listed in the M Axis (see Chapter 2, pp. 76–77), with one exception, highlight crucial areas and try to correlate observable behaviors with brain-based processes. We elaborate on the specific aspects of these domains for children below.

Because of children's fluidity and diverse levels of functioning, we have excluded the capacity for meaning and purpose (capacity 12 in the M Axis; see Chapter 2, pp. 116–117) from our consideration of children. The period covered by this axis represents a developmental period in which rapid cognitive and social-emotional changes take place, creating the foundations of a sense of self that, when development proceeds well, becomes more evident in adolescence. Young children's sense of self evolves over time, becoming increasingly coherent and consistent. A child's sense of self and the narrative that goes with it are inherently fragile, however, and less well differentiated than those of either adolescents or adults.

For children in the 4–11 age group, the influence of others is notable; how they view themselves is mainly a function of identification with parent figures and siblings. A child's dominant culture is the culture of the family. As the child becomes more differentiated and further exposed to influences outside the home, self-representations become increasingly altered and solidified. Still, even young children have a sense of their likes and dislikes and of the kinds of persons they are (e.g., "I am smart, pretty, helpful, naughty"). Their belief systems are typically taken from the adults around them. Particularly at the lower end of this age range, children are far less future-oriented than their adolescent or adult counterparts. Their ability to reflect on the impact of their actions is neither fully developed nor far-reaching. Given the diversity in this age group, and its rapid shifts and variability, we believe that it would only confuse a diagnostician to attempt to explore the dimension of meaning and purpose. Other categories in this axis can help assess a child's current sense of agency.

Empirically Grounded Assessment of MC-Axis Capacities

The assessment of children ages 4–11 is a challenging and comprehensive enterprise, particularly when one tries to create a diagnostic profile that will guide clinical formulation and treatment planning. A thorough assessment requires time and cannot be accomplished in a single interview. In accordance with other chapters of PDM-2, we recommend using a series of validated and nonvalidated tools to help bring together all the pieces of the puzzle of a child's psychodynamic diagnostic profiling.

Meeting with parents or caregivers is essential. It may or may not be appropriate or beneficial for the child to be present at this interview; this issue should be given careful consideration. For example, it may not be appropriate for a child to hear information about dramatic family or parent history that he or she has not previously heard or may be too young to comprehend. The presence of a parent may inhibit a child's play or verbal productions, and while this may be useful information in itself, it also deprives the clinician of information that might otherwise be provided. In addition to the interview, it may be useful to collect observational data as the child plays with the caregiver, or as the clinician plays alone with the child. Observations from school or preschool are valuable as well, as any comprehensive child evaluation is best conducted across settings.

Clinicians may benefit from parent and teacher reports, child self-report rating scales, and clinician-rated scales to compare the perspectives of multiple raters. These empirically based assessment instruments can and should be integrated with information obtained via child and parent interviews. Information gathered should focus on the child's present level of functioning, as well as the child's developmental history and family mental health background. Clinical observations should be made across diverse contexts, such as school, home, and other settings; in addition, informal reports should be obtained from other adults in regular contact with the child, such as grandparents and other relatives, pediatricians, camp counselors, and teachers. (Table 7.1 is an informal checklist of data sources.) When a still more thorough assessment is needed, children should be referred for a comprehensive psychological test battery that includes cognitive, achievement, neuropsychological, projective, and self-report plus parent/teacher report test measures. A comprehensive battery will highlight how each component is affected by others, and will help provide a well-rounded picture of all aspects of the child's present level of functioning.

TABLE 7.1. Checklist of Sources of Data Informing a Child's Mental Functioning Profile

Consulting room (diagnostic session observations)	
Parents/primary caregivers (social and developmental history, checklists, interview)	
Pediatrician (medical history)	
Teacher (checklists, interview)	
Classroom observations	
Formal assessment (e.g., intelligence, achievement, neuropsychological, projective)	
Dyadic observations during diagnostic period	
Other sources of information (child care providers, grandparents/ other extended family members, social services personnel)	

1. Capacity for Regulation, Attention, and Learning

This first capacity allows a child to carry out multiple tasks simultaneously in ways that facilitate growth and development. In the developmental sciences in general and developmental psychopathology in particular, self-regulation and its component skills are viewed as basic capacities that can foster either typical, positive, or atypical developmental outcomes, depending on their articulation with other social, dispositional, and biological resources available. This section attends to a range of cognitive abilities that enable a child to make sense of world and self through a range of information-processing capabilities.

In rating this capacity, a clinician should consider the following and their influence on a child's emerging regulatory capacities within relationships and across a range of contexts (e.g., home vs. school): auditory processing and language, visual–spatial processing, motor planning and sequencing, and sensory modulation; related capacities for executive functioning (problem-solving, sequencing, organization); memory (working, declarative, and nondeclarative); attention; intelligence; and processing of affective and social cues. Different contexts will place unique demands on a child's abilities within this broad domain. There follows a guideline to age-expected attainments in this category for children ages 4–11. This is not intended as a comprehensive guide, but as an outline of the more salient aspects of mental functioning within the category.

Developmental Guideline: Capacity for Regulation, Attention, and Learning in Children Ages 4–11

Age 4

Comprehends two or more connected concepts or ideas. Can talk in full sentences, connecting ideas with words such as "but" and "because." Makes needs known. Gross motor coordination continues to improve (child can run, jump, hop, throw a ball accurately, etc.). Fine motor coordination improves (child can almost tie shoes, draws circles, handles utensils well). Visual abilities are coordinated with motor and information processing (e.g., child can understand pictures/cartoons and simple nonverbal puzzles). May still misinterpret visual cues of emotions. Symbolic capacity is expanded (complex play), as is ability for reality orientation (distinguishing between fantasy and reality); increasing concentration and self-regulation are possible with appropriate context and support. The child displays improved ability for delayed gratification. Noticeable improvement in executive functioning (ability to solve problems, follow a sequence of desired behaviors while inhibiting impulse-driven behavior, etc.). The ability to store, acquire, and recall information (memory) develops with strengths in language-based encoding (e.g., child can retell a story) and recognition over recall.

Ages 5–6

Talks in full complex sentences; begins to show capacity to present ideas. Can begin to comprehend, express, and conceptualize simple reciprocal and inverse relationships between multiple ideas and aspects of physical reality (e.g., figure out degrees of intensity of rage or greed). Gross motor coordination improves, evidenced by more accurate throwing, rhythmic jumping (rope), and kicking. Fine motor coordination improves (child ties shoes, writes letters; draws circles, squares, and triangles). Visual abilities are coordinated with motor and information/affective processing (e.g., child is increasingly able to read facial and social cues). Capacity for self-regulation and concentration is improving, but still subject to context and support. Memory becomes increasingly organized and continuous.

Ages 7–8

Language is used increasingly in comprehending and communicating interrelated ideas and concepts, and in expressing wishes, needs, fantasies, and logic-based efforts to make sense of the world. Gross motor coordination improves further; child can now do most activities (running, jumping, hopping, skipping, throwing, etc.). Fine motor coordination increases, as evidenced by more fluent, improved writing. Visual abilities are coordinated with motor and information/affective processing. Increasing ability to remember and describe visual information or experiences. Capacity for logic in terms of inverse and reciprocal relationships is established. Capacity for self-regulation, following rules, and concentration is established. Ability to manage attention and integrate information about where to look (and minimize effects of conflicting cues) is consolidated. Memory is well organized; rehearsal strategies are used.

Ages 9–11

Language is now used to comprehend and express complex ideas with relationships among a few elements (e.g., "I did this because Alex did that"). Greater muscle strength enhances gross motor coordination: gradual further improvement in all areas, with the capacity for complex activities. New learning is more established. Fine motor coordination improves, with more fluid writing and the capacity to take things apart skillfully. Visual abilities are coordinated with motor and information/affective processing. Child uses logic to understand gradations in feelings or aspects of physical reality and more complex inverse and reciprocal relationships. Tendency for logical exploration to dominate fantasy; greater sense of morality; increased interest in rules and orderliness; increased capacity for self-regulation; and well-established ability to concentrate.

Rating Scale

For this and each of the other MC-Axis capacities, a 5-point rating scale, in which each mental function can be assessed from 5 to 1, is provided in Table 7.2a at the end of the chapter. Descriptions of the anchor points for levels 5, 3, and 1 are provided for each capacity in the text.

5. The child can be focused, calm, organized, and able to learn most of the time, even under stress, in a developmentally expected fashion. There is age-appropriate ability to express thoughts, affects, and other inner experiences, both verbally and nonverbally. Memory, attention, and executive function are all working at age-expected levels in an integrated way.
3. The child can be focused, organized, calm, and able to learn except when over- or understimulated (i.e., in a noisy, active, or very dull setting); when challenged to use a vulnerable skill (e.g., when a child with weak fine motor skills is asked to write rapidly); or when ill, anxious, or under stress. The child's capacity to learn is sometimes restricted to short periods (concentration span is not consistent and is highly dependent on context and support); the child shows problems of language, motor, or visual processing that explain the uneven regulatory profile. The child seems to learn only when very interested, motivated, or captivated.
1. The child has fleeting attention (a few seconds here or there), is very active or agitated, is mostly self-absorbed, and/or is lethargic or passive. Learning capacity is severely limited by multiple processing difficulties. The child's verbal expressions may be compromised, impoverished, or peculiar.

Most Relevant Assessment Tools

Process Assessment of the Learner—Second Edition: Diagnostics for Math

Process Assessment of the Learner—Second Edition (PAL-II): Diagnostics for Math (Berninger, 2007) measures the development of cognitive processes critical to learning math skills and performance. It is appropriate as a Tier 1, Tier 2, or Tier 3 evaluation tool. It introduces novel quantitative and spatial working memory tasks associated with math computation skills; provides evidence-based diagnostics for dyscalculia; and guides early identification/intervention planning by customizing evaluation. It provides brief application and interpretation based on referral concern or as a follow-up to an earlier assessment.

Naglieri Nonverbal Ability Test—Second Edition

The individual administration version of the Naglieri Nonverbal Ability Test—Second Edition (NNAT-2; Naglieri, 2008) assesses general reasoning ability in children and adolescents, including nonverbal reasoning and general problem-solving abilities. Because of the simplicity of directions and minimal use of language required to solve the items, it is ideal for use with examinees from culturally and linguistically diverse backgrounds. It also has minimal motor requirements. It uses progressive matrices, which are fair for all examinees (including minorities, those with hearing impairments, and those with impaired color vision). The NNAT-2 is ideal for children who do not speak English as their first language, since it requires no reading, writing, or speaking.

Battelle Developmental Inventory, Second Edition

The Battelle Developmental Inventory—Second Edition (BDI-2; Newborg, 2005) is designed for screening, diagnosis, and evaluation of children's development from birth through age 8. Designed to identify children with special needs and to assess their functional abilities, it assesses five domains: personal–social, adaptive, motor, communication, and cognitive. There are two components: a screening consisting of 96 items, and an assessment composed of 341 items. The screening test includes 2–3 items for each subdomain; thus the entire personal–social domain (including adult interaction, self-concept/social growth, and peer interaction) is measured with fewer than 10 items. Three different administration methods can be used (direct child assessment, observation, and a parent/professional interview), all of which can be administered by paraprofessionals who have received supervision. The examiner can choose a combination of methods to obtain complete information. The complete BDI-2 requires 1–2 hours; the screening takes approximately 10–30 minutes. CD-ROM and Web-based scoring options are available.

Conners Parent–Teacher Rating Scale—Revised

The Conners Parent–Teacher Rating Scale—Revised (Conners, 1997) assesses attention-deficit/hyperactivity disorder (ADHD) and related problems in children ages 3 through 17 years. There are a short and a long version; both include parent, teacher, and self-report forms with subscales. Although the long version requires more time to complete, it corresponds more closely to the *Diagnostic and Statistical Manual of Mental Disorders*, fourth edition (DSM-IV). In addition to measuring ADHD, the subscales provide information useful for assessing problems of conduct, learning, cognition, family relationships, emotion, anger control, and anxiety. The Conners can be used for screening, for treatment monitoring, as a research instrument, and as a clinical diagnostic aid. Computer programs are available for scoring, calculating standardized *T* scores from raw scores, and providing a graphic display and report of results. The long version's scales take about 20 minutes to complete; the short version's scales take approximately 5 minutes.

Multifactor Emotional Intelligence Scale—Short Version

The Multifactor Emotional Intelligence Scale—Short Version (MEIS; Mayer, Caruso, & Salovey, 1999) measures emotional intelligence prior to implementation and again after the conclusion of the authors' Connecting program. It includes eight tasks divided into components representing three levels of emotional reasoning ability: perceiving, understanding, and regulating emotions. The scale yields four scores: an overall score of general emotional intelligence, and a score for each emotional reasoning ability. The short version consists of 258 items and is scored by an "expert scoring" method, in which each response is compared with an expert answer, or one that MEIS experts believe is the most accurate assessment of a particular ability.

Wechsler Preschool and Primary Scale of Intelligence—Fourth Edition

The Wechsler Preschool and Primary Scale of Intelligence—Fourth Edition (WPPSI–IV; Wechsler, 2012) is an innovative measure of cognitive development for children ages 4:0 to 7:7, rooted in contemporary theory and research. Extensive enhancements benefit both children and examiners. In response to current literature and feedback from experts and clinicians, the WPPSI–IV includes extensive content changes, including new processing speed measures, the addition of working memory subtests, and an expanded factor structure that includes new and separate visual–spatial and fluid reasoning composites. Two new working memory subtests, picture memory and zoo locations, provide age-appropriate, engaging tasks for children as young as 2½. These reliable, child-friendly measures are designed to detect emerging working memory difficulties for early intervention. The primary index scales include a verbal comprehension index, visual–spatial index, working memory index, fluid reasoning index, and processing speed index. Ancillary index scales include a vocabulary acquisition index, nonverbal index, general ability index, and cognitive proficiency index.

Comprehensive Executive Function Inventory

For a description of the Comprehensive Executive Function Inventory (CEFI; Naglieri & Goldstein, 2013), see the section on capacity 1 in Chapter 4 (pp. 265–269).

2. Capacity for Affective Range, Communication, and Understanding

For a broader definition of the second capacity, see Chapter 2 (pp. 84–88).

This category includes the child's capacity for emotional regulation, which is related to but distinct from the impulse regulation described in the context of executive functioning. Acceptance of and pleasure in one's body are included in this domain. A clinician should attend to tension states, how they are manifested, and how they are dealt with. Does a child express specific states of mind through the body? To what extent does the child feel ownership of the body and its functions (e.g., verbal and nonverbal language)?

During this age period (4–11 years), the range and degrees of specific affects are broad. In the aggressive domain, for example, one finds gradations from assertive behaviors, to competitive behavior, to mildly aggressive behavior, to explosive and uncontrolled aggressive behavior. The same is true in the affection and caring domain, which ranges from uninhibited emotional hunger, to mild affection, to a sincere sense of warmth, to compassion, to the developmentally advanced emotion of empathy. The clinician should observe and describe not only the range of affects, but their richness and depth. Is the child genuinely seeking to connect, or simply imitating someone, or expressing what he or she thinks the therapist wants?

In pretend play, does the child express congruent verbal affects? In more elaborate pretend play, are subplots logically connected to one another? Do themes of excitement, longing, and fear of separation suggest the ways the child manages the feelings accompanying them? For example, during pretend play, does a child doll figure ignore the mother doll when the mother leaves for work?

There follows a developmental guideline to age-expected attainments for children ages 4–11.

Developmental Guideline: Capacity for Affective Range, Communication, and Understanding in Children Ages 4–11

Ages 4–6

Further emergence of pride and pleasure in psychological and bodily self. Increased interest in power; feelings of shame and humiliation begin to emerge. Increased feelings of jealousy and envy; more differentiated sadistic and masochistic trends. Emerging capacity for sharing and concern for others. Increasing capacity for empathy and tenderness. Affect system is well organized, showing many states of the emerging sense of self. Many individual affects are present in a relatively stable pattern: Expansiveness, curiosity, pride, and gleeful excitement related to discovery of bodily self and family patterns are balanced with coyness, shyness, fearfulness, jealousy, and envy. Shame and humiliation are still dominant; child is vulnerable to peer response and position vis-à-vis visible capabilities (comparing self to peers). Capacity for empathy and love is developed, but fragile and easily lost if competitive or jealous strivings are on the upsurge. Anxiety and fears related to bodily injury and loss of respect, love, and emerging self-esteem are present; self-esteem may vacillate between extremes. Guilt feelings are emerging and at first severe; self-management breaks down and requires support.

Ages 7–8

Pleasure in approval, success, and mastery emerge. Expansive and competitive affects exist, alongside fears of failure and humiliation. There is some instability between attempts to keep self in order and on track, and earlier expansive and rivalrous affects. Concern for others, empathy, and even worry are growing. Anxiety is occasionally disruptive, usually serving a signal function, and can be dealt with via shifts in fantasy or changes in meanings.

Ages 9–11

Well-developed capacity for empathy, love, compassion, and sharing; emerging capacity for sadness and loss in context of concrete rules. Internal self-esteem is very important. Feelings of guilt and internalized fears are present. New affects around sexual differences are beginning to emerge (excitement and shyness in relation to sexual themes). Cross-gender identifications are fluid. An increase in orgasmic responses to sexual stimulation by ages 10–11. Fantasy life is important for managing sexual and aggressive feelings. Changing emotional states influence gender roles and a fluidity of identifications (e.g., mourning, loss, and loneliness in response to greater separateness from parents). Dreams are prominent in management of sexual and aggressive feelings, conflicts, and fears.

Rating Scale

5. A child uses a wide range of subtle emotions and wishes in a purposeful manner most of the time, even under stress. The child reads and responds to interpersonal communications (both verbal and nonverbal) flexibly and accurately, even under stress. The child also uses symbolic means of communicating affect and accompanying wishes; for example, after an event that triggers intense emotions, the child uses symbolic play to express and process the experience. The child has the self-awareness to recognize his or her emotional state and the need to seek out others for warmth and support when necessary.
3. A child at this level is often purposeful and organized, but does not show a full range of emotional expressions (e.g., seeking others for closeness and warmth with appropriate glances, body postures). The child often accurately reads and responds to a range of emotional signals, except in circumstances involving selected emotions and wishes, or when emotions and wishes or stresses are intense (e.g., becomes fragmented, inhibited, or chaotic when angry). No cohesive larger integrated emotional patterns.
1. A child is mostly aimless or fragmented, without purposeful emotional expressions. The child distorts the intentions of others, misreads cues, and therefore feels suspicious, mistreated, unloved, angry, or the like. The child is unable to verbalize feelings and becomes easily frustrated when someone attempts to verbalize them for him or her. Lack of symbolic capacity; play often has a poor, rigid, and limited quality.

Most Relevant Assessment Tools

Where indicated below, measures (or their adolescent versions) are discussed in the "Most Relevant Assessment Tools" section for capacity 2 in Chapter 4 (pp. 269–274).

Children's Apperception Test

The Children's Apperception Test (CAT; Bellak & Bellak, 1949) is a projective personality measure for children ages 3–10 years. It consists of a series of pictures; a child is asked to describe the situation and make up stories about the animals or people in the picture. The test usually takes 20–30 minutes to administer. Interpretations of test results consider aspects such as who is the protagonist of the story; what is felt by that character; what relationships exist among the characters; and what anxieties, fears, and psychological defenses are expressed. The CAT gives a picture of the child's ability to fantasize and tell coherent narratives.

Positive and Negative Affect Schedule for Children

The Positive and Negative Affect Schedule for Children (PANAS-C; Laurent et al., 1999) comprises two mood scales, one measuring positive affect and the other negative affect. Used as a psychometric scale, it can show relations between positive and negative affect with personality states and traits. Ten descriptors are used for each affect scale (positive and negative) to define the affects' meanings. Participants respond to the 20-item test by using a scale from 1 (very slightly or not at all) to 5 (extremely).

Emotion Regulation Checklist

The Emotion Regulation Checklist (ERC; Shields & Cicchetti, 1997) is described in Chapter 4. The Q-Sort version of the tool (Emotion Regulation Q-Sort) is related to the ERC, both of which are directly applicable to the measurement of emotional regulation. The Q-Sort measures reactivity, empathy, and socially appropriate expressions. Though administration is somewhat cumbersome, it is suitable for a wide age range, and is useful for longitudinal research.

Behavioral and Emotional Rating Scale

The Behavioral and Emotional Rating Scale (BERS; Epstein & Sharma, 1998) (see Chapter 4) is suitable for children ages 5–18.

Social Skills Improvement System

The Social Skills Improvement System (SSIS) Rating Scales (Gresham & Elliott, 2008) enables targeted assessment of individuals and small groups to help evaluate social skills, problem behaviors, and academic competence. Teacher, parent, and student forms help provide a comprehensive picture across school, home, and community settings. The multirater SSIS Rating Scales help measure:

- *Social Skills:* Communication, Cooperation, Assertion, Responsibility, Empathy, Engagement, Self-Control
- *Competing Problem Behaviors:* Externalizing, Bullying, Hyperactivity/Inattention, Internalizing, Autism Spectrum
- *Academic Competence:* Reading Achievement, Math Achievement, Motivation to Learn

3. Capacity for Mentalization and Reflective Functioning

For broader definitions of the third capacity, see Chapters 2 (pp. 88–91) and 4 (pp. 274–278).

Although the ability to develop a mentalizing capacity is innate, its development is highly correlated with a history of secure caregiver–infant attachment—specifically, with the caregiver's ability to imagine and interpret the child's internal experience, and to give this back to the child in a congruent, marked way. Via such mirroring from the adult, the infant starts organizing self-experience and eventually learns to identify and understand self-states. As the caregiver responds to the infant's emotional cues, the infant feels some control over the interaction and in turn feels increasingly agentic. The experience of control is crucial for the development of the senses of agency and self-coherence, which are both important factors for the capacity to mentalize. The caregiver's capacity to treat the child as a psychological agent, whose actions are motivated by mental states, largely depends on the caregiver's own mentalizing capacity.

In assessing this capacity, the following questions are relevant: How is the child able to understand the mental states of others and self? What is the child's capacity for perspective taking? Are there indications that the child can differentiate between psychic (internal) and external reality? How does the child give meaning to his or her actions and the people in his or her world? Is the child able to explore personal intentions, thoughts, and feelings, and to differentiate them from those of others (e.g., "I feel sad, but that does not mean that my friends are sad")? Or is the child operating at a level of "psychic equivalence," meaning that if the child feels a certain way, the whole world must feel that way (e.g., "I am angry and I feel like hurting someone, so I hurt others before I get hurt")? When invited to imagine what a friend is thinking or feeling, can the child regulate his or her own feelings and accept the invitation to think about the other? A strong relationship exists between the capacity to regulate one's feelings and the ability to mentalize. Interpersonal and other environmental stressors challenge the developmental capacity to mentalize. Under stress, is the child able to mentalize with the support of a mindful, mentalizing adult who is displaying a curious, wondering attitude (explicit mentalizing)?

A clinician should observe a child's ability to notice and respond to nonverbal affective shifts in both the clinician and the caregiver (leaning forward, frowning, smiling). The child's ability to respond to nonverbal cues in ways appropriate to age and culture has a major effect on reflective functioning. For children with a history of chronic relational trauma, one should assess their capacity to mentalize in a containing predictable environment. Observations must be made across observers (clinical and others) and settings. Early caregiver–infant history is highly relevant to assessing functioning in this domain.

The following is a developmental guideline to the age-expected attainments for children ages 4–11.

Developmental Guideline: Capacity for Mentalization and Reflective Functioning in Children Ages 4–11

Ages 4–6

There is evidence of theory of mind in the child, and with it the capacity to think about another's perspective as separate. The child displays ability to make meaningful links between people's interior states and their manifest behavior. The child shows the capacity for imitation, shared attention (the ability to look at the same object as another person and to perceive the sameness; this allows for common ground for interacting about what is looked upon), and empathy in the context of relationships. An improvement in capacity for affect regulation is visible as the child is able to make a differentiation between his or her own inner states and the world outside. Increasing executive functioning capacities, as a result of more structure in the schooling environment, allow for higher levels of impulse control and of overall attention and regulation. Empathic responses to peers have initially more of a "state-matching" feeling, which develops into genuine concern for the other. The beginnings of genuine perspective-taking skills appear.

Ages 7–11

There is a consolidation of the child's reflective functioning capacities as a result of exposure to multiple social contexts. An increased sense of agency and flexibility is evident in responding to stressful and unexpected interpersonal scenarios. As development unfolds, there is evidence of more complex mentalization abilities, such as the understanding of subtle social deceptions like bluffs and white lies. There seems to be an understanding of the opaque nature of mental states (one really never knows what is in others' minds) and a curiosity and motivation to understand others' perspectives (inquisitive stance). There is a capacity to interpret ambiguous events (irony and sarcasm). The child can verbalize feelings and respond contingently to nonverbal cues.

Rating Scale

5. The child demonstrates a capacity to understand why people might be reacting in particular ways, is able to consider the intentions behind the behaviors of others in deciding how to react to these behaviors, and is able to anticipate how people may react given specific social contexts. The child shows the capacity to mentalize even when emotionally activated, or may be able to do this after the activating event, especially when some support is offered. There is an ability to identify own emotional reactions, fears, and worries accurately, and to think about this with others. The child is able to assert his or her own needs and wants, while showing interest in what the other thinks and feels. He or she shows curiosity, interest, or concern about why others do what they do, develops ideas about this, is curious about his or her own reactions, and can consider discrepancies between his or her actual and desired behaviors.

3. The child demonstrates a basic capacity to understand what others feel but struggles to anticipate how they may feel in specific circumstances or how they may react in interpersonal contexts. This basic capacity fails when he or she is confronted by more complex or difficult social and interpersonal interactions, is emotionally aroused, or is faced with new challenges. Although the child may have a basic capacity to identify personal affects and mental states, the process lacks complexity and nuance. Without outside scaffolding, the child cannot understand his or her reactions. At first the child may struggle to respond to supportive invitations from mentalizing adults or caregivers, but he or she is able eventually to think with the other, regain affect regulation, reflect on mental life, connect interpersonal events with inner states, and attempt to predict people's actions.

1. The child either does not think about the feelings and intentions of others, showing no interest or curiosity, or adopts an attitude of certainty in attributing inaccurate feelings and intentions to others. There may be evidence of frequent nonverbal miscuing and inappropriate reactions as a result. The child lacks empathy and seems unable to think about the impact of his or her behavior on others' thoughts and feelings. Perspective-taking abilities seem virtually absent across all contexts. The child is unable to label personal affects or describe what he or she is feeling and why, and is unable to give a self-description. The child may describe the self only in terms of behavioral or physical characteristics, or may describe the self in extremely distorted or bizarre terms.

Most Relevant Assessment Tools

Denham's Affect Knowledge Test

Denham's Affect Knowledge Test (Denham, 1986) is a puppet interview assessing social-emotional understanding in preschool children. In a series of vignettes of emotionally charged situations, the child is asked to identify puppet faces that are happy, sad, angry, and afraid.

Test of Emotional Comprehension

The Test of Emotional Comprehension (TEC; Pons & Harris, 2005) is an easily used measure assessing affective understanding and theory of mind in children ages 3–11. It covers nine components of emotional understanding: recognition of basic emotions; understanding of the mixed nature of emotions; the role of external causes, reminders, desires, beliefs, and moral values; ability to distinguish apparent and felt emotion; and regulation of current experience of emotions. It consists of a book with cartoon scenarios on each page, at the bottom of which are four possible emotional outcomes illustrated by facial expressions. The child is read a short story while looking at the cartoon scenario and is then asked to point to the appropriate facial expression. The test has a cognitive focus and may be more useful in clinical settings than outcome research, as it measures generic mentalization capacities.

Affect Task

The Affect Task (Fonagy, Target, & Ensink, 2000) assesses affective understanding in interpersonal contexts. It involves 12 vignettes of children in social interactions with family or friends. The child is asked to identify the child characters' emotions and explain the reason for them. Its tested reliability and validity are good.

Kusche Affective Interview—Revised

The Kusche Affective Interview—Revised (KAI-R; Kusche, Beilke, & Greenberg, 1988) is a popular interview that assesses affective understanding in children. It consists of open-ended questions, assessing understanding of cues for emotions (e.g., "How do you know when you are feeling [happy, sad, jealous, proud . . .]?"), understanding of multiple emotion combinations (e.g., "Can you feel sad and mad at the same time?"), knowledge of the possibility of hiding feelings (e.g., "How do you hide your feelings from others?"), and knowledge about the possibility of changing emotions (e.g., "Can you change your feelings? How?"). Answers are recorded and coded. This measure has been successfully used in outcome studies.

Happé's Strange Stories Test

Happé's Strange Stories Test (Happé, 1994) is a measure assessing cognitive–linguistic aspects of theory of mind. The task consists of 24 short stories comprising pretense, joke, like, white lie, misunderstanding, persuasion, appearance versus reality, figure of speech, irony, double bluff, contrary emotions, and forgetting. After each story, the child is asked questions about the story, typically "Was it true what *X* said?" and "Why did *X* say that?"

Child Reflective Functioning Scale

The Child Reflective Functioning Scale (CRFS; Ensink, Target, & Oandason, 2013), applied to the Child Attachment Interview (Shmueli-Goetz, Target, Fonagy, & Datta, 2008), is a measure of mentalization in children. The interview asks children to reflect on themselves and on their relationship with their primary caregivers and provides a measure of mentalization for both these areas. Children's narratives are coded on an 11-point scale ranging from –1 to 9. A global score of reflective functioning is obtained. The measure can also be used to calculate reflective functioning regarding self and others separately.

Reading the Mind in the Eyes Test

The Reading the Mind in the Eyes Test (RMET; Baron-Cohen, Wheelwright, Hill, Raste, & Plumb, 2001) is sensitive to implicit nonverbal theory of mind. The test consists of 36 pictures of eye regions, for which the respondent is asked to choose the most suitable word out of four, describing what the person in the picture is thinking or feeling. The RMET can be used with children of various ages, and also with adolescents and adults.

4. Capacity for Differentiation and Integration (Identity)

The fourth capacity involves the child's ability to distinguish internal representations, motives, and affect states from external events and experiences, along with the capacity to make links between the internal representations of wishes, affects, self, and others. The child's cognitive maturation catalyzes the transformation of his or her mental life. There is increasing capacity for mental, rather than action-based, thinking. As children begin to plan, organize, and control their behavior, their capacity for affect regulation is linked with the quality of self-representations within relationships (e.g., "I am a boy who is liked by teachers" vs. "Grownups really don't like me"). Early relational experiences and attachment style play a role here in terms of a child's capacity to explore self and others in the context of safety and trust.

The following is a developmental guideline to age-expected attainments for children ages 4–11.

Developmental Guideline: Capacity for Differentiation and Integration (Identity) in Children Ages 4–11

Ages 4–6

There is a great deal of growth and maturation during this period, resulting from rapid evolution of the child's cognition, theory of mind, affect tolerance, language development, and reality orientation. There is evidence of new strong identifications with external figures (superheroes, teachers), which help the child in the process of separation and individuation from parents. There is an emerging capacity to mentalize others' behaviors, as well as integration and differentiation between what is internal and what is external. This progress still remains fragile, particularly when the child is faced with strong feelings of guilt or shame about increasing genital sensations and excitement about the body (which are characteristic of this age group).

Ages 7–8

As guilt and shame recede, there is less externalization, provocation, and focus on others' mistakes. There is also less shame and embarrassment in response to performance demands. Rigidity softens by late latency, and impulsiveness decreases even when the child is aroused. Insight increases, and there is a greater tolerance of internal responsibility.

Ages 9–11

The capacity for self-regulation is still shaky at the beginning of this phase, but consolidates as it progresses. This later period of latency is characterized by greater flexibility and more intense peer socialization. Grandiose fantasies such as "I belong to a different family, so I am better than all of you" may compensate for the loss of idealized parental images and for fears of inadequacy during this period. Gender lines become more delineated as the child moves toward preadolescence. A number of typical gender-segregated latency games and pastimes reveal the use of ritual and symbolization to manage "freshly repressed desires." Group socialization reinforces a sense of identity.

Rating Scale

5. The child at this level can identify and manage the separateness and relatedness of different affect states, motives, and wishes, even when these are nuanced and ambiguous, and can organize varieties of experience and social-emotional demands over time and across contexts with contrasting role demands (e.g., peer, student, sibling, son/daughter). The child can interact with an increasingly complex and demanding environment while using defenses that maximize enjoyment of tasks and increase self-confidence and sense of agency. The child shows a spontaneous and flexible interpersonal style, which is increasingly shaped by the child's sense of self in the world.

3. The child is able to differentiate and integrate experience, but with some constriction and rigidity, especially under stress. Strong emotions or wishes, both general and context-specific, can lead to the temporary fragmentation or polarization (all-or-nothing attitude) of internal experience (the child seems "stuck"). Capacities of differentiation and integration are limited to a few emotional realms (e.g., no real peer relationships). Overall, the child seems to want to find a place in the world, but his or her capacity to do so seems restricted.

1. Internal experience is fragmented most of the time or is rigidly compartmentalized and oversimplified; in extreme cases, internal experience may be detached from external context. There is little ability to move through a range of emotional states, either alone or in interactions with others, without anxiety. The child seems

developmentally stuck in an earlier state of dependency, where an adult must actively manage his or her emotional states. Behaviors or defenses belonging to earlier stages of development (e.g., splitting) lead to feelings of anger and impaired reality testing.

Most Relevant Assessment Tool

Story Stem Completion Task

The Story Stem Completion Task (Hodges et al., 2004) assesses attachment in children, mainly between ages 4 and 9. They are asked to respond to beginnings of stories, displayed with small dolls, each of which involves an inherent dilemma. For each story, the children are asked, "Show and tell me what happens next." The measure allows for attachment classification and gives a clinician a picture of a child's expectations of relationships and family roles.

5. Capacity for Relationships and Intimacy

The next capacity is the child's capacity for relationships and their impact on identity formation. It includes the child's characteristic style of relating or nonrelating (withdrawn, autistic), dyadic relating, capacity for group relating and sharing, and egocentric styles of relating. Information about the child's relationships to parents, siblings, teachers, coaches, and other significant people are all important for building a portrait of the child in the context of relationships across different settings.

The quality of attachment, as manifested in observable behavior and symptomatology and as reported by the child, parents, teachers, and others, is relevant here. Although the child will have different experiences of individual attachment relationships, there will be a consistent attachment pattern that characterizes them. These patterns are underpinned by the child's cognitive internal working models. The child's sense of safety in relationships is central to his or her capacity to explore the world and engage in relationships in an age-adequate manner that fosters the development of trust and intimacy.

The clinician should try to assess the child's sense of safety within relationships by addressing questions such as these: Does the child's behavioral attachment style offer safety when necessary? To whom does the child turn to enhance a sense of safety? What or who makes the child feel afraid? Is the child's relational focus on dyadic or triadic relationships? What is the child's level of investment in others? Does the child seek to engage others? What is the overall affective tone of the child's relationships (e.g., is the child controlling or overly submissive)? Does the child seek or extend affection toward others? Does the child seek assistance from others and, if so, from whom? To what degree? Appropriately, excessively?

The following is a developmental guideline to age-expected attainments for children ages 4–11.

Developmental Guideline: Capacity for Relationships and Intimacy in Children Ages 4–11

Ages 4–6

Relationship patterns become more complicated in content (language, symbolic modes) and in form, as dyadic patterns begin to recede and as capacities for dealing with triangular and other, more complicated patterns emerge (rivalries, intrigues, secrets, two against one). Greater sense of security, capacity for separation, and capacity for carrying a sense of the "other" inside are relatively well established by the end of the fourth year. Anger and other strong feelings do not compromise secure capacity for separation. Capacity for intimacy (not simply need fulfillment) in relationships emerges. Complex triangular modes dominate family life as relationships take on "soap opera" dimensions (intrigue, rivalry, alliance, etc.). A simple, need-fulfilling, two-person relationship pattern is less dominant. Capacity to relate comfortably with others (peers, teachers) grows. There is increased capacity for separation and internal security; the ability to carry a sense of "self" and "other" inside is well established and not easily compromised by separations or strong affects. Self-management still breaks down and requires support. Greater demands to get along with peers and learn in groups arise; increased shame and guilt can disrupt peer relationships, causing provocation and blame; there may be heightened "tattling."

Ages 7–8

Interest in relationships outside family groups (i.e., peers) and capacity for organized, orderly patterns of relating to others (e.g., games with rules) emerge. Some aspects of earlier patterns are still present (power struggles, passive helplessness, family intrigues, rivalries, triangles). Capacity for "buddy" relationships and intimacy with a few "best friends" emerges more fully. Gender-preference peer groups form and are often concrete and categorical. Reactions to criticism from peers and adults is less harsh than the self-condemnation of earlier latency.

Ages 9–11

Peer relationships continue to grow in importance and complexity. Family relationships and friendships may be organized around role models (i.e., simplified adult stereotypes). Relaxed capacity for integrating and enjoying family, peer, teacher, and other adult relationships. Possible special relationship with same-sex parent as a role model, with only hints of earlier levels (triangles, power struggles, passive manipulation). Body-based anxieties are often dealt with by forming same-sex peer groups. Preparation begins for adolescent styles of relating, with special patterns of relating to same- and opposite-sex peers. Capacity for long-term relationships with family, peers, and friends (including a "best friend") increases. There is less reactivity to day-to-day peer fluctuations toward the end of the 10th year.

Rating Scale

5. The child has age-appropriate emotional capacity for intimacy, caring, and empathy, even when feelings are strong or when under stress in a variety of expectable contexts (peers, family, other social settings). He or she shows a developmentally expected desire and capacity to seek closeness in relationships.

3. The child has age-appropriate emotional capacity for intimacy, caring, and empathy, but those capacities are disrupted by strong wishes and emotions such as anger or fear, or by stressors such as separation (i.e., the child withdraws or acts out). The child's behaviors indicate a poor basic sense of safety in relationships and low reflective functioning as a result.

1. The child has a superficial, need-oriented capacity for intimacy and caring, distant from age-expected norms; relationships lack intimacy and empathy. At times, there is clear indifference to others or a more or less complete withdrawal from them.

Most Relevant Assessment Tools

Machover Draw-a-Person Test

The Machover Draw-a-Person Test (Machover, 1949) asks the child to draw two persons, one of each gender. The child is then interviewed about the persons—for example, about their families, wishes, and good and bad sides. Both the quality of the drawings and the answers to the questions are assessed.

Story Stem Completion Task

The Story Stem Completion Task (Hodges et al., 2004) has been described above in regard to capacity 4.

Roberts Apperception Test for Children–2

The Roberts Apperception Test for Children–2 (Roberts-2; Roberts, 2005) helps to evaluate a child's social understanding via a free narrative storytelling format. Appropriate for children between ages 6 and 18, it assesses two independent dimensions: adaptive social perception (development measure) and maladaptive or atypical social perception (clinical measure). This second edition has been updated to reflect current trends and includes new age- and gender-specific normative data. There are now three versions of the pictures: European American, African American, and Hispanic children. The Roberts-2 can be used to document changes as a child grows older and more socially experienced.

6. Capacity for Self-Esteem Regulation and Quality of Internal Experience

Early relationships with caregivers provide a young child with the tools to interact effectively with others while building an internal sense of self as separate and as an active agent of change in relationships. The belief that one can be an active and effective partner in this "relational dance" begins with early, "good-enough" affective attunement. Such experiences are characterized by moments of rupture and repair that build the child's capacity to interact with the external world in a flexible, effective way. This experience of self as an effective agent in relationships is the fuel for the child's self-esteem and sense of self-regard (e.g., "My mommy really loves me, and I love my mommy").

In constructing a diagnostic profile, the clinician should consider questions such as these: Is the psychic self a source of pleasure or pain and conflict for the child (e.g., "I am a likable boy" vs. "Nobody likes me")? How does the child see him- or herself in relationships, and how does the child feel about that (e.g., "My friends like to play with me" vs. "Nobody wants to be my friend")? Do aspects of self suggest incorporation of features of a problematic relationship, such as parental hostility, or of the nature of parental investment (parental narcissistic investment) (e.g., "I am really mean and proud of it")?

Difficulties in language, perceptual–motor, memory, or attentional capacities often influence a child's self-esteem. For example, both clinical and empirical data show that learning delays during the preschool years affect the experience of separation, autonomy, and self-regulation. Deficits in language or motor coordination can prove challenging to the emerging awareness of self–other differentiation. Parents' internal experiences (inferred during clinical interview) of themselves influence their capacity for reflective functioning, and therefore their ability to model effective ways of coping with constitutional and environmental sources of stress that may affect the child's emerging level of confidence.

The following is a developmental guideline to age-expected attainments for children ages 4–11.

Developmental Guideline: Capacity for Self-Esteem Regulation and Quality of Internal Experience in Children Ages 4–11

Ages 4–6

The child's self-esteem and sense of competence are fragile during this period, but maturational changes strengthen them. The emergence of narrative capacities transforms the child's internal world as it expands the capacity for communication and self-understanding. The child displays the capacity for more elaborate stories in play. The child starts to explore and understand his or her mental states and those of others, while still maintaining a certain egocentric stance. There is increased capacity for self-regulation through self-expression and organization of complex feelings.

Ages 7–8

The child displays symbolic play, and with it the capacity to organize complex feelings and conflicts via imaginative stories. The child shows increasing interest in sharing his or her "own stories," thus furthering the sense of self. The child also shows pride in those stories and seeks opportunities to share them with interested adults. Children with a history of secure attachment tend to share richer, more complex make-believe scenarios.

Ages 9–11

The child is increasingly engaged in reality-based events and challenges such as learning goals; clubs and peer relationships become sources of self-esteem. Maturation of the child's ego capacities (self-regulation and impulse control) allows him or her to feel and appear more competent, independent, and secure. There is an internal evolution away from attachments to the primary caregivers and family, and toward the external world of peers. The child shows an increased confidence and a more realistic, less idealized view of parents. The child manages the unpredictable and frustrating aspects of group situations with greater flexibility and increasing reflective function. There is a shift from pretend play to more structured activities.

Rating Scale

5. The child shows age-appropriate capacity to maintain a stable sense of well-being, confidence, and realistic (not grandiose) self-esteem (e.g., "I am good, but I am not better than everyone all the time"). Self-esteem is balanced with, and appropriate to, internal and external situations. The child shows a developmentally adequate level of confidence in his or her capacity to deal with a broad array of tasks and challenges, including novel situations. These characteristics positively influence the way the child thinks, feels, and relates to others and the larger world.

3. The child's sense of well-being, confidence, vitality, and self-esteem is generally adequate, but may be easily disrupted by strong emotions (internally) and stressful situations (externally). The child often expresses (in words, play, behavior) feelings of vulnerability and inadequacy, showing diminished confidence in his or her

capacity to deal with certain situations (e.g., peer activities), to achieve desired results, or to act effectively in the world (sense of agency).

1. The child shows feelings and behaviors indicating a low sense of self-regard (e.g., the figure in the dollhouse is lonely and has no friends, even though he or she is nice). Defensive maneuvers to manage low feelings of confidence are evident, as in the use of grandiose omnipotence and denial in fantasy (e.g., "I don't want to play sports because I am good at all that stuff; the other kids are bad at it, and it's frustrating"). He or she shows a diminished capacity to cope with frustration and engage in age-appropriate activities; play is often restricted. There may be a discrepancy between the child's internal experience and external behavior, diminishing adaptation and resilience.

Most Relevant Assessment Tool

Pictorial Scale of Perceived Competence and Social Acceptance for Young Children

The Pictorial Scale of Perceived Competence and Social Acceptance for Young Children (Harter & Pike, 1984) uses picture plates to assess multidimensional self-concept of children ages 4–7. Designed as a downward extension of the Self-Perception Profile for Children (SPPC), it assesses four domains of self-concept: cognitive competence, physical competence, peer acceptance, and maternal acceptance. See also the SPPC and the Self-Perception Profile for Adolescents (SPPA) described in Chapter 4 (p. 288).

7. Capacity for Impulse Control and Regulation

During childhood, deficiencies in the seventh capacity may lead to unmodulated displays of aggressiveness and lack of age-appropriate inhibition in one or more settings (e.g., home, school, play). Lack of adequate controls can lead to disruptions in learning and relationships with peers and/or authorities. At the other end of this spectrum, children conflicted about expressing aggression and desire may become rigid and overly controlled. Extreme attempts at adaptation of this sort may interfere with relationships and learning. High functioning in this capacity involves the ability to tolerate frustration when necessary and to recognize and describe one's impulses as a means of supporting self-regulation. For further elaboration, see the discussions of capacities 1 and 2 in this chapter, as well as Chapters 8 and 9 (specifically the section on ADHD in Chapter 9, pp. 586–588).

Many of the capacities involved in self-regulation appear to have a temperamental basis. Temperamental self-regulatory capacities are often labeled as "effortful control," defined as the efficiency of executive functioning—including the ability to inhibit a dominant response, activate a subdominant response, plan, and detect errors. In other words, effortful control includes the abilities to shift and focus attention as needed, to inhibit inappropriate behavior, to act when there is a strong tendency to avoid, and to carry out some executive functioning skills involved in integrating information and planning. Effortful control plays a role in self-regulation and also has a significant effect on personality functioning.

Effortful control has been linked conceptually to the development and maintenance of children's externalizing problems (e.g., aggression, defiance). It is believed to be involved via its roles in processing information and modulating emotion. In other words, a child who is having difficulty with executive functioning may also have difficulty with tolerating negative affect (e.g., sadness, anxiety, guilt) and will tend to manage those affective experiences through externalizing behaviors (e.g., attributing blame to others), which can impinge on both his or her learning process and social-emotional development.

The following is a developmental guideline to age-expected attainments for children ages 4–11.

Developmental Guideline: Capacity for Impulse Control and Regulation in Children Ages 4–11

Ages 4–6

Children develop increasing capacities to control their affective and behavioral responses to social interactions and developmental tasks. This promotes their functioning on new tasks requiring sustained attention, rule compliance, and cooperative social behavior. They can inhibit specific behaviors (e.g., running into the street, touching a hot stove). There is an initial ability to carry out simple tasks with multistep instructions and to resist distraction.

Ages 7–8

In school and other social settings, children use social cues to monitor and regulate behavioral and affective responses (e.g., raising a hand before talking, respecting other children's property and personal space). Prosocial behavior increases, and physical aggression decreases. Children increasingly rely on past experience and anticipatory planning to guide their responses. Increased frustration tolerance and delay of gratification are promoted by environmental experience and constitutional factors.

Ages 9–11

Children use their ability to think about consequences to guide their actions (e.g., speaking kindly, following rules when not under direct supervision), guided by an increasing awareness of others' thoughts and feelings and by an internalized sense of the rules. They are more able to inhibit their initial responses in favor of responses that will lead to a better outcome. They are increasingly able to develop self-sufficiently and to draw consciously upon structures to help them modulate behavior over time (e.g., distraction, making a plan).

Rating Scale

5. The child regularly and spontaneously considers the probable consequences of actions before acting. In the face of challenges or distress, he or she can consider how past experience and factors in the current context should inform behavior. The child can plan ahead and rely on self-developed techniques to help regulate behavior. While a strong awareness of the contextual and social norms helps inform decisions, the child has an internalized sense of how to respond, and has an internal locus of control.

3. The child is generally able to delay initial responses in consideration of the probable consequences of actions, including their impacts on the feelings of others. There may be more difficulty inhibiting responses and regulating behavior in the absence of a clear outside authority. In more developmentally challenging or frustrating experiences, such children may have less ability to regulate behavior and may respond in ways that have negative consequences for themselves or others.

1. The child's inability to inhibit responses and to sustain developmentally appropriate attention leads to maladaptive behaviors with negative consequences to self and others. The child lacks the ability to consider the probable consequences of actions before responding. Initial reaction may be aggressive, disruptive, or uncooperative.

Most Relevant Assessment Tools

Child Behavior Checklist

The Child Behavior Checklist (CBCL; Achenbach & Rescorla, 2001) is a checklist that a parent completes to detect emotional and behavioral problems in a child or adolescent. It is part of the Achenbach System of Empirically Based Assessment (ASEBA). There are two other components of the ASEBA: the Teacher's Report Form (TRF), to be completed by a teacher, and the Youth Self-Report (YSR), to be completed by a child or adolescent.

Children's Behavior Questionnaire

The Children's Behavior Questionnaire (CBQ; Rothbart, 1991) is a highly differentiated assessment of temperament in early to middle childhood. Dimensions for which CBQ scales have been developed have been adapted from those studied in both adults and infants. Three factors have been reliably recovered from this instrument, labeled negative affectivity, extraversion, and effortful control.

Conners Parent–Teacher Rating Scale—Revised

The Conners Parent–Teacher Rating Scale—Revised (Conners, 1997) has been described earlier in regard to capacity 1.

8. Capacity for Defensive Functioning

For broader definitions of the eighth capacity, see Chapters 2 (pp. 103–107) and 4 (pp. 292–295).

The first danger situation faced by an infant is helplessness. Freud assumed that defensive processes emerge during the earliest stages of mental development, and that they have one or more of three functions: blocking or inhibition of mental contents, distortion of mental content, and/or screening and covering of mental content by the use of opposing content. Anna Freud (1966) introduced the idea of a developmental hierarchy of defenses. From this perspective, "primitive" defenses are used very early in life, whereas "higher-level" defenses appear after object constancy is established (when a child can keep a mental image of a caregiver that makes the child feel safe even when the caregiver is not present). She demonstrated that defenses can address mental states stimulated from inside (e.g., guilt) and outside (e.g., fear). A developmental view of defenses allows for understanding the relational context in which they arose and provides a framework from which to explain observable defensive behaviors, affects, and ideas.

A developmental view of defenses is particularly useful in helping clinicians consider a child's specific defensive strategy in the context of his or her current developmental stage. The age period of 4–11 years includes rapid maturational shifts, which culminate in an autonomous sense of self in the context of relationships (e.g., with siblings) that may be sources of both support and psychic pain. Effective defenses allow children to navigate rough waters on their own, using their current capacities while retaining maturational gains. A child's style of defense is central to the organization of his or her personality.

The following is a developmental guideline to age-expected attainments for children ages 4–11.

Developmental Guideline: Capacity for Defensive Functioning in Children Ages 4–11

Ages 4–6

The child struggles with the internalization of parental standards of right and wrong. Much of the child's anxiety thus comes from within—from the conflict between internal wishes and needs, and the new standards applied to them. Guilt and shame are common sources of distress. Many children this age still use the defense of denial in fantasy, word, or act to cope with these conflicts and the strength of the feelings attached to them. Management of aggression may be quite a challenging task—one that endangers the fragile balance the child is striving for with all his or her new cognitive and emotional capacities. A move toward defensive strategies in dealing with reality is visible, however. Reversal of affect is a common strategy (e.g., "I love my baby sister"). Identification with the aggressor (turning passive into active) is already in use. A less effective way of coping, often seen at this age, is turning aggression against the self (e.g., "I hit myself before someone tells me off"). Ritualistic and repetitive activities (e.g., songs and rhymes) are common.

Ages 7–8

Children this age show a newfound love affair with the world similar to that observed in toddlers. Sublimation is a central defensive strategy during this period. There is evidence of a relative freedom from immediate inner pressures as a result of opportunities for sublimation. Despite the cognitive advance of this phase, however, a latency-age child still remains rigid and concrete in some cognitive areas; there is a tendency to think categorically about other people (e.g., "Parents are unfair"). Reaction formation and reversal of affect are often still used in dealing with highly conflictual feelings and wishes (e.g., a child who is conflicted about aggressive impulses may take a rather submissive stance in the context of peer relationships).

Ages 9–11

By late latency, provocation and rationalization are often accompanied by decreases in denial. Isolation, reaction formation, undoing, and intellectualization become prominent defenses. Inhibition of such functions as speech, memory, intelligence, and secondary-process thinking can still occur, in addition to obsessional defensive patterns. The child who is functioning well can stop and think with support from a reflective adult and use effective defenses to adjust flexibly and manage challenging situations.

Rating Scale

5. Developmentally appropriate defensive strategies predominate. Their use allows the child to experience a broad range of affects, as well as to be aware of and manage thoughts and feelings in ways that permit continued growth and exploration in relationships and the world at large in adaptive, flexible, and creative ways. When earlier defenses (splitting, projection) are used, they do not significantly impair functioning, as the child typically reverts to more adaptive defenses (e.g.,

sublimation, denial in fantasy, word, and act, displacement, humor) when anxiety, conflict, and stress diminish.

3. At this level, children often respond to internal or external sources of stress by viewing problems as external, and minimizing or ignoring internal sources (developmental expectations are important in determining this). There may be evidence of modest distortion of reality, more than developmentally expected. These children may seem defensive and may disavow aspects of their own experience through denial and projection. Or they may resort to omnipotence as a defense against feelings of shame, powerlessness, and disappointment (to assess how maladaptive this is, one should observe whether a child can abandon this stance in other contexts). Overall, the use of defenses seems somewhat unpredictable and fluctuating, and often relies on early forms of defense such as splitting and projection.

1. The child is easily overwhelmed by anxiety, fear of psychological annihilation, and physical harm or death. These fears are not based in reality; they come from the child's difficulties in dealing with internal conflicts while coping with external demands. The child grossly distorts external reality, but anxiety is poorly contained and adaptation is highly impaired. Defenses such as splitting and projection predominate. Capacity to function in relationships or on one's own is severely restricted and impaired.

Most Relevant Assessment Tools

Children's Play Therapy Instrument

The Children's Play Therapy Instrument (CPTI; Chazan, 2002) assesses therapy process and outcome. The rating scale divides the therapy session into segments of nonplay, pre-play, play activity, and play interruption. The longest segment of play activity within a session is analyzed on three levels: descriptive, structural, and functional. Two sessions are analyzed, one early in treatment and another after 7 months.

Comprehensive Assessment of Defense Style

The Comprehensive Assessment of Defense Style (CADS; Laor, Wolmer, & Cicchetti, 2001) is described in the "Most Relevant Assessment Tools" section for capacity 8 in Chapter 4 (pp. 292–295).

9. Capacity for Adaptation, Resiliency, and Strength

For a broader definition of the ninth capacity, see Chapter 2 (pp. 107–110).

In childhood, "resiliency" can be defined as reduced vulnerability to environmental risk experiences, the overcoming of stress or adversity, or a relatively good outcome despite adversity. The capacity to mentalize others' needs and feelings empathically, the ability to take perspective, and appropriate assertiveness (linked to the child's emerging sense of agency) can all be viewed as strengths. From a transactional viewpoint, the child influences the context, and the context influences the child. Evidence for this long-standing clinical observation can be found in the field of epigenetics.

In this category, a clinician must consider all aspects of a child, seeking to identify both protective and risk factors in the context of stress. We invite clinicians to use a strength-based lens when assessing children's capacity to adapt and respond with behavioral and emotional flexibility to challenges. There is no table of developmentally expected behaviors for this category, as resiliency is a dynamic and global concept that needs to be assessed in the context of individual differences and across contexts.

Observations of a child's functioning and response to stress across settings as reported by teachers, parents, and others are extremely valuable when rating the child's resiliency. The diagnostic process in itself represents for many children a source of significant stress; observing how the child adapts to it is relevant to this area. Identifying potential or current protective and risk factors in the child's relational environment is particularly important, especially for treatment planning.

Rating Scale

5. Children at this level can adapt and respond flexibly to unexpected, stressful situations in an age-appropriate fashion that does not significantly compromise overall functioning and ongoing development. They seem implicitly aware of their strengths and vulnerabilities, have a repertoire of flexible behavioral responses to stressful situations, and can ask for support when necessary. They do not succumb to states of disorganization or fragmentation, and they lead with strengths (e.g., "I can use humor or fantasy to distract myself and cope with this painful experience").

3. At this level, children can adapt and respond flexibly to most unexpected, stressful situations in an age-appropriate fashion. At times, however, they succumb to states of anxiety and use maladaptive defenses that reduce feelings of competence and confidence. At other times, they can rely on strengths in the service of ego functioning and can return to a baseline capacity of thinking about feelings, regaining the capacity for self-regulation. These experiences do not significantly restrict their overall functioning and growth. Mild forms of symptomatology may be present.

1. Children at this level seem extremely vulnerable and at the mercy of the external world for their mental state and even physical survival. When they encounter unpredictable and stressful situations, their responses are maladaptive. They tend to regress to early modes and to try compulsively to regain some internal balance by exerting control on the external world in nonadaptive ways.

Most Relevant Assessment Tools

Where indicated below, measures (or their adolescent versions) are discussed in the "Most Relevant Assessment Tools" section for capacity 9 in Chapter 4 (pp. 295–298).

Child and Youth Resilience Measure–28

The Child and Youth Resilience Measure–28 (CYRM-28; Liebenberg, Ungar, & LeBlanc, 2013) assesses overall resiliency, plus three subcategories that may influence resiliency processes: individual traits, relationship to caregiver(s), and contextual factors that facilitate a sense of belonging. The measure was established via interviews with youth and adults in several countries. Their reflections about obstacles and resources produced a 58-item measure. Pilot testing with 1,451 youth in 14 communities in 11 countries enabled a reduction to a 28-item version. A 12-item version is also available.

Information on the measure's emerging reliability and validity is available in several publications.

Devereux Early Childhood Assessment

The Devereux Early Childhood Assessment (DECA; LeBuffe & Naglieri, 1998), with versions for parents and teachers, was developed as part of an intervention program (the Devereux Early Childhood Initiative) for 2- to 5-year-olds. It promotes teacher–parent collaboration in recognizing children's strengths and protective factors. In 37 items organized into four subscales, it identifies "resilience" and "protective" factors: (1) initiative (child's capacity to use independent thought and actions to meet needs); (2) self-control (child's ability to experience a wide range of feelings and express them in socially appropriate words and actions); (3) attachment (persistent relationships between child and significant adults); and (4) behavior concerns. It provides an individual and classroom profile with specific strategies for a given child and for the class as a whole. The DECA-C (clinical version) is a 62-item questionnaire for mental health and special education professionals dealing with behavioral concerns. It contains the same strengths-based items, plus 25 items that deal with problems of aggression, attention, emotional control, withdrawal/depression, and so on. A DECA program for infants and toddlers has recently been developed.

Resiliency Scales for Children and Adolescents

The Resiliency Scales for Children and Adolescents (RSCA; Prince-Embury, 2005, 2006) is described in Chapter 4 (p. 296).

Penn Interactive Peer Play Scale

The Penn Interactive Peer Play Scale (PIPPS; Fantuzzo et al., 1995) is a 36-item measure to be completed by preschool teachers of 3- to 5-year-olds. It contains items on emotional behavior, desirable social actions, and lack of social connectedness. Its major drawback is the length of time required to administer it.

Strengths and Difficulties Questionnaire

The Strengths and Difficulties Questionnaire (SDQ; Goodman, 1997) is described in Chapter 4 (p. 298).

10. Self-Observing Capacities (Psychological Mindedness)

For a broader definition of the 10th category, see Chapters 2 (pp. 110–113) and 4 (pp. 298–300).

Psychological mindedness develops in response to a child's increasing ability for abstraction, understanding of the self, experience of mixed emotions, and taking the perspective of others. As for capacity 9, there is no table of developmentally expected behaviors for this category, as this is a dynamic and global concept that should be assessed in terms of individual differences and across contexts.

It is hard to stipulate age-related ways in which this set of capacities manifests itself. Clinicians should look for signs of emerging or consolidated interpersonal curiosity and capacity to link different relational experiences in a meaningful way. For younger children, clinicians should pay attention to the stories communicated during play. Do they reflect, via displacement, an emerging capacity for self-observation and emotional insight? For example, if a doll wants to go into the parents' room but must not in a child's story, the child is referencing a wish and its associated emotional needs along with a counteractive reality.

Rating Scale

5. The child can reflect on a full range of feelings or experiences of self and other, including subtle variations in feelings, and can compare them to a longer-term view of self, values, and goals. The child can reflect on multiple relationships between feelings and experiences, and can be reflective across the full range of age-expected experiences in the context of new challenges. The child shows a genuine interest in understanding the feelings and thoughts of others.
3. The child can reflect on feelings or experiences of self and others in the present, and can compare them to a longer-term view of self, values, and goals for some age-expected experiences, but not others. The child cannot be reflective when feelings are strong or when he or she is under significant stress. There is intermittent capacity to reflect on moment-to-moment experiences. Interest is dependent on the child's affective state.
1. The child is unable to reflect on feelings or experiences, even in the present. Self-awareness may be limited to polarized feeling states, or simple basic feeling states, or simple basic feelings without an appreciation of emotional subtlety. On occasion, self-awareness is lacking, and there may be a tendency toward fragmentation and lack of interest on others in general.

Most Relevant Assessment Tools

The Child and Adolescent Mindfulness Measure (CAMM; Greco, Baer, & Smith, 2011) is a recently developed questionnaire that assesses present-moment awareness and nonjudgmental, nonavoidant responses to thoughts and feelings in children and adolescents (e.g., "I keep myself busy so I don't notice my thoughts or feelings"). Its 10 items are each rated on a 5-point scale.

11. Capacity to Construct and Use Internal Standards and Ideals

When assessing this category, a clinician should observe the degree of harshness or rigidity in a child's superego (e.g., a harshly self-critical child tears up work after completing it, whereas a rigid child erases and redoes work in a compulsive manner). There are children for whom superego functioning is uneven, meaning that their reactions depend on the meaning ascribed to a given circumstance. In such cases, clinicians should observe the balance, if it exists, between benign (e.g., "I can do it again") and punitive (e.g., "I always do everything wrong") superego manifestations.

The following is a developmental guideline to age-expected attainments for children ages 4–11.

Developmental Guideline: Capacity to Construct and Use Internal Standards and Ideals in Children Ages 4–11

Ages 4–6

Moral feelings are increasingly integrated into the sense of self. The child begins to internalize more abstract parental values and interpersonal standards. Prohibited behaviors and impulses evoke feelings of shame and guilt. As self-punishments and internal prohibitions substitute for external (parental) enforcement, the child's self-regulatory capacities begin to become more autonomous. Relationships between child and caregivers are complicated by rivalry and hostility, and by any problematic role of parents in addressing a child's destructive or sexual inclinations.

Ages 7–8

To preserve the relationship, the child adapts to parents' demands. In fantasy, the child may vent anger and resentment by momentarily wishing the parents dead or gone. There is still a tendency toward shame, which typically leads to retreat and/or attempts to externalize blame. At times of vulnerability, splits between the ideal and denigrated appear—for example, during play in themes of "good guy versus bad guy" and in sibling relationships (what is right and wrong, fair and unfair). Anxiety related to skills increasingly visible to peers can result in defenses to protect self-worth (e.g., "I don't play four-square because it is boring and stupid").

Ages 9–11

Through identification and internalization, the child's capacity to direct, limit, punish, and reward the self has been consolidated. An increasingly advanced mental organization includes a more gendered self-representation and an internalized sense of right and wrong. The capacity for guilt is strongly established, and with it the need for reparative efforts. Role model behavior and positive regard have been more stably internalized. A more integrated, less harsh "inner voice" replaces earlier internalizations of parents, teachers, and others.

Rating Scale

5. Internal standards are flexible and integrated with a realistic sense of a child's capacities and social contexts. They provide opportunities for meaningful striving and feelings of self-esteem. Developmentally appropriate feelings of guilt function as signals for reappraising the child's behavior.
3. Internal standards and ideals tend to be rigid and insufficiently sensitive to the child's own capacities and social contexts. Feelings of guilt are experienced more as self-criticism than as a signal for reappraising the child's behavior.
1. Internal standards, ideals, and sense of morality are based on harsh, punitive expectations. Feelings of guilt are denied and associated with internalizing and externalizing behaviors. Or the child seems to have no internal standards, ideals, or sense of morality in many or all areas of experience.

Summary of Basic Mental Functioning

Following the approach taken in Chapter 2 on the M Axis and Chapter 4 on the MA Axis, we recommend that clinicians summarize basic mental functioning quantitatively (see Table 7.2).

(text resumes on page 494)

TABLE 7.2. Summary of Basic Mental Functioning: MC Axis

To obtain a quantitative rating of a child patient's overall mental functioning, a clinician should add up the 1–5 point ratings assigned to each of the 11 capacities (Table 7.2a), yielding a numerical index of overall functioning ranging from 11 to 55, with higher scores reflecting healthier functioning. This index allows the clinician to assign the child to one of the seven categories outlined in Table 7.2b, which provides short qualitative descriptions of seven levels of mental functioning.

TABLE 7.2a. MC-Axis Functioning: Total Score

MC-Axis capacities	Rating scale				
1. Capacity for regulation, attention, and learning	5	4	3	2	1
2. Capacity for affective range, communication, and understanding	5	4	3	2	1
3. Capacity for mentalization and reflective functioning	5	4	3	2	1
4. Capacity for differentiation and integration (identity)	5	4	3	2	1
5. Capacity for relationships and intimacy	5	4	3	2	1
6. Capacity for self-esteem regulation and quality of internal experience	5	4	3	2	1
7. Capacity for impulse control and regulation	5	4	3	2	1
8. Capacity for defensive functioning	5	4	3	2	1
9. Capacity for adaptation, resiliency, and strength	5	4	3	2	1
10. Self-observing capacities (psychological mindedness)	5	4	3	2	1
11. Capacity to construct and use internal standards and ideals	5	4	3	2	1
	Total score = __				

TABLE 7.2b. Levels of Mental Functioning

Healthy

MC1. Healthy/optimal mental functioning (range = 50–55)

The child shows optimal or very good functioning in all or most mental capacities, with modest, expectable variations in flexibility and adaptation across life contexts.

Neurotic

MC2. Good/appropriate mental functioning with some areas of difficulty (range = 43–49)

The child shows an appropriate level of mental functioning, with some specific areas of difficulty (e.g., in three or four mental capacities). These difficulties can reflect conflicts or challenges related to specific life situations or events.

MC3. Mild impairments in mental functioning (range = 37–42)

The child shows mild constrictions and areas of inflexibility in some domains of mental functioning, such as self-esteem regulation, impulse and affect regulation, defensive functioning, and self-observing capacity.

Borderline

MC4. Moderate impairments in mental functioning (range = 30–36)

The child shows moderate constrictions and areas of inflexibility in most or almost all domains of mental functioning, affecting quality and stability of relationships, sense of identity, and range of affects tolerated. Functioning at this level reflects significantly impaired adaptation.

(continued)

TABLE 7.2. *(continued)*

MC5. Major impairments in mental functioning (range = 24–29)
The child shows major constrictions and alterations in almost all domains of mental functioning (e.g., tendencies toward fragmentation and difficulties in self–object differentiation), along with limitation of experience of feelings and/or thoughts in major life areas (i.e., love, school, play).
MC6. Significant defects in basic mental functions (range = 17–23)
The child shows significant defects in most domains of mental functioning, along with problems in the organization and/or integration–differentiation of self and other.
Psychotic
MC7. Major/severe defects in basic mental functions (range = 11–16)
The child shows major and severe defects in almost all domains of mental functioning, with impairment in reality testing; fragmentation and/or difficulties in self–object differentiation; disturbances in perception, integration, and regulation of affect and thought; and defects in one or more basic mental functions.

Given the wide range of ages covered in this chapter, we have mentioned specific characteristics expected for subgroups in the sets of guidelines provided in the chapter text. Many of the descriptions are based on Stanley Greenspan's work on the clinical interview of the child. Others are based on our own efforts to integrate contemporary clinical and empirical findings that can guide the comprehensive, developmentally informed clinical assessment of children.

BIBLIOGRAPHY

1. Capacity for Regulation, Attention, and Learning

Bauer, P. J., & Fivush, R. (Eds.). (2014). *The Wiley handbook on the development of children's memory.* Chichester, UK: Wiley-Blackwell.

Berninger, V. (2007). *PAL-II user's guide.* San Antonio, TX: Pearson.

Bliss, S. L. (2007). [Review of the Battelle Developmental Inventory—Second Edition.] *Journal of Psychoeducational Assessment, 25*(4), 409–415.

Clarebout, G., Horz, H., & Schnotz, W. (2010). The relations between self-regulation and the embedding of support in learning environments. *Educational Technology Research and Development, 58*(5), 573–587.

Conners, C. K. (1997). *Conners' Rating Scales—Revised: Technical manual.* North Tonawanda, NY: Multi-Health Systems. (Read more: *www.minddisorders.com/Br-Del/Conners-Rating-Scales-Revised.html#ixzz3X6vn6bnv*)

Crone, E. A., Ridderinkhof, K. R., Worm, M., Van Der Molen, M. W., & Somsen, R. J. M. (2004). Switching between spatial stimulus–response mappings: A developmental study of cognitive flexibility. *Developmental Science, 7,* 443–455.

Dennis, T. A., Brotman, L. M., Huang, K. Y., & Gouley, K. K. (2007). Effortful control, social competence, and adjustment problems in children at risk for psychopathology. *Journal of Clinical Child and Adolescent Psychology, 36,* 442–454.

Eisenberg, N., Haugen, R., Spinrad, T. L., Hofer, C., Chassin, L., Zhou, Q., . . . Liew, J. (2010). Relations of temperament to maladjustment and ego resiliency in at-risk children. *Social Development, 19,* 577–600.

Fan, J., McCandliss, B. D., Fossella, J., Flombaum, J. I., & Posner, M. I. (2005). The activation of attentional networks. *NeuroImage, 26,* 471–479.

Gilliom, M., Shaw, D. S., Beck, J. E., Schonberg, M. A., & Lukon, J. L. (2002). Anger regulation in disadvantaged preschool boys: Strategies, antecedents, and the development of self-control. *Developmental Psychology, 38,* 222–235.

Kester, S., Rakoczy, K., & Otto, B. (2010). Promotion of self-regulated learning in classrooms: Investigating frequency, quality, and consequences for student performance. *Metacognition and Learning, 5*(2), 157–171.

Leon-Carrion, J., García-Orza, J., & Pérez-Santamaría, F. J. (2004). Development of the inhibitory component of the executive functions in children and adolescents. *International Journal of Neuroscience, 114,* 1291–1311.

Lillas, C., & Turnbull, J. (2009). *Infant/child mental health, early intervention, and relationship-based therapies: A neurorelational framework for interdisciplinary practice*. New York: Norton.

Mayer, J. D., Caruso, D., & Salovey, P. (1999). Emotional intelligence meets traditional standards for an intelligence. *Intelligence, 27*(4), 267–298.

Montalvo, F. T., & Torres, M. C. (2008). Self-regulated learning: Current and future directions. *Electronic Journal of Research in Educational Psychology, 2*(1), 1–34.

Naglieri, J. A. (2008). *Naglieri Nonverbal Ability Test—Second Edition*. San Antonio, TX: Pearson.

Naglieri, J. A., & Ford, D. (2003). Addressing underrepresentation of gifted minority children using the Naglieri Nonverbal Ability Test (NNAT). *Gifted Child Quarterly, 47*, 155–160.

Naglieri, J. A., & Goldstein, S. (2013). *Comprehensive Executive Function Index*. Toronto: Multi-Health Systems.

Newborg, J. (2005). *Battelle Developmental Inventory, Second Edition*. Itasca, IL: Riverside.

Rothbart, M. K., Ahadi, S. A., Herhey, K. L., & Fiher, P. (2001). Investigations of temperament at three to seven years: The Children's Behavior Questionnaire. *Child Development, 72*, 1394–1408.

Rueda, M. R., Fan, J., McCandliss, B. D., Halparin, J. D., Gruber, D. B., Lercari, L. P., & Posner, M. I. (2004). Development of attentional networks in childhood. *Neuropsychologia, 42*, 1029–1040.

Schunk, D. H. (2001). Social cognitive theory and self-regulated learning. In B. J. Zimmerman & D. H. Schunk (Eds.), *Self-regulated learning and academic achievement: Theoretical perspectives*. Mahwah, NJ: Erlbaum.

Wechsler, D. (2012). *Wechsler Preschool and Primary Scale of Intelligence—Fourth Edition*. San Antonio, TX: Pearson.

2. Capacity for Affective Range, Communication, and Understanding

Bamford, C., & Lagattuta, K. H. (2012). Looking on the bright side: Children's knowledge about the benefits of positive versus negative thinking. *Child Development, 83*(2), 667–682.

Bellak, L., & Bellak, S. S. (1949). *Children's Apperception Test*. Gracie Station, NY: Consulting Psychologists Press.

Bucci, W. (2001). Pathways of emotional communication. *Psychoanalytic Inquiry, 21*, 40–70.

Denham, S. A., & Weissberg, R. P. (2004). Social-emotional learning in early childhood: What we know and where to go from here? In E. Chesebrough, P. King, T. P. Gullotta, & M. Bloom (Eds.), *A blueprint for the promotion of prosocial behavior in early childhood* (pp. 13–50). New York: Kluwer Academic/Plenum.

Diaconu, I. (2009). The influence of late adoption on maltreated children's non-verbal behavior and display of affect. *Revue Roumaine de Psychanalyse, 2*, 154–167.

Epstein, M., & Sharma, J. (1998). *Behavioral and Emotional Rating Scale: A strength-based approach to assessment*. Austin, TX: PRO-ED.

Gresham, F., & Elliott, S. N. (2008). *Social Skills Improvement System Rating Scales*. San Antonio, TX: Pearson.

Kårstad, S. B., Kvello, O., Wichstrøm, L., & Berg-Nielsen, T. S. (2014). What do parents know about their children's comprehension of emotions?: Accuracy of parental estimates in a community sample of preschoolers. *Child: Care, Health and Development, 40*(3), 346–353.

Katan, A. (1961). Some thoughts about the role of verbalization in early childhood. *Psychoanalytic Study of the Child, 16*, 184–188.

Koch, E. (2003). Reflections on a study of temper tantrums in older children. *Psychoanalytic Psychology, 20*, 456–471.

Kromm, H., Färber, M., & Holodynski, M. (2015). Felt or false smiles?: Volitional regulation of emotional expression in 4-, 6-, and 8-year-old children. *Child Development, 86*(2), 579–597.

Krystal, H. (1978). Trauma and affects. *Psychoanalytic Study of the Child, 33*, 81–116.

Laurent, J., Catanzaro, S. J., Joiner, T. E., Jr., Rudolph, K. D., Potter, K. I., Lambert, S., . . . Gathright, T. (1999). A measure of positive and negative affect for children: Scale development and preliminary validation. *Psychological Assessment, 11*(3), 326–338.

Mayer, J. D., Caruso, D., & Salovey, P. (1999). Emotional intelligence meets traditional standards for an intelligence. *Intelligence, 27*(4), 267–298.

Mayer, J. D., & Salovey, P. (1997). What is emotional intelligence? In P. Salovey & D. Sluyter (Eds.), *Emotional development and emotional intelligence: Educational implications* (pp. 3–31). New York: Basic Books.

Morton, J. B., & Trehub, S. E. (2001). Children's understanding of emotion in speech. *Child Development, 72*(3), 834–843.

Novick, J., & Novick, K. K. (2001). Two systems of self-regulation. *Psychoanalytic Social Work, 8*, 95–122.

Russ, S. (Ed.). (1999). *Affect, creative experience, and psychological adjustment*. Philadelphia: Brunner/Mazel.

Shields, A., & Cicchetti, D. (1997). *Emotion Regulation Checklist*. Princeton, NJ: Educational Testing Service.

Slochower, J. (2004). But what do you want?: The location of emotional experience. *Contemporary Psychoanalysis, 40*, 577–602.

Taumoepeau, M., & Ruffman, T. (2006). Mother and infant talk about mental states relates to desire language and emotion understanding. *Child Development, 77*(2), 465–481.

Thorlacius, O., & Gudmundsson, E. (2015). Assessment of children's emotional adjustment: Construction and validation of a new instrument. *Child: Care, Health and Development, 41*(5), 641–776.

3. Capacity for Mentalization and Reflective Functioning

Astington, J. (2001). The future of theory-of-mind research: Understanding motivational states, the role of language, and real-world consequences. *Child Development, 72*, 685–687.

Baron-Cohen, S., Wheelwright, S., Hill, J., Raste, Y., & Plumb, I. (2001). The "Reading the Mind in the Eyes" Test Revised Version: A study with normal adults, and adults with Asperger syndrome or high-functioning autism. *Journal of Child Psychology and Psychiatry, 42*(2), 241–251.

Bassett, H. H., Denham, S. A., Mincic, M. M., & Graling, K. (2012). The structure of preschoolers' emotion knowledge: Model equivalence and validity using an SEM approach. *Early Education and Development, 23*, 259–279.

Begeer, S., Malle, B. F., Nieuwland, M. S., & Keysar, B. (2010). Using theory of mind to represent and take part in social interactions: Comparing individuals with high functioning autism and typically developing controls. *European Journal of Developmental Psychology, 7*, 104–122.

Bellak, L., & Bellak, S. (1949). *Children's Apperception Test.* Gracie Station, NY: Consulting Psychologists Press.

Carlson, S. M., Moses, L. J., & Brenton, C. (2002). How specific is the relationship between executive functioning and theory of mind?: Contributions of inhibitory control and working memory. *Infant and Child Development, 11*, 73–92.

Carpendale, J. I., & Lewis, C. (2004). Constructing and understanding of mind: The development of children's social understanding within social interaction. *Behavioral and Brain Sciences, 27*, 79–151.

Denham, S. A. (1986). Social cognition, prosocial behavior, and emotion in preschoolers: Contextual validation. *Child Development, 57*, 194–201.

Denham, S. A., Bassett, H. H., Way, E., Mincic, M., Zinsser, K., & Graling, K. (2012). Preschoolers' emotion knowledge: Self-regulatory foundations, and predictions of early school success. *Cognition and Emotion, 26*, 667–679.

Ensink, K. (2003). *Assessing theory of mind, affective understanding and reflective functioning in primary school-aged children.* Unpublished doctoral dissertation, University College London.

Ensink, K., Target, M., & Oandasan, C. (2013). *Child Reflective Functioning Scale scoring manual: For application to the Child Attachment Interview.* Unpublished manuscript, Anna Freud Centre, University College London.

Epstein, M. H., & Sharma, H. M. (1998). *Behavioral and Emotional Rating Scale: A strength-based approach to assessment.* Austin, TX: PRO-ED.

Fonagy, P., & Target, M. (1997). Attachment and reflective function: Their role in self-organization. *Development and Psychopathology, 9*(4), 679–700.

Fonagy, P., & Target, M. (2003). *Psychoanalytic theories: Perspectives from developmental psychopathology.* London: Whurr.

Fonagy, P., & Target, M. (2006). The mentalization-focused approach to self-pathology. *Journal of Personality Disorders, 20*(6), 544–576.

Fonagy, P., & Target, M. (2007a). The rooting of the mind in the body: New links between attachment theory and psychoanalytic thought. *Journal of the American Psychoanalytic Association, 55*, 411–456.

Fonagy, P., & Target, M. (2007b). Playing with reality: IV. A theory of external reality rooted in intersubjectivity. *International Journal of Psychoanalysis, 88*, 917–937.

Fonagy, P., Target, M., & Ensink, K. (2000). *The Affect Task.* Unpublished measure and coding manual, Anna Freud Centre, University College London.

Fonagy, P., Target, M., & Gergely, G. (2006). Psychoanalytic perspectives on developmental psychopathology. In D. Cicchetti & D. J. Cohen (Eds.), *Developmental psychopathology: Vol. 1. Theory and method* (2nd ed., pp. 701–749). Hoboken, NJ: Wiley.

Fonagy, P., Target, M., Steele, H., & Steele, M. (1998). *Reflective-functioning manual for application to Adult Attachment Interviews (Version 5).* Unpublished manual, Psychoanalysis Unit, University College London.

Happé, F. (1994). An advanced test of theory of mind: Understanding of story characters' thoughts and feelings by able autistic, mentally handicapped, and normal children and adults. *Journal of Autism and Developmental Disorders, 24*, 129–154.

Hughes, C., & Leekam, S. (2004). What are the links between theory of mind and social relations?: Review reflections and new directions for studies of typical and atypical development. *Social Development, 13*, 590–619.

Katznelson, H. (2013). Reflective functioning: A review. *Clinical Psychology Review, 34*, 107–117.

Kusche, C. A., Beilke, R. L., & Greenberg, M. T. (1988). *Kusche Affective Interview—Revised.* Unpublished measure, University of Washington, Seattle, WA.

Mayer, J. D., Caruso, D., & Salovey, P. (1999). Emotional intelligence meets traditional standards for an intelligence. *Intelligence, 27*(4), 267–298.

Mayer, J. D., & Salovey, P. (1997). What is emotional intelligence? In P. Salovey & D. Sluyter (Eds.),

Emotional development and emotional intelligence: Educational implications (pp. 3–31). New York: Basic Books.

Meltzoff, A. (2007). "Like me": A foundation for social cognition. *Developmental Science, 10*, 126–134.

Norris, C., Chen, E., Zhu, D. C., Small, S. L., & Cacioppo, J. T. (2004). The interaction of social and emotional processes in the brain. *Journal of Cognitive Neuroscience, 16*, 1818–1829.

Pons, F., & Harris, P. L. (2005). Longitudinal change and longitudinal stability of individual differences in children's emotion understanding. *Cognition and Emotion, 19*(8), 1158–1174.

Pons, M. F. D., Lafortune, L., Doudin, P. A., & Albanese, O. (Eds.). (2006). *Toward emotional competences.* Aalborg, Denmark: Aalborg University Press.

Shmueli-Goetz, Y., Target, M., Fonagy, P., & Datta, A. (2008). The Child Attachment Interview: A psychometric study of reliability and discriminant validity. *Developmental Psychology, 44*, 939–956.

Siegal, M., & Varley, R. (2002). Neural systems involved in theory of mind. *Nature Reviews Neuroscience, 3*, 463–470.

Sterck, E., & Begeer, S. (2010). Theory of mind: Specialized capacity or emergent property? *European Journal of Developmental Psychology, 7*, 1–16.

Sugarman, A. (2006). Mentalization, insightfulness, and therapeutic action: The importance of mental organization. *International Journal of Psychoanalysis, 87*, 965–998.

Target, M., Fonagy, P., Shmueli-Goetz, Y., Schneider, T., & Datta, A. (2000). *Child Attachment Interview (CAI): Coding and classification manual, Version III.* Unpublished manuscript, University College London.

4. Capacity for Differentiation and Integration

Alvarez, A. (2006). Some questions concerning states of fragmentation: Unintegration, underintegration, disintegration, and the nature of early integrations. *Journal of Child Psychotherapy, 32*, 158–180.

Bergman, A. (2000). Merging and emerging: Separation–individuation theory and the treatment of children with disorders of the sense of self. *Journal of Infant, Child and Adolescent Psychotherapy, 1*, 61–75.

Denham, S. A. (1986). Social cognition, prosocial behavior, and emotion in preschoolers: Contextual validation. *Child Development, 57*, 194–201.

Fonagy, P., Target, M., & Ensink, K. (2000). *The Affect Task.* Unpublished measure and coding manual. Anna Freud Centre, University College London.

Happé, F. (1994). An advanced test of theory of mind: Understanding of story characters' thoughts and feelings by able autistic, mentally handicapped, and normal children and adults. *Journal of Autism and Developmental Disorders, 24*, 129–154.

Hodges, J., Hillman, S., Steele, M., & Henderson, K. (2004). *Story Stem Assessment rating manual.* Unpublished manuscript, Anna Freud Centre, University College London.

Kusche, C. A., Beilke, R. L., & Greenberg, M. T. (1988). *Kusche Affective Interview—Revised.* Unpublished manuscript, University of Washington, Seattle, WA.

Jemerin, J. M. (2004). Latency and the capacity to reflect on mental states. *Psychoanalytic Study of the Child, 59*, 211–239.

Lane, R. D., & Garfield, D. A. (2005). Becoming aware of feelings: Integration of cognitive-developmental, neuroscientific, and psychoanalytic perspectives. *Neuropsychoanalysis, 7*, 5–30.

Martin-Vallas, F., & Kutek, A. (2005). Towards a theory of the integration of the other in representation. *Journal of Analytical Psychology, 50*, 285–293.

Pons, F., & Harris, P. L. (2005). Longitudinal change and longitudinal stability of individual differences in children's emotion understanding. *Cognition and Emotion, 19*, 1158–1174.

Schore, A. N. (2003). *Affect dysregulation and disorders of the self.* New York: Norton.

Steiner, A. (2004). Containment, enactment, and communication. In E. Hargreaves & A. Varchevker (Eds.), *Pursuit of psychic change: The Betty Joseph Workshop* (pp. 136–150). London: Brunner-Routledge.

Winnicott, D. W. (1965). *The maturational processes and the facilitating environment.* London: Hogarth Press.

5. Capacity for Relationships and Intimacy

Berlin, N. G. (2005). Tripartite treatment of childhood aggression: A view from attachment theory. *Journal of Infant, Child and Adolescent Psychotherapy, 4*, 134–155.

Forsyth, D. W. (1997). Proposals regarding the neurobiology of oedipality. *Psychoanalysis and Contemporary Thought, 20*, 163–206.

Gilmore, K. (2011). Pretend play and development in early childhood (with implications for the oedipal phase). *Journal of the American Psychoanalytic Association, 59*, 1157–1181.

Hodges, J., Hillman, S., Steele, M., & Henderson, K. (2004). *Story Stem Assessment rating manual.* Unpublished manuscript, Anna Freud Centre, University College London.

Knight, R. (2011). Fragmentation, fluidity, and

transformation: Nonlinear development in middle childhood. *Psychoanalytic Study of the Child, 65*, 19–47.

Machover, K. (1949). *Personality projection in the drawing of the human figure.* Springfield, IL: Charles C Thomas.

Roberts, G. E. (2005). *Roberts Apperception Test for Children–2.* Los Angeles: Western Psychological Services.

Steele, M., Hodges, J., Kaniuk, J., & Steele, H. (2010). Mental representation and change: Developing attachment relationships in an adoption context. *Psychoanalytic Inquiry, 30*, 25–40.

Target, M., Shmueli-Goetz, Y., & Fonagy, P. (2002). Attachment representations in school-age children: The early development of the Child Attachment Interview (CAI). *Journal of Infant, Child and Adolescent Psychotherapy, 2*, 91–105.

6. Capacity for Self-Esteem Regulation and Quality of Internal Experience

Bornstein, B. (1951). On latency. *Psychoanalytic Study of the Child, 6*, 279–285.

Buhs, E. S., Ladd, G. W., & Herald, S. L. (2006). Peer exclusion and victimization: Processes that mediate the relation between peer group rejection and children's classroom engagement and achievement? *Journal of Educational Psychology, 98*, 1–13.

Friedman, R. C., & Downey, J. I. (2000). The psychobiology of the late childhood: Significance for psychoanalytic developmental theory and clinical practice. *Journal of the American Academy of Psychoanalysis, 28*, 431–448.

Harter, S., & Pike, R. (1984). The Pictorial Scale of Perceived Competence and Social Acceptance for Young Children. *Child Development, 55*, 1969–1982.

Hodges, J., Hillman, S., & Steele, M. (2004). *Little Piggy Narrative Story Stem coding manual.* Unpublished manuscript.

Knight, R. (2005). The process of attachment and autonomy in latency: A longitudinal study of ten children. *Psychoanalytic Study of the Child, 60*, 178–210.

Loewald, H. W. (1979). The waning of the oedipal complex. *Journal of American Psychoanalytic Association, 27*, 751–775.

Machover, K. (1949). *Personality projection in the drawing of the human figure.* Springfield, IL: Charles C Thomas.

Novick, J., & Novick, K. K. (1996). A developmental perspective of omnipotence. *Journal of Clinical Psychoanalysis, 5*, 129–173.

Roberts, G. E. (2005). *Roberts Apperception Test for Children–2.* Los Angeles: Western Psychological Services.

Seligman, S. (2003). The developmental perspective in relational psychoanalysis. *Contemporary Psychoanalysis, 39*, 477–508.

Veronneau, M. H., Vitaro, F., Brendgen, M., Dishion, T. J., & Tremblay, R. E. (2010). Transactional analysis of the reciprocal links between peer experiences and academic achievement from middle childhood to early adolescence. *Developmental Psychology, 46*, 773–790.

7. Capacity for Impulse Control and Regulation

Achenbach, T. M., & Rescorla, L. A. (2001). *Manual for ASEBA School-Age Forms and Profiles.* Burlington: University of Vermont, Research Center for Children, Youth, and Families.

Bronson, M. (2000). *Self-regulation in early childhood: Nature and nurture.* New York: Guilford Press.

Conners, C. K. (1997). *Conners' Rating Scales—Revised: Technical manual.* North Tonawanda, NY: Multi-Health Systems.

Dawson, P., & Guare, R. (2010). *Executive skills in children and adolescents: A practical guide to assessment and intervention* (2nd ed.). New York: Guilford Press.

Denham, S. A., Wyatt, T. M., Bassett, H. H., Echeverria, D., & Knox, S. S. (2009). Assessing social-emotional development in children from a longitudinal perspective. *Journal of Epidemiology and Community Health, 63*(Suppl. 1), i37–i52.

Eisenberg, N., Smith, C. L., Sadovsky, A., & Spinrad, T. L. (2004). Effortful control: Relations with emotion regulation, adjustment, and socialization in childhood. In R. F. Baumeister & K. D. Vohs (Eds.), *Handbook of self-regulation: Research, theory, and applications* (pp. 259–282). New York: Guilford Press.

Harter, S., & Pike, R. (1984). The Pictorial Scale of Perceived Competence and Social Acceptance for Young Children. *Child Development, 55*, 1969–1982.

Kopp, C. B. (1982). Antecedents of self-regulation: A developmental perspective. *Developmental Psychology, 18*(2), 199–214.

Olson, S. L., Sameroff, A. J., Lunkenheimer, E. S., & Kerr, D. (2009). Self-regulatory processes in the development of disruptive behavior problems: The preschool-to-school transition. In S. L. Olson & A. J. Sameroff (Eds.), *Biopsychosocial regulatory processes in the development of childhood behavioral problems* (pp. 144–185). New York: Cambridge University Press.

Posner, M. I., & Rothbart, M. K. (2000). Developing mechanisms of self-regulation. *Development and Psychopathology, 12*(3), 427–441.

Rothbart, M. K. (1991). Temperament: A developmental framework. In A. Angleitner & J. Strelau (Eds.), *Explorations in temperament: International perspectives on theory and measurement* (pp. 61–74). New York: Plenum Press.

Rothbart, M. K., & Ahadi, S. A. (1994). Temperament and the development of personality. *Journal of Abnormal Psychology, 103*(1), 55–66.

Rothbart, M. K., Ellis, L. K., & Posner, M. I. (2004). Temperament and self-regulation. In R. F. Baumeister & K. D. Vohs (Eds.), *Handbook of self-regulation: Research, theory, and applications* (pp. 357–370). New York: Guilford Press.

8. Capacity for Defensive Functioning

Benveniste, D. (2005). Recognizing defenses in the drawings and play of children in therapy. *Psychoanalytic Psychology, 22*, 395–410.

Bonfiglio, B. (2014). Analyzing defenses or the first glimmer of development? *Psychoanalytic Dialogues, 24*, 691–705.

Chazan, S. (2002). *Profiles of play.* London: Jessica Kingsley.

Chazan, S. E., & Wolf, J. (2002). Using the Children's Play Therapy Instrument to measure change in psychotherapy: The conflicted player. *Journal of Infant, Child and Adolescent Psychotherapy, 2*(3), 73–102.

Cramer, P. (2015). Change in children's externalizing and internalizing behavior problems: The role of defense mechanisms. *Journal of Nervous and Mental Disease, 203*, 215–221.

Egan, J., & Kernberg, P. F. (1984). Pathological narcissism in childhood. *Journal of the American Psychoanalytic Association, 32*, 39–62.

Freud, A. (1966). *The ego and the mechanisms of defense.* New York: International Universities Press. (Original work published 1936)

Laor, N., Wolmer, L., & Cicchetti, D. V. (2001). The comprehensive assessment of defense style: Measuring defense mechanisms in children and adolescents. *Journal of Nervous and Mental Disease, 189*(6), 360–368.

Tallandini, M. A., & Caudek, C. (2010). Defense mechanisms development in typical children. *Psychotherapy Research, 20*(5), 535–545.

9. Capacity for Adaptation, Resiliency, and Strength

Donnon, T., & Hammond, W. (2007). A psychometric assessment of the self-reported Youth Resiliency: Assessing Developmental Strengths Questionnaire. *Psychological Reports, 100*, 963–978.

Fantuzzo, J., Sutton-Smith, B., Coolahan, K. C., Manz, P. H., Canning, S., & Debnam, D. (1995). Assessment of preschool play interaction behaviors in young low-income children: Penn Interactive Peer Play Scale. *Early Childhood Research Quarterly, 10*, 105–120.

Goodman, R. (1997). The Strengths and Difficulties Questionnaire: A research note. *Journal of Child Psychology and Psychiatry, 38*, 581–586.

LeBuffe, P. A., & J. A. Naglieri (1998). *The Devereux Early Childhood Assessment (DECA).* Villanova, PA: Devereux Foundation.

Liebenberg, L., Ungar, M., & LeBlanc, J. C. (2013). The CYRM-12: A brief measure of resilience. *Canadian Journal of Public Health, 104*(2), 131–135.

Liebenberg, L., Ungar, M., & Van de Vijver, F. (2012). Validation of the Child and Youth Resilience Measure-28 (CYRM-28) among Canadian youth. *Research on Social Work Practice, 22*(2), 219–226.

Prince-Embury, S. (2005). The Resiliency Scales for Children and Adolescents as related to parent education level and race/ethnicity in children. *Canadian Journal of School Psychology, 24*(2), 167–182.

Prince-Embury, S. (2006). *Resiliency Scales for Children and Adolescents: Profiles of personal strengths.* San Antonio, TX: Harcourt Assessment.

Rutter, M. (2012). Resilience as a dynamic concept. *Development and Psychopathology, 24*, 335–344.

Rutter, M., & The ERA Research Team. (1998) Developmental catch-up, and deficit, following adoption after severe global early privation. *Journal of Child Psychology and Psychiatry, 39*, 465–476.

10. Self-Observing Capacities (Psychological Mindedness)

Baer, R. (2003). Mindfulness training as a clinical intervention: A conceptual and empirical review. *Clinical Psychology: Science and Practice, 10*(2), 125–142.

Bartsch, K., & Wellman, H. M. (1995). *Children talk about the mind.* Oxford, UK: Oxford University Press.

Burke, C. A. (2010). Mindfulness-based approaches with children and adolescents: A preliminary review of current research in an emergent field. *Journal of Child and Family Studies, 19*(2), 133–144.

Carpendale, J. I. M., & Lewis, C. (2004). Constructing an understanding of mind: The development of children's social understanding within social interaction. *Behavioral and Brain Sciences, 27*, 79–151.

Farrell, L., & Barrett, P. (2007). Prevention of childhood emotional disorders: Reducing the burden of suffering associated with anxiety and depression. *Child and Adolescent Mental Health, 12*(2), 58–65.

Galantino, M., Galbavy, R., & Quinn, L. (2008). Therapeutic effects of yoga for children: A systematic review of the literature. *Pediatric Physical Therapy, 20*(1), 66–80.

Goodman, R. (1997). The Strengths and Difficulties Questionnaire: A research note. *Journal of Child Psychology and Psychiatry, 38*, 581–586.

Greco, L., & Hayes, S. C. (2008). *Acceptance and mindfulness treatment for children and adolescents: A practitioner's guide.* Oakland, CA: New Harbinger.

Greco, L. A., Baer, R. A., & Smith, G. T. (2011). Assessing mindfulness in children and adolescents: Development and validation of the Child and Adolescent Mindfulness Measure (CAMM). *Psychological Assessment, 23*, 606–614.

Greenspoon, P. J., & Saklofske, D. H. (2001). Toward an integration of subjective well-being and psychopathology. *Social Indicators Research, 54*, 81–108.

King, A. (2013). Healing childhood trauma: Connecting with present experience and body-based insights. *Attachment: New Directions in Psychotherapy and Relational Psychoanalysis, 7*, 243–258.

Liebenberg, L., Ungar, M., & LeBlanc, J. C. (2013). The CYRM-12: A brief measure of resilience. *Canadian Journal of Public Health, 104*(2), 131–135.

Liehr, P., & Diaz, N. (2010). A pilot study examining the effect of mindfulness on depression and anxiety for minority children. *Archives of Psychiatric Nursing, 24*(1), 69–71.

Perner, J., & Wimmer, H. (1985). John thinks that Mary thinks that: Attribution of second-order beliefs by 5- to 10-year-old children. *Journal of Experimental Child Psychology, 39*, 437–471.

Prince-Embury, S. (2006). *Resiliency Scales for Children and Adolescents: Profiles of personal strengths.* San Antonio, TX: Harcourt Assessment.

Siegel, D. J., & Bryson, T. (2011). *The whole-brain child.* New York: Delacorte Press.

Silverman, W., Pina, A., & Viswesvaran, C. (2008). Evidence-based psychosocial treatments for phobic and anxiety disorders in children and adolescents. *Journal of Clinical Child and Adolescent Psychology, 37*(1), 105–130.

Symons, D. K. (2004). Mental state discourse, theory of mind, and the internalization of self-other understanding. *Developmental Review, 24*, 159–188.

Twemlow, S., Sacco, F., & Fonagy, P. (2008). Embodying the mind: Movement as a container for destructive aggression. *American Journal of Psychotherapy, 62*(1), 1–33.

Varni, J. W., Seid, M., & Rode, C. A. (1999). The PedsQ: Measurement model for the pediatric quality of life inventory. *Medical Care, 37*, 126–139.

Williams, J. M. G. (2010). Mindfulness and psychological process. *Emotion, 10*(1), 1–7.

11. Capacity to Construct and Use Internal Standards and Ideals

Baldwin, E. (2014). Recognizing guilt and shame: Therapeutic ruptures with parents of children in psychotherapy. *Psychoanalytic Social Work, 21*, 2–18.

Barish, K. (2006). On the role of reparative processes in childhood: Pathological development and therapeutic change. *Journal of Infant, Child and Adolescence Psychotherapy, 5*, 92–110.

Bernstein, P. P. (2004). Mothers and daughters from today's psychoanalytic perspective. *Psychoanalytic Inquiry, 24*, 601–628.

Bird, H. R. (2001). Psychoanalytic perspectives on theories regarding the development of antisocial behavior. *Journal of the American Academy of Psychoanalysis, 29*, 57–71.

Drexler, P. F. (2001). Moral reasoning in sons of lesbian and heterosexual parent families: The oedipal period of development. *Gender and Psychoanalysis, 6*, 19–51.

Freud, A. (1952). The mutual influences in the development of ego and id: Introduction to the discussion. *Psychoanalytic Study of the Child, 7*, 42–50.

Greco, L. A., Baer, R. A., & Smith, G. T. (2011). Assessing mindfulness in children and adolescents: Development and validation of the Child and Adolescent Mindfulness Measure (CAMM). *Psychological Assessment, 23*, 606–614.

Lampl-de Groot, J. (1957). The role of identification in psychoanalytic procedure. *Psychoanalytic Quarterly, 26*, 581–582.

Loewald, H. W. (1985). Oedipus complex and development of self. *Psychoanalytic Quarterly, 54*, 435–443.

Oppenheim, D., Emde, R. N., Hasson, M., & Warren, S. (1997). Preschoolers face moral dilemmas: A longitudinal study of acknowledging and resolving internal conflict. *International Journal of Psychoanalysis, 78*, 943–957.

Rangell, L. (1972). Aggression, Oedipus, and historical perspective. *International Journal of Psychoanalysis, 53*, 3–11.

Stapert, W., & Smeekens, S. (2011). Five year olds with good conscience development. *Psychoanalytic Study of the Child, 65*, 215–244.

CHAPTER 8

Emerging Personality Patterns and Difficulties in Childhood

PC Axis

CHAPTER EDITORS

Norka Malberg, PsyD **Larry Rosenberg, PhD** **Johanna C. Malone, PhD**

CONSULTANTS

Kenneth Barish, PhD
Karin Ensink, PhD
Alexandra Harrison, MD
Howard Lerner, PhD
Karin Lindqvist, MSc
Hun Millard, MD
John Stokes, PhD
Kirkland Vaughans, PhD

Introduction

Young children do have personalities and traits that may persist over time and that can and should be assessed, even if these are not placed into the personality disorder categories of recent editions of the *Diagnostic and Statistical Manual of Mental Disorders* (DSM). It is worth noting that the stated reasons for referral of most children for mental health services are not personality problems. Rather, children are most often referred with stated reasons having to do with behavioral or learning difficulties. Yet personality variables are often very much associated with behavioral, interpersonal, and school-related difficulties and may shape their treatment and clinical presentation in specific ways. Because the personalities of children are evolving, we talk here only about *emerging* personality patterns. Personality patterns are the characteristic ways of engaging with others and coping with the opportunities and challenges presented by the environment. They also include the ways in which strengths are utilized and vulnerabilities are contended with at different stages of life. These patterns or styles begin to form in childhood and continue to develop throughout life.

This chapter provides practitioners with a clinical guide to the assessment and treatment of children ages 4–11. By separating this period from adolescence, we recognize the uniqueness of each developmental stage and its impact on our understanding of symptomatology in the context of a child's emerging personality organization. On the basis of existing research, theory, and clinical experience with children (Caspi, Roberts, & Shiner, 2005; Shiner & Caspi, 2003; Roberts & DelVecchio, 2000), the PDM-2 work group concluded that it is unreasonable to diagnose personality disorders in children within this age cohort, or even to isolate particular traits that might be expected to develop into a specific personality disorder at some later point in time. As stated elsewhere in this manual, whereas the DSM approach to diagnosis has been categorical, the PDM-2 approach is dimensional. Personality development, conceived in terms of dimensions rather than discrete categories, involves ways of coping and relating to others that either enhance or impede a child's success in life—the ability to work productively, to form satisfying interpersonal relationships, and to actualize innate creative potential. Our tack is not atheoretical, as DSM's tries to be, but integrated. The question of how and why to consider emerging personality styles in this age cohort is a complex one, but one that we believe can be valuable for training, supervision, formulation, and treatment delivery.

Research in developmental psychopathology finds that personality traits in early and middle childhood are not necessarily predictive of the later development of personality pathology or of a specific personality disorder as defined by either DSM-5 (American Psychiatric Association, 2013) or the *International Classification of Diseases*, 10th revision (ICD-10; World Health Organization, 1992). As Caspi and colleagues (2005) point out, young children experience "rapid and wide-ranging" developmental changes (p. 456). For example, although a child's level of cognitive functioning can remain fairly stable over time, psychological assessments of children discretely specify the child's current level of intellectual functioning and do not presume to predict future IQ scores. We apply this same consideration to diagnosing personality disorders in children. Notwithstanding the issue of predictability, children with vulnerabilities and risk factors—inherited, environmentally determined, or both—may have difficulty meeting developmental milestones or have an increased vulnerability to psychopathology that would meet diagnostic criteria for a lower-level personality disorder (Bleiberg, 2001; see also Cicchetti, 2006; Geiger & Crick, 2010; Price & Zwolinski, 2010; Sroufe, 1997). Thus, while certain factors *may* increase the chances for development of psychopathology, it need not be said that all children having the same vulnerabilities and risk factors *will* develop severe psychopathology (Kraemer, Stice, Kazdin, Offord, & Kupfer, 2001; Price & Zwolinski, 2010). Development is complicated and not amenable to reliable predictions.

It is important to look beyond symptoms and describe a child's emerging personality and its impact on his or her psychological adjustment, keeping in mind that children have personalities that evolve slowly, often not demonstrating remarkable changes unless intruded upon by some significant family, environmental, or physical health disruption. Some children typically respond to challenges with defensiveness and rigidity, others with openness and flexibility. Others have begun to react to authority figures with defiant attitudes and an unwillingness to compromise. Still others are perfectionistic and preoccupied with the approval and disapproval of their parents and teachers. Some children, even before age 10, show a lack of empathy and a disregard for the feelings of others. Others, in contrast, are often unable to express their own needs and have become overly concerned with making sure that others are happy. Some children demonstrate attitudes of superiority and arrogance in their peer relationships; others show patterns of shyness, withdrawal from challenges, and difficulty engaging with peers. And some children already show a tendency toward suspiciousness and blaming of others, beyond what is age appropriate.

Whereas these individual responses may be identified and may acquire continuity over time, they also have meaning in the context of a child's life experience, in combination with unique temperamental and developmental features. For example, defensiveness and rigidity may be associated with a "high-reactive" temperament that predisposes a child to perceive ordinary life experiences as threats. Defiance of authority may emerge from a "hard-to-read" child whose parents unwittingly persist in setting unrealistic expectations. A child who lacks empathy may have neurodevelopmental difficulties with social engagement that interfere with learning about others' affective experience in reciprocal exchanges. Regardless, correlated with an emerging personality pattern is an emerging defensive style: unconsciously determined characteristic behavioral, cognitive, and affective adaptations to any level of perceived threat.

Whatever the origin of these personality patterns, if unchecked they may lead—usually as a result of repeated negative exchanges with adults and peers—to increasingly severe difficulties in a child's social and emotional adjustment. They are therefore appropriate and important targets for assessment and therapeutic intervention. Life circumstances, experiences, and maturation can substantially alter the nature of an emerging personality pattern in a child; these emerging patterns and their corresponding behaviors evoke varying responses from those caring for the child, which in turn further shape personality development. The dynamic family constellation around the child, not limited to siblings and parents, has direct implications for the child's development of representations of both self and others. A clinician should aim to understand the child in the context of the family system and the larger sociocultural context.

Some children's experiences or exposures elevate the likelihood that personality difficulties or disorders will develop. Some of these risk factors (e.g., poverty, maltreatment, exposure to violence, trauma, parental substance misuse) might be loosely described as matters of "nurture" that serve to elevate stress and increase the likelihood of actualizing an existing vulnerability. Endogenous vulnerabilities might include traits related to cognition, neurobiology, genetic factors, matters of temperament, and so on. Readers will recognize that any of these variables can serve as either protective factors or areas of vulnerability for a child (Luthar & Zigler, 1991; Rutter, 1987). Personality development and the development of psychopathology are no longer to be considered matters of nature versus nurture, but rather matters of their epigenetic interaction. This intersection of vulnerability, risk, and protective factors is at the center of our developmental approach (cf. Cicchetti & Cohen, 2006).

In line with these considerations, and in keeping with the work of Cohen (2008) and Cicchetti and Cohen (2006), we discuss the role of epigenetics, temperament, neurobiology, attachment style, sociocultural factors, and defensive style, as well as risk and protective factors, in the personality development of young children. We offer clinical illustrations intended to show how these variables can be integrated with the evaluation of mental functions into the assessment of personality organization in young children. Although we do not tie personality traits to specific personality disorders, we attempt to provide profiles of children who present at levels of personality organization consistent with those outlined by P. F. Kernberg, Weiner, and Bardenstein (2000) and others (O. F. Kernberg, 1975; Lerner, 1991; McWilliams, 2011), ranging from healthy to psychotic. Finally, we describe instruments useful for assessing personality in children.

We encourage clinicians to consider the current functioning of each child through multiple lenses. Our goal is to support recognition of emerging personality traits, styles, and difficulties that need to be assessed to develop a clear portrait of a child and to map effectively the direction of treatment. More specifically, we approach assessing and describing personality development in young children in a way that:

- Helps clinicians to appreciate their strengths and weaknesses more fully.
- Is useful in treatment planning and case formulations.
- Assists in the communication and collaboration that must transpire between a child's clinician and parents, to foster a deeper understanding, improve relationships, and maximize possibilities for treatment success. We prioritize assisting parents in developing a clearer sense of who their child is and how he or she sees self, others, and the world, over attempting to fit the child into a diagnostic category that is not fully accurate and has implications for future functioning that may not prove warranted.

We further propose that the same insights that allow for improved treatment planning by the clinician will assist parents in adapting to their child and will increase the chances for the formation of a treatment alliance essential to successful child psychotherapy. Similarly, the ability to offer a comprehensive description of the child's capacities and inner workings should prove valuable to teachers, pediatricians, and other professionals invested in helping the child.

Developing a Profile of Emerging Personality Patterns and Difficulties

Emerging personality patterns in children exist on a continuum from relatively healthy to compromised. The severity of personality difficulties in children may be evaluated via the MC Axis (see Chapter 7, especially Table 7.2, pp. 493–494). Using the components of the MC Axis, a clinician can locate a child's personality on a single continuum of severity reflecting overall distress and impairment. According to P. F. Kernberg and colleagues (2000) and others, these domains of severity include healthy, neurotic, borderline, and psychotic. It is insufficient, however, to think of personality functioning without contextualizing mental functioning within the endogenous and exogenous factors that affect the developing child. In the following section, we describe the significance of such factors in shaping personality development in children. These include (1) epigenetics, (2) temperament, (3) neuropsychology, (4) attachment style, (5) defensive style, and (6) sociocultural factors. Each factor can be directly linked to the components of the MC Axis.

Factors Influencing Emerging Personality Patterns and Difficulties

A growing body of empirical literature has provided an increased understanding of the interactions of genetic and psychosocial variables that create the risk and protective factors informing the emergence of internal organization and structure of children's subjective experiences, coping styles, and relationship patterns. The following is a brief review of factors that should be taken into consideration in trying to understand a child's emerging personality.

Epigenetics

In historical debates about the relative influence of "nature" and "nurture," the field of child development has recognized both sets of causalities. Nevertheless, perhaps because nurture seems more subject to clinical influence, there has been a greater emphasis on "nurture"—that is, the postnatal family environment as the primary determinant of individual differences. In contrast, developmental biology and neuroscience tend to view development through a "nature" lens. A review of research on genetic influence on the "Big Five" traits shows that heritability plays a role in each (Bouchard & Loehlin, 2001). And as we consider cognitive functioning to be a key component of personality, we note that genetics play a considerable role in IQ and neurobiology, especially early on, just as environment and childrearing practices do.

The emerging field of epigenetics offers the potential to unite these divergent perspectives in surprising and exciting ways. Historically, the term "epigenetics" described the dynamic interplay between genes and environment, leading to variations in phenotype. Variation in gene expression rather than gene sequence is the key concept in the study of epigenetics. There have been numerous studies examining epigenetic effects on psychological disorders. Epigenetics may play a role in schizophrenia, bipolar disorders, depression, anxiety disorders, and attention-deficit/hyperactivity disorder (ADHD).

A number of studies in neuroscience and neuropsychology suggest the utility of the epigenetic model for the development of self-regulation and executive functions in children (Bridgett, Burt, Edwards, & Deater-Deckard, 2015; Nahum, 1994). The quality of caregiving has been shown to be a key mediator of links between children's exposure to adversity (e.g., poverty, abuse, trauma) and subsequent physiological, neurobiological and psychological development (Schore, 2003). In this process, stress hormone levels constitute a primary mechanism through which cognitive and social-emotional development in early childhood is shaped by experience, with specific reference to the development of neural systems critical to self-regulation, including attention, emotion, and working memory. The epigenetic model has provided a basis for studies on the intergenerational transmission of individual differences in stress reactivity and resilience. The issue is not one of inheritance, but rather the mode of inheritance.

Epigenetic research indicates that chronic exposure to adversity actively shapes the physiological and behavioral developments that are adaptive to that context. Personality adaptation within adversity and compromised caregiving results in short-term beneficial adaptations but harmful long-term consequences. A central implication of these tradeoffs is that self-regulation can be altered; that is, the shaping of development by experience offers opportunities for repair and reversal. From a developmental psychobiological perspective, experiential and biological influences are highly intertwined.

Working with parents is a central dimension of treatment from this point of view. Supporting caregivers in maintaining high levels of warmth, responsiveness, sensitivity, and consistency has been shown to lead to more flexible regulation of stress physiology, which directly affects a child's executive functioning and capacity for self-regulation. This should be done with the understanding that a child's genetically determined traits will influence the manner in which the child is parented (Ge et al., 1996). Child treatment outcomes associated with early interventions have regularly correlated with changes in parental behavior. In cases where parental behavior proves resistant to alteration, treatment outcomes are more limited. From this perspective, early intervention and a focus on parenting are significant for positive outcomes not only in the child of interest, but also for subsequent generations.

Temperament

Over the past decades, developmental psychology has conclusively established what most parents have always intuitively known (and what all child therapists quickly learn): Children begin life with very different temperaments. Some are "easy," and some are "difficult"; some are inhibited, and others are exuberant and impulsive. Temperament can be broadly defined as "biologically rooted, relatively stable individual differences in an infant's behavioral tendencies" (Wachs, 2006, pp. 28–29). These behavioral styles influence how individuals respond to their environments and are thought to be increasingly stable over time (Caspi et al., 2005; Nigg, 2006; Shiner, 2006; Zeanah & Fox, 2004). Contrary to early perspectives, contemporary approaches emphasize that temperament can in fact be influenced by the environment (Shiner & Caspi, 2003). In fact, the importance of environment is explicit in the definition of temperament because the environment provides the stimuli necessary for a child to show characteristic patterns of response.

Beginning with the classic New York Longitudinal Study (Thomas & Chess, 1977), some temperament descriptions (e.g., the "slow-to-warm-up" child) have become part of our common cultural vocabulary. Although different perspectives on temperament exist, Mervielde, De Clercq, De Fruyt, and Van Leeuwen (2005) identified three consistent dimensions across research teams: "emotionality," "extraversion," and "activity." A fourth dimension, common only to Thomas and Chess (1977), was labeled "persistence." Emotionality addresses negative emotionality, negative affectivity, and distress/anger. Extraversion captures issues such as shyness, inhibition, social fear, and positive emotionality. Activity represents a child's levels of activity, and persistence signifies effortful control and ability to persist on tasks.

Within the field of developmental psychology, the relationship between personality and temperament is unclear. Some argue that temperament dimensions measured in childhood overlap largely with personality dimensions in adulthood (Mervielde et al., 2005), and that both are primarily determined by genetics (Goldsmith, 1983; Plomin & Caspi, 1999). This position is supported by findings that temperament in preschool-age children shows relatively modest stability into adulthood, according to measures of personality (Caspi & Roberts, 1999; Roberts & DelVecchio, 2000). Others see temperament as one dimension of personality (Kernberg & Caligor, 2005). One perspective suggests that temperament represents the entire personality in infancy, but only a portion of personality in childhood, adolescence, and adulthood (Shiner & Caspi, 2003). Contemporary research emphasizes a biobehavioral perspective, providing an understanding of neural systems that represent both behavioral responses and the regulation of responses elicited by the environment (Depue & Lenzenweger, 2005; Nigg, 2006).

Research examining personality traits with the widely utilized five-factor model (FFM, also known as the "Big Five") consistently highlights potential overlaps between childhood and temperament and adult traits. (The five factors include extraversion, agreeableness, conscientiousness, neuroticism, and openness to experience.)

For example, Shiner and Caspi (2003) propose a taxonomy of higher- and lower-order personality traits for children and adolescents that integrates findings from both the FFM and temperament literature. This taxonomy is based in part on the research of Rothbart, Ahadi, Hersey, and Fisher (2001), which emphasizes that negative emotionality maps onto neuroticism, positive emotionality maps onto extraversion, and constraint maps onto conscientiousness. Rothbart and colleagues identified a fourth trait of agreeableness. Whereas research on temperament began with the study of infancy and now extends into studies of adulthood, the FFM originally identified five domains of adult personality and now applies this research to the understanding of children and adolescents (John, Caspi, Robins, Moffitt, & Stouthamer-Loeber, 1994).

Temperament research has had enormously beneficial impacts on child psychotherapy and parent guidance. Our understanding that children are often "difficult" in many ways ameliorates parents' guilt and allows a much richer (and more valid) understanding of the multiple factors that influence the development of children's symptoms and personality. The era when parents were routinely blamed for children's emotional and behavioral problems is, fortunately, past.

Recognition of the importance of temperament does not negate the importance of a child's life experience. A child's temperament interacts in complex (often cyclical) ways with early experience. This interaction was originally conceptualized as the "goodness of fit" between caregiver and child (Chess & Thomas, 1991). Children with a shy or inhibited temperament, given supportive and encouraging help, can become less shy; impulsive children can develop improved behavior regulation and self-control (or, in a punitive environment, can become increasingly impulsive and defiant). Thomas, Chess, Birch, Hertzig, and Korn (1963) also emphasized the importance of the caregiver's warmth and flexibility when interacting with a child who shows difficult temperament, therefore proposing the mutability of temperament depending on a responsive environment (cf. Shiner, 2006).

An important part of our work as child therapists is helping parents understand and respond to their children's temperaments in constructive ways—with a balance of supportive and appropriately challenging practices that promote the children's security and self-confidence, and help prevent the development of increasingly dysregulated, defiant, or withdrawn modes of thought, feeling, and behavior.

Neuropsychology

The capacities to inhibit impulses when necessary, to regulate one's level of activity and attentiveness to facilitate learning, to regulate one's mood, to communicate effectively, and to engage competently in age-appropriate physical activities are all relevant to personality and are all directly related to a child's neuropsychology. Insofar as personality in childhood reflects relatively stable ways of thinking, feeling, perceiving, and relating to others, it will come as no surprise that these functions enjoy multiple and complex linkages to the brain and its functions. As Lewis (2001) has pointed out, childhood is a period not only of rapid physical and social changes, but of major cognitive changes as well.

Brain development, particularly frontal lobe development, continues significantly in children between ages 4 and 10. These changes are linked to increased emotional self-regulation, driven by the development of higher-order language and executive functioning abilities. A child's growing facility with language and conceptual thought plays a significant role in establishing and articulating personal identity. It allows the child greater flexibility in the organization of self, greater continuity of experience, and especially an increased ability to take perspective on negative experiences, which previously were experienced as irreconcilable. The emergence versus absence of these capacities is often key to the quality of relationships and how they inform a child's internal representation of self. Parents may struggle when their child's capacity for emotional self-regulation does not seem to improve with development. Their experience with the child's siblings may play a big role here; parents of a child with regulation issues who have older children functioning at more appropriate levels will tend to make stronger negative attributions to the younger child.

Executive functions promote preparedness and resilience; they permit greater adaptability and more flexible negotiation of adversity. The host of skills subsumed under executive functioning—including, but not limited to, initiation, planning, attention, working memory, self-monitoring, and negotiating novelty—allow children to generate an ever-expanding array of problem-solving strategies, along with the capacity to modify them in real time when necessary. When these changes are joined with enhanced conceptual language ability, a child is better positioned to take perspective on emotions, contextualize them, and hence integrate them into judgments with a greater tolerance for ambiguity and frustration

Deficits in executive functioning are prominent in disorders such as ADHD; frontal lobe abnormalities have been found in conduct disorder and other behavior disorders. Poor executive functioning leaves children more vulnerable to dissociative and externalizing defenses and to disorders in which impulsive behaviors play a prominent role. Parents and teachers need to be made aware of the impact of executive functioning difficulties on children's behavior and emotional development. Parents, teachers, and therapists working with these children may experience them as dependent, avoidant, anxious, or oppositional, without recognizing that such behaviors may be manifestations of the children's attempts to compensate for as-yet-undetected neuropsychological deficits.

Another primary way in which poor executive functioning may burden personality development is by undermining a child's experience of caregiving. One basis for the phase-specific idealization of parents is their capacity to protect the child from danger, both external and internal. Not only does this fortify the child's efforts at affect regulation, but it also strengthens attachment bonds and assists the child in developing inner capacities for self-regulation. Depending on the type and severity of executive functioning problems, the soothing and containing function of a parent's ministrations may be experienced as ineffective, even nonexistent—a kind of psychic abandonment that is distressing rather than reassuring. The child may feel that the parent is unavailable and uninterested, and this may give rise to self-perceptions (both conscious and unconscious) of oneself as unloved and unlovable. Healthy self-esteem depends in part on the parent's capacity for attunement, but also on the child's ability to process what is offered.

Attachment Style

The attachment system, inborn in all children, is central to personality development. Bowlby (1973) construed it as the motivational force behind children's drive to seek proximity and comfort from attachment figures when they are frightened or when they perceive the need for protection and safety. When children feel grounded in what attachment theorists call "a secure base," their attachment system is deactivated, and the exploration of the world feels safe and enticing. This experience encapsulates the impact of parents' capacities, whatever their own hopes and dreams are for a child, to imagine him or her as a separate being with separate feelings, thoughts, and intentions. This "capacity to mentalize" begins with parents and develops in children as ongoing immersion in a caregiving system, guided by a parent's capacity to provide a secure base that enables a child to grow and develop from a place of safety.

Awareness of attachment patterns and how they influence emerging personality patterns aids significantly in the development of a clinical formulation. Creating an opportunity for separation and reunion during a diagnostic process may provide extensive valuable information, not only about the child's pattern upon reunion but also about the parent's capacity and willingness to observe, contain, and buffer the child. A number of valuable instruments that have been produced during the last 30 years in the context of attachment theory may informally aid in assessment. Items from the Parent Development Interview (Slade, 2005), for example, may help to assess a parent's reflective functioning capacities and inform therapeutic goals for working with parents as well as the child.

Having discussed in Chapter 7 the role of attachment in the development of a child's psychological capacities, we examine here some research and clinical evidence from contemporary attachment theory, emphasizing how it informs our understanding of emergent personality patterns in the context of relationships. We begin by looking at existing evidence relevant to emerging borderline organization.

Although most research on personality and attachment focuses on adults and adolescents, links between personality pathology and attachment disruptions in early childhood have been empirically established. Crick, Murray-Close, and Woods (2005) found, in a sample of fourth- through sixth-grade students, four indicators predictive of borderline features: cognitive sensitivity, emotional sensitivity, exclusivity with a best friend, and relational and physical aggression. Yet without prospective longitudinal studies, it remains unclear whether borderline features in preadolescent children are indicative of the same psychopathology found in adolescents and adults. In an adolescent sample, Nakash-Eisikovits, Dutra, and Westen (2003), using clinician-reported data, found that all 10 DSM-IV personality disorders were inversely related to secure attachment. Using the Adult Attachment Interview with adolescents, Kobak and Sceery (1988) found that secure attachment was associated with ego resilience and the ability to regulate emotions, preoccupied attachment was related to higher levels of anxiety, and dismissing attachment was related to increased levels of hostility and a maladaptive self-reliant style.

Findings from a number of studies suggest that the vast majority of adults diagnosed with borderline personality disorder have insecure attachment styles (more than 90%) or are unresolved with regard to trauma (Agrawal, Gunderson, Holmes, & Lyons-Ruth, 2004; Levy, Meehan, Weber, Reynoso, & Clarkin, 2005). More specifically, most borderline patients (60–100%) have anxious–preoccupied attachment styles or have unresolved trauma (50–88%). Individuals with preoccupied attachment may become absorbed by anger about past transgressions. Descriptions of relationships with caregivers are characterized by helplessness, passivity, immaturity, or pervasive fearfulness even when there is no objective danger. The association between unresolved trauma and borderline personality disorder can be understood in terms of unresolved trauma as an index of cognitive and affective disorganization, extreme defensive processes, and dissociation when faced with trauma-related triggers. In a sense, the traumatogenic event becomes an organizer around which the personality develops. Unresolved trauma, as well as lack of mentalization regarding trauma, has been shown to be associated with dysregulation in interpersonal relationships when intense affects such as anger and fear are evoked.

Infant attachment "disorganization" refers to an apparent disorganization and confusion when the infant's attachment needs are activated, even though the child is in the caregiver's presence. It has been linked to frightening or frightened behavior on the part of the parent, so that the infant is trapped in a state that Main (1999) called "fright without solution," in which the parent who should provide a safe haven becomes instead the source of fear. Attachment disorganization has been associated in longitudinal studies and meta-analytic reviews with child behavior problems such as aggression (van IJzendoorn, Schuengel, & Bakermans-Kranenburg, 1999), with posttraumatic stress disorder (PTSD) in middle childhood (Macdonald et al., 2008), and with dissociation in adolescents (Carlson, 1998). Infant attachment disorganization has also been associated with elevated cortisol levels, which may increase the risk of developing later internalizing and externalizing psychopathology (Lyons-Ruth & Jacobvitz, 2008).

Attachment disorganization commonly occurs in the context of trauma, neglect, maltreatment, and loss. There is evidence from microanalytic studies of mother–infant communication that attachment disorganization is linked to maternal failures in responding to infant emotional distress, either via withdrawal or via responses denying a child's state—for example, laughing when the infant shows distress (Beebe et al., 2012). This may contribute to difficulties in understanding and predicting emotional reactions in self and others, and to a feeling of not being sensed or known, especially when distressed. It may contribute over time to the contradictory interpersonal communications (Beebe & Steele, 2013) characteristic of borderline personality disorder. Clinically, these findings have significant implications for assessment and treatment in terms of how a child responds to a clinician's verbal and nonverbal communications. They matter as well for treatment recommendations. The feelings these children evoke in clinicians during assessment and intervention may convey intensely the nature of their difficulties. Their levels of proximity, for example, and the unpredictability of their emotional and behavioral reactions to "ordinary caregiving responses" in adults (including mental health professionals), may be powerfully diagnostic.

There is evidence that infant attachment security is particularly important for later self-regulation in infants with the short 5-HTTLPR (serotonin-transporter-linked polymorphic region) allele (Kochanska, Philibert, & Barry, 2009), suggesting that attachment is implicated in the expression of genes associated with self-regulation. From a neurobiological perspective, Moutsiana and colleagues (2014), in a remarkable longitudinal study, have demonstrated that infant attachment at 18 months alters the neural circuitry of emotion regulation 20 years later. Adults who were classified as insecurely attached as infants showed relative inefficiency in the neural regulation of positive affect. Furthermore, anxious attachment has been empirically associated with hyperactivity in the amygdala in response to images of angry faces, suggesting hypervigilance about possible social punishment (Vrtička, Andersson, Grandjean, Sander, & Vuilleumier, 2008). Avoidant attachment has been associated with hypoactivity in the ventral tegmentum and striatal areas in response to images of smiling, thought to suggest a blunted response to social reward. These findings are consistent with observations that individuals with anxious states of mind are hyperreactive to emotionally salient social cues (Mikulincer & Shaver, 2007; Rom & Mikulincer, 2003; van Emmichoven, van IJzendoorn, de Ruiter, & Brosschot, 2003), whereas those with avoidant states of mind minimize the importance of emotionally relevant information (Dozier & Kobak, 1992).

In summary, in assessing children, clinicians need to explore the quality of the children's relationships to their primary caregivers and to other adults, peers, and siblings. The relational history of parents, when available, can help with the understanding of their reactions to their children and how those reactions influence both the parents' internal representations of the children and the children's representations of self in relationships. For a preliminary understanding of children's images of self and how these are communicated, clinicians should also pay close attention to their own affects during assessment sessions.

Defensive Style

In children, as in adolescents and adults, mental functions such as the capacity to deal with stress, manage impulses, and negotiate conflict are greatly influenced by "defensive styles"—a term that refers to habitual modes of dealing with perceived or anticipated conflicts or stresses. One's defensive style is intimately related to one's level of personality functioning. Relevant conflicts may be internal, between aspects of self (e.g., impulse vs. conscience) or external (self vs. other). In either case, defenses are nonconscious processes distinct from learned skills and conscious coping mechanisms. Even when they are maladaptive (e.g., a projection of rage that results in unwarranted fear and avoidance of others), defenses originate in adaptation and have adaptive aims; they make it possible to cope with life's stresses (Shafer, 1954). Children and adults are similar with respect to the adaptive purpose of defensive operations.

Assessing a child's defensive style is a critical component in helping a clinician understand what is stressful to the child and how the child manages that stress. Understanding a child's defenses has bearing on the content and timing of clinical interventions. Communicating the ways in which a given child's defenses influence his or her thinking, feelings, and behaviors can be of great assistance to parents in reframing their understanding of, and reactions to, their child.

As is true for an adult, the way a child's defenses cluster does in part define the structure of the child's personality. For example, some children tend to approach the world avoidantly, being sensitive or overly sensitive to perceived or imagined threats. Others tend toward risk taking and adventurousness, feeling self-confident, or perhaps being unable to anticipate danger. The child therapist will recognize that avoidant defenses are consistent with more internalizing behaviors, while counteractive defenses are more consistent with externalizing behaviors.

Otto Kernberg (1975) construes personality organization on a continuum extending from healthy, through neurotic, borderline, and psychotic levels of functioning. Lerner (1991) makes similar distinctions among high, low, and intermediate levels of functioning. Within these frameworks, personality organization is viewed as structured by the defensive style of the individual. Paulina Kernberg and colleagues (2000) have focused specifically on children and adolescents and categorized personality at the same levels of organization, delineating the variables that contribute to personality (i.e., temperament, identity, affect, gender, neuropsychology, defense mechanisms). Here, too, defenses are seen as correlated with level of personality organization. That is, the defenses typically employed by someone in the neurotic range would be distinct from those of someone functioning at the borderline level, and so on.

We are talking here about the defenses more dominantly employed by someone at a given level, and not defenses exclusive to that level of functioning. We all use splitting as a defense under some circumstances, but someone with a borderline personality structure may use splitting as a prevailing strategy. Because of developmental distinctions between age groups, the defenses of children described by Kernberg and colleagues (2000) are not precisely those associated with adult levels of functioning.

In keeping with Anna Freud's (1936/1966) developmental approach and the research findings of Cramer (1987, 2015), defense mechanisms can be conceptualized as being of a lower or higher order, depending on when in development they first appear. For example, denial can be categorized as a more primitive defense because it emerges at a younger age and is used more frequently by younger children. Its use typically fades with maturity. Higher-level defenses (e.g., sublimation, intellectualization, humor) characterize healthy and neurotic patients, whereas lower-level defenses (e.g., splitting, projective identification, denial) are often used by borderline and psychotic patients. While all defenses involve some distortion of reality, the more primitive defenses distort reality to the greatest degree. Because their use of relatively primitive defenses is developmentally appropriate, one cannot diagnose personality disorders in young children on the basis of their defensive structure. But, just as it is in adults, excessive use of age-inappropriate defenses is associated with psychopathology in children (Cramer, 2015).

For parents and others working with a child, it is important to recognize that certain problematic behaviors serve a defensive function. A child's apparent indifference to learning, or difficulty in taking responsibility for things that go wrong, or risk-taking actions are behaviors that can be usefully conceptualized as helping the child keep troubling feelings or thoughts from consciousness. Reformulating a child's motives in this way can be helpful not only to the child, but to the parents in the service of more empathic and appropriate responses to the child's problem behavior.

Sociocultural Influences

Personality is shaped epigenetically by both genes and environment. Among the most important environmental determinants are cultural influences. Culture is transmitted through language and the modeling of behavior. Formulating clearly the relationship between culture and personality development is a complex task that can be approached from multiple perspectives. There is a certain stability to culture, but cultures are not static. We can thus ask about the adaptive aims that cultural values serve, about why maladaptive traits may be maintained, and about whether cultural adaptations can carry negative consequences (Serafica & Vargas, 2006).

One can make diagnostic inferences that consider factors such as cultural influences on how affect is displayed, attitudes toward child rearing and childrearing practices, attitudes about gender and sexual expression, and attitudes about violence. Cultural variables need to be considered in how we define and assess pathology, and perhaps in how we treat it. Consider the challenges faced by an immigrant child and parent, for example, when the former has adapted to a culture to which the latter has not yet adapted, and the effects of those differences for the relationship and the development of the child's personality.

A growing movement in psychodynamic thinking urges clinicians to consider the complex interaction of culture with clinical formulation and intervention (see, e.g., Akhtar, 2011; Altman, 2010; Tummala-Narra, 2015). Ryder, Dere, Sun, and Chentsova-Dutton (2014) emphasize that clinicians who are unaware of or fail to consider cultural expectations when assessing personality run the risk of misdiagnosing symptoms. They suggest that clinicians should consider the ways in which certain cultural groups might be exposed to increased environmental stressors (in both the past and the present), and how cultural variations might occur with or without distress or impairment. Clinicians need to be continually reflective about ways in which their own sociocultural backgrounds influence how they perceive, and are perceived when working with, children and their families. To ignore cultural influences on early child development leaves us subscribing to the dubious notion of the "universal child," which, when we engage clinically with cultural others, runs the risk of cultural misattunement—or, worse, cultural impingement.

Shore (1996) notes that in the "universal child" assumption, "Culture is conceived as one of the contents of mind rather than as a defining attribute of mind" (p. 22). We need to be especially attentive to lack of awareness of the inherent cultural bias in our theories of development and pathology. Asking about the cultural meaning of food, sleeping arrangements, toilet training, and other developmentally related matters during the diagnostic process opens the door to better communication with parents. It also allows us to explore more openly issues such as unresolved loss, mourning, and shame in the parents' lives that might be hampering their capacity to "see" their child as a separate individual. Discussing issues of culture openly with parents, teachers, and other involved professionals allows us to reconsider our assumptions about the child's functioning. Cultural bias can either frame a culturally normative behavior as pathological or can blur our capacity to see a child's behavioral pattern as problematic.

Personality Assessment Instruments

The clinical assessment of personality psychopathology in childhood must address at least two diagnostic issues. The first is the identification of the type and severity of problematic personality features, behaviors, and/or relational problems that are interfering with adjustment. The *second* pertains to identification and amelioration of features that pose increased risk for developing future psychopathology, including personality disorder. Both issues can be approached from either categorical or dimensional perspectives, and from numerous theoretical vantage points. Both require careful consideration of a child's developmental level and the severity of the child's problematic traits. Tackett (2010) argues that dimensional conceptualizations provide a better opportunity to examine continuity between child and adult manifestations of personality disorders.

Although personality traits have been found to be moderately stable during childhood and adolescence (e.g., Roberts & DelVecchio, 2000), personality disorder diagnoses are typically less stable. There is, however, some evidence that children experiencing more severe personality difficulties, or compromised levels of personality organization, demonstrate increased vulnerability to longer-term problems. Longitudinal follow-ups of categorical diagnoses provide evidence that children diagnosed with emerging borderline personality features such as reliance on primitive, brittle defenses; lack of a flexible, adaptive approach to stressors; intolerance for negative affect; moments of impaired reality testing and/or disorganized thought processes; impaired interpersonal relationships; and high levels of emotionality show an increased likelihood of developing any personality disorder 10–15 years later (Lofgren, Bemporad, King, Linden, & O'Driscoll, 1991; Thomsen, 1996). There is also evidence that Cluster B (dramatic, emotional) personality disorders identified at ages 10–14 are stable to young adulthood (Crawford, Cohen, & Brook, 2001) (see also Chapter 5 on the PA Axis).

Geiger and Crick (2010) have traced the possible relationship between a range of personality features (hostile, paranoid world view; intense, unstable inappropriate relationships; restricted, flat affect; impulsivity; rigidity; excessive concern with relationships; avoidance of relationships; negative sense of self; lack of coherent thought or exaggerated, peculiar thought processes; lack of concern for social norms and needs of others) and the development of adult personality disorders.

There is general agreement that a multimethod approach to personality assessment is most desirable. For children, this would typically involve some combination of interview, self-report measures, observer ratings, and performance-based measures. The latter might include the Rorschach; storytelling techniques (e.g., the Roberts Apperception Test for Children–2 [Roberts-2], Tell-Me-a-Story [TEMAS], and the Thematic Apperception Test [TAT], all discussed in more detail below); assessment of play (e.g., Chazan, 2000; Kernberg, Chazan, & Normandin, 1998; Perry & Landreth, 2001; Russ, 2004; Westby, 2000); and other measures. Carrying out multimethod assessment for children offers challenges that are not encountered in older populations.

Methods Based on Interview, Self-Report, and Observer (Parent/Teacher) Ratings

With respect to interviews, those attempting to understand child self-report (e.g., Caplan, Guthrie, Fish, Tanguay, & David-Lando, 1989; Harter, 1999, 2006) have outlined difficulties created by lack of insight and failure to distinguish between actual and ideal selves that characterizes developing personalities. Interviewing methods that decrease reliance on insight and self-reflection, and focus more on evoking behaviors of interest, have advantages for this age group. For example, both Caplan and colleagues (1989), employing the Kiddie Formal Thought Disorders Scale (KFTDS), and Viglione (1996), utilizing the Childhood Unusual Beliefs Scale (CUBESCALE), have developed semistructured procedures to evaluate eccentric beliefs and thinking problems in children. Others (e.g., Poorthuis et al., 2014) have designed brief behavioral tests of the Big Five traits of conscientiousness (i.e., number of times a child turned off an entertaining video during a task) and agreeableness (i.e., quality of helping behavior) for sixth graders and found that these predicted academic achievement and social acceptance in the transition to secondary school. Unfortunately, such procedures have not been normed extensively, and their psychometric properties in community populations are uncertain.

As to observer ratings (e.g., parent or teacher ratings), research consistently finds only moderate levels of agreement between child and parent ratings, and between parent ratings across similar constructs (De Los Reyes & Kazdin, 2005). Parents may have differing degrees of awareness of a child's impulse-control problems leading to disruptive behavior, depending upon whether problematic behaviors are occurring in the home or in the school setting, and may have differing levels of understanding of the causes of these behaviors, depending upon the child's ability and/or willingness to communicate distress. Parents may also be unaware of internal preoccupations, distress, or unusual thinking in the child. Assessments in clinical contexts often occur with children whose relationships with their parents have become strained, or with parents who are motivated either to be "defensive" and deny problems, or to exaggerate them in an effort to obtain help for their children (in either case, observer ratings are saturated with parent response bias). In other family situations, clinical personality assessment may involve children in foster care; the foster parents may have little knowledge of the developmental trajectory of the children's problems, and may not be able to distinguish behaviors that are reactive accommodations to parental loss and placement from behaviors indicating more long-standing personality issues. In all these cases, validity indices assessing parental desire to under- or overreport problematic personality features are important in evaluating the results of observer ratings. Additionally, Tackett (2011) found that discrepancies between mothers and fathers on ratings of neuroticism, agreeableness, and conscientiousness were important predictors of internalizing problems.

With respect to self-report, problems may arise because of developmental issues related to reading ability, language comprehension (e.g., understanding how to respond to "true" and "false" in negatively worded questions), developmental limitations in ability to distinguish between real and ideal selves (Harter, 2006), problems related to developmental or characterological lack of insight, and desires either to minimize problems defensively (e.g., the child is rigidly defended or wishes to externalize blame) or to exaggerate problematic personality features (e.g., the child wishes to draw attention to problems that might not be taken seriously if presented in a more matter-of-fact fashion).

Geiger and Crick (2010) have noted that there are relatively few instruments for assessing personality disorders in childhood, and that the few existing ones have involved either downward extensions of adult personality measures or design of new instruments for children based on adult criteria. Those based on downward extension of adult personality disorder constructs would include the Millon Pre-Adolescent Clinical Inventory (MPACI; Millon, Tringone, Millon, & Grossman, 2005) and the Coolidge Personality and Neuropsychological Inventory for Children (CPNI; Coolidge, 2005). Other such downward extensions have been developed for the Child Behavior Checklist (CBCL; Achenbach & Rescorla, 2001). Kernberg and colleagues (2000) identified items within the CBCL that assessed general personality disorder traits, as well as borderline, narcissistic, antisocial, histrionic, paranoid, schizoid, avoidant, and dependent personality disorders in children, but normative and validity evidence for these scales is still lacking. Others (e.g., Kim et al., 2012) have developed configurations that they believe relate to a CBCL dysregulation profile. The manual for the Devereux Scales of Mental Disorders (DSMD; Naglieri, LeBuffe, & Pfeiffer, 1994) identifies sets of items representing criteria for personality disorders. There are also more circumscribed measures of specific personality features that correlate with poorer outcomes for certain DSM-IV-TR Axis I disorders. One example is the Inventory of Callous and Unemotional Traits (ICU; Frick, Stickle, Dandreaux, Farrell, & Kimonis, 2005; Frick & White, 2008), which predicts poor outcome in children with disruptive behavior disorders.

Methods Involving Performance-Based Measures

Although self-report and observer ratings are important sources of information, they may frequently fail to capture information about developmental level, object relatedness, defensive structure, and personality attributes, as well as implicit cognitive, relational, and affective factors that may sustain maladaptive behaviors. For this reason, psychologists often employ "projective measures." It has been suggested that the terms "objective" and "projective" have misleading connotations and need to be discarded to advance the field of personality assessment (Meyer & Kurtz, 2006). Instruments that have typically been subsumed under the "projective" label include the Rorschach Inkblot Test, storytelling techniques, sentence completion measures, and various drawing tasks. These techniques might be better referred to as "performance-based measures" or "constructive measures."

Rorschach Inkblot Test

Descriptions of clinical use of the Rorschach with children and adolescents predate Exner's (1974) Comprehensive System (CS) (e.g., Ames, Learned, Metraux, & Walker, 1952; Ames, Metraux, & Walker, 1971; Halpern, 1953). The CS makes use of different cutoff scores for some variables for which the normative data demonstrate significant developmental changes (i.e., Egocentricity Index, WSUM6, Affective Ratio). Because it has not been demonstrated to be effective, the CS does not employ the Suicide Constellation (SCON) below the age of 16.

Data for the CS have been collected on more than 90 youth ages 5–16. It has been found to have acceptable reliability, and meta-analytic studies have demonstrated validity effect sizes within the range of self-report measures such as the Minnesota Multiphasic Personality Inventory for Adolescents (MMPI-A) (e.g., Hiller, Rosenthal, Bornstein, Berry, & Brunell-Neuleib, 1999; Mihura, Meyer, Dumitrascu, & Bombel, 2013), although most of these studies were conducted with adolescent and adult populations.

Rorschach research has identified constellations of variables that assess difficulties with reality testing and thinking, hypervigilance, difficulties with self-image or relationships, high levels of affective distress, difficulties with controls and stress tolerance, and difficulties with affect regulation. Validity studies based on these configurations have established that elements within those constellations related to thinking and reality testing (i.e., SCZI and PTI) can differentiate children (Stokes, Pogge, Grosso, & Zaccario, 2001) and adolescents (Hilsenroth, Eudell-Simmons, DeFife, & Charnas, 2007) with psychotic disorders. The Ego Impairment Index (EII) is a broad measure of impaired adjustment that weights elements such as those related to reality testing, thinking problems, object relations, and occurrence of critical thought content to provide an overall index of impaired functioning. This index seems to be a measure of personality structure apart from symptom status and has been found to be predictive of poor long-term outcome in psychiatric inpatients across a range of psychopathology, including thinking problems. Children and preadolescents who obtain elevated EII scores do not differ significantly in response to initial intensive treatment, but are at significantly higher risk of long-term recurrence of symptoms (Stokes et al., 2003). Donahue and Tuber (1993) found that the ability of children to withstand severe environmental stressors was related to their ability to provide adaptive fantasy images on the Rorschach. Other validation studies for personality psychopathology in children have involved children with PTSD (Armstrong & Lowenstein, 1990; Holaday, 2000) and ADHD symptomatology (Meehan et al., 2008). Acklin (1995) has outlined the Rorschach assessment of the borderline child. Exner and Weiner (1995) have provided a construct-focused way to explore for the presence of signs of a faltering personality development.

In addition to the Ego Impairment Index (EII-3) and other Rorschach variables that have demonstrated empirical validity, the Rorschach Performance Assessment System (RPAS; Meyer, Viglione, Mihora, Erard, & Erdberg, 2011) includes scales such as the Mutuality of Autonomy Scale, the Oral Dependent Language Scale, and Aggressive Content Scales, which might be of use with latency-age children. Normative data on the RPAS for latency-age children are currently being collected.

Storytelling Techniques

Among the most commonly used storytelling techniques with children are the TAT (Bellak, 1993; Murray, 1943), TEMAS (Costantino, Malgady, & Rogler, 1988), and Roberts-2 (Roberts & Gruber, 2005), as mentioned earlier.

The TAT, despite over 50 years of clinical applications, lacks well-developed normative data. Critics have raised concerns about the absence of figures from diverse cultures, and validity data with children are sorely lacking. Cramer (1982, 1990) developed a scoring system for TAT defenses (denial, projection, identification); proposed a developmental theory of defenses and demonstrated that children exposed to trauma who demonstrated the greatest use of defenses, and especially age-appropriate defenses, showed least emotional impairment (Dollinger & Cramer, 1990). Kelly (1997) has applied the Social Cognition and Object Relations Scale (SCORS; Westen, Lohr, Silk, Kerber, & Goodrich, 1985) to the TAT records of children and adolescents.

TEMAS, designed to be a multiculturally sensitive instrument for children between ages 5 and 18, consists of 23 cards (with parallel sets for minority and nonminority children). A quantitative system evaluates 18 cognitive functions, 9 personality functions (interpersonal relationships, aggression, anxiety/depression, achievement motivation, delay of gratification, self-concept, sexual identity, moral judgment, and reality testing), and 7 affective functions (happy, sad, angry, fearful, neutral, ambivalent, and inappropriate affect). The scoring system was standardized on a regionally homogeneous group of 642 children (281 boys, 361 girls) from the New York City area.

The Roberts-2 was developed from a standardization sample of 1,060 children (518 males, 542 females) ages 6–18, whose demographic features roughly matched 2004 U.S. Census figures. Like TEMAS, the Roberts-2 has parallel sets of cards for minority and nonminority populations. Interrater reliability generally falls in the good to excellent range across the scales provided. These include theme overview, available resources, problem identification (five levels), problem resolution (five levels), emotions (anxiety, aggression, depression, and rejection), outcome scales (unresolved, nonadaptive, maladaptive, and unrealistic), and unusual or atypical responses (nine categories). Validity was attained by establishing the instrument's ability to document developmental differences and distinguish between non-referred and referred samples. Although all variables showed statistically significant ability to differentiate by age and clinical group, there are as yet limited findings on whether variables distinguish among different clinical samples.

Other Performance-Based Measures

Other instruments traditionally regarded as cognitive or neuropsychological in nature may be useful in assessing personality in children. They may assist with formulating a comprehensive understanding of how a child thinks, acts, and feels, contextualizing the findings obtained from "traditional" personality tests. Broadly conceived, abilities like intelligence, executive functioning, and language processing influence the range of defenses and coping strategies available to the child, mediate issues relevant to self-esteem, and provide further data relevant to treatment planning.

Wechsler Intelligence Scale for Children—Fifth Edition

The Wechsler Intelligence Scale for Children—Fifth Edition (WISC-V; Wechsler, 2014) was normed on children ages 6 years, 0 months to 16 years, 11 months. It yields standard scores with a mean of 100 and a standard deviation of 15. It includes three new primary subtests: visual puzzles (visual processing), figure weights (quantitative reasoning and induction), and picture span (visual working memory). It has the following primary scales: a verbal comprehension index, visual–spatial index, working memory index, fluid reasoning index, and processing speed index. It also has five ancillary scales (a quantitative reasoning index, auditory working memory index, nonverbal index, general ability index, and cognitive proficiency index) and three new complementary index scales (a naming speed index, symbol translation index, and storage and retrieval index).

Wechsler Preschool and Primary Scale of Intelligence—Fourth Edition

The Wechsler Preschool and Primary Scale of Intelligence—Fourth Edition (WPPSI-IV; Wechsler, 2012) was normed on children ages 2 years, 6 months to 7 years, 7 months. It yields standard scores with a mean of 100 and a standard deviation of 15. It contains the same five primary scales as the WISC-V, and four ancillary scales: a vocabulary acquisition index, nonverbal index, general ability index, and cognitive proficiency index.

NEPSY—Second Edition

The NEPSY—Second Edition (Korkman, Kirk, & Kemp, 2007) is a battery of neuropsychological tests based on Luria's neuropsychological system, normed on children ages 3 years, 0 months through 16 years, 11 months. It contains 32 subtests and assesses neuropsychological functioning across six domains: executive functioning/attention; language; memory and learning; sensorimotor functioning; visuospatial processing; and social perception.

Clinical Evaluation of Language Functions—Fifth Edition

The Clinical Evaluation of Language Functions—Fifth Edition (CELF-5; Wiig, Semel, & Secord, 2013) assesses a variety of language functioning in youth ages 5–21 years. It contains 16 subtests that assess language abilities (expressive and receptive), plus reading comprehension, writing, and communication pragmatics.

Levels of Emerging Personality Organization for Children Ages 4–11

Within the psychodynamic literature, personality can be conceptualized and measured in a number of different ways. In addition to considering severity and level of personality organization, Chapter 1 on the P Axis examines specific adult "syndromes" organized by externalizing and internalizing features. In this section, we adopt a different approach, to be most clinically useful and attuned to the varying ways personality characteristics might appear during childhood.

We recommend using the MC Axis (see Chapter 7, especially Table 7.2, pp. 493–494) to place a child's current presentation on a continuum of severity spanning the domains of healthy, neurotic, borderline, and psychotic. In applying these categories, we must consider elements of culture, temperament, neurobiology, attachment, and defensive styles, as each plays a significant role in shaping the child's capacity and manner of presentation for each mental function.

We begin in the next section by outlining a sample profile of a child functioning at the "healthy" level of personality, using the MC Axis as a guide. "Healthy" or "normal" represents wide ranges of functioning; most children will show greater strengths in some areas than others. Indeed, each subsequent level of emerging personality organization, though here described as an overall domain (i.e., neurotic, borderline, psychotic), may also embrace varying levels of specific mental functions, much as a child assessed as having overall intelligence (full-scale IQ) in the average range may have pockets of intellectual functioning (e.g., abstract reasoning ability, visual–motor skill, working memory) at levels above or below that overall score.

Following the sample profile of the healthy child, we offer baseline descriptions of children functioning at the neurotic, borderline, and psychotic personality levels. After each of these descriptions is a clinical illustration of a child at that level of functioning, followed by an evaluation of that child in terms of the MC Axis.

Sample Profile of a Child at a Healthy Level of Personality Functioning

In keeping with the structure set forth in Chapter 7 on the MC Axis, and similar to the assessment strategies described by Selzer and colleagues (1987) and Kernberg and colleagues (2000), we first offer a sample profile of a child at the "healthy" level of personality functioning.

COGNITIVE AND AFFECTIVE PROCESSES

1. Capacity for regulation, attention, and learning

The child has adequate fine and gross motor capacities, feels competent, and is on par with the peer group. The child is secure enough with motor functions to enjoy age-appropriate school and play activities. The child's ability to communicate verbally and nonverbally and comprehend verbal and nonverbal communications from others is commensurate with the child's age group. The child's level of cognitive functioning is at a level sufficient to allow for communication and learning at an expectable level, which allows the child to feel competent and capable of success.

The child is school-ready: He or she is able to attend and concentrate in an age-appropriate way. The child can sustain an appropriate level of effort toward work, and can stay calm enough and controlled enough to do so. The child can follow instructions both because he or she is not so oppositional toward authority that the ability to do so is compromised, and because he or she has the cognitive capacity to retain a sequence of instructions appropriate for a child of that age.

2. Capacity for affective range, communication, and understanding

The child has a full range of affects and can express affects at an age-appropriate level. The child has fears, but they are age-appropriate and manageable. They do not interfere with the child's ability to form relationships, enter into age-appropriate activities, attend school, or participate in important activities.

3. Capacity for mentalization and reflective functioning

The child shows emerging or established theory of mind (i.e.,, the ability to imagine others' states of mind as separate from one's own). There is evidence of age-appropriate belief in self as an intentional agent (e.g., "I am able to negotiate with my friends; my behaviors have an impact on others' responses and affective states"). The child shows an emerging capacity for reflective functioning, characterized by the ability to consider the opaqueness of others' states of mind ("What you see is not always what is true"); uses humor appropriately in the context of relationships; has behavioral flexibility (perspective taking), and can deal with overwhelming affective states by using symbolization and verbal expression. In general, the child makes age-appropriate use of interpersonal verbal and nonverbal cues, and allows for experiences of interpersonal rupture and repair.

IDENTITY AND RELATIONSHIPS

4. Capacity for differentiation and integration (identity)

The child has a reasonably well-developed sense of self that does not change radically from one time period or setting to the next. The child can easily distinguish between what is coming from him- or herself and what is the perspective of another person.

5. Capacity for relationships and intimacy

The child can have friendships that feel close and can be made without adult assistance. Friendships have a sense of reciprocity (the feeling that something is being shared and mutually felt). The child can read social cues sufficiently well to allow the other to have this sense. He or she feels that he or she can understand his or her interactions and have a sense of belonging in social experience.

The child's view of others is relatively positive. He or she is trusting where trust is deserved. The child can increasingly tolerate the idea that people are neither all good nor all bad.

6. Capacity for self-esteem regulation and quality of internal experience

The child's view of self is reasonably positive. It is not exaggerated in either a positive or negative way. The child is generally hopeful and confident. The child's sense of self is not easily or severely altered by negative comments or events. The child can rely on a stable, basic sense of self regard.

DEFENSE AND COPING

7. Capacity for impulse control and regulation

The child is in control of aggressive impulses, but is not passive. The child is constructively aggressive, capable of appropriate self-assertion, competition, and ambition.

The child can tolerate anxiety and other negative affects without either behavioral or cognitive disorganization. When emotional equilibrium is temporarily lost, the child is responsive to caregivers' attempts to soothe. The child reconstitutes reasonably quickly and can reflect, either with support or independently, on the disruptive experience.

8. Capacity for defensive functioning

The child's reality testing is intact. He or she can distinguish reality from fantasy, and can identify his or her own thoughts and feelings versus those of another. The child perceives things as others of the same age would generally perceive them. He or she employs defenses that distort reality only to minor degrees.

9. Capacity for adaptation, resiliency, and strength

The child is reasonably flexible in both thinking and ability to adjust to new or unanticipated situations. The child has some degree of adaptability to adversity. He or she does not just tolerate or survive adverse events, but comes away from them better to some degree.

SELF-AWARENESS AND SELF-DIRECTION

10. Self-observing capacities (psychological mindedness)

The child has a sense of curiosity and interest in learning about his or her world. The child is in touch with his or her thoughts and feelings. Furthermore, the child displays curiosity about him- or herself and the impact of own feelings, thoughts, and actions on others and the surrounding world. He or she is aware of the interaction between the inner world and the outside world in a way that motivates his or her sense of agency.

11. Capacity to construct and use internal standards and ideals

The child shows the beginnings of a sense of morality and a value system in keeping with the immediate and larger surrounding cultures. The child is interested in fairness, to others as well as to self. The child can play cooperatively by the rules of games.

The child feels guilt and remorse for wrongdoing; inappropriate or hurtful behavior is ego-dystonic. The child is not overly harsh with either self or others when mistakes are made, and understands that healthy children misbehave at times. The child has the capacity to forgive both self and others.

Other Levels of Personality Functioning: Descriptions, Clinical Illustrations, and Evaluations

Below are depictions of child patients at neurotic, borderline, and psychotic levels of functioning, respectively. Preceding each clinical illustration is a description of typical personality characteristics of a child functioning at that level, with the rationale for the classification. Following each illustration, we use the MC Axis to formulate the child's personality structure. Given the age of each child, the classification should be understood as the child's *current* or *emerging* level of personality organization.

Neurotic Level of Personality Organization

Children functioning at the neurotic level of personality organization are logical and thoughtful. They tend to adapt well to new and challenging circumstances. When they do become upset or dysregulated, they can regain equilibrium, sometimes via their internal resources for self-soothing, and sometimes with help. They can be impulsive, oppositional, or disruptive at times, but when dealt with reasonably and sensitively, they can regain control, reflect on the role they played in what went wrong, and appreciate the perspective of the other. Neurotic-level children are capable of remorse and guilt. At this stage of development (ages 4–10), they have an increasingly clearly defined, if not overly invested, sense of fairness and of right and wrong. They have typically adopted the values of their caregivers and the surrounding culture without undue questioning. Their defenses, which are internalizing as well as externalizing, operate effectively to maintain reality testing.

These children have a pretty good sense of who they are and can make reasonable assessments of others. Neurotic-level children in this age range are capable of simultaneously seeing good and bad in people. They can also be demanding or self-centered, but are capable of empathy and are sensitive to the motives and wishes of others. They tend to have close relationships with both peers and adults in authority. Their boundaries between self and others are reasonable. Relational difficulties that arise are usually resolved without excessive effort. They can reflect on their behavior and take responsibility for much of what may go wrong, and they experience as ego-dystonic the behaviors that they and their parents see as problematic. Their affective range is wide, and the affect they show is appropriate to content.

Ways in Which Children in This Category Tend to Be Experienced Clinically

There is generally a sense of mutuality in play and conversation with a neurotic-level child. It is not that the child would necessarily rather be with a therapist than with friends, but there is the sense that the child likes to be there and finds something warm and pleasant in the relationship. They usually consider therapy as helpful, and both parties to it feel they are on the same team, working toward the same goals. Neurotic-level children are interested in the therapist; they are curious, want to know the clinician better, and may ask about the therapist's thoughts. Play with a neurotic-level child is representational/symbolic. They are creative and tend to welcome the therapist in co-creating their stories, whether in conversation or play.

Neurotic-level children are forgiving. They may have negative transferences, but they feel resolvable. If a clinician's intervention is premature or off base, they either correct it or allow a second try by replaying the same theme in a different form rather than by raging, regressing, or forcefully interrupting the play or conversation. It is easy to empathize with neurotic-level children, and they easily empathize with the therapist. They show a capacity for guilt and a sense of fairness. They are typically not hard to be with; they make a therapist feel confident and effective, or at least like a nice person who is helpful. Their defenses allow therapists to find them accessible. They will play out or talk out themes that are fairly understandable, providing a therapist with a vivid sense of such a child's experience of self and of those closest to the child. Even when they portray relationships as troubled or punitive, they do not typically view them as sadistic or cruel, and they do not view the therapist in this way either.

Clinical Illustration

Nathan was a 6-year-old boy referred because of his parents' concerns about his tendency to become dysregulated to the point of throwing himself on the floor, screaming, and crying for prolonged periods. Some of these rageful episodes included throwing objects, hitting his younger brother, or hitting a parent. Time outs proved unsuccessful; he would refuse to go to his room or any other time-out location. His parents' attempts to walk away from him only led to his pursuing them angrily. These outbursts never occurred outside the home or with his grandparents. When Nathan would finally calm down from these explosions of tense aggression, he would become alternately defensively indifferent and spontaneously remorseful, clearly conveying a sense of shame about his behavior. During sessions he would carry on with this pattern of avoidance, preferring to play games at which he could either succeed or alter the rules to suit himself. He responded to his therapist most often as if she were another parental figure. As such, he would conceal things he felt guilty about, or tell her what he thought she wanted to hear, or turn away from her with a downward glance if told about something that his mother had reported to the therapist. He did not seek help for what troubled him and preferred to feign an air of invincibility, as evidenced in the fantasies explored during play. These seemed age-appropriate on the one hand, but expressive on the other hand of his wishes to impress his therapist and to defend vigorously against feelings of self-disappointment and inadequacy. His therapist found Nathan easy to empathize with, but difficult to get close to.

Nathan came from an intact family, with well-educated European American parents of working-class backgrounds. His father had been diagnosed with major depression, and his mother was in treatment for anxiety, marital issues, and the challenges of parenting. Nathan's father was often absent from family conflicts both physically and emotionally. His mother showed a tendency to yield to her son, partly to avoid his outbursts, but also because of guilt over her negative feelings toward him and her experience of him as being very much like her husband.

Nathan's milestones had all been reached within expected time frames. His history was unremarkable for aversive events. There had been no prolonged separations from caregivers, no marital discord of significant proportion, and no serious physical illnesses in him or other family members. He was described as a happy baby, easy to feed and affectionate. He responded to his brother's emerging toddlerhood with difficulties in being soothed, and he was becoming increasingly competitive and aggressive.

Preschool brought no major separation issues: he enjoyed playing with other children, and his teachers enjoyed him. With the start of kindergarten, however, Nathan became increasingly less fond of school. He did well enough, but as demands for working independently increased, they became a clear source of stress for Nathan. He would be compliant during the school day, but would return home in a moody, tense state. He did not seem intellectually curious even about subjects that interested him.

Nathan's fights with his brother were frequently precipitated by his sense that things were easier for his brother; there were fewer demands placed upon him, and he had other privileges of which Nathan felt jealous. Play between the two of them was possible only if Nathan could win without challenge. Loving gestures toward his brother were counteracted by too-frequent episodes of teasing and bullying.

Nathan had weak fine motor skills, but strong gross motor skills. He enjoyed playing team sports, but was somewhat passive in his style of play and easily became upset when his team (or a team that he was rooting for) was losing. He had limited frustration tolerance and poor self-esteem, and he tended to defend himself against feelings of failure by avoiding things that intimidated him and by exaggerated boastfulness and grandiose fantasies about things at which he would most like to succeed. These were distortions of reality, but not out of keeping with what might be expected from a child his age. He was not aggressive or defiant with peers or teachers. With people outside the family, he showed more capacity for empathy and guilt. Outside his home, he also tended to behave less impulsively and could contain his emotions more successfully. Although he was not self-confident, Nathan wanted very much to be part of the group. He showed no breaks with reality and seemed to have a pretty clear sense of himself.

Nathan showed no signs of notable sensory issues. He ate and slept well. While he could be somewhat tangential when anxious, his verbal productions were otherwise unremarkable. He tended to view other people with some degree of apprehension, but he had several friends with whom he had fun. He showed a full range of emotions, though at home he tended to "go from 0 to 60" rather quickly.

Part of the difficulty Nathan had with both school and self-regulation seemed related to neurobiological factors. Psychological testing revealed deficits in the areas of executive functioning and expressive language. More specifically, his capacity to remain attentive and process information made independent learning and problem solving somewhat taxing. This deficit, combined with expressive language difficulties, served to make verbal mediation of his anger and frustration difficult. Witnessing things that came more easily to his closer friends and his younger brother added to his frustration and jealousy.

Evaluating the Case

Cognitive and Affective Processes

1. *Capacity for regulation, attention, and learning:* Weak fine motor/strong gross motor abilities; regulation of sleep and eating good, no sensory issues; good verbal abilities when anxiety is low; weaknesses in executive functioning and expressive language (on neuropsychological testing).
2. *Capacity for affective range, communication, and understanding:* Full range of emotions, but emotions can become intense quickly; difficulty in effectively communicating affective experience.
3. *Capacity for mentalization and reflective functioning:* Failure at times to recognize how his actions affect others (particularly family members).

Identity and Relationships

4. *Capacity for differentiation and integration (identity):* Clear sense of who he is—although not comfortable with self.
5. *Capacity for relationships and intimacy:* Some apprehension of others, yet enjoys other children and gets along with teachers. Enjoys being part of group. Jealous of sibling. In conflict with parents.
6. *Capacity for self-esteem regulation and quality of internal experience:* Self-esteem challenged by struggles in school and competition with brother.

Defense and Coping

7. *Capacity for impulse control and regulation:* Behavioral and emotional dysregulation, aggression, limited frustration tolerance.
8. *Capacity for defensive functioning:* Avoidant defensive style, sense of invincibility, boastful/grandiose tendencies. Good reality testing.
9. *Capacity for adaptation, resiliency, and strength:* Difficulty adjusting after brother's birth.

Self-Awareness and Self-Direction

10. *Self-observing capacities (psychological mindedness):* Seems to lack curiosity about world.
11. *Capacity to construct and use internal standards and ideals:* Evidence at times (inconsistent) of shame and guilt about actions. Can recognize right from wrong.

Other Factors

Epigenetics: Parental anxiety and depression.

Temperament: Evidence of negative emotionality, despite having been a happy, easy-going baby.

Neuropsychology: Weaknesses in executive functioning and expressive language (on neuropsychological testing).

Attachment style: Behavioral attachment style characteristic of avoidant insecure attachment, characterized by fluctuation in proximity/avoidance indicated in the case description. However, some basic sense of safety is present, as he seems comfortable expressing aggression in the context of the family environment. Avoidant pattern seems the result of parents' apparent lack of predictability and investment in helping him develop effective ways of managing anxiety and frustration.

Sociocultural factors: Difficulties are primarily observed at home with family, but not at school.

Countertransference/Transference Manifestations

Child is connected with and interested in impressing the therapist, while at the same time reluctant to seek support for what he is struggling with. Therapist feels empathy, but because of the nature of the child's defenses, frustrated and shut out at moments. Child also evokes feelings of competitiveness.

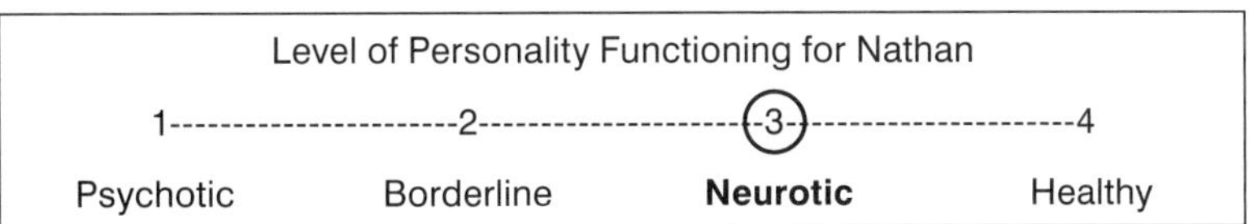

Borderline Level of Personality Organization

Children functioning at a borderline level of personality organization tend to be rigid and inflexible in their thinking. Taking another person's point of view is hard for them. They fail to see nuances and perceive events, people, and interactions in all-good and all-bad terms. Those with trauma histories may become dissociative under stress. They may show evidence of thought disturbance (e.g., loosening of associations, tangentiality, concrete thinking). They may find it difficult to differentiate what is coming from within from what is coming from another. Under stress they may become disorganized, sometimes to the point of short breaks with reality; however, they have the capacity to reconstitute when they are assisted, or when an alternative stimulus is provided. They are difficult to soothe once they become dysregulated. Tantrums, raging, or sobbing may persist for extended periods of time, seemingly regardless of attempts by caregivers to be empathic, supportive, and comforting. Borderline-level children show little capacity for self-reflection.

Histories of maltreatment, including neglect and abuse, are not uncommon among children functioning at this level, though there are clearly children with such histories who do not later develop borderline personality disorders or exhibit the emerging personality deficits highlighted here. Sexually abused children are often found to function at a borderline level of personality organization, particularly when the abuse was perpetrated by caregivers. For some children, however, early and/or persistent empathic failures on the part of caregivers (sometimes interacting with temperamental predispositions toward reactivity) often result in a disorganized attachment style; a tendency to express emotions through action; and impairments in neuropsychological development, symbolic capacity, and capacity for reflective functioning. These children have great difficulty discerning what is on their own minds, or on the minds of others. They tend to show intense shifts in emotion, and emotion is most often acted out rather than given verbal expression. They have little curiosity about themselves and may find it difficult to maintain a consistent sense of who they are. They may relate to others in terms of the function they serve (in psychoanalytic terms, part-object relating), but there is little appreciation or understanding of who the others are, or what motivates them. Rapid shifts in how people are perceived and related to are not uncommon. Borderline-level children can be truly empathic at one moment (or in one setting), but equally callous at the next.

Ways in Which Children in This Category Tend to Be Experienced Clinically

Borderline-level children can be exhausting. Life with them is a roller-coaster ride of intense emotions, with rapid and unanticipated shifts in the nature of the relationship. A therapist is called upon to be a container of those intense emotions, to experience deeply a child's intense mental state while remaining outwardly on an even keel. Reactions to the therapist are frequently at extremes of love and hate, dependence and rejection. These children's affective displays are extreme, and they tend to be unforgiving. They can make therapists feel incompetent. Because of their self-esteem issues and their reliance on primitive defenses, they tend to communicate their state of mind not by words, but by creating their experience within others. There are moments when a therapist feels it is impossible to "get it right," and other moments of feeling as if one is the greatest therapist who ever lived.

Whatever state of affairs exists in the room with a borderline-level child at any time is tenuous at best. Characters in play are often portrayed as unempathic, cold, abusive, or outright sadistic; as using or manipulating others for their own purposes; or as targets of such attitudes. Children with these themes can treat a therapist in extremely hurtful ways, showing little empathy or concern, and being even gleeful about the therapist's suffering. Maintaining boundaries with children in the borderline range can be challenging. They tend to push limits of physical distance, sexuality, demands, and aggression. They may ask inappropriate questions about the therapist, or show no interest at all. Because of either misperception or lack of empathy, they find it difficult to appreciate others' perspectives. As noted above, these children tend to be more about acting than thinking—either about themselves or about what might be in the mind of another.

Clinical Illustration

Ana was an 8-year-old Hispanic girl living with her mother and maternal grandmother in low-income housing. She was referred for rageful behavior at home and school. Her gait, speech, and fine and gross motor skills were age-appropriate. She ate and slept well; her intelligence was estimated as low-average. Ana was an untrusting child who anticipated negative, if not hostile, reactions from other children and adults. Her mother was similarly distrustful and guarded, secretive about her own past and about aspects of Ana's history. She revealed only that Ana had been born in the United States and raised by her mother and grandmother. Unlike her daughter, Ms. J was notably passive and apparently depressed. She described Ana's infancy tersely as being "normal," though she also commented that her child had "always been this way." Little color or detail was provided. When Ana was first seen for evaluation, Ana's mother had been separated from her husband for 2 years. Ana's father was, contrastingly, extremely aggressive. Although both verbally and physically aggressive to his former wife, he had not physically abused his daughter.

Ana was a cute-looking child, but was hard to understand or get close to. Her play was idiosyncratic and often solitary, with thematic content that was repetitive, dry, and disorganized. The disjointed, symbolically stark nature of her play allowed no clear sense to emerge of how she viewed herself. She was often content to exclude her therapist from play activities. When she did show interest in engaging the therapist, she would be demanding and controlling, and not in a playful way. The therapist came to feel that Ana used her rather than played with her. She understood that Ana was suffering, but found herself neither enjoying the child nor feeling enjoyed by her. According to her mother, Ana's changes in attitude and behavior would occur suddenly and forcefully, typically in response to Ms. J's refusing a request or asking Ana to do something she did not want to do. Her therapist similarly reported that the child moved from moments of cooperativeness to moments of extreme oppositionality and physical aggression, with no identifiable precipitant. These mood and behavioral changes seemed more internally than externally determined. The therapist felt as if she were suddenly with another child, or as if the child were suddenly experiencing her in an entirely different way. Also making Ana difficult to understand were peculiar verbal productions marked by loose associations and tangential thinking. Following the sequence of her thoughts was not always possible.

Ana's teacher observed similar tendencies at school, where Ana showed little interest in the work. She had no close friends at school or in her neighborhood, and she had difficulty reading social cues. Her play at school showed little indication of an ability to appreciate the experience of other children, and when peers responded to her negatively, she felt bullied. Ana reacted to her world in a detached manner, or as if she was the undeserving target of its hostility. Her defenses were entirely externalizing. She showed little ability to appreciate her contribution to the conflicts in which she found herself. Her perceptions of others could be grossly distorted, often at variance with perceptions of others. She showed little normal 8-year-old ability or willingness to think about herself; her reactions were nearly entirely reflexive and not reflective. Her thinking was largely inflexible. Ana was impulsive and uninhibited to the point of throwing objects at people, pulling hair, hitting, and cursing. She was neither able to soothe herself nor to allow others to soothe her. Her range of affect was limited. She did not overtly express much sadness or joy; an intense anger was most prominent.

Following bouts of explosiveness, she typically expressed no remorse, only a callous indifference. Yet at other times she could reflect on her mother's sense of loneliness with compassion.

Evaluating the Case

Cognitive and Affective Processes

1. *Capacity for regulation, attention, and learning:* Gait, speech, motor skills all unremarkable. Good sleeping and eating patterns. Intellectual functioning low-average. Lacking in curiosity.
2. *Capacity for affective range, communication, and understanding:* Affective range limited. Unable to communicate emotions in age-appropriate manner.
3. *Capacity for mentalization and reflective functioning:* Unable to read social cues. Reflective capacity extremely limited. No clear interest in understanding others.

Identity and Relationships

4. *Capacity for differentiation and integration (identity):* Difficulty in determining what comes from her and what comes from another. Sense of self not defined in any apparent way.
5. *Capacity for relationships and intimacy:* Untrusting, hard to get close to. Guarded.
6. *Capacity for self-esteem regulation and quality of internal experience:* Internal experience appears disjointed.

Defense and Coping

7. *Capacity for impulse control and regulation:* Poor impulse control. Easily dysregulated. Destructively aggressive.
8. *Capacity for defensive functioning:* Externalizing defenses dominate; unsuccessful in alleviating distress. Reality testing somewhat impaired.
9. *Capacity for adaptation, resiliency, and strength:* Can sometimes feel compassion for mother. Lacks adaptability across settings.

Self-Awareness and Self-Direction

10. *Self-observing capacities (psychological mindedness):* Child is not psychologically minded as yet. Shows little capacity for self-observation. Lacking in self-awareness.
11. *Capacity to construct and use internal standards and ideals:* Largely uninhibited. Can strike out at others without regard for consequences and without apparent remorse.

Other Factors

Epigenetics: Family history not yet revealed.

Temperament: Little information provided, but nothing remarkable reported.

Neuropsychology: Disorganized, inattentive.

Attachment style: Child shows disorganized attachment pattern, as characterized by sudden and unpredictable shifts in affect and extreme episodes of dysregulation. Lack of behavioral flexibility characteristic of overall uneconomical defensive strategies (often succumbs to states of despair and confusion).

Sociocultural factors: Poverty; family and neighborhood violence.

Countertransference/Transference Manifestations

Child is experienced as uncooperative, demanding, and controlling. Therapist has sense of being used. Sense of mutuality and mutual enjoyment difficult to achieve.

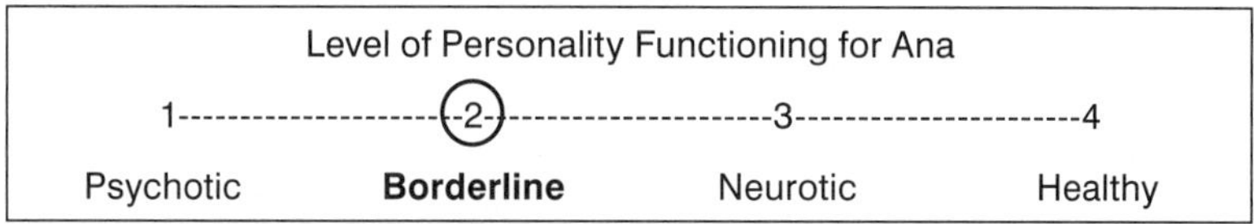

Psychotic Level of Personality Organization

A psychotic level of personality organization in children is characterized by verbal productions that are odd, difficult to follow, and sometimes unrelated to the conversation or situation at hand. Changes in level of cognitive functioning may be noted. Breaks with reality occur consistently and are not subject to correction. Delusions and hallucinatory experiences may be present. Somatization and bodily concerns are not uncommon. Affect is inappropriate to content. Affective reactions, behaviors, and verbal productions may reflect a child's response to internal rather than external stimuli. Psychotic-level children may laugh or become frightened for no discernible reason. Affect may be flat or blunted, or at times extremely intense, but in either case it is out of proportion with circumstances. These children have difficulty discriminating internal from external stimuli and may show confusion about what distinguishes one person from another. Others may be experienced as threatening without apparent justification.

Peers tend to experience these children as "weird" or "crazy." They are frequently bullied or avoided. Their play tends to be idiosyncratic, with strange, rapidly changing, and hard-to-follow themes. They may lose the boundary between self and other and between play and reality. As opposed to having a defined perception of the therapist or the therapeutic relationship, a psychotic-level child is often not mindful of the therapist at all. There is little capacity for, or interest in, self-reflection. Attempts to enter the child's world, or to know the child better, may be seen as intrusive or motivated by hostility, or may be met with indifference. These children frequently have significant family mental health histories.

Ways in Which Children in This Category Tend to Be Experienced Clinically

When therapists find themselves listening to or playing with children and being completely unable to make logical sense of what the children are talking about, their experience may be an important diagnostic indicator. Psychotic-level children have great difficulty communicating their thoughts. There are moments when they seem to disappear from the room, having gone to some other place in their minds, attending to some voices other than their therapists' or their own. Their reactions may seem entirely inconsistent with what has just been said or done, as they either are unable to process the information adequately or are responding to internal stimuli rather than what is coming from the therapists. A clinician can often feel the extreme anxiety that grips a psychotic-level child—a terror of extraordinary intensity. At times one gets the sense of a world entirely out of control, unpredictable, incomprehensible. Psychotic-level children can be hypervigilant. They may have peculiar interests, see the world in unique ways, and easily and often lose track of what is real and what is not. Working with such a child can be confusing, intense, and frightening, but also rewarding. These children are sometimes accepting of help. Because they feel themselves to be different and find themselves rejected by peers, they may be turn to their therapists for assistance.

Clinical Illustration

Paul was a 9-year-old European American boy living with both parents in an upper-middle-class home. He had no siblings. He had previously been seen for mental health services when he was 6. At that time he was having learning difficulties and problems with peers, and he was picking at his skin to the extent of causing bleeding. Paul had met developmental milestones in a timely fashion, with the notable exception of speech: He did not begin to speak fluently until midway through his fourth year. His speech was now clear, with no articulation difficulties. As an infant, Paul reportedly had smiled easily, made good eye contact, and related well. Striking to his parents, then and at the time of referral, was Paul's total lack of anxiety around strangers. The parents described him as overly trusting, relating to all people as if he had known them for a long time. They experienced this as a worrisome rather than as an appealing trait. Both parents were alert to possible difficulties for Paul; there was a history of schizophrenia on one side of the family and of bipolar disorder on the other. There was no history of potentially traumatizing events.

Paul's overall level of intelligence was in the average range, but his performance on his most recent testing was a standard deviation lower than it had been on a previous assessment. His teachers remarked that while he could be attentive, he had difficulty organizing his thoughts and was somewhat concrete and inflexible in his thinking. Paul could memorize things far better than he could think his way through novel situations. All of this added up to problems in learning and in relating, despite his being a rather curious child. Ms. P stated that she had always imagined that her son's learning difficulties were as much related to psychological deficits as they were to cognitive deficiencies. She and her husband described Paul as having always been a very emotional and hard-to-understand little boy.

Although he was not oppositional, Paul's parents would struggle in getting him to switch gears from whatever he was working on or wanting to discuss. Neither could they get him to think about things in a different way when his thoughts were irrational, unrealistic, or frightening. He would get involved in things that were not interesting to other children, in an excessively intensive way that limited other interests and activities. He did what he wanted and said what he wanted without any apparent filter. Paul was not aware that his style of play was not reciprocal, or that his productions existed apart from what other persons were doing or saying. He was somewhat physically awkward. Others would often find his behavior insensitive and inappropriate, as he would laugh at things that did not amuse others, or would seem to ignore others' reactions. He could be friendly and cooperative, but would blurt out random associations without any degree of self-consciousness. His friendships were shallow for a child his age. He had no close friends and belonged to no social group. Paul did not choose to participate in any team sports or engage much with classmates during lunch or recess.

Although his mood was typically upbeat, there was an intensity to his presentation. Some of his interests were not typical for a boy his age; for example, he was fascinated with *The Little Mermaid* and with how to repair laptops. Though intense, his interests did not remain interests for long. Paul would say that he was different from others, but could not say how. He frequently thought that there were things wrong with him, but located them physically and not in the ways he behaved or viewed things. Such physical concerns and complaints would often lead to days of school refusal. These concerns, along with his sense of having no friends and being picked on without provocation, led to moments of unhappiness, confusion, and agitation. Paul was uncomfortable with how things were, but seemed unable to take in any help that was offered. Adults found it easy to sympathize with his obvious struggles. His peers did not.

Paul's thinking and reality testing were both compromised. Loose associations, tangentiality, and concrete thinking were all present. He tended to misperceive and misinterpret. He reacted impulsively, without much contemplation, as he seemed inclined to discharge any intense emotion rather than be able to tolerate it or think about its cause. He would react more often to things going on inside him than to those going on around him. While he seemed sincerely interested in others, he was unable to recognize their experience accurately or differentiate between what might be coming from them or from himself. Although it had not been reported until the time of his referral, Paul mentioned hearing an ambiguous voice that would make sounds with no words. He had described being bothered by this, but as with other things, his reactions were intellectualized, rationalized (however irrationally), or compartmentalized.

Paul's focus was on details of experiences rather than on their emotional valence. In this respect, too, his affect was inappropriate to content. When unable to detach himself from his emotions, Paul became quickly disorganized and increasingly illogical. His play would often be solitary, with more interest in the characters he created than in the therapist. Thematic content could be bizarre and illogical. Alternative themes or outcomes were difficult or impossible for him to integrate into his play. The therapist would feel at times superfluous or intrusive, and yet there remained something endearing about the child.

Evaluating the Case

Cognitive and Affective Processes

1. *Capacity for regulation, attention, and learning:* Child can become emotionally dysregulated. Attention becomes intently fixed. This and disorganized thinking are related to difficulties in learning.
2. *Capacity for affective range, communication, and understanding:* Affect is inappropriate to content. Speech delay.
3. *Capacity for mentalization and reflective functioning:* Lacks capacity to mentalize or reflect on his own behavior.

Identity and Relationships

4. *Capacity for differentiation and integration (identity):* No developed sense of who he is.
5. *Capacity for relationships and intimacy:* No intimate relationships outside his immediate family.
6. *Capacity for self-esteem regulation and quality of internal experience:* Child is aware of being seen as different, but does not understand why. Has a sense of things being wrong with him, but sees them as somatic.

Defense and Coping

7. *Capacity for impulse control and regulation:* Uninhibited and without the capacity to filter what he says or does.
8. *Capacity for defensive functioning:* Defenses fail to prevent primitive thoughts and maintain reality testing.
9. *Capacity for adaptation, resiliency, and strength:* Paul is inflexible and unaware, but nonetheless likable.

Self-Awareness and Self-Direction

10. *Self-observing capacities (psychological mindedness):* No capacity for reasonably accurate self-observation.
11. *Capacity to construct and use internal standards and ideals:* Internal standards are hard to assess.

Other Factors

Epigenetics: Significant family mental health history.

Temperament: Always inflexible and intensely emotional.

Neuropsychology: Rigid and confused thought patterns. Delayed speech.

Attachment style: Evidence of significant difficulties of theory-of-mind functioning, as results of what seem like troubles with reality testing and maintaining a logical flow of ideas. In terms of behavioral attachment style, this child's behavior falls into the disorganized category.

Sociocultural factors: Upper-middle-class, European American family. No sibs.

Countertransference/Transference Manifestations

Feeling of disconnection on both sides. Great difficulty in integrating what is provided. Child remains endearing, even though often detached.

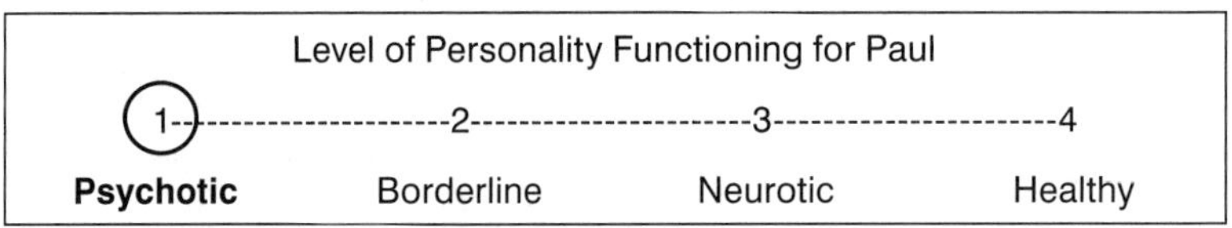

BIBLIOGRAPHY

Achenbach, T. A., & Rescorla, L. A. (2001). *Manual for ASEBA School-Age Forms and Profiles.* Burlington: University of Vermont, Research Center for Children, Youth, and Families.

Acklin, M. (1995). Rorschach assessment of the borderline child. *Journal of Clinical Psychology, 51*(2), 294–302.

Agrawal, H. R., Gunderson, J., Holmes, B. M., & Lyons-Ruth, K. (2004). Attachment studies with borderline patients: A review. *Harvard Review of Psychiatry, 12*(2), 94–104.

Akhtar, S. (2011). *Immigration and acculturation: Mourning, adaptation, and the next generation.* Lanham, MD: Aronson.

Altman, N. (2010). *The analyst in the inner city: Race, class, and culture through a psychoanalytic lens* (2nd ed.). New York: Routledge.

American Psychiatric Association. (2013). *Diagnostic and statistical manual of mental disorders* (5th ed.). Arlington, VA: Author.

Ames, L. B., Learned, J., Mitraux, R. W., & Walker, R. W. (1952). *Childhood Rorschach responses.* New York: Hoeber.

Ames, L. B., Metraux, R. W., & Walker, R. N. (1971). *Adolescent Rorschach responses: Developmental trends from ten to sixteen years* (2nd ed.). New York: Brunner/Mazel.

Armstrong, J. G., & Loewenstein, R. J. (1990). Characteristics of patients with multiple personality and dissociative disorders on psychological testing. *Journal of Nervous and Mental Disease, 178,* 448–454.

Barkley, R. A. (1999a). Response inhibition in attention deficit hyperactivity disorder. *Mental Retardation and Developmental Disabilities Research Reviews, 5,* 177–184.

Barkley, R. A. (1997b). *ADHD and the nature of self-control.* New York: Guilford Press.

Barkley, R. A. (2001). The executive functions and self-regulation: An evolutionary neuropsychological perspective. *Neuropsychology Review, 11,* 1–29.

Barkley, R. A. (2010). Deficient emotional self-regulation is a core component of ADHD. *Journal of ADHD and Related Disorders, 1,* 5–37.

Beebe, B., Lachmann, F. M., Markese, S., Buck, K. A., Bahrick, L. E., Chen, H., . . . Jaffe, J. (2012). On the origins of disorganized attachment and internal working models: Paper II. An empirical microanalysis of 4-month mother–infant interaction. *Psychoanalytic Dialogues, 22*(3), 352–374.

Beebe, B., & Steele, M. (2013). How does microanalysis of mother–infant communication inform maternal sensitivity and infant attachment? *Attachment and Human Development, 15*(5–6), 583–602.

Bell, M. (2003). Bell Object Relations Inventory for Adolescents and Children: Reliability, validity, and factorial invariance. *Journal of Personality Assessment, 80,* 19–25.

Bellak, L. (1993). *The T.A.T., C.A.T., and S.A.T. in clinical use* (5th ed.). Boston: Allyn & Bacon.

Belsky, J., & Pluess, M. (2009). Beyond cumulative risk: Distinguishing harshness and unpredictability as determinants of parenting and early life history strategy. *Developmental Psychology, 48,* 662–673.

Belsky, J., Schlomer, L., & Ellis, B. J. (2012). Beyond diathesis stress: Differential susceptibility to environmental influences. *Psychological Bulletin, 135,* 885–908.

Biederman, J., Rosenbaum, J. F., Bolduc-Murphy, E. A., Faraone, S., Chaloff, J., Hirschfeld, D. R., & Kagan, J. (1993). Behavioral inhibition as a temperamental risk factor for anxiety disorders. *Child and Adolescent Psychiatric Clinics of North America, 2,* 667–684.

Blair, C., & Rawer, C. C. (2012a). Child development in the context of adversity: Experiential canalization of brain and behavior. *American Psychologist, 10,* 1–10.

Blair, C., & Rawer, C. C. (2012b). Individual development and evolution: Experiential canalization of self-regulation. *Developmental Psychology, 48,* 647–657.

Blatt, S. (1974). Levels of object representation in anaclitic and introjective depression. *Psychoanalytic Study of the Child, 29,* 107–157.

Bleiberg, E. (2001). *Treating personality disorders in children and adolescents: A relational approach.* New York: Guilford Press.

Block, J. H., & Block, J. (1980). The role of ego control and ego-resiliency in the organization of behavior. In W. A. Collins (Ed.), *Development of cognition, affect and social relations* (Vol. 13, pp. 39–101). Hillsdale, NJ: Erlbaum.

Bouchard, T. J., Jr., & Loehlin, C. (2001). Genes, evolution, and personality. *Behavior Genetics, 31*(3), 243–273.

Bowlby, J. (1973). *Attachment and loss: Vol. 2. Separation: Anxiety and anger.* New York: Basic Books.

Bridgett, D. J., Burt, N. M., Edwards, E. S., & Deater-Deckard, K. (2015). Intergenerational transmission of self-regulation: A multidisciplinary review and integrative conceptual framework. *Psychological Bulletin, 141*(3), 602–654.

Caplan, R., Guthrie, D., Fish, B., Tanguay, P. E., & David-Lando, G. (1989). The Kiddie Formal Thought Disorder Rating Scale: Clinical assessment, reliability and validity. *Journal of the American Academy of Child and Adolescent Psychiatry, 28*(3), 408–416.

Carlson, E. A. (1998). A prospective longitudinal study of attachment disorganization/disorientation. *Child Development, 69*(4), 1107–1128.

Carlson, E. A., Egeland, B., & Sroufe, L. A. (2009).

A prospective investigation of the development of borderline personality symptoms. *Development and Psychopathology, 21*(4), 1311–1334.

Caspi, A., & Roberts, B. W. (1999). Personality continuity and change across the life course. In L. Pervin & O. John (Eds.), *Handbook of personality: Theory and research* (pp. 300–326). New York: Guilford Press.

Caspi, A., Roberts, B. W., & Shiner, R. L. (2005). Personality development: Stability and change. *Annual Review of Psychology, 56*, 453–484.

Caspi, A., & Shiner, R. L. (2006). Personality development. In W. Damon & R. M. Lerner (Series Eds.) & N. Eisenberg (Vol. Ed.), *Handbook of child psychology: Vol. 3. Social, emotional, and personality development* (6th ed., pp. 300–365). Hoboken, NJ: Wiley.

Caspi, A., & Shiner, R. L. (2008). Temperament and personality. In M. Rutter, D. V. M. Bishop, D. S. Pine, S. Scott, J. Stevenson, E. Taylor, & A. Thapar (Eds.), *Rutter's child and adolescent psychiatry* (5th ed., pp. 182–198). Oxford, UK: Blackwell.

Champagne, F. D. (2010). Epigenetic perspectives on development: Evolving insights on the origins of variations. *Developmental Psychology, 52*, 3–10.

Chapman, B. P., & Goldberg, L. R. (2011). Replicability and 40-year predictive power of childhood ARC types. *Journal of Personality and Social Psychology, 101*, 593–606.

Chazan, S. W. (2000). Using the Children's Play Therapy Instrument (CPTI) to measure the development of play in simultaneous treatment. *Infant Mental Health Journal, 21*, 211–221.

Chess, S., & Thomas, A. (1991). Temperament and the concept of goodness of fit. In J. Srelau & A. Angleitner (Eds.), *Explorations in temperament* (pp. 15–28). New York: Plenum Press.

Cicchetti, D. (2006). Development and psychopathology. In D. Cicchetti & D. Cohen (Eds.), *Developmental psychopathology: Vol. 1. Theory and method* (2nd ed., pp. 1–23). Hoboken, NJ: Wiley.

Cicchetti, D., & Cohen, D. (Eds.). (2006). *Developmental psychopathology: Vol 1. Theory and method.* Hoboken, NJ: Wiley.

Cicchetti, D., & Rogosch, F. A. (2009). Adaptive coping under conditions of extreme stress: Multilevel influences on the determinants of resilience in maltreated children. *New Directions for Child and Adolescent Development, 124*, 47–59.

Cohen, P. (2008). Child development and personality disorder. *Psychiatric Clinics of North America, 31*(3), 477–493.

Coolidge, F. L. (2005). *Coolidge Personality and Neuropsychological Inventory for Children manual.* Colorado Springs, CO: Author.

Costantino, G., Malgady, R. G., & Rogler, I. H. (1988). *TEMAS (Tell-Me-A-Story) manual.* Los Angeles: Western Psychological Services.

Cramer, P. (1982). *Defense mechanism manual.* Unpublished manuscript, Williams College, Williamston, MA.

Cramer, P. (1987). The development of defense mechanisms. *Journal of Personality, 55*(4), 597–614.

Cramer, P. (1990). *The development of defense mechanisms: Theory, research, and assessment.* New York: Springer-Verlag.

Cramer, P. (1996). *Storytelling, narrative, and the Thematic Apperception Test.* New York: Guilford Press.

Cramer, P. (2015). Defense mechanisms: 40 years of empirical research. *Journal of Personality Assessment, 97*(2), 114–122.

Cramer, P., & Blatt, S. J. (1990). Use of TAT to measure changes in defense mechanisms following intensive psychotherapy. *Journal of Personality Assessment, 54*, 236–251.

Cramer, P., Blatt, S., & Ford, R. (1988). Defense mechanisms in the anaclitic and introjective personality configuration. *Journal of Consulting and Clinical Psychology, 56*(4), 610–616.

Crawford, T. N., Cohen, P., & Brook, J. S. (2001). Dramatic–erratic personality disorder symptoms: I. Developmental pathways from early adolescence to late adulthood. *Journal of Personality Disorders, 13*, 319–335.

Crick, N. R., Murray-Close, D., & Woods, K. (2005). Borderline personality features in childhood: A short-term longitudinal study. *Development and Psychopathology, 17*, 1051–1070.

Deal, J., Halverson, C. F., Martin, R. P., Victor, J., & Baker, S. (2007). The Inventory of Children's Individual Differences: Development and validation of a short version. *Journal of Personality Assessment, 89*, 162–166.

Deckel, A., Hesselbrock, V., & Bauer, L. (1998). Antisocial personality disorder, childhood delinquency, and frontal brain functioning: EEG and neuropsychological findings. *Journal of Clinical Psychology, 52*(6), 639–650.

De Clercq, B., & De Fruyt, F. (2012). A five factor model framework for understanding childhood personality disorder antecedents. *Journal of Personality, 80*(6), 1533–1563.

De Clercq, B., Van Leeuwen, K., Van Den Noortgate, W., De Bolle, M., & DeFruyt, F. (2009). Childhood personality pathology: Dimensional stability and change. *Development and Psychopathology, 21*(3), 853–869.

De Haan, A. D., Dekovic, M., van der Akker, A. L., Stoltz, S. E. M., & Prinzie, P. (2013). Developmental personality types from childhood to adolescence: Associations with parenting and adjustment. *Child Development, 84*(6), 2015–2030.

De Los Reyes, A., & Kazdin, A. E. (2005). Informant discrepancies in the assessment of childhood psychopathology: A critical review, theoretical framework, and recommendations for further study. *Psychological Bulletin, 131*, 483–509.

Dennisen, J. J. A., Asendorpf, J. B., & Van Aken, M. A. G. (2008). Childhood personality predicts long-term trajectories of shyness and aggressiveness in the context of demographic transitions in emerging adulthood. *Journal of Personality, 76*, 67–99.

Depue, R. A., & Lenzenweger, M. F. (2005). A neurobehavioral dimensional model of personality disturbance. In M. F. Lenzenweger & J. F. Clarkin (Eds.), *Major theories of personality disorder* (2nd ed., pp. 391–453). New York: Guilford Press.

Digman, J. M., & Shmelyov, A. G. (1996). The structure of temperament and personality in Russian children. *Journal of Personality and Social Psychology, 71*, 341–351.

Dollinger, S., & Cramer, P. (1990). Children's defensive responses and emotional upset following a disaster: A projective assessment. *Journal of Personality Assessment, 54*, 55–62.

Donahue, P. J., & Tuber, S. B. (1993). Rorschach adaptive fantasy images and coping in children under severe environmental stress. *Journal of Personality Assessment, 60*(3), 121–434.

Dozier, M., & Kobak, R. R. (1992). Psychophysiology in attachment interviews: Converging evidence for deactivating strategies. *Child Development, 63*(6), 1473–1480.

Ensink, K., Biberdzic, M., Normandin, L., & Clarkin, J. (2015a). A developmental psychopathology and neurobiological model of borderline personality disorder in adolescence. *Journal of Infant, Child, and Adolescent Psychotherapy, 14*, 46–69.

Ensink, K., Normandin, L., Target, M., Fonagy, P., Sabourin, S., & Berthelot, N. (2015b). Mentalization in children and mothers in the context of trauma: An initial study of the validity of the Child Reflective Functioning Scale. *British Journal of Developmental Psychology, 33*(2), 203–217.

Exner, J. E. (1974). *The Rorschach: A comprehensive system* (Vol. 1). New York: Wiley.

Exner, J. E., & Weiner, I. B. (1995). *The Rorschach: A comprehensive system: Vol. 3. Assessment of children and adolescents* (2nd ed.). New York: Wiley.

Feldman, R., & Blatt, S. (1996). Precursors of relatedness and self-definition in mother–infant interaction. In J. Masling & R. Bornstein (Eds.), *Psychoanalytic perspectives on developmental psychology* (pp. 1–42). Washington, DC: American Psychological Association.

Freud, A. (1966). *The ego and the mechanisms of defense.* New York: International Universities Press. (Original work published 1936)

Frick, P. J., Stickle, T. R., Dandreaux, D. M., Farrell, J. M., & Kimonis, E. R. (2005). Callous–unemotional traits in predicting the severity and stability of conduct problems and delinquency. *Journal of Abnormal Child Psychology, 33*, 471–487.

Frick, P. J., & White, S. F. (2008). The importance of callous–unemotional traits for developmental models of aggressive and antisocial behavior. *Journal of Child Psychology and Psychiatry, 49*(4), 359–375.

Ge, X., Conger, R. D., Cadoret, R., Neiderhiser, J., Yates, W., Troughton, E., & Stewart, M. (1996). The developmental interface between nature and nurture: A mutual influence model of child antisocial behavior and parent behaviors. *Developmental Psychology, 32*(4), 574–589.

Geiger, T. C., & Crick, N. R. (2010). Developmental pathways to personality disorders. In R. E. Ingram & J. E. Price (Eds.), *Vulnerability to psychopathology* (2nd ed., pp. 57–108). New York: Guilford Press.

Germeijs, V., & Verschueren, K. (2011). Indecisiveness and Big Five personality factors: Relationship and specificity. *Personality and Individual Differences, 50*, 1023–1028.

Goldsmith, H. H. (1983). Genetic influences on personality from infancy to adulthood. *Child Development, 54*, 331–355.

Habermas, T., & Köber, C. (2015). Autobiographical reasoning in life narratives buffers the effect of biographical disruptions on the sense of self-continuity. *Memory, 23*(5), 664–674.

Halpern, F. (1953). *A clinical approach to children's Rorschachs.* New York: Grune & Stratton.

Halverson, C. F., Havill, V. L., Deal, J., Baker, S. R., Victor, J. B., Pavloupolos, V., . . . Wen, L. (2003). Personality structure as derived from parental ratings of free descriptions of children: The Inventory of Child Individual Differences. *Journal of Personality, 71*, 995–1026.

Hampson, S. E., & Goldberg, L. R. (2006). A first large cohort study of personality trait stability over the 40 years between elementary school and midlife. *Journal of Personality and Social Psychology, 91*(4), 763–779.

Harris, J. (1998). *The nurture assumption: Why children turn out the way they do.* New York: Free Press.

Harter, S. (1999). *The construction of the self: A developmental perspective.* New York: Guilford Press.

Harter, S. (2006). The self. In W. Damon & R. M. Lerner (Series Eds.) & N. Eisenberg (Vol. Ed.), *Handbook of child psychology: Vol. 3. Social, emotional, and personality development* (6th ed., pp. 505–570) Hoboken, NJ: Wiley.

Hill, J., Stepp, S. D., Wan, M. W., Hope, H., Morse, J. Q., Steele, M., . . . Pilkonis, P. A. (2011). Attachment, borderline personality, and romantic relationship dysfunction. *Journal of Personality Disorders, 25*(6), 789–805.

Hiller, J. B., Rosenthal, R., Bornstein, R. F., Berry, D. T. R., & Brunell-Neuleib, S. (1999). Comparative meta-analysis of Rorschach and MMPI validity. *Psychological Assessment, 11*(3), 278–296.

Hilsenroth, M. J., Eudell-Simmons, E. M., DeFife, J.

A., & Charnas, J. W. (2007). The Rorschach Perceptual and Thinking Index (PTI): An examination of reliability, validity and diagnostic efficiency. *International Journal of Testing, 7*(3), 269–291.

Holaday, M. (2000). Rorschach protocols from children and adolescents diagnosed with posttraumatic stress disorder. *Journal of Personality Assessment, 71*, 306–321.

Hudziak, J. J., Achenbach, T. M., Althoff, R. R., & Pine, D. S. (2007). A dimensional approach to developmental psychopathology. *International Journal of Methods in Psychiatric Research, 16*, S16–S23.

Jang, K. L., McCrae, R. R., Angleitner, A., Rieman, R., & Livesley, W. J. (1998). Heritability of facet level traits in a cross-cultural twin sample: Support for a hierarchical model of personality. *Journal of Personality and Social Psychology, 74*, 1556–1565.

John, O., Caspi, A., Robins, R. W., Moffitt, T. E., & Stouthamer-Loeber, M. (1994). The "Little Five": Exploring the nomological network of the five-factor model of personality in adolescent boys. *Child Development, 65*, 160–178.

Kelly, F. D. (1997). *The assessment of object relations phenomena in adolescents' TAT and Rorschach measures*. Mahwah, NJ: Erlbaum.

Kelly, F. D. (2007). The clinical application of the Social Cognition and Object Relations Scale with children and adolescents. In S. Smith & L. Handler (Eds.), *The clinical assessment of children and adolescents: A practitioner's handbook*. Mahwah, NJ: Erlbaum.

Kernberg, O. F. (1975). *Borderline conditions and pathological narcissism*. New York: Aronson.

Kernberg, O. F., & Caligor, E. (2005). A psychoanalytic theory of personality disorders. In M. F. Lenzenweger & J. F. Clarkin (Eds.), *Major theories of personality disorder* (2nd ed., pp. 114–156). New York: Guilford Press.

Kernberg, P. F., Chazan, S. E., & Normandin, L. (1998). The Children's Play Therapy Instrument (CPTI): Description and development and reliability studies. *Journal of Psychotherapy Theory and Research, 7*(3), 196–207.

Kernberg, P. F., Weiner, A., & Bardenstein, K. (2000). *Personality disorders in children and adolescents*. New York: Basic Books.

Kim, J., Carlson, G. A., Meyer, S. E., Bufferd, S. J., Dougherty, L. R., Dyson, M. W., . . . Klein, D. N. (2012). Correlates of the CBCL dysregulation profile in preschool-aged children. *Journal of Child Psychology and Psychiatry, 52*(9), 918–926.

Kobak, R. R., & Sceery, A. (1988). Attachment in late adolescence: Working models, affect regulation, and representations of self and others. *Child Development, 59*, 135–146.

Kochanska, G., Philibert, R. A., & Barry, R. A. (2009). Interplay of genes and early mother–child relationship in the development of self-regulation from toddler to preschool age. *Journal of Child Psychology and Psychiatry, 50*(11), 1331–1338.

Korkman, M., Kirk, U., & Kemp, S. (2007). *NEPSY—Second Edition*. San Antonio, TX: Pearson.

Kraemer, H., Stice, E., Kazdin, A., Offord, D., & Kupfer, D. (2001). How do risk factors work together?: Mediators, moderators, and independent, overlapping, and proxy risk factors. *American Journal of Psychiatry, 158*(6), 848–856.

Lerner, P. (1991). *Psychoanalytic theory and the Rorschach*. Hillsdale, NJ: Analytic Press.

Levy, K. N., Meehan, K. B., Weber, M., Reynoso, J., & Clarkin, J. F. (2005). Attachment and borderline personality disorder: Implications for psychotherapy. *Psychopathology, 38*, 64–74.

Lewis, L. (2001). Issues in the study of personality development. *Psychological Inquiry, 12*, 67–83.

Liotti, G. (2004). Trauma, dissociation, and disorganized attachment: Three strands of a single braid. *Psychotherapy: Theory, Research, Practice, Training, 41*(4), 472–486.

Lofgren, D. P., Bemporad, J., King, J., Linden, K., & O'Driscoll, G. (1991). A prospective follow-up study of so-called borderline children. *American Journal of Psychiatry, 148*, 1541–1547.

Luthar, S., & Zigler, E. (1991). Vulnerability and competence: A review of research on resilience in childhood. *American Journal of Orthopsychiatry, 61*(1), 6–22.

Luyten, P., & Blatt, S. (2009). A structural-developmental psychodynamic approach to psychopathology: Two polarities of experience across the life span. *Development and Psychopathology, 21*(3), 793–814.

Lyons-Ruth, K., Bureau, J., Holmes, B., Easterbrooks, A., & Brooks, N. H. (2013). Borderline symptoms and suicidality/self-injury in late adolescence: Prospectively observed relationship correlates in infancy and childhood. *Psychiatry Research, 206*(2–3), 273–281.

Lyons-Ruth, K., & Jacobvitz, D. (2008). Attachment disorganization: Genetic factors, parenting contexts, and developmental transformation from infancy to adulthood. In J. Cassidy & P. R. Shaver (Eds.), *Handbook of attachment: Theory, research and clinical applications* (2nd ed., pp. 666–697). New York: Guilford Press.

Maccoby, E. E. (2000). Parenting and its effects on children: On reading and misreading behavior genetics. *Annual Review of Psychology, 51*, 1–27.

Macdonald, H. Z., Beeghly, M., Grant-Knight, W., Augustyn, M., Woods, R. W., Cabral, H., . . . Frank, D. A. (2008). Longitudinal association between infant disorganized attachment and childhood posttraumatic stress symptoms. *Development and Psychopathology, 20*(2), 493–508.

Main, M. (1999). Epilogue: Attachment theory:

Eighteen points with suggestions for future studies. In J. Cassidy & P. R. Shaver (Eds.), *Handbook of attachment: Theory, research, and clinical applications* (pp. 845–888). New York: Guilford Press.

Main, M., & Hesse, E. (1990). Parents' unresolved traumatic experiences are related to infant disorganized attachment status: Is frightened and/or frightening parental behavior the linking mechanism? In M. Main & R. Goldwyn (Eds.), *Attachment in the preschool years: Theory, research, and intervention* (pp. 161–182). Chicago: University of Chicago Press.

McCrae, R. R. (2000). Trait psychology and the revival of personality-and-culture studies. *American Behavioral Scientist, 44*, 10–31.

McCrae, R. R., & Costa, P. T., Jr. (1997). Personality trait structure as a human universal. *American Psychologist, 52*, 509–516.

McCrae, R. R., Costa, P. T., Jr., del Pilar, G. H., Rolland, J.-P., & Parker, W. D. (1998a). Cross-cultural assessment of the five factor model: The revised NEO Personality Inventory. *Journal of Cross-Cultural Psychology, 29*, 171–188.

McCrae, R. R., Costa, P. T., Jr., Ostendorf, F., Angleitner, A., Hrebickova, M., Avia, M. D., . . . Smith, P. B. (2000). Nature over nurture: Temperament, personality, and lifespan development. *Journal of Personality and Social Psychology, 78*, 173–186.

McCrae, R. R., Costa, P. T., Jr., Pedroso de Lima, M., Simoes, A., Ostendorf, F., Angleitner, A., . . . Piedmont, R. L. (1999). Age differences in personality across the adult life span: Parallels in five cultures. *Developmental Psychology, 35*, 466–477.

McWilliams, N. (2011). *Psychoanalytic diagnosis: Understanding personality structure in the clinical process.* New York: Guilford Press.

Meany, M. (2001). Maternal care, gene expression, and the transmission of individual differences in stress reactivity across generations. *Annual Review of Neuroscience, 24*, 1161–1192.

Meany, M., & Szyf, M. (2005). Environmental programming of stress responses through DNA methylation: Life at the interface between a dynamic environment and a fixed genome. *Dialogues in Clinical Neuroscience, 7*(2), 103–123.

Meehan, K. B., McHale, J. Y., Reynoso, J. S., Harris, B. H., Wolfson, V. M., Gomes, H., & Tuber, S. B. (2008). Self-regulation and internal resources in school aged children with ADHD symptomatology: An investigation using the Rorschach inkblot method. *Bulletin of the Menninger Clinic, 72*(4), 259–282.

Mervielde, I., De Clercq, B., De Fruyt, F., & Van Leeuwen, K. (2005). Temperament, personality, and developmental psychopathology as childhood antecedents of personality disorders. *Journal of Personality Disorders, 19*, 171–201.

Meyer, G. J., & Kurtz, J. E. (2006). Advancing personality assessment terminology: Time to retire "objective" and "projective" as personality test descriptors. *Journal of Personality Assessment, 87*(3), 223–225.

Meyer, G. J., Viglione, D. J., Mihora, J. L., Erard, R. E., & Erdberg, P. (2011). *Rorschach Performance Assessment System: Administration coding, interpretation and technical manual.* Toledo, OH: Rorschach Performance Assessment System.

Meyer, S. E., Carlson, G. A., Youngstrom, E., Ronsaville, D. S., Matinez, P. E., Gold, P. W., . . . Radke-Yarrow, M. (2009). Long term outcomes of youth who manifested the CBCL-pediatric bipolar disorder phenotype during childhood and/or adolescence. *Journal of Affective Disorders, 113*, 227–235.

Mihura, J. L., Meyer, G. J., Dumitrascu, N., & Bombel, G. (2013). The validity of the individual Rorschach variables: Systematic reviews and meta-analyses of the comprehensive system. *Psychological Bulletin, 136*, 548–605.

Mikulincer, M., & Shaver, P. R. (2007). Boosting attachment security to promote mental health, prosocial values, and inter-group tolerance. *Psychological Inquiry, 18*(3), 139–156.

Millon, T., Tringone, R., Millon, C., & Grossman, S. (2005). *Millon Pre-Adolescent Clinical Inventory Manual.* Minneapolis, MN: Pearson.

Moutsiana, C., Fearon, P., Murray, L., Cooper, P., Goodyer, I., Johnstone, T., & Halligan, S. (2014). Making an effort to feel positive: Insecure attachment in infancy predicts the neural underpinnings of emotion regulation in adulthood. *Journal of Child Psychology and Psychiatry, 55*(9), 999–1008.

Murray, H. A. (1943). *Thematic Apperception Test.* Cambridge, MA: Harvard University Press.

Naglieri, J. A., Lebuffe, P., & Pfeiffer, S. I. (1994). *The Devereux Scales of Mental Disorders—Manual.* San Antonio, TX: Psychological Corporation.

Nahum, J. P. (1994). New theoretical vistas in psychoanalysis: Louis Sander's theory of early development. *Psychoanalytic Psychology, 11*(1), 1–19.

Nakash-Eisikovits, O., Dutra, L., & Westen, D. (2003). The relationship between attachment patterns and personality pathology in adolescents. *Journal of the American Academy of Child and Adolescent Psychiatry, 41*, 1111–1123.

Neppl, T. K., Donnellan, M. B., Scaramella, L. V., Widaman, K. F., Spilman, S. K., Ontai, L. L., & Conger, R. D. (2010). Differential stability of temperament and personality from toddlerhood to middle childhood. *Journal of Research in Personality, 44*(3), 386–396.

Nigg, J. T. (2006). Temperament and developmental psychopathology. *Journal of Child Psychology and Psychiatry, 47*, 395–422.

Olson, S. L., Bates, J. E., Sandy, J. M., & Lanthier, R.

(2000). Early developmental precursors of externalizing behavior in middle childhood and adolescence. *Journal of Abnormal Child Psychology, 28*, 119–133.

Olson, S. L., Schilling, E. M., & Bates, J. E. (1999). Measurement of impulsivity: Construct coherence, longitudinal stability, and relationship with externalizing problems in middle childhood and adolescence. *Journal of Abnormal Child Psychology, 27*, 151–165.

Palombo, J. (2001). The therapeutic process with children with learning disabilities. *Psychoanalytic Social Work, 8*, 143–168.

Pennington, B. F. (2009). *Diagnosing learning disorders: A neuropsychological framework*. New York: Guilford Press.

Pennington, B. F., & Ozonoff, S. (1996). Executive functions and developmental psychopathology. *Journal of Child Psychology and Psychiatry, 37*, 51–87.

Perry, L. H., & Landreth, G. L. (2001). Diagnostic assessment of children's play therapy behavior. In G. L. Landreth (Ed.), *Innovations in play therapy: Issues, process and special populations* (pp. 155–178). New York: Brunner-Routledge.

Plomin, R., & Caspi, A. (1999). Behavioral genetics and personality. In L. Pervin & O. John (Eds.), *Handbook of personality: Theory and research* (pp. 251–276). New York: Guilford Press.

Poorthuis, A. M. G., Thomaes, S., Denissen, J. J. A., van Aken, M. A. G., & Orobio de Castro, B. (2014). Personality in action: Can brief behavioral personality tests predict children's academic and social adjustment across the transition to secondary school. *European Journal of Psychological Assessment, 30*(3), 169–177.

Price, J. M., & Zwolinski, J. (2010). The nature of child and adolescent vulnerability: History and definitions. In R. Ingram & J. Price (Eds.), *Vulnerability to psychopathology: Risk across the lifespan* (2nd ed., pp. 18–38). New York: Guilford Press.

Pulve, A., Allik, J., Pulkkinen, L., & Haemaelaeinen, M. (1995). A Big Five personality inventory in two non-Indo-European languages. *European Journal of Personality, 9*, 109–124.

Roberts, B., & DelVecchio, W. (2000). The rank-order consistency of personality traits from childhood to old age: A quantitative review of longitudinal studies. *Psychological Bulletin, 126*(1), 3–25.

Roberts, G. E., & Gruber, C. (2005). *Roberts-2: Manual*. Los Angeles: Western Psychological Services.

Rom, E., & Mikulincer, M. (2003). Attachment theory and group processes: The association between attachment style and group-related representations, goals, memories, and functioning. *Journal of Personality and Social Psychology, 84*(6), 12–20.

Rose, L. T., & Fischer, K. W. (2009). Dynamic development: A neo-Piagetian approach. In U. Muller & J. I. M. Carpendale (Eds.), *The Cambridge companion to Piaget* (pp. 400–423). Cambridge, UK: Cambridge University Press.

Rothbart, M. K., Ahadi, S. A., Hersey, K. L., & Fisher, P. (2001). Investigations of temperament at three to seven years: The Children's Behavior Questionnaire. *Child Development, 72*, 1394–1408.

Rourke, B. P. (2000). Neuropsychological and psychosocial subtyping: A review of investigations within the University of Windsor laboratory. *Canadian Psychology, 41*, 34–51.

Russ, S. W. (2004). *Play in child development and psychotherapy: Toward empirically supported practice*. Mahwah, NJ: Erlbaum.

Rutter, M. (1987). Psychosocial resilience and protective mechanisms. *American Journal of Orthopsychiatry, 57*(3), 316–331.

Ryder, A. G., Dere, J., Sun, J., & Chentsova-Dutton, Y. E. (2014). The cultural shaping of personality disorder. In F. T. L. Leong, L. Comas-Díaz, G. C. Nagayama Hall, V. C. McLoyd, & J. E. Trimble (Eds.), *APA handbook of multicultural psychology: Vol. 2. Applications and training* (pp. 307–328). Washington, DC: American Psychological Association.

Salomonsson, B. (2004). Some psychoanalytic viewpoints on neuropsychiatric disorders in children. *International Journal of Psychoanalysis, 85*, 117–136.

Salomonsson, B. (2006). The impact of words on children with ADHD and DAMP: Consequences for psychoanalytic technique. *International Journal of Psychoanalysis, 87*, 1029–1044.

Salomonsson, B. (2011). Psychoanalytic conceptualizations of the internal object in an ADHD child. *Journal of Infant, Child and Adolescent Psychotherapy, 10*(1), 87–102.

Schore, A. (2003). *Affect dysregulation and disorders of the self*. New York: Norton.

Selzer, M. A., Koenigsberg, H. W., & Kernberg, O. F. (1987). The initial contract in the treatment of borderline patients. *American Journal of Psychiatry, 144*, 927–930.

Serafica, F. C., & Vargas, L. A. (2006). Cultural diversity in the development of child psychopathology. In D. Cicchetti & D. Cohen (Eds.), *Developmental psychopathology: Vol. 1. Theory and method* (2nd ed., pp. 588–626). Hoboken, NJ: Wiley.

Shafer, R. (1954). *Psychoanalytic interpretation in Rorschach testing: Theory and application*. New York: Grune & Stratton.

Shiner, R. L. (2005). A developmental perspective on personality disorders: Lessons from research on normal personality development in childhood and adolescence. *Journal of Personality Disorders, 19*(2), 202–210.

Shiner, R. L. (2006). Temperament and personality in

childhood. In D. K. Mroczek & T. D. Little (Eds.), *Handbook of personality development* (pp. 213–230). Mahwah, NJ: Erlbaum.

Shiner, R. L., & Caspi, A. (2003). Personality differences in childhood and adolescence: Measurement, development, and consequences. *Journal of Child Psychology and Psychiatry, 44*(1), 2–32.

Shore, B. (1996). *Culture in mind: Cognition, culture, and the problem of meaning.* New York: Oxford University Press.

Slade, A. (2005) Parental reflective functioning: An introduction. *Attachment and Human Development, 7,* 269–281.

Sroufe, A. (1997). Psychopathology as an outcome of development. *Development and Psychopathology, 9*(2), 251–268.

Stokes, J. M., Pogge, D. L., Grosso, C., & Zaccario, M. (2001). The relationship of the Rorschach SCZI to psychotic features in a child psychiatric sample. *Journal of Personality Assessment, 76*(2), 209–228.

Stokes, J. M., Pogge, D. L., Powell-Lunder, J., Ward, A. W., Bilginer, L., & DeLuca, V. A. (2003). The Rorschach Ego Impairment Index: Prediction of treatment outcome in a child psychiatric population. *Journal of Personality Assessment, 81,* 11–20.

Tackett, J. L. (2010). Measurement and assessment of child and adolescent personality pathology: Introduction to the special issue. *Journal of Psychopathology and Behavior Assessment, 32,* 463–466.

Tackett, J. L. (2011). Parent informants for child personality: Agreement, discrepancies and clinical utility. *Journal of Personality Assessment, 93,* 539–544.

Thomas, A., & Chess, S. (1977). *Temperament and development.* New York: Brunner-Mazel.

Thomas, A., Chess, S., Birch, H., Hertzig, M., & Korn, S. (1963). *Behavioral individuality in early childhood.* New York: New York University Press.

Thomsen, P. H. (1996). Borderline conditions in childhood: A register-based follow-up study over a 22-year period. *Psychopathology, 29,* 357–362.

Tummala-Narra, P. (2015). Cultural competence as a core emphasis of psychoanalytic psychotherapy. *Psychoanalytic Psychology, 32*(2), 275–292.

van Emmichoven, I. A. Z., van IJzendoorn, M. H., de Ruiter, C., & Brosschot, J. (2003). Selective processing of threatening information: Effects of attachment representation and anxiety disorder on attention and memory. *Development and Psychopathology, 15*(1), 219–237.

van IJzendoorn, M. H., Schuengel, C., & Bakermans-Kranenburg, M. J. (1999). Disorganized attachment in early childhood: Meta-analysis of precursors, concomitants, and sequelae. *Development and Psychopathology, 11*(2), 225–250.

Viglione, D. J. (1996). Data and issues to consider in reconciling self-report and the Rorschach. *Journal of Personality Assessment, 67*(3), 579–588.

Vrtička, P., Andersson, F., Grandjean, D., Sander, D., & Vuilleumier, P. (2008). Individual attachment style modulates human amygdala and striatum activation during social appraisal. *PLoS ONE, 3*(8), e2868.

Wachs, T. (2006). The nature, etiology, and consequences of individual differences in temperament. In L. Balter, & C. S. Tamis-LeMonda (Eds.), *Child psychology: A handbook of contemporary issues* (2nd ed., pp. 27–52). New York: Psychology Press.

Wechsler, D. (2012). *Wechsler Scale of Preschool and Primary Intelligence—Fourth Edition.* San Antonio, TX: Pearson.

Wechsler, D. (2014). *Wechsler Intelligence Scale for Children—Fifth Edition.* San Antonio, TX: Pearson.

Weinberger, D. A., Kohler, M., Garner, E. H., & Steiner, H. (1997). Distress and self-restraint as measures of adjustment across the life span: Confirmatory factor analyses in clinical and nonclinical samples. *Psychological Assessment, 9,* 132–135.

Westby, C. (2000). A scale for assessing children's play. In K. Gitlin-Weiner, A. Sangrund & C. Schaefer (Eds.), *Play diagnosis and assessment* (2nd ed., pp. 15–57). New York: Wiley.

Westen, D., Lohr, N., Silk, K., Kerber, K., & Goodrich, S. (1985). Object relations and social cognition in borderline personality disorder and depression: A TAT analysis. *Psychological Assessment, 2,* 355–364.

Wiig, E. H., Semel, E., & Secord, W. A. (2013). *Clinical Evaluation of Language Fundamentals—Fifth Edition.* San Antonio, TX: Pearson.

World Health Organization. (1992). *The ICD-10 classification of mental and behavioural disorders: Clinical descriptions and diagnostic guidelines.* Geneva: Author.

Yang, J., McCrae, R. R., Costa, P. T., Dai, X., Yao, S., Cai, T., & Gao, B. (1999). Cross-cultural personality assessment in psychiatric populations: The NEOPI-R in the People's Republic of China. *Psychological Assessment, 11,* 359–368.

Zeanah, C. H., & Fox, N. E. (2004). Temperament and attachment disorders. *Journal of Clinical Child and Adolescent Psychology, 33,* 32–41.

Zimmermann, P., Mohr, C., & Spangler, G. (2009). Genetic and attachment influences on adolescents' regulation of autonomy and aggressiveness. *Journal of Child Psychology and Psychiatry, 50*(11), 1339–1347.

CHAPTER 9

Child Symptom Patterns: The Subjective Experience

SC Axis

CHAPTER EDITORS

Norka Malberg, PsyD **Larry Rosenberg, PhD**

CONSULTANTS

Kenneth Barish, PhD
Thomas Barrett, PhD
Alexandra Harrison, MD
Leon Hoffman, MD
Howard Lerner, PhD
Eirini Lympinaki, MsC
Ronald Naso, PhD
Tim Rice, PhD
Ionas Sapountzis, PhD
Lea Setton, PhD
Steven Spitz, PhD
Miriam Steele, PhD

Introduction

Symptom patterns in children, as in adults, are best viewed in a developmental, dynamic context. Clinicians who work with children are reminded daily of the multiple factors that contribute to different symptomatology. Consider, for example, a child with anxiety. Recent events in the family or at school, a biologically based vulnerability to anxiety, a history characterized by frightening experiences, and insufficient opportunities to learn to cope with conflict may all contribute, in varying degrees, to the child's current mood and behavior. Children feel and report anxiety in many ways; each child's sense is unique. One may experience anxiety as "My tummy's gurgling" or as "My muscles hurt," while another may say, "I'm scared of being kidnapped." In addition, children develop rapidly, with consequent changes in their behaviors, feelings, thoughts, fantasies, and symptoms. The meaning of a symptom pattern may be quite different for a child at different developmental stages.

This chapter covers the most common symptom patterns of children (see Table 9.1 for an overview). Many of these are also included in the *Diagnostic and Statistical*

TABLE 9.1. Child Symptom Patterns: The Subjective Experience—SC Axis

SC0	**Healthy responses**		
	SC01	Developmental crises	
	SC02	Situational crises	
SC2	**Mood disorders**		
	SC22	Depressive disorders	
	SC24	Bipolar disorder	
	SC27	Suicidality	
	SC29	Prolonged mourning/grief reaction	
SC3	**Disorders related primarily to anxiety**		
	SC31	Anxiety disorders	
		SC31.1	Phobias
	SC32	Obsessive–compulsive and related disorders	
		SC32.1	Obsessive–compulsive disorder
SC4	**Event- and stressor-related disorders**		
	SC41	Trauma- and stressor-related disorders	
		SC41.1	Adjustment disorders (other than developmental)
SC5	**Somatic symptom and related disorders**		
	SC51	Somatic symptom disorder	
SC8	**Psychophysiological disorders**		
	SC81	Feeding and eating disorders	
		SC81.1	Anorexia nervosa
		SC81.2	Bulimia nervosa
SC9	**Disruptive behavior disorders**		
	SC91	Conduct disorder	
	SC92	Oppositional defiant disorder	
	SC93	Substance-related disorders	
SC11	**Disorders of mental functions**		
	SC111	Tic disorders	
	SC112	Psychotic disorders	
	SC113	Neuropsychological disorders	
		SC113.1	Motor skills disorders
		SC113.2	Visual–spatial processing disorders
		SC113.3	Language and auditory processing disorders
		SC113.4	Memory impairments
		SC113.5	Attention-deficit/hyperactivity disorder
		SC113.6	Executive function difficulties
		SC113.7	Severe cognitive deficits
	SC114	Learning disorders	
		SC114.1	Reading disorders
		SC114.2	Mathematics disorders
		SC114.3	Disorders of written expression
		SC114.4	Nonverbal learning disabilities
		SC114.5	Social-emotional learning disabilities

(continued)

TABLE 9.1. *(continued)*

SC12	**Developmental disorders**	
	SC121	Regulatory disorders
	SC122	Feeding problems of childhood
	SC123	Elimination disorders
		SC123.1 Encopresis
		SC123.2 Enuresis
	SC124	Sleep-wake disorders
	SC125	Attachment disorders
	SC126	Autism spectrum disorders
		SC126.1 Autism
		SC126.2 Asperger syndrome
SCApp	**Appendix: Psychological experiences that may require clinical attention**	
	SCApp3	Gender incongruence

Manual of Mental Disorders, fifth edition (DSM-5; American Psychiatric Association, 2013). Some appear only in the DSM-5 adult sections. Because of the developmental processes influencing children's experience and expression of symptoms, we believe that childhood manifestations deserve separate consideration. At the end of this chapter, we include a table (Table 9.2) of the concordance between PDM-2 on the one hand, and DSM-5 and the *International Classification of Diseases*, 10th revision (ICD-10; World Health Organization, 1992), with respect to symptom patterns. Because of divergent preferences of the different PDM-2 work groups, and because of some differences between children and adults, we have put the disorders in this chapter in a different order from those in Chapters 3 and 6 on the S and SA Axes, respectively.

To capture better the "emerging" nature of some of the symptomatology described, PDM-2 separates the child and adolescent disorders into different axes and different chapters. In this chapter, we explore how symptoms may manifest themselves between ages 4 and 11. This school-age period presents children with multiple challenges that may test for the first time their capacities for adaptation and their overall emotional and behavioral flexibility (e.g., challenges in the school environment, challenges from peers). Early experiences of caregiving (as described in Chapter 10 on infancy and early childhood) have set the stage for many of the symptom patterns described here. Thus, even when assessing a child of 8, a clinician should take into account the considerations described in Chapter 10. In this way, the clinician can integrate into a formulation both a developmental and dynamic view of categorical symptoms such as those described here.

SC0 Healthy Responses

SC01 Developmental Crises

Development is a fluid and disharmonious process. Traditionally, child psychoanalysis conceptualized children's mental health in terms of a harmonious interaction among the ego, superego, and id; among the different subsystems of each; and between these agencies and outside influences. Such harmony can be achieved, however, only if the inner agencies have reached and can maintain comparable levels of development, and if the external influences on them reflect an "average expectable environment" (Hartmann, 1939). The internal agencies are always in latent dispute once adequate internal organization has occurred. One indicator of the level of such structuralization in a child is the type of defenses used to manage anxiety states (see Chapter 7 on the MC Axis for further elaboration). For children, even the most normal developmental shifts may not feel harmonious. Every move forward from a phase that is familiar, safe, and gratifying can feel uncertain and even dangerous to a child's well-being.

Anna Freud's (1965) concept of "developmental lines" highlights the back-and-forth process of development. In a healthy response to a developmental challenge, maturational progress is interrupted, with no obvious external precipitant, by an arrest or regression to a prior phase. Such reactions follow a stable period of adjustment and are time-limited. Developmental crises are normal aspects of maturation and vary in how visible they are to others. In efforts to resolve earlier unresolved crises before moving on, children typically regress to the psychological issues associated with earlier phases.

The Subjective Experience of Developmental Crises in Childhood

Affective States

Affective states may include shame and/or blaming self or others for painful feelings. Anger, sadness, and shame may be expressed in outbursts. A child's mood may be subdued or highly charged, inappropriate or euphoric. Acute distress may be expressed by crying, rage, or destructive behavior. The child may understand what has occurred but be upset nevertheless, or may refuse to acknowledge the meaning of the developmental event and yet come to terms with it over time.

Thoughts and Fantasies

Thoughts and fantasies may include the child's puzzlement at the destabilization of a previously unproblematic sense of self. The child may deny or disavow the existence of a problem, or project and displace feelings onto others.

Somatic States

In terms of somatic states, the child's sleep patterns may be disturbed. He or she may complain of not feeling well. Appetite may either increase or be suppressed.

Relationship Patterns

The quality of the primary relationships supporting the child's developmental journey is of great importance during these times. A caregiver's capacity to identify and reflect on changes in a child's behavior as purposeful and meaningful is critical to developmental restoration. Children's behavioral and affective manifestations are highly variable, depending on their age, their resilience, the nature of the developmental problem, the support from caregivers, and other factors.

In a healthy response to a developmental challenge, the child's capacity for relationships is intact and age-appropriate. However, the child may become clingier and more demanding while struggling with the imbalance created by the crisis. There may be bouts of resentment and anger at caregivers who are felt to be unhelpful. Siblings may become targets of displaced anger and hostility.

Clinical Illustration

Marian, 6 years old, was referred because of aggression toward her older sister and mother. Her parents reported an increase in nightmares and a sudden clinginess toward both her mother and father. There had been no previous incidence of such behaviors. During the diagnostic sessions, Marian played with dolls in a school setting, enacting a little girl who was reprimanded by a teacher. When the clinician wondered about the doll's feelings, Marian replied, "She does not like big-girl school. It makes her sad and very scared." During the classroom observation, it became evident that Marian was anxious about her new first-grade teacher, a stern older woman with a rigid behavioral approach. Her kindergarten teacher had also been mature and authoritative, but in contrast to the newer teacher, she was also warm and reflective. Marian also typically tried to emulate her 10-year-old sister, known in the family as the "smart one." It seemed that the demands of the new teacher, coupled with the internal pressure Marian felt to prove she was as good as her sister, increased her levels of anxiety and put intense pressure on her ego capacities. Her clinginess toward her parents and her aggression toward her sister were the only ways she could communicate her anxiety and fear. After 6 months of once-weekly child psychotherapy, with concurrent parent sessions, Marian began to regain her capacity to verbalize feelings. Her externalizing behavior and her nightmares disappeared, and she was able to rejoin after-school activities.

SC02 Situational Crises

In a situational crisis, a child's development is interrupted by a relatively minor precipitant. The child's reaction follows a stable period of adjustment and is time-limited. Examples of precipitants of normal situational crises include a mother's pregnancy, the arrival of a sibling, the first day of day care, the loss of a transitional object, illness, medical procedure, separation at the beginning of school, a caregiver's withdrawal following the death of a relative, and other stresses that fall short of constituting significant traumas. Affective states, thoughts and fantasies, somatic states, and relationship patterns are all similar to those found in children with developmental crises.

Clinical Illustration

Jeremy, age 4, was referred for chronic constipation. He had twin brothers, born when he was 3 years old. Jeremy came across as shy and well mannered. Although small for his age, he seemed keen to show his physical abilities during diagnostic sessions (e.g., jumping and throwing a ball). Jeremy's symptoms had begun 6 months after his brothers were born. His parents understood the behavior as a response to the birth of the twins. A year later, however, he continued to suffer from chronic constipation and refused to use the toilet, defecating only in a diaper. Further evaluation showed that he struggled with new places and situations, and that he was extremely concerned about his mother's well-being (she had been very ill during the second pregnancy). Parent sessions were critical in this case. His mother and father were able to discuss ways of encouraging Jeremy to verbalize his feelings and to promote management of his body in an age-appropriate way. They were invited to think about the meaning behind Jeremy's behaviors and to assume a less rigid approach to toileting. Jeremy attended once-weekly child psychotherapy sessions, the aim of which was to help him use his capacity for symbolic play to express his frustration and anger over the twins' birth and to explore his fears about his mother's health. After 8 months of treatment, Jeremy began to use the toilet, declaring that his siblings now needed to do so "and not do disgusting poos in their pants." His development had gotten back on track. He remained a somewhat rigid child, but he was now able to use the help of his caregivers in facing new situations and social challenges.

SC2 Mood Disorders

SC22 Depressive Disorders

Clinical depression in children manifests itself as a spectrum disorder, with symptoms ranging from subclinical to syndromal. Children can present with sadness, irritability, temper tantrums, low frustration tolerance, somatic complaints, and social withdrawal, as well as anhedonia. Depressed children have more symptoms of separation anxiety and phobias than adolescents do. Parents and teachers are less able to detect depressed feelings in children than in adolescents, especially in children who also have more externalizing difficulties. Children themselves are often not capable of seeking help or support for their depressive symptoms and feelings; they can convey a sense of lethargy, discouragement, and unhappiness. Epidemiologically, depression is more common in adolescents than in prepubertal children. The prevalence rate of depression in children is estimated as 1–2%, with a male-to-female ratio of 1:1 in childhood and 1:2 in adolescence. The risk of depression increases by a factor of 2 to 4 after puberty, especially in females. The prevalence of depression in young children appears to be increasing, with age of onset becoming younger. It is important for clinicians to be able to recognize the symptoms and often masked presentations of depression, to be aware of the distinction between child and adult forms of the disorders, to make sense of the symptoms in a developmental context, to distinguish and identify comorbid disorders, and to identify the protective and risk factors.

There are major conceptual issues in understanding depression in children. The role of gender and age, the impact of genetic/biological/hormonal differences, and psychological processes are all important. The constellation of symptoms and presenting problems involved in depressive spectrum disorders occur frequently in other disorders of childhood. Lack of concentration, impulsivity, and oppositionality appear in attention-deficit/hyperactivity disorder (ADHD) and oppositional defiant disorder (ODD), for example. Anxiety disorders in children often accompany depression, but can also be difficult to distinguish from depression. In an assessment and clinical context, it is important to determine whether depression is primary or secondary to another disorder. For example, obsessive symptoms and ruminations may be a feature of a depressive disorder, or depression may develop secondary to obsessive–compulsive disorder (OCD).

In most community and clinical settings, 40–90% of children with depressive symptomatology also show other psychopathology, with up to 50% having two or more comorbid diagnoses—most commonly anxiety disorders, followed by disruptive behavior disorders and ADHD. There is also an increased risk for obesity, problematic family and peer relationships, and educational underachievement.

Depression in children is likely to result from a constellation of complex interactions between psychological and biological vulnerabilities and environmental factors. Although studies indicate strong heritability and neuroendocrine factors in adolescent depression, these are not major influences on childhood depressions, which have consistently been found to be related to family factors. Some studies indicate that children with demonstrated deficits in memory and cognitive control (executive) functions may be more predisposed to depression. Interestingly, twin studies have shown that there is a greater role for the "shared environment" in explaining depressive symptoms in prepubertal children than in adolescents, for whom the nonshared environment has a much larger role. Family discord, maternal depression, and difficulties in the mother–child relationship have all been associated with childhood depression. Physical and sexual abuse are among the most powerful family-environmental risk factors for the onset and reoccurrence of depression in children. Specific parenting factors, such as consistent communicative mismatches, cumulative empathic failures, and lack of warmth, also contribute significantly to depression and demoralization in children. Bullying, bereavement, and early parent loss have been identified as additional risk factors.

Depression in children seems more heterogeneous than adult depression. Some children with a strong family history of mood disorders are at higher risk for depression, as well as the development of bipolar disorders and behavioral problems, especially substance misuse in adolescence. If untreated, depression can seriously impede the development of a child's emotional, cognitive, and social skills, and can significantly affect family relationships as well. A comprehensive clinical evaluation that includes both the child and caregivers is the single most useful tool for assessing depressive disorders in children.

The Subjective Experience of Depressive Disorders in Childhood

Affective States

Depressive disorders in children are first and foremost affective disorders—they involve the children's feelings. Children either act on or suffer from dysphoric feelings they cannot control: helplessness, hopelessness, vulnerability, and fragility. Discouragement and demoralization can be expressed through irritability and crankiness. Depressed children can be less interested in activities, hobbies, and friends, and seem "not to care" as they once did. Social withdrawal and absence of pleasure can also be observed, as well as self-blame, guilt, and a sense of worthlessness. Depressed children have been found to be sensitive (especially rejection-sensitive), lacking in energy, and nonresilient or lacking in stamina. They are not as gratifying to siblings, teachers, and peers as other children. They have difficulty with self-regulation and frequent episodes of dysregulation as a result. A depressed child often feels assaulted by environmental demands, unsupported, misunderstood, and victimized.

Thoughts and Fantasies

The thoughts and fantasies of depressed children parallel their affective states, tending to be inhibited and somber. Depressed children are prone to negative cognitions about themselves, the world, and their future. Some harbor fantasies drenched with blood and violence, and their play may reflect preoccupations with injury and death. School performance suffers, and learning is inhibited; a precipitous drop in grades can stem from poor concentration and an inner preoccupation. A child who used to play often with friends may now spend most of the time engaged in solitary activities. Many depressed children complain of boredom.

Somatic States

Depressed children tend to see themselves as ill and unable to do much. Somatic complaints are common; changes in appetite may involve either an increase or a reduction in food intake. Sleep disturbance can take the form of either difficulty sleeping or sleeping excessively. Children suffering from sleep disturbance often end up in bed with parents. Increased psychomotor agitation or retardation can occur. Aside from irritability, decreased energy, tiredness, and fatigue are common.

Relationship Patterns

Depressed children, whether through intense need or avoidance, are relatively unavailable for relationships. They feel both provoked by and failed by significant others. The link between interpersonal conflict and depression is bidirectional, in that depression can make a child irritable, avoidant, and unavailable, thereby increasing interpersonal dissonance; this causes others to distance themselves from the child, who then feels rejected, lonely, and lacking support. These children can be remarkably anhedonic, experiencing as well as providing little pleasure. It is not uncommon for depressed children to come from depressed families in which caregivers lack warmth, awareness, and availability, as if there are "not enough supplies to go around."

Clinical Illustration

A sturdy-looking 8-year-old boy was referred for long-standing difficulty with emotional regulation and out-of-control behavior. Previous testing had found him in the superior range of intellectual functioning. Despite being placed part-time in a classroom for emotionally impaired children, he skipped from second to fourth grade; teachers reported he performed well above grade level. His sensory-perceptual skills were normal, and his executive functioning was solid. He was removed from general education classes because of outbursts of verbal and physical aggression toward peers and staff. He resisted rules, and teachers tried to accommodate him. The mother complained that everyone "walked on eggshells" around him. He had previously been diagnosed with generalized anxiety disorder (GAD) and ODD; there was some thought of an autism spectrum disorder.

His brother, 2 years older, suffered from congenital abnormalities and consequent atypical development. There was anxiety and depression on both sides of the family. Labor and delivery had been unremarkable, but he seemed serious from birth on; his mother worried that he would never smile. His outbursts dated from about age 4, when it appears he was painfully neglected at home, especially in comparison with his needier brother. He held grudges and resented the attention his brother got at his expense. Over time, he was put on behavioral programs both at home and at school.

He related tensely to the therapist and would not make eye contact, but became more enlivened while playing ball with him. He would typically become hypercompetitive, get enraged both at himself and the therapist, and melt down into a whimpering state of hopeless, helpless despair. He showed over-the-top aggressive reactions to frustration and seemed to feel ashamed of his loss of control. In states of quiescence, such as when building an impenetrable bank with Legos, he would be quiet, a bit sullen, and capable of unusual concentration and focus. Interactive games provoked the need to win at all costs. His drawings revealed a more depressive state. He seldom experienced fun or excitement and appeared strikingly anhedonic.

Eventually he was able to bond with his therapist via humor, teasing him about being a Yankees fan. He began to take pleasure in his knowledge of sports trivia and began asking the therapist how he did and whether he was clever. A "middle ground" began to open between his lacerating competitiveness and his encapsulated, somber states. His intense anger masked a fairly severe depression. His need for control tended to alienate others and provoked attempts to mediate his behavior through consequences and rewards, but he evoked little empathy or recognition of his deep unhappiness.

SC24 Bipolar Disorder

Recent years have witnessed a growing number of studies and popular interest in bipolar disorder in children. The absence of a more sophisticated developmental perspective is evident in the grouping of children and adolescents together under the misnomer "pediatric bipolar disorder." Nonetheless, the number of children receiving the diagnosis has increased considerably in recent years. Once considered primarily an adult-onset disorder, diagnosed bipolar illness in children has doubled since 2001 and is seen equally between boys and girls. Bipolar children suffer enormously and are difficult to soothe and comfort. Even in infancy, there can be sensory sensitivities, tantrums, sleep disturbance, and separation difficulties. There is a consistency in the symptomatic presentation and diagnostic comorbidity of the disorder. Periods of increased energy are reported in nearly 90% of cases, and grandiosity is identified in nearly 80%. Fluctuating, inflated self-esteem beyond what is age-appropriate is another warning signal. Because of their capacity to fantasize as part of developmentally appropriate imaginativeness, clinical grandiosity in young children may be hard to see.

Bipolar disorder is increasingly being thought of as a spectrum disorder comprising different levels of mania, intensity, episodicity, and cycling. Developmentally inappropriate episodes of elevated mood and irritability are considered "cardinal" symptoms. Irritability appears to be the complement to elated mood. Because it can resemble other diagnoses in children, specifically the new DSM-5 diagnosis of disruptive mood dysregulation disorder, bipolar disorder can be difficult to assess. Considerations of deviation from typical behavior in the form of episodes, and the presence of elevated and expansive mood are pivotal to the diagnosis.

Aggression is often the main presenting problem and the most disruptive to adjustment. In fact, aggression that is markedly episodic and co-occurs with other symptoms of mania indicates the need for careful assessment, including identification of any family history of mood disorder. Along with a decreased need for sleep, another symptom may be "hypersexuality," especially with mania and in the absence of sexual abuse. Clinicians must distinguish between normal sexual behavior in children and excessive sexual behavior and interest in an at-risk population. For example, normal preschool children show interest in the genitals and breasts of familiar adults and children. But surreptitious touching of adults and forcefully demanding to touch or be touched is a signal for clinical concern. For young school-age children, playing games related to sexuality is common, whereas coercing others to play is a clinical signal. Hypersexuality is characterized not only by its frequency in some bipolar children, but also by features of precocity, boundary intrusion, compulsiveness, and aggression.

There is considerable evidence for a strong genetic component in bipolar disorder. The spectrum of this disorder runs in families, and it is one of the most heritable of all psychiatric disorders. There is a four- to sixfold increased risk of the disorder in first-degree relatives of affected individuals, and the degree of familiarity is higher with early onset. Premorbid difficulties are common with early-onset (e.g., preschool), especially problems with disruptive behavior, irritability, and dysregulation. Clarifying the characteristic features of bipolar disorder in children is a critical clinical concern because of its confusion with other disorders (ADHD, anxiety, depression, and conduct disorder [CD]), its strong association with aggression and suicide, the trend toward earlier onset and earlier suicide, and often a longer and more severe course of the condition. Bipolar disorder can be comorbid with several common and well-established children's disorders: ADHD, OCD, depressive disorders, CD, and anxiety-related disorders, including panic disorders. Bipolar disorder and ADHD share inattentiveness, impulsivity, motoric overactivity, talkativeness, and disorganized thinking.

The bandwidth for diagnostic criteria and the continuity of child bipolar disorder with the adult version are critical issues. Some evidence suggests than an overly broad definition of bipolar disorder in children can lead to overdiagnosis and to premature, overly aggressive use of medication. The validity of diagnosing bipolar disorder in preschool children has not been well established. What are euphemistically labeled "mood-stabilizing" medications are essentially "antimania" pharmaceuticals, which, along with lithium, have adverse side effects and have not been adequately studied longitudinally in young children. Like many bipolar adults, bipolar children can resist being "in relationship to medication"; they do not want to need it. Given these concerns, early and careful diagnosis of child bipolar disorder is essential. The risk factors of family genetics, comorbidity, and predictable life course favor early diagnosis, which in turn can lead to earlier treatment on individual, family, and educational levels.

The Subjective Experience of Bipolar Disorder in Childhood

Affective States

Bipolar disorder is a severe affective disorder featuring fluctuating states of mood and emotion, with extreme feelings that occur without pleasure or a sense of well-being. Bipolar children suffer as they are continually bombarded with affect that they are unable to regulate or make sense of. Because of the heritability of the disorder, families are at risk for being unable to deal with unpredictable and prolonged episodes of rage, irritability, and despair. Bipolar children have recurring problems with parents, siblings, peers, and teachers. Features of the disorder are disruptive: grandiosity, negative self-appraisals, being overly self-referential and insensitive to others, and being overly reactive to sensory stimuli. They are prone to be driven by impulse, hypersexuality, and poor social judgment.

Thoughts and Fantasies

Bipolar youth are more easily characterized through their actions and intense feelings than through the fantasies and thoughts that accompany their mood swings. Thinking as well as social judgment can be disrupted and distorted by episodic bursts of energy. Grandiose fantasies and expansive thoughts can alternate with negative self-regard and feelings of hopelessness and lack of control. For bipolar children, grandiose fantasies are too readily converted into unrealistic, inappropriate actions and coercive attempts to enlist others to comply. Running into traffic or jumping from a tree can be less a matter of impulsivity than of the belief that nothing bad will happen to them.

Somatic States

Many bipolar children appear to be restless, irritable, and uncomfortable in their own bodies. Sleep and appetite can be disrupted. They can be injury-prone and overly reactive to injuries and normative medical conditions of childhood. These children have immense difficulty in regulating both their feelings and their bodies.

Relationship Patterns

There is considerable clinical and research evidence indicating that bipolar children experience immense difficulty in psychosocial functioning. They experience less maternal warmth, more tension in their relations with their parents, and more impaired peer relationships. Greater family, social, and school impairment is also reported. These children display greater novelty seeking, consistent with reports of greater creativity in bipolar adults; however, they also feel less pleasure, have lower resilience and self-direction, and have less capacity to cooperate in relationships than other children. Bipolar children are at serious risk for adverse outcomes as they move into adolescence, including suicide, substance abuse, psychotic postpartum depression in young women, and borderline personality disorder. Minority youth are at risk for inaccurate diagnosis and treatment with older, outdated medications. Worse course and outcome are associated with early age of onset, low socioeconomic status, more mixed and more rapid-cycling episodes, exposure to negative life events, and family psychopathology. Early identification, accurate diagnosis, and ongoing treatment are all protective factors.

Clinical Illustration

An intense, wiry 5-year-old was seen for psychotherapy during his parents' high-conflict divorce and custody dispute. Problems included aggression, cruelty to animals, episodic preoccupations with death and killing, and hypersexuality. There were allegations of sexual abuse and a history of disruptive behavior in preschool, leading to expulsion—an ominous sign in a child his age. He and his 8-year-old brother had normal birth histories and a developmental context featuring parental acrimony punctuated by numerous moves. He was described from birth as hyperactive, in contrast to his brother. He already carried an ADHD diagnosis; the parents fought about whether to medicate him. He frequently tried to coerce his brother into aggressive sexual acts. Much of their play was unsupervised. He made many references to pornography. There were substance abuse and bipolar illness on the father's side, and depression on the mother's.

After considerable clinical work with both parents, the child began treatment. From the outset, he appeared out of control, hyperactive, and in continual need of limit setting and restraint. His immature speech and expressive language complicated the situation. Receptive language was also a concern; he appeared not to understand what was said to him, but rather reacted to internal cues, or to what he quickly guessed was being asked. The therapist was struck by his efforts to control all aspects of every interaction. He would dart out of the office to check on the person waiting for him, demand water and food, and ask to take toys home. When told that the toys needed to stay in the office, he tried to steal them. When the therapist prevented the theft, he expressed dislike, called him "mean," said he hated him and planned to kill him, and threatened to leave. Most early sessions devolved into battles for control.

Sessions featured almost no frustration tolerance. The slightest mistake in drawing or building led to meltdowns and tantrums; he would throw things, curse, and crumble papers. He seemed inconsolable. If solutions did not come quickly, he gave up angrily and hopelessly. Many behaviors were sexualized, including masturbating, as well as sucking the tail of a toy dinosaur and putting it into a heating vent with much frenzy. Themes of killing and torturing animals permeated his play and verbalizations. He seemed terribly uncomfortable in his own body, constantly stimulated himself, and (in his own way) demanded limits, support, and nurture. His mother felt that his behavior in sessions was typical of his behavior at her home, but his father tended to minimize its occurrence at his home and did not find it especially problematic. Both parents said that he was accident-prone and in need of constant supervision. He would often lie in the middle of a rural road when frustrated, threatening to kill himself.

SC27 Suicidality

The death of a child is universally felt to be one of the most poignant and tragic events imaginable. It is even more tragic when a child chooses suicide to escape unbearable pain. Suicide is currently the fourth leading cause of death among youngsters between ages 10 and 14; several hundred children kill themselves each year in the United States. Suicide among young children is likely to be underreported. It is seldom officially noted as a cause of death, and figures on suicide in children under 10 years old are not reported. A key rationale for underreporting is the general belief that children lack a sufficient cognitive understanding of death to contemplate suicide. In fact, one's concept of death is intimately connected to suicidal ideation and suicide attempts. Research indicates, however, that there is a developmental sequence in how children think about and discuss death. Death-related experiences are common in childhood. Understanding death is an important issue for children, who begin at an early age to try to understand it. Four components of the biological-scientific concept of death have been identified: universality, irreversibility, nonfunctionality, and causality.

It is important when assessing suicidality to keep in mind developmental norms. The consensus of research studies is that children under age 5 do not recognize death as final, but think of it as reversible. Likewise, children between 5 and 9 years of age tend to consider death temporary, although by age 7 children are thought to be cognitively capable of seeing death as irreversible and permanent. Age is not the only or even the central factor in how death is conceived of by children. Clinical reports indicate that some children as young as 4 or 5 realize the finality of death. Some younger children can recognize the irreversibility of death, but are relatively unable to verbalize or bear the associated pain for more than brief periods. Children can conceive of death, and young children can better accept the finality of death, if provided with empathically imparted honest information.

Suicidal thoughts are not uncommon in children; more than 12% of children 6–12 years of age, of both genders, report having had suicidal thoughts. A major distinction is made between "suicide attempts" with the intention of dying and "suicide gestures," understood as communication without the intent to kill oneself. Gender differences have been found in rates of suicide attempts, gestures, and deliberate self-harm, except for children between ages 4 and 11. Suicide attempts at other ages occur predominantly in boys, while suicide gestures and deliberate self-harm are seen mostly in girls. Suicide attempts early in life are particularly ominous because they significantly lower the threshold for, and increase the probability of, subsequent attempts though the life cycle.

Research indicates that suicidal behavior runs in families, and that the risk of such behavior is transmitted across generations. Youth with predominantly fearful or preoccupied attachments are more likely to engage in suicidal thoughts than those with more secure or dismissive attachment styles. Serious adversities during childhood, such as physical and sexual abuse, neglect, violence in the family, physical illness, and financial strain, significantly increase the risk and persistence of suicidality from childhood through adulthood. Such adversities have been linked to suicidal ideation, suicide attempts, and suicide gestures in children under 18. Specifically, a history of childhood sexual abuse increases the probability of a suicide attempt in children between the ages of 4 and 12 by a factor of 11. Extrapolations to children from findings in adults on the suicide spectrum suggest that school difficulties and psychiatric diagnoses (especially those with affective, impulsive, and aggressive symptoms, such as depressive episodes, CD, and antisocial personality disorder) increase the risk of later suicide attempts. The presence of mania increases the likelihood ninefold. One particularly consistent finding is that repeated traumatic events increase the risk of suicide attempt.

The Subjective Experience of Suicidality in Childhood

Affective States

Children's expressions of intense feelings of rage, sadness, and shame can alert clinicians to the possibilities of suicidal feelings. Such children have a lower tolerance for affect and a lower threshold for distress than others. They frequently explain their actions in terms of wanting to stop unbearable feelings or escape from painful situations. Risk factors include hopelessness, anhedonia, impulsiveness, and high emotional reactivity. They can struggle with feelings of omnipotence, manifested by a need for power and control of others, as well as the opposite—profound feelings of hopelessness and helplessness. Children can express an attitude of "I don't care" or "It doesn't matter," which barely conceals underlying feelings of rage and dysphoria. These feeling states often vary in relationship to feeling cared about. It is important to inquire into a child's feelings about death, as well as specific thoughts of suicide. Children's tolerance for pain is limited and strongly defended against. Parents of children and adolescents with suicidal ideation may behave with considerable denial about the seriousness of their children's struggle with suicidal feelings and intentions.

Thoughts and Fantasies

Thoughts and fantasies of children struggling with suicide are intimately tied to tolerating and managing painful feelings. Obsessive, hopeless ruminations about painful relationships with family and peers are common. Suicidal children have often been victims of bullying, exclusion, and shaming. They may see themselves as a burden, unwanted and uncared about. Fantasies that follow a loss can center on themes of reunion, restoration, and remorse. The act of killing oneself is inherently aggressive; it often has the quality of retaliation and revenge toward family members, authorities, and peers. Anticipated acts of suicide invariably carry particular meanings, including thoughts about how others will feel at the funeral. In-depth case histories frequently reveal that a suicidal child was curious about death of people and/or animals, and asked questions about what happens after death. Some suicidal children are remarkably accident-prone, often to a point where parents either deny injury or become emotionally blunted to the suicidal intentions in these "accidents."

Somatic States

The presence of a psychiatric diagnosis involving abuse and/or an atypical or incipient mood disorder suggests that somatic states in some suicidal children can be linked to mood and to the physiological responses associated with physical intrusion, fear, rage, and despair. Many children with sensory sensitivity disorders feel that there is "something wrong" with their bodies, as they suffer from allergic reactions, sleep disturbance, and eating difficulties. One senses that "nothing is quite right" for these children, and that suicide can be a desperate way to "end it all."

Relationship Patterns

Perceptions of family and social support, as well as the experience of parental warmth, have been empirically noted as protective factors against suicide attempts. Conversely, a child's sense of rejection can often serve as a risk or precipitating factor. Suicidality always takes place within the context of relationships. Numerous clinical studies of the sequence of events leading to suicide attempts implicate the early developmentally formative relationships, especially the mother–child relationship. Core conflicts revolve around issues of soothing/containment, separation, the pleasure economy, and pathological modes of relating and communicating. The documented risk factors for suicide, including attachment style, transgenerational transmission of suicidality, comorbid diagnoses, the spectrum of abuse, and lack of parental warmth, all bear significantly on relationships. The pervasive cultural denial of suicide makes it difficult for both parents and professionals to discuss it openly and truthfully. Few schools acknowledge suicide as the cause of a student's death, in stark contrast to protocols for addressing children's deaths from other causes. Clinically, it is important to discuss suicide and death with both parents and children in an empathic, developmentally informed, and unvaryingly truthful way. This is especially the case when there is a family history of suicide, which has often become a "family secret."

Clinical Illustration

A 10-year-old girl was brought by her mother after a potentially lethal suicide attempt with aspirin. Despite her daughter's preoccupations with death, paralyzing anxiety, and bouts of depression, the mother had no idea that she had either the wish or capacity to kill herself. Her naiveté was perplexing. Both parents reported that as an infant their daughter had been difficult to soothe, intolerant of changes in her environment, and bothered by sensory sensitivities. She was colicky and prone to "sudden, unpredictable movements," and began having "serious tantrums" at 14 months. The parents attempted to cope by indulging her demands, which began a pernicious pattern leading to home schooling (to give her a break from school stress), excessive dependence on parents, and numerous ill-fated attempts at therapy, never lasting more than two sessions. The parent–child relationship appeared reversed, with the child "calling the shots" and the parents complying. One quickly forgot that she had a 14-year-old brother.

The mother reported a normal prenatal history and birth. Her daughter was nursed until age 3, when she was abruptly weaned because her mother developed a thyroid condition. On formula, she had intense pain and vomiting. This seemed to set a pattern for subsequent adaptations, which were experienced as overwhelming. Until recently, she had wet her bed once or twice a week.

In preschool, interactions with peers were immensely anxiety-arousing for her; birthdays were stressful until her mother took over all planning. She struggled with a tendency toward triangular relationships in which she felt "left out" and intensely reactive to perceived slights. Yet she was not without strengths. She was extremely intelligent, and although she was perfectionistic, she did well academically. She could read other people accurately and was capable of empathy. She characterized herself as shy, as having "performance anxiety," and as feeling extremely lonely with other people.

She had a sad, waif-like appearance and made poor eye contact, saying, "I've threatened to kill myself. No, I tried to kill myself, not just threatened." She said she worried about everything from homework to friends and "social stuff." She reported experiencing "severe anxiety" her whole life, but said that her depression began a few months after the end of fifth grade. Once it "set in," she could not cope and wanted to kill herself. When the school year ended, she had a "bad mood" and lost interest in everything. What once excited her left her "sad and almost crying." She was determined to kill herself.

Assessment revealed a girl who came into the world with an insecurely attached temperament expressed in tantrums. Her intense feelings and needs were more than her parents could manage. They abdicated their role by acceding to her omnipotent demands and were unable to help her negotiate adversities. Her virulent tantrums forced them to take care of her in ways that were adaptive only for the moment. She met criteria for several diagnoses, including GAD, major depressive disorder, incipient dependent personality disorder, and, most of all, suicidality.

Her suicide attempt was neither situational nor impulsive; it was the culmination of a lifetime of severe pain, discomfort, and alienation from her family and her body. It occurred during a transition out of school and constituted a way of permanently ending her own pain while inflicting pain on others for failing her. The attempt emboldened her, contributing to a pathological self-esteem based on power over others, especially her parents. She had serious risk factors for both suicide and substance misuse: at least two comorbid psychiatric diagnoses; a recent serious suicide attempt; and early-onset sensory sensitivity, anxiety, and depression. Protective factors included high intelligence, a well-educated and caring family, and financial means and willingness to afford residential treatment.

SC29 Prolonged Mourning/Grief Reaction

Children's reactions to separation and loss include cycles of intense distress, emotional retreat, anger, and detachment. Such episodes may reappear periodically for an extended period of time. There are immense individual variations in the appearance, duration, and intensity of these reactions, as a function of a child's developmental stage, communication skills, and capacity for self-regulation. "Bereavement" is the state of loss, whereas "mourning" is the process children go through in their ongoing struggle to adapt. In this context, "grief" refers to a child's personal experience, thoughts, and feelings about the loss of a parent or other caregiver through death, divorce, or extended separation. A caregiver's death is the most commonly reported adverse life event, especially in childhood.

Research evidence suggests that there are typical reactions for children within the first 2 years of the death of a major love object: generalized anxiety, depression, separation anxiety, posttraumatic stress, and behavioral problems, associated with social withdrawal, irritability, somatic complaints, and increased risk of physical illness. Developmentally, there is a shift from predominantly anxiety-related symptoms in younger children to depression toward adolescence. Studies consistently report significant adjustment and behavioral problems in a large minority of bereaved children (28% in community and 40% in clinically based samples) during the first and second years following the death of a parent, sibling, or peer. Children are most likely to exhibit the most severe pathological grief reactions within the first 3 months of a death.

Adaptation depends on both intrinsic and extrinsic factors. Given the normative dependency on the caregiver, the loss of a primary attachment figure is inherently traumatic for a child. The pervasively disorganizing and destabilizing impact of the caregiver's physical absence upon the child's capacity to self-regulate and carry out daily functions is compromised even when the circumstances of the death may not contain "objectively traumatizing" elements.

Stressful events in childhood, including death of a loved one, activate attachment-related proximity seeking to reduce anxiety and to reestablish routine and self-regulation. Children's grief reactions are co-constructed and facilitated by caregivers. When a surviving caregiver's facilitation of grief and mourning is disrupted (by parental depression or maladaptive grief), a child is at higher risk for clinically significant distress, alterations of biological stress systems, and derailment from a normative developmental trajectory. Conversely, higher functioning of the surviving caregiver, parental warmth, high quality of parent–child communication, and stability of positive family routines are all important protective factors. "Emotional blunting," when parents fail to express pain over the loss, is problematic, as children need a model for appropriate emotional expression and a context for safe expression of their own feelings. Interestingly, research indicates that bereaved children exposed to an anticipated death undergo higher levels of posttraumatic stress than children exposed to sudden or natural deaths.

The Subjective Experience of Prolonged Grief/Mourning Reaction in Childhood

Affective States

The range of feelings experienced by a bereaved child depends on the child's age, developmental demands, and resilience, and on the role of the surviving caregiver. Because their understanding of the nature and permanence of death is evolving, children express marked variations of feelings in words, play, and actions. Intense sorrow and emotional pain may be difficult to recognize when disguised as irritability, protest, or tantrums. Accepting the reality and permanence of death is difficult for young children, prompting behavior such as lethargy, withdrawal, and lack of interest. Developmental regressions around speech and toileting, acquisitions of new fears, and disruptions of sleep and appetite both disguise and express intense feelings associated with the death of a loved one.

Thoughts and Fantasies

Children can develop preoccupations not only with the person who died but also with the circumstances of death. Children often have fantasies characterized by themes of personal responsibility, prevention, protection, and reparation in which they imagine what they or others might have done to prevent the death, intervene effectively, or repair fatal conditions. Self-blame, maladaptive self-appraisals, and blame toward self or others are important indicators of problematic grief. Likewise, the avoidance of thoughts and feelings about the deceased or about death itself are risk factors for prolonged grief, poor health outcomes, and posttraumatic stress disorder (PTSD). Bereaved children who can think and talk about feelings, particularly with a caregiver, fare better than those who cannot.

Somatic States

Bereaved children are at greater risk for developing somatic symptoms or actual physical illness, and are more accident-prone than those not experiencing loss. Somatic complaints and disruptions in appetite and sleep are clear "red flags" for professional evaluation.

Relationship Patterns

Losses during childhood have a profound impact on both immediate and future relationships. They create major discontinuities in a child's life, not the least of which is difficulty with peer relationships and interactions. The death of a loved one, or loss of an intact family, makes children feel different—often at a time when they want to be the same as everyone else. Strong defenses against loss can be built up, which, through the course of development, can propel individuals either toward or away from intimate relationships. Perhaps the most important long-term impact of parent loss is the perpetual "presence" of the lost parent, transformed developmentally through the life cycle. Despite adequate parenting and adjustment, making meaning of the loss is an ongoing process. Later losses rekindle feelings associated with earlier ones. As Dylan Thomas noted, "After the first death, there is no other." If an early loss is responded to in a sensitive, caring, and loving way, it can provide a valuable life lesson for the child, increasing his or her sense of valuing the present.

Clinical Illustration

A 4½-year-old boy came to therapy a year after his father, a popular high school teacher, died tragically in a fiery car crash. There was a tremendous outpouring of sympathy and support for him, his mother, and sisters, ages 7, 9, and 12. He was described as having been "a bit cranky" and "a fussy eater" before the loss, yet he was involved with other boys. Since the death, he had had trouble going to sleep, often ending up in his mother's bed. Teachers reported increasing social withdrawal, inattentiveness, and overall demeanor of sadness, drowsiness, and being "spaced out." A scrawny, withdrawn, internally preoccupied boy with a perpetual runny nose and whiny tone, he clung to his mother and glanced furtively at the therapist and his office, particularly the windows. He had immense difficulty separating from his mother.

His play in therapy involved elaborate crashes involving cars, boats, planes, and buses, followed by frantic attempts to repair what was broken. He could not understand why his father could not be repaired if vehicles could be. At night, he pleaded with God to return his father. Over time, the theme of crashes was interpreted. Ensuing play was interrupted by his frequent running to the window to observe traffic. Discussions ensued about how he was waiting for his father to return.

After a year, he gradually began to feel perkier and to engage with friends again. Mourning, however, was just beginning. As with any parental loss, clinical work with the surviving parent was essential. His mother was sensitive to her son's separation distress, which she handled with consistent patience. She addressed his feeling different from other kids by joining a family grief program and coming into his class to discuss death with his classmates—an important step that facilitated his reintegration with friends. Both school personnel and his mother reported that he was gradually catching up with his peers developmentally.

SC3 Disorders Related Primarily to Anxiety

SC31 Anxiety Disorders

Fear and anxiety are universal human emotions that evolved as signals of danger and uncertainty about our ability to control important events and to maintain bonds with important others. Emotion theorists often distinguish between "fear" and "anxiety": Fear motivates immediate escape or avoidance, whereas anxiety concerns unavoidable events (for example, an examination). Panksepp and Biven (2012) locate fear and anxiety in different areas of the brain, mediated by different neurotransmitters. The former (the *fear* system) concerns external stimuli seen as dangerous, the latter (the *panic* system) concerns separation from a needed attachment figure. Analysts have called the former "annihilation anxiety" or "paranoid anxiety," and the latter "separation anxiety."

For both children and adults, the experience of anxiety depends, decisively, on an appraisal of coping potential—whether an individual feels able to master the threat or challenge. In its most adaptive function, fear motivates caution and preparedness. Mild to moderate anxiety often stimulates constructive problem solving. Severe anxiety, however, typically disrupts concentration and other cognitive processes, including perspective taking and long-term planning. Like all emotions, anxiety has characteristic cognitive, affective, physiological, and behavioral components. Anxiety is characterized by increased autonomic arousal, a narrowing of attention, increased vigilance, and an inhibition of exploratory behavior. Chronic anxiety is likely to have significant consequences for all aspects of a child's life and is a risk factor for many other emotional and behavioral disorders.

Anxiety has a central role in the history of psychoanalytic theory and remains a fundamental principle of a psychodynamic understanding of both symptoms and character. Some degree of anxiety is present in almost everything we humans do. Anxiety is more than a symptom; it is a dynamic process, a feeling state that sets in motion both adaptive coping responses and maladaptive actions. Throughout life, how well we are able to cope with anxiety determines, to a large extent, our emotional health.

In recent decades, there has been extensive research into children's anxiety. Biological risk factors for developing anxiety disorders in childhood, evident in children's temperament early in life, have been reliably established. There is a strong genetic influence on anxiety disorders; specific genes and gene–environment interactions that may predispose children to anxiety are being investigated. Neuroscience research has mapped brain regions and neural pathways associated with fear and anxiety. Family risk factors have also been studied. Insecure attachment, marital conflict, and high levels of parental criticism and overcontrol are associated with increased risk of childhood anxiety disorders. Less often studied, but of critical importance, are experiences outside the home—especially the impact of learning disorders, peer rejection, and bullying.

The Subjective Experience of Anxiety Disorders in Childhood

Affective States

Anxious children not only worry excessively. In their attempts to avoid situations that make them anxious, they may also make urgent and insistent demands. A child may then be described as clingy, controlling, defiant, or stubborn. When parents (or clinicians) regard a child's behavior as demanding or controlling (rather than as anxious), they often respond with excessive anger, criticism, or punishment. This common misunderstanding then sets in motion a vicious cycle of negative interactions, leading to both continued anxiety and escalating family conflict.

Thoughts and Fantasies

With increasing maturity, children learn to tolerate the normal anxieties of living. This achievement—the ability to "regulate" anxiety—is accomplished gradually and is an essential prerequisite for emotional health. In healthy development, children are able to face anxiety-provoking situations with a minimum of avoidance and inhibition, and as a result to engage in life with interest and enthusiasm. When children are chronically anxious, or when their anxiety is easily evoked, their thoughts, imagination, behavior, and relationships are all drawn into the orbit of their anxious mood. Anxious children expect or imagine that bad things will happen; in their behavior, they avoid or withdraw from common activities, or they may fly toward them counterphobically.

Somatic States

Psychodynamic theory emphasizes the conscious and unconscious strategies children use to reduce felt anxiety, as well as the multitude of ways a child's anxiety may be expressed. Anxiety may be more varied in its expression than any other emotion. Frequent nightmares, eating and sleeping disorders, and regressive behaviors, for example, are common expressions of anxiety in children. In addition to avoidance and inhibition, children make use of defense mechanisms (e.g., denial, repression, displacement, selective inattention, and dissociation) to minimize their experience of anxiety. They often deny that they are anxious, but complain instead of physical symptoms (e.g., stomachaches, headaches, nausea, or frequent urination). A child's anxiety may also be masked by oppositional behavior or an attitude of indifference. At times, children may be unaware of the situation causing their anxiety. Or they may know what they are worried about, but refuse to say what it is.

Relationship Patterns

Anxiety is a daily experience in the lives of children, as they anticipate their interactions with their parents, teachers, and peers. Children may be anxious in any new situation (e.g., the first day of school or summer camp). They are anxious about possible criticism and punishment; about separation from attachment figures; about possible illness, injury, pain, and death; and about experiences that evoke feelings of shame (e.g., social rejection or academic failure).

An anxiety disorder is diagnosed when a child's experience of anxiety causes significant distress over an extended period of time and/or interferes with the child's ability to participate in normal activities of daily life. DSM-5 identifies seven anxiety disorders—separation anxiety disorder, selective mutism, specific phobia, social anxiety disorder, panic disorder, agoraphobia, and GAD—with diagnostic criteria for each. Current research indicates a high co-occurrence of these disorders in individual children. There is also evidence, however, that these symptom patterns occur separately with sufficient frequency to justify their identification as distinct syndromes.

The assessment of any anxious child (or any child who, for extended periods of time, avoids normal, age-appropriate activities) must include an exploration of the situations or demands in the child's current life that may be contributing to anxiety or avoidance. Is this child having difficulties in learning? Is there bullying or exclusion by peers? Is there an atmosphere of family conflict, parental anxiety, excessive criticism, or overcontrol? Have there been traumatic events in this child's life? Because of the many factors that may contribute to children's anxiety, the question "Why is this child unusually anxious?" is often difficult, perhaps impossible, to answer with any degree of certainty in any given case. In clinical practice, it is therefore wise to consider all possible determinants of a child's anxiety as avenues for exploration and therapeutic intervention.

Clinical Illustration

The following case illustrates the escalating, cyclical effects of anxious moods on both a child's and a family's functioning. When children are unable to regulate anxiety, their moods and behavior may set destructive family interactions in motion, putting them at risk for worse symptoms.

An exceptionally bright 9-year-old girl excelled in schoolwork and had many friends, but also had frequent tantrums. When it was time to do homework, she would "freak out" and find excuses to procrastinate, telling her parents, "I need a different pencil," or "I need to sit in a different chair." If she made a mistake, she would become dramatically upset. She had meltdowns in reaction to other minor frustrations and disappointments, as when her parents said it was time to stop using her iPad. She would complain, "No! I have to; I need to . . ." On school days, she kept changing her mind about what to wear and so was usually late. She had a tantrum—about something—every Sunday night. She had difficulty falling sleep and was often tired. On weekends, she was hard to wake up and would miss activities (e.g., skiing) that she greatly enjoyed. Her behavior caused frequent, severe family stress. Her parents had lost their patience—first with her, then with each other. Now she was not only anxious; she was also angry and defiant, and at times depressed and withdrawn. Her parents understood that many of her unmanageable behaviors resulted from her inability to regulate her anxiety. They were at their wits' end, however, and often regarded her as spoiled, demanding, bossy, and controlling.

Treatment combined individual psychotherapy and family counseling, focusing on helping the child develop improved anxiety tolerance and affect regulation. Her parents were helped to respond to her anxiety in more useful ways, and thereby to arrest malignant cycles of family interactions.

SC31.1 *Phobias*

A phobia can develop early in life. Although many children experience excessive fearfulness at some time during childhood, a severe or prolonged phobia may lead to serious complications in a child's overall emotional adjustment. Risk factors for a child's developing a phobia include an anxious temperament, family psychopathology (especially an anxiety disorder in a first-degree relative), and early developmental difficulties. Specific phobias may develop following a traumatic event (e.g., being attacked by an animal or trapped in an elevator).

In the famous case of Little Hans, Freud (1909) presented a theory of the formation of phobias that remains influential. Psychodynamic clinicians regard phobias as symbolizing unconscious anxieties about separation, injury, or death. Anxiety about these basic dangers is displaced onto an object that is less threatening, either because it is inherently less dangerous or because of its decreased proximity. The process by which the phobic object becomes associated with danger is generally not accessible; children are rarely able to explain how they became afraid of a benign object. A phobia resolves when a child is able to master the original anxiety, making the displacement no longer necessary.

The Subjective Experience of Phobias in Childhood

Affective States

A child's phobia is usually limited to a specific situation (e.g., flying, heights, animals, infections, or the sight of blood). In some cases, however, the child's anxiety may spread from one object to many. The course of children's phobias is extremely variable, lasting from days to years. If there is fear or intense anxiety in one or more social situations in which a child feels exposed to others, a sense of rejection or humiliation may affect schoolwork and disable the child in other areas. As long as a child is able to avoid the phobic stimulus, there is minimal anxiety. When the feared object or situation becomes unavoidable, however, the child characteristically feels severe anxiety that can escalate into panic. No amount of reassurance diminishes it. Children may express their intense fear by crying or having tantrums that may persist for long periods. Some phobic children, even in the absence of phobic objects, are hypervigilant with respect to their environment.

Thoughts and Fantasies

A child's thoughts and fantasies may be dominated by the phobic object and strategies to elude it, or the child may avoid thinking about the topic entirely. Overall, the ideational life of phobic children may be characterized by constrictions in certain age-expected emotional themes, such as competition and aggression, and by an intensification of other themes, such as dependency relationships.

Somatic States

Phobic children often develop somatic symptoms associated with the anticipation of exposure to the phobic object: tightening in the chest, stomachaches or a hollow feeling in the stomach, rapid heartbeat, loss of appetite, frequent urges to urinate or defecate, nausea, and vomiting. The intensity of these physical complaints depends upon the level of a child's fear. The feelings dissipate if the phobic object is removed or the situation is avoided.

Relationship Patterns

Phobic children often approach relationships with caution. New situations and people may be assimilated only gradually. The capacity for attachment relationships, however, tends to be unimpaired in phobic children, who are often quite dependent on their caregivers.

Clinical Illustration

A 4-year-old girl was hospitalized with a life-threatening illness. Her parents told her that she had to fight the "little bugs" that were making her ill. During her recovery, she had to stay in the hospital for several months and at home for several more. During this time, she developed a phobia of bugs (all insects: ants, flies, mosquitos, etc.), for which she was treated for 8 months with psychodynamic psychotherapy. Her favorite game was to imagine that she was Princess Rapunzel, trapped in a tower by an evil witch who kept her away from her parents. Through this game, she was able to symbolically express and process her feelings of anger and frustration toward her mother (and her therapist), the "evil witch" who kept her confined. She talked about her fear of being killed by bugs associated with her illness, and her fear of retaliation from her parents because of her anger.

SC32 Obsessive–Compulsive and Related Disorders

SC32.1 *Obsessive–Compulsive Disorder*

The hallmark symptoms of obsessive–compulsive disorder (OCD) are unwanted intrusive thoughts (obsessions), compulsively repeated behaviors (rituals), or both. Recent research has identified at least three OCD symptom clusters: fear of contamination, concern with symmetry, and doubt and checking. It is unclear whether a fourth cluster, hoarding behaviors, should be included in the diagnosis. On the basis of current research, DSM-5 identifies hoarding disorder as distinct from OCD.

Obsessive and compulsive symptoms can occur in children as young as 4, but more commonly first appear between ages 6 and 9. Early adolescence and young adulthood are other common periods for new or recurring OCD. In many individuals, symptoms wax and wane over the course of a lifetime. An OCD spectrum, including tic disorders and hair pulling, has recently been explored. In DSM-5, obsessive–compulsive and related disorders are no longer classified as anxiety disorders, though the presence of anxiety is a core feature of OCD symptoms. Most researchers and clinicians now regard OCD as a neurological disorder, and thus feel that psychodynamic therapy is not the best treatment for children so diagnosed.

The Subjective Experience of OCD in Childhood

Affective States

Obsessional ideas and compulsive rituals may be mild and transient (thus not meeting criteria for an OCD diagnosis), or, in severe cases, may result in profound impairment in a child's functioning in many aspects of life. Many children with OCD are aware that their fears are unrealistic, but still feel compelled to perform compulsive actions. Initially, most are deeply distressed by their unwanted thoughts, and they actively, even urgently, seek help. Over time, however, especially if untreated, children may become more secretive and hide their obsessional thoughts and compulsive rituals. The avoidances and compulsions of OCD may take up a great deal of a child's time and mental energy, even when symptoms are not overt. In severe cases, when OCD symptoms have become extensive, children may express thoughts that seem psychotic (e.g., the idea that they change identities when they walk through different rooms, or that they are living in an alternate universe). Such ideas are essentially elaborations of obsessional thoughts and do not require a new diagnosis.

Thoughts and Fantasies

The classical psychoanalytic understanding of OCD focuses on a child's efforts to expiate guilt feelings over sexual or aggressive wishes (or actions). Freud presented this theory in his early papers on the mechanisms of defense (e.g., Freud, 1894) and, most famously, in his case of the "Rat Man," who suffered from OCD in both childhood and adulthood (Freud, 1909). Even more famous is Shakespeare's Lady Macbeth, who woke at night, unable to wash the guilt of murder off her hands.

Common obsessive thoughts in OCD include the following:

- Fear of being contaminated by germs or dirt, or of contaminating others.
- Fear of causing harm to oneself or others.
- Intrusive, sexually explicit or violent thoughts and images.
- Excessive focus on religious or moral ideas.
- Fear of losing or not having things one might need.
- Order and symmetry: the idea that everything must line up "just right."
- Superstitions; excessive attention to something considered lucky or unlucky.

Somatic States

Sensory overresponsivity (exaggerated behavioral responses to sensory stimuli) is relatively common among children with OCD. These include tactile, visual/auditory, and gustatory/olfactory hypersensitivity. Sensory overresponsivity seems more common in younger children. In some cases, particularly during adolescence, there is evidence of hyperawareness of particular bodily processes, urges, or sensations such as focus on breathing and tongue movement.

Relationship Patterns

When children are not preoccupied by obsessional fears, they often function well; they participate actively in life and are capable of warm, close relationships. When prevented from performing a compulsive behavior, they experience severe anxiety or panic. Children with OCD therefore often attempt to rigidly control situations and relationships because of their underlying panic. Their behavior may be misunderstood as "controlling" (rather than as efforts to prevent severe anxiety). As with other anxious children, this misunderstanding frequently creates family tension and conflict, with no reduction in the children's symptoms.

Clinical Illustration

A 9-year-old girl was referred for severe anxiety, especially at bedtime. Her symptoms included perfectionism, a need to keep rearranging items on her dresser and desk, and a preoccupying fear of vomiting. She was the younger of two girls from a middle-class, professional family. Beginning at age 5, she experienced extreme separation anxiety at bedtime and insisted on elaborate bedtime rituals. Every night, she would ask her parents four times, "What if I throw up?" They were required to respond four times, "You're not going to throw up, we love you, and good night." Her fear was accompanied by "gross images of guts and body parts," and she would feel nauseated as her parents were leaving her room. Her fear of vomiting made her finicky about food; she was consequently quite thin.

She also showed heightened tactile sensitivity (e.g., to tags on her clothes). She was an exceptionally bright, model student, liked by peers. Her parents were eager to help their daughter, whom they described as often controlling, demanding, and difficult to please. Her complicated birth history was an important part of the clinical picture. During delivery, she went into fetal distress, necessitating an emergency C-section. As the family story was told, the mother's "guts were laid out on a table." This gory description of her birth starkly contrasted with her parents' tidy and proper demeanor.

The child's strengths included being psychologically minded and open to exploring where her "big feelings" came from. Early in therapy, she did a lot of artwork and enjoyed being messy, but she needed permission to express "ugly feelings" (anger, hatred, disgust). One picture showed her mother in a forest, being murdered. In discussing her drawing, she expressed fear that her mother might be killed. She then spontaneously mentioned how the mother had almost died giving birth to her. She seemed to worry that her "ugly feelings" could kill her mother. Over time, she connected her preoccupation with guts, body parts, and throwing up to her birth story.

Her anxiety and need for bedtime rituals diminished. She gradually became less anxious and perfectionistic. Work with her parents was crucial. Her mother came to realize that she was quite demanding and perfectionistic herself, and gave her daughter greater latitude to be messy. Her father came to recognize how he idealized her. Helping the child own and channel aggressive feelings went a long way to reduce her anxiety, need for rituals, and perfectionism to more normative, realistic levels.

SC4 Event- and Stressor-Related Disorders

SC41 Trauma- and Stressor-Related Disorders

Childhood trauma is defined by a child's experience in reaction to an event or series of events perceived to pose catastrophic danger to life or self. Particularly in young children, a perceived threat to a primary caregiver can be experienced as posing such a threat. Such experiences produce overwhelming affect that leaves a child feeling helpless, paralyzed, unable to organize thoughts, and unable to cope. Defensive operations fail, and dissociative responses are typical.

The field has become far more "trauma-sensitive" in recent decades. Clinicians are now more likely to be properly alert to childhood trauma as contributing to myriad symptom constellations and diagnoses, including mood disorders, disruptive behavior disorders, depression, intermittent explosive disorder, and issues related to physical health. Additionally, there has been an increased awareness that continuous, cumulative, aversive events (such as exposure to violence, domestic violence, sexual abuse, physical abuse, neglect, maternal depression, chronic affective misattunement, and the like) can have a significant effect on both neuropsychological and ego development. These are events that, taken individually, may or may not lead to symptoms consistent with the diagnosis of posttraumatic stress disorder (PTSD), and may or may not lead to a child's becoming overwhelmed or developmentally disrupted by the affective intensity associated with these events. Sustained exposure to overwhelming events has been referred to in the literature by various names, including "strain trauma," "cumulative trauma," "relational trauma," "complex trauma," and "developmental trauma." Importantly, these early and persistent aversive experiences are risk factors in the development of defensively determined personality traits, including severe personality disorders, emergent in adolescents and fixed in adults. These traits are consistent with those listed within the Cluster B grouping of personality disorders listed in DSM-5. Indeed, traumatogenic events can serve as organizers of personality and identity. Thorough history taking is essential to understanding the experiences that may contribute to symptom constellations of this sort; it is equally essential for treatment planning.

"Episodic trauma" refers to a single occurrence, leading to symptoms consistent with the diagnosis of PTSD. The full array of PTSD symptoms may or may not be instantaneously felt by the child or observed by others. Nonetheless, traumatogenic events of this sort are experienced as overwhelming, leaving a child unable to manage the intensity of affect they generate, and often interfering with the child's capacity to continue to develop, make use of symbolic capacities, or mentalize.

Coinciding with the field's heightened sensitivity to trauma, there remains the long-standing caution that the term "trauma" should not lose its meaning and clinical utility because of overuse, or that we should not inadvertently diminish the intensity and singularity of suffering of victims of actual psychic trauma. It has been argued that too often, events are categorized as "traumatic" without consideration of their actual effects on a child. In other words, children exposed to seemingly identical stressors (e.g., death of a parent, earthquake, domestic violence, physical or sexual abuse, painful medical treatments) may not all be traumatized by the event in question. Aversive events present a risk for trauma but do not guarantee its occurrence. Children may be greatly stressed, grief-stricken, or temporarily disrupted, but not necessarily traumatized. Previously existing risk factors (e.g., prior traumatization, attachment style) and protective factors (e.g., family support, community resources, inherent resiliency traits), in addition to a child's cognitive and emotional capacities, are mediating variables in determining the ultimate impact of a potentially traumatizing event for any given child.

Of particular importance to a child's ability to avoid developing PTSD, or to reduce its duration, is the support of primary caregivers. The benefit derived from having a parent who is able to tolerate hearing what has occurred and its impact on the child, and being empathic and comforting in response, cannot be overstated. When a parent is the victim of trauma, or suffers from other mental health issues, the capacity to provide such support may be compromised. Helping the child to avert or attenuate traumatic symptoms will involve helping both child and parent recognize the impact of a traumatogenic event, and facilitate communication between the child and parent about that event and its consequences. This therapeutic role may involve empathically addressing impediments to the parent's ability to respond helpfully to the child's needs.

Single-episode psychological trauma in children can create disturbances similar to those found in adults. There is some evidence that girls are more vulnerable to posttraumatic stress syndromes, but that boys are more disabled by their symptoms. Regressive responses to trauma are particularly visible in childhood, especially in younger children. For example, a previously confident child may cling to a caregiver, or a child who was able to sleep alone may stop being able to do so. Older children may withdraw from social contact, appear hyperactive, or show other behavioral difficulties. Traumatized children may also show hyperalertness and an increased startle response. Increased volatility, poor concentration, poorer attention and distractibility, and more labile affect are all possible consequences of a child having been traumatized. So too are disturbances in eating and sleeping (including disturbing dreams), as well as interference with learning and memory functioning. Other common responses include the defensive/adaptive use of superheroes in attempts to avoid stimuli associated with the traumatic events or to gain a sense of mastery over them. Similarly, children may develop ritualistic behaviors, or label events as omens and predictors of future adversity.

A list of instruments for assessing childhood trauma can be found at the website of the National Child Traumatic Stress Network (*www.nctsn.org/resources/topics/trauma-informed-screening-assessment/resources*).

The Subjective Experience of Trauma- and Stressor-Related Disorders

Affective States

Affective response patterns will emanate in part from the sense of loss of control, power, and identity that result from a traumatic experience. Responses may range from anxiety and panic to obsessive preoccupation and fear, which may appear most vividly in nightmares. Avoidant or phobic behaviors may appear, often accompanied by somatic concerns and complaints. Some children become irritable and/or angry as a way of turning passive into active responding, and in an unconscious effort to ward off feelings of helplessness and despair. Others may be overtaken by exhaustion, sadness, and/or shame. Traumatized children may have a level of emotional lability out of keeping with their premorbid condition.

Thoughts and Fantasies

Thoughts and fantasies may involve the preoccupation described above, compulsive ruminations, fragmented thinking, "all-or-nothing" thinking, and escapist fantasies (including a degree of magical thinking beyond what is age-appropriate). If the nature of the traumatic event is interpersonal, children may come to think of themselves as bad, dirty, or unlovable. A newfound belief in omens may serve the defensive function of allowing a child the sense of knowing when danger is to be anticipated, rather than contending with the unpredictability of life. In some children, we see denial as a dominant defense in response to the experienced threat. In the play of children who have been traumatized, the drama may be compulsively reenacted, often in a distorted form that seeks to prevent the return of traumatic memories and help the children gain mastery over the event. Nondirected, symbolic play of this sort might be thought of as a child's self-directed, naturalistic version of exposure therapy. At the same time, traumatized children may develop difficulty maintaining the boundary between fantasy and reality—something that can be observed in their play and in other manifestations of their extreme anxiety.

Somatic States

Somatic states follow affective patterns, most notably those associated with anxiety, such as rapid heart rate, tense muscles, gastrointestinal symptoms, headaches, and muscle aches. If the traumatic experience involved physical pain, this may be reexperienced in dissociative ways. Trauma resulting from sexual abuse, molestation, or exposure to sexualized material is particularly likely to trigger both somatic symptoms and hypersexualized behaviors.

Relationship Patterns

Relationships may become needy and dependent, characterized by seeking relief from the traumatic anxiety. But children may likewise become withdrawn and avoidant even with close friends, as well as fearful of contact with strangers, who become seen as potentially harmful. Indeed, any stimulus (sounds, smells, etc.) that reminds a child of a traumatizing event can trigger an anxious, aggressive, or avoidant reaction. In children whose somatic complaints become the vehicles for achieving closeness and support, relationships may come to have a manipulative cast.

Clinical Illustration

A 6-year-old boy was brought to treatment for behavior beyond his parents' control. He was of average height and thin, with angular features and large, wide-open eyes. Disheveled-looking, he exuded a sense of dyscontrol and fragility. His mother seemed either overly or appropriately involved with him, depending on one's perspective. She was herself unmodulated and hyperreactive, and could be intensely angry or overwhelmingly sad. His father seemed the polar opposite: withdrawn, passive, blunted in his affect. A sister 2 years older was similarly disheveled-looking, but did not engage in similar emotional storms, defiance, and clingy dependency. At school, he had angry outbursts when asked to do anything he objected to. He was overly sensitive to perceived aggression, had no real buddies, and acted as if friendships were unimportant to him.

He had been diagnosed at age 4 with a rare abdominal cancer. For over a year, he underwent surgery, painful invasive procedures, chemotherapy, and periods of physical isolation that saved his life but caused him intense suffering, drained his vitality, and deprived him of any normative childhood experiences. Through it all, his mother was in his hospital room or bedroom, or had him in her bed. She fought with doctors about procedures they administered, and fought with her son to allow procedures to be completed. While his symptoms met diagnostic criteria for a number of disruptive behavior disorders and for childhood bipolar disorder, one could not rule out trauma from his medical experiences. Having parents and teachers view him through this lens was essential to his improvement.

SC41.1 *Adjustment Disorders (Other Than Developmental)*

As described in the introductions to this chapter and to Chapter 7 on the MC Axis, children's path of progressive development can be impinged upon by sudden stressors that pose additional strain on their sense of safety and well-being. Exposures to such stressors may result in states of developmental disharmony characterized by sudden regressions in functioning or in temporary inhibitions of aspects of the children's ordinary functioning (e.g., peer relationships).

The Subjective Experience of Adjustment Disorders in Childhood

Adjustment disorders in children can be characterized by a wide range of affective states. They may feel anxious or depressed, angry or impulsive, or bereft and defeated. A child's thoughts and fantasies will reflect whatever emotional pattern is triggered by the loss, illness, family problem, or school problem to which the child is reacting. The child's relationships may become more dependent and clingy or more distant and aloof. Children with adjustment disorders may also experience a variety of somatic discomforts, sleeping problems, and eating difficulties. In short, the subjective states accompanying adjustment disorders are similar to those accompanying other childhood disorders. There is a critical difference, however: In adjustment disorders, the reaction is temporary and related to a specific situation or event. Helping a child understand the subjective reaction in relationship to the current challenge, along with providing extra support and opportunities for mastery, can favorably influence the child's subjective state. Helping the parent or caregiver understand the context of the child's experience will benefit the parent and subsequently the child. No single pattern characterizes adjustment disorders, as children's affective states, thoughts and fantasies, somatic states, and relational patterns vary widely.

Clinical Illustration

An 8-year-old boy was brought for evaluation by his parents, who were concerned about his severe nightmares, which had started 9 months previously. They described his needing a parent to be with him while he fell asleep and his waking in the middle of the night to crawl into their bed, too frightened to sleep alone. These symptoms had begun when a fire alarm salesman had come to their apartment to demonstrate his product and showed a graphic video of a devastating fire. The boy was transfixed. About a week later, he developed the sleep disorder. Upon further exploration with the boy, the therapist became aware of an unresolved separation problem that had been reactivated by the incident.

SC5 Somatic Symptom and Related Disorders

SC51 Somatic Symptom Disorder

DSM-IV included the category of somatoform disorders. DSM-5 has eliminated this category and substituted somatic symptom and related disorders. All the disorders in this category share a common characteristic: the importance of the somatic symptoms, associated with a malaise that causes major problems in everyday life. In children, the most common somatic symptoms are abdominal pain, headaches, fatigue, and nausea; one symptom usually predominates. How parents respond to a child's symptoms helps determine the level of anguish associated with them. Parents influence the child's interpretation of the symptoms, their duration, how often the child misses school, and how quickly medical and psychological help is sought. We concentrate here on somatic symptom disorder.

The Subjective Experience of Somatic Symptom Disorder

Affective States

The affective states of children with somatic symptom disorder are often characterized by anxiety, neediness, and feelings of loneliness. A child appears distressed and in pain, especially if caregivers seem to question the reality of the illness. Feeling disbelieved, the child is likely to protest loudly, to feel injured, and to become enraged. The child's thoughts often focus on a particular somatic symptom; the child may feel seriously ill and in danger of dying.

Thoughts and Fantasies

It is critical not to ignore the possibility of undiagnosed medical illness. Taking the child's pain and anxiety seriously may prevent an escalation of complaints designed to prove how real the child's suffering is. The child may become excessively fearful of separating from caregivers, or may become withdrawn and isolated. There is often avoidance of new relationships, especially those requiring exploration and curiosity.

Somatic States

Children with somatic symptom disorder complain about a variety of physical symptoms for which no medical cause can be found. They may suffer from stomachaches, headaches, nausea, urgency to urinate or defecate, and other physical complaints. Although the symptoms usually appear in situations that evoke anxiety, children often do not recognize or accept that their physical symptoms are associated with stressful life events.

Relationship Patterns

Somatization tends to occur in families that have difficulty integrating physical sensations, feelings, and thoughts. The symptoms, which are not produced intentionally, may begin spontaneously or after a minor illness. Most often, a child is convinced that the ailment is purely physical. A pattern ensues in which the child increasingly uses physical symptoms in the service of avoidance. In severe cases, this pattern may become generalized to the point where the child is so debilitated by physical complaints that most everyday activities are disrupted.

Clinical Illustration

A 9-year-old girl complained of abdominal pain and recurrent vomiting, although she would vomit mostly saliva. This seemed to occur mostly when her parents would argue. Because of her vomiting, they worried about her and kept her out of school. Medical evaluation revealed no physiological reasons for the vomiting. It was later revealed that prior to the onset of the vomiting, the parents had been threatening to divorce. Since the vomiting, however, they had come together to care for her.

SC8 Psychophysiological Disorders

SC81 Feeding and Eating Disorders

Anorexia nervosa and bulimia nervosa are psychophysiological disorders involving both psychological and biological functioning. They occur in less than 1% of the prepubertal population, though the rate of occurrence is rising. These patients suffer pathological thoughts and feelings about food, eating, and body appearance. Cultural factors such as the idealization of being thin influence such preoccupations, which are prominent features of both anorexia and bulimia nervosa. Multidimensional interactions of psychological, biological, familial, and cultural factors are implicated in the etiology, identification, and treatment of eating disorders. Although more common in adolescent girls and adult women, they do occur in males and young children. Eating disorders in children have characteristics similar to those in adolescents and adults, but include a number of distinguishing features.

1. The uniformity of anorexic and bulimic symptoms in adulthood is not present in childhood. Eating disorder symptoms differ for children of different ages and genders. A child's stage of cognitive development must be considered in diagnosing an eating disorder. Young children without the capacity for abstract thinking may not formulate their distress in terms of excessive fear of weight gain.
2. In regard to gender, boys tend to be pickier or more selective eaters early on, but girls tend to develop symptoms of anorexia nervosa or bulimia nervosa in adolescence. This factor and others suggest that eating disorders arise from dysfunction in multiple developmental domains. Gender difference has been noted in the characteristics of mothers of children with eating disorders. One study (Jacobi, Agras, & Hammer, 2001) found that 8-year old girls were more

likely than similarly diagnosed 8-year-old boys to have mothers with disturbed eating behaviors and attitudes.

3. Familial factors play a critical role. Problematic relational patterns between mothers and daughters, especially mutual overcontrol and mothers' critical comments about weight and shape, are commonly observed. Fathers also play an important role in the development of their daughters' subjective experience of their weight and shape.
4. Being teased by peers is often mentioned as precipitating an eating disorder in a prepubertal child.
5. Sexual abuse is a risk factor for bulimia nervosa, with significant comorbidity.
6. Early eating problems such as "infantile anorexia"—a serious feeding disorder in infants that has been related to child temperament, sensory sensitivity, and maternal factors—may predispose older children to develop eating disorders. So far, however, this has not been demonstrated, and it is more likely that eating disorders follow multiple pathways in their development.
7. Treatment of eating disorders in children requires an active family therapy component. It is important to include a pediatrician and a nutritionist, as well as an individual psychotherapist.

From a therapeutic perspective, children with anorexia and bulimia nervosa may be experienced differently. An anorexic child tends to deny all dependency needs, while a bulimic child tends to show extreme ambivalence about such needs. These differences can play themselves out within the therapeutic alliance and the nature of the transference and countertransference experience of the clinician.

Clinical Illustration

A 7½-year-old girl was brought by parents because of her being bullied at school. They described her as intellectually gifted and highly sensitive, with trouble making friends because the other girls did not share her interest in books and science. She was fearful of certain movies and books, and ran from the room when those books were read in class. Her classmates would sometimes tease her and call her a "baby." Her history was remarkable for feeding difficulties and gastric reflux, plus severe colic in the newborn period and fearfulness and separation anxiety as a toddler. When she was 2, her mother had a complicated pregnancy with her younger brother and almost died. After the birth, her mother had many painful physical sequelae that affected her energy, gait, and posture.

Therapy seemed to go well at first. The girl began to make friends with whom she played fantasy games, mostly of her invention. When she was 9, however, her friends began to move on in their interests, and she was not yet ready to do so. She began having meltdowns at home, threatening to run away. Her parents felt helpless and unable to set effective limits on her noncompliant and aggressive behavior. In the context of a family wedding in which she played a starring role, she became preoccupied with her weight. She felt her dress was too tight; she began to restrict food intake and exercise excessively. The result was an alarming drop in her weight. Although she seemed pleased with her new body, stretching and displaying her concave belly to the therapist, she continued to insist that she was fat. Her pediatrician instituted a weight plan, but she became enraged when her parents addressed her eating behavior, saying that it was her own body and she would decide what and how much she was going to eat.

SC81.1 Anorexia Nervosa

In addition to the adult and adolescent symptom patterns for anorexia nervosa described in the corresponding sections of Chapters 3 and 6, respectively, please see the discussion above.

SC81.2 Bulimia Nervosa

In addition to the adult and adolescent symptom patterns for bulimia nervosa described in the corresponding sections of Chapters 3 and 6, respectively, please see the discussion above.

SC9 Disruptive Behavior Disorders

SC91 Conduct Disorder

Children with behavior disorders have been a long-standing concern of psychiatry and psychoanalysis. Psychoanalytic theory attempts to describe the mental mechanisms through which antisocial behaviors develop and supports the notion that these in fact constitute psychiatric disturbances rather than entirely volitional misdeeds. From a psychoanalytic perspective, the understanding of the development of antisocial behaviors must be grounded on those parts of the theory that deal with the development of the superego and of conscience (for elaboration on this matter, refer to Chapter 7 on the MC Axis). A child whose behaviors suggest emerging antisocial tendencies is one in whom these mental structures have not developed normally. In such a child, the equilibrium that needs to exist between different hypothesized mental agencies is temporarily, or sometimes permanently, unbalanced.

"Conduct disorder" (CD) is the umbrella term for a complicated group of provocative behavioral and emotional problems in youngsters. The hallmarks of CD are indifference toward others, impulsivity, and affective instability. Children and adolescents with conduct disorder have great difficulty following rules and behaving in a socially acceptable way.

Among the behaviors manifested by a child with CD are these:

- Aggression toward people and animals (the child bullies, threatens, or intimidates; initiates physical fights; has used a weapon that could cause serious harm; is cruel to people or animals; steals from victims while assaulting them; or forces someone into sexual activity).
- Destruction of property (the child defaces buildings, damages automobiles, or sets fires intended to destroy others' property).
- Deceitfulness, lying, or stealing (the child breaks into someone's building, house, or car; lies to obtain goods or favors or to avoid obligations; or steals items without confronting a victim).
- Serious violations of rules (the child stays out at night despite parental objections or is consistently disruptive at school).

The Subjective Experience of CD in Childhood

Affective States

These children are remarkably unaware of their own affective states and are also remarkably unresponsive to the feelings of others. Neuropsychiatric studies demonstrate that, in contrast to the dysfunctional connectivity within the implicit emotion regulation subsystem hypothesized to be primary in ODD, children and adolescents with CD may have disrupted structural connectivity between these structures. Structural deficits (what psychoanalysts call a weak superego) have been hypothesized to be the product of initial functional deficits and may be influenced by several chemical and hormonal factors, including testosterone and oxytocin.

Thoughts and Fantasies

Recent findings underlie the difficulty these children demonstrate in theory-of-mind tasks and in understanding their own emotions. Because of this quality of being emotionally out of touch, some clinicians describe children with CD as enjoying hurting others, as lacking remorse, and as being greedy and opportunistic. Some children fit this description, but many do not. Socialized and asocialized children with CD were described in early editions of DSM; the former seem to be children who remain in greater touch with their emotions and who are capable of attachment. In DSM-5, these children may be classified as having "callous–unemotional" traits. They have been carefully studied by some psychodynamic clinicians, particularly Paulina Kernberg and Saralea Chazan.

Somatic States (as States of Dysregulation)

In children with this diagnosis, affect in general is labile and not well regulated; they are usually not able to tolerate even small amounts of frustration or delay of gratification. They rarely express underlying affect through somatization, however, especially if they are males. Children with CD tend to act out their emotions rather than internalize them. They may rage when they do not get their way and express satisfaction when they succeed. At times they express feelings of fear, and they may also admit to feelings of pain and resentment at being neglected or mistreated by others. For some, the sense of being uncared for and mistreated speaks to an underlying depression. They commonly express a defeated attitude of having given up on people.

Relationship Patterns

Some patterns of early parent–child interaction have been empirically implicated in CD. These include parental uninvolvement and neglect; lack of warmth and emotional support; overly harsh treatment; inability to establish reasonable expectations and enforce limits; reinforcement of inappropriate behavior; and inconsistent, erratic, or inappropriate discipline. Research shows that children with CD are likely to have ongoing problems if they and their families do not receive early and comprehensive treatment. Many youngsters with CD are unable to adapt to the demands of adulthood and continue to be antisocial, to have problems with relationships, to lose jobs, and to break laws.

Clinical Illustration

A 10-year-old boy would climb under or on top of his classroom desk, ostentatiously drooling, especially after being asked to quiet down by his teacher. At bedtime he would whisper in his 8-year-old brother's ear, "I'll kill you while you're asleep." Frequently he would pack the family's water spigots with fecal matter. After the failure of outpatient daily psychotherapy, medication, family therapy, and various individualized education programs, he was institutionalized.

SC92 Oppositional Defiant Disorder

Children ages 4–11 are often referred to child and adolescent psychiatric services because parent or teachers are disturbed and worried by their oppositional, aggressive, and disruptive behavior. In some cases, such problems can be resolved or outgrown; in others, they are serious enough to meet the diagnostic criteria for oppositional defiant disorder (ODD). These children are a quite heterogeneous group. Many children so diagnosed have other disorders, such as psychiatric or neuropsychiatric problems, learning difficulties, family problems, school problems, and social problems. Recent efficacy studies of psychodynamic child psychotherapy (e.g., Winkelmann et al., 2005) have found that short-term psychodynamic therapy is an effective intervention for children and adolescents with behavioral disorders. ODD is among the most common childhood disorders. As the presence of ODD increases the risk of multiple diverse disorders of childhood, adolescence, and adulthood, we consider it the primary and progenitor childhood disorder.

Symptoms of ODD within the "irritable" subcluster include that a child (1) often loses his or her temper, (2) is often touchy or easily annoyed, and (3) is often resentful or angry. Symptoms within its "headstrong" subcluster include that the child (1) often argues with adults or other authority figures, (2) often actively defies or will not comply with requests from authority figures or with rules, (3) often intentionally annoys other persons, and (4) often blames others for his or her behavior or mistakes. The main symptom within the "vindictive" subcluster is that the child has been vindictive or spiteful at least twice in the past 6 months.

The Subjective Experience of ODD in Childhood

Affective States

Whereas ODD has been traditionally defined as a behavior disorder of childhood, recent empirical studies have found a strong association between ODD and disorders of mood. In fact, ODD has lately been termed a disorder of emotional dysregulation (Cavanagh, Quinn, Duncan, Graham, & Balbuena, 2014). Children whose symptoms are predominantly within the irritable subcluster tend to develop mood disorders, whereas children with symptoms predominantly within the headstrong and vindictive subclusters tend to develop CD. These findings suggest that many children diagnosed with ODD may be responsive to an affect-oriented treatment targeted to the neurobiological deficits of the disorder. The emotion regulation subsystem of the functional central nervous system may be considered a top-down control mechanism to promote adaptive and survival behaviors. Inhibitory input to the limbic system from the prefrontal cortex subsequently reduces excitatory output to the brainstem structures and autonomic nervous system controlling the fight-or-flight state. Children with ODD may be considered to have deficits in the emotion regulation subsystem, creating a propensity toward explosive outbursts and disruptive, ultimately self-defeating behaviors.

Thoughts and Fantasies

Most children with this diagnosis are unaware that they have a problem. From their perspective, the problem lies in the demands for conformity that others make on them. Their impulsivity leads to behaviors that adults find unacceptable, yet they seem oblivious to the consequences of those behaviors. Although expressions of remorse or contrition may follow some defiant actions, children with ODD more often feel justified and see themselves as victims of injustice. Recurrent disapproval from others may erode the sense of self-cohesion in oppositional children, making them more vulnerable to narcissistic injury and fragmentation. Their inability to demonstrate their competence leads such youngsters to feel especially vulnerable to criticism and to failure.

Somatic States

The heterogeneous nature of the diagnosis makes prediction of specific somatic concerns unreasonable. But the high level of comorbidity associated with the disorder, including anxiety and underlying depression, suggests that somatic concerns may be present. Stomachaches, headaches, sensory sensitivity, and sleep difficulties are, therefore, not uncommonly found among children with oppositional defiant disorder.

Relationship Patterns

Social and family relationships are usually impaired because of these children's disruptiveness, bossiness, and oppositional behaviors. In a vicious cycle, the disapproval to which they are regularly subjected may lead oppositional children to be more rebellious and defiant. These responses and their related tendency to associate with peers on the fringe may crystallize into delinquent patterns. In other cases, oppositional symptoms can appear in reaction to a child's feeling overly controlled, or in situations where parents are unable to provide adequate or consistent limits. ODD symptoms may also appear as a reflection of family aggression and stress, particularly when related to conflict between parents.

Clinical Illustrations

An 8-year-old boy was insulted by his sister, whom he impulsively slapped. When his mother confronted him, he began to argue, blame his sister for his misbehavior, and refuse to take a time-out, throwing himself on the floor in a tantrum. His parents responded by denying him dessert at dinner. This illustration demonstrates the quick-to-anger temper of children with ODD. We may hypothesize that the failure of the child's underdeveloped prefrontal cortex to inhibit subcortical structures associated with rage led to the production of more automatic behaviors influenced by subcortical striatothalamic and sympathetic arousal in the form of a slap. The child's ongoing failure to tolerate and regulate his negative state led to headstrong and dysregulated behaviors, which ultimately were not adaptive (he liked dessert). A clinician should consider addressing the child's immature implicit emotion regulation system via his defense mechanisms. The child's headstrong behaviors may be formulated as maladaptive defenses against full recognition of the negative and painful affects induced by his mother's confrontation. To reduce the operation of maladaptive defenses, the clinician should attend to them, point out their negative consequences, and ultimately help the child bear the raw feelings and their associated implications that he tries so hard to avoid.

In another case, an active, athletic 7-year-old boy was disruptive in school, needing disciplinary actions. One parent was anxious, overindulgent, and inconsistent, and the other was rigid, punitive, and emotionally unavailable. Play in psychotherapy sessions consisted of a variety of ball games, often kickball. Like most children, he wanted to win. Unlike other children, however, he reacted to the clinician's occasional point or win with dramatic hysterics and accusations that the clinician was cheating (in other words, he denied his own wishes and actions and projected them onto the other person: "I am not cheating; *you* are cheating"). His parents behaved similarly. He was being threatened with suspension from school, leading the parents to be dissatisfied with the treatment.

In sessions, his cheating during games was rampant. Often the clinician felt provoked by it. When the clinician discussed one session with colleagues, he became aware that his response was a result of countertransference feelings of which he was unaware during the session. He had said to the boy, "You know, I really don't understand why it's so difficult for you to ever lose a point, even though you win every game." These words expressed his own frustration, disguised aggression, and wish that the boy would "shape up." The child ran out of the playroom to his mother and screamed inconsolably that the clinician was cheating. "He wants to cheat all the time and stops me from winning." He refused afterward to come into the office alone. Eventually, the treatment was interrupted.

This vignette highlights a common circumstance when a clinician may not be aware of an affective response and communication to the patient, and hence cannot appropriately address the child's emotional state. In this instance, the clinician was engaged in a communication in the cognitive sphere, without being aware of the emotional state that was affecting the child's cognitions. A psychodynamic, affect-oriented approach shares many features with the predominant cognitive-behavioral approaches to disorders of childhood. Behaviors that place a child at risk of harm to self or others are the immediate focus. But, unlike a cognitive-behavioral therapist, a psychodynamic clinician encourages a child to employ "bad" behavior as a means of understanding and ultimately defusing the strength of this maladaptive emotion regulation process.

A child with ODD symptoms should have a comprehensive evaluation, as other disorders (e.g., difficulties with attention and hyperactivity, learning disabilities, mood disorders, and anxiety disorders) may be present. Social and family relationships are usually impaired as a result of the child's behaviors. The disapproval to which they are regularly subjected may lead oppositional children to be more rebellious and defiant. These responses, and their related tendency to associate with peers on the fringe, may crystallize into delinquent patterns. CD may result. Yet a child with ODD presents a valuable opportunity for a clinician to intervene prior to the establishment of more entrenched psychopathology.

SC93 Substance-Related Disorders

Substance-related disorders are described in greater detail in the corresponding sections of Chapters 3 and 6. Substance misuse patterns are not infrequently found in children and, to a much greater extent, in adolescents. When children under age 10 use substances, the use is typically limited to tobacco, alcohol, and/or marijuana. Children with substance-misusing parents and with self-regulatory difficulties are most vulnerable to early substance use.

The Subjective Experience of Substance-Related Disorders in Childhood

Affective States

A variety of affective states may be involved, including excitement associated with experimentation; anxiety about developmental and social challenges; and attempts to counteract feelings of numbness, emptiness, embarrassment, humiliation, and rage.

Thoughts and Fantasies

Thoughts and fantasies leading up to the substance misuse often relate to the motives inherent in the affective states just mentioned. Once the substance is used, resultant cognitive patterns reflect the effect of the substance on the nervous system. These range from agitated, fragmented, and paranoid thinking, to fantasies of specialness and brilliance, to wish-fulfilling convictions of desirability, potency, and invulnerability.

Somatic States

Somatic states accompany both the affects described above and the substances used. They range from arousal and agitation to numbness and tranquility. Use of alcohol and other drugs also has consequences, both immediate and long-term, for many organ systems and physiological processes.

Relationship Patterns

Relationships range from active involvement in a social group where the substance abuse pattern is ritualized, to isolated, self-absorbed states of solitary withdrawal. The sense of belonging to a group may be pursued via substance misuse. Once a child is involved in regular substance use, relationships tend to be valued as a means of obtaining the substance and thus take on a manipulative quality. Interestingly, many young adult males report that their first experiences with alcohol were with fathers, whom they describe as having offered infrequent opportunities for closeness. Some children report being "pulled into" a pattern of drug use by a substance-using parent; in such instances, they tend to have had little or no experience with sincere and intimate relationships.

SC11 Disorders of Mental Functioning

SC112 Tic Disorders

Tics are brief, stereotypical, nonrhythmic movements and/or vocalizations. They are not uncommon in childhood: about 5% of all children will have transient tics that resolve within 12 months. A smaller number will have a diagnosable motor or vocal tic disorder, and a smaller number still will have Tourette syndrome (TS), involving both motor and vocal tics. Our understanding of the prevalence of TS has recently changed, in light of the recognition of many undiagnosed cases of TS. Recent epidemiological studies have demonstrated prevalence figures between 0.4 and 3.8% for youngsters between 5 and 18 years old.

The Subjective Experience of TS and Other Tic Disorders in Childhood

Affective States

Affective states include anxiety and shame related to the tics, but a poor sense of self related to other conditions, such as learning and behavior problems, may be the most salient affective factor.

Thoughts and Fantasies

Thoughts and fantasies may involve fears of loss of control, especially of aggressive and sexual feelings and impulses. Children with tic disorders can come to think of themselves as different, defective, or "weird." Their self-concepts may become colored by the reactions of family, teachers, and peers.

Somatic States

TS usually begins in children at about ages 8–9, with eye-rolling tics, and may progress to head, limb, and trunk movements and vocalizations. Vocal tics usually occur in the form of throat clearing or grunts, and sometimes in the form of swearing. It is common for children with tic disorders to have other psychiatric disorders, especially in severe cases. Chief among the comorbid conditions is ADHD; others include learning disabilities, OCD, anxiety disorders, depression, and CD. Often children suffer more from these associated conditions than from the tics.

Although tic disorders were originally thought to be psychological in origin, they are now understood to be behavioral expressions of a developmental neuropsychiatric disorder with childhood onset that is highly influenced by environmental and behavioral factors. Advances in understanding the underlying neurobiology of tics have been made through *in vivo* neuroimaging and neurophysiology techniques. In addition, twin studies have demonstrated that like other neurodevelopmental conditions, TS and other tic disorders have an important heritable component. There are most likely multiple genes involved, but no specific gene or genes have been identified. On rare occasions, tics are found to be sequelae of a streptococcal infection; such tics have been termed "pediatric autoimmune neuropsychiatric disorders associated with streptococcal infections" (PANDAS).

Tics are exacerbated by stress or excitement, such as everyday psychosocial stress, a birthday party, or simply fatigue. Typically, they are transiently extinguished by activities requiring focus and fine motor control, such as reading aloud or playing a musical instrument. Although an individual usually has some control over the tic behavior, there is a compelling urge to discharge the premonitory tension antecedent to the tic. Ignoring tics—long a recommended strategy—is now not thought to be the best practice. Instead, it is important for the child and family to understand the role of reinforcement patterns, and to adopt positive and proactive procedures to manage the tics.

Recommended treatments are behavioral and include developing strategies specific to the individual child and family. These interventions first require exploring the factors influencing the occurrence or frequency of tics, such as doing homework or being the focus of social attention. Then a competing behavior, such as reading aloud or deep breathing, can be initiated. Children with tics may also benefit from psychodynamic treatments that help them become more aware of, and able to monitor better, their internal states, and to assist them in creating a more adaptive and positive sense of self and relationship to the world. Medication is also an option. Stimulant medications for comorbid ADHD are now not thought to worsen tics. Alpha-2 agonists or atypical antipsychotics may also be helpful.

Relationship Patterns

Relationship patterns often revolve around inadvertent reinforcement of tics when family members allow a child to avoid situations that elicit them. Sometimes the affected child becomes the focus of anxious attention in a way that controls the family's life. The sometimes inappropriate and involuntary nature of the behavior can create anxiety for peers in this age cohort. Relationships with peers may hence be affected, as other children may avoid or tease the child with the disorder.

Clinical Illustration

An 8-year-old boy with a history of ADHD was seeing a therapist for impulsive behavior and problems at home and school related to inattention and noncompliance. His parents said that for several months he had been rolling his eyes upward and to the side of his head, and that now he was beginning to turn his head in the same direction. His teacher had complained that he was making disruptive noises in class. He felt chronically misunderstood and mistreated by his teachers, and sometimes by his parents, but he liked school because of his many friends and sports activities. Now, suddenly, he was anxious about going to school and often told his mother he did not feel well and wanted to stay home.

When his therapist gently explored the situation with him, he admitted that his friends had asked him why he was doing "that funny thing with his eyes," and that kids at school had recently told him he was "weird." His therapist empathized with his feelings and inquired more about his behavior. He said that he did not understand why he did that thing with his eyes, but he just had a feeling he should do it, and after he did it he felt better for a while. Then he would start to feel bad again and would repeat the behavior. The therapist asked if he could tell when he got that feeling. Over the next few weeks, he and his parents were able to determine that when he was doing his homework—especially assignments that required him to write something—his tic behavior increased. The boy also told the therapist that when one of his friends said something funny and got in trouble with the teacher, he began to have the tic.

The therapist worked with him to become more familiar with the feeling he got before he felt he had to roll his eyes. Then he helped the boy learn how to "hold it" for 1 minute with a stop watch and see if he could make it go away. Sometimes this worked well, but sometimes when he was doing his homework it stopped being effective. The therapist and patient found that at those times, a brief period of reading a favorite comic aloud would take away the urge. These techniques made they boy feel stronger and more masterful, and he began to have an easier time going to school. He told the kids in his carpool that his eyes "just did that sometimes," but that he was learning to control it. His parents also explained his symptoms to his teacher, so that she would not interpret his vocal tics as intentional disruptions.

The therapist also was aware of the boy's long-standing conflicts about aggression. His chronic impulsivity made him anxious that he would strain his relationships with his parents. Stories he told in therapy revealed his fantasies that they preferred his younger sister and wanted to get rid of him. The tics made him feel even more defective than he had before, and the anxiety generated by these conflicts made him all the more vulnerable to his tics. Over time, he was able to appreciate both his mastery over his tic symptoms and his distorted perspective of his parents' feelings toward him. He and his therapist worked to correct his parents' sense of him as vulnerable, and to help them recognize strengths they had not known he had. This diminished their anxiety and led them to focus less on their son's symptoms and more on his competence in sports and friendship. They hired a tutor to help him with remedial academic tasks; they also got him accommodations for his attentional and organizational problems.

SC112 Psychotic Disorders

Psychotic disorders are characterized by loss of reality testing, by the inability to distinguish between internal and external sources of information, and often by delusions and/or hallucinations. The condition may be chronic, as is often the case in schizophrenia, or transient, as in psychotic depression, bipolar illness, and dissociative disorders. Loss of reality testing may have an organic etiology, may result from severe trauma or narcissistic injury with consequent psychological fragmentation, or may be complexly and epigenetically determined. Childhood-onset psychotic disorders are considered quite rare (they have an incidence rate of 0.04%, based on a National Institute of Mental Health cohort), and the presence of psychotic symptoms in childhood *does not* necessarily indicate the presence of a full psychotic disorder.

The capacity to separate reality from fantasy and to organize thoughts into successively higher-level organizations develops gradually in children. Typically, by age 4, children have a reasonably stable capacity to differentiate fantasy from reality and to appreciate increasingly subtle distinctions. A healthy 10-year-old is capable of commenting, "I only think other kids are being unfair to me when I am really upset." Not infrequently, however, children persist in confusing reality and fantasy—either during fairly circumscribed challenges or chronically, in which case the child may have highly organized and elaborate delusions. For example, a 7-year-old child insisted that he was having conversations with creatures from outer space, and that only he knew their plans for poisoning the planet.

It is often difficult to distinguish whether a child with a psychotic disorder has never developed age-expected reality testing or has developed this capacity and then lost it. The developmental histories of psychotic children vary considerably. Some children, for example, have difficulty in modulating sensation and/or processing auditory and visual–spatial experiences, while other children have a history of severe emotional distress; still others have both. Thought disorders may not emerge fully until adolescence, when the capacity for formal operational thought normally emerges. However, these children may display loosening of associations and concrete or tangential thinking.

Parents and clinicians may first become aware of persistent difficulties or changes in children's behavior, including language, motor, and social functioning. Academic functioning may decline. Given the possibility of misdiagnosis, clinicians should be cautious about diagnosing and treating childhood psychotic disorders (e.g., what appears as childhood psychosis may be an anxiety, mood, trauma, autism spectrum, or receptive and expressive language disorder). Once a diagnosis is made, it is important that interventions continue to address the child's psychosocial functioning across domains (family, school, and other settings), emotional experience (e.g., anxiety) and other developmental issues (e.g., language delays), and not focus narrowly on the psychotic symptoms.

The Subjective Experience of Psychotic Disorders in Childhood

Affective States

The affective states of children with reality-testing problems vary considerably, depending on the nature of their difficulties. Anxiety, depression, and combinations of the two are common; such feelings may be intense and disorganizing. Relationship patterns of children with early onset psychosis often show a lack of flexibility and capacity to incorporate the minds of other children cooperatively into pretend play. These children may become increasingly isolated and have trouble fitting in.

Thoughts and Fantasies

Thoughts may reflect poor judgment, extreme impulsivity, marked social withdrawal, disorganized or illogical thinking, and unrealistic beliefs and experiences. Affect may be inappropriate to the content of what is being articulated. Fantasies, especially of specialness, may not be experienced as products of imagination but as self-evident truths. They may also contain bizarre content.

Somatic States

Somatic states, consistent with the existence of intense affective states, may include a range of somatic complaints and bodily concerns despite an absence of medical findings.

Relationship Patterns

Relationship patterns may be either excessively dependent or excessively aloof. As a result of their idiosyncratic behaviors and odd productions, psychotic children are often picked on, made fun of, or avoided by peers. They will also erroneously experience themselves at times as being negatively judged, criticized, or antagonized.

Clinical Illustration

A 9-year-old girl with a diagnosis of bipolar disorder came to treatment for serious behavior problems. Her mood and affect were intense and fluctuated unpredictably. The parents said that she was sometimes pleasant and engaging, but at other times irritable and despondent. Her behavior difficulties and mood fluctuations had subsided a bit when she was prescribed medication at age 6, but over the past year she had become increasingly suspicious and angry. She began to express fears of the dark and of being around people she did not know. Unless she was soothed, the fears would increase in intensity to almost panic level. She had no friends in school and had retreated into herself. Her teachers and parents reported that when she became agitated, she would talk to herself and seem to be in her own world. She did follow the routine in the classroom, but the teachers felt that any provocation could set her off. When in an agitated mood, she would show looseness of association and disorganized thinking.

SC114 Neuropsychological Disorders

The following disorders should be considered in the context of the MC-Axis categories.

SC114.1 Motor Skills Disorders

Motor skills disorders in children are variously described as "problems with motor planning," "vestibular disorders," "developmental apraxia," "perceptual–motor dysfunction," "coordination disorders," and an assortment of other terms. The multiplicity of terms created to describe gross and fine motor problems in children suggests a lack of specificity in this area of dysfunction, as well as a lack of knowledge about their etiology. DSM-5 now classifies developmental coordination disorder (DCD) in the category of neurodevelopmental disorders; this may be the best general term for purposes of definition. Although extreme cases of DCD occur at a frequency of approximately 5% in 7-year-old children, the frequency of milder forms of coordination problems approaches 9%.

The Subjective Experience of DCD in Childhood

Affective States

Because young children's cognition is relatively concrete and body-focused, it is hard for a child with significant DCD to feel confident and masterful. In more severe cases of DCD, children may experience significant insecurity of their bodies in space, causing them to bump into objects or fall, and consequently to feel excessively vulnerable to injury and loss.

Somatic States

DCD is sometimes identified in infants by delays in sitting, crawling, or walking. It is often not diagnosed, however, until a child enters school and begins to show difficulties keeping up with other children, or with getting dressed, writing, or drawing. Children with DCD are often clumsy and awkward in their physical approach to their peers, which can cause problems in relationships. Some children have DCD alone, but most have DCD in association with other developmental problems. There is a large overlap between children with DCD and ADHD, and also an overlap between DCD and autism spectrum disorder, learning disabilities, and language disorders.

Relationship Patterns

Children who lack competence in motor skills are at risk of withdrawing from athletic activities and interactions with peers. This avoidance of activities that are hard for them may in turn increase their relative weakness. Especially in the early school years, and particularly in boys, valuation of status among peers emphasizes agility, strength, and speed. A child who cannot keep up may suffer from low self-esteem and may withdraw from active peer play. Children's responses to DCD vary widely and are heavily influenced by cultural values in families and communities.

Clinical Illustration

Seven-year-old Jack was always the last child to leave the classroom when it was time for recess. This was because he struggled with the zipper on his jacket, had a hard time fitting his feet into his boots, and frequently could not find his hat. Even in the summer—when he did not have to wear a jacket, boots, or a hat—he would lag behind because he tended to have trouble leaving what he was doing and making the transition to another activity. When Jack appeared on the playground, he would frequently take some time to survey the scene and then try to approach a group of boys. If they were clustered together in some kind of group play, he would seem to "crash the party" by squashing his body into the others, which did not meet with approval. If they would (as they often did) suddenly jump up and take off running across the playground, Jack would attempt to run with them, but would quickly fall behind and lose the group. He was also unable to master the monkey bars or the swings. He rarely talked about these experiences, but once he sadly told his mother that he was the slowest runner in the class, and that was why he didn't have any friends.

SC114.2 *Visual–Spatial Processing Disorders*

Disorders of visual–spatial processing are marked by limitations in the ability to use visual–spatial information to perceive, analyze, synthesize, think, and/or solve problems. The diagnosis of such a disorder is established when (1) one or more aspects of a child's visual–spatial processing, as measured by individually administered, standardized tests of cognitive/intellectual functioning, falls substantially below the mean performance of children of the same age or grade, or below the child's verbal comprehension index on an IQ test and/or other measures of verbal-language ability; and (2) the disorder significantly affects the child's academic functioning and/or activities of daily living. Caution should be used in interpreting age- and grade equivalents for diagnostic and/or placement purposes. Generally speaking, standard scores, scaled scores, stanines, and percentiles interpreted within the context of confidence intervals offer more direct ways of comparing performances across a wide range of tasks and skills.

When the primary impact of a visual–spatial processing disorder is limited to a specific academic skill, such as reading or mathematics, an additional diagnosis of a learning disorder is warranted. Excluded from the diagnosis of visual–spatial processing disorders are disorders of social perception that fail to meet the criteria above. In this circumstance, a diagnosis on the autism spectrum should be considered. Also excluded from this diagnosis are problems of visual acuity and blindness.

Disorders of visual–spatial processing range occur on a spectrum from primary sensory deficits to higher-order processing that disrupts the interpretation of visual information and/or its integration into higher-order problem solving. Children with visual–spatial processing disorders may have difficulty identifying or manipulating visual patterns or orientation of lines, interpreting charts and graphs, tracing paths, making accurate judgments about spatial orientation of objects or locating them in space, and constructing figures in three-dimensional space. These disorders may also underlie some forms of learning disorders in mathematics, reading, and written expression, as suggested above.

When not identified early, many children suffering from visual–spatial processing disorders are badly wounded in the traditional school system. They are often made to feel stupid, lazy, defiant, and unworthy. The damage to their self-esteem can be healed through work with caring, sensitive teachers who see their strengths and understand their weaknesses. Lack of understanding and support from school and family may lead to social isolation and other relational difficulties (e.g., being bullied, being aggressive toward peers to defend oneself against feelings of being lost in the social environment).

Clinical Illustration

A 10-year-old girl presented with a history of difficulties with mathematics, as well as problems with slow processing speed, reading delay, and what appeared to be symptoms of ADHD. Her written expression was weak, despite her ability to convey ideas eloquently in verbal form. Understandably, she found schoolwork particularly challenging and functioned only with a great deal of support. Although she had longstanding friendships and a capacity to empathize with others, she frequently misinterpreted or failed to notice important visual cues and struggled to infer mental states from facial expressions, causing her sometimes to miss the "big picture" or to have difficulty distinguishing irony from serious comments.

She met criteria for disorders in reading, mathematics, and written expression, but further evaluation revealed that her learning difficulties were undergirded by a visual–spatial processing disorder. That is, her reading was not uniformly impaired, but was weakened by difficulties with visual tracking and spatial reversals; her mathematics performance was derailed by her inability to align columns in her computations, notice the signs of operations, and other details. Her understanding of math concepts and retention of math facts was intact. Her written expression suffered from poor spatial planning and spelling. She sometimes could not read her own handwriting.

SC114.3 *Language and Auditory Processing Disorders*

Language and auditory processing disorders have traditionally been divided into two broad categories: disorders of expressive language and disorders of receptive language. Often deficits in both aspects of language are present; in this case, a diagnosis of mixed receptive–expressive language disorder as defined by DSM-IV would be warranted (this diagnosis has been dropped from DSM-5). Expressive language disorders are characterized by dysfluency, word repetition difficulties, and dysnomia. Children with these problems have limited expressive vocabulary and struggle to generate verbiage of developmentally appropriate length, complexity, and grammatical competence. Comprehension of verbal information is generally preserved in an expressive language disorder. It is diagnosed when dysfluency, word repetition difficulties, and dysnomia, as measured by individually administered, standardized tests of language functioning, fall substantially below the mean performance of children of the same age or grade, or below the child's perceptual reasoning index on an IQ test and/or measures of visual–spatial processing skills.

Children with expressive language disorders also may show problems in one or more of the following areas: general language functioning (simplified, nonspecific speech); grammar (word order and agreement); semantics (poor vocabulary and circumlocution); pragmatics (conversational skills—problems with these are not associated exclusively with autism spectrum disorders); and discourse (organization and expression of ideas). As in diagnosing visual–spatial processing disorders, caution should be taken in interpreting age and grade equivalents for diagnostic and/or placement purposes. Generally speaking, standard scores, scaled scores, stanines, and percentiles interpreted within the context of confidence intervals offer more direct ways of comparing performances across a wide variety of tasks and skills.

In receptive language disorders, verbal fluency is preserved. Typically, children with these disorders show few or no deficits in speech production, although paraphasia (inaccurate syllables, words, and/or phrases) and, in severe cases, neologisms may occur. A diagnosis of a receptive language disorder is made when picture naming, word repetition, and comprehension of language, as measured by individually administered, standardized tests of language functioning, fall substantially below expectations based on the mean performance of children of the same age or grade, or from the child's perceptual reasoning index on an IQ test and/or measures of visual–spatial processing skills.

Children with receptive language disorders may also may demonstrate problems in one or more of the following areas: general language functioning (comprehension); grammar (interpretation of complex sentences); semantics (limited vocabulary; difficulty understanding conversation); pragmatics (difficulty distilling, inferring, and generalizing ideas from conversations—not associated exclusively with autism spectrum disorder); and discourse (comprehension of complex narrative information). The cautions described above should be taken in interpreting age and grade equivalents for diagnostic and/or placement purposes, and the alternative scores and statistics suggested above should be considered.

Language disorders typically emerge at 15–18 months of age, when language acquisition occurs. Delayed negotiation of language milestones, particularly in the area of expressive language, is common. Because of differences in development, however, diagnosis is often deferred until age 3 or 4 years. Because communicative competence is essential to social discourse, a disorder of expressive and/or receptive language may contribute to a child's relationship problems. Without early remediation, such a disorder usually becomes increasingly problematic as the child matures. Prevalence rates for language disorders range between 5 and 8%. No single pattern of affect, cognition, somatic involvement, or relationships characterizes language disorders, as children's responses to them vary widely.

Clinical Illustration

A 9-year-old fourth grader was referred for reevaluation because of continuing difficulties with speech and language processing. She had long-standing difficulties with mathematics, reading comprehension, and sustained attention as well. Expressive language difficulties had grown more pronounced; she struggled to formulate and express her ideas. She appeared increasingly disorganized and confused in the classroom, seeming to "zone out" and simply shut down during group instruction.

Because she was adopted at birth, relatively little was known about her prenatal care. Despite grossly normal motor milestones, there were significant delays in her use of language; she did not speak clearly and comfortably until about 42 months. Fluency continued to be problematic. Otherwise she negotiated all developmental milestones within normal limits. She was referred to the local Birth to Three program, where she received speech and language therapy services. She struggled to learn her letters in preschool, and despite ongoing support, she was consistently among the weakest readers in her classes. She struggled socially, her spelling was poor, and her written expression skills were delayed.

SC114.4 *Memory Impairments*

Memory includes a variety of processes broadly subsumed by the terms "working memory," "declarative memory," and "nondeclarative memory." Working memory connotes processes in which a limited amount of information is actively maintained over a short period of time, so that it is available for further use and mental manipulation. Conceptually, it can be further divided into short-term storage memory systems, dedicated to holding visual and auditory information.

Declarative or explicit memory refers to processes for holding information consciously in the mind. It is divided into episodic and semantic memory. The former subsumes one's conscious memory of facts and events, including autobiographical data. Typically, it is evaluated in the auditory sphere by list or story learning; in the visual sphere, by design learning. By contrast, semantic memory describes one's semipermanent store of facts, subsuming one's knowledge of words, concepts, and meanings. It is evaluated through a variety of tasks, including word fluency, category fluency, vocabulary, naming, and tests of general knowledge.

Implicit or nondeclarative memory contains nonconscious material. It consists of processes such as procedural memory, priming, and associative and nonassociative learning. Working memory and procedural memory problems are quite common in children with learning disabilities, ADHD, and executive function difficulties. Significant memory problems, however, particularly those involving declarative or explicit memory, are often associated with either traumatic brain injury or innate factors, as well as selective recall of traumatic experiences. Memory dysfunctions caused by innate factors emerge early during development; those resulting from a traumatic brain injury may sometimes be traced to the location and developmental phase of the injury. Although these dysfunctions are often irreversible, the child may be able to compensate for the deficits. In making this diagnosis, it is important to determine whether the child's memory deficits are better explained by reference to another disorder. For example, symptoms of poor working memory in a child diagnosed with ADHD and executive function difficulties may be better explained by reference to difficulties with sustained, selective, and/or alternating attention. The clinician must be sensitive to the multifactorial structure of memory and the range of neuropsychological and learning disorders that may affect the clinical picture. No single pattern of affect, cognition, somatic states, or relationships characterizes memory impairments.

Clinical Illustration

A third-grade boy with a long history of school evaluations was referred by a teacher, who was concerned about his difficulty keeping up with classroom demands despite substantial individual assistance, especially in math and written language. His performance was variable, marked by distractibility, difficulty remaining on task, and poor comprehension of oral directions. He tired easily and required one-to-one assistance both to initiate and to complete tasks. The therapist noted relative strengths in verbal reasoning, word knowledge and usage, social reasoning, attention to visual details, and part-to-whole synthesis, and relative weaknesses in tasks involving manipulation of information in working memory, retrieval of factual information, attention, and visual–motor integration within a structured format. Visual-perceptual skills were variable, with sequential memory falling in the low-average range. He also had a word retrieval problem, which inhibited his capacity to communicate fluidly.

SC114.5 *Attention-Deficit/Hyperactivity Disorder*

According to DSM-5, the three core features associated with a diagnosis of attention-deficit/hyperactivity disorder (ADHD) are inattention, impulsivity, and hyperactivity. Depending on how these features are manifested clinically, a diagnosis of ADHD can be categorized as falling into one of three subtypes: combined presentation, predominantly inattentive presentation, and predominantly hyperactive/impulsive presentation. Among the three subtypes, the predominantly hyperactive/impulsive subtype is associated with a noticeably higher level of activity than that exhibited by a child's peers and is typically diagnosed early. The combined subtype is associated with both inattentiveness and impulsivity and is likely to be more noticeable with the onset of the school years, when difficulties with sustaining attention, completing tasks, and not interrupting others become more noticeable. The predominantly inattentive subtype is likely to be diagnosed after the early grades of elementary school, when tasks get harder and a child's effort does not always lead to adequate performance.

Academic performance may be impaired in all three subtypes, but the impairment is secondary to impulsivity and inattentiveness. The expression of symptoms varies, depending on context and setting. They may be minimal or absent when a child is in a novel setting and under close supervision, or is engaged in highly absorbing activities (such as video and electronic games), but can be elevated when the child is in a large-group situation and expected to be involved in an activity in which he or she has no interest. Although there is consensus that children with ADHD have poor self-regulation and organization skills, there is also a growing awareness that ADHD is not a uniform diagnostic entity, but one that includes considerable individual and subgroup variation. Emotional conflict, neglect, cultural dynamics, mourning and/or depression, and growing up with a severely depressed or absent mother have been found to contribute to symptoms consistent with an ADHD diagnosis.

Academic deficits, school-related problems, and peer neglect tend to be more closely associated with elevated symptoms of inattention and impulsivity, whereas peer rejection and, to a lesser extent, accidental injury are more closely associated with hyperactivity. Although there is great variability, individuals with ADHD obtain, on average, less schooling and have poorer vocational achievement than their peers. In its more severe form, the disorder is markedly impairing, affecting social, familial, and scholastic/occupational adjustment. In adolescence, some of the hyperactivity that was evident at an earlier age subsides, but the overall fidgetiness and restlessness remains.

The Subjective Experience of ADHD in Childhood

Affective States

The affective states of children with ADHD vary widely, depending on subtype and contextual factors. Typically, the combination of impulsivity and agitated mood makes them come across as overreactive and on the brink of being out of control. Furthermore, their difficulty relying on secondary-process functions to organize their thoughts and make sense of what is happening can leave them unable to contain intense emotions and thus more prone to act out. Their inadequate or poor application to tasks that require sustained effort often masks an underlying anxiety over task demands, and is often interpreted by others as laziness, irresponsibility, and failure to cooperate. Contributing to their seeming lack of motivation, and even to their impulsive reactions, is their negative perception of themselves. A punitive internal object may make it very hard to contain wishes and intense affects.

Thoughts and Fantasies

The thoughts of hyperactive children are notably unruly. Their play and modes of engagement reflect states of mind that are often disorganized and overexcited. Although they are able to sustain attention if an object or activity is sufficiently stimulating, their impulsivity affects their thinking, and they may consequently move from topic to topic or activity to activity with no apparent connective thread. Their sudden shifts or random statements may seem triggered by excitement or impulsivity, but may also be caused by an underlying anxiety or agitation they cannot contain or express with words.

Somatic States

Somatic states may include feelings described by comments such as "I have to move" or "My muscles are exploding." A child with ADHD may also have a sense that the body has its own imperatives, in the face of which the child is helpless ("My legs just do what they need to").

Relationship Patterns

The interpersonal relationships and modes of engagement of children with ADHD are inconsistent, and interactions that are mutual and continuous may be hard to maintain. Their difficulty in attending to social cues and organizing their behavior accordingly provokes negative interactions at home and in school, leading them to experience peer rejection, neglect, and teasing. Their impulsive, restless demeanor may cause family discord, exacerbated by their difficulty in using verbal symbols to communicate their experiences and convey their internal states. The fragility of these children and their highly critical internalizations cause them to experience interactions with others, especially those that involve the sharing or exploring of feelings, as disruptive and disorganizing.

Clinical Illustration

A 9-year-old boy whose pediatrician had diagnosed ADHD and prescribed Ritalin was referred to a therapist by his mother, who reported that he had nightmares, difficulty with separation, and oppositional behaviors, especially around morning and bedtime routines. His emotions alternated between intense reactions and seeming indifference to others. He and his mother got into frequent power struggles that required the father's intervention. Although he seemed content to play by himself, he seemed to need others to be available and willing to play at the level of his own interests.

The boy had always seemed a bit slow to react and would spend many hours watching cartoons. He was very close to his mother, and although he had many play dates, he never seemed to have a close friend. His language appeared delayed. His school troubles began in first grade and had continued since. His teachers complained that he would not listen, was easily distracted, had problems concentrating, failed to complete assignments, and failed at tasks that required sustained attention. Although his distractibility and restlessness subsided after he was prescribed Ritalin, he still had difficulty completing assignments and seemed more withdrawn and apathetic. Getting him to accept taking the pill each morning was a struggle, and the parents reported prolonged agitation in the evening when the effects of the medication wore off. Completing homework was also a challenge. He would express his frustration in self-deprecating statements such as "I hate myself" and "I can't do this."

The boy expressed confusion about what was happening between him and his mother. He felt generally uncomfortable in the school setting, but could not articulate why. He seemed to lose interest in any discussions aimed at exploring his experiences and emotions or linking internal states and external demands. He would become fidgety and switch topics or activities, as if what was happening was of no interest. He did seem, however, to respond to the therapist's efforts to point out disjunctive moments in the session and to empathize with his difficulty tolerating or understanding what he had experienced. When the therapist was able to share a narrative that made him feel understood and recognized, the boy's attitude would visibly change, and he would become more engaged in the discussion.

SC114.6 *Executive Function Difficulties*

The diagnosis of executive function disorders was included in the first PDM to denote a complex and overlapping set of difficulties in areas that are critical to a child's ability to succeed academically and socially. They include managing time and organizing resources effectively, making realistic plans and carrying them out, remembering details and attending to the task at hand, monitoring one's efforts or progress, and self-regulation. Most researchers and clinicians, however, do not associate difficulties in these areas with a distinct executive function disorder. Instead, they are likely to regard executive functions as a significant set of skills that are instrumental in a child's ability to perform well in school, feel self-esteem, and relate well with others. As a result, although difficulties with executive functions are not regarded as distinct *disorders* in PDM-2, the significant role of difficulties with these skills in a child's development and adjustment merits their inclusion here.

Difficulties with executive functions are particularly prevalent in children with an ADHD diagnosis, who typically have similar difficulties in their ability to plan, organize, attend to details, switch focus, self-monitor, and self-regulate. However, although almost all children diagnosed with ADHD have difficulties with executive skills, not all children with executive function difficulties are diagnosable as having ADHD. Children with other learning disabilities, such as math or reading problems, show difficulty in organizing information, initiating strategies, developing plans that take into account what they are expected to do, monitoring their performance, and adjusting their efforts or strategies when necessary. Executive function difficulties are prevalent in children with emotional problems, including those diagnosed with bipolar disorder and those who have experienced trauma and neglect.

Typically, a child with executive function difficulties has poor study skills, is inefficient in doing class assignments, is scattered and disorganized, and tends to procrastinate. Problems do not emerge until the school years, when demands are made to undertake tasks whose complexity is greater than the child's capabilities. As these demands increase and executive function breaks down, the child's ability to complete work-related tasks, function independently, learn from class activities, and feel involved in school life is affected. Children with this problem typically know what they have to do, but cannot take the initiative or implement their knowledge.

For many children with executive function difficulties, the learning process can be experienced as especially demoralizing, leading them to develop a negative attitude toward school and toward themselves and their capacities. Their failure to self-regulate and to organize academic information in an effective manner can prevent them from developing a sense of agency and mastery. In their social relationships, children with executive difficulties are less likely to be as aware of themselves in relation to others as their peers might be and may display poor social self-regulation. Their insight about themselves and their ability to understand the perspective of others is also likely to be compromised.

No single pattern of affect, thoughts, somatic states, or relationships characterizes the executive function difficulties.

Clinical Illustration

A 10-year-old boy was referred for treatment because of inappropriate behavior in school. Despite notable intellectual skills, he had a history of attentional and social difficulties that interfered with his peer relationships, general social-emotional adjustment, and schoolwork. His mother depicted him as always passive, needing constant prompting to do his work and to follow up with assigned tasks. His room and desk were reportedly cluttered with papers, notebooks, clothes, and toys. He had difficulty organizing his belongings, was forgetful, and would become easily overwhelmed when he felt he had a lot to do. Because of his forgetfulness, he needed constant monitoring and prompting. In instances where he lost track of time or forgot to take work to school or plan for an assignment ahead of time, he would typically collapse and would need his mother's or tutors' encouragement and help to complete his work. He was a rather shy boy, slow to do his work, and would quickly become frustrated when he made mistakes or felt that the task was too demanding.

As the complexity of academic tasks increased, his somatic complaints increased, and he made frequent statements of self-resignation. His parents and tutors helped him with the demands of particular tasks and offered him strategies for organizing the material. Once he was able to perform a task, his level of agitation would subside, but not his negative statements about himself. His perception of himself affected his peer relationships and his sense of accomplishment, and he began to refuse to go to school. Despite his considerable talents and good language skills, he appeared fragile, filled with anxiety and frustration, and convinced that he was simply not as good he should be. Because of his poor time management skills, he seemed to need repeated prompts to be able to follow through with his chores. He had particular difficulty adjusting to novel situations and would complain whenever there was a change in his routine. His dependency on others and their ongoing monitoring of him confirmed his perception of himself as someone who was defective, and reinforced his frustration and resignation. Getting him up to go to school in the morning had become an increasingly tense time for the family, and getting him out of the house on time was a battle. Working with him required tolerating his passivity without becoming overly reactive in return, and engaging with him in exchanges that were not framed exclusively in terms of what he was failing to do.

SC114.7 *Severe Cognitive Deficits*

See also the discussions above of the other neuropsychological disorders, as well as the discussions in Chapter 10 of regulatory–sensory processing disorders (pp. 674–677) and neurodevelopmental disorders of relating and communicating (pp. 687–689).

Traditionally, IQ tests have been used to evaluate the extent of cognitive deficits. A condition of severe cognitive deficits, intellectual disability, or intellectual developmental disorder reflects significant subaverage intellectual functioning. Areas of deficits typically include (but are not limited to) reasoning, planning, problem solving, communication, judgment, and learning. In the past, these deficits had to be documented by full-scale IQ scores on standardized testing falling below 70 or two standard deviations below the mean for children of the same age, although DSM-5 has dropped these specific cutoffs. In addition to IQ testing, it is important to evaluate the child's adaptive functioning. The latter deficits also must be significant, preventing the child from negotiating age, developmental, and sociocultural milestones appropriately. Adaptive skills include (but are not limited to) self-care, home living, social-interpersonal skills, self-direction, and health/personal safety.

Current research suggests that children with severe cognitive deficits may have strengths of various kinds that are not necessarily identified by IQ testing. For this reason, clinicians must carefully evaluate adaptive functioning, broadly construed. While learning disorders are common in children diagnosed with severe cognitive deficits, the diagnostic concept excludes these diagnoses. A framework for describing a child's individual differences is presented in Chapter 10. The child's subjective experience of cognitive deficit depends on his or her level of self-awareness. Prevalence rate for severe cognitive deficits is approximately 2%. No single pattern of affect, thought, somatic states, or relationships characterizes severe cognitive deficits.

Clinical Illustration

A 6-year-old girl was having difficulty learning to read, do math, and communicate logically with peers. Her teachers suspected a severe cognitive deficit after testing showed a full-scale IQ of 65, with little differentiation between verbal comprehension and perceptual reasoning abilities. Further clinical evaluation revealed that despite severe difficulties in auditory processing, her level of conceptual understanding was higher when she was given instructions in a highly animated form combining short verbal explanations with gesturing and concrete visual guides (pictures). Once she had information to work with, her verbal reasoning was stronger than suggested by her IQ test results. She showed better ability on rote, repetitive tasks after repeated exposure, direct instruction, and supervised practice.

An individualized education program was developed for this child that focused on using her relative strengths in conceptual reasoning and response to repetition and supervised practice to improve her memory and academic functioning. Her progress with this program further confirmed the diagnostic profile constructed from a comprehensive clinical evaluation and functional assessment.

SC115 Learning Disorders

SC115.1 *Reading Disorders*

Reading disorders are diagnosed when reading achievement, as measured by individually administered, standardized tests of reading, falls substantially below the mean performance of children of the same age or grade, or below what is expected from a child's IQ. Again, caution should be used in interpreting age and grade equivalents for diagnostic and/or placement purposes. Generally speaking, standard scores, scaled scores, stanines, and percentiles interpreted within the context of confidence intervals offer the best way of comparing performances across a wide variety of tasks and skills.

Reading disorders are not diagnosed in children who carry a concomitant diagnosis of severe cognitive deficits or intellectual disability, or in whom the disparate reading scores result directly from (1) primary impairments in vision, hearing, or motor functioning; (2) emotional disturbance; (3) limited English proficiency; or (4) environmental, cultural, or economic disadvantage, specifically lack of appropriate instruction in the essential components of reading. These disorders are seen in approximately 9% of the population.

Reading achievement should be understood to include any and all of the following: reading pace/fluency, phonological processing and decoding, and reading comprehension. To be considered a diagnosable disorder, a reading deficit must interfere significantly with academic achievement or activities of daily living that require reading skills. As a practical matter, this inference has traditionally been made by one or more of the following: (1) a reading achievement score that falls one standard deviation below the mean performance of children of the same age or grade, or below the child's IQ; or (2) a reading achievement score that falls one standard deviation below the child's scores for other academic abilities. Although a comprehensive psychoeducational or neuropsychological assessment is the preferred means of making the diagnosis, the child's grades, response to instruction, and teacher observations and ratings may be used to establish presumptive evidence of a disorder. Clinicians are encouraged to draw on multiple data sources to establish the diagnosis.

Development is usually unremarkable in children with reading problems, and no social problems are associated with reading disorders until children are required to complete reading tasks. Their embarrassment at not being able to do what other children do easily may then interfere with peer relationships. Shame is associated with this type of learning disability. The repeated embarrassment of children with reading difficulties may eventually lead to self-esteem problems.

Clinical Illustration

A 7-year-old second grader in a large public elementary school came for assessment because his reading skills did not keep pace with his mathematical and conceptual reasoning abilities. He was an obviously bright boy with fine communication skills and a facility with conceptual thinking. Listening comprehension and ability to follow directions were excellent. He was able to identify all of the letters and their sounds, but struggled to decode and had a very limited sight vocabulary. Neuropsychological evaluation findings included a full-scale IQ of 115 (84th percentile), with real-word and pseudoword decoding scores at approximately the 16th percentile. A product of an uncomplicated pregnancy, he was presently in good health, although his mother reported that he was a colicky infant who seemed to cry all night for the first 3 months of his life. All developmental milestones were negotiated in a timely fashion, however, and he did not come to the attention of the school psychologist until his parents and teacher grew concerned that at the end of first grade he was still a nonreader.

SC115.2 *Mathematics Disorders*

Mathematics disorders are diagnosed when mathematical achievement, as measured by individually administered, standardized tests, falls substantially below the mean performance of children of the same age or grade, or below what is expected from a child's IQ. The usual cautions and recommendations about the use of test scores for diagnostic and/or placement purposes apply to mathematics disorders.

Like reading disorders, mathematics disorders are not diagnosed in children who carry a concomitant diagnosis of severe cognitive deficits/intellectual disability, or in whom the disparate mathematical achievement scores result directly from (1) primary impairments in vision, hearing, or motor functioning; (2) emotional disturbance; (3) limited proficiency in the language of the culture; or (4) environmental, cultural, or economic disadvantage, specifically lack of appropriate instruction in the essential components of mathematics. These disorders are diagnosed in 3–6.5% of the population.

Mathematical achievement includes any and all of the following: slow, inaccurate, or impoverished retrieval of math facts; slow or inaccurate generation and execution of computational procedures; difficulty with recognizing and conceptualizing number sets and generating estimates; and/or difficulties counting and representing numbers spatially. The last may include the alignment of columns, or place value. To be considered a diagnosable disorder, a mathematics deficit must interfere significantly with academic achievement or activities of daily living that require math skills. As a practical matter, this inference has usually been made by one or more of the following: (1) a mathematics achievement score one standard deviation below the mean performance of children of the same age or grade, or below the child's IQ; or (2) a mathematics achievement score that falls one standard deviation below the child's scores for other academic abilities. Again, although a comprehensive psychoeducational or neuropsychological assessment is the preferred means of making the diagnosis, the child's grades, response to instruction, and teacher observations and ratings may be used to establish presumptive evidence of a disorder. Clinicians are encouraged to derive the diagnosis from multiple data sources.

Development is usually unremarkable in children with mathematics problems, and no social problems are associated with this learning disorder until children are required to complete mathematics tasks. Their embarrassment at not being able to do what other children do easily may then interfere with peer relationships and eventually lead to self-esteem problems.

Clinical Illustration

A delightful 9-year-old fourth grader was referred for an evaluation of her inconsistent school performance, as well as of her subpar performances in mathematics and language arts on state-required mastery tests. She had had tutoring since first grade on a twice-weekly basis; thus one would thus expect her to have consolidated her basic academic skills and to have handled the majority of her work without difficulty. This was not the case. She frequently appeared distracted in class, did not enjoy school, and had difficulty retaining what she learned—word spellings, math facts, and mathematical procedures. Despite these concerns, she was performing at an average level, and her problems were not particularly evident on her report cards. She was well behaved and popular, clearly deriving pleasure from the social-interpersonal dimension of school. Nevertheless, she struggled to make connections and got bogged down in unnecessary details.

SC115.3 *Disorders of Written Expression*

A disorder of written expression is diagnosed when written production, as measured by individually administered, standardized tests of writing, falls substantially below the mean performance of children of the same age or grade, or below what would be expected from the child's IQ. The usual cautions and recommendations about the use of test scores for diagnostic and/or placement purposes apply to disorders of written expression.

Disorders of written language are not diagnosed in children with a concomitant diagnosis of severe cognitive deficits/intellectual disability or in whom the disparate written expression achievement scores result directly from (1) primary impairments in vision or hearing; (2) neurological conditions affecting movement, such as cerebral palsy, muscular dystrophy, or a degenerative disorder; (3) emotional disturbance; (4) limited proficiency in the language of the culture; or (5) environmental, cultural, or economic disadvantage, specifically lack of appropriate instruction in the essential components of writing. They may, however, be diagnosed in children who have been identified with DCD (see the earlier discussion of DCD); who have difficulties with fine motor coordination and exhibit clumsiness; or who lack age-appropriate proficiency in motor skills, such as tying shoelaces, using scissors or cutlery, or handwriting. These disorders are diagnosed in approximately 5–10% of the population. Comorbidity with ADHD is 30–50%.

Importantly, written expression deficits should be interpreted broadly to include any and all of the following: low rate and volume of written production; illegible, transposed, or spatially disorganized writing (including letter formation quality, size, spacing, slant, and alignment); inaccurate spelling, grammar, or punctuation; and organization, coherence, and logical communication of ideas. To be considered a diagnosable disorder, the writing deficit must interfere significantly with academic achievement or activities of daily living that require written expression. As a practical matter, this inference has usually been made by one or more of the following: (1) a written expression achievement score one standard deviation below the mean performance of children of the same age or grade, or below the child's IQ; or (2) a written expression achievement score one standard deviation below the child's other academic abilities. Once again, although a comprehensive psychoeducational or neuropsychological assessment is the preferred means of making the diagnosis, the child's grades, response to instruction, and teacher observations and ratings may be used to establish presumptive evidence of a disorder. The clinician is encouraged to draw from multiple data sources to establish the diagnosis.

Clinical Illustration

A seventh-grade boy of above-average intelligence was chronically late with written assignments and sometimes would not bother to hand them in. In sessions, he described having particular difficulty with English assignments and essay writing in general. When asked to write a brief essay, he had difficulty initiating it; he often stared at the computer screen or paper, unable to get started, let alone produce much verbiage. Sometimes he simply gave up in frustration, unable to produce more than a few sentences, with many words misspelled and multiple punctuation errors. By contrast, when his mother offered to be his "secretary" and allowed him simply to dictate his thoughts, his production increased dramatically. Neuropsychological testing revealed a boy of high-average intelligence, with writing skills within the low-average range. Although his language processing was strong, his visual–motor coordination was poor, again rating in the low-average range.

SC115.4 *Nonverbal Learning Disabilities*

Children with nonverbal learning disabilities have a complex set of neurocognitive strengths and weaknesses. Their strengths include rote verbal memory, reading decoding, and spelling; their weaknesses include tactile and visual perception and attention, concept formation, reading comprehension of complex materials, problem solving, and dealing with novel materials. They may have problems in math and science, as well as social-emotional difficulties involving the reception and expression of modulated affects and nonverbal modes of communication. They typically have poor handwriting and are deficient in arithmetic skills. Their reading comprehension is not on a par with their verbal skills; although they are good readers, they have great difficulty with art assignments. They also have problems with attention, novel materials, and new situations.

As infants, children with these disabilities are passive, fail to engage in exploratory play, and do not respond as expected. They appear clumsy and poorly coordinated. They have difficulties interacting with other children in groups. They are unable to form friendships or to be with other children even for brief periods without erupting. They usually interact well with adults, but not with peers. They are unable to decode social cues, failing to "read" other people's body language, facial expressions, and vocal intonations.

The Subjective Experience of Nonverbal Learning Disabilities in Childhood

Affective States

With respect to their affective states, children with nonverbal learning difficulties have problems in the reception, expression, and processing of affective communication. Their self-esteem may be damaged by recurrent failures to complete tasks that appear simple to others and by their lack of success in social relationships. They may suffer chronic anxiety and have trouble with self-regulation.

Thoughts and Fantasies

Thoughts and fantasies may focus on being "a failure," being "different," or feeling lost. Thinking may be piecemeal or fragmented, especially in situations that require "big-picture" or synthetic thinking. As a result of efforts to reduce fragmentation, thinking can be narrow and rigid.

Somatic States

Somatic states may include a diffuse physical clumsiness, especially in fine motor skills.

Relationship Patterns

In their relationship patterns, children with these problems may appear out of step. They lack the ease and fluidity in social discourse that we associate with social competence. They may make people anxious or uncomfortable, yet they appear to have little awareness of the impact they have on others. Some such children appear socially disconnected and out of touch with what goes on around them. In group situations, they tend to withdraw into silence; if they attempt to engage others, they speak in ways that show a lack of understanding of the subtleties of the group's interactions.

Clinical Illustration

A third-grade boy was referred for trouble with nonverbal communication. He did not make good eye contact or show emotions in his facial expression, and he seemed stiff and wooden. He could not process visual–spatial information, despite being highly verbal and capable of expressing himself at a level beyond his chronological age. Because of his visual–spatial processing problems, he had academic difficulties, especially in math and art. He was acutely aware of these difficulties and of his relative isolation in school. His fragile sense of self and low self-esteem provided a filter through which he understood interpersonal situations; he not only misinterpreted them, but also presumed that the poorly understood pieces constituted negative commentary about him. In conversations, he could become easily confused; had a difficult time integrating ideas to develop a synthesized meaning; and, when overwhelmed, would fall into a daydreaming, nonresponsive, wide-eyed gaze. He seemed unable to determine the relevant aspects of a situation and decode their meanings conventionally.

Stimulating situations disorganized his thinking, leading to heightened emotional arousal until he would explode in helpless anger. Although he seemed unaware of his contribution to interpersonal conflicts, he seemed to perceive at some level that most of his relationships were dysfunctional and unrewarding—a fact that undermined his self-esteem. His organizational difficulties were greatly exacerbated by anxiety, which would increase in proportion to his level of visual stimulation. His anxiety about relationships kept him more attentive to other people's feelings than most children with nonverbal learning disabilities. He was often unhappy and anxious, prone to mood fluctuations, and in need of reassurance. Although he was not good at understanding and responding to affective states in other children, he had some capacity to accommodate to adult emotional displays, perhaps because such expressions are more controlled and at times more obvious. He also had trouble expressing his own feelings.

SC115.5 *Social-Emotional Learning Disabilities*

Children with social-emotional learning disabilities have difficulties interacting with peers in groups. They are unable to be with other children even for brief periods of time without great distress; consequently, they rarely make friends, though they may interact reasonably with adults. They fail to "read" other people's body language, facial expressions, and vocal intonations, and are therefore socially inept. While they have many of the social features of children with nonverbal learning disabilities, they do not have the same cognitive or academic deficits.

These children appear unimpaired during their early development; it is only when they begin to interact with others that their problems emerge. Their self-help skills do not develop comparably to those of other children their age. Because they do not seem to know how to play with others, they are eventually excluded from social groups. Their consequent isolation deprives them further of opportunities to develop socially, and thus compounds their difficulties. Although they may have one or two individual friends, by adolescence they are typically rejected by peers and excluded from group activities.

The Subjective Experience of Social-Emotional Learning Disabilities in Childhood

Affective States

With respect to their affective states, children with social-emotional learning difficulties understand the world of emotions only intellectually. Feelings are like a foreign language. Only when their feelings reach a threshold of explosive intensity can they experience their own affective states. Most often, these are frustration, rage, and terror.

Thoughts and Fantasies

With respect to their thoughts and fantasies, these children seem to have a diminished capacity to develop a theory of mind. They seem unaware that others have beliefs, desires, and intentions. Consequently, they appear to disregard others' thoughts and feelings. Their capacity for pretense, whether imaginative play or intentional deception, is greatly limited.

Somatic States and Relationship Patterns

There are no typical somatic states that characterize children with social-emotional learning disabilities. In regard to relationships, for these children the world is unrewarding, unpredictable, and unintelligible. They try to memorize rules that would explain how people are supposed to behave, but then they are mystified as to when these rules apply and when they do not. They long for contact with others, yet when they occasionally make efforts to befriend someone, they are disappointed at being met with indifference. For reasons inexplicable to them, their relationships fall apart. They appear immature or inappropriate and are socially disconnected when with others. Their behavior may become socially dysfunctional, as they become argumentative, disruptive, or disrespectful. They are not successful in maintaining peer relationships; have no close friendships; and are rejected, teased, or bullied by peers.

Clinical Illustration

A 9-year-old boy was somewhat awkward with ordinary social interactions; although he apparently had learned rules for behavior, he applied them so repeatedly and mechanically that they lost their meaning. He showed little emotional responsivity to social cues and jokes. Because of his difficulty in negotiating the reciprocal nature of play and other social interactions, he had few friends and was seldom included in games at school. His caregivers said that he was sometimes unresponsive when other children would speak to him; he talked mainly about his own interests and had problems changing topics. In addition, he asked inappropriate personal questions, made people uncomfortable by standing too close to them or touching them, failed to grasp abstract ideas, and took jokes too literally.

This boy could not always perceive and interpret situations as most others would. Sometimes his perceptions were accurate, but he would focus upon peripheral details. At other times, especially in complex situations, he would develop idiosyncratic interpretations of an occurrence, the factors leading up to it, and its meaning. His marked difficulty in reading other people's emotional expressions prevented his appreciating the impact of his behavior on others, and he seemed to lack feelings such as guilt and empathy that are predicated upon knowledge of others' feelings toward oneself.

SC12 Developmental Disorders

SC121 Regulatory Disorders

Each child has a unique pattern of regulating emotion and processing sensory stimuli. There is a broad continuum of functional variability expressing individual differences in children's healthy development of social, emotional, and intellectual functioning. Some children, however, have such aberrant response and regulation patterns that these significantly interfere with functioning at home, in school, and in relationships.

Regulatory disorders are generally recognizable in infancy or early childhood and may continue into latency or adolescence. They are described in the *Diagnostic Classifications of Mental Health and Developmental Disorders of Infancy and Early Childhood*, revised edition (DC: 0–3R; Zero to Three, 2005, pp. 28–34). For infants and toddlers, three subtypes are identified: (1) hypersensitive, (2) hyposensitive/underresponsive, and (3) sensory stimulation-seeking/impulsive. The hypersensitive category is subdivided into Type A, fearful/cautious, and Type B, negative/defiant. Identifying a child as having a particular subtype is difficult because in clinical practice children with mixed features are often encountered.

Regulatory–sensory processing disorders are described (with case illustrations) by the the Interdisciplinary Council on Developmental and Learning Disorders (ICDL) in its *Diagnostic Manual for Infancy and Early Childhood* (ICDL-DMIC; ICDL, 2005, pp. 73–112). These include sensory modulation challenges (Type I), sensory discrimination challenges (Type II), and sensory-based motor challenges (Type III). These regulatory–sensory processing variations can extend into the school years, affecting school performance. To diagnose a regulatory–sensory processing disorder, "both a distinct behavioral pattern and a sensory modulation, sensory-motor, sensory discrimination or attentional processing difficulty" must be present. See Chapter 10 for further discussions of these disorders.

Latency-age children with regulatory disorders may be hypersensitive to sounds, sight, and touch; seem easily distracted; and have problems with emotional regulation/modulation. Descriptions by parents and caregivers contribute to the diagnosis of regulatory disorders, and standardized assessments may yield signs of gross and fine motor skill difficulties. Sensory tolerance varies widely even across subtypes and variations. Long-term difficulties with social interactions and behavior problems may occur. While such disorders are thought to originate from multiple factors (e.g., endowment, temperament, and "parent–infant fit") physiological, parasympathetic, and neurological indicators of differences between typically developing children and those with regulatory disorders have been noted (e.g., in electrodermal activity, vagal tone, and white matter microstructure). Although studies in these areas have identified correlations, causation, including clear evidence of genetic links, remains undetermined. Children with prenatal exposure to teratogens (including drugs and alcohol), children with postnatal histories of trauma, and even some children with neurotic defensive inhibitions or ego restrictions may also show similar symptoms. They are also seen in children diagnosed with separation anxiety, ADHD, ODD, and autism spectrum disorder.

SC122 Feeding Problems of Childhood

Feeding behavior disorder in infancy and early childhood is described in DC: 0–3R (Zero to Three, 2005). In ICDL-DMIC (ICDL, 2005, pp. 73–112), eating disorder is included among interactive disorders, and eating problems are listed among regulatory–sensory processing disorders.

During infancy and toddlerhood, difficulties with eating may have physiological origins (e.g., pyloric stenosis, reflux, or other gastrointestinal difficulties). Even when such problems are rectified, residual apprehension in the child or the caregiver(s) may influence ongoing difficulties. Similarly, eating may lack pleasure for children with sensory over- or underresponsiveness and/or sensory discrimination challenges. For young children, food refusal (or vomiting) may follow a traumatic event. For children with such histories, eating difficulties and/or conflicts and/or a lack of pleasure associated with food intake may extend into the school years (and may continue to involve conflicted interactions with primary caregivers). Even without trauma histories, prelatency-age children may feel conflict about eating certain foods that they associate with particular animals or whose type or texture causes them disgust. Such feelings frequently resolve by middle childhood. Should they not, or should such conflicts reappear, intervention may prove necessary. When there is no history of difficulties in infancy or early childhood, and an eating or feeding problem emerges during latency, it is important to rule out a physiological cause or recent traumatic precipitant. If none is identified, and if bulimia and anorexia nervosa are also ruled out, defensive inhibitions or ego restrictions may be suspected. Should the latter be determined, treatment considerations should involve the dynamics of eating for the child and family. Parental/caregiver behaviors may be contributory (e.g., parental insecurity about being a "nurturer," family or marital discord, patterns of parental eating difficulties) and should be evaluated.

SC123 Elimination Disorders

Elimination disorders in infancy and early childhood are described in more detail in Chapter 10 (pp. 641–643). In ICDL-DMIC (ICDL, 2005, pp. 73–112), elimination disorder is included among interactive disorders, and elimination problems are listed among regulatory–sensory processing disorders.

Elimination disorders include encopresis and enuresis. A distinction is made between a "primary" form (in which mastery of urinary or bowel control has never been achieved) and a "secondary" form (in which mastery has been attained but later is lost). Some children who have poor sensory responsiveness (e.g., low muscle tone) or sequencing or motor planning challenges, or who are overresponsive and/or crave greater sensory stimulation, may be delayed in attaining elimination mastery. Young children experiencing conflicts with affects—both quality and quantity (including conflicts with control, aggression, shame, and/or guilt, vacillating with feelings of insecurity and/or inadequacy)—may also be delayed in attaining mastery. For such children, episodes of withholding (feces and/or urine) may occur, as may episodes of noncontrol. Conflicts in relationships with caregivers are often observed. Such conflicts may have contributed to an elimination disorder and/or may be responsive to it.

When primary enuresis or encopresis extends into latency or middle childhood, even in instances when regulatory–sensory processing challenges are felt to be contributory, work with parents to support patience, understanding, and empathy can prove helpful. A critical reason for working with parents is that dynamic problems between parents and children with elimination disorders can intensify. Parental expressions of frustration and anger can contribute to reduced self-esteem in a child, but they may also provide some secondary gratification in the form of attention.

Working with parents is equally important in situations where an elimination disorder has emerged in a child with previous bladder and bowel mastery. In such a secondary elimination disorder, it is important to rule out physical or medical causes, as well as to check for trauma. If such precipitants can be eliminated, the emergence of enuretic or encopretic symptoms may be understood as a regressive response to a developmental (often unconscious) conflict within the child and/or conflicts within the child's environment (marital/parental discord, alteration in life circumstances, including separation, loss, bereavement, etc.). In their secondary form, elimination disorders (especially enuresis) are more frequently nocturnal. Secondary encopresis often takes the form of "soiling," which results in fecal staining of clothing, caused by the intermittent release of small amounts of feces that may also be drawn back up into the rectum. This pattern may symbolize ambivalence in the child and/or may relate to conflicts over affects and impulses, particularly aggression.

Both enuresis and encopresis are more common among younger children, with steadily decreasing frequency as they age. It is at younger ages that instances of "spontaneous cure" are more often reported. At all ages, males are more frequently diagnosed than females, and co-occurrence of enuresis with hyperactivity in males has been noted.

SC123.1 *Encopresis*

Please refer to the discussion of encopresis in Chapter 10's section on elimination disorders.

SC123.2 *Enuresis*

Please refer to the discussion of enuresis in Chapter 10's section on elimination disorders.

SC124 Sleep–Wake Disorders

Difficulties with sleeping are common in infancy and childhood. Many factors can contribute to problems in the establishment of healthy sleep patterns. Sleeping difficulties can result from a variety of stresses and can also reflect difficulties with attachment and separation. Trauma, anxiety, depression, and adjustment to different transitions may be contributing factors as well. Sensory overresponsivity, along with self-regulation problems, are sometimes components of sleep difficulties. Psychosocial considerations, especially family dynamics and the family culture around sleep, can be further elements in a sleep problem. Sleep difficulties can be quite subjective.

Three types of frequently seen sleep disturbances are insomnia, nightmares, and night terrors. Each of these difficulties may be part of other presenting problems with a child. These difficulties are often not part of the presenting picture and only come to light during a clinical interview with the parents or the child. Such disorders typically result in compromised functioning in different areas and have been linked to poor daytime behavior, anxiety, and depression.

Insomnia

Insomnia can be expressed in a variety of ways. A child may experience difficulty in falling asleep or maintaining sleep. Early morning awakenings without the ability to fall back asleep can be a problem. Children often go into their parents' bedroom to resume sleep. Again, these difficulties can be somewhat subjective; factors such as family culture and interference in daytime functioning are relevant considerations in determining the presence of a disorder. Insomnia may last for a few nights and be self-limiting or may persist in the long term.

Nightmares

Nightmares involve the repeated occurrence of intensely felt dreams, vividly experienced and remembered, which usually involve threats to one's survival or physical integrity. A child is usually oriented and alert quickly after waking.

Sleep Terror Disorders (Night Terrors)

Night terrors typically occur in children between ages 3 and 12. They usually happen later in the nighttime sleep cycle. Night terrors are distinguished from nightmares in that they are not well remembered, and a dreamer often cannot be awakened when in the throes of the experience.

These episodes may be characterized by intense fear and crying while the child is asleep. Elevated heart rate and dilated pupils are common physical reactions during night terrors. While night terrors may be quite frightening to the family, they are not inherently harmful events. Stressful life events, sleep deprivation, fever, and medications may contribute to their occurrence.

SC125 Attachment Disorders

Attachment disorders connote a distinct class of adjustment difficulties—namely, problematic behavior underpinned by core deficits in self and social development, seemingly specific to children growing up in, or removed from, contexts of impersonal institutional rearing or chronically maltreating environments. The disturbed behaviors characteristic of attachment disorders are assumed to be responses to extreme deviations from average expectable environments. Most institutional rearing (given its regimentation, high child-to-caregiver ratios, multiple shifts, and frequent changes of caregivers) deprives children of reciprocal interactions with stable caregivers and thus involves structural neglect. Many studies have shown that children growing up in orphanages are at risk in various domains of functioning, including physical, social-emotional, and cognitive development.

Catch-up rates by children adopted into families after early institutional rearing have been studied extensively, and meta-analytic reviews have been published (Juffer & van IJzendoorn, 2009; van IJzendoorn & Juffer, 2006). The results suggest that catch-up is usually observed first in the domain of physical development, with children assuming a place on normal growth curves within 6 months of receiving appropriate nutrition and stimulation. Developmental catch-up typically takes longer in the domain of cognition, with some persisting language and cognitive delays evident for years in a substantial group of children adopted out of institutions.

The DSM-IV-R (American Psychiatric Association, 2000) criteria for reactive attachment disorder (RAD) stipulated that it:

- Must be differentiated from pervasive developmental disorders.
- Is likely to occur in relation to abusive or impoverished child care.
- Has an age of onset before 5 years.
- Involves markedly disturbed and developmentally inappropriate social relatedness.

RAD was split into two subtypes, inhibited and disinhibited. The inhibited subtype was characterized by hypervigilant, excessively inhibited, highly ambivalent, and contradictory responses to attachment figures. The disinhibited subtype described children with diffuse attachments, marked by indiscriminate sociability and inability to make appropriate selective attachments. These children would go still or frozen on reunion with a caregiver, and appear flat and frightened emotionally in that person's presence. Yet these children (judged to have a disorganized attachment style) would often, either on their own or with a stranger, become animated and even playful. Zeanah and Gleason (2010) proposed changes to the RAD diagnosis that have been incorporated into DSM-5, which now distinguishes two separate syndromes with distinctive phenotypic characteristics, correlates, course, and response to intervention, despite their close connection as deriving from pathogenic care. The disinhibited type, often referred to as showing indiscriminate friendliness, is now termed disinhibited social engagement disorder (DSED), while the inhibited type retains the name of RAD. In the latter case, a child is thought to best merit the RAD label in cases when a reliable and sensitive caregiver has become available, but the child appears to inhibit the usual response of forming a selective attachment. DSED occurs in children with and without selective attachment, even among children with secure attachments; it is also far more persistent over time and less amenable to intervention, which distinguishes it from RAD as defined by DSM-5.

Both RAD and DSED are relatively rare in the population at large, but are common among abandoned or previously institutionalized children. Although the overall prevalence of these disorders is less than 1% in the overall population, this figure soars to 40% or more when institutionalized children, radically deprived of consistent and sensitive early care, are later studied.

Clinical Illustrations

Case 1: Reactive Attachment Disorder

Susan was 3 years old when her parents sought help. She had been adopted from South America at the age of 18 months, having been, according to her parents, cared for in a well-run orphanage. Her parents were devoted and invested in their daughter's development. They described Susan as easygoing, eating and sleeping well, and enjoying social activities. However, they also described her as "sad at times or irritable for no apparent reason." When her parents attempted to comfort her at these times, she seemed to prefer being on her own and resisted their attempts. They tended to comply with what seemed her wish to be left alone and hoped that if they followed her lead, she would feel more comfortable and would eventually be more accepting of their care. The immediate impetus for seeking treatment was Susan's difficulty settling in at nursery school, where the staff described her as "a solitary child." Indeed, upon meeting Susan, it felt to the clinician as if she was a miniature adult who watched the clinician's every move, creating mutual uneasiness. Treatment focused on forging a therapeutic relationship (which came about slowly) by closely following her play, which most often included themes of mothers and babies. Over time, she was able to turn to her parents when she was distressed, but she continued to display a hypervigilant stance; her seeking of help or protection from adults was still constrained.

Case 2: Disinhibited Social Disengagement Disorder

Karl was a 6-year-old boy adopted from an Eastern European orphanage at age 3 by a couple who had previously adopted a girl and boy from Asia. Karl's parents described him as the "darling of the orphanage," who seemed to stand out among the nearly 100 children with his "sparkling eyes and ready smile." Karl entered the orphanage at age 6 months, when his substance-misusing teenage mother was deemed unfit to care for him. When his parents brought him home, they were struck by how readily he adapted, establishing seemingly close relationships with his adopted siblings and especially with both sets of grandparents. According to his parents, however, his behavior would swing from overly compliant (when he wanted something) to "creatively unkind" (when frustrated). His friendships with peers were characterized by intensely close and quick-forming relationships that would then fade, leaving Karl perplexed as to why no one wanted to play with him. In his cognitive evaluations, he performed in the above-average range, though with marked unevenness in his scores. He scored especially highly on the Wechsler block design subtest, and much lower on the comprehension subscale. In treatment, it first appeared easy to engage Karl, as his ability to play (most often with animal figures and small cars) was well organized; however, his play was rather concrete, and attempts to address the meaning of relationships, even in a displaced form, were often rebuffed. He had difficulty leaving a session or even saying goodbye to the therapist. Treatment progressed slowly, with nuanced changes mainly in his relationship with his father, who began to invest more effort in following Karl's lead in play or activities.

SC126 Autism Spectrum Disorders

SC126.1 *Autism*

Autism is a developmental disorder broadly affecting all areas of a child's development, including social relationships, language and communication, cognition, and sensory and motor functioning. The severity of this disorder varies widely in terms of its impact on thinking, relating, and communicating. Personality variations can be quite pronounced as well.

Deficits in social relationships and a circumscribed range of interests are hallmark features of this diagnostic group. Repetitive behavior in a circumscribed interest area is common. This category incorporates the full range of what was previously categorized as pervasive developmental disorders, including what DSM-5 refers to as autism spectrum disorder.

At one end of the spectrum are children who are dependent, show little capacity for attention and reciprocal interactions, and often seem in their "own world." They appear unresponsive to attempts to engage them. Intellectual and adaptive functioning are usually significantly compromised, with tested IQ scores below 70 and very poor self-care skills. Affective expression may be flat; they move clumsily and perseverate in their interests. These children are likely to require ongoing and highly specialized behavioral and educational programs with personal aides to help them manage in school settings. Progress is quite slow, and long-term prognosis is poor.

At the other end of the spectrum are children with what DSM-IV labeled as Asperger's disorder, and what we refer to as Asperger syndrome. Their overall functioning is compromised in many of the same areas, but it is also not too divergent from normal functioning. Distinguishing them from others on the autism spectrum are their intact intelligence and the nature of their communication difficulties, which are considerably more circumscribed (e.g., prosody, tone, missing subtleties) than is the case for typical same-age children.

Children diagnosed with Asperger syndrome are often described as "odd" or "quirky." They typically have friends and often relate well to adults, but they miss many social cues, including nonverbal signifiers essential to reciprocal relating. Many can eventually function fairly independently as adults, working and living on their own.

All the disorders in this category are thought of as having a significant biological and constitutional genesis, although environment, including trauma and stress, are also relevant. Sensory and motor functioning is significantly compromised, and many of these children have language delays (or regressions) and sensorimotor integration difficulties, including tactile and other sensory sensitivities. They sometimes crave stimulation; at other times, they seem completely unresponsive to stimulation.

DSM-5 has eliminated Asperger's disorder as a separate diagnostic entity. However, both before and since its publication, considerable research—including extensive meta-analyses (Kulage, Smaldone, & Cohn, 2014; Tsai, 2013; Tsai & Ghaziuddin, 2014)—has suggested that the distinction between Asperger's disorder/Asperger syndrome and high-functioning autism (HFA) is real, measurable, and valid.

Researchers have explored both quantitative and qualitative ways in which individuals with HFA and those with Asperger syndrome can be distinguished. Many have cited the lack of early language delay in Asperger syndrome; such delay is present and significant in HFA. Noterdaeme, Wriedt, and Höhne (2010) and others have noted the higher verbal IQ in Asperger syndrome. Woodbury-Smith and Volkmar (2009) highlighted the consistent pattern of superior verbal IQ compared with performance IQ in Asperger syndrome, a pattern that seems reversed in HFA. Instead, the relationship between verbal and performance IQ in Asperger syndrome is very similar to the one observed in nonverbal learning difficulties. Finally, executive functioning has been studied with the Behavior Rating Inventory of Executive Function (BRIEF) to distinguish between the two diagnoses (Blijd-Hoogewys, Bezemer, & van Geert, 2014). This survey is hardly exhaustive.

The social/communication domain has seen considerable exploration, with some research highlighting greater social seeking behavior in Asperger syndrome in contrast with social isolation in HFA. Children with Asperger syndrome may be socially clumsy, but they tend to be much more interested is social relations than children with HFA; in fact, some have characterized Asperger syndrome as socially motivated autism. Conversational patterns have been studied, including variables such as topic management, gaze management, intonation, and reciprocity.

Although the current research is not unequivocal, it seems to us premature to eliminate the Asperger diagnosis. It continues to have considerable face validity. Existing research has been hampered by inconsistent starting definitions and diagnostic procedures, small sample sizes, and circular logic. At this juncture, it makes sense to treat Asperger syndrome as a valid diagnostic entity whose varied dimensions merit further study and delineation.

Clinical Illustration

A 6-year-old boy was diagnosed at age 3 by a developmental pediatrician as having autism. When he appeared for the update evaluation, he approached the examiner cautiously, with head down. His affect was flat, and his face lacked any expression. He did not make eye contact. He did, however, enter the examination room with little hesitation. He was intermittently responsive to requests from the examiner, but lacked any self-initiated interest in interaction. At times, his lack of response made it appear that he had not heard the question. He was motorically active, fidgety, and at times self-stimulating. Some hand flapping was noted. His overall presentation made valid administration of the Wechsler Intelligence Scale for Children impossible. His play seemed purposeless and random.

His developmental history was characterized by significant delays in language, motor functioning, and social interaction. He made no eye contact and had no comprehensible words until age 4, and gross motor milestones were all significantly delayed. His gait was awkward, and he seemed clumsy at simple gross motor tasks such as jumping, skipping, and hopping. Motor sequencing and planning were clearly compromised. At times, he seemed sensorily unresponsive; at other times, he seemed to seek sensory stimulation. He was difficult to soothe. He received in-home services from the local public Birth to Three program, including speech and language therapy, occupational therapy, and applied behavioral analysis. He was eventually evaluated by his school district and placed in a specialized preschool program, and subsequently a special program for kindergarten. He had a one-on-one aide with him in the classroom, and other school accommodations that were expected to continue throughout his school years.

SC126.2 Asperger Syndrome

As noted above, individuals diagnosed with Asperger syndrome are often described as "odd" or "quirky." Their difficulties in social relationships and communication, though present and apparent, are more subtle than those seen in HFA. These children may have friends and often relate well to adults, but miss many social cues that are essential to reciprocal social interaction. Many of these individuals may be able to function fairly independently as adults in terms of working and living on their own. Again, although DSM-5 has eliminated Asperger's disorder as a separate diagnosis, we feel that it remains real, measurable, and valid as an entity distinct from HFA. See the discussion of HFA versus Asperger syndrome above for more details.

Clinical Illustration

A 6-year-old boy greeted the examiner with a smile and had no difficulty separating from his mother to enter the evaluation room; in fact, he barely noticed the separation. He made erratic eye contact and seemed, at least superficially, to be interpersonally related. He was chatty and a bit anxious. Most of his scores on intelligence and development assessments fell into the average range. Verbal intelligence was stronger than nonverbal intelligence. He spoke in a sing-song voice.

He was responsive to directions and suggestions from the examiner, but he did not seek or seem to welcome external involvement. His play was active, and he was more than happy to play by himself. In general, his mood was upbeat. He showed some nonverbal cues associated with reciprocal relating, but was not able to sustain ongoing dialogue in a meaningful way. Conversation quickly deteriorated into a monologue. During the evaluation, he played with a variety of objects, including cars, animals, and cooking items. He could stick with play materials for a while and did not appear too distracted. His activity generally consisted of organizing the materials. For example, he lined up the cars, broke down the lineup, and then lined them up again in a ritualized, perseverative manner. He did not use the cars symbolically in his play.

His developmental history was characterized by limited ability to participate in routine, reciprocal social interactions. He displayed little empathy, seeming self-absorbed and unaware of his impact on others. He was described as overresponsive to sound and touch and as highly active. He had low muscle tone. He made self-stimulatory sounds while lining up his cars. He disliked changes in his routines. His parents found his memory for certain facts remarkable. Because of his unusual behaviors, his pediatrician referred him for early intervention. He received ongoing in-home services and was eventually diagnosed by a developmental pediatrician as having Asperger syndrome.

With continual help, the boy began to seem less eccentric, though not entirely without some quirky behavior. He made better eye contact, could sustain longer social interactions, and became an expert on car brands and models. He related adequately, if superficially, to peers and did well academically in his regular classroom. On weekends, he had few play dates and showed no interest in having them.

SCApp Appendix: Psychological Experiences That May Require Clinical Attention

For issues relevant to demographic minority populations, see Chapter 6 (pp. 440–442).

SCApp3 Gender Incongruence

Gender incongruence with early onset in childhood differs from gender incongruence that first appears in adolescence and adulthood. Most children with gender incongruence do not grow up to be transgender; most (termed "desisters") grow up to be gay, bisexual, and cisgender (non-transgender) adults. A few may become heterosexual, cisgender adults. When childhood gender dysphoria continues into adolescence ("persisters"), individuals may undergo puberty suppression and then later seek cross-hormonal and surgical treatment. In some cases, gender incongruence desists after puberty suppression, treatment is stopped, and the child goes on to have a delayed puberty. Incongruence with late onset (adolescence) is unlikely to desist; gender reassignment is often the treatment of choice.

Gender incongruence designations are controversial, and in childhood they are even more so. While there is almost universal support among clinical experts for retaining adolescent and adult diagnoses as a means of obtaining access to health care, opinions are divided regarding retention of the child diagnosis. Some argue that gender incongruence or gender variance (both nonpathologizing terms) is not a mental disorder and that all the gender diagnoses should be expunged, as homosexuality was in the past. This position regards a diagnosis in childhood as unnecessarily stigmatizing and fulfilling no medical need. Those who support retaining a child diagnosis argue that while gender-incongruent children do not need medical treatment, they and their families often require considerable psychosocial support from mental health professionals.

Clinical approaches to treating prepubescent children with gender incongruence are also controversial and may vary, depending on the protocols of a particular clinic and the wishes of a child's parents. One traditional approach involves working with the child and caregivers to lessen dysphoria over gender incongruence and decrease cross-gender behaviors and identification. The assumption is that this decreases the likelihood that incongruence will persist into adolescence and culminate in adult transsexualism, which is considered an undesirable outcome both because of social stigma and because of the risks and costs of likely hormonal and surgical procedures. Since many children's gender incongruence desists without interventions, critics of this approach say there is no empirical evidence that such treatment reduces the rate of persistence and prevents adult transsexualism. They liken it to "reparative therapy," a term for efforts to change homosexuality in adults or prevent it in "prehomosexual" children.

An alternative approach, pioneered by the Dutch, makes no direct effort to lessen gender incongruence or gender-atypical behaviors. As incongruence diagnosed in childhood usually does not persist into adolescence, and there are no reliable markers to predict in whom it will or will not persist, there is no therapeutic target with respect to gender identity outcome. The developmental trajectory of gender identity is allowed to unfold naturally, without anyone's pursuing or encouraging a specific outcome. Puberty suppression is offered to those children who become anxious about impending body changes, but full social transition is done only after a puberty-suppressed child's gender incongruence persists. Critics of this approach fault it for not allowing social transition in childhood.

A third approach affirms a child's cross-gender identification by social (not medical) transitioning to a cross-gendered role, also with the option of endocrine treatment at puberty to suppress the development of unwanted secondary sex characteristics. This approach eschews diagnoses, referring to the children simply as gender-variant. Proponents assume that children who make the transition can revert to their originally assigned gender if incongruence desists, since the transition is made solely at a social level and without medical intervention. Critics believe that supporting gender transition in childhood increases the likelihood of persistence and of a lifetime of medical treatment, and also downplays the complexity of transitioning back to the natal gender in a child whose incongruence desists.

In DSM-IV-TR, having a disorder of sexual development was an exclusionary criterion for making a gender identity disorder diagnosis (as it was then called). DSM-5 recognizes, in contrast, that some intersex children develop what it now calls gender dysphoria; it has added a fifth-digit specifier for patients with both dysphoria and disorders of sexual development.

The Subjective Experience of Gender Incongruence in Childhood

Gender incongruence is characterized by marked and persistent lack of alignment between an individual's subjectively experienced gender and birth-assigned (natal) gender. Some children reject their assigned gender as early as age 2. DSM-5 requires six out of eight criterion A symptoms for a diagnosis of gender dysphoria in childhood, including wanting strongly to be the other gender or declarating that one is the other gender. This A1 requirement is intended to distinguish children with gender dysphoria from those who merely have gender-atypical interests, such as playing with other-sex playmates or preferring the toys and activities associated with children of the other gender.

Affective States

Affective states include anxious and depressed moods, usually from frustration of the child's efforts to play or identify as the nonassigned gender. It is standard practice in gender identity clinics to evaluate children for comorbid anxiety and depression.

An inability to express the child's experienced gender may lead to rage directed at the child's own body or at external factors or individuals seen as obstructing gender expression. Children generally report satisfaction and pleasure when permitted, either privately or publicly, to express their experienced gender.

Thoughts and Fantasies

Cognitive patterns include preoccupations with gender, bordering on the obsessional. Young children are less likely to verbally express anatomic dysphoria. Autism spectrum disorder may be present in children presenting with gender incongruence.

Somatic States

Somatic states are characterized by discomfort with the natal body. Only a small minority of young children openly express discomfort with their sexual anatomy or state the desire to change their gender. Expressions of gender incongruence are more commonly behavioral; for example, natal boys may insist on urinating in a sitting position, while natal girls may urinate standing up.

Relationship Patterns

Relationship patterns vary. Children may encounter social difficulties as they try to balance their own experienced gender with the gender expectations of their peers. Gender-atypical interests may lead to social isolation.

Clinical Illustration

A 4-year-old natal boy, healthy and with no disorders of sexual development, had been trying on his mother's jewelry and shoes since age 2. He often wore a towel as a skirt and colored his fingernails with crayons. When told not to do so, he would cry and become withdrawn. He preferred playing with girls and avoided roughhousing with boys. The father discouraged his cross-gender interests; the mother saw them as a harmless, passing phase. She thought he might grow up to be gay, which was not a problem for her. After the boy kept insisting on sitting while urinating and hiding his penis, tensions between the parents about the "proper" response increased. They researched the various clinical approaches online and discussed them with their pediatrician. Neither wished to have the child make the social transition to being a girl (involving a name change and using the girl's bathroom at school). Although the father would have preferred consulting a clinic that discouraged cross-gender behaviors, he acquiesced to his wife's wish to follow a more permissive path that would help them come to terms with the child's cross-gender interests without a social transition.

TABLE 9.2. Concordance of PDM-2 and ICD-10/DSM-5 Diagnostic Criteria for Children

PDM-2
SC0 Healthy responses
SC01 Developmental crises
SC02 Situational crises

PDM-2	
SC2 Mood disorders	
SC22 Depressive disorders	
SC24 Bipolar disorder	
SC27 Suicidality	
SC29 Prolonged mourning/grief reaction	
ICD-10	**DSM-5**
F30–39. Mood (affective) disorders	Depressive disorders
F32. Depressive episode	F32. Major depressive disorder
F33. Recurrent depressive disorder	F34.1. Persistent depressive disorder (dysthymia)
F34. Persistent mood [affective] disorders	F34.8. Disruptive mood dysregulation disorder
F31. Bipolar affective disorder	Bipolar and related disorders
F92.0. Depressive conduct disorder	*Conditions for further study.* Suicidal behavior disorder
	Conditions for further study. Persistent complex bereavement disorder

PDM-2	
SC3 Disorders related primarily to anxiety	
SC31 Anxiety disorders	
SC31.1 Phobias	
SC32 Obsessive–compulsive and related disorders	
SC32.1 Obsessive–compulsive disorder	
ICD-10	**DSM-5**
F40–48. Neurotic, stress-related, and somatoform disorders	Anxiety disorders
F41.1. Generalized anxiety disorder	F41.1. Generalized anxiety disorder
F42. Obsessive–compulsive disorder	F40.2x. Specific phobias
F93.1. Phobic anxiety disorder of childhood	Obsessive–compulsive and related disorders
NB: Phobic anxiety disorder of childhood is included in F90–98. Behavioral and emotional disorders with onset usually occurring in childhood and adolescence.	F42. Obsessive–compulsive disorder

PDM-2	
SC4 Event- and stressor-related disorders	
SC41 Trauma- and stressor-related disorders	
SC41.1 Adjustment disorders (other than developmental)	
ICD-10	**DSM-5**
F43. Reaction to severe stress, and adjustment disorders	Trauma- and stressor-related disorders
F43.1. Posttraumatic stress disorder	F43.1. Posttraumatic stress disorder (includes posttraumatic stress disorder for children 6 years and younger)
F43.2 Adjustment disorders	F43.2. Adjustment disorders

(continued)

TABLE 9.2. *(continued)*

PDM-2	
SC5 Somatic symptom and related disorders SC51 Somatic symptom disorder	
ICD-10	**DSM-5**
F45. Somatoform disorders F45.0. Somatization disorder	Somatic symptom and related disorders F45.1. Somatic symptom disorder
PDM-2	
SC8 Psychophysiological disorders SC81 Feeding and eating disorders SC81.1 Anorexia nervosa SC81.2 Bulimia nervosa	
ICD-10	**DSM-5**
F50. Eating disorders F50.0. Anorexia nervosa F50.2. Bulimia nervosa	Feeding and eating disorders F50.0–.02. Anorexia nervosa F50.2. Bulimia nervosa
PDM-2	
SC9 Disruptive behavior disorders SC91 Conduct disorder SC92 Oppositional defiant disorder SC93 Substance-related disorders	
ICD-10	**DSM-5**
F90–98. Behavioral and emotional disorders with onset usually occurring in childhood and adolescence F91. Conduct disorders F91.3. Oppositional defiant disorder F10–19. Mental and behavioral disorders due to psychoactive substance use	Disruptive, impulse-control, and conduct disorders F91.1. Conduct disorder (childhood-onset type) F91.3. Oppositional defiant disorder Substance-related and addictive disorders
PDM-2	
SC11 Disorders of mental functioning SC111 Motor skills disorders SC112 Tic disorders SC113 Psychotic disorders SC114 Neuropsychological disorders SC114.1 Visual–spatial processing disorders SC114.2 Language and auditory processing disorders SC114.3 Memory impairments SC114.4 Attention-deficit/hyperactivity disorder SC114.5 Executive function difficulties SC114.6 Severe cognitive deficits SC115 Learning disorders SC115.1 Reading disorders SC115.2 Mathematics disorders SC115.3 Disorders of written expression SC115.4 Nonverbal learning disabilities SC115.5 Social-emotional learning disabilities	

(continued)

TABLE 9.2. *(continued)*

ICD-10	DSM-5
F82. Specific developmental disorder of motor function	Motor disorders F82. Developmental coordination disorder
F95. Tic disorders	Tic disorders
F95.1. Chronic motor or vocal tic disorder	F95.1. Persistent (chronic) motor or vocal tic disorder
F95.2. Combined vocal and multiple motor tic disorder (de la Tourette's syndrome)	F95.2. Tourette's disorder
F20–29. Schizophrenia, schizotypal and delusional disorders	Schizophrenia spectrum and other psychotic disorders
F80. Specific developmental disorders of speech and language	Communication disorders F80.9. Language disorder
F80.0. Specific speech articulation disorder	F80.0. Speech sound disorder
F80.1. Expressive language disorder	
F80.2. Receptive language disorder	
F90.0. Disturbance of activity and attention	F90. Attention-deficit/hyperactivity disorder
F70–79. Mental retardation	F70–79. Intellectual disability (intellectual developmental disorder)
F81. Specific developmental disorders of scholastic skills	F81. Specific learning disorder
F81.0. Specific reading disorder	F81.0. With impairments in reading
F81.2. Specific disorder of arithmetical skills	F81.2. With impairments in mathematics
F81.1. Specific spelling disorder	F81.81. With impairments in written expression

PDM-2

SC12 Developmental disorders
- SC121 Regulatory disorders
- SC122 Feeding problems of childhood
- SC123 Elimination disorders
  - SC123.1 Encopresis
  - SC123.2 Enuresis
- SC124 Sleep disorders
- SC125 Attachment disorders
- SC126 Pervasive developmental disorders
  - SC126.1 Autism
  - SC126.2 Asperger syndrome

ICD-10	DSM-5
F98.2. Feeding disorder of infancy and childhood	F98. Elimination disorders
F98.0. Nonorganic enuresis	F98.0. Enuresis
F98.1. Nonorganic encopresis	F98.1. Encopresis
F51. Nonorganic sleep disorders	Sleep–wake disorders
F51.0. Nonorganic insomnia	G47.00. Insomnia disorder
F51.4. Sleep terrors (night terrors)	F51.4. Non-rapid eye movement sleep arousal disorder, sleep terror type
F51.5. Nightmares	F51.5. Nightmare disorder
F94. Disorders of social functioning with onset specific to childhood and adolescence	Trauma- and stressor-related disorders F94.1. Reactive attachment disorder
F94.1. Reactive attachment disorder of childhood	F94.2. Disinhibited social engagement disorder
F84. Pervasive developmental disorders	F84.0. Autism spectrum disorder
F84.0. Childhood autism	
F84.5. Asperger's syndrome	
F84.8. Other pervasive developmental disorders	

(continued)

TABLE 9.2. *(continued)*

PDM-2	
SCApp Appendix: Psychological experiences that may require clinical attention SCApp3 Gender incongruence	
ICD-10	**DSM-5**
F64.2. Gender identity disorder of childhood	F64.2. Gender dysphoria in children

BIBLIOGRAPHY

General Bibliography

American Psychiatric Association. (2000). *Diagnostic and statistical manual of mental disorders* (4th ed., text rev.). Washington, DC: Author.

American Psychiatric Association. (2013). *Diagnostic and statistical manual of mental disorders* (5th ed.). Arlington, VA: Author.

Interdisciplinary Council on Developmental and Learning Disorders (ICDL). (2005). *Diagnostic manual for infancy and early childhood*. Bethesda, MD: Author.

Panksepp, J., & Biven, L. (2012). *The archaeology of mind*. New York: Norton.

World Health Organization. (1992). *The ICD-10 classification of mental and behavioural disorders: Clinical descriptions and diagnostic guidelines*. Geneva: Author.

Zero to Three. (2005). *Diagnostic classification of mental health and developmental disorders of infancy and early childhood* (rev. ed.). Washington, DC: Zero to Three Press.

SC0 Healthy Response

Freud, A. (1965). *The writings of Anna Freud: Vol. 6. Normality and pathology in childhood: Assessments of development*. New York: International Universities Press.

Hartmann, H. (1939). Psycho-analysis and the concept of mental health. *International Journal of Psycho-Analysis, 20*, 308–321.

SC2 Mood Disorders

SC22 *Depressive Disorders*

Barish, K. (2006). On the role of reparative processes in childhood: Pathological development and therapeutic change. *Journal of Infant, Child, and Adolescent Psychotherapy, 5*, 92–110.

Bhardwaj, A., & Goodyer, I. M. (2009). Depression and allied illness in children and adolescents: Basic facts. *Psychoanalytic Psychotherapy, 23*, 176–184.

Birmaher, D., & Brent, D. (2007). Practice parameter for the assessment and treatment of children and adolescents with depressive disorders. *Journal of the American Academy of Child and Adolescent Psychiatry, 46*, 1503–1526.

Costello, A., Mustillo, A., Erkanli, A., Keeler, A., & Angold, A. (2003). Prevalence and development of psychiatric disorders in childhood and adolescence. *Archives of General Psychiatry, 60*, 837–844.

Dunn, I. M., & Goodyer, I. M. (2006). Longitudinal investigation into childhood and adolescence onset depression: Psychiatric outcome in early adulthood. *British Journal of Psychiatry, 188*, 216–222.

Nolen-Hoeksema, S. (2000). The role of rumination in depressive disorders and mixed anxiety/depressive symptoms. *Journal of Abnormal Psychology, 109*, 504–511.

Scourfild, P., Rice, P., Thapar, P., Harold, P., & McGuffin, P. (2003). Depressive symptoms in children and adolescents: Changing etiological influences with development. *Journal of Child Psychology and Psychiatry, 44*, 968–976.

SC24 *Bipolar Disorders*

Adelson, S. (2010). Psychodynamics of hypersexuality in children and adolescents with bipolar disorder. *Journal of the American Academy of Psychoanalysis and Dynamic Psychiatry, 38*(1), 27–35.

Akiskal, H. S. (1998). The childhood roots of bipolar disorder. *Journal of Affective Disorders, 51*, 75–76.

Axelson, D., Birmaher, B., Strober, M., Gill, M. K.,Valeri, S., Chiappetta, L., . . . Keller, M. (2006).

Phenomenology of children and adolescents with bipolar spectrum disorders. *Archives of General Psychiatry, 63*, 1139–1148.

Axelson, D., Findling, R. L., Fristad, M. A., Kowatch, R. A., Youngstram, E. A., Horwitz, S. M., . . . Birmaher, B. (2012). Examining the proposed disruptive mood dysregulation disorder diagnosis in the Longitudinal Assessment of Manic Symptoms Study. *Journal of Clinical Psychiatry, 10*, 1342–1350.

Birmaher, B. (2013). Bipolar disorder in children and adolescents. *Child and Adolescent Mental Health, 18*(3), 140–148.

Faedda, G. I., Baldessarini, R. J., Glovinsky, I. P., & Austin, N. B. (2004). Pediatric bipolar disorder: Phenomenology and course of illness. *Bipolar Disorders, 6*, 305–313.

Henin, A., Biederman, J., Mick, E., Sachs, G. S., Hirshfield-Becker, D. R., Siegal, R. S., & Nierberg, A. A. (2005). Psychopathology in the offspring of parents with bipolar disorder: A controlled study. *Biological Psychiatry, 58*, 554–561.

Hunt, J., Birmaher, B., Leonard, M., Strober, M., Axelson, D., Ryan, N., & Keller, M. (2009). Irritability without elation in a large bipolar youth sample: Frequency and clinical description. *Journal of the American Academy of Child and Adolescent Psychiatry, 48*, 730–739.

McClellan, J., Kowatch, R., Findling, R. L., & Work Group on Quality Issues. (2007). Practice parameters for the assessment and treatment of children and adolescents with bipolar disorders. *Journal of the American Academy of Child and Adolescent Psychiatry, 46*(1), 107–125.

Youngstrom, E. A., Birmaher, B., Axelson, D., Williamson, D. E., & Findling, R. L. (2008). Pediatric bipolar disorder: Validity, phenomenology, and recommendations for diagnosis. *Bipolar Disorders, 10*, 194–214.

SC27 *Suicidality*

Brent, D. A. (2011). Preventing youth suicide: Time to ask how. *Journal of the American Academy of Child and Adolescent Psychiatry, 50*(8), 738–740.

Bruffaerts, R., Demyttenaere, K., Borges, G., Haro, J. M., Chiu, W. T., Hwang, I., . . . Nock, M. K. (2010). Childhood adversities as risk factors for onset and persistence of suicidal behavior. *British Journal of Psychiatry, 197*(1), 20–27.

Cavanagh, J. T., Carson, A. J., Sharpe, M., & Lawrie, S. M. (2003). Psychological autopsy studies of suicide: A systematic review. *Psychological Medicine, 33*(3), 395–405.

Gureje, O., Oladeji, B., Borges, G., Bruffaerts, R., Haro, J. M., Hwang, I., . . . Nock, M. K. (2011). Parental psychopathology and the risk of suicidal behavior in their offspring: Results from the World Mental Health surveys. *Molecular Psychiatry, 16*, 1221–1233.

Nock, M. K. (2012). Future directions for the study of suicide and self-injury. *Journal of Clinical Child and Adolescent Psychology, 41*(2), 255–259.

Nock, M. K., Borges, G., Bromet, E. J., Alonso, J., Angermeyer, M., Beautrais, A., . . . Williams, D. (2008). Cross national prevalence and risk factors for suicidal ideation, plans, and attempts. *British Journal of Psychiatry, 192*(2), 98–105.

Nock, M. K., & Kessler, R. C. (2006). Prevalence of and risk factors for suicide attempts versus suicide gestures: Analysis of the National Comorbidity Survey. *Journal of Abnormal Psychology, 115*(3), 616–623.

Spence, M. K. (1995). Children's concept of death. *Michigan Family Review, 1*(1), 57–69.

SC29 *Prolonged Mourning/Grief Reaction*

American Psychiatric Association. (2012). Proposed criteria for the persistent complex bereavement-related disorder. Retrieved from *www.dsm5.org/ProposedRevison/Pages/proposedrevision.aspx?rid=577.*

Brown, E. J., Amaya-Jackson, L., Cohen, J., Handel, S., Thiel De Bocanergra, H., Zatta, E., . . . Mannarino, A. (2008). Childhood traumatic grief: A multi-site empirical examination of the construct and its correlates. *Death Studies, 32*, 899–923.

Dowdney, L. (2000). Childhood bereavement following parental death. *Journal of Child Psychology and Psychiatry, 41*(7), 819–830.

Harris, T., Brown, G. W., & Bifulco, A. (1986). Loss of parent in childhood and adult psychiatric disorder: The role of adequate parental care. *Psychological Medicine, 16*, 641–659.

Kaplow, J. B., Howell, K. H., & Layne, C. M. (2014). Do circumstances of the death matter?: Identifying socio-environmental risks for grief-related psychopathology in bereaved youth. *Journal of Traumatic Stress, 27*(1), 42–49.

Kaplow, J. B., Layne, C. M., Pynoos, R. S., Cohen, J. A., & Lieberman, A. (2012). DSM-V diagnostic criteria for bereavement-related disorders in children and adolescents: Developmental considerations. *Psychiatry, 75*(3), 243–265.

Kaplow, J. B., Prossin, A. R., Shapiro, D., Wardecker, B., & Adelson, J. (2011). Cortisol, posttraumatic stress, and maladaptive grief reactions in parentally bereaved children. In J. B. Kaplow (Chair),

Cortisol and mental health out-comes in infants and children. Symposium presented at the 58th Annual Meeting of the American Academy of Adolescent and Child Psychiatry, Toronto, ON, Canada.

Layne, C. M., Beck, C. J., Rimmasch, H., Southwick, J. S., Moreno, M. A., & Hobfoll, S. E. (2009). Promoting "resilient" posttraumatic adjustment in childhood and beyond: "Unpacking" life events, adjustment trajectories, resources, and interventions. In D. Brom, R. Pat-Horenczyk & J. Ford (Eds.), *Treating traumatized children: Risk, resilience, and recovery* (pp. 13–47). New York: Routledge.

Lieberman, A. F., Compton, N. C., Van Horn, P., & Ghosh Ippen, C. (2003). *Losing a parent to death in the early years: Guidelines for the treatment of traumatic bereavement in infancy and early childhood.* Washington, DC: Zero to Three Press.

Nader, K. O., & Layne, C. M. (2009). Maladaptive grief in children and adolescents: Discovering developmentally linked differences in the manifestation of grief. *Stress Points, 23*(5), 12–15.

Shapiro, D. N., Howell, K. H., & Kaplow, J. B. (2014). Associations among mother-child communication: Quality, childhood maladaptive grief, and depressive symptoms. *Death Studies, 38*(1–5), 172–178.

Shear, M. K., Simon, N., Wall, M., Zisook, S., Neimeyer, R., Duan, N., . . . Keshaviah, A. (2011). Complicated grief and related bereavement issues for DSM-5. *Depression and Anxiety, 28*(2), 103–117.

Spence, M. K. (1995). Children's concept of death. *Michigan Family Review, 1*(1), 57–69.

SC3 Disorders Related Primarily to Anxiety

SC31 *Anxiety Disorders*

Beesdo, K., Knappe, S., & Pine, D. S. (2009). Anxiety and anxiety disorders in children and adolescents: Developmental issues and implications for DSM-V. *Psychiatric Clinics of North America, 32*(3), 483–524.

Beesdo, K., Lau, J. Y. F., Guyer, A. E., McClure-Tone, E. B., Monk, C. S., Nelson, E. E., . . . Pine, D. S., (2009). Common and distinct amygdala function perturbations in depressed vs. anxious adolescents. *Archives General of Psychiatry, 66*(3), 275–285.

Biederman, J., Rosenbaum, J. F., Bolduc-Murphy, E. A., Faraone, S., Chaloff, J., Hirschfeld, D. R., & Kagan, J. (1993). Behavioral inhibition as a temperamental risk factor for anxiety disorders. *Child and Adolescent Psychiatric Clinics of North America, 2*, 667–684.

Chorpita, B. (2001). Control and the development of negative emotions. In M. W. Vasey & M. R. Dadds (Eds.), *The developmental psychopathology of anxiety* (pp. 112–142). New York: Oxford University Press.

Freud, S. (1926). Inhibitions, symptoms, and anxiety. *Standard Edition, 20*, 77–178.

Higa-McMillan, C. K., Francis, S. E., & Chorpita, B. F. (2014). Anxiety disorders. In E. J. Mash & R. A. Barkley (Eds.), *Child psychopathology* (3rd ed., pp. 345–428). New York: Guilford Press.

Jovanovic, T., Nylocks, K. M., & Gamwell. K. L. (2013). Translational neuroscience measures of fear conditioning across development: Applications to high-risk children and adolescents. *Biology of Mood and Anxiety Disorders, 3*, 17.

Joyce, A. F. (2011). Interpretation and play: Some aspects of the process of child analysis. *Psychoanalytic Study of the Child, 65*, 152–168.

Knappe, S., Lieb, R., Beesdo, K., Fehm, L., Low, N. C. P., Gloster, A. T., & Wittchen, H. U. (2009). The role of parental psychopathology and family environment for social phobia in the first three decades of life. *Depression and Anxiety, 26*(4), 363–370.

Midgley, N., & Kennedy, E. (2011). Psychodynamic psychotherapy for children and adolescents: A critical review of the evidence base. *Journal of Child Psychotherapy, 37*(3), 232–260.

Ohman, A. (2000). Fear and anxiety: Evolutionary, cognitive, and clinical perspectives. In M. Lewis & J. M. Haviland-Jones (Eds.), *Handbook of emotions* (2nd ed., pp. 573–593). New York: Guilford Press.

Pine, D. S., Helfinslein, S. M., Bar–Haim, Y., Nelson, E., & Fox, N. A. (2009). Challenges in developing novel treatments for childhood disorders: Lessons from research on anxiety. *Neuropsychopharmacology, 34*(1), 213–228.

Reiss, S., Silverman, W., & Weems, C. (2001). Anxiety sensitivity. In M. W. Vasey & M. R. Dadds (Eds.), *The developmental psychopathology of anxiety* (pp. 92–111). New York: Oxford University Press.

SC31.1 *Phobias*

Beidel, D., & Turner, S. (1998). *Shy children, phobic adults: Nature and treatment of social phobia.* Washington, DC: American Psychological Association.

Freud, S. (1909). Analysis of a phobia in a five-year-old boy. *Standard Edition, 10*, 5–149.

Greenacre, P. (2010). The predisposition to anxiety: Part II. *Psychoanalytic Quarterly, 79*, 1075–1101.

Schneider, F. R., Blanco, C., Antia, S. X., & Liebowitz, M. R. (2002). The social anxiety spectrum. *Psychiatric Clinics of North America, 25*(4), 757–774.

Yorke, C., Wiseberg, S., & Freeman, T. (1989). *Development and psychopathology: Studies in psychoanalytic psychiatry*. New Haven, CT: Yale University Press.

SC32 Obsessive–Compulsive and Related Disorders

SC32.1 Obsessive–Compulsive Disorder

Chused, J. F. (1999). Obsessional manifestations in children. *Psychoanalytic Study of the Child, 54*, 219–232.

Esman, E. H. (1989). Psychoanalysis and general psychiatry: Obsessive–compulsive disorder as paradigm. *Journal of the American Psychoanalytic Association, 37*, 319–336.

Esman, E. H. (2001). Obsessive–compulsive disorder: Current views. *Psychoanalytic Inquiry, 21*, 145–156.

Freud, S. (1894). The neuro-psychoses of defence. *Standard Edition, 3*, 45–68.

Freud, S. (1907). Obsessive actions and religious practices. *Standard Edition, 9*, 117–127.

Freud, S. (1909). Notes upon a case of obsessional neurosis. *Standard Edition, 10*, 153–252.

Piacentini, J., Chang, S., Snorrason, I., & Woods, D. W. (2014). Obsessive–compulsive spectrum disorders. In E. J. Mash & R. A. Barkley (Eds.), *Child psychopathology* (3rd ed., pp. 429–475). New York: Guilford Press.

SC4 Event- and Stressor-Related Disorders

SC41 Trauma- and Stressor-Related Disorders

Bleiberg, E. (2001). *Treating personality disorders in children and adolescents: A relational approach*. New York: Guilford Press.

Briere, J., & Elliott, D. (1994). Immediate and long-term impacts of child sexual abuse. *The Future of Children, 4*, 54–69.

Cook, A., Spinazzola, J., Ford, J., Lanktree, C., Blaustein, M., Cloitre, M., & van der Kolk, B. (2005). Complex trauma in children and adolescents. *Psychiatric Annals, 35*, 390–398.

De Bellis, M. (2001). Developmental traumatology: The psychobiological development of maltreated children and its implication for research, treatment and policy. *Development and Psychopathology, 13*, 539–564.

Fellitti, V., Anda, R., Nordenberg, D., Williamson, D., Spitz, A., & Edwards, V. (1998). Relationship of childhood abuse and household dysfunction to many of the leading causes of death in adults: The Adverse Experiences (ACE) Study. *American Journal of Preventative Medicine, 14*(4), 245–258.

Foa, E. B., Keane, T. M., Friedman, M. J., & Cohen, J. A. (Eds.). (2009). *Effective treatments for PTSD* (2nd ed.). New York: Guilford Press.

Fonagy, P., Gergely, G., Jurist, E., & Target, M. (2002). *Affect regulation, mentalization, and the development of self.* New York: Other Press.

Furman, E. (1986). On trauma: When is the death of a parent traumatic? *Psychoanalytic Study of the Child, 41*, 191–208.

Furst, S. (1978). The stimulus barrier and the pathogenicity of trauma. *International Journal of Psychoanalysis, 59*, 345–352.

Hesse, E. (1999a). *Unclassifiable and disorganized responses in the Adult Attachment Interview and in the infant Strange Situation procedure: Theoretical proposals and empirical findings*. Unpublished doctoral dissertation, Leiden University, Leiden, The Netherlands.

Hesse, E. (1999b). The Adult Attachment Interview: Historical and current perspectives. In J. Cassidy & P. R. Shaver (Eds.), *Handbook of attachment: Theory, research, and clinical applications* (pp. 395–433). New York: Guilford Press.

Hesse, E., & Main, M. (1999). Second-generation effects of unresolved trauma in non-maltreating parents: Dissociated, frightened, and threatening parental behavior. *Psychoanalytic Inquiry, 19*, 481–540.

Jurist, E., Slade, A., & Bergner, S. (Eds.). (2008). *Mind to mind: Infant research, neuroscience and psychoanalysis*. New York: Other Press.

Kestenberg, J. S., & Brenner, I. (1996). *The last witness: The child survivor of the Holocaust*. Washington, DC: American Psychiatric Press.

Khan, M. R. (1963). The concept of cumulative trauma. *Psychoanalytic Study of the Child, 18*, 286–306.

Kris, E. (1956). The recovery of childhood memories in psychoanalysis. *Psychoanalytic Study of the Child, 11*, 54–88.

Krystal, H. (1978). Trauma and affects. *Psychoanalytic Study of the Child, 33*, 81–116.

Marans, S. (1996). Psychoanalysis on the beat: Children, police and urban trauma. *Psychoanalytic Study of the Child, 51*, 522–541.

Marans, S. (2014). Intervening with children and families exposed to violence (Part I). *Journal of Infant, Child, and Adolescent Psychotherapy, 13*, 350–357.

Marans, S., & Adelman, A. (1997). Experiencing violence in a developmental context. In J. Osofsky (Ed.), *Children in a violent society* (pp. 202–222). New York: Guilford Press.

Osofsky, J. D. (2003). Psychoanalytically based treatment for traumatized children and families. *Psychoanalytic Inquiry, 23*, 530–543.

Parker, B., & Turner, W. (2013). Psychoanalytic/psychodynamic psychotherapy for sexually abused children and adolescents: A systematic review. *Cochrane Database of Systematic Reviews, 31*(7), CD008162.

Pruett, K. D. (1984). A chronology of defensive adaptations to severe psychological trauma. *Psychoanalytic Study of the Child, 39*, 591–612.

Pynoos, R., Frederick, C., Nader, K., Arroyo, W., Steinberg, A., Eth, S., . . . Fairbanks, L. (1987). Life threat and posttraumatic stress in school-age children. *Archives of General Psychiatry, 44*, 1057–1063.

Riviere, S. (1996). *Memory of childhood trauma: A clinician's guide to the literature*. New York: Guilford Press.

Schore, A. (2001). The effects of early relational trauma on right brain development, Affect regulation, and infant mental health. *Infant Mental Health Journal, 22*(1–2), 201–269.

Schwartz, E. D., & Kowalski, J. M. (1991). Malignant memories: PTSD in childhood and adults after a school shooting. *Journal of the American Academy of Child and Adolescent Psychiatry, 30*, 936–944.

Shengold, L. L. (1979). Child abuse and deprivation: Soul murder. *Journal of the American Psychoanalytic Association, 27*, 533–559.

Steele, B. F. (1994). Psychoanalysis and the maltreatment of children. *Journal of the American Psychoanalytic Association, 42*, 1001–1025.

Sugarman, A. (2008). The use of play to promote insightfulness in the analysis of children suffering from cumulative trauma. *Psychoanalytic Quarterly, 77*, 799–833.

Terr, L. C. (1991). Childhood traumas: An outline. *American Journal of Psychiatry, 148*, 10–20.

van der Kolk, B. (2005). Developmental trauma disorder: Toward a rational diagnosis for children with complex trauma histories. *Psychiatric Annals, 35*, 401–410.

SC5 Somatic Symptom and Related Disorders

SA51 *Somatic Symptom Disorder*

Bonnard, A. (1963). Impediments of speech: A special psychosomatic instance. *International Journal of Psycho-Analysis, 44*, 151–162.

Kradin, R. L. (2011). Psychosomatic disorders: The canalization of mind into matter. *Journal of Analytical Psychology, 56*, 37–55.

Merskey, H. A., Evans, P. R. (1975). Variations in pain complaint threshold in psychiatric and neurological patients with pain. *Pain, 1*, 73–79.

Milrod, B. (2002). A 9-year-old with conversion disorder, successfully treated with psychoanalysis. *International Journal of Psychoanalysis, 83*(3), 623–631.

Schulte, I. E., & Petermann, A. (2011). Somatoform disorders: 30 years of debate about criteria!: What about children and adolescents? *Journal of Psychosomatic Research, 70*(3), 218–228.

SC8 Psychophysiological Disorders

SC81 *Feeding and Eating Disorders*

Agras, W., Bryson, S., Hammer, L., & Kraemer, H. (2007). Childhood risk factors for thin body preoccupation and social pressure to be thin. *Journal of the American Academy of Child and Adolescent Psychiatry, 46*(2), 171–178.

Chatoor, I., Ganiban, J., Hirsch, R., Borman-Spurrell, E., & Mrazek, D. (2000). Maternal characteristics and toddler temperament in infantile anorexia. *Journal of the American Academy of Child and Adolescent Psychiatry, 39*(6), 743–751.

Chatoor, I., Ganiban, J., Surles, J., & Doussard-Roosevelt, J. (2004). Physiological regulation and infantile anorexia: A pilot study. *Journal of the American Academy of Child and Adolescent Psychiatry, 43*(8), 1019–1025.

Eddy, K., Le Grange, D., Crosby, R., Hoste, R., Doyle, A., Smyth, A., & Herzog, D. (2010). Diagnostic classification of eating disorders in children and adolescents: How does DSM IV-TR compare to empirically-derived categories? *Journal of the American Academy of Child and Adolescent Psychiatry, 49*(3), 277–287.

Jacobi, C., Agras, W., & Hammer, L. (2001). Predicting children's reported eating disturbances at 8 years of age. *Journal of the American Academy of Child and Adolescent Psychiatry, 40*(3), 364–372.

Steiner, H., & Lock, J. (1998). Anorexia nervosa and bulimia nervosa in children and adolescents: A review of the past 10 years. *Journal of the American Academy of Child and Adolescent Psychiatry, 37*(4), 352–359.

Wonderlich, S., Brewerton, T., Jocic, Z., Dansky, B., & Abbot, D. (1997). Relationship of childhood sexual abuse and eating disorders. *Journal of the American Academy of Child and Adolescent Psychiatry, 36*(8), 1107–1114.

SC9 Disruptive Behavior Disorders

SC91 *Conduct Disorder*

Bird, H. R. (2001). Psychoanalytic perspectives on theories regarding the development of antisocial behavior. *Journal of the American Academy of Psychoanalysis, 29*, 57–71.

Blair, R. J. R., Budhani, S., Colledge, E., & Scott, S. (2005). Deafness to fear in boys with psychopathic tendencies. *Journal of Child Psychology and Psychiatry, 46*, 327–336.

Kendziora, K. T., & O'Leary, S. G. (1993). Dysfunctional parenting as a focus for prevention and treatment of child behavior problems. In T. H. Ollendick & R. J. Prinz (Eds.), *Advances in clinical child psychology* (Vol. 15, pp. 175–206). New York: Plenum Press.

Patterson, G. R. (1982). *Coercive family process.* Eugene, OR: Castalia.

Patterson, G. R., DeBaryshe, B. D., & Ramsey, E. (1989). A developmental perspective on antisocial behavior. *American Psychologist, 44*(2), 329–335.

Pettit, G. S., Bates, J. E., & Dodge, K. A. (1993). Family interaction patterns and children's conduct problems at home and school: A longitudinal perspective. *School Psychology Review, 22*, 401–418.

SC92 *Oppositional Defiant Disorder*

Bambery, M., & Porcerelli, J. H. (2006). Psychodynamic therapy for oppositional defiant disorder: Changes in personality, object relations, and adaptive function after six months of treatment. *Journal of the American Psychoanalytic Association, 54*(4), 1334–1339.

Cavanagh, M., Quinn, D., Duncan, D., Graham, T., & Balbuena, L. (2014). Oppositional defiant disorder is better conceptualized as a disorder of emotional regulation. *Journal of Attention Disorders.* [Epub ahead of print]

Gross, J. J. (1998). The emerging field of emotion regulation: An integrative review. *Review of General Psychology, 2*(3), 271–299.

Gross, J. J. (Ed.). (2014). *Handbook of emotion regulation* (2nd ed.). New York: Guilford Press.

Hoffman, S. G. (2007). Cognitive factors that maintain social anxiety disorder: A comprehensive model and its treatment implications. *Cognitive Behaviour Therapy, 36*, 193–209.

Rice, T. R., & Hoffman, L. (2014). Defense mechanisms and implicit emotion regulation: A comparison of a psychodynamic construct with one from contemporary neuroscience. *Journal of the American Psychoanalytic Association, 62*(4), 693–708.

Stringaris, A., & Goodman, R. (2009a). Longitudinal outcome of youth oppositionality: Irritable, headstrong, and hurtful behaviors have distinctive predictions. *Journal of the American Academy of Child and Adolescent Psychiatry, 48*, 404–412.

Stringaris, A., & Goodman, R. (2009b). Three dimensions of oppositionality in youth. *Journal of Child Psychology and Psychiatry, 50*, 216–223.

Winkelmann, K., Stefini, A., Hartmann, M., Geiser-Elze, A., Kronmüller, A., Schenkenbach, C., . . . Kronmüller, K. T. (2005). Efficacy of psychodynamic short-term psychotherapy for children and adolescents with behaviour disorders. *Praxis der Kinderpsychologie und Kinderpsychiatrie, 54*(7), 598–614.

SC11 Disorders of Mental Functions

SC111 *Motor Skills Disorders*

Fliers, E., Vermeulen, S., Rijsdijk, F., Altink, M., Buschgens, C., Rommelse, N., . . . Franke, B. (2009). ADHD and poor motor performance from a family genetic perspective. *Journal of the American Academy of Child and Adolescent Psychiatry, 48*(1), 25–34.

Kadesjo, B., & Gillberg, C. (1999). Developmental coordination disorder in Swedish 7-year old children. *Journal of the American Academy of Child and Adolescent Psychiatry, 38*(7), 820–828.

van Meel, C., Oosterlaan, J., Heslenfeld, D., & Sergeant, J. (2005). Motivational effects on motor timing in attention-deficit/hyperactivity disorder. *Journal of the American Academy of Child and Adolescent Psychiatry, 44*(5), 451–460.

SC112 *Psychotic Disorders*

Burgin, D., & Meng, H. (2004). *Childhood and adolescent psychosis.* Basel, Switzerland: Karger.

Carlson, G. A. (2013). Affective disorders and psychosis in youth. *Child and Adolescent Psychiatric Clinics of North America, 22*, 569–580.

Driver, D. I., Gogtay, N., & Rapoport, J. L. (2013). Childhood onset schizophrenia and early onset schizophrenia spectrum disorders. *Child and Adolescent Psychiatric Clinics of North America, 22*(4), 539–555.

McClellan, J., & McCurry, C. (1999). Early onset psychotic disorders: Diagnostic stability and clinical characteristics. *European Child and Adolescent Psychiatry, 8*(1), 13–19.

Rutter, M., Bishop, D., Pine, D., Scott, S., Stevenson, J., Taylor, E., & Thapar, A. (2008). *Rutter's child and adolescent psychiatry* (5th ed.). Malden, MA: Blackwell.

SC114 Neuropsychological Disorders

SC114.1 Tic Disorders

Bennett, S., Keller, A., & Walkup, J. (2013). The future of tic disorder treatment. *Annals of the New York Academy of Sciences, 1304*, 32–39.

Bloch, M., Panza, K., Landeros-Weisenberger, A., & Leckman, J. (2009). Meta-analysis: Treatment of attention-deficit hyperactivity disorder in children with comorbid tic disorders. *Journal of the American Academy of Child and Adolescent Psychiatry, 48*(9), 884–893.

Khalifa, N., & von Knorring, A. L. (2006). Psychopathology in a Swedish population of school children with tic disorders. *Journal of the American Academy of Child and Adolescent Psychiatry, 45*(11), 1346–1353.

Robertson, M. (2008). The prevalence and epidemiology of Gilles de la Tourette syndrome: Part 1. The epidemiological and prevalence studies. *Journal of Psychosomatic Research, 65*(5), 461–472.

Spencer, T., Biederman, J., Harding, H., Wilens, T., & Faraone, S. (1995). The relationship between tic disorders and Tourette's syndrome revisited. *Journal of the American Academy of Child and Adolescent Psychiatry, 34*(9), 1133–1139.

Swain, J., Scahill, L., Lombroso, P., King, R., & Leckman, J. (2007). Tourette syndrome and tic disorders: A decade of progress. *Journal of the American Academy of Child and Adolescent Psychiatry, 46*(8), 947–968.

SC114.2 Visual–Spatial Processing Disorders

Greene, J. D. (2005). Apraxia, agnosias, and higher visual function abnormalities. *Journal of Neurology, Neurosurgery & Psychiatry, 76*, 25–34.

Rourke, B. P. (2000). Neuropsychological and psychosocial subtyping: A review of investigations within the University of Windsor laboratory. *Canadian Psychology, 41*, 34–51.

Solan, H. A., Larson, S., Shelley-Tremblay, J., Ficarra, A., & Silverman, M. (2001). Role of visual attention in cognitive control of oculomotor readiness in students with reading disabilities. *Journal of Learning Disabilites, 34*, 107–118.

Vidyasagar, T. R., & Pammer, K. (1999). Impaired visual search in dyslexia relates to the role of the magnocellular pathway in attention. *NeuroReport, 26*, 1283–1287.

SC114.3 Language and Auditory Processing Disorders

Beitchman, J. H., & Brownlie, E. (2014). *Language disorders in children*. Boston: Hogrefe.

Bishop, D. V., & Snowling, M. J. (2004). Developmental dyslexia and specific language impairment: Same or different? *Psychological Bulletin, 130*, 858–886.

SC114.4 Memory Impairments

Baddeley, A. D. (1993). Short-term phonological memory and long-term learning: A single case study. *European Journal of Cognitive Psychology, 5*, 129–148.

Baddeley, A. D., Gathercole, S. E., & Papagno, C. (1998). The phonological loop as a language learning device. *Psychological Review, 105*, 158–173.

Baddeley, A. D., & Wilson, B. A. (1993). A developmental deficit in short-term phonological memory: Implications for language and reading. *Memory, 1*, 65–78.

Cornoldi, C., Barbieri, A., & Gaiani, C. (1999). Strategic memory deficits in attention deficit disorder with hyperactivity participants: The role of executive processes. *Developmental Neuropsychology, 15*, 53–71.

SC114.5 Attention-Deficit/Hyperactivity Disorder

Gilmore, K. (2000). A psychoanalytic perspective on attention-deficit/hyperactivity disorder. *Journal of the American Psychoanalytic Association, 48*, 1259–1293.

Leuzinger-Bohleber, M., Laezer, K. L., Pfennig-Meerkoetter, N., Fischmann, T., Wolff, A., & Green, J. (2011). Psychoanalytic treatment of ADHD children in the frame of two extra clinical studies: The Frankfurt Prevention Study and the EVA Study. *Journal of Infant, Child, and Adolescent Psychotherapy, 10*, 32–50.

Martin, N. C., Piek, J. P., & Hay, D. A. (2006). DCD

and ADHD: A genetic study of their shared etiology. *Human Movement Science, 25*, 110–124.

Migden, S. (1998). Dyslexia and self-control: An ego-psychoanalytic perspective. *Psychoanalytic Study of the Child, 53*, 282–299.

Palombo, J. (1993). Neurocognitive deficits, developmental distortions, and incoherent narratives. *Psychoanalytic Inquiry, 13*, 85–102.

Palombo, J. (2001). The therapeutic process with children with learning disabilities. *Psychoanalytic Social Work, 8*, 143–168.

Pitcher, T. M., Piek, J. P., & Hay, D. A. (2003). Fine and gross motor ability in males with ADHD. *Developmental Medicine and Child Neurology, 45*, 525–535.

Salomonsson, B. (2004). Some psychoanalytic viewpoints on neuropsychiatric disorders in children. *International Journal of Psychoanalysis, 85*, 117–136.

Salomonsson, B. (2006). The impact of words on children with ADHD and DAMP: Consequences for psychoanalytic technique. *International Journal of Psychoanalysis, 87*, 1029–1044.

Salomonsson, B. (2011). Psychoanalytic conceptualizations of the internal object in an ADHD child. *Journal of Infant, Child, and Adolescent Psychotherapy, 10*(1), 87–102.

SC114.6 *Executive Function Difficulties*

Barkley, R. A. (2012). *Executive functions: What they are, how they work and why they evolved.* New York: Guilford Press.

Denckla, M. B. (2007). Executive function: Binding together the definitions of attention-deficit/hyperactivity disorder and learning disabilities. In L. Meltzer (Ed.), *Executive function in education: From theory to practice* (pp. 5–18). New York: Guilford Press.

Gioia, G. A., Isquith, P. K., Kenworthy, L., & Barton, R. M. (2002). Profiles of everyday executive function in acquired and developmental disorders. *Child Neuropsychology, 8*, 121–137.

Meltzer, L., & Krishnan, K. (2007). Executive function difficulties and learning disabilities: Understandings and misunderstandings. In L. Meltzer (Ed.), *Executive function in education: From theory to practice* (pp. 77–105). New York: Guilford Press.

Pennington, B. F. (2009). *Diagnosing learning disorders: A neuropsychological framework.* New York: Guilford Press.

SC114.7 *Severe Cognitive Deficits*

Ellison, Z., van Os, J., & Murray, R. (1998). Special feature: Childhood personality characteristics of schizophrenia: Manifestations of, or risk factors for, the disorder? *Journal of Personality Disorder, 12*, 247–261.

Hodapp, R. M., & Dykens, E. M. (1996). Mental retardation. In R. J. Mash & R. A Barkley (Eds.), *Child psychopathology* (pp. 362–389). New York: Guilford Press.

Pennington, B. F. (2009). *Diagnosing learning disorders: A neuropsychological framework.* New York: Guilford Press.

SC115 *Learning Disorders*

SC115.1 *Reading Disorders*

Gletcher, J. M., Foorman, B. R., Shaywitz, S. E., & Shaywitz, B. A. (1999). Conceptual and methodological issues in dyslexia research: A lesson for developmental disorders. In H. Tager-Flusberg (Ed.), *Neurodevelopmental disorders* (pp. 271–305). Cambridge, MA: MIT Press.

Migden, S. (2002). Self-esteem and depression in adolescents with specific learning disability. *Journal of Infant, Child, and Adolescent Psychotherapy, 2*(1), 145–160.

Pennington, B. F. (2009). *Diagnosing learning disorders: A neuropsychological framework.* New York: Guilford Press.

SC115.2 *Mathematics Disorder*

Geary, D. C. (1993). Mathematical disabilities: Cognitive, neuropsychological, and genetic components. *Psychological Bulletin, 114*, 345–362.

Pennington, B. F. (2009). *Diagnosing learning disorders: A neuropsychological framework.* New York: Guilford Press.

Shalev, R. S., & Gross-Tsur, V. (2001). Developmental dyscalculia. *Pediatric Neurology, 24*, 337–342.

SC115.3 *Disorders of Written Expression*

Beeson, P. M., & Rapcsak, S. Z. (2010). Neuropsychological assessment and rehabilitation of writing disorders. In J. M. Gurd, U. Kischka, & J. C. Marshal (Eds.), *The handbook of clinical neuropsychology* (2nd ed., pp. 323–348). New York: Oxford University Press.

Beeson, P. M., Rising, K., Kim, E. S., & Rapcsak, S. Z. (2008). A novel method for examining response to spelling treatment. *Aphasiology, 22,* 707–717.

SC115.4 *Nonverbal Learning Disabilities*

Little, S. S. (1993). Nonverbal learning disabilities and socio-emotional functioning: A review of the recent literature. *Journal of Learning Disabilities, 26,* 653–665.

Molenaar-Klumper, M. (2002). *Non-verbal learning disabilities: Characteristics, diagnosis and treatment with an educational setting.* London: Jessica Kingsley.

Pally, R. (2001). A primary role for nonverbal communication in psychoanalysis. *Psychoanalytic Inquiry, 21,* 71–93.

Palombo, J. (1996). The diagnosis and treatment of children with nonverbal learning disabilities. *Child and Adolescent Social Work, 13,* 311–333.

Palombo, J. (2006). *Nonverbal learning disabilities: A clinical perspective.* New York: Norton.

Rourke, B. P. (1989). *Nonverbal learning disabilities: The syndrome and the model.* New York: Guilford Press

Rourke, B. P., & Tsatsanis, K. D. (2000). Nonverbal learning disabilities and Asperger syndrome. In A. Klin, F. R. Volkmar, & S. S. Sparrow (Eds.), *Asperger syndrome* (pp. 231–253). New York: Guilford Press.

Stein, M. T., Klin, A., Miller, K., Goulden, K., Coolman, R., & Coolman, D. M. (2004). When Asperger's syndrome and a nonverbal learning disability look alike. *Journal of Developmental and Behavioral Pediatrics, 25,* 190–195.

Tanguay, P. B. (2001). *Nonverbal learning disabilities at home: A parent's guide.* London: Jessica Kingsley.

Tanguay, P. B. (2002). *Nonverbal learning disabilities at school: Educating students with NLD, Asperger syndrome, and related conditions.* London: Jessica Kingsley.

SC115.5 *Social-Emotional Learning Disabilities*

Adolphs, R. (2003a). Cognitive neuroscience of human social behavior. *Nature Reviews Neuroscience, 4,* 165–178.

Adolphs, R. (2003b). Investigating the cognitive neuroscience of social behavior. *Neuropsychologia, 41,* 119–126.

Bryan, T. (1991). Assessment of social cognition: Review of research in learning disabilities. In H. L. Swanson (Ed.), *Handbook on the assessment of learning disabilities: Theory, research, and practice* (pp. 285–312). Austin, TX: PRO-ED.

Palombo, J. (1996). The diagnosis and treatment of children with nonverbal learning disabilities. *Child and Adolescent Social Work, 13,* 311–333.

Palombo, J. (2006). *Nonverbal learning disabilities: A clinical perspective.* New York: Norton.

SC12 Developmental Disorders

SC125 *Attachment Disorders*

Juffer, F., & van IJzendoorn, M. H. (2009). International adoption comes of age: Development of international adoptees from a longitudinal and meta-analytical perspective. In G. M. Wrobel & E. Neil (Eds.), *International advances in adoption research for practice* (pp. 169–192). Chichester, UK: Wiley-Blackwell.

O'Connor, T., & Zeanah, C. H. (2003). Attachment disorders: Assessment strategies and treatment approaches. *Attachment and Human Development, 5*(3), 223–244.

Richters, M. M., & Volkmar, F. R. (1994). Reactive attachment disorder of infancy or early childhood. *Journal of the American Academy of Child and Adolescent Psychiatry, 33*(3), 328–332.

Steele, H., & Steele, M. (2014). Attachment disorders. In M. Lewis & K. Rudolph (Eds.), *Handbook of developmental psychopathology* (3rd ed., pp. 357–370). New York: Springer.

van IJzendoorn, M. H., & Juffer, F. (2006). The Emanuel Miller Memorial Lecture 2006: Adoption as intervention: Meta-analytic evidence for massive catch-up and plasticity in physical, socioemotional, and cognitive development. *Journal of Child Psychology and Psychiatry, 47*(12), 1228–1245.

Zeanah, C. H., & Gleason, M. M. (2010). *Reactive attachment disorders: A review for DSM-V.* Report presented to the American Psychiatric Association.

SC126 *Pervasive Developmental Disorders*

Blijd-Hoogewys, E. M., Bezemer, M. L., & van Geert, P. L. (2014). Executive functioning in children with ASD: An analysis of the BRIEF. *Journal of Autism and Developmental Disorders, 44*(12), 3089–3100.

Byars, K., & Simon, S. (2014). Practice patterns and insomnia treatment outcomes from an evidence-based pediatric behavioral sleep medicine clinic. *Clinical Practice in Pediatric Psychology, 2*(3), 337–349.

Greenspan, S., & Shanker, S. (2004). *The first idea: How symbols, language and intelligence evolved from our primate ancestors to modern humans.* Boston: Da Capo Press.

Kulage, K. M., Smaldone, A. M., & Cohn, E. G. (2014). How will DSM-5 affect autism diagnosis?: A systematic literature review and meta-analysis. *Journal of Autism and Developmental Disorders, 44*(8), 1918–1932.

Levy, A. J. (2011). Psychoanalytic psychotherapy for children with Asperger's syndrome: Therapeutic engagement through play. *Psychoanalytic Perspectives, 37,* 72–91.

Noterdaeme, M., Wriedt, E., & Höhne, C. (2010). Asperger's syndrome and high-functioning autism: Language, motor and cognitive profiles. *European Child and Adolescent Psychiatry, 19*(6), 475–481.

Paul, R., Orlovski, S. M., Marcinko, H. C., & Volkmar, F. (2009). Conversational behaviors in youth with high-functioning ASD and Asperger syndrome. *Journal of Autism and Developmental Disorders, 39*(1), 115–125.

Tsai, L. Y. (2013). Asperger's disorder will be back. *Journal of Autism and Developmental Disorders, 43,* 2914–2942.

Tsai, L. Y., & Ghaziuddin, M. (2014). DSM-5 ASD moves forward into the past. *Journal of Autism and Developmental Disorders, 44*(2), 321–330.

Volkmar, F. R., State, M., & Klin, A. (2009). Autism and autism spectrum disorders: Diagnostic issues for the coming decade. *Journal of Child Psychology and Psychiatry, 50*(1–2), 108–115.

Woodbury-Smith, M. R., & Volkmar, F. R. (2009). Asperger syndrome. *European Child and Adolescent Psychiatry, 18*(1), 2–11.

SCApp Appendix: Psychological Experiences That May Require Clinical Attention

SCApp3 *Gender Incongruence*

Byne, W., Bradley, S. J., Coleman, E., Eyler, A. E., Green, R., Menvielle, E. J., . . . Tompkins, D. A. (2012). Report of the American Psychiatric Association Task Force on Treatment of Gender Identity Disorder. *Archives of Sexual Behavior, 41*(4), 759–796.

Cohen-Kettenis, P. T., & Pfäfflin, F. (2010). The DSM diagnostic criteria for gender identity disorder in adolescents and adults. *Archives of Sexual Behavior, 39*(2), 499–513.

Drescher, J. (2014). Controversies in gender diagnoses. *Journal of Lesbian, Gay, Bisexual and Transgender Health, 1*(1), 9–15.

Drescher, J., & Byne, W. (2013). *Treating transgender children and adolescents: An interdisciplinary discussion.* New York: Routledge.

Drescher, J., Cohen-Kettenis, P., & Winter, S. (2012). Minding the body: Situating gender diagnoses in the ICD-11. *International Review of Psychiatry, 24*(6), 568–577.

Drescher, J., & Pula, J. (2014). Ethical issues raised by the treatment of gender variant prepubescent children. *Hastings Center Report, 44*(Suppl. 4), S17–S22.

Meyer-Bahlburg, H. F. (2010). From mental disorder to iatrogenic hypogonadism: Dilemmas in conceptualizing gender identity variants as psychiatric conditions. *Archives Sexual Behavior, 39,* 461–476.

Zucker, K. J. (2010). The DSM diagnostic criteria for gender identity disorder in children. *Archives of Sexual Behavior, 39*(2), 477–498.

Zucker, K. J., Cohen-Kettenis, P. T., Drescher, J., Meyer-Bahlburg, H. F. L., Pfäfflin, F., & Womack, W. M. (2013). Memo outlining evidence for change for gender identity disorder in the DSM-5. *Archives of Sexual Behavior, 42,* 901–914.

PART IV

Infancy and Early Childhood

CHAPTER 10

Mental Health and Developmental Disorders in Infancy and Early Childhood

IEC 0–3

CHAPTER EDITORS

Anna Maria Speranza, PhD **Linda Mayes, MD**

CONSULTANTS

Fabia E. Banella, MA
Tessa Baradon, MA
Irene Chatoor, MD
Jack Drescher, MD
Leon Hoffman, MD
Marianne Leuzinger-Bohleber, PhD
Loredana Lucarelli, PhD
Sandra Maestro, MD
Steven Marans, PhD
Filippo Muratori, MD
Timothy Rice, MD
Theodore Shapiro, MD
Gabrielle H. Silver, MD
Fred Volkmar, MD
Charles H. Zeanah, MD

Introduction

Mental development during infancy and early childhood reflects dynamic relationships among many dimensions of human functioning, including emotional, social, language, cognitive, regulatory–sensory processing, and motor capacities. Challenges in these areas and in relationship patterns need to be considered for a comprehensive classification of infancy and early childhood disorders.

Infant researchers and clinicians in developmental psychopathology, relational psychoanalysis, attachment theory, and neuroscience have contributed to this domain, describing the interplay among the biological, psychological, and social-contextual aspects of development across the lifespan. As suggested by Sameroff's (2009) transactional model, infant mental health and disorders are the results of ongoing and interactive developmental changes between a child and the environment. Appreciating the bidirectional nature of these influences is crucial to understanding various disorders, tracing their developmental pathways, and making meaningful case formulations and treatment plans.

A biopsychosocial model of early development as described in the seminal work of Greenspan (1992, 1996, 2004) is proposed here. It includes the infant's (1) developmental level of emotional, social, and intellectual functioning; (2) constitutional and biologically based individual processing differences; and (3) relationships, including child–caregiver–family and other patterns. Infant experiences (as well as those throughout the course of life) can only be understood in the context of a relational, social, and cultural framework. Moreover, the developmental process is understood in terms of the interplay among genetic factors; environmental factors; developmental history; and current challenges in physiological, neuropsychological, cognitive, social, emotional, and representational domains. Disorders and maladaptive patterns of development assume specific forms that reflect both the history of the preceding forms of adaptive organization and the developmental task characteristic of each phase.

The Infancy and Early Childhood (IEC) classification presented in this chapter covers the most common disorders of infants and young children. Our main sources have been the Interdisciplinary Council on Developmental and Learning Disorders (ICDL) *Diagnostic Manual for Infants and Young Children* (ICDL-DMIC; ICDL, 2005) and the *Diagnostic Classification of Mental Health and Developmental Disorders of Infancy and Early Childhood,* revised edition (DC: 0–3R; Zero to Three, 2005), as they are the best-known classification systems for infancy and early childhood. We have followed ICDL-DMIC in terms of both general structure and approach to disorders and clinical formulation.

While this chapter was already in draft, the DC: 0–5™ (Zero to Three, 2016) had been published. We did not have the possibility to integrate all the cues provided by the DC: 0–5, however, we tried to point out, as key points, the innovations of this system and put them in dialogue with our approach.

The IEC classification takes a developmental, comprehensive, multiaxial approach that primarily includes functional emotional developmental capacities (Axis II), regulatory–sensory processing capacities (Axis III), relational patterns and disorders (Axis IV), and other medical and neurological diagnoses (Axis V) as determinant components of a multiaxial diagnosis for infant disorders (Axis I) (see Figure 10.1).

We have made some changes to the IEC classification from that in the first PDM. First, we have given more emphasis to the contribution of the different axes to the diagnostic profile. Assessment of a symptomatic pattern in childhood is not possible without an accurate evaluation of a child's sensory processing abilities, functional emotional developmental capacities, and prevalent relational patterns.

For these reasons, the axes for the IEC classification have a different organization and different constructs from the PDM-2 axes for older children, adolescents, and adults. We have maintained the different multiaxiality of this chapter in recognition of the special nature of this period and its theoretical and clinical framework. Where possible, we have tried to reduce conceptual gaps by cross-referencing between axes. For example, significant changes in an infant's social, cognitive, and emotional functioning (Axis II) tend to lead to specific mental functions in that child when older, in continuity with the MC Axis (see Chapter 7). PDM-2 thus tries to indicate developmental pathways toward symptomatic patterns of older children and adolescents. At the same time, both constitutional sensory processing abilities (Axis III) and relational patterns and disorders (Axis IV), though contributing to emerging personality development, are not easily superimposable on the PC Axis (see Chapter 8).

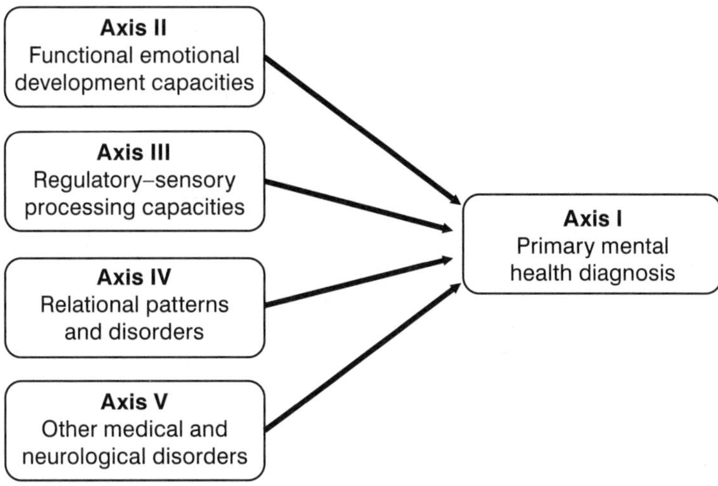

FIGURE 10.1. The IEC classification's multiaxial approach.

We have also introduced user-friendly assessment scales whereby a clinician can formulate a clinically relevant profile of an infant or child, and have listed other relevant assessment tools.

Overview of the Multiaxial System

The classification of infancy and early childhood disorders requires a comprehensive assessment that captures the unique qualities of each individual. Presenting problems and symptomatology are described in IEC Axis I (primary mental health diagnoses), beginning with disorders of psychophysiological functioning, followed by affective disorders, disorders related to traumatic events, behavioral disorders, and so on. We felt that this choice would maintain greater continuity with the MC Axis (see Chapter 7) and the SC Axis (see Chapter 9). In addition to the primary diagnoses, clinicians should capture the unique qualities of each young child and family on a multiaxial developmental profile that includes descriptions of six basic functional emotional developmental capacities (Axis II); constitutional and maturational variations (regulatory–sensory processing patterns, Axis III); caregiver–infant or caregiver–child and family interaction patterns and disorders (Axis IV); and other medical or neurological diagnoses (Axis V).

Brief descriptions of the five axes now follow.

- *Axis I: Primary mental health diagnoses.* This axis describes the main diagnostic categories and types of disorders observed in infancy and early childhood. When appropriate, it can augment other existing diagnostic systems, such as the *International Classification of Diseases,* 10th revision (ICD-10; World Health Organization, 1992), the *Diagnostic and Statistical Manual of Mental Disorders,* fifth edition (DSM-5; American Psychiatric Association, 2013), DC: 0–3R, and DC: 0–5.

- *Axis II: Functional emotional developmental capacities.* This axis describes the young child's emotional and social functioning, including shared attention and regulation; engagement and relating; two-way intentional, affective signaling and communication; long chains of co-regulated emotional signaling and shared social problem solving; creation of symbols and ideas; and building of bridges between ideas and logical thinking.

- *Axis III: Regulatory–sensory processing capacities.* This axis describes the child's regulatory–sensory processing profile in terms of sensory modulation, sensory discrimination, and sensory-based motor abilities, including postural control and motor planning. Each child presents a unique profile of sensory processing regulation. The different observed patterns exist on a continuum from relatively normal variations to disorders. These latter occur when the individual sensory differences are sufficiently severe to interfere with daily living abilities and with age-expected emotional, social, cognitive, or learning capacities.
- *Axis IV: Relational patterns and disorders.* This axis describes characteristics of infant/child–caregiver interactive patterns and family patterns. Parent–infant relationships are assessed in terms of caregiving patterns, interactive styles, and subjective experiences, and are placed along a continuum from well-regulated interactions to relational disorders.
- *Axis V: Other medical and neurological diagnoses.*

It is critical to consider the contribution of each axis to comprehensive evaluation. Each helps a clinician not only to form an overall view of a child's functioning, but to understand the role it plays in pathogenesis. A feeding disorder, for example, could be influenced by a specific sensory processing problem (Axis III) that makes the child vulnerable to the introduction of new foods; or it could be determined by a medical condition such as gastroesophageal reflux (Axis V); or it could express a conflictual relational pattern between child and caregiver (Axis IV). Each dimension could be the unique or prevalent factor, but the interweaving of different dimensions is most significant. Accordingly, we suggest that clinicians not focus on primary diagnoses alone, but complete the clinical evaluation of all five axes.

A Comprehensive Approach to Clinical Evaluation

Clinical assessment in infancy and early childhood is a dynamic and ongoing process involving several key steps. The initial stages include the diagnosis of one or more specific disorders—a diagnosis that captures a child's unique development and individual differences in motor, sensory, language, cognitive, affective, and interactive patterns. The clinician should consider constitutional and maturational features; levels of emotional, cognitive, and social functioning; family system functioning; and adult–child relationships and patterns of interaction.

During infancy and early childhood, not only is the brain (and consequently the mind) growing more rapidly than it ever will again, but it is also literally forming the relationships among its different components. Attending to these interrelated components is vital in conceptualizing disorders that can be meaningfully treated and researched.

The IEC classification system integrates all components of development and functioning in infancy and early childhood. It can be used as a road map to understanding the interactions among the different components of the child's development, family, and environment, and as a guide to clinical interventions. It provides a systematic approach to depicting each child's unique pattern of functioning. A primary diagnosis is made via a clinical judgment about the predominant contributing factor. Before deciding on a primary diagnosis, a clinician must fully evaluate all axes to determine the various dimensions contributing to the presenting problems. Once all this information is considered, clinical reasoning guides the clinician in selecting the predominant pattern.

Clinicians may develop their individual ways of evaluating infants and young children. Any assessment, however, requires several sessions to understand how a child is functioning in each developmental area. The clinical evaluation therefore implies consideration of a large number of contexts and assessment tools, which can be summarized as follows:

- *Observation of infant or child functioning.* Level and quality of social-emotional, cognitive, linguistic, relational, sensory, and motor abilities can be investigated through observational techniques, ranging from free play to structured observations or assessments.
- *Observation of caregiver–infant or caregiver–child interactive patterns.* Direct observation of family functioning (e.g., family and parental dynamics, the caregiver–child relationship, and interaction patterns) is important. Unstructured observations and/or standardized procedures can be used to assess the quality of interactions.
- *Clinical interviews with parents.* Such interviews should include evaluation of the child's developmental history, nature of the child's strengths and difficulties, parental representations of the child and of themselves as caregivers, and quality of parents' reflective function. The clinician should obtain two levels of information: "objective" data, such as the child's medical history, and "subjective" data, comprising parental emotional and affective states and mental representations of themselves and of their child, subjective experience of the caregiver, and quality of the relationship with the child.

Assessment tools for clinical use are listed at the ends of the sections on Axes II–IV.

Axis I: Primary Diagnoses

Axis I describes the main diagnostic categories and types of disorders observed in infancy and early childhood (see Table 10.1). In contrast to what was done in the first PDM, "interactive disorders" are not put under this label. Although it is often clear that infant/child–caregiver interaction patterns play the major role in these challenges, there may be many different pathways to adaptive and maladaptive patterns. Clinician should consider the role of social-emotional development, conflicts, constitutional and maturational variations, and experience with caregivers and family members to understand the meaning of each observed pattern in a particular child. Since biological, constitutional, or relational components can affect all disorders, all primary diagnoses have been put on this axis.

In our revision of primary diagnoses, we have put both developmental anxiety disorders and selective mutism under anxiety disorders, and have considered attentional

TABLE 10.1. Main Diagnostic Categories and Types of Disorders Observed in Infancy and Early Childhood

- IEC01 Sleep disorders
- IEC02 Feeding and eating disorders
- IEC03 Elimination disorders
- IEC04 Anxiety disorders
- IEC05 Disorders of emotional range and stability
- IEC06 Depressive disorders
- IEC07 Mood dysregulation: A unique type of interactive and mixed regulatory–sensory processing disorder characterized by bipolar patterns
- IEC08 Prolonged grief reaction
- IEC09 Adjustment disorders
- IEC10 Traumatic stress disorders
- IEC11 Reactive attachment disorders
- IEC12 Disruptive behavior and oppositional disorders
- IEC13 Gender incongruence
- IEC14 Regulatory–sensory processing disorders
  - IEC14.01 Hypersensitive or overresponsive disorder
    - IEC14.01.1 Hypersensitive or overresponsive: Fearful, anxious pattern
    - IEC14.01.2 Hypersensitive or overresponsive: Negative, stubborn pattern
  - IEC14.02 Hyposensitive or underresponsive: Self-absorbed pattern
    - IEC14.02.1 Pattern A: Self-absorbed and difficult-to-engage type
    - IEC14.02.2 Pattern B: Self-absorbed and creative type
  - IEC14.03 Active, sensory-seeking pattern
  - IEC14.04 Inattentive, disorganized pattern
    - IEC14.04.1 With sensory discrimination difficulties
    - IEC14.04.2 With postural control difficulties
    - IEC14.04.3 With dyspraxia
    - IEC14.04.4 With combinations of all three
  - IEC14.05 Compromised school and/or academic performance pattern
    - IEC14.05.1 With sensory discrimination difficulties
    - IEC14.05.2 With postural control difficulties
    - IEC14.05.3 With dyspraxia
    - IEC14.05.4 With combinations of all three
  - IEC14.06 Mixed regulatory–sensory processing patterns
    - IEC14.06.1 Mixed regulatory–sensory processing patterns with evidence of somatic complaints and attentional, emotional, and behavioral problems
    - IEC14.06.2 Mixed regulatory–sensory processing patterns without evidence of behavioral or emotional problems
- IEC15 Neurodevelopmental disorders of relating and communicating
  - IEC15.01 Type I: Early symbolic, with constrictions
  - IEC15.02 Type II: Purposeful problem solving, with constrictions
  - IEC15.03 Type III: Intermittently engaged and purposeful
  - IEC15.04 Type IV: Aimless and unpurposeful

problems as symptoms of different disorders specified within regulatory–sensory processing disorders. In conformity with ICDL-DMIC, we describe each Axis I disorder in terms of its presenting pattern, developmental pathways, and therapeutic implications.

"Presenting pattern" describes the symptomatic patterns as well as the subjective experience of a child in terms of wishes, feelings, motives, and thoughts. Even before young children can represent or symbolize experience, they can organize affects and behaviors into differentiated groups, such as those associated with warmth and dependency and those associated with assertiveness and anger.

"Developmental pathways" describe both risk factors and basic mechanisms that can lead to a specific disorder and its developmental trajectories. Where possible, PDM-2 highlights homotypic and heterotypic continuities. "Homotypic continuity" defines conditions of substantial uniformity of disorders over time (i.e., the same diagnosis continues from childhood to adulthood). In "heterotypic continuity," instead, behaviors or traits assume a different phenomenology over time. In cases of the latter, a developmental process is assumed to connect the different maladaptive behavioral manifestations, such that while they have an apparently different clinical meaning, they are underpinned by the same developmental and psychopathological processes. Identifying developmental pathways of psychopathology, by considering mental functioning, personality, and developmental dynamics, enables more accurate diagnostic predictions for an individual. In reporting empirical and clinical studies on continuity in this chapter, we refer to relevant chapters/axes on older children, adolescents, and adults.

"Therapeutic implications" for each disorder are indicated according to the clinical literature.

Before we begin presenting detailed descriptions of the Axis I disorders, a preliminary note on the first three categories—sleep, feeding and eating, and elimination disorders—may be in order. Difficulties with sleeping or eating, and difficulties with toilet training and elimination in older children, are common in infancy and early childhood. Sometimes they appear to be the only challenges a child faces. Often such difficulties arise in response to interactive challenges, including trauma, anxiety, adjustment reactions to transitions, illness, and psychosocial stress. The choice of the symptoms is often determined by underlying sensory and/or motor vulnerabilities, in combination with developmental anxieties and/or interactive patterns. Difficulties with sleeping, eating, toilet training, and elimination may also be related to regulatory–sensory processing disorders. A child's developmental profile always reflects the relative contributions of constitutional–maturational variations, child–caregiver interactions, and family and environmental factors.

IEC01 Sleep Disorders

Establishing sleep–wake cycles is a core developmental task of the first 3 years of life. Infants often experience either transitory or longer-lasting disturbances in their sleep during this period. Both regulation and timing of sleep undergo substantial developmental changes; not only does diurnal rhythmicity emerge, but changes also occur in the proportions of time young children spend in each sleep state and in total time asleep. Although many of these changes are maturational, the environmental context to which they must adapt affects the development of sleep and waking patterns. The affective and social regulation provided by the environment—the primary caregiver(s) and family—is responsible for facilitating the development of self-regulation of sleep patterns. Numerous transitions occur each day between sleep and waking, and each one offers an opportunity for homeostatic (hunger, temperature, dryness) and affective (separation, reunion, comfort, security) regulation. During these transitions, a caregiver's contingent responsiveness supports the development of self-regulation and fosters a secure attachment relationship. A caregiver's failure to respond consistently and predictably to support a child during these transitions leads to poor regulation or dysregulation.

Many factors may contribute to problems in this area. Disruptions in sleep patterns can occur secondary to illness, changes in location, transitions in development, and other stressors, but the patterns usually get reestablished with the resumption of security and soothing relationships. Sometimes, however, healthy sleep routines have not been established in the first place because of inconsistent times or settings for sleep, or parental difficulties in helping children learn to fall asleep on their own. Some infants rely on nursing or sucking from a bottle to initiate sleep. Parents do not always learn other techniques to help a child become calm and fall asleep independently. Some infants maintain disorganized tendencies that originated in fussy, irritable periods of early infancy, even after maturation appears to have resolved other issues from these periods. In other cases, the environment is too chaotic to sustain routines and security, resulting in disorganized sleep patterns.

Another factor to consider is the culture of the family. Sleep disorders exist to some extent in the eye of the beholder. Complaints of a sleep disorder can reflect the perceptions and feelings of caregivers, who may have varying tolerance for irregular or disrupted sleep patterns, or who may have similar patterns themselves. In cultures where sleeping with children is acceptable or normative, it may be an alien idea to help a child learn to go to sleep separately. What presents as a sleep disturbance for one parent may not be a sleep disturbance for another. Therefore, a large degree of individual variability marks the development of sleep, making it somewhat complicated to assume what is "normal."

Presenting Pattern

Infants and young children may have difficulty settling into sleep when they first go to bed, or they may wake up and be unable to fall asleep again on their own. Some restless, sensitive sleepers wake frequently throughout the night. Many children have difficulties in both settling into sleep (sleep-onset dyssomnia) and night waking (night-waking dyssomnia), and thus a clear distinction between subtypes is not always feasible. Sleep disruption can also occur when a child who is becoming more symbolic awakens from a nightmare and is not sure what is real and not real. Nightmares, anxiety dreams that awaken the sleeping child, occur during active (rapid-eye-movement or REM) sleep and result in a fully awake and oriented child who remembers and recounts the content of the dream. Dream content before age 8 is usually short and concrete. Nightmares (REM parasomnia) should be distinguished from night terrors (NREM parasomnia), which occur at the transition out of deep sleep (NREM Stages 3–4) and often involve cognitive disorientation, autonomic processes, and skeletal muscle disturbances. Night terrors, the most common parasomnias among preschool-age children, appear to decrease with age—a phenomenon believed to be related to central nervous system maturation.

Because young children rarely meet strict criteria for diagnosis, the term "protodysomnias" (sleep-onset protodysomnia/night-waking protodysomnia) is used to suggest a potential precursor of a later full-blown dysomnia (DC: 0–3R). A protodysomnia cannot be diagnosed before 1 year of age. Duration criteria are subdivided: "Perturbations" (one episode per week for at least 1 month) are considered variations within normal development; "disturbances" (two to four episodes per week for at least 1 month) are considered possible risk conditions that may be self-limiting; "disorders" (five to seven episodes per week for at least 1 month) are likely to continue and require intervention. There are certainly children with problematic sleep before 1 year of age; however, the infant–caregiver relationship, family, and environmental contexts may require more attention than the infant's sleep problem. It is important with the youngest children to rule out medical causes for sleep problems, such as middle-ear infections, congestion, gastroesophageal reflux, allergies, atopic dermatitis, and asthma. Sometimes, even after successful medical treatment, however, a sleep problem may persist because of the parent–infant interaction patterns that have emerged during the course of the acute illness.

Interactions between caregivers and children may contribute to sleep disorders. Relationships of children with these problems are often characterized by neediness, negativism, and impulsivity, with different parts of this pattern dominating in different children and families. Some parents feel inadequate upon learning that their child can fall asleep with others but not with them. Especially if there are preexisting conflicts between the parents, parents may blame each other for not getting the baby to sleep. Conflicts may also maintain a sleep disorder, as the child picks up tension between the caregivers.

Developmental Pathways

Studies (Anders & Dahl, 2007; Anders, Goodlin-Jones, & Sadeh, 2000; Goodlin-Jones & Anders, 2004) have demonstrated that night awakenings per se are not problematic. Typically, infants average one to three awakenings each night throughout the first year of life. By 12 months, 70% of infants are able to return to sleep on their own without alerting their parents. Thus nearly 30% of infants cry out for their parents and appear to need their support to return to sleep; these children have been called "signalers." Other babies, referred to as "self-soothers," are much better able to put themselves to sleep after awakening. Even among toddlers, very few sleep through the whole night.

As infants mature, however, most gradually switch from signaling to self-soothing. Interestingly, follow-up studies have found that consistent signalers between ages 6 and 12 months (33% of the sample) were more likely to meet criteria for a sleep-onset disorder and to be co-sleeping at age 2 years. Sleeping in the parents' room at 12 months of age was predictive of night waking at 2 years of age. Approximately 25% of children were reported to be co-sleeping at each follow-up, but only 33% of their parents saw this behavior as problematic (Goodlin-Jones & Anders, 2004; Goodlin-Jones, Burnham, Gaylor, & Anders, 2001; Tikotzky & Sadeh, 2009).

Sleep patterns develop largely through transactions between a child's characteristics and the caregiving environment. To understand how sleep patterns develop, it is important to consider all components of the transactional model, including the child's behavior and characteristics; parent–child interactions; and parents' expectations, cultural values, and psychological well-being. Research on mothers of sleep-disordered children classifies them as insecure with respect to attachment, compared with control group mothers. The role that parental characteristics, particularly maternal mood disorders, play in the development of infantile sleep problems has received a great deal of attention; various studies (Goodlin-Jones & Anders, 2004; Gregory et al., 2005; Tikotzky & Sadeh, 2009; Warren, Howe, Simmens, & Dahl, 2006) suggest that maternal depression may be related to infants' sleeping difficulties. Maternal depression was more common for 8-month-old to 3-year-old children with sleep problems than for children without sleep problems, and higher levels of maternal depressive feelings were correlated with fewer instances of self-soothing during the middle of the night in infants under 1 year of age. In addition, high levels of separation anxiety in mothers of 1-year-olds were significantly related to their children's night waking. When parents are highly anxious, apart from sometimes missing the baby's signals because they are preoccupied with their worries, they may focus their anxiety on the child. They may worry about the child's ability to cope with ordinary challenges and find it hard to give the baby opportunities to self-regulate, feeling they need to overprotect the child or encourage the child to avoid difficult experiences. In these cases, the child's increasing tendency to be fearful and avoid challenges can further reinforce an anxious parent's perception of the child's vulnerability, and the parent may try even harder to protect the child.

Maternal depressive symptoms were also found to predict longer duration of child awakenings, both for the 3-year trajectory and across the 15- to 24-month and 24- to 36-month age periods. These periods have been described as times of increasing autonomy, self-awareness, and self-regulation for children, and may represent an important time of sleep consolidation. Research on children with depressed mothers has found that such mothers behave in a more withdrawn or intrusive fashion with their children. Such behaviors may interfere with external calming strategies and thus may not foster the development of internal self-soothing tactics. Maternal depression has been shown to correlate with living in adverse circumstances and experiencing more marital conflict and less support. There is also a high incidence of paternal depression and/or psychosomatic symptoms under such circumstances (Goodlin-Jones & Anders, 2004; Gregory & O'Connor, 2002; Warren et al., 2006).

Research has shown that, without effective interventions, children who have sleep problems in early childhood continue to have sleep problems later (Anders & Dahl, 2007; Gregory et al., 2005; Gregory & O'Connor, 2002; Warren et al., 2006). Sleep difficulties can shape affect, attention, cognitive, and language development, and have been found to predict later behavior regulation problems. Separation anxiety disorder (often associated with early childhood sleep problems) becomes less common at older ages, but generalized anxiety disorder and social phobia become more frequent. Longitudinal studies up to adolescence and adulthood (Gregory et al., 2005; Gregory & O'Connor, 2002) have found that children with persistent sleep problems in childhood are at significantly increased risk for developing a subsequent anxious and/or depressed condition. These studies highlight the complex and bidirectional relation between sleep and affective disorders.

Therapeutic Implications

Approximately 10–47% of parents of children presenting to an infant psychiatry clinic reported symptoms of sleep disturbances. Interestingly, the average age of the children at the time of evaluation was over 30 months. Although pediatricians have opportunities for prevention and intervention during the first 5 years of child's life, some professionals (and parents) rely on the "wait-and-see approach." Therefore, clinicians often first address disordered sleep during the preschool years.

When evaluating children with sleep problems, one should obtain a careful sleep history. But one should also inquire about sleep habits in all children with behavior problems. Some attention-deficit and hyperactivity symptoms may be manifestations of disordered sleep rather than actual syndromes; growth retardation also may be associated with sleep disorders. There are four areas to assess: (1) the specifics of the sleep problem and for whom it is a problem; (2) infant characteristics, such as temperament and illness; (3) parent–child interaction patterns; and (4) contextual factors, including both proximal factors (parental characteristics and family context) and more distal factors, such as culture and environment.

The impact of parent–child interaction as a critical "regulator" of sleep–wake transitions on the process of consolidation is one of the most consistent findings about sleep problems in early childhood. From the perspective of the transactional model, interventions should be relationship-based and focused on the factors that affect optimal parent–child regulation; that is, each intervention should be individually tailored to the particular child and family. There are, however, some general guidelines that benefit all children with sleep-onset problems. It is important to help parents to establish a regular bedtime and a regular sleep routine. For a young child, this would mean that after a bath, a parent sits with the child in the room and reads one or two books. Parents should decide ahead of time how many books they are willing to read because children like to put off getting into bed by requesting more and more books. It is also helpful to have a child choose a stuffed animal to hold while a parent reads and for the parent to include the stuffed animal in the reading. For example, the parent can say, "Your little rabbit is listening with you." When the story is over, the parent can tell the child, "Now hold your little rabbit friend tightly because you are both slipping under the cover to go to sleep." For many children, it is helpful to play soft music when they lie down to sleep, which will serve as a conditioner for sleep onset. It is important that parents explain this routine to the child before they start it, and that they tell the child they will leave the room after they put the child down to sleep.

Clinical Illustration

Maria, a 2-year-old girl, had a serious night waking problem and was refusing to go to bed. Both parents felt helpless when Maria struggled at bedtime and refused to settle down, crying and protesting for periods that lasted from 1 to 3 hours each night. Her father said that he could not put his daughter in a supine position because she resisted; he was concerned that he might break her back if he persisted. Her mother associated Maria's sleep disorder with possible organic problems resulting from her own depression during pregnancy; she therefore tried her best to provide relief to her, emphasizing physical comfort rather than effective reassurance. Maria was showing signs of separation anxiety, including temper tantrums, excessive crying, and clinging in response to separation from her mother, along with refusal to take naps at day care. Her mother admitted feeling guilty and fearful when she left her daughter at the day care center. Maria usually won all of the battles with her parents. Both parents were increasingly angry and frustrated with their daughter's control over them.

When these issues were addressed in treatment, the mother revealed her own sense of incompetence and inability to assert herself. This understanding was used in processing and changing the interactive patterns with Maria that had been sustaining the child's sense of omnipotence, control, and demandingness. The treatment involved both education about the importance of autonomy for Maria and redefinition of what had happened during the mother's pregnancy, directed at exploring her guilty belief that she had damaged her daughter during that time. Psychodynamic inference revealed that the father was preoccupied with aggression and competition. In his mind, limit setting was aggressive; thus he refrained from asserting himself with his daughter. He was helped to understand his own feelings of vulnerability, which had colored his view of Maria as vulnerable and fragile. A 2-year follow-up revealed improvement in all areas of relationship functions, including sleep–wake regulation.

IEC02 Feeding and Eating Disorders

Eating disorders, like sleep disorders, can be symptomatic of many of the interactive disorders. Or they may represent regulatory disorders with sensory hypersensitivities and oral–motor difficulties. They may also reflect residual anxiety from resolved biological problems, such as gastrointestinal difficulties, reflux, and other illnesses that create anxiety and lack of pleasure around eating. Feeding is a relationally embedded phenomenon: Infants become increasingly able to self-regulate their feeding, and parents provide the context for these normative transitions to occur. Yet many of the diagnostic criteria for feeding and eating disorders focus solely on the infant, not the feeding relationship. A failure to incorporate relational phenomena ignores strong evidence linking aspects of the caregiving environment with infant feeding and eating disorders. Approximately 25% of otherwise normally developing infants, and up to 80% of those with developmental disabilities, have been reported to have feeding problems. In addition, 1–2% of infants have been found to have serious feeding difficulties associated with poor weight gain. Feeding disorders not only disrupt an infant's early development; they have also been linked to later deficits in cognitive development, behavioral problems, anxiety, and eating disorders during childhood, adolescence, and young adulthood. Interactions between caregivers and children may contribute significantly to eating disorders. For example, in the absence of appropriate nurturance, eating can become an overrelied-on source of comfort and self-soothing. In the absence of symbolic expression, fear, anger, or rejection can be expressed in food refusal.

Presenting Pattern

An eating disorder may involve poor or irregular intake, food refusal, vomiting, restricted eating, or insatiable eating. Because a baby's health and weight are often seen as indicative of "good" parenting, problems in a child's eating can become an enormous source of worry, stress, and feelings of inadequacy in a caregiver. In the past, the term "failure to thrive" (FTT) was used as a catch-all diagnosis for all feeding disorders. Clinicians initially distinguished between two forms: "organic" and "nonorganic" FTT. Organic FTT represented growth failure traceable to a diagnosable medical cause. Nonorganic FTT was thought to reflect maternal deprivation or parental psychopathology. A third category was later added to describe growth failure related to a mix of organic and environmental factors. In recent years, the use of FTT has been sharply criticized. A primary concern is that not all infants with feeding disorders demonstrate growth failure. Consistent with this view, some clinicians have argued that FTT represents a symptom rather than a diagnostic category. To address the question of how to differentiate various severe feeding problems from each other and from transient or milder feeding difficulties, a classification system has been developed in DC: 0–3R that describes the phenomenology and provides operational diagnostic criteria for six subtypes of feeding disorders. It is not all-inclusive, but covers the most common feeding disorders associated with behavioral symptoms:

- *Feeding disorder of state regulation* begins in the postnatal period and is characterized by irregular, poor, and inadequate food intake. Infants exhibit difficulties in state regulation: Some are too irritable, cry excessively, and cannot calm themselves for feeding; others are too sleepy and cannot wake up or stay awake long enough to feed adequately. A parent is often stressed by an infant's irritability and difficulty feeding and may be anxious or depressed, or both, or may show more severe psychopathology. Longitudinal studies indicate that early problems in regulation of state and feeding may predispose infants to continue having eating problems.

- *Feeding disorder of caregiver–infant reciprocity* is characterized by a lack of engagement between caregiver and infant, leading to inadequate food intake and growth failure of the infant; the main problem here seems to lie in the caregiver's inability to connect with the infant. Between 2 and 6 months, most of the infant's interactions with the caregiver occur around feeding, and the regulation of food intake is closely linked to the baby's emotional engagement with the caregiver. If the infant and caregiver are not engaged with each other, feeding and growth will suffer, and the infant's emotional and social development will be impaired.

- *Infantile anorexia* becomes evident before a child is 3 years old, when the transition to self-feeding is being made, and when issues of autonomy and dependency have to be negotiated between parents and child. Anorexic children take only a few bites of food and then refuse to open their mouths for more. They throw food and utensils, and may try to climb out of their high chairs and run around. Most parents report that these children are active, playful, curious, and engaging, but show hardly any signals of hunger and are not interested in eating. These children are described as going for hours or all day long without signaling that they are hungry. Some parents become so anxious that they try to feed the children whenever they are willing to open their mouths, and some become so desperate that they resort to force-feeding. Toddlers with infantile anorexia have been found to have a higher level of physiological arousal and more difficulty down-regulating their arousal. This may explain why they have so little awareness of hunger: They seem very excited by their play and enjoy talking, but they have difficulty turning away from these pleasurable activities. Studies from different centers have found significant correlations among difficult child temperament, irregular feeding and sleeping patterns, negative and willful behaviors by toddlers, and mother–child conflict during feeding. At the same time, mothers' insecure attachment to their own parents; their drive for thinness; and maternal bulimia, anxiety, and depression have also correlated significantly with mother–child conflict during feeding. Finally, feeding conflicts have been correlated strongly with a child's weight: The more conflict between a mother and child, the less the child weighed.

- *Sensory food aversions* involve food refusal related to the taste, texture, temperature, or smell of particular foods. When an infant is fed specific foods, aversive reactions may range from grimacing, to spitting the food out and wiping the tongue or mouth, to gagging and vomiting. Most commonly, infants begin to show aversive reactions when introduced to baby foods with different flavors and textures, or in the second year of life, during the introduction of different table foods. In addition to their sensory food aversions, many of these children experience hypersensitivities in other areas as well (e.g., not wanting to touch wet food, resisting having their hair washed or wearing clothing with labels, refusing to walk on sand or grass). If parents do not understand the child's food refusal and try too hard to get their child to accept the foods by coaxing, bargaining, threatening, or force-feeding, the child will become increasingly fearful and restrictive in accepting foods.

- *Feeding disorder associated with a concurrent medical condition* is characterized by a combination of organic problems and psychological difficulties, and leads to severe feeding problems and growth failure. For example, feeding problems, including choking/gagging, food refusal, arching, and maternal distress are seen in the observation of mother–infant interactions during feeding in infants with gastroesophageal reflux. The infants associate feeding with pain and may cry in anticipation of feeding, refuse all feedings, and develop a posttraumatic feeding disorder.

- *Feeding disorder associated with insults to the gastrointestinal tract* (also termed *posttraumatic feeding disorder of infancy*) is a condition in which food refusal follows a traumatic experience to the oropharynx or gastrointestinal tract. After an incident of choking, gagging, vomiting, or oropharyngeal impingement, an infant or child becomes fearful of eating and refuses to drink from the bottle or eat any solid food, depending on what dangerous experience the child associates with eating. Often such children experienced some underlying anxiety before the incident, and then their anxiety became focused on the danger of eating. A child's food refusal can be so intense that it causes severe anxiety in parents, who may try to coax and distract the child, offer various foods, and try to feed the child day and night without success. Some very young infants who are afraid to drink from the bottle when awake may drink when asleep. If they wake and see the bottle, however, they usually push it away and cry.

Developmental Pathways

The acquisition of autonomous internal regulation of feeding is an important developmental achievement in the first years of life. An infant becomes increasingly aware of hunger and satiety cues, and responds by communicating interest in eating when hungry and ceasing to accept food when full. This development of autonomous internal regulation unfolds in three stages: (1) state regulation, (2) dyadic reciprocity, and (3) transition to self-feeding and regulation of emotions.

Most infants have a distinct cry when hungry, in contrast to other cries, such as those indicating pain, fear, or tiredness. Ideally, these distinct cries become increasingly distinguishable for parents during the first weeks of life, and thereby a communication system develops that allows the infant to express needs. To feed successfully, however, an infant must attain a state of calm alertness. If infants cannot calm themselves for feeding, or, on the other hand, if they are too sleepy to suckle, the result will be inefficient and stressful feedings for both infants and parents.

The mutually regulated caregiver–infant feeding process may not develop or may be derailed when an infant's hunger signals are weak or difficult to read, or when the parents are preoccupied with their own needs and unable to tune in to those of their infant. Parent and child may not develop a reciprocal relationship, and the infant may be at risk for a feeding disorder of failed reciprocity.

Between 6 months and 3 years of age, motor and cognitive maturation enables the infant to become physically and emotionally more independent. Autonomy versus dependency has to be negotiated daily during the parent–infant feeding interactions. As infants become more competent, their parents need to facilitate their learning to feed themselves. During this transition to self-feeding, an infant needs not only to understand the difference between hunger and satiety, but also to differentiate the physical sensations of hunger and fullness from emotional experiences (e.g., comfort, affection, anger, frustration). If a parent misinterprets an infant's emotional cues and responds to wishes for comfort with feeding, the infant may confuse hunger with emotional experience and associate eating with emotional calming. Infants who give weak hunger cues often raise parents' anxiety. Out of concern for an infant's nutritional needs, a parent may try to override the infant's cues by feeding the baby, even if the infant is not interested and not opening his or her mouth. This may result in battles of will about eating, which only exacerbate the infant's food refusal. Conversely, if an infant gives weak signals of satiety and is easily comforted by food when distressed, parents may be contributing to their child's learning to eat when emotionally distressed or when seeking pleasure.

During each developmental stage, the infant's and caregiver's characteristics can interfere with the mutual regulation of feeding versus the development of internally regulated feeding. When this occurs, maladaptive feeding patterns emerge.

To date, few studies (Bryant-Waugh, Markham, Kreipe, & Walsh, 2010; Chatoor, 2002, 2009) have followed children with feeding disorders over time. With the exception of two studies of infantile anorexia (Ammaniti, Lucarelli, Cimino, D'Olimpio, & Chatoor, 2012; Chatoor, 2005, 2009), other longitudinal studies focusing on the development of children with feeding problems have not attempted to differentiate between subtypes of feeding disorders. As a result, it is not well known how specific feeding disorders in early childhood are related to eating disorders in adolescence and adulthood.

Infantile anorexia is the most investigated and best-known feeding disorder in the recent literature. Cross-sectional studies (Ammaniti, Lucarelli, Cimino, D'Olimpio, & Chatoor, 2010; Chatoor, 2002, 2005, 2009; Lucarelli, Cimino, D'Olimpio, & Ammaniti, 2013) have highlighted dysfunctional mother–child interactions during feeding, especially dyadic conflict; "difficult temperament" and emotional regulation difficulties in the children; and a psychopathological profile of their mothers, characterized by depression and dysfunctional eating attitudes. This pattern of disturbed eating behavior and emotional symptoms in both children and mothers supports recent findings showing that dyadic interactional conflict, maternal psychopathology, difficult child temperament, and child emotional problems are reciprocally involved in the origin and persistence of infantile anorexia. A large longitudinal Italian study (Ammaniti et al., 2012) followed toddlers with infantile anorexia, matched with healthy controls, at 5, 8, and 11 years of age. The anorexic children had minimal interventions and consequently presented more of the natural course of this feeding disorder. About 70% of the children with infantile anorexia at follow-up showed ongoing eating problems and higher scores in anxiety, moodiness, aggressive behaviors, and somatic complaints, compared to the controls. This study also showed significant correlations between maternal eating and children's psychopathology and internalizing problems. A treatment study from Washington, D.C. (Chatoor, 2002, 2005, 2009) of toddlers ranging in age from 1 to 3½ years was based on these findings. The treatment model "facilitating internal regulation of eating" involved parent training: helping parents establish regular mealtimes, refrain from distractions and from coaxing the children to eat, and set limits on inappropriate mealtime behaviors. The follow-up study (Chatoor, 2005, 2009), when the children were 7–13 years of age, demonstrated that two-thirds of the children had outgrown their feeding and growth problems, whereas the other third continued to show poor appetite, lack of interest in eating, and poor growth, and had developed sleep and anxiety disorders. Both lack of regular family meals and not eating lunch at school significantly differentiated the poor-growth group from the recovered group.

Therapeutic Implications

Assessment of an infant's feeding problems should begin with an extensive clinical interview with caregivers to evaluate the infant's feeding difficulties, developmental history, medical history, and family history. This interview is critical for establishing when feeding problems began, as well as identifying medical conditions that may be interfering with feeding or traumatic experiences that may have triggered feeding problems. This interview should be followed by direct observations of the child with the primary caregiver during feeding and play. The purpose is to evaluate when and how feeding interactions go awry. Such observations are key to the clinician's understanding of how to foster mutually regulated feeding interactions. Observations of play interactions enable the clinician to determine whether problematic feeding interactions reflect more fundamental problems in the infant–parent relationship. For example, maternal intrusiveness and dyadic conflict during play indicate a serious problem that needs to be taken into consideration in making the diagnosis and planning treatment.

Above all, more studies of infant and parent characteristics associated with various feeding disorders are needed to improve prevention and treatment (Bryant-Waugh, Markham, Kreipe, & Walsh, 2010; Chatoor, 2002, 2005, 2009; Cooper, Whelan, Woolgar, Morrell, & Murray, 2004; Lucarelli et al., 2013). Preliminary studies show that a treatment that is effective for one type of feeding disorder may be ineffective or even contraindicated for another. In particular, in the case of infantile anorexia, the therapeutic approach should have a dual focus on the child and on the parents. Moreover, facilitating internal regulation of eating through parent training is an effective intervention for toddlers with infantile anorexia. Conversely, in feeding disorders associated with insults to the gastrointestinal tract, the treatment should feature desensitization interventions for the child and psychological support for the parents. In the case of sensory food aversions, which have been confirmed as less severe feeding disorders with respect to the interactional and individual variables involved, helping parents to understand their child's sensory difficulties in regard to the taste, texture, temperature, or smell of certain foods may be effective.

Clinical Illustration

Albert was 15 months old when he was referred because of food refusal and faltering growth. His mother reported that she started to get worried about Albert's eating when he was 8 months old. He was very precocious in his motor development and was already walking along the furniture at that time. He wanted to move around and protested being put in the high chair. When his mother got him settled there, he would refuse to open his mouth, grab the spoon from her, and throw it away. She then gave up on the high chair and tried to feed him while he was walking around and playing with his toys. At the time of assessment, the mother was exhausted and felt trapped by Albert's feeding pattern. The interview of the parents revealed that Albert's mother had been a poor eater as a child; she remembered "food battles" with her parents throughout her childhood and adolescence. She admitted that she often forgot to eat when she got very busy, and that she could not eat when distressed. The father stated that he had a good appetite, and that he had always been tall and athletic.

The parents were helped to understand that Albert was a bright little boy who seemed too busy exploring the world to pay attention to his inner signals of hunger, and that the therapeutic challenge was to help Albert become aware of his hunger and learn to sit in the high chair until his tummy was full. The parents were helped to develop a daily schedule of three regular meals and one snack, with nothing but water in between, to allow Albert to feel hungry. The parents found that giving him small portions of food seemed to keep him interested in eating. The father started to look forward to coming home in the evening for a family meal, and seemed more comfortable with setting limits for Albert. Albert seemed to feel hungry at some of the meals, but his usual pattern was a good meal followed by eating much less during the next one. Overall, his food intake improved, and he became calmer during meals. The parents were encouraged by the progress they had made in helping Albert to respond to his inner signals of hunger and fullness, and reported that they had started to have enjoyable dinners together.

IEC03 Elimination Disorders

Elimination disorders include functional enuresis and encopresis. There is a primary type, in which expected urinary or bowel control has not been reached by an age-expected outer limit of normal development, and a secondary type, in which control has been reached but has been subsequently lost. Children who withhold stools or urine are considered to have elimination disorders. Secondary enuresis has repeatedly been found to be associated with a high incidence of distressing events, including parental separation and disharmony. Some parents may hold the belief that wetting or soiling is under the child's control, leading to intolerance, and aggravation of the child's symptoms.

Presenting Pattern

Children with elimination disorders may experience a range of affective states. Fear, shame, and embarrassment over the "accident" are readily observed. At a deeper subjective level, a child often feels unsure about his or her body. There is a pervasive sense of insecurity about bodily functioning, with significant anxiety over "not being in control" of unexpected urges. Because of this apprehensiveness, some children defend against perceiving the bodily signals to eliminate and may hide or deny their bodily needs. They may compensate by trying to "control" everyone else. Some children are not sufficiently aware of needing to urinate or defecate until it is "too late." They may have poor sensory registration of their bodies' signals, coupled with reduced muscle tone, leaving them confused and embarrassed. For others, mastery of toileting implies demanding expectations of being "big" that conflict with wishes to remain a baby. This conflict may originally be either the child's or the parent's, but it usually becomes a mutual theme as caregiver and child struggle with fears of loss and separation, incompetence, changes in alliances (e.g., "Babies belong to Mom, but big boys go to Daddy"), or other conflicts. The child's mental content in play and conversation tends to mirror the affective patterns described above. Play themes may be characterized by avoidance of strong affect, explosive bursts of affective content, and alternations between the two. The child often verbalizes a wish to "do better" and please caregivers, coupled with less conscious negativism and intermittent impulsivity. An examination of functional developmental capacities can help identify the constrictions contributing to these problems and the specific dynamic formulation that may be relevant. A psychodynamic understanding of the ego-syntonic nature and purpose of the symptom is essential for appropriate treatment.

Developmental Pathways

Before a child can achieve independent toileting, there must have been adequate development in various domains: communication skills, social and emotional development, fine and gross motor development, and cognitive development. Thus an overall evaluation of developmental readiness is the first step in assessing any child's toileting problems. In particular, communication skills are required to convey to caregivers that an elimination need is present. Social and emotional development must have reached the point where the child recognizes the necessity of adhering to parental and societal expectations. Fine and gross motor skills are needed to manipulate clothing, assume the required body positions, use toilet paper, and so on; cognitive skills are needed to understand the meaning of relevant bodily sensations, and to exhibit planfulness and self-control when it comes to satisfying elimination needs. Underlying sensory and/or motor vulnerabilities, combined with interactive challenges, may contribute to elimination difficulties. For example, some children may have low muscle tone, poor motor planning, and sensory underreactivity, making it difficult to sense and then execute motor control over basic bodily functions. Others may be too sensitive to or fearful of flushing the toilet. Somatic states also tend to express the particular type of affects and physical challenge a child is evidencing. For some children, withholding can become a way to express anger and/or opposition in the absence of more symbolic use of words or play to communicate feelings. Relationships are often characterized by vacillations among neediness, negativism, and impulsivity, with different parts of this pattern dominating in different children and families.

Therapeutic Implications

Prevalence rates show that an elimination disorder will "take care of itself" by age 9 in just over half of those children suffering from it (Fishel & Liebert, 2000). On average, an elementary-school-age child with a toileting problem has only about a 15% chance of its resolving by itself within the succeeding 12 months (Butler, 2008; Fishel & Liebert, 2000). Given this information, most parents and children should not wait for a spontaneous remission. This is especially so because elimination disorders cause serious embarrassment, lowered self-esteem, and social withdrawal. Increasing numbers of studies are finding evidence for increased levels of psychological problems in children who wet the bed compared to those who do not, including more internalizing and externalizing problems, attention-deficit/hyperactivity disorder (ADHD), and reduced self-esteem. In particular, a recent cohort of over 8,000 children averaging 8 years of age, enrolled in the population-based Avon Longitudinal Study (Joinson, Heron,

Butler, von Gontard, & the Avon Longitudinal Study of Parents and Children Study Team, 2007), showed that combined (day and night) wetting conferred an increased risk for externalizing problems (oppositional behavior, attention and conduct problems). Moreover, psychological differences between children with and without chronic encopresis showed that children with encopresis had more anxiety and depression symptoms, less parental warmth and organization, more attention problems, greater social problems, more disruptive behavior, and poorer school performance (Cox, Morris, Borowitz, & Sutphen, 2002). Such problems may interfere with a plan of symptom-focused intervention. One should screen for such issues and address them with a broader treatment program.

Early treatment programs may help children to deal with uncertainty and insecurity about how the body functions. Sensory and motor processing can be supported to facilitate a child's sense of bodily competence through a mix of sensory, motor, visual, and spatial activities. It is critical to help the parents deal with their feelings about elimination—what it means to them and how they feel, and what may allow them to implement an effective approach to support the child. It is also important to help the child work through fears about anger or assertiveness, and to help caregiver and family provide an emotional climate that supports both security and initiative.

Clinical Illustration

Pauline, a 4-year-old girl, presented with ongoing secondary enuresis, having previously been dry by 2½ years of age. Onset coincided with the birth of her younger brother. The parents also expressed concern about her aggressive behaviors and angry mood. Intervention by the enuresis nurse was initially helpful, and Pauline responded to conditioning techniques with the pad-and-buzzer approach. The problems recurred, however, and for 1 year, Pauline was wetting the bed several times each week. After her birth, Pauline's mother had suffered from postpartum depression for nearly 2 years. When depressed, she said she often came close to hitting Pauline, and would leave her in the room and walk away when angry with her. Pauline's father described her as pleasant and sweet. He felt that his wife overtly disliked Pauline, and that Pauline often did not warrant the negative responses she elicited from her mother. Although Pauline mostly wanted "cuddles" from her mother, she had learned to engage her mother with mutually aggressive outbursts. The ongoing enuresis established an overt contact and a sense of intimacy between them in an otherwise barren relationship. The regressive act of bedwetting proved ego-syntonic and reparative, with echoes of infantile intimacy.

This pattern of seeking intimacy through maladaptive behaviors was interpreted to the parents as related to Pauline's experiences with maternal postpartum depression and the failure of early intimacy and attachment. Thereafter, each follow-up session brought reports of decreasing aggression and decreasing episodes of enuresis. This improvement was the result of changes in her mother's attitude toward Pauline. She became more available to her—placing her needs first when appropriate, differentiating between Pauline and her brother, and providing her with more contact and time. While Pauline's mother initially accepted the need to change on a cognitive level (realizing that intimacy was less destructive than either conflict or enuresis), she slowly adopted these behaviors in a more affective way, such that Pauline had to initiate intimate contacts less often. Pauline's parents also reported less marital tension and better capacity to work together in a unified way.

IEC04 Anxiety Disorders

Anxiety is a normal and necessary emotional state with an adaptive role in human development, serving the purpose of increased self-protective action. Infants and young children display normative patterns of anxiety, as well as atypical excessive, misplaced, or persistent forms that can interfere with daily functioning and normal development. Anxiety is closely related to evolutionarily based mammalian fear and can alert a child to threatening or dangerous situations.

In typical development, fear of strangers and distress at separation from caregivers between ages 6 and 12 months are adaptive responses to danger represented by unfamiliar adults or being alone. Such anxieties, which decrease for most children by about 30 months of age, reflect a child's attachment to caregivers and ability to distinguish loved ones from strangers.

Anxiety may become symptomatic when it limits developmentally adaptive behavior. In this case, it leads a child to develop specific fears or excessive worries, obsessions, or preoccupations, as well as atypical behaviors: excessive tantrums, compulsions, physical overactivity, or avoidance (including mutism, clinging, and poor self-regulation). Children may also express anxiety by developing somatic symptoms, such as aches and pains or alterations in appetite. "Good-enough" caregiving allows an infant to establish a secure attachment base from which to explore novel, unfamiliar experiences. Insensitive relationships with primary caregivers may evolve into insecure relationships, difficulty in emotional regulation, and anxiety symptoms. Infants and children may be even less able than adults to identify the source(s) of their anxiety, and may be quite distressed when unable to explore and seek new experiences because of disabling anxiety. It is well documented that up to 80% of anxious children have anxious parents, implicating both heredity and environment.

Unlike the corresponding section in the first PDM, this section includes "developmental anxieties," such as separation anxiety and fear of strangers, which should be considered anxiety disorders only when they persist over time and impair a child's functioning or development. It also includes selective mutism as one possible symptom or expression of an anxiety disorder, and not as a disorder in its own right.

Presenting Pattern

Early in infancy with a "good-enough parent," who can appreciate a child's emotional life and reflect it to the child, typical development includes attachment to primary caregivers and the attainment of an awareness of self and other, as well as a sense of connectedness to primary caregivers and a wariness of others, expressed in normative separation anxiety, in which a 5- to 8-month-old will express distress when separating from a primary caregiver. Atypically, a child may express more generalized distress and be either unable to separate from a parent or separate too easily. Their less developed capacity for language and abstract reasoning may lead children to express distress through excessive tantrums, agitation, avoidance, and worries. Because of the interrelatedness of anxiety and physiological fear responses of children of all ages, one can regard the behavioral presentations as "fight, flight, or freeze" reactions. As children develop, they may evolve counterphobic reactions in which they approach or provoke what they fear, to alleviate the anxiety they cannot control via mastery.

The fight-or-flight system activation may lead to a kind of hyperfocus or hypervigilance, which can cause even very young infants to be on near-constant alert.

Functioning at this heightened level can greatly impede interactions and experiences necessary for normal development. Children may present with various disruptions in their development and in their interactions with others, such as feeding and eating disorders, sleep difficulties, apprehensiveness about playing with peers, overly aggressive responses to perceived threats in play, school refusal, difficulty separating from parents to participate in activities, somatic preoccupations, and elimination disorders.

Childhood anxiety disorders commonly present first as separation anxiety and specific phobias, followed by the onset of social phobia. This may follow the development of insecure attachment patterns, or be related to strain that emerges when a highly anxious or depressed mother (or other primary caregiver) cannot sufficiently soothe or comfort the child, or when a temperamental mismatch leads to poor understanding of the child's needs by the caregiver.

Because of the irrational, fantasy-based nature of anxiety, usual parental attempts to explain away the described source of a child's anxiety are generally fruitless. Often caregivers are also anxious and responding in a vigilant or hypersensitive fashion to their children, or to the caregivers' internal experiences of the children and of themselves as "failing in parenting."

DC: 0–3R identifies the following criteria for the most important anxiety disorders in early infancy:

- *Separation anxiety disorder.* The child may worry to the point of being reluctant or refusing to go to school, be alone, or sleep alone. The child may also experience repeated nightmares and may complain of physical symptoms such as headaches, stomachaches, nausea, or vomiting.
- *Specific phobia.* The child either avoids the phobic situation or object, or shows intense anxiety or distress when contact is unavoidable. Exposure to the phobic stimulus provokes an immediate anxiety response, such as panic, crying, tantrums, freezing, or clinging.
- *Social anxiety disorder (social phobia).* The child exhibits marked and persistent fear of one or more social or performance situations involving unfamiliar people or possible scrutiny by others.
- *Generalized anxiety disorder.* The child experiences excessive anxiety that is not linked to any one event or situation. He or she feels significantly distressed over any number of things—from the health of family members to performance at school and future events.

In addition to those listed above, DC: 0–5 defines criteria for a new anxiety disorder, *inhibition to novelty disorder.* The child shows an overall and pervasive difficulty to approach new situations, toys, activities, and persons. He or she exhibits fearful symptoms in the presence of novel/unfamiliar objects, people, and situations, with freezing, withdrawn, or pervasive negative affects. This disorder appears to increase risk for later emerging anxiety disorders.

As noted above, selective mutism, instead of being considered a disorder in itself, is seen as a complex anxiety disorder characterized by the child's inability to speak and communicate effectively in select social settings, such as school. Children with this disorder are able to speak and communicate in settings where they are comfortable, secure, and relaxed. Almost all children with selective mutism also have social phobia or social anxiety. As with mutism, research confirms a high co-occurrence of these disorders.

A clinician should first assess whether a processing impairment, such as sensory, motor, or other processing difficulties, interferes with a child's ability to deal with unknown situations. In this case, an infant could be irritable, anxious, and overly responsive, but anxiety is primarily related to a regulatory–sensory processing disorder. Second, the clinician should assess whether anxiety is primarily related to expected developmental transitions or to a task the child is having difficulty mastering (developmental anxiety disorder). Finally, anxiety related to the infant–caregiver relationship should be considered.

To achieve better accuracy in the clinical evaluation, one must consider not simply symptoms, but impairments in emotional functioning and in the child's subjective and interpersonal experience.

Developmental Pathways

A review of the main factors that may predispose or contribute to the onset and persistence of anxiety syndromes suggests multiple developmental pathways and complex transactions among biological, genetic, environmental, and relational factors.

There is moderately strong evidence that a temperamentally inhibited infant or toddler tends to become a separation-anxious or phobic child, who may evolve into a socially anxious child and then a generally anxious adult. The anxious temperament may reflect a biological predisposition to low-threshold anxiety in response to environmental stressors, behaviorally expressed as a slow-to-warm-up, cautious, hypervigilant pattern, or, in a more extreme presentation, as behavioral inhibition. The expression of anxiety reflects the developmental stage of the child. The preverbal child whose experience of the world is less defined and comprehensible will present with irritability, tantrums, disruptions in eating or sleeping, and poor engagement in age-appropriate activities. As the child matures and develops more complex verbal skills, he or she will be increasingly able to describe worries, fears, and phobias, and may become more avoidant and regressed. Parsing out contributing factors, both constitutional–maturational and interactional–situational, is critical in developing a diagnosis.

A secure attachment to a primary caregiver has been found to build resiliency and provide infants and toddlers the resources to respond to stressful experiences. Conversely, insecure–resistant attachment may be a risk factor for depressive and anxiety disorders in children and adolescents. Preschool children with insecure–resistant attachment are described as tense, anxious, fearful, easily frustrated, passive, and oriented to adults. They are not able to take comfort and reassurance, and often show anger, emotional distress, and anxiety. Insecure attachment can intensify avoidant traits, especially in a sensitive child, who may avoid feared situations or react to frustration with oppositionality.

There is also evidence for the increased risk for anxiety in a child whose mother is anxious. Caregivers who, either for mismatch reasons or because of their own difficulties, cannot provide opportunities for their children to develop self-regulatory capacities, and who cannot create an environment that feels safe and secure to the children, will be unable to prevent the development of anxiety in the children. Dysfunctional parenting style, characterized by preoccupation, intrusiveness, criticism, "catastrophism," poor emotional warmth, negative affects, and a tendency to inhibit a child's initiatives hinders emotional development toward autonomy and may lead to anxiety disorders.

Anxiety disorders represent a significant clinical risk for a psychopathological continuity in subsequent phases of development. This finding has emerged in longitudinal data, which consistently attest to the heterotypic continuity from anxiety to depression, even when comorbidity is controlled for. This heterotypic continuity is more frequent among girls.

Therapeutic Implications

Given that anxiety in later childhood and adulthood is often preceded by early childhood anxiety or temperamental predisposition to it, early identification and intervention may be protective. And given the role of the environment and the caregiver in helping a child to develop self-regulatory capacities, there is a fine opportunity for therapeutic intervention. Anxious children will benefit greatly from a safe, soothing environment—one that includes stable and reliable rituals such as waking up each morning to the same music, or going to sleep every evening to a familiar ritual such as bath, reading, and lights out. They can benefit from understanding where their fears come from and becoming better able to differentiate fantasy and reality. They also benefit from the ability to separate and individuate from their primary caregivers, and from those caregivers' ability to help with the separation process. Both through the relationship with a therapist who can provide a new model for interacting, and through parent–child treatment, much symptom relief and restoration of a developmental trajectory can be obtained.

Clinical Illustration

Nina was a 2-year-old girl whose immigrant parents brought her to the hospital because she refused to eat. Parents described a normal pregnancy and delivery, followed by typical growth and development. Nina had nursed and made the transition to foods with no difficulties. She was described as a happy, bright child until the last few months. Her medical history was notable for a gastrointestinal infection 3 months earlier, during which time she had been vomiting and quite miserable for a few days. One week before admission, she became ill again with a viral illness and nausea. She stopped eating and expressed a fear that she would vomit again. Her social history was notable for her having become an older sister at about the time of the first illness. During her hospitalization, she continued to refuse to eat and ultimately was given a G-tube because of excessive weight loss. Nina seemed quite content to be fed by tube. On discharge she began twice-weekly therapy, coincident with weekly parental therapy. She was initially quite resistant to separating from her mother, and so the mother would leave the baby with a sitter and come in with Nina. As treatment progressed, it became clear that Nina had a great deal of anger and resentment toward this new sibling and the parents who had brought her into their home, though she was unwilling to say so. Through play, which was first aggressive and then more verbally expressive, she was able to express some of the anger. She became more able to leave her mother and participate in school and other activities, and she began to eat. The G-tube was removed.

IEC05 Disorders of Emotional Range and Stability

Infants experience and express emotion from birth (Brazelton, 1979; Oster, 2005), in the service of establishing a communicative, cooperative relationship with their caregivers (Trevarthen, 1993). Because their emotions are felt intensely, infants and young children are reliant on their primary caregivers for help regulating emotional states of both over- and underarousal (Fonagy, Gergely, Jurist, & Target, 2002; Hobson, 2002; Schore & Schore, 2007; Stern, 1985). From early infancy into the preschool years, children experience a gradual increase in their emotional range (differentiation) and stability. A 2- to 3-month-old infant shows global emotions—joy, distress, rage, fear—and can shift rapidly from one state to another. A highly distressed baby may be quickly consoled by a sensitive parent, and will soon be smiling and babbling. An infant who feels a caregiver's efforts to apprehend and scaffold his or her emotional experience, to give it meaning, will grow into a toddler who can differentiate and express more nuanced emotions (Schore, 1994). As a 16-month-old, this baby may evidence warmth, delight, curiosity, excitement, caution, fear, annoyance, assertiveness, sympathy, sadness, and other more subtle emotional states. The adaptive toddler experiences and expresses emotions in a relatively predictable and moderated manner in relationship to expectable experiences (e.g., happiness when a smiling parent appears, and anger when a favorite toy is put on the shelf because it is bedtime).

A child's capacity to experience the full range of age-expected emotions and to regulate them in stable ways is an important foundation of that child's future social and intellectual development (Lyons-Ruth, 1999). Because of their potential long-term consequences, it is important to recognize difficulties with age-expected emotional range and stability.

To determine whether a child has difficulty with age-appropriate emotional range and stability, a clinician must have a road map of expected emotional development in infants and young children. Their emotional development can be observed in their body expressions, relationships, and interactions with others, as well as in their age-appropriate capacity to play (Hobson, 2002; Stern, 1985). Earliest expressions of emotion relate to bodily states (satiated, dry, warm, not tired) and social-emotional experiences (security, pleasure, playfulness) with caregivers. Negative emotion in infancy appears to be largely responsive (e.g., to the pain of hunger or to feelings of not being safe when put down too quickly). More negative emotions emerge as children encounter limitations inherent in, or set by, the reality around them in relation to others and to their own capacities. They may feel anger, jealousy, sibling rivalry, competition, aggression, and a wish for control and power over others. They may feel humiliation at their own lack of prowess and success. These "negative" emotions can challenge caregiver–child interactions if the caregiver does not understand the emotional underpinnings of the child's behaviors and if the relationship does not embrace the full range of human feelings (Woods & Pretorius, 2011). As the child masters reality testing, accommodating to compromise in line with possibilities, and reaches higher developmental levels, emotions expand to friendship, loyalty, justice, and morality. They become increasingly differentiated as a child is able to describe complex feelings, including ambivalence and conflicting emotions and the reasons for them. A 2-year-old boy may hit his baby sister. At 3, he may make a verbal claim on her toy. At 4, he may say that his mommy never spends time with him and the baby always comes first, while noting his love for the baby. Between 5 and 6, he may be protective and helpful, but also able to talk about his jealousy.

It is thus the lack of normal differentiation, range, and stability of emotions that characterizes disorders of emotional range and stability. In contrast to children with developmental anxieties, children who are appropriately given this diagnosis present with a narrow range of affects or interests, and their experience may lack the full-blown intensity of anxiety reactions.

Presenting Pattern

Disorders in this category may manifest themselves in a variety of ways. An infant may show a very limited range of emotions of apparently low-key intensity (dull), or very rapid escalation of negative emotion, or abrupt collapse. A toddler may not recognize emotions or emotional cues, or may confuse discrete emotions (such as excited and angry), or reverse affect (e.g., laughing when the mother is hurt)—therein displaying inappropriate emotion. An older child may have trouble answering questions about feelings and may seem unable to reflect on the connections among thoughts, feelings, and behavior.

The functioning of such children can be quite severely limited. Their developing capacity for emotional regulation can be disrupted by their limited ability to understand emotional states and tolerate frustration and distress in an age-expectable manner. Executive functioning, such as the ability to pay attention, engage in social learning, and make links between cause and effect, can be affected. For example, emotional lability may affect even a baby's ability to focus for any length of time; a toddler's interests may be limited to a few areas, and the emotional drama that could accompany such interests seems absent. Interpersonal relationships can be affected by the narrow range of emotions in the child's repertoire, such that play with other children is affected—for example, as the child has fewer emotionally based ideas and is less interested in the symbolic play of others. The young child's developing theory of mind may be affected by lack of differentiation between his or her own emotions and those of others, as this differentiation affects range, authenticity, and stability/predictability.

In sum, the clinician may observe (1) a notable absence of age-expectable fears, concerns, or anxieties; and/or (2) disturbed intensity of affect, reversed affect, or affect inappropriate to the situation. Both of these can lead to (3) interference with appropriate functioning.

Developmental Pathways

A child may develop disorders of range and stability along different pathways. However, environmental factors play the central role.

Deficit can be a factor, in that a child who has not had the mind-to-mind scaffolding required to understand emotional states may fail to develop the capacities to recognize, name, understand and regulate emotions (Alvarez, 2012; Fonagy et al., 1993; Hurry, 1998). Additionally, the infant may have learned to exclude certain emotions from dialogue with a parent. Parents and infants communicate about emotions both verbally and nonverbally. For example, a baby may learn that negative emotions are unacceptable to a parent through admonitions such as "There is nothing to be afraid of!" or "Don't feel sad," or through parental withdrawn facial expression, cold tone of voice, or bodily turning away. Parents who are conflicted about recognizing or expressing their own emotions avoid those feelings in their children and may, for example, share only happy times. When a parent suppresses the safe expression of a full range of emotions, or finds only certain emotions acceptable, the child has fewer opportunities to explore and navigate his or her emotional world. Because parents may be unaware of the cues they are giving a child, this "arrangement" may occur outside consciousness and thus become inbuilt as a pattern of being and relating. Adaptation and defense on the part of the infant or young child can also play a role in the development of this disorder. For example, if negative states in the baby are not moderated by an adult, the infant may struggle for self-regulation by using precocious defenses. The infant may inhibit emotions and behaviors, thus showing a limited range of affect; or a toddler may reverse *affect,* thereby displaying inappropriate emotion (see studies by Fraiberg, 1982; A. Freud & Burlingham, 1943, 1944; Spitz, 1961).

Parental communications and parent–infant accommodations may interact with sensory modulation challenges (under- or overresponsivity, or a mixed pattern; see Axis III), as these make it more difficult to negotiate the functional emotional developmental capacities in a stable, regulated manner (see Axis II for a description of these latter capacities). For example, a child may be underresponsive to bodily sensations of emotion (e.g., not feeling the tightening of muscles during anger, or the pit in the stomach during fear).

Therapeutic Implications

The key intervention is to provide the infant or young child with experiences of stable relationship with receptive and sensitively responsive adults. If possible, the primary caregiver(s) should be helped to engage with the infant in this way. The parents can be offered interventions that develop their capacities to recognize, reflect on, and respond to their child's particular emotional cues, and to support the child's awareness and expression of those feelings. To broaden their emotional range and ability to support their child, parents also need help to explore their own discomfort with or conflicts about feelings and the meanings emotions have had in their lives (Baradon, Biseo, James, & Joyce, 2016; Beebe, Knoblauch, Rustin, & Sorter, 2005; Fonagy & Target, 1997; Midgley & Vrouva, 2012).

In cases where a parent is unable to take on this aspect of relationship with a child, an alternative relational environment should be provided.

Clinical Illustration

Zita, age 6 months, was described as a "good baby" because she made few demands on her mother. Her father had left the family shortly after her birth, and her mother described feeling overwhelmed at finding herself a single parent, but pleased to have a daughter. The health professionals were not concerned about the infant's achievement of developmental milestones, but referred the dyad for parent–infant psychotherapy because of Zita's avoidance of eye contact with her mother.

In the first session, the therapist observed Zita's extreme passivity. She sat where placed at the edge of her mother's lap for an extended period, without seeking to make contact with the mother; she also showed no anxiety about or interest in the therapist, who was new to her. She did not look around at the unfamiliar room or reach out for the toys laid out invitingly next to her. The therapist actively reached out to engage Zita, using "motherese," gestures, and toys to interest her. Zita watched impassively. The therapist's impression was that Zita was inhibiting the range of her emotions, including anxiety in a new situation, as well as reliance on her mother for safety, curiosity, pleasure, or passion for a new relationship. In a later session, her mother expressed surprise at the degree of liveliness the therapist had shown in interactions with Zita, saying that she mostly just sat with Zita on her lap, as she remembered her mother doing with her younger sister. The therapist encouraged her to engage face-to-face with Zita, using her face and voice to hold Zita's attention. She explained the importance of drawing Zita into an emotional exchange with her, and asked her to notice and respond to even the smallest expressions of emotion—pleasure, surprise, or discomfort—in the baby. Over time, Zita became more lively and expressive; at times, she even became demanding of her mother's engagement. Her mother found her daughter interesting and amusing. Zita also became interested in relating with the clinic's receptionist as well as the therapist.

IEC06 Depressive Disorders

In healthy development, infants and young children gradually expand their capacities for emotional expression and the experience of a range of feelings. There is a growing sense of one's own uniqueness as a beloved, specific human being. These gradually expanding capacities emerge from the infant–caregiver relationship. Adaptive interactive patterns enable infants to negotiate each of the functional emotional developmental capacities, and thereby to experience, by the time of toddlerhood, a wide range of emotions—from joy, pleasure, and enthusiasm to transient sadness and fear. They are also able to enjoy assertiveness, exploration, and a growing curiosity about their mental, moral, and social capacities. A basic feeling of trust in the self and the other (a "good object") is developing.

Presenting Pattern

Since Spitz's (1965) famous pictures of very small infants suffering from anaclitic depression or even "hospitalism," and the impressive films of Robertson and Robertson in the 1970s, it is well known that early neglect and trauma may cause depression very early in childhood. Depressed babies or toddlers show a variety of psychosomatic symptoms, such as eating and sleeping disorders, infections, and diffuse pain due to stress. Their emotional, cognitive, and social development breaks down. The growing capacity for emotional expression and experiences is lost. By the time they are toddlers, their range of emotions is limited. Sadness and fear predominate; joy, pleasure, enthusiasm, and the gratifications of exploration and social exchange are missing.

Depressed infants and young children begin to show a consistent mood pattern, rather than the range of emotional states expected for their age and developmental stage. Some toddlers and preschoolers display persistently sad or depressed affect. They may say that they are sad or well up with tears when asked about feelings or when they see someone else feeling sad or crying. They show little pleasure or interest in activities that are usually enjoyable, and they do not initiate fun activities. They may have difficulty showing or verbalizing sadness in situations that would ordinarily elicit it, or they may insist that they are happy even as they cry or look very sad. As they become symbolic, they may play out and talk about depressive themes. Preschoolers may, for example, play out and/or verbalize persistent feelings of being bad. Slightly older children may even talk about wishing they were not alive, or, despite a lack of bereavement or trauma, present themes of dying in their play.

Infants and young children may also evidence persistent agitation and irritability; nothing can please them. Or they may move very little, show little energy, and turn down activities they may have once enjoyed. Other children have sleep or eating difficulties (with weight loss or gain), which are common symptoms related to various sources of stress.

The severity of the mood disorder may be reflected in the intensity of just a few of the behaviors described above, or in the increasing number of challenges as the child feels depressed for longer. Infant–caregiver interaction patterns may play a major role in the child's difficulties in mood regulation. A child may feel a loss of love or support when a parent cannot accept the child's full range of behavior and feelings, whether because of the parent's own traumatic experiences, severe depressions, or other psychic or psychosocial restrictions. Parents may be very loving in response to compliance and good behavior, but may pull away when the child is angry or aggressive. They may not be able to respond to the child when their own conflicts are triggered.

Developmental Pathways

Depressive mothers have a strong impact on the early development of narcissistic and affective self-regulation because they are not able to create a joyful, responsive, holding, and containing relationship with their babies. Stern (1995, p. 100 ff.) describes different characteristic "schemas-of-being-with," or sustainable psychic structures that are built into interactions with a depressed mother: (1) an infant's experience of repeated "microdepression" (favoring the development of a depressive disorder); (2) the infant's experience of being a "reanimator" (favoring the development of parentification); (3) the experience of "mother as a background context in seeking stimulation elsewhere" (favoring the development of ADHD or oppositional defiant disorder [ODD]); and (4) the experience of an inauthentic mother and self (favoring the development of a false self).

Tronick and Reck (2009) showed that the infant of a depressed mother continuously faces a climate of negative affect that disrupts the flow of mother–child interaction. The child experiences a repeating loss or rupture in the relationship, sometimes only for a few seconds. This brief sense of loss becomes associated with strong affect. As expectations are formed and patterns constructed, the child expects loss and/or emptiness in response to the child's strong feelings. As the child becomes more symbolic, this pattern can be experienced in terms of images of loss and, later on, "I must have caused the loss by being bad or angry or demanding." Instead of an internal security blanket of warm, soothing, comforting images and expectations, the child experiences emptiness, loss, and sadness.

The depression becomes apparent over time when the child experiences some loss or conflict with others and is unable to rely on an internalized, nurturing image to soothe and comfort. If unaddressed, such difficulties can persist into adulthood (see, e.g., Leuzinger-Bohleber, 2015).

There are numerous pathways into depression (see, e.g., Bleichmar, 1996). Many studies have shown that early neglect or abuse increases the probability of developing a depressive disorder. Growing up with a traumatized, depressed, psychically ill, or violent parent is a well-known risk factor, particularly in combination with genetic factors on the one hand and social factors (poverty, migration, persecution, war, etc.) on the other. As research on resiliency and epigenetics impressively shows, however, alternative intensive relationships are essential for these "children at risk" and often enable the children to overcome their depressive disorders (see Emde & Leuzinger-Bohleber, 2014).

Therapeutic Implications

One aspect of therapeutic work with small children (particularly babies) with depressive tendencies is helping their caregivers maintain co-regulated, affective, empathetic interactions—taking up their infants' signals appropriately, and pulling the children in with warm enthusiasm as needed, rather than temporarily withdrawing or freezing. At the same time, one should help a caregiver understand what might have created these tendencies. The goal is to help an infant become able to experience, express, and explore a broad range of affects, including feelings of anger, entitlement, and fear of loss. Helping the child learn to visualize the nurturing parent helps alleviate the sense of loss, and encourages self-soothing and adaptive responses even in very early interactions.

Schechter and Rusconi Serpa (2014) work with severely traumatized teenage mothers. They show the traumatized mothers video-recorded sessions of how their babies (or toddlers) react when they leave the room, or when the infants desperately need them during their unregulated, emotionally overloaded states of mind. The mothers cannot stand the crying infants in despair because the intensive negative emotions unconsciously remind them of their own traumas. The therapists help the mothers to understand their (unconsciously determined) behavior and to build up more appropriate behavior, helping the babies to regulate their own intensive negative affects. Thus they try to interrupt the transgenerational transmission of trauma and depression.

The clinical illustration below (adapted from a case described by Sandell, 2014) summarizes a course of therapy with 22-month-old Hilda and her mother. It shows how valuable the empathic, affect-regulating relationship with the therapist was for Hilda and her parents, along with the value of the therapist's effort to understand what had gone wrong.

With an older child, the more differentiated symbolic inner world can be observed in the transference relationship with the therapist. But even while working with more mature depressed patients, one must still understand and work through their specific fantasies, conflicts, and experienced traumatizations in the therapeutic relationship. Depressed patients have to understand their (often traumatic) early relationship experiences and regain a feeling of trust in an active, coherent self and a reliable, empathic "good object."

Clinical Illustration[1]

Hilda was 22 months old when the therapist met her for the first time. Her mother had called the therapist and briefly related her concerns. Hilda had a brother 11 months older. The mother described him as being more robust—more resilient and patient. There had never been any particular problems with him, she said. She told the therapist that Hilda had never seemed calm, secure, or peaceful, not even in the presence of her mother. She never seemed to surrender herself to a relaxed calmness, and much less to secure, trustful sleep. During Hilda's first 6 months, the mother always had to carry her around, but still she was never calm. At 6–7 months, it was possible to put her

[1]This case is adapted from Sandell (2014).

down without her screaming, but she just lay there, staring into nothingness. Whenever the parents checked on her, day and night, she appeared the same. Her brother needed as much care as Hilda, and the parents were exhausted.

It did not help that Hilda usually slept with her parents. She lay still, just staring. The unhappy parents found this behavior lonely, incomprehensible, and uncanny. Hilda had a tendency to withdraw into herself and shut everything out, in a disturbing way. She was difficult to reach. She was often caught up in monotonous, aimless picking and sorting of things. At home, instead of eating, she sorted the cutlery or the food on her plate. In preschool, she sorted Lego pieces. Instead of building, she put them in piles. She was then hard to contact; she just went on sorting. Although sorting objects can be normal for a young child, Hilda did it in a way that made the day care personnel worried.

Hilda's life had had a traumatic start: The mother had almost died when Hilda was born, and it was some weeks before she recovered. The poor father had been shocked and utterly distressed, feeling completely powerless and terrified as he found himself with the newborn Hilda and another baby at home.

IEC07 Mood Dysregulation: A Unique Type of Interactive and Mixed Regulatory–Sensory Processing Disorder Characterized by Bipolar Patterns

In recent years, there has been growing interest in early identification and treatment of bipolar-type mood dysregulation in children (Blader & Carlson, 2007; Leibenluft & Rich, 2008; McClellan, Kowatch, Findling, & Work Group on Quality Issues, 2007; Renk et al., 2014; Van Meter, Moreira, & Youngstrom, 2011). In the youngest sufferers, manic or hypomanic states often cause aggressive behavior or agitation, rather than the frantic, grandiose thinking commonly seen in adults. The switch between manic and depressed states may be much more frequent and dramatic than in older children and adolescents. Their behavior is consequently often misdiagnosed as lack of early affect regulation and interpreted as signs of developing ADHD. Diagnosing bipolar patterns in children is difficult (Carlson & Klein, 2014; Mitchell, Loo, & Gould, 2010). We lack a clear understanding of the antecedent variables, although a host of neuropsychological vulnerabilities or deficits have been suggested, including problems in language, motor development, perception, executive functioning, and social functioning. Furthermore, a comprehensive intervention program that addresses family interactions and educational issues, as well as biochemical treatments, has not been formulated.

More research is needed to develop clear criteria for distinguishing between early bipolar patterns on the one hand and precursors of ADHD and disruptive mood dysregulation disorder (DMDD) on the other hand, both of which should be diagnosed only after age 6 (see Chapter 6 on the SA Axis and Chapter 9 on the SC Axis).

Presenting Pattern and Developmental Pathways

Greenspan and Glovinsky (2002) see bipolar patterns in children as arising from a unique configuration of antecedents involving sensory processing and motor functioning, early child–caregiver interaction patterns, and early states of personality organization. Specifically, they suggest that children at risk for developing bipolar-type mood dysregulation share the following characteristics:

1. A rare processing pattern in which overresponsivity to sound, touch, or both coexists with a craving for sensory stimulation, particularly movement (most overresponsive children are more fearful and cautious). Sensory craving is usually associated with high activity and aggressive, agitated, or impulsive behavior. When overloaded with stimuli, children with this unusual combination of processing differences cannot self-regulate by withdrawing, as a cautious child might. Instead, they become agitated, aggressive, and impulsive, thereby overloading themselves even more.

2. An early pattern of interaction, continuing into childhood, characterized by a lack of fully co-regulated reciprocal affective exchanges. In particular, caregivers are unable to interact with these infants or children in ways that help them up-regulate and down-regulate moods to modulate states of despondency and agitation. (This inability is often seen when mothers suffer from severe depression or trauma.)

3. A personality organization in which the fifth and sixth functional emotional levels of development have not been mastered (see Axis II). Emotions either are not addressed at the symbolic level, instead remaining at the level of behavior or somatic experience; or are represented as global, polarized affect states rather than in integrated form.

Another plausible explanation comes from experimental sleep research (e.g., Weinstein & Ellman, 2012). Genetic factors may make the level of endogenous stimulation of babies very different in determining sleep–wake cycles and REM sleep. Parents need to respond in an empathic and efficient way to an infant's idiosyncratic biological rhythm. Mismatch and misinterpretation of the baby's needs may lead to early failure in affect regulation, increasing bipolar-type mood dysregulation.

Therapeutic Implications

A careful assessment of a child and family determines whether such circumstances apply. A developmentally based intervention program must address all issues mentioned above. It can be designed to head off the interactive experiences that intensify the child's sensory processing difficulties, and the child can be helped to understand his or her particular processing challenges and to prepare for situations in which these are likely to pose a problem. A child with constrictions at the early, presymbolic level of two-way affective interaction can be helped to master the capacity for long sequences of co-regulated affective exchanges, which are necessary for stabler mood. For example, when an infant girl begins to show more agitation in her voice and movement, the therapist might shift to a more soothing tone to down-regulate the intensity of affect. When she becomes more apathetic and self-absorbed, the therapist might use a more energetic rhythm of preverbal and verbal exchange, speaking faster and with more animated gestures to up-regulate the child's mood. With a verbal child, the therapist might also explore how she feels during these shifts of affective rhythm and intensity. During such discussions, the child can be helped to symbolize and reflect on the feelings she is experiencing.

A child who can use words for actions but not emotions can be helped to move through the levels of development described in Axis II: first, to use words to describe feelings as concrete mental states demanding action ("I'm mad," "I'm hungry"); and, second, to use affects as signals of internal experience ("I feel mad," "I feel hungry"), thus making reflection and problem solving possible.

A developmentally based treatment program for a child with patterns suggesting a bipolar disorder might involve several components: individual psychotherapy for the child, perhaps twice a week; weekly sessions with her parents to help them create a family environment that facilitates her development; and work with the school to help staff understand and adapt to her. It might also include specialized educational programs to strengthen processing weaknesses and facilitate social and emotional growth in the school setting.

By ensuring that parents fully understand their child's developmental profile and therapeutic goals, the therapist can increase the likelihood that they support the long-term, comprehensive approach necessary to help a child with bipolar patterns. Having very specific goals that are easily understood, but that nonetheless embrace complex psychological processes (e.g., the child begins naming, and later reflecting upon, intense feelings), helps the parents to participate effectively and to monitor their child's progress. The therapist also needs to help the parents work through whatever conflicts may previously have precluded a commitment to long-term therapy.

One such comprehensive approach is that of therapists working in "Outpatient Services for Crying Babies," using video recordings of caregiver–baby interactions (Emde & Leuzinger-Bohleber, 2014). Watching and discussing the interactions with mothers proves helpful in their understanding and monitoring the idiosyncratic rhythms and problems of their babies. Case studies suggest that this approach helps the mothers to cope with the emerging bipolar patterns of their infants.

Clinical Illustration

Ahib was 12 months old when his mother, full of despair, told a research team that she was about to lose her apartment: Ahib was crying for hours and hours during the night. The neighbors had called the police and demanded that the refugee family be moved to another place. She stated that Ahib had panic attacks during the nights. He would cry again and again, "Mom, Mom, Mom . . . where are you, Mom?"—even if she was holding him in her arms.

The researchers finally understood that Ahib was right: His mother was not "there." She was psychically absent, in a state of paralysis, in a severe dissociative state due to her traumatic experiences. Her husband had been killed before her eyes in Eritrea. The next day she gave birth to Ahib and succeeded in escaping to Germany. She had not been capable of containing the early emotions and impulses of her baby son. As a result, his development was retarded, with repetitive and bizarre behavior during the days and panic attacks at night. He was not capable of calming himself down. Neither was his mother.

A psychoanalytic crisis intervention following the treatment model of Daniel Schechter and his team was highly successful.

IEC08 Prolonged Grief Reaction

The loss of a primary caregiver in early childhood is a profound calamity with a devastating impact on a child's developmental trajectory. When such a loss occurs, the basic security, integrity, and continuity of the child's sense of self is threatened. Younger children are at greater risk because they rely almost entirely on parents for their sense of security and their physical and mental well-being. In addition, they are yet not able to use adequate emotional and coping mechanisms or to seek assistance from others while going through the grieving process.

In the mourning process, children experience overlapping stages of grief. A child who is well supported will, in time, gradually abandon the illusory hope that the dead parent will return and will be able to integrate the memories of the parent into an ongoing sense of self. Such a child will also be able to turn to another attachment figure for support, affection, and stability. Children of different ages show grief in varying ways, but the severity of reactions and the impact on the individual child require clinical attention because they clearly depend on multiple external and internal circumstances.

In addition to losing a family member, a bereaved child usually experiences profound changes in the surviving parent's behavior, in family life, and in everyday routines, which may have additional negative effects on development. Such secondary aspects of bereavement may lead to the co-occurrence of other disorders, such as anxiety, depression, and traumatic stress disorders.

Presenting Pattern

Reactions to significant loss take many forms and may progress over time. Loss of a caregiver may be temporary or permanent, but from a young child's point of view, it is the incomprehensible absence of an integral part of the child's security and sense of continuity.

Prolonged grief reaction is distinguished from normal mourning by its persistence and/or multiplicity of symptoms. The child's age and developmental profile determine the length of normal mourning, and thus the temporal criteria for whether to regard the child's emotional state as a prolonged grief reaction or disorder. Whether the loss is temporary or permanent is a relevant diagnostic issue. It may be easier to identify grief over a temporary loss as a disorder because the reappearance of the lost caregiver does not bring relief and reassurance. When the child experiences a permanent loss, it may be harder to know the time frame for this child's natural mourning response.

Robertson and Bowlby (1952) documented young children's responses to temporary loss of their mothers and described three phases of response to separation characterized initially by protest, then despair, and ultimately denial or detachment. Most often, when an infant or young child loses a primary caregiver, the initial reaction is to search for the lost person and protest the caregiver's absence. The child may also withdraw, become more passive and self-absorbed, and avoid expected or pleasurable activities. Fear, anxiety, and agitation after the loss may give way to despondency and self-absorption, depending on the length of the loss, the intensity of the child's response, and the supports available. Some children appear not to react and may take on the role of comforting or distracting other family members from their grief, either by being entertaining or by becoming demanding.

In a permanent loss, differences in the manifestation, duration, and intensity of reactions are influenced by factors including whether or not the death is unexpected, whether the child witnessed the event, and the quality of emotional support available in the child's environment. These factors interact with individual's characteristics, such as the child's developmental stage, temperament, and capacity to regulate affects and communicate.

DC: 0–3R describes eight symptoms of prolonged bereavement/grief reaction (crying and searching for the absent caregiver, refusal of others' attempts to provide comfort, emotional withdrawal, regression or arrest in development, narrow range of affects, disruptions in sleeping and eating patterns, and marked disturbance in the face of reminders of the loss). A diagnosis of this disorder is given when three or more of those symptoms are present for at least 2 weeks.

Manifestations of prolonged grief reaction include other reactions as well, such as increased separation anxiety and new fears (e.g., of strangers, dark, being alone, loud noises). Some children cling to the remaining caregiver and cannot tolerate separation. Some express their anger and aggression at the surviving parent and idealize the missing parent. In some cases, children appear to "carry on" in one environment (e.g., at preschool or day care) but not in another (e.g., at home).

Younger children have limited capacity to tolerate continued negative affect and may express sadness for the loss alternately with periods of engagement in other activities. Many suffer sleep and eating disruptions, weight loss or gain, illness and somatic symptoms, reduced frustration tolerance, or regression in recently mastered skills. In some cases the grief can be so intense that it involves somatic disruptions and traumatic responses, such as re-experiencing, avoidance, affective numbness, and increased autonomic arousal to any stimulus associated with the loss. It is not unusual for a verbal child to express expectations of a parent's return, assumptions that the dead caregiver is alive elsewhere, or fantasies of reunion. Some children show marked distress at reminders of a missing caregiver, while others seek reminders to the extent of wanting nothing changed or moved.

Parents and others may be puzzled over how infants may experience loss: What could they possibly remember? Infants, toddlers, and children with significant developmental delays who may have many of the reactions described above are frequently misunderstood as too young to remember the loss and therefore as not devastated by it. It is now well known that even though very young children have not yet developed the concept of the permanence of loss, they may be nevertheless severely affected by it. The memories that a child has of a parent are visceral, implicit, and interactive, based on the ways the parent and infant used to do things together. Loss of the physical experiences of solace and stimulation deeply and permanently affects infants' sense of themselves and their security.

Developmental Pathways

Premature grief can be considered an inherently traumatic event because it occurs before a child has established an autonomous, coherent, and organized sense of self. Making meaning of the loss is an ongoing process. The course of grief can be particularly unpredictable in the first years of life because the child's reactions are profoundly affected by multiple factors (strengths and vulnerabilities, changes in the family, availability of an alternative caregiver and environmental supports). The variability of responses is even greater if the death is violent and unexpected, and if relationships within the family are severely disrupted. Bereaved children may have delays in development and in several areas of functioning, showing major disruption in the emotional, social, and cognitive domains.

When a child's work of mourning the loss of a parent is not adequately supported and secondary stresses occur, the child's emotional health is at greater risk for concurrent conditions, such as depression, traumatic stress disorders, and anxiety. When grief reactions are ignored, or when a child has multiple losses—as in neglectful families and in serial foster care placements—a coping strategy marked by impersonal relationship patterns, aggressive behavior, or both may gradually set in.

Dissociative processes and trajectories might be expected to occur among children traumatized by the death of a parent. There is research and clinical evidence that dissociative responses in the first years of life may occur when a child feels no protection from the parent and is not capable of engaging in self-protective responses of flight or fight.

Therapeutic Implications

The treatment of prolonged grief reactions in children should be flexible and multifocal, taking into account the age of each child. It must include an evaluation of the child's level of development, the circumstances of the loss, and the child's reaction to it. To inform and guide treatment, one should evaluate the strengths and limitations of the child's primary relationships and daily environment.

Whatever the reaction of the child to the loss of a parent or primary caregiver, and however the child tries to comprehend its meaning, it is important to help the child, in age-appropriate ways, to understand the reasons for the loss and to appreciate its finality. Whether the loss of a caregiver is permanent or temporary, it is essential to include a nurturing substitute caregiver to help the child reestablish a sense of security.

When the loss of a caregiver is permanent, a dyadic treatment model is required that keeps the focus on the unit of the child and the surviving caregiver. Emotional support needs to be provided to the surviving parent, who is also experiencing a devastating loss. Guidance to caregivers on how to recognize grief reactions and talk about the loss from a developmental perspective is essential. When a death is expected, as from a long terminal illness, valuable preparatory work can be done with the child—talking, making arrangements for a new primary caregiver if necessary, and supporting the building of this bond.

Therapeutic factors include the opportunity for the child to express the full range of feelings and to play out emerging fears as well as feelings of loss. The therapist can suggest activities that foster the restoration of hope and openness to emotional intimacy and pleasurable experiences. The child should not be expected to "forget" the lost love object; the child needs to know that the absent person is not lost from memory, and that feelings, thoughts, and recollections can be shared with others. Despite the importance of a substitute caregiver, a bereaved child cannot be expected to "replace" the lost object. The new person, even if gradually accepted and loved, will always be different and other.

Family members should be advised about the importance of daily comfort, stability in routines and playtime, and the value of increased symbolic play and talk time. If possible, they should not make abrupt moves. Psychotherapy for the child and surviving family members may be necessary.

IEC09 Adjustment Disorders

Like older children and adults, infants and young children may have difficulty adapting to change, loss, and stress. Experiences such as a change of caregiver, the beginning of school, conflicts with peers, illness of a family member, birth of a sibling, separation and divorce of parents, or moving from one home to another may trigger an adjustment reaction. In infants and young children, adjustment disorders are inferred from behaviors that are notably at variance with their prior adaptation.

An adjustment disorder in infancy and early childhood is essentially defined by the exclusion of a major disorder (e.g., an anxiety disorder or traumatic stress disorder), by its relationship to a stressful life event or change, and by its onset (within 1 month after the event) and duration (symptoms persist for more than 2 weeks) (DC: 0–3R).

Presenting Pattern

An adjustment disorder occurs when an infant or young child is unable to adjust to an identifiable psychosocial or environmental challenge. The child's coping strategies are counterproductive or maladaptive; the overwhelmed child conveys distress through emotional and/or behavioral symptoms.

In addition to easy-to-observe temporary shifts in sleeping and eating, minor regressions in language and behavior, mood shifts, poor frustration tolerance, increased anxiety or fears, oppositional behaviors, or impulse control patterns, a clinician must look for subtle changes in a child's ongoing mastery of each of the functional emotional developmental capacities (refer to the later discussion of Axis II). In making this diagnosis, it is critical to identify the source of the challenge (e.g., a parent's absence on a business trip); the changes in behavior and mood relative to prior functioning; and the way in which the challenge is disrupting the child's mastery of functional emotional developmental capacities (e.g., the child's typical optimism and happiness). To qualify as a disorder, symptoms of an adjustment reaction have to involve a clinically significant impairment in the child's functioning.

Developmental Pathways

Adjustment reactions can have different developmental pathways, depending on a child's temperament and prior adaptation. There may be a disruption in a recently mastered developmental task, such as separation or toilet training. A child–caregiver interaction pattern characterized by a caregiver's overresponse to a child's expectable feelings may set the stage for fear over temporary challenges. A child with an adjustment disorder may show features of a disordered relationship with a caregiver, particularly an anxious/tense or overinvolved relationship.

Therapeutic Implications

We lack substantial data on treatment for adjustment disorders, especially in childhood. Removing or minimizing the impact of the stressful situation would seem appropriate, but most important is understanding the effects of the stress on the child and supporting child and caregivers to reduce the severity of the challenge and to find flexible coping strategies.

In general, increasing caregiver availability, security, interactive opportunities, and time for symbolic play can help the child cope with new concerns. When persistent measures to support the child do not alleviate the problem, other primary diagnoses should be considered.

Clinical Illustration

An example of a childhood adjustment disorder is found in the case of Steven (available online; see the box at the end of this manual's table of contents).

IEC10 Traumatic Stress Disorders

We use the term "traumatic stress disorders," rather than "posttraumatic stress disorder" (PTSD) because infants and young children may respond immediately to trauma or severe stress. The reaction may then continue, depending on several factors discussed below. Traumatic stress can severely disrupt children's emotional, social, language, and intellectual development. Such stresses may include the witnessing of terrifying events (e.g., accidents, animal attacks, fires, war, natural disasters) or overwhelmingly frightening interpersonal events (e.g., experiencing severe abuse of self or a loved one, witnessing the murder of a parent, witnessing rape of a caregiver or the sexual activity of a drug-addicted parent).

For decades, literature on childhood trauma has focused primarily on the impact of specific types of abuse (e.g., sexual abuse). There is now an increased awareness that "trauma" needs to be more broadly defined as the impact of multiple and chronic traumatic experiences. Differences between episodic trauma and continuous, cumulative, aversive events (which have been variously named "strain trauma," "cumulative trauma," "relational trauma," "complex trauma," and "developmental trauma") are described for adolescents and adults in the sections of Chapters 3 and 6 describing trauma- and stressor-related disorders on the S and SA Axes (pp. 171–180 and 413, respectively).

Complex trauma is defined as multiple and chronic interpersonal traumatic experiences, typically occurring within the caregiving system, such as emotional abuse and neglect, sexual abuse, physical abuse, witnessing of domestic violence, and maternal depression. These aversive events can happen in combination or in sequence. Because they are continuous and cumulative, they can have a profound impact on a child's development.

Cumulative traumatic experiences can result in severe physical and mental health outcomes over time; these are not adequately captured, especially in childhood, by the PTSD diagnosis in existing diagnostic formulations such as DSM-5 (American Psychiatric Association, 2013). Many chronically traumatized children fail to meet full diagnostic criteria for PTSD, yet show a combination of behavioral, emotional, and relational problems and have symptoms of several other mental health diagnoses, such as depression, ADHD, ODD, conduct disorder, anxiety disorders, disorders of eating and sleep, communication disorders, separation anxiety disorder, and reactive attachment disorder. A developmental trauma framework can more adequately capture the complex constellation of symptoms shown by children exposed to chronic interpersonal trauma because it considers the complexity of a child's self-regulatory and relational impairment in several domains.

Whenever a known trauma or series of traumatic events is associated with immediate or delayed disruption in a child's age-expected emotional, social, language, and/or cognitive capacities, the diagnosis of a traumatic stress disorder should be considered. It is important to consider both the immediate and long-term consequences of children's exposure to traumatic experiences. There are three phases of traumatic reaction: acute (immediate, within the first 36–48 hours after the event); peritraumatic (from within days of a potentially traumatic event to 4–6 weeks afterward); and longer-term (beyond 6 weeks—typically designated as PTSD or a related disorder) in children and adults of all ages. It may be useful to designate these phenomena in phase-specific ways and provide a more accurate and clinically relevant set of diagnostic descriptors than the criteria for the DSM diagnosis of longer-term PTSD.

Presenting Pattern

The effects of a traumatic experience are multifaceted, encompassing reactions of many types, depending on a child's age, developmental stage, and other external and internal circumstances. In DC: 0–3R, a diagnosis of PTSD is given when the child has been exposed to a traumatic event and shows, for at least 1 month, evidence of reexperiencing the event(s) (e.g., posttraumatic play, recurrent and intrusive recollections of the traumatic event outside play, nightmares, physiological distress, recurrent episodes of flashbacks or dissociation); at least one symptom of numbing or developmental problem (increased social withdrawal, restricted affect, diminished interest in activities, efforts to avoid activities, places, people, thoughts, feelings, and conversations associated with the trauma); and at least two symptoms of increased arousal (difficulties in concentration or sleeping, hypervigilance, exaggerated startle response, increased irritability).

In addition to DC: 0–3R, the trauma- and stressor-related disorders for adults (again, see the discussion of these in Chapter 3) may be valuable for understanding children's manifestations of "complex PTSD." A review of the literature identifies seven major domains of impairment in young sufferers of complex trauma: attachment, biology, affect regulation, dissociation, behavioral regulation, cognition, and self-concept.

Manifestations of traumatic stress disorders include disruption in basic capacities such as sleeping, eating, elimination, attention, impulse control, and mood. Physiological disruption, common in traumatized children, reflects the powerful impact of trauma on a young child's autonomic functions and regulation of basic states (as evidenced in startle responses, increased heart rate, heavy breathing, shaking, or sweating). Any prior regulatory–sensory processing challenges, whether in auditory processing, visual–spatial processing, or motor planning, may become exacerbated and disrupt the functioning of the child—who may have difficulty following directions, feel lost or confused in space, or be unable to sequence problem-solving interactions. These experiences can contribute to further anxiety and insecurity, and may increase depressive feelings or aggressive behavior. Some children become sick and needy after a traumatic experience. They may find it hard to focus and may be so vigilant, anxious, or avoidant that typical routines and activities become impossible. Traumatized young children may become more clinging and demanding, or, alternatively, more withdrawn from their primary relationships and from activities that normally offer pleasurable opportunities to master developmental challenges. In the wake of traumatic disruption, the skills most recently attained are typically the first lost.

Fears that were not present before the trauma may emerge as a child becomes more worried in general and displaces fears of recurrence of the traumatic event onto other objects. These fears may be accompanied by nightmares. Some children ask relentless questions about the event, repeating questions to which they already know the answers. Children who play symbolically may reenact the trauma in their play over and over, in an unchanging, ritualized manner.

Even when a child's initial reactions to trauma are tempered by a parent's ability to help the child quickly feel safe again, traumatic reactions may surface later. There may be a disruption in ongoing mastery of the functional emotional developmental capacities. Difficulties with concentration and/or hypervigilance may make it hard for the child to attend and engage after trauma and ensuing insecurity. The child either may feel distrustful or angry about not having been protected, or may become more clingy, frightened, or sad. Some traumatized children slowly become less communicative and more helpless, unable to sustain the longer back-and-forth problem-solving interactions of ongoing development. As noted above, a child who is able to play symbolically may reenact a version of the trauma, with the child as either the victim or the perpetrator. Reality testing can get derailed as the child resorts to denial, becomes confused about what is remembered, or regresses to magical thinking.

Attachment can be severely compromised when the child–caregiver relationship is itself the source of trauma. A wealth of clinical and neuroscientific studies show that the majority of maltreated children develop attachment disorganization—an array of contradictory, confused, fearful, odd, or overtly conflicted behaviors, leading to vulnerability to dissociative psychopathology. This disorganized–disoriented attachment pattern hampers the development of integrative mental functions and impairs the right brain's capacity to process and regulate emotion.

Complex trauma responses include affect and impulse dysregulation; difficulties in self-perception, somatization, attachment, and interpersonal relations; alterations in attention and consciousness; and challenges with systems of meaning. They are also associated with both undercontrolled and overcontrolled behavior patterns, observed as early as the second year of life. Overcontrolled patterns may encompass rigid controlling behaviors, compulsive compliance with adult requests, resistance to changes in routine, inflexible bathroom rituals, and rigid control of food intake. Either overcontrolled or undercontrolled behaviors may have several functions, such as reenacting specific aspects of traumatic experiences, automatic behavioral reactions to reminders, attempts to gain a sense of mastery, avoidance of intolerable levels of emotional arousal, or attempts to achieve acceptance and intimacy.

The familial context is an important mediating factor in determining symptomatology and outcome. Familial support and parental emotional functioning can foster a child's resources and capacities to deal with adverse experiences. When caregivers themselves are distressed and unable to manage their own emotional response or respond adequately to children's needs and feelings, the children will be affected. In such situations, children may attempt to avoid caregivers, suppress their own feelings and behaviors, or engage in caregiving behaviors to reduce the distress of the parents.

Developmental Pathways

Traumatic stress disorders in childhood do not quickly remit, and the developmental effects of trauma take many forms in terms of homotypic and heterotypic continuity. Studies suggest that exposure to complex interpersonal trauma puts children at greater risk for lifelong functional and mental health problems, and for additional trauma exposure and cumulative impairment that may extend from childhood through adolescence and adulthood. Complex trauma in childhood is specifically linked to increased incidence of affect and impulse dysregulation, aggressive behaviors, and interpersonal difficulties.

As noted above, complex trauma often involves the caregiving system itself. When attachment is severely disrupted, there is increased vulnerability to stress—especially difficulties in attention and arousal; inability to regulate emotions without external assistance; and either excessive help seeking and dependency or social isolation and disengagement. The continuous and repetitive interpersonal traumatic experience contributes to the development of a sense of self as powerless, deficient, and unlovable. When children have established a sense of self as defective, they are more likely to perceive themselves as incompetent and to expect rejections by others. This in turn will lead them to have problems eliciting and responding to social support, and to blame themselves for negative experiences.

Traumatized children are at increased risk for major depression and suicide attempts. They may fail to develop brain capacities necessary for modulating emotional responses to stress. Effects on affect regulation extend into the long term. Complex childhood trauma is also associated with dissociation and alterations in consciousness, which place children at risk for further victimization, other forms of trauma, and learning difficulties. The sensory and emotional deprivation associated with complex trauma seems linked with impairment in cognitive development, delays in expressive and receptive language development, and deficits in overall IQ. These children show less creativity and flexibility, and have poorer scores on standardized tests and other indices of academic achievement.

Therapeutic Implications

Reestablishing the security of traumatized children is paramount. This includes securing the basic safety of the family members, who can then try to quickly restore the safety of their children. Young children are particularly sensitive to the mental states of their caregivers. When a traumatic event occurs, optimal interaction may be difficult for a caregiver who has also experienced the trauma and is very anxious.

To be of optimal help to young children, clinicians need to assess the reactions of caregivers, identifying areas of symptomatology and changes in daily routines that reflect caregivers' distress and interfere with the children's recovery. Systematic assessment of symptoms, daily routines, mood and feelings, and presence of ongoing stressors is critical for planning treatment or intervention. This process can introduce the structure and self–other observation that are casualties of traumatic dysregulation. Other relationships may be needed to help the family members and children to feel secure and to deal with fears. Caregivers or their substitutes must provide stable and nurturing environmental conditions, regulate affective interactions, and set firm but gentle limits if needed. Opportunities for play and conversation may help the children work through the trauma and strengthen overall developmental capacities.

Finding words for traumatic reactions is critical for both a caregiver and a child. Working through trauma requires increased nurturing and reciprocal affective interactions, as well as regulation and calm soothing, with gradual support of the child's initiative. Designations of acute, peritraumatic, and longer-term reactions may guide clinicians in placing differential emphasis on focused intervention strategies that are most helpful at each phase. In the acute and peritraumatic periods, clinical interventions focusing on pretend play are contraindicated.

In longer-term treatment, in the context of a broader trauma-focused caregiver–child therapy, pretend play may emerge as the most age-appropriate opportunity for increased understanding of the child's experience and as the forum in which words can be found to articulate affects, impulses, and sequences of traumatic reminders and reactions. Parents and other caregivers can involve children in soothing communications that enable them to ponder, give names to feelings, and be assured that all is being done to help them feel safe again. They need to help the children with fears, conveying that the children can calm down, can be protected, and can gradually express and explore feelings, including fears. Children who are more sensitive to sensations require a high degree of soothing and regulation.

The Complex Trauma Workgroup of the National Child Traumatic Stress Network has identified six core components of complex trauma intervention, which build on one another in a sequential, phase-oriented way: safety, self-regulation, self-reflective information processing, integration of traumatic experiences, relational engagement, and positive affect enhancement. The implementation of these core components can be successful only through a flexible adaptation of treatment strategies characterized by a systems approach and multiple types of intervention.

Psychodynamic and attachment-based intervention—whether addressed to a traumatized parent who may be frightening a child, or to the child–parent relationship—can be helpful in interrupting the intergenerational transmission cycle and providing new experiences of safety.

IEC11 Reactive Attachment Disorders

Forming an emotionally trusting relationship is a well-established basis of healthy emotional development. In extreme conditions of deprivation or deficient caregiving, children are at risk for serious alterations in developmental trajectories and for compromises in forming or sustaining healthy relationship patterns. These damaged relationship patterns have been called "attachment disorders."

To identify disorders of attachment, one must understand the construct of attachment. By 7–9 months of age, a young child begins to direct attachment behaviors selectively toward a parent figure in times of stress or distress. This process occurs cross-culturally; a large literature describes variations and perturbations in attachment under species-typical rearing conditions. When securely attached, a young child approaches the parent for comfort, support, nurturance, or protection, and is effectively calmed by physical proximity to the parent. Secure attachment is more likely to develop with more sensitive and responsive caregiving. Securely attached children are more likely to have normal physiological status and more positive psychological outcomes. Conversely, although disorganized attachment patterns are not per se evidence of psychopathology and occur in 15% of low-risk dyads, such patterns are closely associated with risk for psychopathology. This classification describes behaviors demonstrating that a child lacks a coherent strategy for eliciting comfort from a caregiver. Extreme violations of the expectable environment, such as institutional rearing that prevents a child from forming reliable attachments, create conditions in which disorders of attachment may develop.

Presenting Pattern

Attachment problems include a wide range of difficulties. Some infants and young children are not able to engage in social and emotional reciprocity; do not seek or respond to comfort; and seem despondent, withdrawn, or self-absorbed. Others are diffusely promiscuous in their relationships. Still others show more subtle variations in degrees and qualities of intimacy, empathy, and capacities for negotiating and sustaining relationships.

There is now a broad consensus that in early childhood, attachment disorders result from inadequate caregiving environments. The most severe versions of these reactions are seen in children who grow up in orphanages that do not provide sufficient emotional nurturance, and in children who experience extensive neglect within their families. We should emphasize, however, that only some children reared in contexts of deprivation or maltreatment develop attachment disorders; deprivation or pathological caregiving seems necessary but not sufficient to produce these disorders.

Attachment disorders encompass two clinical patterns: an emotionally withdrawn/inhibited phenotype and an indiscriminately social/disinhibited phenotype. In both, emotions and behaviors in relationships are so disturbed as to indicate the presence of a serious and persistent alteration of psychic functioning (Zeanah, Mammen, & Lieberman, 1993). Other than their similarity in arising in conditions of social neglect, the two types of reactive attachment disorder represent separate clinical entities and differ in important ways, including phenotypic characteristics, correlates, course, and response to intervention (Rutter, Kreppner, & Sonuga-Barke, 2009; Zeanah & Smyke, 2015). Indeed, they are now classified as two separate disorders in DSM-5 as well as in DC: 0–5: reactive attachment disorder and disinhibited social engagement disorder.

Core features of emotionally withdrawn/inhibited reactive attachment disorder in young children include the absence of focused attachment behaviors directed toward a preferred caregiver; failure to seek and respond to comforting when distressed; reduced social and emotional reciprocity; and disturbances of emotion regulation, including reduced positive affect and unexplained fearfulness or irritability. The essence of the emotionally withdrawn/inhibited disorder is lack of selective attachment. It shares some clinical signs with depression, but can occur independently of a depressive disorder. For children who remain in conditions of deprivation, signs of the disorder are quite stable and are associated with substantial functional impairment at all ages (Gleason et al., 2011).

Core behavioral features of what is now defined in DSM-5 and in DC: 0–5 as disinhibited social engagement disorder (formerly indiscriminately social/disinhibited reactive attachment disorder) include inappropriate approach to unfamiliar adults, lack of wariness toward them, and a willingness to wander off with strangers. Children in this subtype also demonstrate unmodulated and indiscriminate social behavior, and a lack of appropriate social and physical boundaries. They may interact with adult strangers in overly close proximity (experienced by the adults as intrusive) and seek close physical contact. What is disinhibited is children's behavior with unfamiliar adults, not with their putative attachment figures, for whom they may show focused attachment behaviors and preferential comfort seeking. This socially disinhibited behavior must be distinguished from the impulsivity that accompanies ADHD because several lines of evidence suggest that some signs of ADHD and of disinhibited social engagement disorder overlap. It is clear that children may have ADHD without socially indiscriminate behavior, or socially indiscriminate behavior without ADHD, but there are often moderately strong correlations between the two symptom profiles (Gleason et al., 2011; Roy, Rutter, & Pickles, 2004).

When extreme, disruptions in early attachment may be associated with compromises in language, cognitive, and social difficulties. In many cases, however, attachment and relationship problems in infancy and early childhood are not extreme. There are many subtle variations within which the early relationship lacks emotional depth, range, and optimal levels of trust and security. In looking at the more subtle attachment and relationship problems of infants and young children, clinicians should consider the implications of infant–caregiver attachment in light of the infants' capacity to master each of the functional emotional developmental capacities. The attachment relationship needs to be viewed from the perspective of the full range and stability of age-expected feelings.

These disorders are described not only by DSM-5 (American Psychiatric Association, 2013), but also by ICD-10 (World Health Organization, 1992). DC: 0–5 recognizes reactive attachment disorder and disinhibited social engagement disorder.

Though there is a consensus about the phenotypic pictures of reactive attachment disorder and disinhibited social engagement disorder, the question of whether the latter actually represents an attachment disorder is unresolved (Lyons-Ruth, Zeanah, & Gleason, 2015). Disturbances in a child's early attachment relationship seem necessary for the disorder to develop, but unlike the signs of reactive attachment disorder, signs of the disinhibited disorder may continue even after the child forms a secure attachment following placement in a better caregiving environment. Thus, whereas reactive attachment disorder seems to represent the absence of attachments in a child capable of forming them, disinhibited social engagement disorder may be present in children with no attachments, in children with insecure attachments, and even in those with secure attachments (Bakermans-Kranenburg, Dobrova-Krol, & van IJzendoorn, 2011a; Bakermans-Kranenburg et al., 2011b; Zeanah & Gleason, 2015).

Several studies have shown that classifications derived from the Strange Situation procedure do not preclude high levels of indiscriminate behavior. Children with fully formed selective attachments do not appear to show signs of reactive attachment disorder. Children with reactive attachment disorder exhibit few or minimal behaviors, suggesting that they have not formed selective or organized attachments to anyone. Although children with avoidant attachments may seem to lack comfort seeking, and children with resistant attachments show emotion regulation problems, neither shows the pervasive lack of preference, affective disturbance, and lack of responsiveness seen in reactive attachment disorder. One should not, in any case, base a diagnosis solely on a child's behavior in a brief, contrived laboratory paradigm. What distinguishes *disorders* of attachment from *classifications* or patterns of attachment is that the former are clinical conditions evident cross-contextually and involving profound disturbances in a child's behavior with both caregiving and unfamiliar adults (O'Connor & Zeanah, 2003; Zeanah, Berlin, & Boris, 2011; Zeanah et al., 1993). Insecure or disorganized attachments may be associated with interpersonal difficulties concurrently or subsequently, but they are relationship-specific; a child's pattern with one adult may be secure, and with another insecure. Signs of attachment disorders may have fluctuations of intensity, but they are seen across interactions with different individuals and in different situations. Essentially, attachment disorders are risk factors for maladjustment, not labels connoting intrinsic maladjustment.

Developmental Pathways

Little is known either about mechanisms by which insufficient caregiving leads to the two phenotypes or about the long-term sequelae of these disorders. Early experiences of deprivation seem necessary for the disorders to develop, but the issue deserves further study.

The best evidence of the course of attachment disorders in early childhood comes from the Bucharest Early Intervention Program, in which signs of reactive attachment disorder and disinhibited social engagement disorder were associated with concurrently assessed lack of social competence at 30 and 42 months and with functional impairment at 54 months. For those children who remained continuously in institutions, stability of signs was even greater (Gleason et al., 2011).

The long-term consequences of attachment disorders may be a pervasive lack of affect regulation, poor impulse control, poor self-control, hyperactivity, and low frustration tolerance, but also violent behavior, lack of empathy, personality disorders (Kay Hall & Geher, 2003), and significant academic difficulties (Schwartz & Davis, 2006). A number of longitudinal studies of children raised in institutions, many of whom have signs of reactive attachment disorder, have implicitly described functional impairment years later, particularly with respect to problematic interpersonal relationships (Chisholm, 1998; Hodges & Tizard, 1989; Rutter et al., 2007).

Toddlers whose behavior was indiscriminate with strangers showed more aggressive and hyperactive behavior problems in kindergarten (Lyons-Ruth, Bureau, Riley, & Atlas-Corbett, 2009). For children adopted out of institutions, signs of disinhibited social engagement disorder persist in a minority of children, even years after adoption (Chisholm, 1998). This disorder is associated with functional impairment, difficulties with close relationships, and increased need for special education and mental health services (Gleason et al., 2011; Rutter et al., 2007). In formerly institutionalized children, there is some stability in indiscriminate social behavior and attention-seeking behavior from early to middle childhood and adolescence; moreover, once established, indiscriminate behavior seems especially resistant to change (Tizard & Hodges, 1978; Tizard & Rees, 1975). In adolescence, indiscriminate behavior with caregivers is less apparent, but may be evident with peers. Relations with peers are more likely to be superficial (e.g., naming a recent acquaintance as a best friend) and conflicted (Hodges & Tizard, 1989).

The extant literature indicates that developmental delays explain the signs of neither subtype. In the Bucharest study, reactive attachment disorder was only modestly associated with developmental quotient/IQ in children at 22, 30, and 42 months, and not associated at 54 months. Conditions of deprivation lead to cognitive delays as well as to disturbances of attachment, but either can occur without the other.

Generally, in studies of disinhibited social engagement disorder, cognitive development has been either not associated or only modestly associated with indiscriminate behaviors in young children (Bruce, Tarullo, & Gunnar, 2009; Chisholm, 1998; O'Connor, Bredenkamp, & Rutter, 1999). Given the emotional impairments in reactive attachment disorder and the intrusive behaviors in disinhibited social engagement disorder, we may suspect convergence between the former and internalizing problems, and between the latter and externalizing problems. Several studies have identified modest to moderate correlations in those directions (O'Connor & Zeanah, 2003; Smyke, Dumitrescu, & Zeanah, 2002; Zeanah, Smyke, & Dumitrescu, 2002).

Therapeutic Implications

Studies designed as interventions for these two types of attachment disorders are limited. Since signs of attachment disorders have been noted in young children being reared in institutions (Smyke et al., 2002; Tizard & Rees, 1975; Zeanah, Smyke, Koga, Carlson, & the BEIP Core Group, 2005), it is reasonable to hope that fostering or adoption will slowly eliminate or substantially reduce signs of the disorders. Implicit is the notion that the enhanced caregiving following adoption will ameliorate signs of attachment disorders.

There are different prognostic implications for the two types of attachment disorders. For example, reactive attachment disorder resolves nearly completely with access to an adequate attachment figure, whereas disinhibited social engagement disorder can persist in the context of adequate caregiving and a selective attachment relationship. In the Bucharest Early Intervention Project, well-supported foster care led to rapid and complete elimination of signs of reactive attachment disorder (Smyke et al., 2012). Once children with reactive attachment disorder receive adequate care, their symptoms seem to diminish substantially and usually disappear. Adoption or foster care by sensitive caregivers would thus be a treatment of choice for children with reactive attachment disorder (see Bernard et al., 2012; Hoffman, Marvin, Cooper, & Powell, 2006; Juffer, Bakersman-Kranenburg, & van IJzendoorn, 2007).

Only some children with disinhibited social engagement disorder respond as well to provision of a skilled caregiver. Still, as best we can determine, sensitive and responsive care, in which a caregiver identifies and responds to a child's needs, would also be valuable for children in that group. There is some evidence that the earlier the enhanced caregiving is provided, the greater the reduction in signs of disinhibited social engagement disorder (Smyke et al., 2012). Although adequate caregiving seems both to prevent and to ameliorate this disorder, the persistence of its signs in some children may reflect individual differences in responsiveness to caregiving (see Drury et al., 2012) or incomplete remediation in those who were most severely affected initially. The reduced responsiveness of children with disinhibited social engagement disorder to adequate caregiving suggests that additional strategies and approaches beyond an enhancement of caregiving are needed. Given that social and cognitive abnormalities plausibly underlie the boundary violations and disinhibition that characterize the disorder, interventions that target these features may be appropriate.

IEC12 Disruptive Behavior and Oppositional Disorders

Disruptive and oppositional behaviors in infancy and early childhood may be precursors of the disruptive externalizing disorders of childhood and adolescence. In alignment with the SC Axis of PDM-2 (see Chapter 9), we see these behaviors as products of a disturbed emotion regulation system resulting from unmodified sensory and temperamental difficulties. In the same way, DC: 0–5 has introduced the disorder of dysregulated anger and aggression of early childhood (DDAA) to describe a pattern of irritability and anger as expressions of emotion dysregulation that lead to dysregulated behaviors.

The transition from infancy to toddlerhood to later childhood is a distinctive process wherein the child gradually shifts from a denial-based emotion regulation strategy to a projective-based one. This transition coincides with the emergence of disruptive behavior and oppositional behavior—the "terrible twos"—and warrants special consideration as the platform from which disruptive behavior and externalizing disorders may emerge.

Presenting Pattern and Developmental Pathways

Phebe Cramer (1991, 2006) identified the developmental trajectory of defense mechanisms, based on infant observation and other empirical research. The recent recognition of the similarity of defense mechanisms and the implicit emotion regulation system enables this developmental map to be understood through a dimensional, brain-based paradigm with clear connections to the neurobiological sciences (Rice & Hoffman, 2014). Cramer (2006) determined through factor-analytic studies that the wide array of defense mechanisms could be validly organized into three clusters of defenses: denial, projection, and identification.

The infant observation analyses of Stern (e.g., 1985) and the more recent experiments of Tronick (e.g., 2007) demonstrate the complex use of time-sensitive gaze deviation and detachment in the production of dyadic regulation and the further consolidation and development of denial-based defenses. Distraction and self-soothing mechanisms, such as thumb sucking, lip compression, or knitting the brow, defend against threatening external stimuli via denial. The use of these mechanisms may coincide with parietally mediated neural systems that modulate attention and arousal.

The infant's central nervous system development, through interactions of constitutional and environmental determinants including parental interactions and dyadic scaffolding (Calkins & Hill, 2007), allows for the expansion of the ability to withdraw attention from frustrating stimuli. Crockenberg, Leerkes, and Bárrig Jó (2008) found that

> an infant's tendency to look at a frustrating event is associated with a stronger tendency to engage in aggressive behavior 2 years later, and further that the infant's shifting of attention away from a frustrating event and toward something else is adaptive over time, as demonstrated by its association with less aggressive behavior, albeit only for girls. In addition, the exacerbating effect of maternal behavior provides meaningful information about the conditions under which we can expect both continuity and lawful discontinuity between early temperamental reactivity to frustrating events and later aggressive behavior. Taken together, these findings are congruent with a contextual approach to temperament that emphasizes the fit between infant characteristics and the social environment in predicting developmental outcomes. (p. 52)

Infant observation studies have established that "goodness of fit" between infant and caregiver is critical to the maturation of implicit emotion regulation processes. Some caregivers read and respond to an infant's signal of pleasure or fear with appropriate reciprocal gestures (smiles beget smiles, fear begets comfort, etc.), but may become either nonreactive or overreactive, often because of temporary anxiety, when the child begins to show annoyance and anger. Sometimes caregivers appear almost "stone-faced" as a child becomes increasingly angry and impelled to push or bite. Others quickly become too punitive. Not infrequently, one caregiver "freezes" while another is overly punitive, leaving the child without sensitive reciprocal regulating and limit setting.

This process of dyadic self-regulation drives the child's internalization of self-regulating skills, possibly via activation of relevant neural networks for intrapersonal implicit emotion regulation. A "good-enough" caregiver (Winnicott, 1973) may be sufficient to trigger learning processes (Hebb, 1949) of neuronal plasticity and network strengthening through repeated activation, as captured by the maxim "Use it or lose it." Internalization of regulatory processes and the transition from interpersonal to intrapersonal regulation may be accompanied by a successful separation–individuation process (and may be a prime determinant of such a transition). Caregiver-facilitated developmental gains may provide toddlers with emotion regulation capacities sufficient to avoid maladaptive defenses, including aggressive behaviors and defensive breakdowns (e.g., dysregulated and disorganized tantrums).

In other words, during the first year of life, a caregiver's input is needed as an infant's ability to disengage from disturbing external stimuli gradually develops.

Highly reactive and more easily frustrated infants need more sensitive input to help them develop their emotion regulation techniques, manifested by avoidance (denial) of the frustrating stimulus. Gradually, more complex emotion regulation techniques develop, consistent with Cramer's finding of increasing use of projective defenses as an infant develops to toddlerhood and middle childhood.

This process coincides with the activation of prefrontally mediated limbic attenuation capacities (Lewis, Granic, & Lamm, 2006; Rothbart, Sheese, Rueda, & Posner, 2011). These defenses are more complex, in that they do not simply deny the presence of threatening internal or external stimuli; rather, they reappraise the stimuli by reversing their origin and thus absolving the individual of responsibility for threatening or painful affects. As toddlers attain additional motoric skills and strengths, their normative predilection toward projective defenses encourages aggressive, disruptive, and oppositional behavior: They may go "on the offense" rather than remain "on the defense."

Toddlers' failures to engage emotion regulation processes may lead to maladaptive, uncontrollable aggressive behaviors, including severe tantrums with risk of self-injury. The dimensional nature of aggression makes it difficult to distinguish "normal" disruption during toddlerhood from the precursors of maladaptive disruptive behaviors.

As toddlers mature, their transition from preoperational to concrete-operational processing enables them to understand the process of defense conceptually (Cramer, 2006). By early school age, projection becomes the predominant defense mechanism, owing to the conceptual diminishment of denial in normative, nonpathological development. This makes the therapeutic approach described below a particularly useful one for young school-age children (see also the discussion of the disruptive behavior disorders in Chapter 9 on the SC Axis, pp. 571–573), although it is equally applicable to the 0–3 age range, when projective defenses manifested in disruptive behavior disorders are predominant.

Family system, social system, and community factors affect the maturation of implicit emotion regulation processes, either directly or indirectly. For example, a constitutionally intense or dysregulated child can exhaust a caregiver who is alone for long stretches with the child, especially a single parent with little or no social support. Development can also be understood in relation to experiences with extended family members in the home, or with teachers at the day care center or preschool.

The development of these implicit emotion regulation capacities has wide-ranging effects on multiple other tasks of infancy, toddlerhood, and later life. Disruptive behavior tends to derail maturation toward use of language; ability to negotiate as a self-confident, autonomous being; and capacities to engage in pretend play, express needs and feelings, resolve conflicts, and delay gratification. As such, the processes described here are of great relevance to other sections of PDM-2.

Therapeutic Implications

The understanding of infant and toddler disruptive behavior within this developmental context enables therapeutic strategies for the disruptive disorders of childhood and early adolescence. It can guide parents in helping their young children to develop self-regulating techniques, especially those children who react easily to frustrating stimuli and need to distract themselves. These children are described in greater detail in Chapter 9 of PDM-2, but are also relevant to this chapter.

Clinical Illustration

Johnny, age 2 years and 5 months, was beginning to develop severe problems in aggression. He frequently resorted to biting his mother. In observing their interaction, the clinician noted that Johnny had difficulty managing the "frustrations of daily life." It was difficult for the mother to diaper him or to help him dress when it was time to leave the house, and so on. At those times, seemingly endless screaming bouts alternated with the mother's withdrawal from her toddler.

Observation revealed that the mother had difficulty distracting the child from necessary but unpleasant events. Rather than introduce an attractive toy or other stimulus while changing him, she used only words, expecting the boy to manage his frustration at the imposition of unpleasant stimuli. One could easily conjecture that in later childhood, Johnny, who tended to overreact to frustrating events and had not been helped to develop self-regulating mechanisms to master unpleasant affects, could develop problems with aggression in response to painful stimuli as elaborated in Chapter 9 of PDM-2. A psychodynamic approach to youth with disruptive behavior disorders is depicted there in detail and may be referenced in relation to these problems of infancy and toddlerhood.

Perhaps most important for the 0–3 age range is the incorporation of the caregiver(s) and other family members into the treatment, with a strong emphasis on helping parents help their infants and toddlers through the normative interpersonal emotion regulation process. A comprehensive program needs to involve the family and the educational system, as well as specific therapies, if indicated, to strengthen underlying emotion regulation capacities or abilities to understand feelings.

IEC13 Gender Incongruence

In the mid-20th century, theories of gender identity development grew out of work with children born with disorders of sexual development (historically referred to as "hermaphroditic" or "intersex" conditions). John Money (e.g., 1994) was highly influential in this area. His theory that gender identity was formed by age 3 led to early surgical interventions on intersex children. Also influential was psychoanalyst Robert Stoller (1964), who coined the term "gender identity" based on his work with transsexual individuals.

The present state of research, however, cannot yet explain what causes a child to develop gender dysphoria or gender incongruence (as PDM-2 now refers to this condition). Nor have researchers, psychoanalytic or otherwise, definitively determined how a cisgender (non-transgender or non-gender-variant) identity develops.

The first edition of PDM focused on some hypothetical psychodynamic causes of the phenomenon and made some unsubstantiated recommendations for clinical intervention. For example:

- The first PDM noted a wide range of patterns that are part of "healthy" exploration of gender roles, but identified as going "beyond healthy exploration" children who too strongly and persistently prefer opposite-gender roles and toys, who dislike their genitals and insist that their anatomy is incorrect. PDM claimed that if the preference to be the other gender and rejection of one's natal gender were not addressed, the patterns could persist. There is little empirical support now for the belief that clinical interventions prevent the persistence of gender incongruence.

- The first PDM also claimed that "unique constitutional–maturational variations as well as caregiver–child interactions and family patterns may contribute to a child's gender identity difficulties" (PDM Task Force, 2006, p. 338). It cited as contributing to gender confusion (1) a parent's wish for a child of the opposite sex; (2) perceptions of one parent as weak and devalued; (3) underlying concerns with separation from the primary caregiver; (4) conflicts over aggression and assertiveness; and (5) conflicts in identifying with the parent of the same gender, or the absence of a positive relationship with that parent. These formulations came out of individual and family work with such children. While they may apply in those specific cases, there is no evidence that such formulations explain gender incongruence in what is increasingly seen as heterogeneous clinical populations.

DSM-5 has replaced gender identity disorder with the diagnosis of gender dysphoria in children and adolescents. DSM-5 has no lower age limit for the diagnosis. A diagnosis can only be made, however, in children who meet criteria sets A and B. There are eight potential manifestations of criterion A, of which at least six must be met. Importantly, the A1 criterion, "a strong desire to be of the other gender or an insistence that one is the other gender (or some alternative gender [that is neither conventionally male nor female] different from one's assigned gender)" (American Psychiatric Association, 2013, p. 452), must be met.

The other seven A criteria include preferring cross-dressing and rejecting conventional attire of one's assigned gender; preferring cross-gender roles in make-believe play; preferring toys, games, or activities stereotypically associated with the other gender; and preferring play with children of the other gender. These children frequently express a dislike of their sexual anatomy and may desire the sex characteristics, primary and/or secondary, of the experienced gender.

Criterion B requires clinically significant distress or impairment in social, school, or other important areas of functioning. A notable change from previous editions of DSM is that DSM-5 no longer has a multiaxial system. Whereas in DSM-IV and -IV-TR, a disorder of sexual development was listed on Axis III, in DSM-5 gender dysphoria in children includes a new fifth-digit specifier: "With a disorder of sex development."

The forthcoming ICD-11 will rename gender identity disorder of childhood as gender incongruence of childhood, defined as a marked incongruence between an individual's experienced/expressed gender and the assigned sex in prepubertal children (Drescher, Cohen-Kettenis, & Reed, 2016). The marked incongruence must be manifested by (1) a strong desire on the child's part to be a different gender from the assigned gender, or insistence that he or she belongs to a gender different from the assigned gender; (2) a child's strong dislike of his or her sexual anatomy or anticipated secondary sex characteristics and/or a strong desire for the primary and/or anticipated secondary sex characteristics that match the experienced gender; and (3) make-believe or fantasy play, toys, games, or activities and playmates typical of the experienced rather than assigned gender. ICD-11 will not permit diagnosing infants with gender incongruence, as the incongruence must have persisted for about 2 years. Thus, the diagnosis cannot be made before approximately age 5. DC: 0–3R and DC: 0–5 no longer include gender identity disorder.

Presenting Pattern

In children with gender incongruence, a strong interest in gender-atypical clothing, play, and playmates may occur as early as age 2. It is usually not possible to determine whether such interests will persist. In older children who meet diagnostic criteria for either a DSM or ICD diagnosis, there is strong anatomical dysphoria and rejection of the assigned gender. Chapters 6 and 9, on the SA and SC Axes, respectively, address the subjectivity of gender incongruence.

Developmental Pathways

Research with children appearing at gender clinics finds that most such children do not become transgender as adolescents or adults. The majority grow up to be gay or bisexual adults with cisgender identities. Some become heterosexual and cisgender. Currently, however, there are no agreed-upon evaluative tools to determine, on an individual level, which children's gender incongruence will remit ("desisters") and which children's will not ("persisters"). Recent research in The Netherlands tried to identify which if any factors might lead to persistence of gender dysphoria and found a link between greater intensity of childhood dysphoria and persistence, and a higher probability of persistence among natal girls.

In children whose gender incongruence persists until the onset of puberty, it is increasingly common to suppress unwanted physiological changes with hormone blockers. In some cases, gender incongruence desists after puberty suppression, and treatment is stopped. The child goes on to have a delayed puberty. For those whose incongruence persists, puberty suppression may ease the physical transition with hormones and/or surgery at a later age.

Therapeutic Implications

Treatment for gender-incongruent prepubescent children is a subject of controversy. Chapter 9 outlines three differing treatment approaches offered by gender clinics.

IEC14 Regulatory–Sensory Processing Disorders

Regulatory–sensory processing disorders (see Table 10.2) are constitutionally based maladaptive responses to sensory stimuli that may lead to difficult behaviors and complicate a child's interactions with the environment. Children vary in how they respond to different sensations (e.g., touch, sound), comprehend these sensations, and plan actions. How they gradually learn to perceive and organize information from multiple sensory modalities will determine the subsequent "regulatory–sensory profile" that is unique for each child.

Lester (1998) offers the "four A's" (Arousal, Attention, Affect, and Action) as the core domains of behavioral regulation in young children. Some children, however, have processing differences extreme enough to interfere with daily functioning at home, in school, in other interactions with peers or adults, and with routine functions such as self-care, sleeping, and eating. Understanding individual differences in regulatory–sensory processing can help therapists and families find ways to promote healthy emotional, social, and intellectual functioning in any child.

TABLE 10.2. Regulatory–Sensory Processing Disorders (IEC14)

IEC14.01	Hypersensitive or overresponsive disorder
IEC14.01.1	Hypersensitive or overresponsive: Fearful, anxious pattern
IEC14.01.2	Hypersensitive or overresponsive: Negative, stubborn pattern
IEC14.02	Hyposensitive or underresponsive: Self-absorbed pattern
IEC14.02.1	Pattern A: Self-absorbed and difficult-to-engage type
IEC14.02.2	Pattern B: Self-absorbed and creative type
IEC14.03	Active, sensory-seeking pattern
IEC14.04	Inattentive, disorganized pattern
IEC14.04.1	With sensory discrimination difficulties
IEC14.04.2	With postural control difficulties
IEC14.04.3	With dyspraxia
IEC14.04.4	With combinations of all three
IEC14.05	Compromised school and/or academic performance pattern
IEC14.05.1	With sensory discrimination difficulties
IEC14.05.2	With postural control difficulties
IEC14.05.3	With dyspraxia
IEC14.05.4	With combinations of all three
IEC14.06	Mixed regulatory–sensory processing patterns
IEC14.06.1	Mixed regulatory–sensory processing patterns with evidence of somatic complaints and attentional, emotional, and behavioral problems
IEC14.06.2	Mixed regulatory–sensory processing patterns without evidence of behavioral or emotional problems

The concept of regulatory–sensory processing disorders arose in the 1980s and early 1990s from Greenspan's concept of regulatory disorders (Greenspan, 1992; Greenspan et al., 1987). Ayres's (1963, 1972) concept of sensory processing disorders has been developing along parallel lines for several decades. In the first edition of DC: 0–3 (Zero to Three, 1994), regulatory disorder was included as a diagnostic entity; in DC: 0–3R, to draw attention to particular difficulties that characterize each pattern, the authors renamed the category as regulation disorder of sensory processing. The DC: 0–5 defines them as sensory processing disorders.

In 2004, a new taxonomy of classic patterns and subtypes of sensory processing problems was presented (Miller, Cermak, Lane, Anzalone, & Koomar, 2004). More recently, the Regulatory–Sensory Processing Work Group of the ICDL reformulated and expanded the description of regulatory–sensory processing disorders by integrating the occupational therapy literature with the developmental, individual-difference, relationship-based (DIR) model of infant and early childhood mental health (Greenspan, 1992).

A regulatory–sensory processing disorder should be considered when a child's motor and sensory patterns interfere with age-expected emotional, social, language, cognitive (including attention), motor, or sensory functioning. This disorder is characterized by some of the same symptoms present in other primary diagnoses discussed in Axis I, including nightmares, withdrawal, aggressiveness, fearfulness, and anxiety;

sleeping and eating problems; and difficulty with peers. In contrast to those disorders, regulatory–sensory processing disorders involve clearly identifiable constitutional–maturational factors in children.

Clinical Evidence and Prevalence of Regulatory–Sensory Processing Differences

There is now considerable evidence for the existence of regulatory–sensory processing differences in children with a range of mental health, developmental, and learning difficulties. For an overview of this research, see the ICDL-DMIC (ICDL, 2005) section on regulatory–sensory processing disorders. To understand how regulatory–sensory processing differences affect children's functioning, one must discriminate between research that includes attention to these processes as part of a comprehensive, developmental, biopsychosocial intervention program (Greenspan & Wieder, 2003) and studies that focus only on interventions for specific sensory processing dimensions.

Diagnosis of Regulatory–Sensory Processing Disorders

The diagnosis of regulatory–sensory processing disorders requires both a distinct behavior pattern *and* a sensory modulation, sensorimotor, sensory discrimination, or attentional processing difficulty. When a behavioral and a sensory pattern are not both present, other diagnoses are more appropriate. For example, an infant who is irritable and withdrawn after being abandoned may be suffering from an attachment problem. An infant who is irritable and overly responsive to routine interpersonal experiences, in the absence of a clearly identified sensory, sensorimotor, or processing difficulty, may have an anxiety or mood disorder. The diagnosis of this disorder implies that processing impairment interferes significantly with the child's ability to manage calm, alert, emotionally positive states.

Terms such as "overly sensitive," "difficult temperament," or "reactive" have commonly been used to describe infants and children with atypical motor and sensory processing. But clinicians have tended to use such terms without specifying the sensory system or motor functions involved. There is growing evidence that constitutional and early maturational patterns contribute to the difficulties of such infants, but it is also clear that early caregiving patterns can exert considerable influence on how constitutional–maturational patterns develop and become part of a child's evolving personality. The concept of "goodness of fit" offers a paradigm to illustrate how parents' representations determine the expectations of the "social environment" that may "fit" or not with the constitutional characteristics of the child; parental style in modulating interaction on the basis of a child's communicative cues influences the child's sensory integration, one of the biological roots of personality.

As interest in these children increases, it is important to systematize descriptions of each child's sensory, motor, and integrative patterns, as well as the caregiving patterns presumed to be involved. For a regulatory–sensory processing disorder to be aptly diagnosed, the clinician must observe the way the child develops self-regulation through the integration of the four domains of attention, arousal, affect, and action, and describe the resulting behavioral difficulties, such as a problem with sensory modulation, sensorimotor functioning, sensory discrimination, or attention.

More elaborated materials to orient clinicians' observations are provided at the end of this chapter's section on Axis III.

Presenting Pattern

Below we describe some presenting patterns of regulatory–sensory processing disorders, using three main dimensions: sensory processing impairments, behavior profiles, and caregiver attitudes. Even though these disorders lie on a continuum and co-occur with many other disorders in early childhood, the diagnosis of a specific subtype may provide useful information for treatment and for follow-up. In formulating a diagnosis, clinicians are advised to integrate their assessment with other tools (checklists, questionnaires, parents' reports).

Sensory Modulation Difficulties (Type I)

Sensory Processing Impairments

The first group of regulatory–sensory processing disorders involves difficulties in sensory modulation, characterized by an inability to grade the degree, intensity, and nature of responses to sensory input. Often a child's responses do not fit the demands of a situation. The child therefore has trouble achieving and maintaining an optimal range of performance and adaptation to ordinary challenges. There are three subtypes of sensory modulation problems: hypersensitive or overresponsive disorder (IEC14.01); hyposensitive or underresponsive: self-absorbed pattern (IEC14.02); and active, sensory-seeking pattern (IEC14.03).

IEC14.01 Hypersensitive or Overresponsive Disorder

IEC14.01.1 *Hypersensitive or Overresponsive: Fearful, Anxious Pattern*

Some children have responses to sensory stimuli that are more intense, quicker in onset, or longer-lasting than those of most children facing the same conditions. Their responses are particularly pronounced when a stimulus is not anticipated. They may demonstrate overresponsivity in only one sensory system (e.g., "auditory defensiveness" or "tactile defensiveness"), or they may demonstrate it in multiple sensory systems. Overresponsivity to sensory stimuli in multiple modalities is often referred to as "sensory defensiveness." Children with this problem may be particularly reactive to specific types of sensory stimuli (e.g., in the tactile domain, they respond defensively to light touch but not to deep pressure), rather than to all stimuli within a domain. Responses to sensory stimuli occur along a spectrum. Some children manage their tendency toward overresponsivity most of the time, while other children are overresponsive almost continuously. Responses may appear inconsistent because overresponsivity is highly dependent on context. Although children may attempt to avoid particular sensory experiences, sensitivities may vary throughout the day, and from day to day. Since sensory input tends to have a cumulative effect, a child's efforts to control responses to sensory stimuli may build up and result in a sudden behavioral disruption in response to a seemingly trivial stimulus.

A child's behavioral characteristics when faced with uncomfortable stimuli can fall within a broad range. At one end, the child shows fearfulness and anxiety, often avoiding many sensory experiences. At the other end, the child shows negativity and stubbornness or obstinacy, exemplified by attempts to control the environment. This latter tendency is described as a separate type below. This range of reactions has been termed the "fight, flight, fright, or freeze" response, and is attributed to sympathetic nervous system activation. Secondary behavioral characteristics include irritability, fussiness, poor adaptability, moodiness, inconsolability, and poor socialization. In general, children who are overresponsive to sensation have difficulty with transitions and unexpected changes.

Sensory overresponsivity is often seen with other sensory reaction patterns. For example, children may be overresponsive to tactile stimuli while seeking proprioceptive stimuli. Sensory overresponsivity may coexist with sensory discrimination problems and dyspraxia.

Behavior Profiles

Behavior profiles include excessive cautiousness, inhibition, and fearfulness. These children avoid sensation in an effort to control unexpected incoming stimuli. In early infancy, one sees a restricted range of exploration and assertiveness, dislike of changes in routine, and a tendency to be frightened and to cling. The behavior of toddlers and older preschoolers with sensory overresponsivity is characterized by excessive worrying and shyness in new situations, such as forming peer relationships or engaging with new adults. Occasionally a child behaves impulsively when overloaded or frightened, becoming easily upset, hard to soothe, and slow to recover from frustration or disappointment, especially in environments with multiple or intense sensory stimuli. The fearful, cautious child may have a fragmented rather than an integrated internal representational world, and may therefore be easily distracted by different stimuli.

Caregiver Attitudes

Caregiver attitudes characterized by soothing, regulating interactions, which respect a child's sensitivities and do not convey that the child has "bad behaviors," are helpful. Supportive parents anticipate noxious environments and minimize them or prepare the child for them. Enhancing flexibility and assertiveness in fearful children requires empathy for the children's sensory and affective experience. Caregivers who give low-key support to explore new experiences and also set gentle but firm limits do well with these children. Inconsistent caregiver patterns intensify their difficulties, as when caregivers are overindulgent or overprotective some of the time, and punitive or intrusive at other times.

IEC14.01.2 *Hypersensitive or Overresponsive: Negative, Stubborn Pattern*

Children with an overresponsive, negative, stubborn pattern may show evidence of the same physiological responses described for overresponsive, fearful, and anxious children. These children, however, seek to control their sensory environments and thus may prefer repetition and the absence of change (or, at most, change at a slow, predictable pace). Rather than becoming fearful, anxious, and cautious, they attempt to control their environments to minimize fear and anxiety.

Behavior Profiles

Behavior profiles may appear negative, stubborn, and controlling. A child can become aggressive and impulsive in response to sensory stimulation, often doing the opposite of what is requested or expected. Infants with this pattern tend to be fussy, difficult, and resistant to transitions and changes. Preschoolers tend to be negative, angry, and stubborn, as well as compulsive and perfectionistic. These children can, however, display joyful, flexible behavior in certain situations.

In contrast to the fearful or cautious child, the negative and stubborn child does not become fragmented, but organizes an integrated sense of self around negative patterns. In contrast to the impulsive, sensation-seeking child (described below), the negative and stubborn child is more controlling; tends to be avoidant of, or slow to engage in, new experiences rather than to crave them; and is not generally aggressive unless provoked.

Caregiver Attitudes

Caregiver attitudes that enhance flexibility, offer empathic support, approach change slowly, and avoid power struggles (e.g., by offering a child choices and opportunities for negotiation whenever possible) are helpful. Caregivers' warmth, coupled with gentle, firm guidance and limits—even in the face of negative or impulsive responses that may feel like rejection—is critical to helping an oppositional child. Encouragement of symbolic representation of affects (especially dependency, anger, and annoyance) also helps such children become more flexible. Caregiver patterns that are intrusive, excessively demanding, overstimulating, or punitive tend to intensify negative patterns.

IEC14.02 Hyposensitive or Underresponsive: Self-Absorbed Pattern

Children who are hyposensitive or underresponsive to sensory stimuli are often quiet and passive. They may appear withdrawn, difficult to engage, and/or self-absorbed because they have not registered the sensory input in their environment. The term "poor registration" is often used to describe their behavior, as they do not seem to detect or "register" incoming sensory information. They may also appear apathetic and lethargic, giving the impression of lacking the drive that most children have for socialization and motor exploration. They do not notice the possibilities for action that are around them. Their underresponsivity to tactile and proprioceptive inputs may lead to a poorly developed sense of their bodies, clumsiness, or poorly modulated movement. They may fail to respond to bumps, falls, cuts, scrapes, or objects that may burn or chill them, as they may not notice pain. This aspect of their sensory problem presents a significant danger. Children with sensory underresponsivity also may have sensory discrimination problems and dyspraxia.

Underresponsive children are often deprived of the level of intensity in sensory input required for optimal maturation. Because they fail to make demands on people and things in the environment, children with this pattern may be overlooked as "good babies" or "easy children." They often need high intensity and highly salient input in order to become actively involved in the environment, a task, or an interaction. Some children who are easily overloaded by sensory stimulation may appear underresponsive when in fact they are extremely overresponsive. The observable behavior is one that suggests withdrawal and shutdown, perhaps as a defense mechanism. Some children with an underresponsive pattern are self-absorbed, unaware, and disengaged; others, equally self-absorbed, are very creative and overly focused on their own fantasy lives. Accordingly, PDM-2 describes two subtypes of the underresponsive self-absorbed pattern.

IEC14.02.1 Pattern A: Self-Absorbed and Difficult-to-Engage Type

Behavior Profiles

These children seem uninterested in exploring relationships or engaging with challenging games or objects. They may appear apathetic, easily exhausted, and remote. High affective tone and saliency are required to attract their interest, attention, and emotional engagement. Infants may appear delayed or depressed, lacking in motor exploration and social overtures. Preschoolers may evidence diminished verbal dialogue. Their behavior and play may present a limited range of ideas and fantasies. Sometimes these children seek out desired sensory input by engaging in repetitive sensory activities, such as spinning, swinging, or jumping up and down on a bed. The children need the intensity or repetition of these activities in order to experience them fully.

Caregiver Attitudes

Caregiver attitudes that provide high-energy interactive input help engage a child in activities and relationships, and foster his or her initiative. These involve energized wooing and robust responses to the child's cues, however faint. In contrast, caregiver patterns that are low-key, "laid back," or depressive in tone and rhythm tend to intensify these children's patterns of withdrawal.

IEC14.02.2 Pattern B: Self-Absorbed and Creative Type

Behavior Profiles

Self-absorbed children of the creative type have a tendency to tune into their own sensations, thoughts, and emotions, rather than to attend to communications from others. Infants may become interested in objects through solitary exploration rather than in the context of interaction. They may appear inattentive, easily distracted, or preoccupied, especially when they are not pulled into a task or interaction. Preschoolers with this pattern tend to escape into fantasy when faced with external challenges, such as a demanding activity or competition from a peer. They may prefer to play by themselves if others do not actively join in imaginative play as they have scripted it. In their fantasy lives, they may show enormous imagination and creativity.

Caregiver Attitudes

Caregiver attitudes that are beneficial include efforts to help a child engage in genuine dialogue—that is, to "open and close circles of communication." Caregivers should encourage a good balance between fantasy and reality, and help a child who is attempting to escape into fantasy stay grounded in reality (e.g., by showing sensitivity to the child's interests and feelings; by promoting discussion of daily events, feelings, and other real-world topics; and by making fantasy play a collaborative endeavor between parent and child rather than a solitary activity). Self-absorption in caregivers may intensify a child's difficulties, as may any pattern of confusing family communications.

IEC14.03 Active, Sensory-Seeking Pattern

Some children actively seek sensory stimulation. They seem to have an insatiable desire for sensory input. They energetically engage in activities geared toward adding more intense "feelings." They tend to be constantly moving, crashing, bumping, and jumping; they may want to touch everything and have difficulty inhibiting this behavior; they may play music or television at loud volumes, fixate on visually stimulating objects, or seek out unusual smells and tastes. Their sensory experiences are more intense and longer-lasting than those of children with typical sensory responsivity.

Atypical responses occur along a spectrum; some sensory-seeking behavior is normal. Children at the sensation-seeking end of the continuum prefer a higher level of arousal than adults usually find appropriate in a given situation. For those with reduced awareness of sensation, sensory seeking may be a means to increase their level of arousal. For children who are sensory seekers, the need for constant stimulation is difficult to fulfill and may be particularly problematic in environments (e.g., schools, performances, movies, libraries) where children are expected to sit quietly. When it is unstructured, the sought-after sensory stimulation may increase a child's overall state of arousal and result in disorganized behavior. If directed, however, it can have an organizing effect.

When their sensory needs are not met, these children tend to become demanding and insistent. They may be impulsive, almost explosive, in their attempts to fill their quotas for sensation. Adjectives describing the secondary behavioral characteristics of these children include "overly active or aggressive," "impulsive," "intense," "demanding," "hard to calm," "restless," "overly affectionate," and "attention-craving." Constant or extreme craving of sensory input can disrupt children's ability to maintain attention and learn. Activities of daily living are frequently disrupted. Children with this pattern may have trouble in school because their drive for extra sensory stimulation interferes with their focus on tasks.

Behavior Profiles

Behavior profiles involve high activity and the seeking of physical contact and stimulation—for example, through deep pressure and intense movement. The motorically disorganized child who craves stimulation is notable for disruptive behavior (e.g., breaking things, unprovoked hitting, intruding into other people's physical space). Behavior that begins as a result of craving sensations may be interpreted by others as aggression rather than excitability. Once others react aggressively, the child's own behavior may become aggressive in response. Infants in this group are most satisfied when provided with strong sensation in the form of movement, sound, touch, or visual stimulation. They may be content only when held or rocked. Toddlers may be very active. Preschoolers often show aggressive, intrusive behavior and a daredevil, risk-taking style, as well as preoccupation with aggressive themes in pretend play. Young children who are anxious or unsure of themselves may use counterphobic behaviors, such as hitting another child first in anticipation of being hit, or repeating unacceptable behavior after being asked to stop. When older and capable of self-reflection, the children may describe the need for stimulation as a way to feel alive, vibrant, and powerful. Children with this pattern have a tendency to "get in trouble" as they create situations that others view as bad or dangerous.

Caregiver Attitudes

Caregiver attitudes characterized by continuous, warm relating, nurturing, and empathy, together with clear structure and limits, enhance flexibility and adaptiveness. Caregivers give the child many opportunities to get more stimulation, preferably through interactive, modulated play. Encouraging the use of imagination and verbal dialogue to explore the environment and elaborate feelings further enhances the child's flexibility. Advocacy in settings outside the home may be necessary so that others understand the child's behavior, adopt these caregiver patterns, and avoid labeling the child a "behavior problem." Caregiver patterns that lack warm, continuous engagement (e.g., frequent changing of caregivers); that over- or underestimate the child; that are overly punitive; or that vacillate between harsh consequences and insufficient limit setting may intensify the child's difficulties.

Sensory Discrimination Difficulties (Type II) and Sensory-Based Motor Difficulties (Type III)

Sensory Processing Impairments

In addition to problems of sensory modulation, there are regulatory–sensory processing disorders involving difficulties in sensory discrimination and sensory-based motor skills (e.g., postural control problems, dyspraxia). Children with sensory discrimination difficulties may have trouble determining what they are touching or how close to stand to someone. Children with dyspraxia (motor planning and sequencing problems) may find it hard to carry out a multistep task. These two types of regulatory–sensory processing disorders are associated with inattentive, disorganized behavior patterns and problems in school performance. They may involve combinations of difficulties in sensory discrimination, sensory-based motor performance, or both.

IEC14.04 Inattentive, Disorganized Pattern

IEC14.04.1 *With Sensory Discrimination Difficulties*

IEC14.04.2 *With Postural Control Difficulties*

IEC14.04.3 *With Dyspraxia*

IEC14.04.4 *With Combinations of All Three*

Behavior Profiles

Behavior profiles related to sensory discrimination, motor planning, and/or postural control include a tendency to be inattentive and disorganized. A child may have difficulty following through on tasks. In the middle of a homework assignment or household chore, the child may wander off to some other activity, seemingly unmindful of the original goal. In the extreme, the child's behavior appears fragmented. As others put more pressure on these children, they may become more disorganized. When these challenges continue over time, they can become demoralized, depressed, and/or angry. They may show impulsive or defiant behavior, passivity, avoidance, and preference for activities like video games, which are less demanding of sequencing and organizing complex plans of action.

When such children are expected to attempt difficult tasks, one often sees increasing avoidance, fragmentation, disorganization, and "inattentiveness." It is not unusual for parents to describe a child as "organized" and "attentive" when getting ready to go to the ice cream shop or the video arcade, but as "fragmented," "inattentive," and "disorganized" when attempting a multistep math problem. Clinicians as well as caregivers often ask whether such patterns differ from attentional problems or ADHD. This connection between "motivation" and ability to orient attention for long enough to reach a goal is a criterion for differential diagnosis. Clinicians should observe the relationship between specific regulatory–sensory processing patterns and general attentional abilities, focusing on their variations or fluctuations in different contexts.

Caregiver Attitudes

Caregivers who recognize a child's underlying challenges can help the child strengthen the processing areas that contribute to the difficulties. While the child is working to improve underlying processing skills, caregivers and educators who can help break down complex tasks into manageable steps and provide patient, multisensory support (visual, auditory, and motor cues) can help the child progress. Caregiving patterns that characterize the child as "unmotivated," "bad," or "lazy," and that pressure and punish the child, inevitably intensify the child's problems. The key to constructive caregiver patterns is to understand and strengthen the contributing processing functions described later in this chapter (see the discussion of Axis III, below).

IEC14.05 Compromised School and/or Academic Performance Pattern

IEC14.05.1 *With Sensory Discrimination Difficulties*

IEC14.05.2 *With Postural Control Difficulties*

IEC14.05.3 *With Dyspraxia*

IEC14.05.4 *With Combinations of All Three*

Behavior Profiles

Behavior profiles associated with dyspraxia, postural control problems, and sensory discrimination difficulties include problematic school performance in circumscribed areas. Difficulties with motor planning and postural control may make handwriting difficult. Sensory discrimination problems may make it hard to distinguish shapes or letters. Visual–spatial problems may make it difficult to line up columns in math or to understand graphs or diagrams. Motor planning and sequencing difficulties may interfere with sequencing ideas into sentences. If the processing contributions to these types of problems are not addressed, a child may become avoidant, uninterested, and/or demoralized. School may become viewed as a place of failure, and school activities (or school itself) may be avoided.

Caregiver Attitudes

Caregiver attitudes that recognize the processing contributions to the child's school performance and provide supportive, stepwise help can improve the child's overall functioning. Caregivers who can break the challenge down into small enough steps for the child to experience a sense of mastery 70–80% of the time are especially helpful. Those who are punitive, rejecting, or overly expectant may increase the difficulties. In contrast to a child with natural gifts in an activity, a child who is challenged by a motor or sensory discrimination task has little pleasure in performing it. Support, guidance, incentives, and breaking the challenge down into easily mastered steps are essential to helping the child overcome limitations and feel a sense of pride and accomplishment.

Contributing Sensory Discrimination and Sensory-Based Motor Difficulties

IEC14.06 Mixed Regulatory–Sensory Processing Patterns

IEC14.06.1 *Mixed Regulatory–Sensory Processing Patterns with Evidence of Somatic Complaints and Attentional, Emotional, and Behavioral Problems*

Sensory Processing Impairments

Many children have mixed regulatory–sensory processing patterns. Combinations of subtypes are common, as are differences among sensory domains in the same child. For example, it is not uncommon for a child to have sensory overresponsivity in the tactile system and sensory seeking in the vestibular and proprioceptive systems. Atypical response patterns vary as a function of time of day, context, stress, fatigue, level of arousal, and other factors.

Behavior Profiles

These mixed regulatory–sensory processing patterns sometimes occur with behavioral and emotional complications. Certain symptom patterns, noted in the next paragraph, are associated with mixed types of regulatory–sensory processing problems. We should note first that they may be related to interactive difficulties and/or unique motor and sensory processing problems, instead of (or in addition to) processing problems. When caregiver–child relational patterns seem to be the main sources of difficulty, an interactive or relational disorder may be diagnosed. When the primary contributor seems to be a unique motor or sensory processing pattern, clinicians should consider a regulatory–sensory processing disorder, in which case they should determine whether it constitutes a specific pattern (such as sensory overresponsivity) or a mixed pattern.

The problems commonly associated with this pattern of sensory processing disorders, with different degree of intensity of each symptom based on how the social environment reacts to a child's impairments, include attentional difficulties, disruptive behavior patterns, sleep problems, eating problems, elimination problems, and receptive language difficulties.

IEC14.06.2 *Mixed Regulatory–Sensory Processing Patterns without Evidence of Behavioral or Emotional Problems*

In their earliest years, many children with mixed regulatory–sensory processing problems do not yet show emotional, social, and/or behavioral problems. Their difficulties may be noted by parents, early childhood educators, or primary health care providers who may, for example, see that they are overresponsive to touch and have difficulty sequencing motor responses. The recognition of these challenges provides an opportunity for family guidance geared to improving functioning in such areas, and thus preventing emotional, social, and/or behavioral problems. Many parents and educators implement such strategies intuitively. Identifying these patterns, however, can help systematize these efforts and increase the number of children who are helped.

Developmental Pathways

Some studies have investigated predictive associations between regulatory–sensory processing disorders and children's later difficulties. Kinnealey and Fuiek (1999) found hypersensitve patterns to be linked to social-emotional problems in the internalizing domain (e.g., anxiety, depression, withdrawal). The association between sensory overresponsiveness and internalizing symptoms has also been documented in studies of typically developing individuals across the lifespan (Aron & Aron, 1997; Carter, Briggs-Gowan, Jones, & Little, 2003; Goldsmith, Van Hulle, Arneson, Schreiber, & Gernsbacher, 2006; Kagan & Snidman, 1991), as well as in clinical populations such as children with autism spectrum disorder (e.g., Pfeiffer, Kinnealey, Reed, & Herzberg, 2005).

Although less commonly reported, hypersensitve patterns have been modestly linked with externalizing behaviors (e.g., aggression, activity/impulsivity) in typically developing toddlers (Carter et al., 2003; Goldsmith et al., 2006). Other studies have retrospectively associated regulatory–sensory processing difficulties in school-age children with impairments in academic skills and social participation (Stagnitti, Raison, & Ryan, 1999). The authors suggests that with entry into the more stimulating social environment of school, children may have less control over their abilities to process sensory information, manage environmental challenges, and carry out daily activities.

Other evidence suggests that early symptoms of mixed regulatory–sensory processing problems, such as difficulties with crying, sleeping, and feeding, are associated with parental stress (Calkins & House, 2004) and problematic infant–parent interactions (Lindberg, Bohlin, Hagekull, & Palmerus, 1996). These factors may increase the risk of behavioral dysregulation across childhood, by undermining the development of competent self-regulation (Olson, Bates, Sandy, & Schilling, 2002). The childhood dysregulation syndrome (Althoff, Verhulst, Rettew, Hudziak, & van der Ende, 2010; Holtmann, Becker, Banaschewski, Rothenberger, & Roessner, 2011a; Holtmann et al., 2011b)—operationalized by summing anxious/depressed, impulsive/aggressive, and attentional problem scales from the Child Behavior Checklist (CBCL) (Holtmann et al., 2011b)—predicts negative outcomes in adolescence and adulthood, including anxiety, mood, and disruptive behavior disorders; drug abuse (Althoff et al., 2010); suicidality (Holtmann et al., 2011b); and personality disorders (Halperin, Rucklidge, Powers, Miller, & Newcorn, 2011). The childhood dysregulation profile appears to be stable throughout childhood at 7, 10, and 12 years (Boomsma et al., 2006; Hemmi, Wolke, & Schneider, 2011).

The quality of early parent–child relationships or family organization is one factor via which infant regulatory problems can cascade into later behavioral dysregulation (Kelly, Kelly, & Sacker, 2013; Sroufe, 1997; Wolke, Gray, & Mayer, 1994). Maestro and colleagues (2012), in a follow-up study of 28 children diagnosed in early childhood with regulatory disorders of sensory processes, reported on the basis of DC: 0–3R criteria that 42.8% of school-age participants no longer showed any disturbance; 21.4% had heterogeneous development (anxiety disorders, language disorders, and ADHD); and the rest (35.7%) evolved toward severe autism spectrum disorder and intellectual disability. Retrospectively, this subgroup had worse scores on the CBCL, the Parenting Stress Index, and the parent–infant relationship as assessed by Axis II of DC: 0–3R.

Most studies have investigated predictive associations between regulatory–sensory processing disorders and behavioral disturbance assessed at only one time point; thus the extent to which early disorders are developmental precursors of trait-like behavioral dysregulation over time is unclear. Some longitudinal studies confirm the persistence of sensory integration deficits and poor motor organization in more complex clinical pictures of hyperactivity, attentional disorders, and problems of emotional and behavioral regulation, such as depression, sleeping disorders, somatic complaints, and aggressive behaviors (Briggs-Gowan, Carter, Bosson-Heenan, Guyer, & Horowitz, 2006; DeGangi, Breinbauer, Roosevelt, Porges, & Greenspan, 2000; DeGangi, Porges, Sickel, & Greenspan, 1993). The cascade model of development proposed by Masten and Cicchetti (2010) offers insight into how early regulatory–sensory processing disorders may culminate in different phenotypes at different ages (Shrout & Bolger, 2002).

At this point, we need (1) a valid operational classification system to archive sufficiently homogeneous clinical populations; (2) single-case studies to explore how constitutional impairments affect children's trajectories as they interfere step by step in developmental tasks (e.g., a toddler who is easily overloaded by sensory stimulation may develop apparent separation anxiety when entering preschool); and (3) evidence on how environmental variables (early interactions, parental style), including specific treatments, may correct or accentuate a child's vulnerabilities.

Therapeutic Implications

Self-regulation includes children's abilities in relating to others, preverbal reciprocal affective communication, using symbols to represent emotional conflicts, and verbal competence to express subjectivity. Achieving self-regulation generates self-confidence and so may be considered a biological root of self-esteem. A child's biological endowment also has a role in shaping parental thoughts and beliefs, which, influenced by social and cultural contexts, will determine caregiving style. Treatments of regulatory–sensory processing disorders should be aimed at helping children cope with their vulnerabilities and increase their self-confidence, and at supporting and shaping the social and nonsocial environments to enhance their adaptive skills. From a sensory integrative perspective, it is necessary (1) to help parents and caregivers understand sensory contributions to a child's behavior; (2) to adapt environments to fit the child's special needs; and (3) to provide, when necessary, specialized intervention designed to correct identified problems.

The aim of treatment is to foster successful, satisfactory relationships between the child and significant others, and to increase the child's perception of the impacts of his or her intentions. For an overview of general principles of treatment, see the comprehensive, developmental, biopsychosocial intervention program of Greenspan and Wieder (2003). The occupational therapy field has developed effective behavioral treatments that focus on specific sensory processing dimensions. The Sensory Therapies and Research (STAR) model (Miller et al., 2007b) includes the following elements:

- An intensive model (three to five times a week) for a set, relatively short time (e.g., 20–40 sessions).
- A strong emphasis on parent education (approximately one of every five or six sessions with parents only).
- A multidisciplinary approach, involving a pediatrician, psychologist, speech/language therapist, and occupational therapist.
- An intervention model focused on arousal regulation, relationships and engagement, and sensory integration.

In this approach, the repairing of sensory or motor functioning is a means to an end; the overall treatment goals include social participation, self-regulation, and self-esteem and self-confidence.

Early detection of regulatory–sensory processing disorders can prevent mismatches between a child's constitutional response to sensory stimuli and parents' possible maladaptive interactive patterns; a difficult child may undermine parents' self-confidence and thus increase their anxiety, making caregiving more difficult and intensifying the child's regulation difficulties. A practitioner should observe the child in different contexts, including with parents, in order to assess the role of sensory integration in interactive patterns. Exploration of the parents' representations and interpretations of the child's behaviors and states is fundamental to effective interventions. Checklists and parents' reports should be integrated with clinical observations to provide measures to evaluate outcome and treatments.

IEC15 Neurodevelopmental Disorders of Relating and Communicating

Neurodevelopmental disorders of relating and communicating (NDRC) involve problems in multiple aspects of a child's development, including social relationships, language, cognitive functioning, and sensory and motor processing. This category includes earlier conceptualizations of multisystem developmental disorders, as well as disorders of relating and communicating as characterized in DC: 0–3R. It includes the DSM-5 category of autism spectrum disorder in terms of earlier manifestations. The main distinction between this diagnosis and the other constructs is that the NDRC framework enables clinicians to subtype disorders of relating and communicating more accurately in terms of the young child's level of social, intellectual, and emotional functioning, and associated regulatory–sensory processing profile.

The system proposed here has limited connections to other classification schemes. It is heavily theoretical, relying on Greenspan's (Greenspan & Wieder, 2009) model of psychopathology and intervention. Data supporting this approach are available (National Research Council, 2001), but these data are very limited, compared to those for other treatments (Volkmar, Reichow, & Doehring, 2011). The approach proposed here has potential usefulness as well as many potential limitations. Classification schemes differ in their orientations (e.g., toward clinical work, research, or demographic records). The question of orientation is complex when, as here, the diagnosis includes some aspects of prognosis.

For any diagnostic system, criteria must be clear and widely used. The model proposed here is of theoretical interest, especially for its emphasis on relational issues. It is less specific in terms of actual criteria. Diagnosis is only one aspect of formulation for clinical purposes (Volkmar & McPartland, 2014); a case formulation must include a fuller description of the clinical situation and areas of strength and weakness relevant to intervention. Systems such as DSM and ICD try to strike a balance between being overly broad and too narrow. Major changes in diagnostic approaches will complicate both research (e.g., longitudinal studies, epidemiology) and clinical practice; for example, will a child with the new DSM-5 label of social (pragmatic) communication disorder be able to access the same levels of service as is typically provided to the individual with a DSM-5 autism spectrum disorder label (Rutter, 2011a, 2012)?

The role of theory in the system proposed here differs markedly from that in ICD-10, DSM-IV, and DSM-5. The two earliest editions of DSM (before 1980) were heavily theoretical in nature and, as a practical matter, severely constricted research (see Spitzer, Endicott, & Robins, 1978). The detailed developmental descriptions here do suggest areas for further research, particularly on developmental change. Again, however, we confront issues of theory, specifically the inference of etiology and meaning. For example, early approaches to autism viewed echolalia as a child's attempt to avoid social interaction, whereas subsequent work views it as normative in some respects (typically, children echo when learning language), but also as one part of a more general "gestalt learning style" or tendency toward the repetitive behavior characteristic of autism (Volkmar & Wiesner, 2009).

As for all diagnostic approaches, issues of comorbidity pose substantial problems as children age. This issue was first highlighted in the classic Isle of Wight study (Rutter, Tizard, Yule, Graham, & Whitmore, 1976) and subsequently has posed challenges for DSM and ICD (which adopt rather different approaches with respect to comorbidity and clinical vs. research criteria). Other diagnostic challenges arise as our knowledge of basic neurobiology and genetics advances via genetic studies and brain imaging (Rutter, 2011b, 2012). These issues have already surfaced with respect to different patterns of clinical presentation, course, and associated mental health and behavioral problems in conditions of known etiology (Dankner & Dykens, 2012; Hodapp & Dykens, 2012). Diagnostic systems have differed and changed over time; for example, Rett's disorder was included in DSM-IV, but the discovery of a gene associated with the condition led to its exclusion in DSM-5.

Issues of diagnosis and classification of the neurodevelopmentally based disorders of relating and communicating are complex, particularly in early childhood. But there is some consensus that the severe problems of these types are likely to set the stage for subsequent major problems in many areas (e.g., learning, adaptive skills/generalization, social development) (National Research Council, 2001; Volkmar, Reichow, & McPartland, 2012). The period from 1994 to 2014—two decades of diagnostic stability, with convergent definitions of autism in ICD-10 (World Health Organization, 1994) and DSM-IV (American Psychiatric Association, 1994)—was notable for an explosion of research, with over 30,000 published studies. Somewhat paradoxically, changes in DSM-5 (American Psychiatric Association, 2013) have sparked a major debate about diagnosis, partly because of some evidence that the new criteria may work even *less* well for infants (Barton, Robins, Jashar, Brenna, & Fein, 2013).

At the same time, DC: 0–3R has changed its criteria for multisystem developmental disorder. Unlike autism spectrum disorder, it continues to be seen as curable. The DC: 0–5 has instead introduced the early atypical autism spectrum disorder to define severe social-communication abnormalities and restricted and repetitive symptoms in infants/young children between 9 and 36 months old who have not ever met full criteria for autism spectrum disorder.

We should note that while the diagnosis of autism spectrum disorder in systems like DSM has its challenges (particularly in infancy) it is also clear that new models of intervention that are either developmentally based (e.g., Rogers et al., 2012) or developmentally informed (e.g., Voos et al., 2013) can have a significant impact both on ultimate child outcome, child–parent relationships, and even neurobiological status, with brain changes seen in processing of social stimuli (Dawson et al., 2012).

Although DSM-5 has moved to a single diagnostic label (autism spectrum disorder), it is now clear that the spectrum aspect of the term is somewhat misleading. The system as proposed is actually focused on "classic" autism. Our proposals for NDRC are, in some ways, more akin to the DSM-IV model, which included a range of subtypes. A challenge for neurobiologically based conditions of relating is how best to encompass relationship models, given the presumption that the infant is primarily disordered. As has been noted elsewhere, it is possible that the use of other dimensional models might be helpful in providing an alternative (e.g., in evaluating issues such as parental goodness of fit and severity of social-affective disturbance in the child).

Yet another model might (as is implicit in the current approach) specify stages. Such a model would address levels of child difficulty relative to some well-recognized developmental issues, such as mutual attention, response to social overtures, and so on. This approach might have the additional advantage of guiding treatment—for example, relative to development of joint attention and mutual affective engagement (Mundy, Gwaltney, & Henderson, 2010). As already noted, despite substantial progress (Egger & Emde, 2011), classifications for infants and young children remain a challenge. Such frameworks have to achieve validity and reliability, while also respecting the interdisciplinary nature of infant difficulties and the vital role of infant–caregiver interaction (Fitzgerald, Weatherston, & Mann, 2011).

Children with NDRC tend to evidence very different biologically based patterns of sensory reactivity, processing, and motor planning. These differences may have diagnostic and prognostic value, and therefore it may be helpful to describe them. A child's tendencies can be briefly summarized within the framework outlined in Table 10.3. Almost all children with an NDRC diagnosis have significant difficulties with language and visual–spatial thinking. The patterns described in Table 10.3 on the next page are those that tend to differ among children. It might be useful for the clinician to check all patterns and to indicate the degree to which each characteristic applies on a 1–3 scale (with 1 indicating the minimum and 3 indicating the maximum degree).

Four clinical types of NDRC have been observed (ICDL, 2005). They exist on a continuum and often overlap (see Table 10.4 on page 691 for an overview).

IEC15.01 Type I: Early Symbolic, with Constrictions

Children with Type I NDRC have constricted capacities for shared attention, engagement, initiation of two-way affective communication, and shared social problem solving. They have difficulty maintaining flow of affective interactions and can open and close only 4–10 consecutive circles of communication (see the section on Axis II, below). Perseveration and some self-absorption are common. At initial evaluation, one sees islands of memory-based symbol use, such as labeling pictures or repeating memorized scripts, but the child does not show an age-expected range of affect and has difficulty integrating symbol use with other core developmental capacities and engaging in all processes simultaneously.

TABLE 10.3. Motor and Sensory Processing Profile

	Rating scale (1–3)
Sensory modulation	
Tends to be overresponsive to sensations, such as sound or touch (e.g., covers ears in response to mild sounds, gets dysregulated with light touch)	_____
Tends to crave sensory experience (e.g., actively seeks touch, sound, and different movement patterns)	_____
Tends to be underresponsive to sensations (e.g., requires highly energized vocal or tactile support to be alert and attentive)	_____
Motor planning and sequencing	
Relative strength in motor planning and sequencing (e.g., carries out multiple-step action patterns, such as negotiating obstacle courses or building complex block designs)	_____
Relative weakness in motor planning and sequencing (e.g., can barely carry out simple movements; may simply bang blocks or do other one- to two-step action patterns)	_____
Auditory memory	
Relative strength in auditory memory (remembers or repeats long statements or materials from books, TV, songs)	_____
Relative weakness in auditory memory (difficulty remembering even simple sounds or words)	_____
Visual memory	
Relative strength in visual memory (tends to remember what is seen, such as book covers, pictures, and eventually words)	_____
Relative weakness in visual memory (difficulty remembering even simple pictures or objects)	_____

Clinical Illustration of Type I

David, age 2½ years, was self-absorbed, perseverative, and given to self-stimulation. He did not make eye contact with his parents or show much pleasure in relating to them; nor did he play with other children. During his evaluation, David spent most of his time reciting numbers or letters in a rote sequence, spinning and jumping around randomly, and lining up toys and cars while making self-stimulatory sounds. When extremely motivated, he could blurt out what he wanted. He occasionally showed affection by hugging his parents, and although he never looked at them, he tolerated their hugs. He could imitate actions, sounds, and words, and he recognized pictures and shapes. David's regulatory–sensory processing profile showed both weaknesses and strengths. He was a highly active child, interested in learning about the world, even though he could do so only in a fragmented and fleeting way as he flitted around, flapping his arms, searching for something familiar. His intense movement had increased his muscle tone and energy. When an object captured his attention, he would explore it briefly and sometimes blurt out its label, but with no evident communicative intent. He could recite memorized letters and numbers, but could not process (comprehend) what others said to him. By his third year, he was becoming increasingly self-absorbed and would resort to exciting himself with recitations, but he was unable to respond to his name, much less engage in two-way communication.

David also demonstrated some visual–spatial strengths, in that he could discriminate objects in his environment and later locate them again. As he could not process incoming auditory feedback from others, he sought out mirrors to reflect what he was doing and used them for visual feedback. He manipulated toys and could use them in simple sequences that showed understanding of what they represented (e.g., he would pretend to eat the toy food or push the toy car), indicating that he had the rudiments of connecting purposeful intent to motor planning. This was also seen in his ability to initiate new actions with toys and make ritualized movements to songs. David had strong affect. He showed great pleasure when happy—even in his self-absorbed pursuits—and intense anger or avoidance when thwarted. His ability to initiate and connect affect to intent was his strongest asset. Although his auditory and visual processing capacities were significantly compromised, his relative strengths boded well for him.

IEC15.02 Type II: Purposeful Problem Solving, with Constrictions

When seen initially (often between ages 2 and 4), children with Type II NDRC have significant constrictions in the third and fourth core capacities: (1) purposeful, two-way presymbolic communication and (2) social problem-solving communication. They engage in only intermittent interactions at these levels, completing at most 2–5

TABLE 10.4. Overview of Neurodevelopmental Disorders of Relating and Communicating (NDRC)

IEC15.01 Type I: Early symbolic, with constrictions	Intermittent capacities for attending and relating; reciprocal interaction; and, with support, shared social problem solving and the beginning use of meaningful ideas (i.e., with help, the child can relate and interact and even use a few words, but not in a continuous and stable age-expected manner). Children with this pattern tend to show rapid progress in a comprehensive program that tailors meaningful emotional interactions to their unique motor and sensory processing profile.
IEC15.02 Type II: Purposeful problem solving, with constrictions	Intermittent capacities for attention, relating, and a few reciprocal interactions, with only fleeting capacities for shared social problem solving and repeating some words. Children with this pattern tend to make steady, methodical progress.
IEC15.03 Type III: Intermittently engaged and purposeful	Only fleeting capacities for attention and engagement. With considerable support, occasionally a few reciprocal interactions. Often no capacity for repeating words or using ideas, although the child may be able to repeat a few words in a memory-based (rather than meaningful) manner. Children with this pattern tend to make very slow but steady progress, especially in the basics of relating with warmth and learning to engage in longer sequences of reciprocal interaction. Over long periods of time, they may gradually master some words and phrases.
IEC15.04 Type IV: Aimless and unpurposeful	Similar to Type III above, but with a pattern of multiple regressions (loss of capacities). May also evidence a greater number of associated neurological difficulties (seizures, marked hypotonia, etc.). Children with this pattern tend to make exceedingly slow progress, which can be enhanced if the sources of the regressive tendencies can be identified.

consecutive circles of communication. Other than repeating a few memorized scripts from favorite shows, they exhibit few islands of true symbolic activity. Many show some capacity for engagement, but their engagement has a global, need-oriented, on-their-own-terms quality. They may have moderate processing dysfunctions in multiple areas.

These children face greater challenges than those with Type I NDRC. The slow development of the continuous flow of affective interactions prevents more robust development of symbolic capacities; these also improve, but children tend to rely on imitation of books and videos as a basis for language and imaginative play. As they progress through each new capacity, they begin creating ideas and may even start building bridges between ideas in delimited areas of interest. But they do not show age-appropriate depth and range of affect, and their abstract thinking is limited and focused on real-life needs.

Clinical Illustration of Type II

Three-year-old Joey was extremely avoidant, always moving away from his caregivers and making only fleeting eye contact with them. He displayed considerable perseverative and self-stimulatory behavior, such as rapidly turning the pages of preferred books or pushing his toy train around and around the track. He also chose books and figures from his favorite shows, such as Barney or Winnie-the-Pooh, and had them board his trains. No one dared to touch his figures; he would begin a tantrum instantly when he thought they would be taken away. He could purposefully reach for juice, put out his arms to get dressed, and give his parents an object or take one from them—but despite some vocalizing, he could neither negotiate complex preverbal interactions nor imitate sounds. He showed pleasure with his parents only during roughhousing, tickle games, and his mother's lullabies.

Joey relied on visual information to deal with his environment. His memory for things and places was remarkable. He was underresponsive to words, but overresponsive to sudden, high-pitched or vibrating sounds, which distracted or alarmed him and kept him vigilant. In daily life, he relied on ritualized patterns and protested changes he could not understand. While he could somehow find his favorite books or figures, he did not search for things in any planned way, and was easily subject to frustration and tantrums. Obstacle courses were beyond him; rather than follow other children in the preschool gym, he would collapse on the floor and watch them. These patterns reflected multiple sensory and motor processing difficulties (auditory, visual–spatial, and motor planning), compounded by over- and underresponsiveness and low tone. Life was becoming increasingly challenging for Joey and for his family, as he pulled away from relationships and frustrated the expectations that accompanied his getting older.

IEC15.03 Type III: Intermittently Engaged and Purposeful

Children in the Type III NDRC group are highly self-absorbed. Their engagement with others is extremely intermittent, having an "in-and-out" quality. They display very limited purposeful two-way communication, usually in pursuit of concrete needs or basic sensorimotor experiences (e.g., jumping, tickling). They may be able to imitate or even initiate some rote problem-solving actions, but they usually show little or no capacity for shared social problem solving or for a continuous flow of affective exchange. They can learn to convey simple feelings ("happy," "sad," and "mad"), but the "in-and-out" quality of their relatedness constricts the range and depth of affect they can negotiate. Over time, they can learn islands of presymbolic purposeful and problem-solving behavior.

Some children in this group use toys as if they are real; for example, they try to eat pretend foods or feed a life-size baby doll, or put their feet into a pretend swimming pool as if they could go swimming. They do not usually reach the level of truly representing themselves by using toys or dolls, however. Multiple severe processing dysfunctions—including severe auditory processing and visual–spatial processing difficulties, and moderate to severe motor planning problems—impede the continuous flow of purposeful communication, preventing problem-solving interactions. Some children in this group have severe oral–motor dyspraxia and speak only a few words, if they speak at all; they may, however, learn to use a few signs or to communicate by using pictures or a favorite toy.

Clinical Illustration of Type III

Sarah, age 3 years, ran into the playroom looking for Winnie-the-Pooh. She climbed up on the stool in front of the shelves, but could not move the figures in the basket around to search for her beloved character. She inadvertently pulled the basket off the shelf, causing all the figures to fall out. Neglecting to look on the floor, Sarah began searching in the next basket. Her mother ran over to prevent the second basket from being dropped and offered to help. Sarah echoed, "Help!"; she grabbed her mother's hands and put them in the basket. Her mother had to point to the Pooh figure before Sarah could see it. She grabbed it and ran off to lie on the couch. Her mother then brought Tigger over; Sarah grabbed Tigger and ran to the other side of the room. She held her figures tightly and turned away when her mother joined her. Her mother then took Eeyore and started to sing "Ring around the Rosie" while moving the figure up and down. This time, Sarah looked, and joined in singing "down" to the lyric "We all fall down." She then moved rapidly away and went to the mirror. This pattern of flight and avoidance after getting what she wanted, followed by not knowing what to do next, was typical.

IEC15.04 Type IV: Aimless and Unpurposeful

Children in the Type IV NDRC group are passive and self-absorbed or active and stimulus-seeking; some have both patterns. They have severe difficulties with shared attention and engagement unless involved in sensorimotor play. They tend to make very slow progress. Developing expressive language is extremely challenging for them.

Some children with Type IV profiles learn to complete organized sequences of the sort needed to play semistructured games or carry out self-help tasks, such as dressing and brushing teeth. Many such children can share with others the pleasure they experience when they use their bodies purposefully to skate, swim, ride bikes, play ball, or engage in other motor accomplishments. These meaningful activities can be used to encourage shared attention, engagement, and purposeful problem solving.

Children in this group have the most severe challenges in all processing areas. Many have significant motoric deficits, including oral–motor dyspraxia. They have the most difficulty with complex problem-solving interactions, expressive language, and motor planning. Their progress tends to be periodically interrupted by regressions, the causes of which are hard to discern. Sometimes regressions appear to occur because the environment is not sufficiently tailored to a child's processing profile.

Clinical Illustration of Type IV

Harold progressed only very slowly to imitating sounds and words, even with an intensive program to facilitate imitation. He could say one or two words spontaneously when he felt angry or insistent on getting something, but otherwise he had to be prompted and pushed to speak. Every utterance seemed to defeat him. He would sometimes stare at a caregiver's mouth to try to form the same movements. His severe dyspraxia interfered with his engaging in pretend play, although from his facial expressions, especially the gleam in his eye during playful interactions with his parents, one could infer that he was playing little "tricks." He sometimes used toy objects such as a soft sword or magic wand in ritualized ways, but he could not use toys to sequence new ideas.

He could become engaged and even initiated sensorimotor interactions involving the expression of pleasure and affection. Although games with his brother had to be orchestrated, Harold enjoyed running around the schoolyard and the pool with other children. At age 5, in the second year of intervention, he was able to communicate with three or four back-and-forth exchanges about what he wanted (e.g., pulling his father to the refrigerator and finding the hot dogs). He could even retrieve a few words at such moments: "Hot dog." "What else?" his father would ask. Harold could reply, "French fries." Harold became more consistently engaged over time, developed islands of presymbolic ability, and tuned in to more of what was going on around him. He no longer wandered aimlessly and could be observed picking up trucks to push, putting together simple puzzles, or engaging in other cause-and-effect play. He let others join him, but invariably turned the interaction into sensorimotor play, which brought him great pleasure.

Axis II: Functional Emotional Developmental Capacities

Axis II describes an infant's/young child's emotional and social functioning in a developmental perspective from birth to preschool years. Relying on the accurate descriptions in ICDL-DMIC and DC: 0–3R, and integrating these with clinical and neuroscientific findings, we have aimed to provide the clinician with clear clinical descriptions of infant/child emotional developmental capacities and of useful assessment tools to support a developmentally based approach to the assessment and diagnosis.

Emotional functioning includes capacities for self-regulation; different levels of relating to others; emotional cuing and signaling evident of preverbal affective reciprocity and communication; co-regulated social problem solving; symbolizing or representing wishes and emotions; elaborating emotional themes in pretend play; reasoning about feelings; reflecting on one's own feelings and empathizing with the feelings of others; and reality testing. The infant/child–caregiver interaction experiences determine the child's capacity for relative mastery (or nonmastery) of these six core functional emotional developmental capacities or levels as they are developed and build upon each other in the course of early life.

At birth, an infant has a sophisticated perceptual apparatus that allows him or her to orient attention selectively to the voice and face of the infant's mother, recognizing her as a favored interactive partner. The child has an early behavioral organization, which is expressed in the ability to self-regulate physiological processes such as sensory, attentional, motor, and affective capacities, in order to modulate his or her arousal state in the relationship context. As a complement to self-regulatory ability, the infant has a rich repertoire of expression and communication; this allows the infant to express needs and emotions, to actively propose interactive exchanges, or to limit his or her involvement in the interaction if it is perceived as stressful. The caregiver supports the functionality and the evolution of these innate regulatory processes, through the ability to properly interpret the child signals, in order to adjust his or her behavior according to the appropriate levels of intensity.

Research over the past 30 years on infancy and early childhood has given increasing importance to the concept of regulation, as the capacity to regulate emotional states and to organize experience and appropriate behavioral responses (Lichtenberg, 1989; Sander, 1962, 1987, 1988; Stern, 1985). The regulation process will develop from continuous interweaving between these innate abilities of the child, who organize the myriad of tactile, visual, acoustic, and proprioceptive stimuli, and repeated interactions of the child–caregiver dyad around the achievement of homeostasis (Sroufe, 1997). Strategies for state regulation are initially provided by the caregiver and subsequently internalized by the child; they generalize over time to include the regulation of affective states, arousal, attention, and organization of complex behaviors that include social interactions. In this way, positive infant–caregiver interactions can shape the infant's developmental outcomes through inducing mechanistic changes in brain structure and function (Schore, 2001). According to the mutual regulation process proposed by Tronick (2007), the child has the dual task of regulating his or her emotional state and involvement in dyadic interactions with the caregiver in moments that represent ruptures or changes in the internal state, such as the emergence of hunger or excessive external stimulation. Infants and young children have an overall wealth of biopsychosocial competencies and are able to react to the meanings of others' intentions and emotions. With these biopsychosocial competencies, infants make meaning about their relationships to the world of people and things and about themselves. When aberrant or atypical forms of meaning making persist, they can distort how infants master age-appropriate developmental tasks, such as developing self-regulation, forming attachments with caregivers, or achieving autonomy (Tronick & Beeghly, 2011).

The functional emotional developmental framework of Axis II also serves as an organizing construct for integrating the other aspects of development, including motor, sensory, language, and cognitive functioning. The functional emotional developmental levels provide a way of characterizing emotional functioning and, at the same time, a way of looking at how all the components of development (cognition, language, and motor skills) work together in a functional manner (as a mental team) organized by the designated emotional goals at each level.

Each developmental level involves different tasks or goals. The relative effects of the constitutional–maturational, environmental, or interactive variables, therefore, depend on and can only be understood in the context of the developmental level they relate to.

The goal of Axis II is to enable clinicians to look at child–caregiver interactions at different stages of development, consider what influences their interaction, and determine whether emotional functioning leads to adaptive or maladaptive organizations at each developmental level. It is important, however, to note that other developmental aspects, such as emotional sharing in relationships or sensory processing abilities, are evaluated on other axes, even if they are conceptually linked to this axis.

The Six Developmental Functional Levels

There are six early organizational levels of experience (see Table 10.5). Each is described below, with characteristics of expected emotional functioning and examples of challenges. Reflecting the seminal work of Greenspan and colleagues, the PDM-2 labels and descriptions of functional emotional developmental capacities have been revised and reformulated in a clinician-friendly way.

The assessment of the developmental functional level reached by an infant/child needs to be evaluated in the context of infant/child–caregiver interactions. Such an evaluation provides a rich, nuanced profile of how a very young child experiences his or her physical and human environment, the ways in which the child uses his or her own resources and the support of caregivers to engage with the world, and the challenges that confront the child (Greenspan, 1996).

Level 1: Shared Attention and Regulation (Typically Observable between Birth and 3 Months)

The first level of development involves self-regulation and shared attention—that is, the capacity to attend to multisensory affective experience and, at the same time, organize a calm, regulated state (e.g., looking at, listening to, and following the movements of a caregiver). Homeostasis is the fundamental goal in the first few months of life. The child needs to establish the basic rhythms of sleep, wakefulness, nutrition, and elimination, and to achieve a state of calm alertness (which can be compromised by excessive irritability or persistent drowsiness). Signals of hunger, satiety, interest, or curiosity need to receive contingent and appropriate responses from the caregiver, who supports the child's self-regulatory capacities. This ongoing process, in its constant repetition, allows the child to distinguish different internal states. In the early stages of development, the caregiver normally provides sensory input through play and caretaking experiences such as dressing and bathing, and soothes the young infant when distressed to facilitate state organization. The infant can stay regulated, without over- or underreacting to external or internal stimuli, to attend and interact. It is an interactive process of mutual co-regulation, whereby the infant uses the caregiver's physical and emotional state to organize him- or herself. The early regulation of arousal and

TABLE 10.5. Developmental Levels of Emotional Functioning

Level	Expected emotional function	Developmental level
1	Shared attention and regulation	0–3 months and beyond
2	Engagement and relating	3–6 months and beyond
3	Two-way purposeful emotional interactions	6–9 months and beyond
4	Shared social problem solving	9–18 months and beyond
5	Creating symbols and ideas	18–30 months and beyond
6	Building logical bridges between ideas: Logical thinking	30–48 months and beyond

physiological states is critical for successful adaptation to the environment and for learning self-calming, attention, and emotional responsivity. The optimal level varies considerably and depends on the infant's threshold for arousal, tolerance for stimulation, and ability to self-control arousal. The caregiver needs to tailor interactions to sensory modulation differences (e.g., under- or overresponsivity to touch or sound), as well as the infant's motor planning capacities (e.g., turning to look at the caregiver). The failure of regulation and attention may be due to difficulties in the regulatory–sensory processing capacities or to noncontingent and arbitrary caregiver responses, as when the caregiver is depressed or self-absorbed.

Rating Scale

For this and each of the other five levels of functioning, a 5-point rating scale, in which each mental function can be assessed from 5 to 1, is provided in Table 10.6 on page 703. Descriptions of the anchor points for ratings of 5, 3, and 1 are provided for each level in the text.

5. The infant is attentive to visual, auditory, and tactile sensations, and experiences interest in sight, sound, touch, movement, and other sensory experiences. He or she is able to calm down and to modulate affects and states to maintain a long-lasting flow of interactions. Age-appropriate shared attention and regulation are fully mastered.
3. The infant shows interest in the world, but the ability to remain calm and focused is limited to short periods of time. Attention and responsivity may be affected by some mild regulatory–sensory processing difficulties and/or by excessive over- or understimulation from the caregiving context. Some failure of mutual regulation may delay the achievement of the age-appropriate level of functioning.
1. The infant has difficulty organizing the affective domains of joy, pleasure, and exploration, as well as goal-directed movement or social behaviors. He or she is difficult to calm and may experience uncomfortable states, becoming very upset or distressed; conversely, the infant may be very sleepy and passive and fail to maintain adequate arousal level except with extremely intense stimuli. Age-appropriate shared attention and regulation are deficient.

Level 2: Engagement and Relating (Typically Observable between 3 and 6 Months)

Dyadic reciprocity begins to occur between 2 and 4 months of age, when interaction within the infant–caregiver dyad is characterized by mutual gaze, vocalizations, and physical proximity to each other. The infant becomes more engaged in social and emotional interactions, looking for soothing, security, and pleasure. He or she shows greater ability to respond to the external environment and to form a special relationship with one or more primary caregivers. Engagement is supported by early maturational capabilities for selectively focusing on the human face and voice and for processing and organizing information from senses. By the second month of life, infants are sensitive to reciprocity (timing and turn taking) while interacting with caregivers, and it provides a sense of shared experience or "intersubjectivity." Primary intersubjectivity is also expressed in infant imitation. Infants and mothers show protodialogic behaviors in which they time their behavior in a bidirectional, coordinated way. Innate predispositions to social interactions are gradually organized in an infant's attachment bond to the available caregiver. At the same time, the child experiences a widening range of emerging positive and negative emotions within these interactions; joy, pleasure, assertiveness, curiosity, protest, and anger all progressively become part of the forming relationship. Early engagement has implications for later attachment patterns and behavior, as well as for emotional regulation.

Engagement and reciprocity can be affected by caregiver psychological difficulties (absorbed in affective states of withdrawal or overstimulating) and/or by specific characteristics of the child. Infants with autism showed a specific qualitative deficit in responding to social stimuli, whereas attention paid to objects did not distinguish autistic from normal infants during the first 6 months of life.

Rating Scale

5. The infant shows joint emotional involvement (seen in looking, joyful smiling and laughing, and synchronous arm and leg movements) when interacting with the caregiver. As development proceeds, the infant evidences a growing sense of security and comfort with, as well as interest and curiosity in, the caregiver. The full range of emerging emotions becomes part of this capacity (e.g., protest and anger at the caregiver are tolerated, along with positive affects of pleasure and joy).
3. The infant may turn his or her head away, avert gaze, or appear indifferent and withdrawn in interactions when under stress. The infant may show some constriction in affective range or some difficulty in returning to his or her earlier interest in the primary caregiver if something bothers the infant or if interactive ruptures occur. Limitations are evidenced by flat or shallow affect or are shown under stress.
1. The infant is not able to employ his or her senses to form an affective relationship with a caregiver—such as when sounds, touch, and even scents are avoided, with either chronic gaze aversion, flat affect, or random or nonsynchronous patterns of brightening and alerting. The infant may avoid affective contact with caregiver or may not experience the full range and depth of affects in interactions. The child shows an evident preference for the physical over the interpersonal world.

Level 3: Two-Way Purposeful Emotional Interactions (Typically Observable between 6 and 9 Months)

The next stage involves purposeful communication consisting of intentional, preverbal communications or gestures (i.e., opening and closing a number of circles of communication in a row). These gestures convey affective communication; they may include facial expressions, arm and leg movements, pointing, vocalizations, and postures or movement patterns. This stage indicates processes occurring at the somatic (sensorimotor) and emerging psychological levels once the infant is able to discriminate primary caregivers and differentiate his or her own actions from their consequences. One can see cause-and-effect signaling with the full range of expected emotions. The child is able to interact in a purposeful, intentional, and reciprocal manner, both initiating and responding to the other's signals. For example, the infant initiates looking at an object (opens the circle of communication); the caregiver responds by picking up the object, putting it right in front of the infant with a big smile, and saying, "Here it is!"

When the infant either vocalizes or reaches or changes facial expression in response to the parent, he or she is closing the circle of communication by building on the caregiver's response. This capacity is usually established by 10 months.

Simple gestures of a 10-month-old child, such as pointing, reaching to be picked up, or playing "give and take," become complex sequences of gestures during the second year, and then back-and-forth conversations as the child develops language. These reciprocal, two-way, dialogic interactions are considered a critical step in the development of connections between emotional intent and purposeful action, which can enable the child to begin participating in back-and-forth emotional signaling.

A lack of reciprocal responses from a caregiver, as occurs when the primary caregiver responds in a mechanical, remote, or overstimulating manner, can compromise the full acquisition of this developmental ability. Children with developmental dyspraxia and pervasive developmental delay may engage in stereotypic, aimless, or disorganized actions, suggesting nonmastery of this developmental task.

Rating Scale

5. The infant uses purposeful gestures, such as facial expressions, motor gestures (e.g., showing the caregiver something), or vocalizations, in a reciprocal, back-and-forth manner (including affective interactions), to convey his or her intentions or desires to start the "conversations" needed to participate actively in interactions. The infant may initiate such gestures. For example, the infant may show curiosity and assertiveness in reaching for a rattle; may show anger and protest by throwing food on the floor in an intentional manner and looking at the caregiver as if to say, "What are you going to do now?"; or may respond to the caregiver's countergesturing with a further gesture of his or her own, closing the circle of communication.
3. The infant is able to use purposeful gestures to convey some affects, but not others. For instance, the infant may show pleasure with smiles and love of touching when cuddling, but may not be able to protest as an expression of anger or to show assertiveness. Some limitations of intentional communication are expressed when the infant is not always able to initiate or respond to another's signal.
1. The infant shows only fragmented islands of purposeful interaction. His or her behavior may appear aimless or nonoriented toward interaction with caregivers. The infant shows self-absorbed behavior or may misread another person's cues. All these behaviors are signs of significant challenges at this level.

Level 4: Shared Social Problem Solving (Typically Observable between 9 and 18 Months)

The Level 4 capacity is evidenced by engaging in a continuous flow of circles of communication. These are now complex, organized, problem-solving, affective interactions (e.g., a 14-month-old boy can take his mother's hand, walk her to the refrigerator, bang on the door, and point to the desired food when the door is opened). The toddler now sequences many cause-and-effect units related to wishes and intentions into a chain or organized pattern, and takes a more active role in developing and maintaining the reciprocal relationship with the caregiver's interactions. The child can now use and respond to social cues to achieve a sense of competence and autonomy (i.e., a presymbolic sense of self). At about 1 year of age, joint attention (person–person–object awareness) and the ability to share social context transitions demonstrate the emergence of secondary intersubjectivity—that is, the ability to understand others' intentions and feelings.

The toddler takes a more active role in developing and maintaining the reciprocal relationship with the caregiver, and attachment patterns are organized as goal-directed behaviors, including intentional communications that negotiate security, intimacy, exploration, aggression, and limit setting.

Basic emotional messages of safety and security versus danger, acceptance versus rejection, and approval versus disapproval can all be communicated through facial expressions, body posture, movement patterns, and vocal tones and rhythms. At about 9–11 months of age, children are able to see bodily movements as expressive of emotions and as goal-directed, intentional movements, and to perceive other persons as agents. Words enhance these more basic communications, but gestures convey emotional messages even before a conversation gets started and may discount the words.

The nonverbal, gestural communication system is therefore a part of every dialogue contributing to children's developing sense of who they are and what they perceive. In the second year of life, toddlers can make their intentions known and are learning to comprehend the intentions of others through opening and closing many circles of communication.

A child may not establish this distal communication capacity because a caregiver is overanxious, overprotective, overly symbiotic, intrusive, or withdrawn. The child may have difficulty reading facial gestures or interpersonal distance, and tends to see people only as fulfilling the hunger for physical touch, food, or other concrete satisfactions.

Rating Scale

5. The toddler is able to use emerging motor skills and language to solve problems and to connect many affective-thematic areas in multiple circles of communication. The caregiver and child respond and initiate reciprocal, back-and-forth chains of interactions with each other, stringing together connected circles of communication or units of interaction. Different emotional patterns are organized into integrated, problem-solving affective interactions. Intentional communication and goal-directed behaviors are fully mastered abilities.
3. The toddler shows islands of intentional problem-solving behavior. In some stressful situations, the child regresses from organized behavior patterns to highly fragmented patterns, or becomes withdrawn or rejecting.
1. The toddler shows significant limitations in making the transition to complex emotional and problem-solving interactions. He or she may appear withdrawn and hypoactive, with poor social interaction, and difficulties in eye and emotional contact.

Level 5: Creating Symbols and Ideas (Typically Observable between 18 and 30 Months)

The fifth level is the capacity to represent or symbolize experience, as evidenced in functional use of language, pretend play, and the verbal labeling of feelings for communicating emotional themes and ideas. It involves the creation, elaboration, and sharing of meanings, seen in the toddler's ability to represent experience in pretend play, the verbal labeling of feelings ("I feel happy"), and the functional use of language. Now affect or emotions invest symbols and give them meaning. Pretend play is perhaps an even more reliable indicator than language of the child's ability to represent experience, especially when the child may have language delays. The elaboration of ideas or representations gradually becomes more complex, as does the sense of self, which now involves symbols and not just behaviors. Initially, the elements in the complex drama may not be logically connected, but expand to include a range of themes, including dependency, pleasure, assertiveness, curiosity, aggression, setting limits on the self, and eventually empathy and love.

Over time, the child begins to go beyond the basic needs and simple themes to convey two or more emotional ideas at a time in the service of more complex intentions, wishes, or feelings (e.g., themes of closeness or dependency, separation, curiosity, assertiveness, or anger).

The child begins to express thoughts, ideas, and feelings through symbols, using pretend play and words. A child can communicate what he or she imagines through role play, dress-up games, and play with dolls or action figures, all of which now represent experiences from real life as well as those learned from other sources. These become the child's own as he or she projects feelings into the characters and actions.

Parental anxiety often leads to intrusive, overcontrolling, undermining, overstimulating, withdrawn, or concrete behavioral patterns. As a result, the child may not use ideas to reason, but may regress to a concrete-prerepresentational behavioral pattern of acting out.

Rating Scale

5. The child uses language or pretend play (e.g., playing with dolls or action figures) to communicate needs, wishes, intentions, or feelings. The child projects his or her feelings into the characters and actions, even before achieving the functional use of language.
3. The child may be afraid of emotional fantasy, especially specific themes such as separation, rejection, aggression, or assertiveness. Some areas gain access, but core areas remain at a behavioral level.
1. The child is not getting practice through interactive pretend play and/or functional language use, and deficits or constrictions may occur. The child may never learn to use the representational mode; may show impulsive or withdrawn behavior; or may limit symbolic modes to dominance and aggression, and show little elaboration in the pleasurable or intimate domain.

Level 6: Building Logical Bridges between Ideas: Logical Thinking (Typically Observable between 30 and 48 Months)

The sixth level involves creating logical bridges between ideas and feelings, and differentiating those feelings, thoughts, and events that emanate from within and those that emanate from others through pretend play and reality based conversations. As logical bridges between ideas are established, reasoning and appreciation of reality grow—including distinguishing what's "pretend" from what's believed to be real, distinguishing what's right from what's wrong, and learning to deal with conflicts and finding prosocial outcomes. As children become capable of emotional thinking, they begin to understand relationships between their own and others' experiences and feelings (e.g., "I am mad because you took my toy"). As they develop, they balance fantasy and reality, taking time, space, and causality into account.

Pretend play often begins with feeding or hugging scenes suggesting nurturance and dependency. Over time, however, the dramas the child may initiate (with parental interactive support) may expand to include scenes of separation (e.g., one doll goes off on a trip and leaves the other behind), competition, assertiveness, aggression, injury, death, recovery (e.g., the doctor doll fixes the wounded soldier, since "good guys never die"), and so forth. At the same time, the structure of the fantasy/drama becomes more and more logical and causally related.

It is at this stage that the young child develops the capacity to share differentiated meanings. The child can not only communicate his or her own ideas, but also build on the ideas and comments of another person, whereby he or she explores a wider range of feelings. The child can connect and elaborate ideational sequences in logical ways, taking time and space into account. Realistic conversations and pretend play stories are now made up of logically interconnected ideas. They often may have a beginning, middle, and end, with clear motives and anticipated consequences. The child can now also abstract and reflect on various feelings. In addition, children at this stage begin to negotiate the terms of their relationships with others in more reality-based conversations—for example, "Can I do this?" or "Can I do that?" or "What will you do if I kick the ball into the wall?" They begin to engage in debates, opinion-oriented conversations, and/or more planful and elaborate pretend dramas.

Representational differentiation provides the basis for the capacity to regulate impulse and mood, and to focus attention and concentration.

Caregivers who confuse their own feelings with their children's feelings, or who cannot set limits, may compromise the formation of reality orientation. Deficits in children's sensory processing abilities, such as auditory–verbal or visual–spatial symbolic abstracting capacities, may also affect the achievement of this level of reasoning.

Rating Scale

5. The child uses symbolic communication (pretend play or actual conversations) to convey two or more emotional ideas at a time in the service of more complex intentions, wishes, or feelings that are *logically connected*—for example, themes of closeness or dependency, separation, exploration, fear, assertiveness, anger, aggression, pride in the self, or showing off. The child can distinguish the real from the unreal and is able to switch back and forth between fantasy and reality.

3. The child uses pretend play sequences of two or more ideas that are logically connected and grounded in reality in some areas, but not in others. For instance, anger or sexual curiosity are avoided and may remain relatively undifferentiated.

1. The child's ability to organize impersonal or affective information may be limited or compromised. Simple pretend sequences or islands of symbolic capacities are used, but the child usually is self-absorbed and avoidant. Age-appropriate reciprocal or symbolic capacities are not mastered.

Summary of Expected Emotional Functioning

Axis II provides descriptions for the evaluation of the developmental functional level reached by a child (Table 10.6). Many of the descriptions have been defined by Greenspan and colleagues in IDCL-DMIC. Age-appropriate clinical descriptions have been provided above, and a listing of most relevant assessment tools is provided below, as ways to help a clinician systematically organize observations of a child's strengths and deficits in order to define a clinical diagnostic profile.

Most Relevant Assessment Tools

Functional Emotional Assessment Scale for Infancy and Early Childhood

The Functional Emotional Assessment Scale for Infancy and Early Childhood (FEAS; Greenspan, DeGangi, & Wieder, 2001) enables clinicians, educators, and researchers to observe and measure emotional and social functioning in infants, young children, and their families. It systematically assesses children's primary emotional capacities; their affective and sensorimotor emotional range; and related motor, sensory, language, and cognitive capacities from 3 months to 48 months of age. It was specifically designed for infants and young children who experience problems in self-regulation, attachment, communication, attention, and behavioral control. The scale conceptualizes, operationalizes, and measures in a reliable and valid manner the full range of emotional functioning in infants, young children, and their caregivers; the naturally occurring emotional interactions between infants/children and caregivers in a variety of settings, including home and school; and both easily observable emotional behaviors and the subtle, deeper levels of emotional functioning. These include self-regulation; relationships (attachments); reciprocal emotional interactions; emotional range and stability; social and emotional problem solving; the emergence of a sense of self; the ability to symbolize or represent emotions and emotional experience; imagination and creativity; pretend play; emotional thinking; appreciation of reality; and the wishes, interests, and range of emotional themes that characterize a child's personality and interactions with caregivers. It was validated on four samples of infants and children ranging in age from 7 to 48 months. The FEAS appears to be a reliable and valid measure of social-emotional functioning in young children.

TABLE 10.6. Summary of Expected Emotional Functioning

Level	Expected emotional function	Rating scale				
1	Shared attention and regulation	5	4	3	2	1
2	Engagement and relating	5	4	3	2	1
3	Two-way purposeful emotional interactions	5	4	3	2	1
4	Shared social problem solving	5	4	3	2	1
5	Creating symbols and ideas	5	4	3	2	1
6	Building logical bridges between ideas: Logical thinking	5	4	3	2	1

Greenspan Social-Emotional Growth Chart: A Screening Questionnaire for Infants and Young Children

The Greenspan Social-Emotional Growth Chart: A Screening Questionnaire for Infants and Young Children (Greenspan, 2004) is a 35-item questionnaire completed by a child's parent, educator, or other caregiver. As its name indicates, it is designed as a screening tool to measure social-emotional milestones, deficits, and compromises in young children. The chart identifies six areas of social emotional growth for children from birth to 42 months of age. The six stages incorporate eight functional emotional milestones (0–3 months, 4–5 months, 6–9 months, 10–14 months, 15–18 months, 19–24 months, 25–30 months, and 31–42 months). Administration requires 10 minutes. Items are rated on a 5-point scale, and they are ordered developmentally, according to the age range in which each item is typically mastered. This brief tool is intended to determine the mastery of early capacities and to detect deficits or problems in social-emotional growth and functioning. It can also be used to determine goals and monitor progress in early intervention programs.

Neonatal Behavioral Assessment Scale

The Neonatal Behavioral Assessment Scale (NBAS; Brazelton & Nugent, 1995, 2011) is a multidimensional assessment scale designed to evaluate a baby's behavioral repertoire and use of states to manage his or her responsiveness to environmental stimuli. The NBAS is used to assess babies from 36 weeks gestational age to 2 months after a full-term birth, and consists of 53 items (18 neurological reflexes, 28 behavioral items, and 7 supplementary items). NBAS examiners are trained to get the best performance from each child; by the end of the assessment, an examiner has a behavioral "portrait" of an infant, including the baby's strengths, adaptive responses, and possible vulnerabilities. In order to compare the evaluations of the infant's behavior, the items that interact in similar ways have been grouped into seven clusters describing global functions, following Lester, Als, and Brazelton (1982). The clusters include reflexes (e.g., plantar grasp, Babinski, and ankle tonus); motor system (which includes tonus, motor maturity, pull-to-sit, defensive movements, and level of activity); autonomic stability (which includes tremors, startles, and skin color); habituation (which includes response decrement to light, bell, and tactile stimulation); social-interactive organization (which includes animate and inanimate visual orientation, auditory orientation, and alertness); range of states (which includes peak of excitement, rapidity of buildup, irritability, and lability of states); and regulation of states (which includes cuddliness, consolability, self-quieting activity, and hand-to-mouth activity). The administration of the NBAS requires 20–30 minutes, and scoring takes up to 10–15 minutes. Each of the behaviors is scored on a 9-point scale, and the reflexes are evaluated on a 4-point scale.

Newborn Behavioral Observations System

The Newborn Behavioral Observations (NBO) System (Nugent, Keefer, Minear, Johnson, & Blanchard, 2007) is a structured set of observations designed to help a clinician and parent to observe the infant's behavioral capacities together and identify the kind of support the infant needs for successful growth and development. It is a relationship-based tool designed to foster the parent–infant relationship. The NBO System consists of a set of 18 neurobehavioral observations, which describe a newborn's capacities and behavioral adaptation from birth to the third month of life. The items include observations of the infant's capacity to habituate to external light and sound stimuli (sleep protection); the quality of motor tone and activity level; the capacity for self-regulation (including crying and consolability); the response to stress (indices of the infant's threshold for stimulation); and visual, auditory, and social-interactive capacities (degree of alertness and response to both human and nonhuman stimuli). By providing this behavioral profile of an infant's strengths and challenges, the NBO System can provide a clinician with the kind of individualized guidance that can help parents meet their baby's needs. This, in turn, will help the parents to develop the kind of confidence they need to support their baby's development and enjoy the experience of being new parents. The NBO System, therefore, was designed as a relationship-building method that can be flexibly administered.

NICU Network Neurobehavioral Scale

The NICU Network Neurobehavioral Scale (NNNS; Lester, Tronick, & Brazelton, 2004) is a neurobehavioral assessment scale comprising 45 individual items that are clustered into state-dependent "packages" (with an additional 21 summary items), designed for researchers and clinicians to provide a comprehensive assessment of neurological integrity, behavioral functioning, and stress behavior in term and preterm infants. The NNNS follows a fixed sequence of administration that starts with a pre-examination observation, followed by the neurological and behavioral components. The NNNS items are scored with these 13 summary scores: habituation, attention, arousal, regulation, number of handling procedures, quality of movement, excitability, lethargy, number of nonoptimal reflexes, number of asymmetric reflexes, hypertonicity, hypotonicity, and stress/abstinence signs. The neurological examination includes assessment of active and passive tone, primitive reflexes, the integrity of the central nervous system, and the maturity of the infant. The behavioral component is based on the NBAS (Brazelton & Nugent, 1995; see above) and includes assessment of state, sensory, and interactive responses. The stress component is a checklist of signs observed throughout the examination. The complete NNNS examination should be performed only on a medically stable infant in an open crib or isolette and requires about 30 minutes. It is probably not appropriate for infants under 30 weeks gestational age, and the upper age limit may vary between 46 and 48 weeks (corrected or conceptional age). It has norms based on 125 full-term healthy infants.

Bayley Scales of Infant and Toddler Development—Third Edition

The Bayley Scales of Infant and Toddler Development—Third Edition (Bayley-III; Bayley, 2006) is a revision of the frequently used and well-known Bayley Scales of Infant Development—Second Edition (Bayley, 1993). Like its precedessors, the Bayley-III is an individually administered instrument designed to measure the developmental functioning of infants, toddlers, and young children between 1 and 42 months of age. Administration time ranges from 30 to 90 minutes, depending on a child's age. The Bayley-III provides five scales in the following domains: cognitive, language, motor, adaptive, and social-emotional development. In particular, the Bayley-III social-emotional scale focuses on the acquisition of functional social-emotional milestones that broadly represent social-emotional patterns and significant accomplishments, not just specific or isolated emotions or social skills. Thus the scale assesses the attainment of important age-related milestones, including the capacity to engage and use a range of emotions, experiences, and expressions, as well as to comprehend various emotional signals and to elaborate upon a range of feelings through the use of words and symbols. The assessment focuses on behaviors that occur in naturalistic settings; thus the Bayley-III social-emotional scale relies on information provided by primary caregivers, including parents. The items on this scale are derived from the Greenspan Social-Emotional Growth Chart, a screening questionnaire for infants and young children described above. In addition, the Bayley-III social-emotional scale incorporates an assessment of sensory processing and provides a brief description of selected sensory processing patterns.

Infant–Toddler Social and Emotional Assessment

The Infant–Toddler Social and Emotional Assessment (ITSEA; Carter et al., 2003; Carter & Briggs-Gowan, 2006) is a parent report questionnaire developed to assess a wide array of social-emotional and behavioral problems in 12- to 36-month-old children. The ITSEA includes 166 items and assesses four broad domains of behavior: externalizing, internalizing, dysregulation, and competencies. The externalizing domain is composed of activity/impulsivity, aggression/defiance, and peer aggression scales. The internalizing domain includes scales for depression/withdrawal, general anxiety, separation distress, and inhibition to novelty. The dysregulation domain includes sleep, negative emotionality, eating, and sensory sensitivity scales. Competencies include scales for compliance, attention, imitation/play, mastery motivation, empathy, and prosocial peer relations. The primary caregiver rates each specific aspect of the child's behavior on a 3-point scale (0, not true/rarely; 1, somewhat true/sometimes; and 2, very true/often). A "no opportunity" code allows caregivers to indicate that they have not had the opportunity to observe certain behaviors. Behaviors represented on the ITSEA include both those behaviors that are otherwise part of typical development, but become problems when exhibited either in excess or too infrequently, and infrequently occurring problem behaviors that represent deviations from a normative developmental course.

Brief Infant Toddler Social and Emotional Assessment

A brief 42-item version of the ITSEA (the Brief Infant–Toddler Social and Emotional Assessment, or BITSEA; Briggs-Gowan & Carter, 2006) is available to assess social-emotional and behavior problems or delays and social-emotional competence in young children ages 12–36 months. It includes a 31-item problem scale and an 11-item competence scale. Higher scores indicate more social-emotional or behavior problems or greater social-emotional competence, respectively. Various studies have assessed the psychometric properties of the BITSEA and have found that it has strong internal consistency reliability; good temporal consistency reliability; and content, convergent, discriminant, concurrent, and predictive validity.

Early Social Communication Scales

The Early Social Communication Scales (ESCS; Mundy et al., 2003) is a video-recorded structured observation measure that requires between 15 and 25 minutes of administration time. It has been designed to provide measures of individual differences in nonverbal communication skills that typically emerge in children between 8 and 30 months of age. The video recordings of the ESCS enable observers to classify children's behaviors into one of three mutually exclusive categories of early social communication behaviors: joint attention behaviors, behavioral requests, and social interaction behaviors. Behaviors are also classified as to whether they are child-initiated bids or the child's responses to a tester's bids (initiating/responding to joint attention, initiating/responding to behavioral requests, initiating/responding to social interaction). Finally, a measure of social communication imitation may also be obtained from the ESCS by summing the number of times the child imitates the pointing and/or clapping gestures displayed by the tester.

Ages and Stages Questionnaires: Social-Emotional

The Ages and Stages Questionnaires: Social-Emotional (ASQ:SE; Squires, Bricker, & Twombly, 2002) is a companion tool to the Ages and Stages Questionnaires that specifically examines the social-emotional development of children via parental responses. The ASQ:SE is a series of questionnaires designed for use with a child's parent or other primary caregiver, and has eight separate intervals for children at 6, 12, 18, 24, 30, 36, 48, and 60 months. Each ASQ:SE questionnaire contains items focusing on seven social and emotional areas (i.e., self-regulation, compliance, communication, adaptive behavior, autonomy, affect, and interactions with people). The questionnaires use a standard format that contains simply worded items in which caregivers indicate whether their child does a behavior "most of the time," "sometimes," or "never or rarely." An additional column allows parents to indicate whether they have a concern about the behavior being addressed by a question. A high total score is indicative of risk, while a low score suggests that the child's social and emotional behavior is considered typical and expected for his or her age. Research on the instrument's psychometric properties supports the validity and reliability of the ASQ:SE.

Infant/Toddler Symptom Checklist

The Infant/Toddler Symptom Checklist (ITSC; DeGangi, Poisson, Sickel, & Wiener, 1995) was devised as a parent report measure to obtain valuable information about a child's day-to-day behaviors. The ITSC was developed for infants and toddlers from 7 to 30 months of age who experience problems of self-regulation. There are five age-specific versions of the checklist and a general screening form. The checklist focuses on an infant's responses in the following domains: self-regulation (fussy/difficult behaviors [including crying and tantrums], poor self-calming, inability to delay gratification, difficulties with transitions between activities, and need for other-regulation); attention (distractibility, difficulty initiating and shifting attention); sleep (difficulty staying and falling asleep); feeding (gagging or vomiting that may be related to reflux or other oral–motor problems, food preferences, and behavioral problems during feeding); dressing, bathing, and touch (tactile hypersensitivities related to dressing and bathing, aversion to exploring through the sense of touch, and intolerance of being confined); movement (high activity level and craving for movement, motor planning and balance problems, and insecurity in movement in space); listening, language, and sound (hypersensitivities to sound, auditory distractibility, auditory processing problems, and expressive and receptive language problems); looking and sight; and attachment/emotional functioning (gaze aversion, mood deregulation, flat affect, immaturity in play and interactions, separation problems, difficulty accepting limits, and other behavioral problems).

Cry–Feed–Sleep Interview

The Cry–Feed–Sleep Interview (CFSI; McDonough, Rosenblum, Devoe, Gahagan, & Sameroff, 1998) is an unpublished 56-item measure designed to assess details of an infant's crying or fussiness, feeding, and sleeping patterns, and parents' perceptions of these patterns early in the first year of life. It is designed to assess infants' early emotional and physiological regulation at 3 months to 1 year of age. Scoring of the CFSI is based on researcher aims. The crying and sleeping items are based on two earlier measures. First, the Crying Patterns Questionnaire assesses total crying time in infancy (CPQ; St. James-Roberts & Halil, 1991). A 5-item crying scale assesses the total number of minutes the infant cries at various times of the day (morning, afternoon, evening, and night), and a 3-item feeding problems scale assesses the infant's appetite, picky eating habits, and difficulty to feed using a 3-point response scale (1 indicates no problems, and 3 indicates definite problems). Second, the Sleep Habits Scale (Seifer et al., 1994; Sameroff, Barrett, & Krafchuk, 1994) assesses an infant's sleep problems. A 3-item sleeping problems scale assesses whether the infant sleeps too little, the right amount, and the same amount each day, using a 3-point response scale (1 indicates rarely, and 3 indicates usually).

Achenbach System of Empirically Based Assessment Preschool Forms and Profiles

The Achenbach System of Empirically Based Assessment (ASEBA) Preschool Forms and Profiles (Achenbach & Rescorla, 2000) include a Parent Report Form (Child Behavior Checklist for Ages 1½–5, or CBCL/1½–5), a Caregiver–Teacher Report Form (C-TRF), and a Language Development Survey (LDS). It is an extension of the former CBCL/2–3, based on the CBCL/4–18. The instruments are designed to capture both similarities and differences in how children and youngsters behave and function under different conditions in different social settings. The CBCL/1½–5 and C-TRF are similarly constructed to cover an empirical range of behavioral, emotional, and social functioning problems. Both forms comprise 100 problem items—99 closed items and 1 open-ended item, which requests the respondent to add any problems not previously listed. A parent or other adult living with the child in a family-like setting completes the CBCL/1½–5, whereas a day care provider or other caregiver of the child during the daytime completes the C-TRF. The respondent is requested to rate each item, based on the preceding 2 months, as 0 for not true, 1 for somewhat or sometimes true, and 2 for very true or often true. The C-TRF substitutes 17 items pertinent to family situations for items specific to group situations. The CBCL/1½–5 requests supplementary information about the health of the child. The C-TRF requests information about kind of day care and the role of the respondent in relation to the child, including how well the respondent knows the child and in which context the child is evaluated. For the purpose of relating symptoms to formal diagnostic criteria and for cross-cultural comparisons, five different DSM-oriented scales were constructed: affective problems, anxiety problems, pervasive developmental problems, attention-deficit/hyperactivity problems, and oppositional defiant problems.

Infant Behavior Questionnaire—Revised

The Infant Behavior Questionnaire—Revised (IBQ-R; Gartstein & Rothbart, 2003) is a 191-item measure of temperament in infants ages 3–12 months. Parents rate their infant on each item, using a scale of 0–7 (0, not applicable; 1, never engages in the behavior; and 7, always engages in the behavior). The IBQ-R yields 14 subscales and three higher-order factors: surgency/extraversion, negative affectivity, and orienting/regulation. Surgency/extraversion comprises the subscales of approach, vocal reactivity, high-intensity pleasure, smiling and laughter, activity level, and perceptual sensitivity. Negative affectivity includes the subscales of sadness, distress to limitations, fear, and falling reactivity. Orienting/regulation is the combination of the subscales of low-intensity pleasure, cuddliness, duration of orienting, and soothability.

Early Child Behavior Questionnaire

The Early Child Behavior Questionnaire (ECBQ; Putnam, Gartstein, & Rothbart, 2006) is a 201-item measure of temperament in children ages 18–36 months. A 0–7 rating scale is used for all items, and 18 subscales and three higher-order factors can be derived. The surgency/extraversion factor includes the subscales of impulsivity, activity level, high-intensity pleasure, sociability, and positive anticipation. Negative affectivity includes the subscales of discomfort, fear, sadness, frustration, soothability (reverse-coded), motor activation, perceptual sensitivity, and shyness. The orienting/regulation factor comprises the subscales of inhibitory control, attentional shifting, low-intensity pleasure, cuddliness, and attentional focusing.

Axis III: Regulatory–Sensory Processing Capacities

Axis III describes a child's regulatory–sensory processing profile. There are a number of constitutional–maturational differences in the ways infants and young children respond to and comprehend sensory experiences and then plan actions. The different observed patterns exist on a continuum from relatively normal variations to disorders. The latter occur when the individual sensory differences are sufficiently severe to interfere with daily living abilities and with age-expected emotional, social, cognitive, or learning capacities. When the disorder is isolated, a primary diagnosis of a regulatory–sensory processing disorder is indicated, and the clinicians can search the different patterns described above under Axis I. In other cases, the disordered regulatory–sensory processing can be associated with other primary diagnoses (e.g., autism spectrum disorder or an anxiety disorder). In such a case, Axis III allows the clinician to indicate regulatory differences that can be useful to understand the disease and to plan treatment (e.g., sensory difficulties in feeding disorders, hyposensory processing in autism, sensory seeking in attentional disorders, hypersensory processing in sleep disorders). In many other cases, the regulatory–sensory processing capacities can be described just as normal variations.

The conceptual model for regulatory–sensory processing capacities hypothesizes that, for each sensory system—the five well-known sensory domains (sound, sight, touch, smell, and taste), plus vestibular/movement and proprioceptive/body position functioning, for a total of seven domains—there is a continuous interaction between neurological thresholds and behavioral responses. "Neurological thresholds" are the amounts of stimuli required for a neuron system to respond. At one end of the continuum, thresholds are very high (i.e., it takes a lot of stimuli to meet the thresholds, and children tend to be underresponsive); at the other end of the continuum, thresholds are very low (i.e., it takes very few stimuli to meet the threshold, and children tend to be overly responsive). "Behavioral response" refers to the way people act in regard to their thresholds. At one end of this continuum, children respond in accordance with their thresholds (i.e., they have a tendency to let the nervous system respond very quickly or not respond when the thresholds are too high); at the other end of the continuum, children respond to counteract their thresholds (i.e., they work against their thresholds—searching for stimuli when the neurological thresholds are very high, or not searching when the thresholds are very low).

The high extreme end of a neurological threshold is called "habituation," which is necessary for coping with the myriad of stimuli in the world. Children who have difficulties with habituation may appear distractible, agitated, and inattentive. The low extreme end is called "sensitization," which is necessary for remaining attentive to one's surroundings while engaged in play and other learning. Children who have difficulties with sensitization may appear avoidant. A child must develop a balance of habituation and sensitization to support adaptive behavior and appropriate responses to environmental demands.

The continuous relationships between neurological thresholds and behavioral responses can be organized into four quadrants, as shown in Table 10.7 (based on Dunn, 1997). A clinician using this table will be able to place each child in one of the four quadrants for each sensory system. For example, for some children, music in the background provides sensory support; for other children, background music creates a distraction, interrupting thinking and performance.

Clinical Evaluation of Axis III

Clinical evaluation of Axis III consists of direct observations of the child, supplemented with caregiver interviews and questionnaires. As the observations take place, it is important to keep some principles of sensory functioning in mind. First, sensory functions can be influenced by developmental level. Younger children typically show less ability to self-regulate independently, and their various sensory systems work as a whole. Second, a clinician needs to take into consideration the child's expected behavior within any given environment. A sensation-seeking child may appear a little

TABLE 10.7. Relationships between Behavioral Responses and Neurological Thresholds

	Behavioral response continuum	
Neurological threshold continuum	Responds in ACCORDANCE with threshold	Responds to COUNTERACT the threshold
HIGH (habituation)	Poor registration	Sensation seeking
LOW (sensitization)	Sensitivity to stimuli	Sensation avoiding

Note. Based on Dunn (1997).

rambunctious if observed on a playground, but when the child is observed in a quiet office space, the need for sensation may be played out very differently. Likewise, a child avoidant of sensory stimuli may not demonstrate overly problematic behavior in the confines of an office with only the clinician and caregiver present, but in the classroom, this child's withdrawal may be more apparent. Third, responses to sensory stimuli are influenced by who is creating the stimulus: The clinician should verify the behavioral observations by asking caregivers whether the behavior is typical of that child, or if it is affected by contingent emotional and physiological state.

An observation session should be child-directed, play-based, and flexible. During the observation, the following are required: (1) a playful interaction with the child; (2) reliance on parent/caregiver participation; (3) parent/caregiver feedback regarding whether what the clinician is observing is typical of that child in multiple settings (waiting room, office, playground, classroom, cafeteria, home); (4) assessment of a collection of behaviors rather than a single behavior (e.g., a dislike of having face and hair washed, alone, does not indicate sensory overresponsivity to touch); and (5) observation of the *quality* of the child's response, not simply of the basic skills displayed.

Any clinician can organize a toolbox that might include actual materials (or questions) for observation (or caregiver information) about sensory modulation (over- or underresponsivity), sensory discrimination, and sensory-based motor challenges. Materials for each type of sensory system should be gathered together before testing begins (such as a tactile basket, a visual basket, an auditory basket, a vestibular/proprioceptive basket, and an olfactory basket). Clinicians should use their own judgment to decide which test materials are appropriate for each child.

The observation may be accompanied by a record form that facilitates the examiner's assessment of a child's sensory profile. ICDL-DMIC (ICDL, 2005) includes record forms for recording a clinician's observations on sensory modulation (overresponsivity, underresponsivity, and sensory seeking), sensory discrimination, and sensory-based motor challenges (postural disorder and dyspraxia). A total of six record forms and a summary form are provided; for each item, a mark describes the child's performance as not a problem, a possible problem, or a problem. When all six record forms are completed, the summary record form (a form based on this form is provided in Table 10.8 on the next page) can be used. Each subtype in each category can be rated on a Likert scale of 1–4, where higher scores indicate better performance.

As a complement to the direct observation of the child, a judgment-based caregiver questionnaire can be used.

Most Relevant Assessment Tools

Infant–Toddler Social and Emotional Assessment

The ITSEA (Carter et al., 2003; Carter & Briggs-Gowan, 2006), described in the section on Axis II, provides specific information about sensory processing in one of its subscales. Within the dysregulation domain, four subscales are included (sleep, eating, negative emotionality, and sensory sensitivity). The items in the sensory sensitivity subscale are directed to the investigation of sensory processing: the tactile, hearing, visual, olfactory, and proprioceptive systems; oral sensitivity; and the intensity of response to stimuli. The possible identified difficulties in this subscale mainly describe children with lower thresholds who have more difficulty adapting to new experiences (e.g., they have tantrums every time they need to change clothes because of their tactile defensiveness).

TABLE 10.8. Summary of Regulatory–Sensory Processing Capacities

		Challenge in this area			
Category	Subtype	No indication; never or rarely a problem	Mild problem or only occasionally a problem	Moderate problem or frequently a problem	Severe problem or almost always a problem
Sensory modulation	Sensory underresponsivity	4	3	2	1
	Sensory overresponsivity	4	3	2	1
	Sensory seeking	4	3	2	1
Sensory discrimination	Tactile	4	3	2	1
	Auditory	4	3	2	1
	Visual	4	3	2	1
	Taste/smell	4	3	2	1
	Vestibular/propriocep.	4	3	2	1
Sensory-based motor functioning	Postural challenges	4	3	2	1
	Dyspraxis challenges	4	3	2	1

Note. Based on Interdisciplinary Council on Developmental and Learning Disorders (2005).

Infant/Toddler Sensory Profile

The Infant/Toddler Sensory Profile (Dunn, 2002; Dunn & Daniels, 2002) is a parent questionnaire assessing an infant's or toddler's sensory processing abilities. It consists of 36 items for children from birth to 6 months of age, and 48 items for children ages 7–36 months. It provides scores for the four quadrants illustrated in Table 10.7 (poor registration, sensation seeking, sensitivity to stimuli, sensation avoiding) and for each sensory system (vision, touch, etc.), describing children's sensory processing abilities as follows: typical performance (scores at or less than ±1 *SD* from the mean, for children without disabilities); probable difference (scores ±1–2 *SD* from the mean); and definite difference (scores more than ±2 *SD* from the mean). Thus it allows a clinician to identify either an actual regulatory–sensory processing disorder or normal variations in an individual sensory profile. Reliability analyses were consistent with clusters previously identified in Dunn's (1997) model of sensory processing for older children.

Infant/Toddler Symptom Checklist

The ITSC (DeGangi et al., 1995), also described in the section on Axis II, is a measure enabling parents to provide valuable information about their child's day-to-day behaviors. The checklist focuses on an infant's responses in the following domains: (1) self-regulation; (2) attention; (3) sleep; (4) feeding; (5) dressing, bathing, and touch; (6) movement; (7) listening, language, and sound; (8) looking and sight; and (9) attachment/emotional functioning. The ITSC was developed for infants and toddlers from 7 to 30 months of age who experience problems of self-regulation. There is also a general screening form. The ITSC was validated on 154 normal infants and 67 infants with regulatory disorders.

Test of Sensory Functions in Infants

The Test of Sensory Functions in Infants (TSFI; DeGangi & Greenspan, 1989) is a 24-item test developed to measure sensory processing and reactivity in infants. It focuses on evaluation of responses to tactile deep pressure, visual–tactile integration, adaptive motor skills, ocular motor control, and reactivity to vestibular stimulation. The TSFI was validated on 288 normal infants, 27 infants with developmental delays, and 27 infants with regulatory disorders, all from 4 to 18 months of age. Norms for 18-month-olds were used in interpreting data for subjects in the 19- to 24-month age group. Psychometric studies of the instrument show that the test can be used reliably and validly in guiding clinical decisions for infants with delays or regulatory disorders.

Sensory Experiences Questionnaire

The Sensory Experiences Questionnaire (SEQ; Baranek, David, Poe, Stone, & Watson, 2006) is a 105-item caregiver report instrument designed to characterize sensory features in children ages 2–12 years. The SEQ was developed to match an evolving conceptual model including an enhanced perception construct, sensory response patterns, sensory modalities, and control items. The SEQ 3.0 items measure the frequency of sensory behaviors across sensory response patterns, modalities, and social or nonsocial contexts. The frequency of the first 97 items is measured on a 5-point Likert-type scale, with a higher score indicating more sensory features. The last 8 items ask broader questions about the child's sensory features and allow the caregiver to elaborate with a qualitative response. A factor analysis confirmed the presence of four sensory factors: hyporesponsiveness (HYPO); hyperresponsiveness (HYPER); sensory interests, repetitions, and seeking behaviors (SIRS); and enhanced perception (EP).

First Year Inventory

The First Year Inventory (FYI; Reznick, Baranek, Reavis, Watson, & Crais, 2007) is a questionnaire developed to identify infants at risk of autism. It is composed of 63 items (46 measured on a Likert scale, and 17 multiple-choice items) that can be aggregated into two main domains (a socio-communicative domain and a sensory/regulatory domain). Each domain is composed of four different sets of items. The sensory/regulatory domain includes the following four sets: sensory processing, regulatory patterns, behavioral reactivity, and repetitive behaviors.

Cry–Feed–Sleep Interview

The CFSI (McDonough et al., 1998), described in the section on Axis II, assesses infants' early emotional and physiological regulation involving crying/fussiness, feeding, and sleeping patterns, as well as parents' perceptions of these patterns, at 3 months to 1 year of age. It is an unpublished 56-item measure. Scoring of the CFSI is based on researcher aims. Higher total scores indicate more functional regulatory problems.

Rating Scale

A clinician may use the following rating scale to indicate the degree to which a regulatory–sensory pattern represents a normal variation versus a disorder:

5. *Within a range of normal variation:* The child uses its own regulatory pattern to obtain a good level of attention, to reach goals, and to maintain relationships.
3. *Mild to moderate impairment:* The child allows purposeful actions and communication, except in certain circumstances involving high level of stress for his or her sensory profile; the child presents stable symptoms, such as irritability when he or she has to get dressed, or underresponsivity in a stimulating/learning setting.
1. *Severe impairment:* Sensory difficulties make it difficult for the child to engage in relationships, to form basic patterns of communication, or to learn and to think.

Axis IV: Relational Patterns and Disorders

Axis IV describes the overall functioning of significant relationships in an infant's or child's life, considering both the degree to which the caregiver is able to support the child's functional capacity at each developmental level and the child's unique contribution to these relationships. In assessing caregiver–infant relationship and interactive patterns, the clinician needs to consider the mutuality of this relationship—to which both the child's specific abilities or difficulties and the caregiver's feelings, wishes, and conflicts (past and present) may contribute.

Developmental psychopathology, relational psychoanalysis, and attachment theory all provide support for the idea that the development of the self is not an individual process, but an interpersonal and intersubjective one. A child's personality develops, his or her defenses and capacities to regulate emotions are structured, and representations of self and others are constructed within the child's primary relationships. At the same time, neuroscientific studies have demonstrated that disturbances in early relationships can alter the neural systems that control emotional resilience, leading to long-term vulnerability. Understanding the quality of the infant/child–caregiver relationship thus appears an essential part of the diagnostic process in infancy and early childhood, regardless of a child's symptoms or disorders.

Different caregiving interactive styles will have a strong impact on a child's ability to modulate sensory input, to maintain a calm and positive affective state, and to develop the ability to regulate emotions and behaviors. It is assumed that patterns of irritability and high reactivity are modifiable (at least in part) by sensitive caregiving, and that positive experiences of mutual regulation affect the child's developing brain and personality. Conversely, the child's emotional and social functioning can be disrupted by negative experiences of caregiving, and maladaptive patterns may be increased by unempathic relationships. In looking at the caregiver–child relationship, the clinician should consider the process of mutual regulation (i.e., the interactive pattern of connections and disconnections) as an ongoing process, in which failures followed by reparative efforts may help the child develop self-regulatory skills and resilience for coping with interactive stress. Conversely, miscommunications, interactive failures without repairs, or rigid (withdrawn or intrusive) caregiving styles can reinforce dysfunctional defensive strategies and become the ground for the emergence of psychopathology.

Increasing numbers of studies have now demonstrated the extent to which the quality of early interaction between child and caregiver is constructed reciprocally, starting with the individual and unique characteristics of the partners of the dyad. The process of mutual regulation (Tronick, 1989) thus highlights the behaviors of co-regulation, coordination, and cooperation as the bases for the construction of early relational patterns. Since child and caregiver mutually influence each other, the clinician should consider behavioral and representational levels of influence; the deep links between early interactional maladjustment and later disorders; and the continuity of subjective experiences and relational patterns over time, beyond the observable changes. Regardless of manifest symptomatology, relational processes should be considered as etiological mechanisms for some psychiatric disorders.

In general, the assessment of Axis IV should help the clinician to place the significant alterations of primary relationships along the following continuum:

1. Healthy, reciprocal, and synchronous interactions, in which infant/child and caregiver share pleasant experiences, successfully manage the stresses of everyday life, and are able to promote mutual growth.
2. Situations of perturbation or disturbance (Anders, 1989), characterized by mild alterations with regard to developmental tasks or by dysfunctional interactions whose patterns are not rigidly fixed or are related to one interactive area only (e.g., a sleep disorder).
3. Situations in which the patterns of caregiver–child interaction are generally problematic or steadily dysfunctional, as can happen with patterns of insecure attachment or with relational disorders (Sameroff & Emde, 1989) or even with relationship disorders as defined in DC: 0–5. Such interaction patterns lead to a developmental risk.
4. Finally, situations in which the caregiving context is so problematic or deficient that the caregiver and child are highly unlikely to establish a safe and trustworthy relationship, as in complex trauma disorders or in reactive attachment disorders.

Following this continuum, PDM-2 labels Axis IV as "relational patterns and disorders." This perspective considers difficulties in caregiver–child relationships as phenomena to assess and, when necessary, to diagnose as parameters independent of the presence of child symptomatology. It also emphasizes that assessment should take into account not only observed interactive behaviors, but also the child's and caregiver's subjective experiences and the influence of the dynamic factors at play. Assessment should include the level of global functioning of the relationship; the level of anxiety and the adaptive flexibility of both the child and the parent; the level of caregiver–child conflict and the capacity for its resolution; and the effect that the relationship can have on the child's development.

Compared to its counterpart in the first PDM, Axis IV of PDM-2 is intended to assist clinicians with the following: assessing caregiver–child relationships regardless of children's symptomatology; defining specific features of relationships on the basis of caregiving patterns, quality of affective tone, interactive styles, and subjective experience; indicating the main risk factors, such as parental disease, maternal depression, marital adjustment, stress, or social context, that may interfere with the quality of the relationships; and defining attachment patterns and relationships.

Axis IV is intended to provide clinicians with a broad overview of multiple dimensions that characterize early relationships. For practical reasons, the individual dimensions are discussed separately, but clinicians need to maintain an overall perspective on relational issues. Assessment of infant/child–caregiver relationships must integrate multiple sources, as each source provides unique information about relationship functioning. The sources include direct observations of the interactive patterns, supplemented with caregiver interviews and questionnaires. This section of the chapter also describes a number of assessment tools and observational procedures that can be taken into account.

Again, Axis IV patterns and disorders should be assessed independently of a child's individual symptoms or disorders, to see whether the caregiver–child relationship must be considered as a risk factor or a resource for the child's social-emotional and adaptive functioning. The clinician should consider a dysfunctional caregiver–child relationship as a clinical problem distinct from child psychopathology. Because relational problems are dependent on the quality of fit and interaction between the caregiver and the child, the disorder is thus specific to that relationship. This implies that each child's relationship with a significant caregiver (usually the mother or father, but a foster parent, grandparent, teacher, etc., as appropriate) should be evaluated. Whereas existing diagnostic classifications overemphasize disorders in the individual, Axis IV aims to highlight the importance of considering disorders in relationships.

Assessment of Relational Patterns and Disorders

Given that many dimensions affect the caregiver–child relationship and the partners' mutual influence, it is important to consider these factors in their specificity. Research and clinical studies in the last several decades have identified some important features of caregiving patterns, interactive styles, mental representations, and subjective experiences that influence caregiver–infant interactive patterns and relationships.

As a general observation, it is possible to distinguish between relational environments that recognize infants' needs and respond in ways that promote infant development (growth-promoting environments) and environments that inhibit, perturb, or derail development (growth-inhibiting environments). Caregiver–child relationships that support growth are characterized by a caregiver's sensitivity, reflective capacity, and ability to respond contingently to the infant. For example, when the baby cries, the parent wonders, "What is the matter? Are you tired? Hungry? Had enough of playing by yourself? Missing Daddy?" The parent seeks concrete solutions to the baby's distress, simultaneously giving meaning to the baby's signals. The baby's overriding experience in this relationship is of the adult's trying to understand and to meet his or her distress with empathy and succor; the infant then accrues memories of "feeling better" as a result. This interaction reinforces the baby's sense of self and of agency in influencing his or her world. If the parent's attempts to console the baby do not work in the first instance, it can be expected that they will continue to work together (the parent's reaching out and the baby's guiding and cuing via his or her responses) so that interactive repair takes place.

By contrast, growth-inhibiting environments are characterized by over- or under stimulation without interactive repair. The parent does not recognize the infant's behaviors as communications, or misconstrues their meaning, and responds in ways that distort or even cut off the infant's vital, genuine, and idiosyncratic attachment communications. For example, when the baby cries, the parent's response to the baby is "You have been fed and changed. You are a spoiled child and are crying just to get under my skin." The parent puts a pacifier into the baby's mouth and leaves the room. The infant is flooded by negative emotions such as fear and hopelessness, and resorts to defensive maneuvers to protect the self. In an infant, these may include avoidance, inhibition, freezing, and dissociation. In an older child, externalizing behaviors (more common in boys) and depression (more common in girls) may be underpinned by such early experiences.

Questions to Aid in Assessment

In observations of caregiver–infant interactions, the clinician may consider the questions below. The reader should note that the emphasis here is on caregiver–child–caregiver or child–caregiver–child *sequences*. It is important to consider both the caregiver's and the baby's input into the interaction, since the baby's response will inform the clinician about the infant's mental state and experience.

- How does the caregiver talk about the child? The comments and adjectives used, as well as body-based cues (e.g., tone of voice, gestures), may indicate predominantly positive, ambivalent, or negative *representations of the child*. And how does the child react to the caregiver's voice and comments? With interest? Perplexity? Fear?
- What is the quality of the caregiver and child's *nonverbal engagement,* as much communication takes place nonverbally? Is it engaging? Playful? Intrusive? Rough? How does the child react to the caregiver's touch? Does the child reach out for it? Show anxiety or vigilance? Recoil?
- What is the dominant *interactive style* between the caregiver and the infant/young child? In particular, is it characterized by mutuality, so that the sequence of "serve and return"—the flow of cuing and responding—is structured into interactions? Are adult–child (generational) roles clear, with the caregiver looking after the child rather than the child's taking care of the adult's needs? Are the infant's needs privileged?
- What is the dominant *affective tone* of the caregiver–infant relationship? Is the infant/young child spontaneously and age-appropriately turning to the adult for comfort and social information ("referencing")? Is there shared pleasure? Is a broad range of affects, both positive and negative, acceptable to the caregiver? Are certain emotions not "allowed" (e.g., infant protest, anger)?

Caregiving Patterns and Interactive Styles

Caregiving patterns and interactive styles characterize caregiver–infant relationships in different ways. As proposed in ICDL-DMIC regarding caregiving behaviors, a clinician may consider the following guidelines to observe each caregiver's interaction with the child:

- *The caregiver tends to comfort the infant/child,* especially when the child is upset (e.g., by relaxed, gentle, firm holding or rhythmic vocal or visual contact), rather than tending to make the child more tense (by being overly worried, tense, or anxious, or mechanical, or anxiously over- or understimulating).
- *The caregiver tends to find appropriate levels of stimulation to interest the infant/child* in the world (by being interesting, alert, and responsive, including offering appropriate levels of sound, sights, and touch [including the caregiver's face], appropriate games and toys, etc.), rather than being overstimulating and intrusive (e.g., by picking at and poking or shaking the child excessively to gain his or her attention).

- *The caregiver tends to engage the infant/child pleasurably* in a relationship (by looking, vocalizing, gentle touching, etc.), rather than tending to ignore the infant or child (by being depressed, aloof, preoccupied, withdrawn, indifferent, etc.).

- *The caregiver tends to read and respond to the infant's/child's emotional signals and needs in most emotional areas* (e.g., responds to desire for closeness as well as needs to be assertive, explorative, and independent), rather than either misreading signals or only responding to one emotional need. For example, the caregiver can hug when the baby reaches out, but hovers over the baby and cannot encourage assertive exploration.

- *The caregiver tends to encourage the infant/child to move forward in development,* rather than to misread the child's developmental needs and overprotect, "hold on," infantilize, be overpressured and/or punitive, be fragmented and/or disorganized, or be overly concrete. For example:

  a. The caregiver helps the baby to crawl, vocalize, and gesture by actively responding to the infant's initiative (rather than overanticipating the infant's needs and doing everything for him or her).
  b. The caregiver helps the toddler make the shift from proximal, physical dependency (e.g., being held) to feeling more secure while being independent (e.g., the caregiver keeps in verbal and visual contact with the toddler as he or she builds a tower on the other side of the room).
  c. The caregiver helps the 2- to 3-year-old child shift from motor discharge and gestural ways of relating to the use of "ideas" through encouraging pretend play (imagination) and language around emotional themes (e.g., the caregiver gets down on the floor and plays out dolls hugging each other, dolls separating from each other, or soldiers fighting with each other).
  d. The caregiver helps the 3- to 4-year-old take responsibility for behavior and deal with reality, rather than "giving in all the time," infantilizing, or being overly punitive.

The caregiver characteristics described above cover a number of developmentally based adaptive patterns. If in considering these patterns there is an impression that the caregiver patterns are less than optimal, it may be useful to consider the following characteristics. Does the caregiver tend to be:

- Overly stimulating?
- Withdrawn or unavailable?
- Lacking in pleasure, enthusiasm, or zest?
- Random or chaotic in reading or responding to the infant's signals?
- Fragmented and/or insensitive to context?
- Overly rigid and controlling; trying to get the infant to conform to a rigid agenda?
- Overly concrete in reading or responding to communication?
- Illogical in reading or responding to the infant's communication?
- Avoidant of selected emotional areas (security and safety, dependency, pleasure/excitement, assertiveness and exploration, aggression, love, empathy, limit setting)?
- Unstable in the face of intense emotion?

Interactional Patterns and Representational Level

In assessing the quality of the caregiver–infant relationship, the clinician should consider both interactional patterns and representational level, taking into account that caregiver–infant interactional dyads are mutually regulated systems where all dimensions are intertwined.

It may be useful for the clinician to refer to the following dimensions, which have received attention from clinical research and have been operationalized in different assessment tools (described below).

Interactional Patterns

As regards interactional patterns, the clinician can consider the following (on a scale from 5 to 1, as indicated):

5. *Sensitivity* is the caregiver's ability to perceive and to interpret accurately the signals and communications implicit in the infant's behavior, and, given this understanding, to respond to them appropriately and promptly. This ability is based on the caregiver's awareness, freedom from distortion, and empathy, that is, the ability to see things from the infant's point of view and to interpret communication without distortions due to the caregiver's own needs and defenses.
3. *Lack of sensitivity* can be expressed in different ways, as when the caregiver fails to respond; is preoccupied with other things and/or inaccessible to the infant's signals (understimulation); or shows intrusive, hyperstimulating, and controlling behaviors (overstimulation), aimed to bound the infant's exploratory and autonomous behaviors. Lack of sensitivity has as a consequence negative affective reactions in infants, who can express anger, active avoidance, or passivity. Repeated failures of interactive repair due to under- or overstimulation lead to dysfunctional relationships and psychopathology.
1. Finally, *frightened/frightening behaviors* are threatening and/or frightened behaviors, conflicting behavioral and/or verbal communications ("affective communication errors"); and other indications that a traumatized parent shows a somewhat dissociated state (often associated with fear of the child), such as timid/deferential, sexualized, or disorganized/disoriented behaviors.

A clinician can refer also to *emotional availability* (EA) as the capacity of a dyad to share an emotional connection and to enjoy a mutually fulfilling and healthy relationship. EA describes a dyadic or relational capacity for mutual emotional awareness, perception, experience, and expression.

Various research measures described below under "Most Relevant Assessment Tools" can be used by clinicians to describe caregivers' behaviors and dyads' interactive styles. These empirically validated assessment instruments can be integrated with other clinical information to obtain a more nuanced and detailed picture of a caregiver–child relationship.

Representational Level and Subjective Experience

As regards a caregiver's representational level and subjective experience, a clinician should consider the way the caregiver represents, perceives, and experiences his or her role; the quality of the relationship with the child; and the caregiver's sense of the child's unique and distinctive features—with emphasis on the role that present and past (positive, negative, or traumatic) experiences have played in the construction of the caregiver's representational world and caregiving attitude. Particular emphasis should be given to the caregiver's *reflective capacity* (i.e., the person's ability to understand his or her own and the infant/child's behavior in terms of the mental states underlying that behavior). With a 3- or 4-year-old child, the clinician can use story stem tasks to explore the child's mental representations of self and of significant relationships. Attention should be paid also to the functioning of the couple and family systems, given the impact of these systems on the child's development.

Numerous assessment tools are relevant to the assessment of mental representations; again, many of these are included in the "Most Relevant Assessment Tools" section below. These interviews and questionnaires can help the clinician understand the caregiver's inner world with respect to the caregiving role and infant/child representations. Narrative story stem techniques can be used for children 3 years of age and older.

Rating Scale

The clinician may use the rating scale in Table 10.9 to indicate the degree to which the pattern represents a healthy/adapted relationship versus disorders.

TABLE 10.9. Infant/Child–Caregiver Relationship

Infant/child–caregiver relationship	Rating scale				
Quality and flexibility of caregiver's representation of the child	5	4	3	2	1
Quality of caregiver's reflective functioning	5	4	3	2	1
Quality of caregiver and child's nonverbal engagement	5	4	3	2	1
Quality of interactional patterns (reciprocity, synchrony, interactive repair)	5	4	3	2	1
Affective tone of the caregiver–infant relationship	5	4	3	2	1
Quality of caregiver's behavior (sensitivity vs. threatening and/or frightening behaviors)	5	4	3	2	1
Quality of caregiving patterns (comfort, stimulation, response to infant emotional signals, encouragement vs. withdrawal, overstimulation, controlling behavior, insensitivity)	5	4	3	2	1
Infant/child's ability to engage and form a significant relationship (vs. specific difficulties that impair this ability)	5	4	3	2	1
	Total score = ____				

Risk Factors and Other Conditions Related to Relational Problems

The presence of parental and familial risk factors may have a deep impact on caregiving, which in turn influences the infant's development and functioning; when multiple risk factors exist, they can lead to relational disorders. Some of the main parental risk factors examined in the literature are as follows:

- Maternal and/or paternal depression
- Parental psychopathology (psychosis, etc.)
- Addiction (alcoholism, drug addiction, etc.)
- Deviant behaviors (antisocial personality, incarcerated women, etc.)
- Single parenthood
- Adolescent parenthood
- Marital conflict
- Lack of social support

Each of these parental risk factors, together with the child's characteristics (prematurity, constitutional difficulties such as regulatory–sensory processing disorders, etc.), may interfere with the development of a healthy relationship between child and caregiver. The clinician may refer to the concept of "goodness of fit" between a caregiver's expectations and capabilities on the one hand, and an infant's temperament, aptitudes, and needs on the other, as the way the quality of caregiving may alleviate or exacerbate the child's constitutional difficulties and determine the development of caregiver–child relations (see also the discussion of Axis III, above). The clinician can also refer to the DSM-5 chapter "Other Conditions That May Be a Focus of Clinical Attention," and to Axis IV of DC: 0–3R and of DC: 0–5, to identify the multiple sources of stress that may be experienced by an infant/child and family.

Assessment of Attachment Patterns and Relationships

Compared to its counterpart in the first PDM, Axis IV of PDM-2 includes specific attention to the assessment of attachment—taking into consideration the large amount of observational and representational data, clinical reports, and instruments that have been produced by attachment researchers and theorists. Two significant aspects in the diagnostic assessment of the child have to do with attachment: the *sense of security* (which may be observed in the 1-year-old attachment pattern and progressively assessed through representational measurement of the internal working models), and the *quality of affect regulation* associated with it. The standard tools for assessing attachment (the Strange Situation, the Crowell procedure, narrative story stem techniques) provide important diagnostic indicators of the way the child regulates his or her sense of security and confidence in self and others, the quality of the child's affective relationships and internal working models, and the ways these contribute to defining affect regulation styles.

As emphasized throughout this part of the chapter, the child–caregiver relationship is characterized by many dimensions (intersubjectivity, intentional communication, play, learning, etc.). "Attachment" refers to the specific and circumscribed aspect of the relationship that is involved with making the child feel safe, secure, and protected. The child uses the caregiver as a secure base from which to explore and, when necessary, as a haven of safety and a source of comfort. Typically, the quality of attachment is largely determined by the caregiver's response to the infant when the infant's attachment system is "activated" by internal or external stimuli, such as physical or emotional threats.

Attachment is one of the most powerful predictors of a child's later social and emotional outcome. A wide range of research has shown that attachment is associated with mental capacities such as affective regulation, mentalization, reflective functioning, differentiation, relationship and intimacy, self-esteem, internal experience, defensive functioning, and resiliency (all of which are included on the MA and MC Axes for adolescents and older children, respectively; see Chapters 4 and 7).

Attachment Prototypes

Even if a standardized assessment of attachment is not usually conducted in clinical settings, the clinician should undertake an *attachment-informed* assessment—one that includes the history of the child's attachment (available attachment figures, disruptions in care, abandonment, alternate caregivers, etc.) and information about the child's attachment behaviors (help- or comfort-seeking behaviors, discrimination of attachment figures, ability to use a caregiver for comfort, ability to explore and play in a new setting, quality of interaction with the caregiver, etc.).

Below, patterns of attachment are described as assessed in the Strange Situation procedure (Ainsworth, Blehar, Waters, & Wall, 1978) for a 1-year-old, with some references to later behaviors and internal working models as assessed in reunion procedures and narrative story stems. Clinician may use a 5-point Likert-type scale, with a higher score indicating a better match with the prototype.

Secure

A 1-year-old child who is securely attached to a parent (or other familiar caregiver) explores freely while the caregiver is present, typically engages with strangers, is often visibly upset when the caregiver departs, and is generally happy to see the caregiver return. Distress upon separation decreases almost immediately, and active exploration starts again, upon reunion. Secure attachment is usually associated with sensitive caregiving. This attachment strategy is "organized" because the child "knows" exactly what to do with a sensitive caregiver: seeking proximity to and maintaining contact with the caregiver until he or she feels safe. The balance between attachment and exploration in the child is mirrored by the balance between protectiveness and encouragement of exploration in the caregiver.

A 3-year-old securely attached child is able to explore, and to use pretend play and symbolic communication to convey wishes and feelings. Following a longer separation, the child continues to show a warm and intimate relationship with the caregiver, starting a warm and personal conversation with him or her. At the representational level, the child tends to describe doll family interactions as positive, supportive, and warm, and the self as accepted and valued. Narratives are coherent, and attachment stories have usually a good end: The child is looked after, helped, and taken care of. Positively contributing to a narrative story stem, a secure child is able to recognize the existence of a conflict by facing it, and never refers to him- or herself or to the family as perfect and problem-free.

5 .... 4 .... 3 .... 2 1

Insecure–Avoidant

A 1-year-old child with the insecure–avoidant attachment pattern shows little or no distress upon separation, avoids or ignores the caregiver's efforts to attract attention or establish contact upon reunion, and shows little emotion when the caregiver departs or returns. This apparently unruffled behavior may represent an "organized shift of attention" away from the caregiver and/or his or her absence, but it is in fact a mask for distress—a hypothesis later supported by studies on the heart rates of avoidant infants. Avoidance may be linked to the caregiver's rejection of infant attachment signals. In this case, "organized" strategy leads the child to avoid the caregiver when distressed and to minimize displays of negative emotion.

A 3-year-old avoidantly attached child, who tends to be focused on play and to reduce physical and psychological intimacy on reunion with the caregiver, shows at the same time difficulties in getting involved or interested in narrative stories, especially if they concern attachment issues. The child described in the narratives is often depicted as isolated and unloved, and as frequently punished. At other times, conflicts in the stories are simply not accepted; as a consequence, no action is taken toward possible solutions. On the whole, for an avoidant child, the issues related to attachment seem to raise emotional difficulties that activate defensive mechanisms.

5 .... 4 .... 3 .... 2 1

Insecure–Ambivalent/Resistant

A 1-year-old child with an insecure–ambivalent/resistant attachment pattern typically shows little exploration (in the Strange Situation) and is often wary of strangers, even when the caregiver is present. The child shows preoccupation with the caregiver, intense distress during separation, and heightened emotionality and inability to be settled by the caregiver upon reunion. This attachment strategy is supposed to be a response to unpredictably responsive caregiving, and the displays of anger or helplessness toward the caregiver on reunion can be regarded as a conditional ("organized") strategy for maintaining the caregiver's availability by preemptively taking control of the interaction: Extreme negative emotions draw the attention of an inconsistently responsive caregiver.

A 3-year-old ambivalently attached child may show expressions of irritation or nervousness on reunion and feelings of inadequacy; the child seems to exaggerate the intimacy with the caregiver and the dependence on him or her, showing a relatively immature stance. Evidence of ambivalence may be observed in hostility combined with apparent attempts to pretend intimacy, dependence, and so on. Narrative stories describe the child as characterized by lack of accessibility, excessive dependence, and feelings of rejection and guilt on the part of the child, who implements actions of coercion to get support. The emotional expression is also exaggerated, improper, or inconsistent.

5 .... 4 .... 3 .... 2 1

Disorganized/Disoriented

During the Strange Situation, a 1-year-old child displays disorganized and/or disoriented behaviors in the caregiver's presence, suggesting a temporary collapse of behavioral strategies. The child exhibits a mix of approaching, avoidant, and "trance-like" behaviors, especially upon reunion with the caregiver. This pattern may be linked to maltreatment or to frightening/frightened caregiver behaviors, and it is supposed to be produced by the fear of the caregiver.

A 3-year-old child may show role-inverting or "disorganized/controlling" behavior with the caregiver, being either punitive (doing something to humiliate, embarrass, or refuse the caregiver) or caregiving/solicitous (being caring and protective of the caregiver, showing concern or care in a manner suggesting that the caregiver is dependent on the child), with the aim to direct the caregiver's behaviors. The child also shows a moderate avoidance (e.g., talking to the caregiver with his or her back turned), as well as a subtle or open hostility and occasionally fear or sadness.

Disorganized narrative stories usually have hostile or negative themes. The child or some other member of the family is described as involved in violent, hostile, or bizarre behaviors.

Disorganized attachment in infancy is recognized as a powerful predictor for serious psychopathology and maladjustment in older children and adolescents.

5 .... 4 .... 3 .... 2 1

Summary of Relational Patterns and Disorders

The Summary of Relational Patterns and Disorders (Table 10.10) helps the clinician to capture the overall quality of significant relationships and to reflect on where the challenges lie and where they stem from. The family history and functioning can be described in the clinical narrative along with a clinical formulation of how they contribute to the current relationship. In the assessment of relationship, the clinician may refer to the PIR-GAS (DC: 0–3R; see "Most Relevant Assessment Tools," below) as a scale that considers the behavioral quality of interaction, the affective tone, and the psychological involvement of the infant-caregiver relationship. Compared to the PIR-GAS, Axis IV tries to give due consideration to caregiving patterns, parental interactive styles, child–caregiver interactional patterns, attachment, and quality of mental representations of relationships.

A listing of most relevant assessment tools is provided below as a way to help a clinician systematically organize observations of the child's relationships and to define a clinical diagnostic profile of relational patterns and disorders.

Most Relevant Assessment Tools

This section includes rating scales of the caregiver–child relationship and/or interaction, then some of the most important standardized observational procedures, and finally assessment tools for evaluating the child's and caregiver's affective and representational states.

TABLE 10.10. Summary of Relational Patterns and Disorders

R01. Healthy/adapted relational patterns (range = 36–40)

Caregiver–child relationship is very well adapted and clearly promotes the growth of both child and caregiver. Interactions are enjoyable, and reciprocal and synchronous interactions are observed. The caregiver can fully support the functional ability appropriate to the child's age. Caregiver representations of the child are rich, detailed, and flexible, with a moderate or high level of reflective functioning. Attachment patterns are secure.

R02. Adapted relational patterns with some areas of difficulty (range = 29–35)

Some areas of difficulty may be observed, but nonetheless the caregiver–child relationship is still adapted and shows minor interference. At times caregiver and child may be in conflict, but difficulties do not persist longer than a few days, and relationship mantains adaptive flexibility (e.g., ability to negotiate conflict). The child may show some difficulties (e.g., in separation), or the caregiver may appear overprotective and express some concern regarding the child's well-being, behavior, or development. In other cases, the child has a mild constitutional difficulty that impairs the caregiver's ability to maintain a suitable relationship. Despite these minor difficulties, the caregiver–child relationship is supportive of the child's functioning. Attachment patterns are still secure.

R03. Moderate perturbation or disturbance in relational patterns (range = 22–28)

There is a perturbation or a disturbance in the caregiver–child relationship, but it is restricted to one domain of functioning (feeding, play, regulation, etc.), or the caregiver is unable to support two or more areas of the child's functioning. Consistency is sometimes lacking between the caregiver's expressed attitudes toward the child and the quality of observed interactions (predictability, reciprocity, or both). Interactions are mildly stimulating and controlling, or are lacking in vitality and mutual pleasure. The caregiver may be moderately insensitive and/or unresponsive to the cues of the child, or may not adequately mirror the child's internal affective states. Resolution of conflict is difficult and may lead to caregiver and child distress. Attachment patterns may be insecure–avoidant or insecure–resistant.

R04. Significant disturbance in relational patterns (range = 15–21)

Most child–caregiver interactions are conflicted and associated with distress for both partners. The caregiver often interferes with the child's goals and desires, or neglects the child's physical and emotional needs. The caregiver cannot consider the child as a separate person with individual needs, and some domains of functioning (e.g., assertiveness or autonomy) may be thwarted. Conflicts may spread across multiple domains of functioning. The child's range of affective expressions may be very constricted. Affect in the relationship is flat, constricted, and characterized by withdrawal and sadness; or interactions are tense, with no or little sense of relaxed enjoyment or mutuality. Attachment patterns may be insecure or disorganized.

R05. Major impairments in relational patterns, or relational disorders (range = 8–14)

The relationship shows deeply rooted dysfunctional patterns and is characterized by interactions that are harsh and abrupt; often lacking in emotional reciprocity; or even hostile, angry, or frightening, so that the child may feel in danger. The child may exhibit fearful, vigilant, and avoidant behaviors, or may appear submissive with compliant or defiant behaviors. These major impairments undermine the foundation of the child's healthy functioning. Disorganization of attachment is prevalent.

Parent–Infant Relationship Global Assessment Scale

The Parent–Infant Relationship Global Assessment Scale (PIR-GAS; Zero to Three, 2005) is an additional global assessment tool in DC: 0–3R. Its aim is to evaluate the quality of the relationship between a parent (or another caregiver) and a child from 0 to 5 years old. Three components are assessed by the PIR-GAS: behavioral quality of parent–infant interaction, affective tone, and psychological involvement. Ratings take into account the overall functioning of the dyad, including the level of dyadic distress, the adaptive flexibility of both caregiver and child, and the level of conflict and resolution. A global score on a 90-point scale, from grossly impaired (10) to well adapted (100), is assigned by the evaluator. The scale is primarily a diagnostic tool rather than an evaluation measure.

Ainsworth Maternal Sensitivity Scale

The Ainsworth Maternal Sensitivity Scale (AMSS; Ainsworth, Bell, & Stayton, 1974) is a global measure of maternal sensitivity (i.e., a mother's accuracy in perceiving and interpreting her infant's cues, and her ability to react in a timely and appropriate manner). Four aspects of maternal behavior are evaluated: (1) mother's awareness of her baby's signals, (2) accurate interpretation of them, (3) appropriate response, and (4) prompt response. Ratings are made on a 9-point scale of maternal sensitivity, with five anchor points (1, highly insensitive; 3, insensitive; 5, inconsistently sensitive; 7, sensitive; 9, highly sensitive). The final score represents the degree to which all four of these components are observed during the interaction. To differentiate mothers of insecure–avoidant from those of insecure–ambivalent infants, Ainsworth and colleagues (1974) developed three additional scales (cooperation–interference, acceptance–rejection, and accessibility–ignoring). No guidance on the optimal setting in which to observe and record interactions is provided, and the AMSS can be applied to contexts of variable lengths and interaction tasks, such as free play, feeding, or teaching tasks.

Emotional Availability Scales: Infancy to Early Childhood Version

The Emotional Availability Scales: Infancy to Early Childhood Version (EAS; Biringen, Robinson, & Emde, 1993, 2000) is a global rating system for the assessment of dyadic interactions. It measures the emotional availability of the parent to the child and of the child to the parent. The Infancy to Early Childhood Version is for ages 0–4 years. It is an emotion-focused measure that assesses the overall affective quality of the relationship; it does not quantify distinct behaviors, but analyzes the interactional style of the dyad. The scales consist of four parental dimensions (sensitivity, structuring, non-intrusiveness, and non-hostility) and two infant dimensions (responsiveness and involvement). Data are collected with a video recording of at least 20 minutes of interaction, although the EAS has been used for shorter time periods. Each of the six dimensions is coded on a 9-, 7-, or 5-point Likert scale.

Frightening/Frightened Coding System

The Frightening/Frightened (FR) Coding System (Hesse & Main, 2006; Main & Hesse, 1992a, 1992b) is a scale intended to examine parental behaviors that are thought to be linked with a parent's unresolved loss or trauma in his or her own past experiences. The coding system can be applied to the observation of either parent–infant free-play interactions or structured interactions in different contexts, such as a laboratory or home setting. This coding system comprises six subcategories of FR behaviors. The first three subcategories are seen as the primary forms of FR behaviors, as they are experienced directly by the infant: frightening/threatening behaviors (e.g., looming over or assuming attack postures toward the child); frightened behaviors (e.g., frightened facial expressions, pulling or backing away from the infant); and dissociated behaviors (e.g., stilling, freezing, sudden changes in voice, mood, or state). The other three subcategories are considered secondary, as they are not seen as overtly frightening to the infant: timid/deferential behaviors (e.g., treating the child as an attachment figure, submissive behavior to the infant); sexualized behavior (e.g., extended kissing, sexualized or romantic caressing); and disorganized/disoriented behaviors (e.g., sudden change of affect, contradictory signals, limpness of movement). The level of FR behavior is scored for each occurrence of such a behavior on a 9-point scale, and an overall rating is given to the entire segment of observation, based on the highest score of all occurrences in that segment. Scores above 5 are classified as FR.

Atypical Maternal Behavior Instrument for Assessment and Classification

The Atypical Maternal Behavior Instrument for Assessment and Classification (AMBIANCE; Bronfman, Madigan, & Lyons-Ruth, 2008; Bronfman, Parsons, & Lyons-Ruth, 1993) is a coding scheme that expands on Main and Hesse's FR Coding System and is designed to assess the degree of atypical caregiver-to-infant behaviors that are linked with disorganized attachment in infancy. It was originally designed to assess atypical caregiver behaviors directed toward 2- to 18-month-olds; however, it has since been used with caregivers of 4-month-old infants and 24-month-old toddlers. The AMBIANCE involves recording the number of atypical behaviors displayed by a caregiver during interactions with the infant on five dimensions (affective communication errors, role/boundary confusion, disorganized/disoriented behaviors, negative/intrusive behavior, and withdrawal). Behaviors on each dimension are coded, and an overall score for the level of disruption on a 7-point scale is assigned. Furthermore, the caregiver's behavior can be classified as disrupted or not disrupted in communication with the infant.

Disconnected and Extremely Insensitive Parenting Measure

The Disconnected and Extremely Insensitive Parenting Measure (DIP; Out, Bakermans-Kranenburg, & van IJzendoorn, 2009) is a coding system for maternal behavior. It encompasses two dimensions: disconnected behavior and extremely insensitive behavior. The first dimension, disconnected parental behavior, consists of adapted and rearranged items from Main and Hesse's (1992a, 1992b) coding instrument and includes five categories of parental behavior: frightening and threatening behavior; behaviors indicating fear of the child; dissociative behaviors indicative of absorption or intrusion of an altered state of awareness; interacting with the child in a timid, submissive, and/or deferential manner; sexualized/romantic behaviors; and disoriented/disorganized behaviors. Each behavior is accompanied by specific criteria that need to be fulfilled before a score can be assigned. The second dimension encompasses two forms of extreme parental insensitivity: parental withdrawal and neglect; and intrusive, negative, aggressive, or otherwise harsh parental behaviors. The evaluation is based on the duration, frequency, quality, and severity of the behaviors, as well as the context in which the behavior occurs. This dimension is an adaptation of a selection of items from the AMBIANCE. Discrete disconnected and extremely insensitive behaviors are coded on a 9-point scale every time they occur, and for both dimensions, a final score is assigned.

LoTTS Parent–Infant Interaction Coding System

The LoTTS Parent–Infant Interaction Coding System (LPICS; Beatty et al., 2011) was developed as a brief, simple, and easy-to-teach observational measure of parent–infant interactions during face-to-face free play. It allows for general impressions to be captured along a well-defined continuum, and also allows for the recording of the frequency of specific key behaviors. The LPICS includes three subjective/global scores that capture key elements of the interaction (responsiveness, sensitivity, and warmth) and four behavioral counts of key parent behaviors (looking, touching, talking to, and smiling at the infant). It was developed specifically to require minimal training and to be maximally useful for clinical rather than research settings, and although it is a simplified scale it seems to be a reliable and valid tool.

Coparenting and Family Rating Scale

The Coparenting and Family Rating Scale (CFRS; McHale, Kuersten-Hogan, & Lauretti, 2000) is a measure developed to assess seven dimensions of coparenting and family processes from video-recorded family play sessions. The CFRS comprises, first, four dimensions of coparenting rated on a 5-point Likert scale: competition, cooperation, verbal sparring, and coparental warmth. The competition dimension assesses the frequency with which parents interfere in each other's interactions with the child (e.g., by overriding each other's suggestions or distracting the child). The cooperation dimension measures the degree of support and collaboration between parents. The verbal sparring dimension evaluates the frequency and degree of parents' sarcastic and/or hostile remarks toward each other, ranging from mild teasing to explicit criticism or derogation. The coparental warmth dimension assesses the frequency and intensity of positive affect between parents (e.g., joking, warm glances, and verbal or physical affection). A fifth dimension indicates which family member predominantly shapes the direction of family play, ranging from (1) child-centered to (5) parent-centered; a sixth dimension measures the frequency and intensity of positive affect between each parent and the child, ranging from (1) low to (7) high parent–child warmth. Finally, a dimension of parent–child investment evaluates how active, engaged, interested, and attentive each parent appears with the child, ranging from complete disengagement (1) to overinvolvement (7).

Strange Situation

The Strange Situation procedure (Ainsworth et al., 1978) is a semistructured laboratory procedure designed to elicit and categorize an infant's attachment behaviors and strategy to his or her caregiver in children between ages 12 and 18 months. The infant's behavior is observed during different episodes involving separations and reunions with the caregiver, and interaction with a friendly but unfamiliar female stranger. Each episode lasts 3 minutes, and the infant's behavior is observed in terms of separation anxiety, willingness to explore, stranger anxiety, and reunion behaviors. The infant's reactions to the episodes can be placed into one of three organized attachment groups: secure (B), avoidant (A), or resistant (C). Later work by Main and Solomon (1986) defined a fourth group of disorganized (D) children, who showed inconsistent and confused behaviors.

Attachment Q-Sort

The Attachment Q-Sort (AQS; Vaughn & Waters, 1990; Waters & Deane, 1985) is an alternative measure to the Strange Situation, designed to assess the security of infants' and toddlers' attachment to their parents or caregivers. It can be used with older children (specifically between 12 and 48 months of age) and is not as intrusive and stressful as the Strange Situation. The AQS consists of a large number of cards (75, 90, or 100); on each card, a specific behavioral characteristic of children is described. After several hours of observation of a child and caregiver in the home setting, the observer ranks the cards into several piles (the number of piles and the number of cards that can be put in each pile are fixed), from "most descriptive of the subject" to "least descriptive of the subject." At the end of this process, a score for attachment security can be derived. The AQS can be considered an adequate assessment tool of attachment because it appears to show sufficient validity.

Crowell Procedure

The Crowell procedure (Crowell & Feldman, 1988, 1991; Crowell, Feldman, & Ginsburg, 1988) provides a method of observing caregiver–child interactions in a clinical setting. This procedure involves a series of eight episodes designed to elicit behaviors that allow the clinician to focus on the relationship between a child and caregiver in a setting that is unstructured enough to allow for "real-life" or spontaneous interactions. The Crowell procedure requires 45–60 minutes to complete. The eight episodes include free play, cleanup, a bubble-blowing episode, four increasingly difficult problem-solving tasks, and a separation–reunion episode. These episodes allow the clinician to see how comfortable and familiar the child and caregiver are with each other, how the dyad negotiates transitions, the dyad's ability to solve problems together, the use of shared affect (positive and negative) to communicate, and attachment behaviors. This procedure has been shown to be related to different types of caregivers' representations (Aoki, Zeanah, Heller, & Bakshi, 2002; Crowell & Feldman, 1988), to distinguish between clinic-referred and comparison toddlers (Crowell & Feldman, 1988), to distinguish between delayed and nondelayed toddlers (Crowell & Feldman, 1988), and to be specific for a given dyad (Aoki et al., 2002).

Child–Adult Relationship Experimental Index

The Child–Adult Relationship Experimental (CARE) Index (Crittenden, 2003) is a rating scale used to code the quality of mother–infant interactions, with a particular focus on maternal sensitivity and attachment behaviors. This coding procedure is suitable for infants from birth to 36 months of age. Usually 3–5 minutes of free-play interactions are video-recorded, and the dyad is provided with toys but not forced to play with them. The CARE Index consists of 52 items organized around seven aspects of dyadic behavior: facial expression; verbal expression; position and body contact; affection; turn-taking contingencies; control; and choice of activity. Each adult and each infant are separately evaluated on these seven aspects of interactive behavior. For each aspect, there are three items describing the quality of adult behavior, and four describing infant behavior. For adults, one item describes sensitive behavior, one controlling behavior, and one unresponsive behavior. Four items describe the quality of the infant's interactive behavior—cooperative, compliant, difficult, and passive. Although the adult is scored separately from the infant, mother and infant are each scored from the other's perspective. Although it was developed for research purposes, the CARE Index can be applicable to clinical contexts, and video-recording can be carried out in multiple settings, such as laboratory, clinic, or home.

Lausanne Trilogue Play

Lausann Trilogue Play (Fivaz-Depeursinge & Corboz-Warnery, 1999) allows an assessment of coordination between two parents, coordination within the other two dyadic family subunits (mother–child and father–child), and the family's coordination as a whole. The tool was developed to study families through the first year of life. The central element of the method is the Lausanne Trilogue Play situation. During this situation, parents and their babies are brought together to play in four configurations: mother–infant, father–infant, mother–father, and a single "three-together" configuration where all three partners are active in play.

Narrative Story Stem Techniques

Young children's representations can be assessed with narrative story stem completion tasks. Protocols provide structured story stems depicting typical family situations and conflicts, with the aid of doll figures. The children are asked to respond to a set of narrative beginnings of stories, each with an inherent dilemma. Two protocols were originally developed by Bretherton and colleagues: the Attachment Story Completion Task (Bretherton, Ridgeway, & Cassidy, 1990b) and the MacArthur Story Stem Battery (Bretherton & Oppenheim, 2003; Bretherton, Oppenheim, Buchsbaum, Emde, & the MacArthur Narrative Group, 1990a). Other methods were then developed by many researchers, such as the Story Stem Completion Task (Hodges, Hillman, & Steele, 2004) and the Manchester Child Attachment Task (Goldwyn, Stanley, Smith, & Green, 2000; Green, Stanley, Smith, & Goldwyn, 2000). All these measures allow for attachment classifications and provide a clinical picture of a child's mental representations of self and relationships.

Adult Attachment Interview

The Adult Attachment Interview (AAI; George et al., 1984, 1985, 1996) is a semistructured interview designed to capture a person's experience of attachment with caregivers and his or her current state of mind concerning attachment. The interview takes 1–2 hours to administer. Interviewees are asked to describe their early childhood relationship with their parents; to provide adjectives and examples to describe this relationship; and to recall early separations, losses, and means of comfort seeking. They are also asked to reflect on the reasons behind their parents' behavior, and to describe changes in the parental relationship over time. Category classification on the AAI is based on continuous 9-point scales ranging from low (1) to high (9). The scales relating to the inferred experiences are loving, rejecting, involving/reversing, pressure to achieve, and neglecting. The scales relating to state of mind with regard to attachment figures are idealization, involving anger, and derogation. Other scales concern overall states of mind with regard to attachment, such as overall derogation of attachment, insistence on lack of recall, metacognitive monitoring, passivity of discourse, fear of loss, unresolved loss, unresolved trauma, coherence of mind, and coherence of transcript. After the scoring of the AAI transcript, a rating of secure–autonomous, insecure–dismissing, insecure–preoccupied, unresolved with regard to past loss or trauma, or cannot classify is assigned to the transcript.

Working Model of the Child Interview

The Working Model of the Child Interview (WMCI; Zeanah, Benoit, Hirshberg, Barton, & Regan, 1994) is a 1-hour semistructured interview that has been developed to evaluate a parent's perceptions and subjective experience of an infant's individual characteristics and of his or her relationship with the infant. Initially developed for research purposes, it is now also used in clinical settings. The interview includes questions about the pregnancy, delivery, infant's development, infant's personality and behavior, and parent's relationship with the infant. The interview transcription can be rated on eight 5-point rating scales (richness in perception; openness to change; intensity of involvement; coherence; caregiving sensitivity; acceptance; infant difficulty; and fear for infant safety). From these ratings, parents' representations can be classified as balanced, disengaged, or distorted. The affective tone of the parent's responses can also be rated (i.e., joy, pride, anger, guilt, and other emotions expressed).

Parent Development Interview—Revised

The Parent Development Interview—Revised (PDI-R; Aber, Slade, Berger, Bresgi, & Kaplan, 1985; Slade, Aber, Bresgi, Berger, & Kaplan, 2004a) is a 45-item semistructured clinical interview designed to elicit parents' representations of their child, their perceptions of themselves as parents, and their experiences of their relationship. The interview is aimed to evoke current experiences and memories, and it can be used as a tool to explore the parent–infant relationship and the parent's mental representations of the relationship's different aspects. In the interview, a parent is asked to portray the child's behavior, thoughts, and feelings in various situations, and to provide real-life examples. The parent is also asked to describe responses to the child in these situations, to describe him- or herself as a parent, and to discuss the emotions he or she is experiencing as a parent. The interview takes approximately 90 minutes to administer, and training is required to be able to code the interview.

Reflective Functioning in the Parent Development Interview

"Reflective functioning" (RF) refers to a person's ability to understand his or her own and another's behavior in terms of the mental states underlying that behavior. It is also the capacity to understand the intersubjective nature of mental states. For specific use with the original PDI, Slade, Bernbach, Grienenberger, Levy, and Locker (2004b) developed an addendum to the RF coding manual developed by Fonagy, Target, Steele, and Steele (1998) for use with the AAI. RF on the PDI is assessed in four broad categories (awareness of the nature of mental states; the explicit effort to tease out mental states underlying behavior; recognizing developmental aspects of mental states; and mental states in relation to the interviewer). It is an 11-point scale ranging from negative RF to full or exceptional RF. Scoring is based on a reading of verbatim transcripts from the PDI.

Mind-Mindedness Coding Scheme

The Mind-Mindedness Coding Scheme (Meins & Fernyhough, 2010) was developed to code mothers' speech. It has been applied to mother–infant play sessions transcribed verbatim, and it is aimed to evaluate a mother's tendency to view her infant as an intentional agent with autonomous thoughts, intentions, emotions, and desires. "Mind-related" comments are defined as comments on mental states, such as knowledge, thoughts, desires, and interests; comments on mental processes; references to the infant's level of emotional engagement; comments on the infant's attempts to manipulate people's beliefs; and the mother's "putting words into the infant's mouth" so that her speech takes the form of a dialogue. Each mind-related comment can be classified as an appropriate or not-appropriate mind-related comment.

Parenting Stress Index

The Parenting Stress Index (PSI; Abidin, 1983, 1995) is a self-administered questionnaire for a parent, designed to yield a measure of the relative magnitude of stress in the parent–child relationship. The tool has 47 items within the child domain that measure adaptability, acceptability, demandingness, mood, distractibility/hyperactivity, and reinforcement to parents, and 54 items in the parent domain that measure depression, attachment, restrictions of role, sense of competence, social isolation, relationship with spouse, and parent health. The PSI comprises three subscales: parenting distress, which measures the distress the parent is experiencing in his or her role as a parent; parent–child dysfunctional interaction, which focuses on the parent's perceptions of the child as not meeting the parent's expectations; and difficult child, which evaluates the child's basic behavioral characteristics that render him or her either easy or difficult to manage. Finally, defensive responding, which is not included in the total score, assesses the extent to which a respondent responds truthfully to the questionnaire. A total raw score above 90 indicates a clinically significant level of stress. All subscales show good internal consistency. A short 36-item version is also available.

Revised Dyadic Adjustment Scale

The Revised Dyadic Adjustment Scale (RDAS; Busby, Christensen, Crane, & Larson, 1995) is a self-report questionnaire designed to evaluate marital adjustment. The RDAS consists of 14 items extracted from the 32 items of the original Dyadic Adjustment Scale (DAS; Spanier, 1976). The RDAS can assess three aspects of dyadic adjustment: consensus, satisfaction, and cohesion. The subscales can be summed to create a total score representative of overall dyadic adjustment. It has been used in numerous studies with good reliability and is highly correlated with the DAS. Previous research also indicates that the RDAS is successfully able to distinguish between distressed and nondistressed relationships.

Coparenting Relationship Scale

The Coparenting Relationship Scale (CRS; Feinberg, Brown, & Kan, 2012) is a 35-item self-report measure that yields an overall score for coparenting quality, as well as subscale scores representing each domain of coparenting. Items are chosen and adapted from previous measures of the parenting alliance and coparenting, and additional items were created. It is composed of seven subscales: coparenting agreement, coparenting closeness, exposure to conflict, coparenting support, coparenting undermining, endorsement of partner's parenting, and division of labor. Each item is rated on a 7-point scale ranging from "not true of us" to "very true of us" for the first 30 items, and "never" to "very often" for the last 5 items.

Axis V: Other Medical and Neurological Diagnoses

Frequently children with mental health, developmental, regulatory–sensory processing, language, and/or learning disorders evidence medical disorders that may contribute to their difficulties. For example, children with allergies may evidence behavioral, as well as respiratory or dermatological, reactions. Children with thyroid disorders may evidence over- or underresponsivity to their environments. Gastrointestinal disorders are not uncommon in children with pervasive developmental problems. Whether medical problems are clearly contributing or not, it is important for the clinician to indicate any such disorders that are in evidence. Careful listing of medical disorders facilitates their thorough investigation and the exploration of possible relationships with the child's mental health, developmental, or learning challenges.

BIBLIOGRAPHY

Aber, J., Slade, A., Berger, B., Bresgi, I., & Kaplan, M. (1985). *The Parent Development Interview.* Unpublished protocol, City University of New York.

Abidin, R. R. (1983). *Parenting Stress Index manual.* Charlottesville, VA: Pediatric Psychology Press.

Abidin, R. R. (1995). *Parenting Stress Index: Professional manual* (3rd ed.). Odessa, FL: Psychological Assessment Resources.

Achenbach, T. M., & Rescorla, L. A. (2000). *Manual for ASEBA Preschool Forms and Profiles.* Burlington: University of Vermont, Research Center for Children, Youth, and Families.

Ainsworth, M. D. S., Bell, S. M., & Stayton, D. (1974). Infant–mother attachment and social development: "Socialization" as a product of reciprocal responsiveness to signals. In P. M. Richards (Ed.), *The integration of a child into a social world* (pp. 99–135). Cambridge, UK: Cambridge University Press.

Ainsworth, M. D. S., Blehar, M. C., Waters, E., & Wall, S. (1978). *Patterns of attachment: A psychological study of the Strange Situation.* Hillsdale, NJ: Erlbaum.

Althoff, R. R., Verhulst, F. C., Rettew, D. C., Hudziak, J. J., & van der Ende, J. (2010). Adult outcomes of childhood dysregulation: A 14-year follow-up study. *Journal of the American Academy of Child and Adolescent Psychiatry, 49,* 1105–1116.

Alvarez, A. (2012). *The Thinking Heart: Three levels of psychoanalytic therapy with disturbed children.* London: Routledge.

American Psychiatric Association. (1994). *Diagnostic and statistical manual of mental disorders* (4th ed.). Washington, DC: Author.

American Psychiatric Association. (2013). *Diagnostic and statistical manual of mental disorders* (5th ed.). Arlington, VA: Author.

Ammaniti, M., Lucarelli, L., Cimino, S., D'Olimpio, F., & Chatoor, I. (2010). Maternal psychopathology and child risk factors in infantile anorexia. *International Journal of Eating Disorders, 43,* 233–240.

Ammaniti, M., Lucarelli, L., Cimino, S., D'Olimpio, F., & Chatoor, I. (2012), Feeding disorders of infancy: A longitudinal study to middle childhood. *International Journal of Eating Disorders, 45,* 272–280.

Anda, R. F., Felitti, V. J., Bremner, J., Walker, J. D., Whitfield, C., & Perry, B. D. (2006). The enduring effects of abuse and related adverse experiences in childhood: A convergence of evidence from neurobiology and epidemiology. *European Archives of Psychiatry and Clinical Neuroscience, 256*(3), 174–186.

Anders, T. F. (1989). Clinical syndromes, relationship disturbances and their assessment. In A. J. Sameroff & R. N. Emde (Eds.), *Relationship disturbances in early childhood* (pp. 125–144). New York: Basic Books.

Anders, T. F., & Dahl, R. (2007). Classifying sleep disorders in infants and toddlers. In W. E. Narrow, M. B. First, M. S. Sirovatka, & D. A. Regier (Eds.), *Age and gender considerations in psychiatric diagnosis* (pp. 215–226). Arlington, VA: American Psychiatric Association.

Anders, T. F., Goodlin-Jones, B., & Sadeh, A. (2000). Sleep disorders. In C. H. Zeanah (Ed.), *Handbook of infant mental health* (2nd ed., pp. 326–338). New York: Guilford Press.

Aoki, Y., Zeanah, C. H., Heller, S. S., & Bakshi, S. (2002). Parent–infant relationship global assessment scale: A study of its predictive validity. *Psychiatry and Clinical Neurosciences, 56,* 493–497.

Aron, E. N., & Aron, A. (1997). Sensory-processing sensitivity and its relation to introversion and emotionality. *Journal of Personality and Social Psychology, 73*(2), 345–368.

Ayres, A. J. (1963). Tactile functions: Their relation to hyperactive and perceptual motor behavior. *American Journal of Occupational Therapy, 18,* 6–11.

Ayres, A. J. (1972). *Sensory integration and learning disabilities.* Los Angeles: Western Psychological Services.

Ayres, A. J. (1979). *Sensory integration and the child.* Los Angeles: Western Psychological Services.

Bakermans-Kranenburg, M. J., Dobrova-Krol, N., & van IJzendoorn, M. H. (2011a). Impact of institutional care on attachment disorganization and insecurity of Ukrainian preschoolers: Protective effect of the long variant of the serotonin transporter gene (5HTT). *International Journal of Behavioral Development, 36,* 1–8.

Bakermans-Kranenburg, M. J., Steele, H., Zeanah, C. H., Muhamedrahimov, R. J., Vorria, P., Dobrova-Krol, N. A., & Gunnar, M. R. (2011b). III. Attachment and emotional development in institutional care: Characteristics and catch-up. *Monographs of the Society for Research in Child Development, 76*(4), 62–91.

Bakermans-Kranenburg, M., & van IJzendoorn, M. (2007). Genetic vulnerability or differential susceptibility in child development: The case of attachment. *Journal of Child Psychology and Psychiatry, 48*(12), 1160–1173.

Baradon, T. (Ed.). (2009). *Relational trauma in infancy: Psychoanalytic, attachment and neuropsychological contributions to parent–infant psychotherapy.* London: Routledge.

Baradon, T., with Biseo, M., Broughton, C., James, J., & Joyce, A. (2016). *The practice of psychoanalytic parent–infant psychotherapy: Claiming the baby* (2nd ed.). Abingdon, UK: Routledge.

Baradon, T., & Steele, M. (2008). Integrating the AAI in the clinical process of psychoanalytic parent–infant psychotherapy in a case of relational trauma. In H. Steele & M. Steele (Eds.), *Clinical applications of the Adult Attachment Interview* (pp. 195–212). New York: Guilford Press.

Baranek, G. T. (1994). Tactile defensiveness in children with developmental disabilities: Responsiveness and habituation. *Journal of Autism and Developmental Disorders, 24,* 457–471.

Baranek, G. T. (2002). Efficacy of sensory and motor interventions for children with autism. *Journal of Autism and Developmental Disorders, 32*(5), 397–422.

Baranek, G. T., David, F. J., Poe, M. D., Stone, W. L., & Watson, L. R. (2006). Sensory Experiences Questionnaire: Discriminating sensory features in young children with autism, developmental delays, and typical development. *Journal of Child Psychology and Psychiatry, and Allied Disciplines, 47,* 591–601.

Barton, M. L., Robins, D., Jashar, D., Brenna, L., & Fein D. (2013). Sensitivity and specificity of proposed DSM-5 criteria for autism spectrum disorder in toddlers. *Journal of Autism and Developmental Disorders, 43*(5), 1184–1195.

Bayley, N. (1993). *Bayley Scales of Infant Development—Second Edition.* San Antonio, TX: Psychological Corporation.

Bayley, N. (2006). *Bayley Scales of Infant and Toddler Development—Third Edition.* San Antonio, TX: Harcourt Assessment.

Beatty, J., Stacks, A. M., Partridge, T., Tzilos, G. K., Loree, A., & Ondersma, S. (2011). LoTTS parent–infant interaction coding scale: Ease of use and reliability in a sample of high-risk mothers and their infants. *Children and Youth Services Review, 33*(1), 86–90.

Beebe, B., Knoblauch, S., Rustin, J., & Sorter, D. (2005). *Forms of intersubjectivity in infant research and adult treatment.* New York: Other Press.

Beesdo-Baum, K., & Knappe, S. (2012). Developmental epidemiology of anxiety disorders. *Child and Adolescent Psychiatric Clinics of North America, 21*(3), 457–478.

Beesdo-Baum, K., Knappe, S., & Pine, D. (2009). Anxiety and anxiety disorders in children and adolescents: Developmental issues and implications for DSM-V. *Psychiatric Clinics of North America, 32*(3), 483–524.

Ben-Sasson, A., Carter, A. S., & Briggs-Gowan, M. J. (2010). The development of sensory overresponsivity from infancy to elementary school. *Journal of Abnormal Child Psychology, 38*(8), 1193–1202.

Bernard, K., Dozier, M., Bick, J., Lewis-Morrarty, E., Lindhiem, O., & Carlson, E. (2012). Enhancing attachment organization among maltreated children: Results of a randomized clinical trial. *Child Development, 83,* 623–636.

Berthelot, N., Ensink, K., Bernazzani, O., Normandin, L., Luyten, P., & Fonagy, P. (2015). Intergenerational transmission of attachment in abused and neglected mothers: The role of trauma-specific reflective functioning. *Infant Mental Health Journal, 36,* 200–212.

Biederman, J., Rosenbaum, J. F., Bolduc-Murphy, E. A., Faraone, S. V., Chaloff, J., Hirshfeld, D. R., & Kagan, J. (1993). A 3-year follow-up of children with and without behavioral inhibition. *Journal of the American Academy of Child and Adolescent Psychiatry, 32*(4), 814–821.

Biringen, Z., Robinson, J., & Emde, R. N. (1993). *Emotional Availability Scales*. Unpublished manuscript, Health Science Center, University of Colorado, Denver, CO.

Biringen, Z., Robinson, J., & Emde, R. N. (2000). Appendix B: Emotional Availability Scales (3rd ed., abridged infancy/early childhood version). *Attachment and Human Development, 2*, 256–270.

Blader, J. C., & Carlson, G. A. (2007). Increased rates of bipolar disorder diagnoses among U.S. child, adolescent, and adult inpatients, 1996–2004. *Biological Psychiatry, 62*(2), 107–114.

Bleichmar, H. (1996). Some subtypes of depression and their implications for psychoanalytic treatment. *International Journal of Psychoanalysis, 77*, 935–961.

Boomsma, D. I., Rebollo, I., Derks, E. M., van Beijsterveldt, T. C. E. M., Althoff, R. R., Rettew, D. C., & Hudziak, J. J. (2006). Longitudinal stability of the CBCL-juvenile bipolar disorder phenotype: A study in Dutch twins. *Biological Psychiatry, 60*(9), 912–920.

Bouchard, M. A., Target, M., Lecours, S., Fonagy, P., Tremblay, L. M., Schachter, A., & Stein, H. (2008). Mentalization in adult attachment narratives: Reflective functioning, mental states, and affect elaboration compared. *Psychoanalytic Psychology, 25*(1), 47–66.

Bowlby, J. (1958). The nature of the child's tie to his mother. *International Journal of Psycho-Analysis, 39*, 350–373.

Bowlby, J. (1960). Grief and mourning in infancy and early childhood. *Psychoanalytic Study of the Child, 15*, 9–52.

Bowlby, J. (1979). *The making and breaking of affectional bonds*. London: Tavistock.

Bowlby, J. (1980). *Attachment and loss: Vol. 3. Loss*. New York: Basic Books.

Bowlby, J. (1988). *A secure base: Parent–child attachment and healthy human development*. New York: Basic Books.

Brandt, K. A., Perry, B. D., Seligman, S., & Tronick, E. (Eds.). (2013). *Infant and early childhood mental health: Core concepts and clinical practice*. Arlington, VA: American Psychiatric Publishing.

Brazelton, T. B. (1979). Evidence of communication during neonatal behavioural assessment. In M. Bullowa (Ed.), *Before speech: The beginning of human communication* (pp. 79–88). Cambridge, UK: Cambridge University Press.

Brazelton, T. B., & Nugent, J. K. (1995). *The Neonatal Behavioral Assessment Scale* (3rd ed.). London: MacKeith Press.

Brazelton, T. B., & Nugent, J. K. (2011). *The Neonatal Behavioral Assessment Scale*. Cambridge, UK: MacKeith Press.

Bretherton, I., & Oppenheim, D. (2003). The MacArthur Story Stem Battery: Development, administration, reliability, validity, and reflections about meaning. In R. N. Emde, D. P. Wolf, & D. Oppenheim (Eds.), *Revealing the inner worlds of young children: The MacArthur Story Stem Battery and parent–child narratives* (pp. 55–80). New York: Oxford University Press.

Bretherton, I., Oppenheim, D., Buchsbaum, H., Emde, R. N., & the MacArthur Narrative Group. (1990a). *The MacArthur Story Stem Battery (MSSB)*. Unpublished manual, University of Wisconsin, Madison, WI.

Bretherton, I., Oppenheim, D., Emde, R. N., & MacArthur Narrative Working Group. (2003). The MacArthur Story Stem Battery. In R. N. Emde, D. P. Wolf, & D. Oppenheim (Eds.), *Revealing the inner worlds of young children: The MacArthur Story Stem Battery and parent–child narratives* (pp. 55–80). New York: Oxford University Press.

Bretherton, I., Ridgeway, D., & Cassidy, J. (1990b). Assessing internal working models of the attachment relationship: An attachment story completion task for 3-year-olds. In M. Greenberg, D. Cicchetti, & E. M. Cummings (Eds.), *Attachment during the preschool years* (pp. 272–308). Chicago: University of Chicago Press.

Briggs-Gowan, M. J., & Carter, A. S. (2006). *The Brief Infant–Toddler Social and Emotional Assessment BITSEA)*. San Antonio, TX: Harcourt Assessment.

Briggs-Gowan, M. J., Carter, A. S., Bosson-Heenan, J., Guyer, A. E., & Horwitz, S. M. (2006). Are infant–toddler social-emotional and behavioral problems transient? *Journal of the American Academy of Child and Adolescent Psychiatry, 45*(7), 849–858.

Brisch, K. H. (2012). *Treating attachment disorders: From theory to therapy* (2nd ed.). New York: Guilford Press.

Bronfman, E., Madigan, S., & Lyons-Ruth, K. (2008). *Atypical Maternal Behavior Instrument for Assessment and Classification (AMBIANCE): Manual for coding disrupted affective communication* (2nd ed.). Unpublished manual, Harvard Medical School.

Bronfman, E., Parsons, E., & Lyons-Ruth, K. (1993). *Atypical Maternal Behavior Instrument for Assessment and Classification (AMBIANCE): Manual for coding disrupted affective communication*. Unpublished manuscript, Harvard Medical School.

Bruce, J., Tarullo, A. R., & Gunnar, M. R. (2009). Disinhibited social behavior among internationally adopted children. *Development and Psychopathology, 21*, 157–171.

Bryant-Waugh, R., Markham, L., Kreipe, R. E., & Walsh, B. T. (2010). Feeding and eating disorders in childhood. *International Journal of Eating Disorders, 43*, 98–111.

Busby, D. M., Christensen, C., Crane, D. R., & Larson, J. H. (1995). A revision of the Dyadic Adjustment Scale for use with distressed and non-distressed couples: Construct hierarchy and multi-dimensional scales. *Journal of Marital and Family Therapy, 21*(3), 289–308.

Butler, R. J. (2008). Wetting and soiling. In M. Rutter, D. V. M. Bishop, D. Pine, S. Scott, J. Stevenson, E. Taylor, & A. Thapar (Eds.), *Rutter's child and adolescent psychiatry* (5th ed., pp. 916–929). Malden, MA: Wiley-Blackwell.

Byne, W., Bradley, S. J., Coleman, E., Eyler, A. E., Green, R., Menvielle, E. J., . . . Tompkins, D. A. (2012). Report of the American Psychiatric Association Task Force on Treatment of Gender Identity Disorder. *Archives of Sexual Behavior, 41*(4), 759–796.

Calkins, S. D., & Hill, A. (2007). Caregiver influences on emerging emotional regulation: Biological and environmental transactions in early development. In J. J. Gross (Ed.), *Handbook of emotion regulation* (pp. 229–248). New York: Guilford Press.

Calkins, S. D., & House, R. (2004). Individual differences in self-regulation: Implications for childhood adjustment. In P. Philipot & R. Feldman (Eds.), *The regulation of emotion* (pp. 307–332). Mahwah, NJ: Erlbaum.

Carlson, G. A., & Klein, D. N. (2014). How to understand divergent views on bipolar disorder in youth. *Annual Review of Clinical Psychology, 10*(1), 529–551.

Carter, A. S., Ben-Sasson, A., & Briggs-Gowan, M. J. (2011). Sensory over-responsivity, psychopathology, and family impairment in school-aged children. *Journal of the American Academy of Child and Adolescent Psychiatry, 50*(12), 1210–1219.

Carter, A. S., & Briggs-Gowan, M. J. (2006). *The Infant–Toddler Social and Emotional Assessment (ITSEA) manual.* San Antonio, TX: Harcourt Assessment.

Carter, A. S., Briggs-Gowan, M. J., Jones S., & Little T. D. (2003). The Infant–Toddler Social and Emotional Assessment (ITSEA): Factor Structure, Reliability, and Validity. *Journal of Abnormal Child Psychology, 31,* 495–514.

Casey, P. (2014). Adjustment disorder: New developments. *Current Psychiatry Reports, 16*(6), 1–8.

Chatoor, I. (2002). Feeding disorders in infants and toddlers: Diagnosis and treatment. *Child and Adolescent Psychiatric Clinics of North America, 11,* 163–183.

Chatoor, I. (2005). Diagnostic classification of feeding disorders. In Zero to Three, *Diagnostic classification of mental health and developmental disorders of infancy and early childhood* (rev. ed.). Washington, DC: Zero to Three Press.

Chatoor, I. (2009). *Diagnosis and treatment of feeding disorders in infants, toddlers, and young children.* Washington, DC: Zero to Three Press.

Chatoor, I., & Ganiban, J. (2004). The diagnostic assessment and classification of feeding disorders. In R. DelCarmen-Wiggins & A. Carter (Eds.), *Handbook of infant, toddler, and preschool mental health assessment* (pp. 289–305). New York: Oxford University Press.

Chisholm, K. (1998). A three-year follow-up of attachment and indiscriminate friendliness in children adopted from Romanian orphanages. *Child Development, 69,* 1092–1106.

Cicchetti, D., & Cohen, D. J. (Eds.). (2006). *Developmental psychopathology: Theory and method* (3 vols., 2nd ed.). Hoboken, NJ: Wiley.

Clayden, G. (2001), The child who soils. *Current Paediatrics, 11,* 130–134.

Coates, S., & Wolfe, S. (1995). Gender identity disorder in boys: The interface of constitution and early experience. *Psychoanalytic Inquiry, 51,* 6–38.

Cook, A. C., Spinazzola, J., Ford, J., Lanktree, C., Blaustein, M., Cloitre, M., . . . van der Kolk, B. (2005). Complex trauma in children and adolescents. *Psychiatric Annals, 35*(5), 390–398.

Cooper, P. J., Whelan, E., Woolgar, M., Morrell, J., & Murray, L. (2004). Association between childhood feeding problems and maternal eating disorders: Role of the family environment. *British Journal of Psychiatry, 184,* 210–215.

Costello, E. J., Burns, B. J., Angold, A., & Leaf, P. J. (1993). How can epidemiology improve mental health services for children and adolescents? *Journal of the American Academy of Child and Adolescent Psychiatry, 32,* 1106–1113.

Costello, E. J., Erkanli, A., Fairbank, J. A., & Angold, A. (2002). The prevalence of potentially traumatic events in childhood and adolescence. *Journal of Traumatic Stress, 15,* 99–112.

Costello, E. J., Mustillo, S., Erkanli, A., Keeler, G., & Angold, A. (2003). Prevalence and development of psychiatric disorders in childhood and adolescence. *Archives of General Psychiatry, 60*(8), 837–844.

Cox, D. J., Morris, J. B., Borowitz, S. M., & Sutphen, J. L. (2002). Psychological differences between children with and without chronic encopresis. *Journal of Pediatric Psychology, 27,* 585–591.

Cramer, P. (1991). *The development of defense mechanisms: Theory, research and assessment.* New York: Springer-Verlag.

Cramer, P. (2006). *Protecting the self: Defense mechanisms in action.* New York: Guilford Press.

Crittenden, P. M. (2003). *CARE-Index manual.* Unpublished manuscript, Family Relations Institute, Miami, FL.

Crockenberg, S. C., Leerkes, E. M., & Bárrig Jó, P. S. (2008). Predicting aggressive behavior in the third year from infant reactivity and regulation as moderated by maternal behavior. *Development and Psychopathology, 20*(1), 37–54.

Crowell, J. A., & Feldman, S. S. (1988). Mothers' internal models of relationships and children's behavioral and developmental status in mother–child interaction: A study of mother–child interaction. *Child Development, 59,* 1275–1285.

Crowell, J. A., & Feldman, S. S. (1991). Mothers' working models of attachment relationships and mother and child behavior during separation and reunion. *Developmental Psychology, 27*(4), 597–605.

Crowell, J. A., Feldman, S. S., & Ginsberg, N. (1988). Assessment of mother-child interaction in preschoolers with behavior problems. *Journal of the American Academy of Child and Adolescent Psychiatry, 27*(3), 303–311.

Cuthbert, B. N., Insel, T. R., Charney, D. S., Buxbaum, J. D., Sklar, P., & Nestler, E. J. (2013). Toward precision medicine in psychiatry: The NIMH Research Domain Criteria Project. In D. S. Charney, J. D. Buxbaum, P. Sklar, & E. J. Nestler (Eds.), *Neurobiology of mental illness* (4th ed., pp. 1076–1088). New York: Oxford University Press.

D'Andrea, W., Stolbach, B., Ford, J., Spinazzola, J., & van der Kolk, B. A. (2012). Understanding interpersonal trauma in children: Why we need a developmentally appropriate trauma diagnosis. *American Journal of Orthopsychiatry, 82*(2), 187–200.

Dankner, N., & Dykens, E. M. (2012). Anxiety in intellectual disabilities: Challenges and next steps. In R. M. Hodapp (Ed.), *International review of research in developmental disabilities* (Vol. 42, pp. 57–83). San Diego, CA: Elsevier Academic Press.

Dawson, G., Jones, E. J., Merkle, K., Venema, K., Lowy, R., Faja, S., & Smith, M. (2012). Early behavioral intervention is associated with normalized brain activity in young children with autism. *Journal of the American Academy of Child and Adolescent Psychiatry, 51*(11), 1150–1159.

de Vries, A. L., & Cohen-Kettenis, P. T. (2012). Clinical management of gender dysphoria in children and adolescents: The Dutch approach. *Journal of Homosexuality, 59*(3), 301–320.

DeGangi, G. A. (2000). *Pediatric disorders of regulation in affect and behavior: A therapist's guide to assessment and treatment.* San Diego, CA: Academic Press.

DeGangi, G. A., Breinbauer, C., Roosevelt, J. D., Porges, S., & Greenspan, S. (2000). Prediction of childhood problems at three years in children experiencing disorders of regulation during infancy. *Infant Mental Health Journal, 21*(3), 156–175.

DeGangi, G. A., & Greenspan, S. I. (1989). The development of sensory functions in infants. *Physical and Occupational Therapy in Pediatrics, 8*(4), 21–34.

DeGangi, G. A., Poisson, S., Sickel, R. Z., & Wiener, A. S. (1995). *Infant/Toddler Symptom Checklist: A screening tool for parents.* Tucson, AZ: Therapy Skill Builders.

DeGangi, G. A., Porges, S. W., Sickel, R. Z., & Greenspan, S. I. (1993). Four-year follow-up of a sample of regulatory disordered infants. *Infant Mental Health Journal, 14*(4), 330–343.

Drescher, J. (2014). Controversies in gender diagnoses. *Journal of LGBT Health Research, 1*(1), 9–15.

Drescher, J., & Byne, W. (2013). *Treating transgender children and adolescents: An interdisciplinary discussion.* New York: Routledge.

Drescher, J., Cohen-Kettenis, P. T., & Reed, G. M. (2016). Gender incongruence of childhood in the ICD-11: Controversies, proposal, and rationale. *Lancet Psychiatry, 3,* 297–304.

Drescher, J., & Pula, J. (2014). Ethical issues raised by the treatment of gender variant prepubescent children. *Hastings Center Report, 44*(Suppl. 4), S17–S22.

Drury, S. S., Gleason, M. M., Theall, K. P., Smyke, A. T., Nelson, C. A., Fox, N. A., & Zeanah, C. H. (2012). Genetic sensitivity to the caregiving context: The influence of 5httlpr and BDNF val66met on indiscriminate social behavior. *Physiology and Behavior, 106*(5), 728–735.

Dunn, W. (1997). The Sensory Profile: A discriminating measure of sensory processing in daily life. *SISIS Quarterly, 20*(1), 1–3.

Dunn, W. (2002). *Infant/Toddler Sensory Profile.* San Antonio, TX: Psychological Corporation.

Dunn, W., & Daniels, D. B. (2002). Initial development of the Infant/Toddler Sensory Profile. *Journal of Early Intervention, 25*(1), 27–41.

Dunn, W., Myles, B. S., & Orr, S. (2002). Sensory processing issues associated with Asperger syndrome: A preliminary investigation. *American Journal of Occupational Therapy, 56*(1), 97–102.

Easterbrooks, M., Bureau, J. F., & Lyons-Ruth, K. (2012). Developmental correlates and predictors of emotional availability in mother–child interaction: A longitudinal study from infancy to middle childhood. *Development and Psychopathology, 24*(1), 65–78.

Egger, H. L., & Angold, A. (2006). Common emotional and behavioral disorders in preschool children: Presentation, nosology, and epidemiology. *Journal of Child Psychology and Psychiatry, 47*(3–4), 313–337.

Egger, H. L., & Emde, R. N. (2011). Developmentally sensitive diagnostic criteria for mental health disorders in early childhood. *American Psychologist, 66*(2), 95–106.

Ehrensaft, D. (2012). From gender identity disorder to gender identity creativity: True gender self child therapy. *Journal of Homosexuality, 59*(3), 337–356.

Emde, R. M., & Leuzinger-Bohleber, M. (Eds.). (2014). *Early parenting and prevention of disorder.* London: Karnac.

Fabrizi, A., Costa, A., Lucarelli, L., & Patruno, E. (2010). Comorbidity in specific language disorders and early feeding disorders: Mother–child interactive patterns. *Eating and Weight Disorders, 15,* 152–160.

Feinberg, M. E., Brown, L. D., & Kan, M. L. (2012). A multi-domain self-report measure of coparenting. *Parenting: Science and Practice, 12,* 1–21.

Ferdinand, R. F., & Verhulst, F. C. (1995). Psychopathology from adolescence into young adulthood: An 8 year follow-up study. *American Journal of Psychiatry, 152,* 1586–1594.

Figley, C. R., Bride, B. E., & Mazza, N. (1997). *Death and trauma: The traumatology of grieving.* London: Taylor & Francis.

Finkelhor, D., Ormrod, R. K., & Turner, H. A. (2007). Poly-victimization: A neglected component in child victimization. *Child Abuse and Neglect, 31*(1), 7–26.

Fishel, J. E., & Liebert, R. M. (2000). Disorders of elimination. In A. J. Sameroff, M. Lewis, & S. M. Miller (Eds.), *Handbook of developmental psychopathology* (pp. 625–636). New York: Springer.

Fitzgerald, H. E., Weatherston, D., & Mann, T. L. (2011). Infant mental health: An interdisciplinary frame for early social and emotional development. *Current Problems in Pediatric and Adolescent Health Care, 41,* 178–182.

Fivaz-Depeursinge, E., & Corboz-Warnery, A. (1999). *The primary triangle: A developmental systems view of mothers, fathers, and infants.* New York: Basic Books.

Fonagy, P., Gergely, G., Jurist, E. L., & Target, M. (2002). *Affect regulation, mentalization, and the development of the self.* New York: Other Press.

Fonagy, P., Moran, G. S., Edgcumbe, R., Kennedy, H., & Target, M. (1993). The roles of mental representations and mental processes in therapeutic action. *Psychoanalytic Study of the Child, 48,* 9–48.

Fonagy, P., & Target, M. (1997). Attachment and reflective function: Their role in self-organisation. *Development and Psychopathology, 9,* 679–700.

Fonagy, P., Target, M., Steele, H., & Steele, M. (1998). *Reflective Functioning Manual, Version 5.0, for application to Adult Attachment Interviews.* Unpublished manuscript, University College London.

Ford, J. D., & Courtois, C. A. (Eds.). (2013). *Treating complex traumatic stress disorders in children and adolescents: Scientific foundations and therapeutic models.* New York: Guilford Press.

Ford, J. D., Elhai, J. D., Connor, D. F., & Frueh, B. (2010). Polyvictimization and risk of posttraumatic, depressive, and substance use disorders and involvement in delinquency in a national sample of adolescents. *Journal of Adolescent Health, 46*(6), 545–552.

Fraiberg, S. H. (1982). Pathological defenses in infancy. *Psychoanalytic Quarterly, 51,* 612–635.

Freud, A., & Burlingham, D. (1943). *War and children.* New York: Medical War Books.

Freud, A., & Burlingham, D. (1944). *Infants without families.* New York: International Universities Press.

Frick, S. (1989). Sensory defensiveness: A case study. *Sensory Integration Special Interest Section Newsletter, 12*(2), 1–3.

Gartstein, M. A., & Rothbart, M. K. (2003). Studying infant temperament via the Revised Infant Behavior Questionnaire. *Infant Behavior and Development, 166,* 1–23.

George, C., Kaplan, N., & Main, M. (1984, 1985, 1996). *The Adult Attachment Interview.* Unpublished manuscript, Department of Psychology, University of California, Berkeley, CA.

Gillberg, C., & Kadesjo, B. (2003). Why bother about clumsiness?: The implications of having developmental coordination disorder (DCD). *Neural Plasticity, 10,* 59–68.

Ginsburg, G. S., Kendall, P. C., Sakolsky, D., Compton, S. N., Piacentini, J., Albano, A. M., . . . March, J. (2011). Remission after acute treatment in children and adolescents with anxiety disorders: Findings from the CAMS. *Journal of Consulting and Clinical Psychology, 79*(6), 806–813.

Gleason, M. M., Fox, N., Drury, S. S., Smyke, A. T., Egger, H. L., Nelson, C. A., . . . Zeanah, C. H. (2011). The validity of evidence-derived criteria for reactive attachment disorder: Indiscriminately social/disinhibited and emotionally withdrawn/inhibited types. *Journal of the American Academy of Child and Adolescent Psychiatry, 50,* 216–231.

Goldsmith, H. H., Van Hulle, C. A., Arneson, C. L., Schreiber, J. E., & Gernsbacher, M. A. (2006). A population-based twin study of parentally reported tactile and auditory defensiveness in young children. *Journal of Abnormal Child Psychology, 34*(3), 393–407.

Goldwyn, R., Stanley, C., Smith, V., & Green, J. (2000). The Manchester Child Attachment Story Task: Relationship with parental AAI, SAT and child behaviour. *Attachment and Human Development, 2*(1), 71–84.

Goodlin-Jones, B. L., & Anders, T. F. (2004). Sleep disorders. In R. DelCarmen-Wiggins & A. Carter (Eds.), *Handbook of infant, toddler, and preschool mental health assessment* (pp. 271–288). New York: Oxford University Press.

Goodlin-Jones, B. L., Burnham, M., Gaylor, E., & Anders, T. (2001). Night waking, sleep–wake organization, and self-soothing in the first year of life. *Journal of Developmental and Behavioral Pediatrics, 24,* 226–233.

Grandin, T. (1995). *Thinking in pictures and other reports from my life with autism.* New York: Doubleday.

Green, J., Stanley, C., Smith, V., & Goldwyn, R. (2000). A new method of evaluating attachment representations in young school-age children: The Manchester Child Attachment Story Task.

Attachment and Human Development, 2(1), 48–70.

Green, R. (1987). *The "sissy boy syndrome" and the development of homosexuality.* New Haven, CT: Yale University Press.

Greenspan, S. I. (1992). *Infancy and early childhood: The practice of clinical assessment and intervention with emotional and developmental challenges.* Madison, CT: International Universities Press.

Greenspan, S. I. (1996). Assessing the emotional and social functioning of infants and young children. In S. J. Meisels & E. Fenichel (Eds.), *New visions for the developmental assessment of infants and young children* (pp. 231–266). Washington, DC: Zero to Three.

Greenspan, S. I. (2004). *Greenspan social-emotional growth chart.* Bulverde, TX: Psychological Corporation.

Greenspan, S. I., DeGangi, G., & Wieder, S. (2001). *The Functional Emotional Assessment Scale (FEAS) for infancy and early childhood, clinical and research applications.* Bethesda, MD: Interdisciplinary Council on Developmental and Learning Disorders.

Greenspan, S. I., & Glovinsky, I. (2002). *Children with bipolar patterns of dysregulation: New perspectives on developmental pathways and a comprehensive approach to prevention and treatment.* Bethesda, MD: Interdisciplinary Council on Developmental and Learning Disorders.

Greenspan, S. I., & Wieder, S. (1998). *The child with special needs: Encouraging intellectual and emotional growth.* Reading, MA: Addison-Wesley.

Greenspan, S. I., & Wieder, S. (2003). Infant and early childhood mental health: A comprehensive developmental approach to assessment and intervention. *Bulletin of Zero to Three: National Center for Infants, Toddlers, and Families, 24,* 6–13.

Greenspan, S. I., & Wieder, S. (2009). *Engaging autism: Using the floortime approach to help children relate, communicate, and think.* Cambridge, MA: Da Capo Lifelong Books.

Greenspan, S. I., Wieder, S., Nover, R. A., Lieberman, A. F., Lourie, R. S., & Robinson, M. E. (1987). *Infants in multirisk families: Case studies in preventive intervention* (Clinical Infant Reports No. 3). Madison, CT: International Universities Press.

Gregory, A. M., Caspi, A., Eley, T. C., Moffit, T. E., O'Connor, T. G., & Poulton, R. (2005). Prospective longitudinal associations between persistent sleep problems in childhood and anxiety and depression disorders in adulthood. *Journal of Abnormal Child Psychology, 33,* 157–163.

Gregory, A. M., & O'Connor, T. G. (2002). Sleep problems in childhood: A longitudinal study of developmental change and association with behavioural problems. *Journal of the American Academy of Child and Adolescent Psychiatry, 41,* 964–971.

Halperin, J. M., Rucklidge, J. J., Powers, R. L., Miller, C. J., & Newcorn, J. H. (2011). Childhood CBCL bipolar profile and adolescent/young adult personality disorders: A 9-year follow-up. *Journal of Affective Disorders, 130,* 155–161.

Hebb, D. (1949). *The organization of behavior.* New York: Wiley.

Hembree, W. C., Cohen-Kettenis, P., Delemarre-van de Waal, H. A., Gooren, L. J., Meyer, W. J., 3rd, Spack, N. P., . . . Montoril V. M. (2009). Endocrine treatment of transsexual persons: An Endocrine Society clinical practice guideline. *Journal of Clinical Endocrinology and Metabolism, 94*(9), 3132–3154.

Hemmi, M. H., Wolke, D., & Schneider, S. (2011). Associations between problems with crying, sleeping and/or feeding in infancy and long-term behavioural outcomes in childhood: A meta-analysis. *Archives of Disease in Childhood, 96,* 622–629.

Hesse, E., & Main, M. (2006). Frightened, threatening, and dissociative parental behavior in low-risk samples: Description, discussion, and interpretations. *Developmental Psychopathology, 18*(2), 309–343.

Hill, P. (2002). Adjustment disorders. In M. Rutter & E. Taylor (Eds.), *Child and adolescent psychiatry* (4th ed.). Oxford, UK: Blackwell.

Hobson, P. (2002). *The cradle of thought: Exploring the origins of thinking.* London: Macmillan.

Hodapp, R. M., & Dykens, E. M. (2012). Genetic disorders of intellectual disability: Expanding our concepts of phenotypes and of family outcomes. *Journal of Genetic Counseling, 21*(6), 761–769.

Hodges, J., Hillman, S., & Steele, M. (2004). *Little Piggy narrative story stem coding manual.* Unpublished manual, Anna Freud Centre, London.

Hodges, J., & Tizard, B. (1989). Social and family relationships of ex-institutional adolescents. *Journal of Child Psychology and Psychiatry, 30,* 77–97.

Hofer, M. A. (1996). On the nature and consequences of early loss. *Psychosomatic Medicine, 58,* 570–581.

Hofer, M. A. (2003). The emerging neurobiology of attachment and separation: How parents shape their infant's brain and behavior. In S. Coates, J. L. Rosenthal, & D. S. Schechter (Eds.), *September 11: Trauma and human bonds.* Hillsdale, NJ: Analytic Press.

Hoffman, K., Marvin, R., Cooper, G., & Powell, B. (2006). Changing toddlers' and preschoolers' attachment classifications: The Circle of Security intervention. *Journal of Consulting and Clinical Psychology, 74,* 1017–1026.

Holliday, R. P., Clem, M. A., Woon, F. L., & Surís, A. M. (2014). Developmental psychological trauma, stress, and revictimization: A review of risk and resilience factors. *Austin Journal of Psychiatry and Behavioral Sciences, 1*(7), 5.

Holtmann, M., Becker, A., Banaschewski, T.,

Rothenberger, A., & Roessner, V. (2011a). Psychometric validity of the Strengths and Difficulties Questionnaire–Dysregulation Profile. *Psychopathology, 44,* 53–59.

Holtmann, M., Buchmann, A. F., Esser, G., Schmidt, M. H., Banaschewski, T., & Laucht, M. (2011b). The Child Behavior Checklist–Dysregulation Profile predicts substance use, suicidality, and functional impairment: A longitudinal analysis. *Journal of Child Psychology and Psychiatry, 52,* 139–147.

Houts, A. C., Berman, J. S., & Abramson, H. (1994). Effectiveness of psychological and pharmacological treatments for nocturnal enuresis. *Journal of Consulting and Clinical Psychology, 62,* 737–745.

Hurry, A. (1998). *Psychoanalysis and developmental therapy.* London: Karnac.

Insel, T. R. (2014). Mental disorders in childhood: Shifting the focus from behavioral symptoms to neurodevelopmental trajectories. *Journal of the American Medical Association, 311*(17), 1727–1728.

Interdisciplinary Council on Developmental and Learning Disorders (ICDL). (2005). *Diagnostic manual for infancy and early childhood.* Bethesda, MD: Author.

Ippen, C. G., Lieberman, A. F., & Osofsky, J. D. (2014). My daddy is a star in the sky: Understanding and treating traumatic grief in early childhood. In P. Cohen, K. M. Sossin, & R. Ruth (Eds.), *Healing after parent loss in childhood and adolescence: Therapeutic interventions and theoretical considerations* (pp. 73–93). Lanham, MD: Rowman & Littlefield.

Joinson, C. J., Heron, J., Butler, U., von Gontard, A., & the Avon Longitudinal Study of Parents and Children Study Team. (2007). Psychological differences between children with and without soiling problems. *Pediatrics, 117,* 1575–1584.

Joinson, C. J., Heron, J., Emond, A., & Butler, R. J. (2007). Psychological problems in children with bedwetting and combined (day and night) wetting: A UK population-based study. *Journal of Pediatric Psychology, 32,* 605–616.

Joinson, C. J., Heron, J., & von Gontard, A. (2006). Psychological problems in children with daytime wetting. *Pediatrics, 118,* 1985–1993.

Juffer, F., Bakersmans-Kranenburg, M. J., & van IJzendoorn, M. H. (2007). *Promoting positive parenting: An attachment-based intervention.* Mahwah, NJ: Erlbaum.

Kagan, J., Reznick, J. S., & Snidman, N. (1988). Biological bases of childhood shyness. *Science, 240,* 167–171.

Kagan, J., & Snidman, N. (1991). Temperamental factors in human development. *American Psychologist, 46*(8), 856–862.

Kay Hall, S. E., & Geher, G. (2003). Behavioral and personality characteristics or children with reactive attachment disorder. *Journal of Psychology: Interdisciplinary and Applied, 137,* 145–162.

Kelly, Y., Kelly, J., & Sacker, A. (2013). Time for bed: Associations with cognitive performance in 7-year-old children: A longitudinal population-based study. *Journal of Epidemiology and Community Health, 67,* 926–931.

Kennedy, E., & Midgley, N. (Eds.). (2007). *Process and outcome research in child, adolescent and parent–infant psychotherapy: A thematic review.* London: North Central London Strategic Health Authority.

Kinnealey, M., & Fuiek, M. (1999). The relationship between sensory defensiveness, anxiety, depression, and perception of pain in adults. *Occupational Therapy International, 6,* 195–206.

Kisiel, C. L., Fehrenbach, T., Torgersen, E., Stolbach, B., McClelland, G., Griffin, G., & Burkman, K. (2014). Constellation of interpersonal trauma and symptoms in child welfare: Implications for a developmental trauma framework. *Journal of Family Violence, 29,* 1–14.

Kisiel, C., Fehrenbach, T., Small, L., & Lyons, J. S. (2009). Assessment of complex trauma exposure, responses, and service needs among children and adolescents in child welfare. *Journal of Child and Adolescent Trauma, 2*(3), 143–160.

Kreppner, J., Kumsta, R., Rutter, M., Beckett, C., Castle, J., Stevens, S., & Sonuga-Barke, E. J. (2010). IV. Developmental course of deprivation-specific psychological patterns: Early manifestations, persistence to age 15, and clinical features. *Monographs of the Society for Research in Child Development, 75*(1), 79–101.

Leibenluft, E., & Rich, B. A. (2008). Pediatric bipolar disorder. *Annual Review of Clinical Psychology, 4*(1), 163–187.

Lester, B. M. (1998). The Maternal Lifestyles Study. *Annals of the New York Academy of Sciences, 846*(1), 296–305.

Lester, B. M., Als, H., & Brazelton, T. B. (1982). Regional obstetric anesthetic and newborn behavior: A reanalysis towards synergistic effects. *Child Development, 53,* 687–692.

Lester, B. M., Tronick, E. Z., & Brazelton, T. B. (2004). The Neonatal Intensive Care Unit Network Neurobehavioral Scale procedures. *Pediatrics, 113,* 641–667.

Leuzinger-Bohleber, M. (2015). *Finding the body in the mind: Psychoanalysis, neurosciences and embodied cognitive science in dialogue.* London: Karnac.

Lewis, M. D., Granic, I., & Lamm, C. (2006). Behavioral differences in aggressive children linked with neural mechanisms of emotion regulation. *Annals of the New York Academy of Sciences, 1094,* 167–177.

Lichtenberg, J. D. (1989). *Psychoanalysis and motivation.* Hillsdale, NJ: Analytic Press.

Lieberman, A. F., Compton, N. C., Van Horn, P., & Ghosh Ippen, C. (2003). *Losing a parent to death in the early years: Guidelines for the treatment of traumatic bereavement in infancy and early childhood.* Washington, DC: Zero to Three Press.

Lieberman, A. F., Silverman, R., & Pawl, J. H. (2000). Infant–parent psychotherapy: Core concepts and current approaches. In C. H. Zeanah (Ed.), *Handbook of infant mental health* (2nd ed., pp. 472–484). New York: Guilford Press.

Lindberg, L., Bohlin, G., Hagekull, B., & Palmerus, K. (1996). Interactions between mothers and infants showing food refusal. *Infant Mental Health Journal, 17,* 334–347.

Lucarelli, L., Cimino, S., D'Olimpio, F., & Ammaniti, M. (2013). Feeding disorders of early childhood: An empirical study of diagnostic subtypes. *International Journal of Eating Disorders, 46,* 147–155.

Lyons-Ruth, K. (1999). The two person unconscious: Intersubjective dialogue, enactive relational representation, and the emergence of new forms of relational organization. *Psychoanalytic Inquiry, 19*(4), 576–617.

Lyons-Ruth, K., Bronfman, E., & Parsons, E. (1999). Maternal frightened, frightening, or atypical behaviour and disorganised infant attachment patterns. *Monographs of the Society for Research in Child Development, 64*(3), 67–69.

Lyons-Ruth, K., Bureau, J. F., Riley, C. D., & Atlas-Corbett, A. F. (2009). Socially indiscriminate attachment behavior in the Strange Situation: Convergent and discriminant validity in relation to caregiving risk, later behavior problems, and attachment insecurity. *Development and Psychopathology, 21*(2), 355–372.

Lyons-Ruth, K., Zeanah, C. H., & Gleason, M. M. (2015). Commentary: Should we move away from an attachment framework for understanding disinhibited social engagement disorder (DSED)?: A commentary on Zeanah and Gleason. *Journal of Child Psychology and Psychiatry, 56,* 223–227.

Maestro, S., Felloni, B., Grassi, C., Intorcia, C., Petrozzi, A., Salsedo, H., & Muratori, F. (2012). Regulatory disorders: A follow-up study. *Minerva Pediatrica, 64*(3), 289–301.

Maestro, S., Rossi, G., Curzio, O., Felloni, B., Grassi, C., Intorcia, C., . . . Muratori, F. (2014). Assessment of mental disorders in preschoolers: The multiaxial profiles of Diagnostic Classification 0–3. *Infant Mental Health Journal, 35*(1), 33–41.

Main, M., & Hesse, E. (1992a). Frightening, frightened behavior in low-risk samples: Description, discussion, and interpretations. *Development and Psychopathology, 18*(2), 309–343.

Main, M., & Hesse, E. (1992b). *Frightening, frightened, dissociated or disorganised behavior on the part of the parent: A coding system for parent–infant interaction.* Unpublished manuscript.

Main, M., & Solomon, J. (1986). Discovery of an insecure-disorganised/disorientated attachment pattern. In T. B. Brazelton & M. W. Yogman (Eds.), *Affective development in infancy* (pp. 95–124). Norwood, NJ: Ablex.

Masten, A. S., & Cicchetti, D. (2010). Developmental cascades: Part 1. *Development and Psychopathology, 22,* 491–495.

McClellan, J., Kowatch, R., Findling, R. L., & Work Group on Quality Issues. (2007). Practice parameter for the assessment and treatment of children and adolescents with bipolar disorder. *Journal of the American Academy of Child and Adolescent Psychiatry, 46*(1), 107–125.

McDonough, S. C., Rosenblum, K., Devoe, E., Gahagan, S., & Sameroff, A. (1998). Parent concerns about infant regulatory problems: Excessive crying, sleep problems, and feeding difficulties. *Infant Behavior and Development, 21,* 565.

McHale, J. P., Kuersten-Hogan, R., & Lauretti, A. (2000). Evaluating coparenting and family-level dynamics during infancy and early childhood: The Coparenting and Family Rating System. In P. Kerig & K. Lindahl (Eds.), *Family observational coding systems: Resources for systemic research.* Hillsdale, NJ: Erlbaum.

Meins, E., & Fernyhough, C. (2010). *Mind–mindedness coding manual, version 2.0.* Unpublished manuscript, Durham University, Durham, UK.

Midgley, N., & Vrouva, I. (Eds.). (2012). *Minding the child: Mentalization-based interventions with children, young people and their families.* London: Routledge.

Mikkelsen, E. J. (2001). Enuresis and encopresis: Ten years of progress. *Journal of the American Academy of Child and Adolescent Psychiatry, 40,* 1146–1158.

Miller, L. J., Anzalone, M. E., Lane, S. J., Cermak, S. A., & Osten, E. T. (2007a). Concept evolution in sensory integration: A proposed nosology for diagnosis. *American Journal of Occupational Therapy, 61*(2), 135–140.

Miller, L. J., Cermak, S., Lane, S., Anzalone, M., & Koomar, J. (2004, Summer). Position statement on terminology related to sensory integration dysfunction. *S.I. Focus,* pp. 6–8.

Miller, L. J., Coll, J. R., & Schoen, S. A. (2007b). A randomized controlled pilot study of the effectiveness of occupational therapy for children with sensory modulation disorder. *American Journal of Occupational Therapy, 61*(2), 228–238.

Miller, L. J., Schoen, S. A., James, K., & Schaaf, R. C. (2007c). Lessons learned: A pilot study on occupational therapy effectiveness for children with sensory modulation disorder. *American Journal of Occupational Therapy, 61*(2), 161–169.

Milrod, B., Busch, F., Cooper, A., & Shapiro, T. (1997). *Manual of panic-focused psychodynamic psychotherapy*. Washington, DC: American Psychiatric Press.

Milrod, B., Leon, A. C., Busch, F., Rudden, M., Schwalberg, M., Clarkin, J., . . . Shear, M. K. (2007). A randomized controlled clinical trial of psychoanalytic psychotherapy for panic disorder. *American Journal of Psychiatry, 164*(2), 265–272.

Milrod, B., Markowitz, J. C., Gerber, A. J., Cyranowski, J., Altemus, M., Shapiro, T., . . . Glatt, C. (2014). Childhood separation anxiety and the pathogenesis and treatment of adult anxiety. *American Journal of Psychiatry, 171*(1), 34–43.

Mitchell, P. B., Loo, C. K., & Gould, B. M. (2010). Diagnosis and monitoring of bipolar disorder in general practice. *Medical Journal of Australia, 193,* 10–13.

Money, J. (1994). The concept of gender identity disorder in childhood and adolescence after 39 years. *Journal of Sex and Marital Therapy, 20,* 163–177.

Moran, G., Bailey, H. N., Gleason, K., DeOliveira, C. A., & Pederson, D. R. (2008). Exploring the mind behind unresolved attachment: Lessons from and for attachment-based interventions with infants and their traumatized mothers. In H. Steele & M. Steele (Eds.), *Clinical applications of the Adult Attachment Interview* (pp. 371–398). New York: Guilford Press.

Mundy, P., Delgado, C., Block, J., Venezia, M., Hogan, A., & Seibert, J. (2003). *A manual for the abridged Early Social Communication Scales.* Coral Gables, FL: University of Miami.

Mundy, P., Gwaltney, M., & Henderson, H. (2010). Self-referenced processing, neurodevelopment and joint attention in autism. *Autism, 14*(5), 408–429.

Murray, L., Cooper, P., Creswell, C., Schofield, E., & Sack, C. (2007). The effects of maternal social phobia on mother–infant interactions and infant social responsiveness. *Journal of Child Psychology and Psychiatry, 48*(1), 45–52.

Murray, L., Stanley, C., Hooper, R., King, F., & Fiori-Cowley, A. (1996). The role of infant factors in post-natal depression and mother–infant interaction. *Developmental Medicine and Child Neurology, 38*(2), 109–119.

National Research Council. (2001). *Educating young children with autism.* Washington, DC: National Academy Press.

National Scientific Council for the Developing Child. Harvard University. Available online at *http://developingchild.harvard.edu/activities/council.*

Neuman, I. D., Wigger, A., Krömer, S., Frank, E., Landgraf, R., & Bosch, O. J. (2005). Differential effects of periodic maternal separation on adult stress coping in a rat model of extremes in trait anxiety. *Neuroscience, 132*(3), 867–877.

Nicol-Harper, R., Harvey, A. G., & Stein, A. (2007). Interactions between mothers and infants: Impact of maternal anxiety. *Infant Behavior and Development, 30*(1), 161–167.

Nugent, J. K., Keefer, C. H., Minear, S., Johnson, L. C., & Blanchard, Y. (2007). *Understanding newborn behavior early relationships. The Newborn Behavioral Observations (NBO) system handbook.* Baltimore: Brookes.

Nugent, J. K., Petruaskas, B., & Brazelton, T. B. (2009). *The infant as a person: Enabling healthy infant development worldwide.* Hoboken, NJ: Wiley.

O'Connor, T. G., Bredenkamp, D., & Rutter, M. (1999). Attachment disturbances and disorders in children exposed to early severe deprivation. *Infant Mental Health Journal, 20,* 10–29.

O'Connor, T. G., & Zeanah, C. H. (2003). Assessment strategies and treatment approaches. *Attachment and Human Development, 5,* 223–244.

Olson, S. L., Bates, J. E., Sandy, J. M., & Schilling, E. M. (2002). Early developmental precursors of impulsive and inattentive behavior: From infancy to middle childhood. *Journal of Child Psychology and Psychiatry, 43,* 435–447.

Ornitz, E. M. (1989). Autism at the interface of sensory processing and information processing. In G. Dawson (Ed.), *Autism: Nature, diagnosis, and treatment* (pp. 174–207). New York: Guilford Press.

Oster, H. (2005). The repertoire of infant face expressions: An ontogenetic perspective. In J. Nadel & D. Muir (Eds.), *Emotional development* (pp. 261–292). Oxford, UK: Oxford University Press.

Out, D., Bakermans-Kranenburg, M. J., & van IJzendoorn, M. H. (2009). The role of disconnected and extremely insensitive parenting in the development of disorganized attachment: Validation of a new measure. *Attachment and Human Development, 11*(5), 419–443.

PDM Task Force. (2006). *Psychodynamic diagnostic manual.* Silver Spring, MD: Alliance of Psychoanalytic Organizations.

Pérez-Robles, R., Doval, E., Jané, M. C., da Silva, P. C., Papoila, A. L., & Virella, D. (2013). The role of sensory modulation deficits and behavioral symptoms in a diagnosis for early childhood. *Child Psychiatry and Human Development, 44*(3), 400–411.

Pfeiffer, B., Kinnealey, M., Reed, C., & Herzberg, G. (2005). Sensory modulation and affective disorders in children and adolescents with Asperger's disorder. *American Journal of Occupational Therapy, 59,* 335–345.

Pine, D. S., Cohen, P., Gurley, D., Brook, J., & Ma, Y. (1998). The risk for early adulthood anxiety and depressive disorders in adolescents with anxiety and depressive disorders. *Archives of General Psychiatry, 55,* 56–64.

Ponizovsky, A. M., Levov, K., Schultz, Y., & Radomislensky, I. (2011). Attachment insecurity and psychological resources associated with adjustment disorders. *American Journal of Orthopsychiatry, 81*(2), 265–276.

Porges, S. W. (1996). Physiological regulation in high-risk infants: A model for assessment and potential intervention. *Developmental Psychopathology, 8,* 43–58.

Putnam, S. P., Gartstein, M. A., & Rothbart, M. K. (2006). Measurement of fine-grained aspects of toddler temperament: The Early Childhood Behavior Questionnaire. *Infant Behavior and Development, 29*(3), 386–401.

Pynoos, R. S., Steinberg, A. M., & Piacentini, J. C. (1999). A developmental psychopathology model of childhood traumatic stress and intersection with anxiety disorders. *Biological Psychiatry, 46,* 1542–1554.

Ramsauer, B., Lotzin, A., Mühlhan, C., Romer, G., Nolte, T., Fonagy, P., & Powell, B. (2014). A randomized controlled trial comparing Circle of Security intervention and treatment as usual as interventions to increase attachment security in infants of mentally ill mothers: Study protocol. *BMC Psychiatry, 14*(1), 24.

Reid, H., & Bahar, R. (2006). Treatment of encopresis and chronic constipation in young children: Clinical results from interactive parent–child guidance. *Clinical Pediatrics, 45,* 157–164.

Renk, K., White, R., Lauer, B. A., McSwiggan, M., Puff, L., & Lowell, A. (2014). Bipolar disorder in children. *Psychiatry Journal, 2014,* 928685.

Rescorla, L. A. (2005). Assessment of young children using the Achenbach System of Empirically Based Assessment (ASEBA). *Mental Retardation and Developmental Disabilities Research Reviews, 11,* 226–237.

Reznick, J. S., Baranek, G. T., Reavis, S., Watson, L. R., & Crais, E. R. (2007). A parent-report instrument for identifying one-year-olds at risk for an eventual diagnosis of autism: The First Year Inventory. *Journal of Autism and Developmental Disorders, 37*(9), 1691–1710.

Rice, T. R., & Hoffman, L. (2014). Defense mechanisms and implicit emotion regulation: A comparison of a psychodynamic construct with one from contemporary neuroscience. *Journal of the American Psychoanalytic Association, 62*(4), 693–708.

Robertson, J. (1970). *Young children in hospital* (Vol. 57). New York: Routledge Kegan & Paul.

Robertson, J., & Bowlby, J. (1952). Responses of young children to separation from their mothers: II. Observations of the sequences of response of children aged 18 to 24 months during the course of separation. *Courrier du Centre International de l'Enfance, 2,* 131–142.

Robles, R. P., Ballabriga, M. C. J., Diéguez, E. D., & da Silva, P. C. (2012). Validating regulatory sensory processing disorders using the Sensory Profile and Child Behavior Checklist (CBCL 1½–5). *Journal of Child and Family Studies, 21*(6), 906–916.

Rogers, S. J., Estes, A., Lord, C., Vismara, L., Winter, J., Fitzpatrick, A., . . . Dawson, G. (2012). Effects of a brief Early Start Denver Model (ESDM)-based parent intervention on toddlers at risk for autism spectrum disorders: A randomized controlled trial. *Journal of the American Academy of Child and Adolescent Psychiatry, 51*(10), 1052–1065.

Rogers, S. J., Hepburn, S. L., & Wehner, E. (2003). Parent reports of sensory symptoms in toddlers with autism and those with other developmental disorders. *Journal of Autism and Developmental Disorders, 33,* 631–642.

Rosen, G. M., Lilienfield, S. O., Frueh, C., McHugh, P., & Spitzer, R. L. (2010). Reflections of PTSD's future in DSM-V. *British Journal of Psychiatry, 197*(5), 343–344.

Rosenbaum, J. F., Biederman, J., Gersten, M., Hirshfeld, D. R., Meminger, S. R., Herman, J. B., . . . Snidman, N. (1988). Behavioral inhibition in children of parents with panic disorder and agoraphobia: A controlled study. *Archives of General Psychiatry, 45*(5), 463–470.

Rothbart, M. K. (1981). Measurement of temperament in infancy. *Child Development, 52,* 569–578.

Rothbart, M. K., Sheese, B. E., Rueda, M. R., & Posner, M. I. (2011). Developing mechanisms of self-regulation in early life. *Emotion Review: Journal of the International Society for Research on Emotion, 3*(2), 207–213.

Roy, P., Rutter, M., & Pickles, A. (2004). Institutional care: Associations between overactivity and lack of selectivity in social relationships. *Journal of Child Psychology and Psychiatry, 45,* 866–873.

Rutter, M. (1981). *Maternal deprivation reassessed.* New York: Penguin Books.

Rutter, M. (1993). Resilience: Some conceptual considerations. *Contemporary Pediatrics, 11,* 36–48.

Rutter, M. (2011a). Integrating science and clinical practice. *Journal of the American Academy of Child and Adolescent Psychiatry, 50*(1), 3–5.

Rutter, M. (2011b). Research review: Child psychiatric diagnosis and classification: Concepts, findings, challenges and potential. *Journal of Child Psychology and Psychiatry, 52*(6), 647–660.

Rutter, M. (2012). Gene–environment interdependence. *European Journal of Developmental Psychology, 9*(4), 391–412.

Rutter, M., Colvert, E., Kreppner, J., Beckett, C., Castle, J., Groothues, C., . . . Sonuga-Barke, E. J. (2007). Early adolescent outcomes for institutionally-deprived and nondeprived adoptees: I. Disinhibited attachment. *Journal of Child Psychology and Psychiatry, 48,* 17–30.

Rutter, M., Kreppner, J., & Sonuga-Barke, E. (2009). Emanuel Miller Lecture: Attachment insecurity, disinhibited attachment, and attachment disorders: Where do research findings leave the concepts? *Journal of Child Psychology and Psychiatry, 50,* 529–543.

Rutter, M., Tizard, J., Yule, W., Graham, P., & Whitmore, K. (1976). Research report: Isle of Wight

Studies, 1964–1974. *Psychological Medicine, 6*(2), 313–332.

Sadler, L. S., Slade, A., Close, N., Webb, D. L., Simpson, T., Fennie, K., & Mayes, L. C. (2013). Minding the Baby: Enhancing reflectiveness to improve early health and relationship outcomes in an interdisciplinary home-visiting program. *Infant Mental Health Journal, 34*(5), 391–405.

Sadler, L. S., Slade, A., & Mayes, L. C. (2006). Minding the Baby: A mentalization-based parenting program. In J. G. Allen & P. Fonagy (Eds.), *Handbook of mentalization-based treatment* (pp. 271–288). Chichester, UK: Wiley.

Sameroff, A. J. (Ed.). (2009). *The transactional model of development: How children and contexts shape each other.* Washington, DC: American Psychological Association.

Sameroff, A. J., & Emde, R. N. (Eds.). (1989). *Relationship disturbances in early childhood: A developmental approach.* New York: Basic Books.

Sameroff, A. J., Lewis, M., & Miller, S. M. (Eds.). (2000). *Handbook of developmental psychopathology* (2nd ed.). New York: Kluwer Academic/Plenum.

Sameroff, A. J., McDonough, S. C., & Rosenblum, K. (Eds.). (2004). *Treating parent–infant relationship problems: Strategies for Intervention.* New York: Guilford Press.

Sandell, A. (2014). From nameless dread to bearable fear: The psychoanalytic treatment of a twenty-two-month-old child. In R. M. Emde & M. Leuzinger-Bohleber (Eds.), *Early parenting and prevention of disorder* (pp. 328–343). London: Karnac.

Sander, L. W. (1962). Issues in early mother–child interaction. *Journal of the American Academy of Child Psychiatry, 1*(1), 141–166.

Sander, L. W. (1987). Awareness of inner experience: A systems perspective on self-regulatory process in early development. *Child Abuse and Neglect, 11*(3), 339–346.

Sander, L. W. (1988). The event-structure of regulation in the neonate–caregiver system as a biological background of early organization of psychic structure. In A. Goldberg (Ed.), *Progress in self psychology: Vol. 3. Frontiers in self psychology* (pp. 64–77). Hillsdale, NJ: Analytic Press.

Saunders, B. E. (2003). Understanding children exposed to violence: Toward an integration of overlapping fields. *Journal of Interpersonal Violence, 18*(4), 356–376.

Schechter, D. S., & Rusconi Serpa, S. (2014). Understanding how traumatized mothers process their toddlers' affective communication under stress. In R. M. Emdc & M. Leuzinger-Bohleber (Eds.), *Early parenting and prevention of disorder* (pp. 90–118). London: Karnac.

Scheeringa, M. S., Zeanah, C. H., & Cohen, J. A. (2011). PTSD in children and adolescent: Toward an empirically based algorithm. *Depression and Anxiety, 28,* 770–782.

Schore, A. N. (1994). *Affect regulation and the origins of the self.* Hillsdale, NJ: Erlbaum.

Schore, A. N. (2001). The effects of early relational trauma on right brain development, affect regulation, and infant mental health. *Infant Mental Health Journal, 22*(1–2), 201–269.

Schore, J. R., & Schore, A. N. (2007). Modern attachment theory: The central role of affect regulation in development and treatment. *Clinical Social Work Journal, 36,* 9–20.

Schwartz, E., & Davis, A. S. (2006). Reactive attachment disorder: Implications for school readiness and school functioning. *Psychology in the Schools, 43,* 471–479.

Seifer, R., Dickstein, S., Sameroff, A. J., Hayden, L., Magee, K., & Schiller, M. (1994). Sleep in toddlers whose parents have psychopathology. *Sleep Research, 23,* 145.

Shrout, P. E., & Bolger, N. (2002). Mediation in experimental and nonexperimental studies: New procedures and recommendations. *Psychological Methods, 7,* 422–445.

Silver, G., Shapiro, T., & Milrod, B. (2013). Treatment of anxiety in children and adolescents: Using child and adolescent anxiety psychodynamic psychotherapy. *Child and Adolescent Psychiatric Clinics of North America, 22*(1), 83–96.

Slade, A., Aber, J. L., Bresgi, I., Berger, B., & Kaplan, N. (2004a). *The Parent Development Interview* (rev.). Unpublished manuscript, City University of New York.

Slade, A., Bernbach, E., Grienenberger, J., Levy, D., & Locker, A. (2004b). *Addendum to Fonagy, Target, Steele, and Steele reflective functioning scoring manual for use with the Parent Development Interview.* Unpublished manuscript, City University of New York.

Slep, A. M. S., & Tamminen, T. (2013). Caregiver–child relational problems: Definitions and implications for diagnosis. In H. M. Foran, S. R. H. Beach, A. M. S. Slep, R. E. Heyman, & M. Z. Wamboldt (Eds.), *Family problems and family violence: Reliable assessment and the ICD-11* (pp. 185–196). New York: Springer.

Smyke, A. T., Dumitrescu, A., & Zeanah, C. H. (2002). Disturbances of attachment in young children: I. The continuum of caretaking casualty. *Journal of the American Academy of Child and Adolescent Psychiatry, 41,* 972–982.

Smyke, A. T., Zeanah, C. H., Gleason, M. M., Drury, S. S., Fox, N. A., & Guthrie, D. (2012). A randomized controlled trial comparing foster care and institutional care for children with signs of reactive attachment disorder. *American Journal of Psychiatry, 169,* 508–514.

Spanier, G. (1976). Measuring dyadic adjustment: New scales for assessing the quality of marriage and similar dyads. *Journal of Marriage and the Family, 38,* 15–38.

Spinazzola, J., Ford, J. D., Zucker, M., van der Kolk, B. A., Silva, S., & Smith, S. F. (2005). Survey evaluates complex trauma exposure, outcome, and intervention among children and adolescents. *Psychiatric Annals, 35*(5), 433–439.

Spitz, R. A. (1961). Some early prototypes of ego defenses. *Journal of the American Psychoanalytic Association, 9,* 626–651.

Spitz, R. A. (1965). *The first year of life: A psychoanalytic study of normal and deviant development of object relations.* New York: International Universities Press.

Spitzer, R. L., Endicott, J. E., & Robins, E. (1978). Research Diagnostic Criteria. *Archives of General Psychiatry, 35,* 773–782.

Squires, J., Bricker, D., Heo, K., & Twombly, E. (2001). Identification of social-emotional problems in young children using a parent-completed screening measure. *Early Childhood Research Quarterly, 16*(4), 405–419.

Squires, J., Bricker, D., & Twombly, E. (2002). *Ages and Stages Questionnaires Social-Emotional.* Baltimore: Brookes.

Sroufe, L. A. (1997). *Emotional development: The organization of emotional life in the early years.* New York: Cambridge University Press.

St. James-Roberts, I., & Halil, T. (1991). Infant crying patterns in the first year: Normal community and clinical findings. *Journal of Child Psychology and Psychiatry, 32,* 951–968.

Stagnitti, K., Raison, P., & Ryan, P. (1999). Sensory defensiveness syndrome: A pediatric perspective and case study. *Australian Occupational Therapy Journal, 46,* 175–187.

Steensma, T. D., McGuire, J. K., Kreukels, B. P., Beekman, A. J., & Cohen-Kettenis, P. T. (2013). Factors associated with desistence and persistence of childhood gender dysphoria: A quantitative follow-up study. *Journal of American Academy Child and Adolescent Psychiatry, 52*(6), 582–590.

Stein, S. M. (1998). Enuresis, early attachment and intimacy. *British Journal of Psychotherapy, 15,* 167–176.

Stephens, C. L., & Royeen, C. B. (1998). Investigation of tactile defensiveness and self-esteem in typically developing children. *Occupational Therapy International, 5*(4), 273–280.

Stern, D. N. (1985). *The interpersonal world of the infant.* New York: Basic Books.

Stern, D. N. (1995). *The motherhood constellation.* London: Karnac.

Stoller, R. J. (1964). A contribution to the study of gender identity. *International Journal of Psycho-Analysis, 45,* 220–226.

Tikotzky, L., & Sadeh, A. (2009). Maternal sleep-related cognitions and infant sleep: A longitudinal study from pregnancy through the 1st year. *Child Development, 80,* 860–874.

Tizard, B., & Hodges, J. (1978). The effect of early institutional rearing on the development of eight year old children. *Journal of Child Psychology and Psychiatry, 19*(2), 99–118.

Tizard, B., & Rees, J. (1975). The effect of early institutional rearing on the behaviour problems and affectional relationships of four-year-old children. *Journal of Child Psychology and Psychiatry, 16,* 61–73.

Trevarthen, C. (1993). The function of emotions in early infant communication and development. In J. Nadel & L. Camaioni (Eds.), *New perspectives in early communicative development* (pp. 8–81). London: Routledge.

Trevarthen, C. (2010). What is it like to be a person who knows nothing?: Defining the active intersubjective mind of a newborn human being. *Infant and Child Development, 20,* 119–135.

Tronick, E. (1989). Emotions and emotional communication in infants. *American Psychologist, 44*(2), 112–119.

Tronick, E. (2007). *The neurobehavioral and social emotional development of infants and children.* New York: Norton.

Tronick, E., & Beeghly, M. (2011). Infants' meaning-making and the development of mental health problems. *American Psychologist, 66*(2), 107–119.

Tronick, E., & Reck, C. (2009). Infants of depressed mothers. *Harvard Review of Psychiatry, 17*(2), 147–156.

van der Kolk, B. A. (2005). Developmental trauma disorder: Toward a rational diagnosis for children with complex trauma histories. *Psychiatric Annals, 35*(5), 401–408.

van der Kolk, B. A., Roth, S., Pelcovitz, D., Sunday, S., & Spinazzola, J. (2005). Disorders of extreme stress: The empirical foundation of a complex adaptation to trauma. *Journal of Traumatic Stress, 18*(5), 389–399.

Van Meter, A. R., Moreira, A. L. R., & Youngstrom, E. A. (2011). Meta-analysis of epidemiologic studies of pediatric bipolar disorder. *Journal of Clinical Psychiatry, 71*(9), 1250–1256.

Vasey, M. W., & Ollendick, T. H. (2000). Anxiety. In A. J. Sameroff, M. Lewis, & S. M. Miller (Eds.), *Handbook of developmental psychopathology* (2nd ed.). New York: Kluwer Academic/Plenum.

Vaughn, B. E., & Waters, E. (1990). Attachment behavior at home and in the laboratory: Q-sort observations and strange situation classifications of one-year-olds. *Child Development, 61,* 1965–1973.

Volkmar, F. R. (2014). Editorial: The importance of

early intervention. *Journal of Autism and Developmental Disorders, 44*(12), 2979–2980.

Volkmar, F. R., & McPartland, J. C. (2014). From Kanner to DSM-5: Autism as an evolving diagnostic concept. *Annual Review of Clinical Psychology, 10,* 193–212.

Volkmar, F. R., Reichow, B., & Doehring, P. (2011). Evidence-based practices in autism: Where we are now and where we need to go. In B. Reichow, P. Doehring, D. V. Cicchetti, & F. R. Volkmar (Eds.), *Evidence-based practices and treatments for children with autism* (pp. 365–391). New York: Springer.

Volkmar, F. R., Reichow, B., & McPartland, J. (2012). Classification of autism and related conditions: Progress, challenges, and opportunities. *Dialogues in Clinical Neuroscience, 14*(3), 229–237.

Volkmar, F. R., & Wiesner, L. A. (2009). *A practical guide to autism: What every parent, family member, and teacher needs to know.* Hoboken, NJ: Wiley.

Voos, A. C., Pelphrey, K. A., Tirrell, J., Bolling, D. Z., Vander Wyk, B., Kaiser, M. D., . . . Ventola, P. (2013). Neural mechanisms of improvements in social motivation after pivotal response treatment: Two case studies. *Journal of Autism and Developmental Disorders, 43*(1), 1–10.

Warren, S. L., Howe, G., Simmens, S. J., & Dahl, R. E. (2006). Maternal depressive symptoms and child sleep: Models of mutual influence over time. *Development and Psychopathology, 18,* 1–16.

Warren, S. L., Huston, L., Egeland, B., & Sroufe, L. A. (1997). Child and adolescent anxiety disorders and early attachment. *Journal of the American Academy of Child and Adolescent Psychiatry, 36*(5), 637–644.

Warren, S. L., & Sroufe, L. A. (2004). Developmental issues. In T. H. Ollendick & J. S. March (Eds.), *Phobic and anxiety disorders in children and adolescents: A clinician's guide to effective psychosocial and pharmacological interventions* (pp. 92–115). New York: Oxford University Press.

Waters, E., & Deane, K. (1985). Defining and assessing individual differences in attachment relationships: Q-methodology and the organization of behavior in infancy and early childhood. In I. Bretherton & E. Waters (Eds.), Growing points of attachment theory and research. *Monographs of the Society for Research in Child Development, 50*(1–2, Serial No. 209), 41–65.

Weinstein, L., & Ellman, S. J. (2012). It's only a dream: Physiological and developmental contributions to the feeling of reality. In P. Fonagy, H. Kächele, M. Leuzinger-Bohleber, & D. Taylor (Eds.), *The significance of dreams* (pp. 126–147). London: Karnac.

Williamson, G. G., & Anzalone, M. (1997). Sensory integration: A key component of the evaluation and treatment of young children with severe difficulties in relating and communicating. *Zero to Three, 17,* 29–36.

Winnicott, D. (1973). *The child, the family, and the outside world.* London: Penguin.

Wolke, D., Gray, P., & Meyer, R. (1994). Excessive infant crying: A controlled study of mothers helping mothers. *Pediatrics, 94,* 322–332.

Woods, M. Z., & Pretorius, I. (2011). *Parents and toddlers in groups: A psychoanalytic developmental approach.* New York: Routledge.

World Health Organization. (1992). *The ICD-10 classification of mental and behavioral disorders: Clinical descriptions and diagnostic guidelines.* Geneva: Author.

World Health Organization. (1994). *Diagnostic criteria for research* (10th ed.). Geneva: Author.

Zeanah, C. H., Benoit, D., Hirshberg, L., Barton, M. L., & Regan, C. (1994). Mothers' representations of their infants are concordant with infant attachment classifications. *Developmental Issues in Psychiatry and Psychology, 1,* 1–14.

Zeanah, C. H., Berlin, L. J., & Boris, N. W. (2011). Practitioner review: Clinical applications of attachment theory and research for infants and young children. *Journal of Child Psychology and Psychiatry, 52,* 819–833.

Zeanah, C. H., Boris, N. W., & Lieberman, A. F. (2000a). Attachment disorders of infancy. In A. J. Sameroff, M. Lewis, & S. M. Miller (Eds.), *Handbook of developmental psychopathology* (2nd ed., pp. 293–307). New York: Kluwer Academic/Plenum.

Zeanah, C. H., & Gleason, M. M. (2015). Annual research review: Attachment disorders in early childhood—clinical presentation, causes, correlates, and treatment. *Journal of Child Psychology and Psychiatry, 56,* 207–222.

Zeanah, C. H., Larrieu, J. A., Heller, S. S., & Valliere, J. (2000b). Infant–parent relationship assessment. In C. H. Zeanah (Ed.), *Handbook of infant mental health* (2nd ed., pp. 222–235). New York: Guilford Press.

Zeanah, C. H., Mammen, O., & Lieberman, A. (1993). Disorders of attachment. In C. Zeanah (Ed.), *Handbook of infant mental health* (pp. 332–349). New York: Guilford Press.

Zeanah, C. H., Nelson, C. A., Fox, N. A., Smyke, A. T., Marshall, P., Parker, S. W., & Koga, S. (2003). Designing research to study the effects of institutionalization on brain and behavioral development: The Bucharest Early Intervention Project. *Development and Psychopathology, 15,* 885–907.

Zeanah, C. H., & Smyke, A. T. (2015). Disorders of attachment and social engagement related to deprivation. In A. Thapar, D. Pine, J. F. Leckman, S. Scott, M. J. Snowling, & E. Taylor (Eds.), *Rutter's child and adolescent psychiatry* (6th ed., pp. 795–805). Chichester, UK: Wiley-Blackwell.

Zeanah, C. H., Smyke, A. T., & Dumitrescu, A.

(2002). Disturbances of attachment in young children: II. Indiscriminate behavior and institutional care. *Journal of the American Academy of Child and Adolescent Psychiatry, 41,* 983–989.

Zeanah, C. H., Smyke, A. T., Koga, S., Carlson, E., & the BEIP Core Group. (2005). Attachment in institutionalized and community children in Romania. *Child Development, 76,* 1015–1028.

Zero to Three. (1994). *Diagnostic classification of mental health and developmental disorders of infancy and early childhood.* Washington, DC: Author.

Zero to Three. (2005). *Diagnostic classification of mental health and developmental disorders of infancy and early childhood* (rev. ed.). Washington, DC: Author.

Zero to Three. (2016). DC: 0–5™. *Diagnostic classification of mental health and developmental disorders of infancy and early childhood.* Washington, DC: Author.

Zucker, K. J. (2010). The DSM diagnostic criteria for gender identity disorder in children. *Archives of Sexual Behavior, 39*(2), 477–498.

Zucker, K. J., Cohen-Kettenis, P. T., Drescher, J., Meyer-Bahlburg, H. F. L., Pfäfflin, F., & Womack, W. M. (2013). Memo outlining evidence for change for gender identity disorder in the DSM-5. *Archives of Sexual Behavior, 42,* 901–914.

Zucker, K. J., Wood, H., Singh, D., & Bradley, S. J. (2012). A developmental, biopsychosocial model for the treatment of children with gender identity disorder. *Journal of Homosexuality, 59*(3), 369–397.

PART V
Later Life

CHAPTER 11

Introduction to Part V

CHAPTER EDITORS

Franco Del Corno, MPhyl, DPsych **Daniel Plotkin, MD**

In Part V of PDM-2, we consider older adults. This is the first time a separate section on the elderly has been included in any major diagnostic manual or system (PDM, DSM, or ICD). The first edition of PDM contained only brief mentions of older adults, and when this was brought to the attention of the manual and chapter editors, it resulted in an invitation to develop a section on later life in PDM-2. This anecdote illuminates an important aspect of any endeavor involving older adults in our societies. Almost everyone, including the authors and editors of the first PDM (and many of them were over age 70 at the time, which says something about denial of aging as a general problem), is vulnerable to the powerful biases our youth-oriented societies harbor toward aging and old age. Indeed, in some ways, little has changed since Robert Butler coined the term "ageism" in 1969 or since the 1975 publication of his Pulitzer Prize–winning book, *Why Survive?: Being Old in America.*

What sets Part V of PDM-2 apart, then, is that it, perhaps more than any other section of the manual, involves attitudes. The prevailing attitude in most societies is that older adults are rigid and incapable of change. A special issue of the journal *Science* ("The Aging Brain," October 31, 2014) has suggested otherwise. Another prevalent negative assumption about the elderly is either that they do not have a psychodynamic dimension, or that if they do, it is not relevant. Again, clinical experience suggests otherwise. Thus it is anticipated that this new PDM-2 section will be a template—a work in progress that sheds light on the emotional and psychological aspects of mental conditions in older adults, and that helps to improve attitudes toward them. Although it cannot be the final word, it can serve as a basis and inspiration for future endeavors.

The chapters in this section of the manual build on the basic PDM-2 formulation of multiple axes, to address directly how individuals experience illness in the context of aging minds and brains, as well as in the context of daily life, social networks, cultural expectations, and general societal considerations. Thus we retain the PDM-2 framework of M, P, and S Axes, with modifications for older adults. Specifically, the next three chapters are as follows:

Chapter 12. Profile of Mental Functioning for the Elderly—ME Axis
Chapter 13. Personality Patterns and Syndromes in the Elderly—PE Axis
Chapter 14. Symptom Patterns in the Elderly: The Subjective Experience—SE Axis

It should be noted that certain dimensions were considered for additional axes or subaxes in this section (e.g., cognitive status and level of engagement), but ultimately it was decided to include these aspects in relevant sections of existing axes, rather than to add further complexity to an already complex system. Since PDM-2 seeks to strengthen its connections to DSM-5 and ICD-10, explicit discussions of those diagnostic systems are included whenever they are relevant.

PDM-2 also seeks to include empirical research that informs more operationalized descriptions of the various disorders. Unfortunately, there is a paucity of empirical research on older adults in general, and specifically on psychodynamic aspects of aging. For example, the psychodynamically oriented personality measures such as the Inventory of Personality Organization (IPO), the Structured Interview of Personality Organization (STIPO), and the Karolinska Psychodynamic Profile (KAPP) have not been studied in older age groups. This is due, in part at least, to an unfortunate cycle in which older adults have often been excluded from clinical research studies. Thus we ask readers to indulge us as we present a necessarily incomplete section.

Still, there is an evidence base to support some basic observations:

1. *Heterogeneity.* A literature review on research in aging must begin with recognition that one of the most robust findings is heterogeneity: There is tremendous variability associated with aging. Indeed, some older adults function well as heads of state, while others cannot recognize their own family members or even get out of bed. It should also be noted that the DSM and ICD descriptive approach to diagnosis results in heterogeneous and overlapping diagnostic categories. Indeed, such issues are often cited as a reason why pharmaceutical companies have largely withdrawn from drug development for mental disorders. To provide an alternative framework for research into psychiatric disorders, the U.S. National Institute of Mental Health has recently introduced its Research Domain Criteria (RDoC) project. In the RDoC, each of five domains reflects a brain system in which functioning is impaired, to different degrees, in different psychiatric conditions. The domains are as follows: cognitive systems, systems for social processes, arousal/regulatory systems, negative valence systems, and positive valence systems. The RDoC focuses on neural circuits and uses a dimensional approach rather than the categorical approach of DSM/ICD. It is anticipated that RDoC categorizations will better reflect underlying molecular, genetic, and physiological mechanisms of disorders than do the current descriptive DSM/ICD systems (Casey et al., 2013).

2. *Classification of older adults.* While there is no biological or psychological parameter that defines "old," it has been generally accepted that old age begins at 65

years. For clinical purposes, an accepted cutoff has been even younger, 55 years of age. Indeed, a recent epidemiological study of mental disorders in older adults in the United States (Reynolds, Pietrzak, El-Gabalawy, Mackenzie, & Sareen, 2015) divided the elderly into four groups: "young-old" (55–64 years of age), "middle-old" (65–74 years of age), "old-old" (75–84 years of age), and "oldest-old" (85 years of age and older).

3. *Aging as positive.* Contrary to popular belief, aging is in general associated with positive emotional and mental health benefits, including increased life satisfaction and increased capacity to find meaning in life.

4. *Chronicity and comorbidity.* Aging is associated with chronicity and with comorbidity. That is, medical and emotional conditions tend to be chronic and to coexist and interact in complex ways.

5. *Change is possible.* Neuroscience research has identified the concept of neuroplasticity, finding that brain (and presumably mind) change is possible, even in old age. These data have has obvious implications for hope and possibilities for older adults.

6. *Cultural views and attitudes.* As suggested earlier, cultural views and attitudes on aging are important considerations in any effort to design a classification of mental health conditions, especially one that focuses on a psychodynamic dimension. In general, the older population is becoming increasingly diverse. Ethnic/racial factors have been shown to play roles in physiological/medical dimensions such as blood pressure and sleep, as well as in attitudes and expectations about aging, dependency, and living arrangements. Ethnic groups differ in decision-making processes, disclosure of personal information, and end-of-life care. From an international perspective, there is a wide divergence in people's confidence that they will have an adequate standard of living in their old age (Wickrama, Mancini, Kwag, & Kwon, 2013). Confidence in one's eventual standard of living appears to be related to the rate at which a country is aging and to its economic vitality.

With the aging of modern societies and further advances in health care delivery (Wang & Nussbaum, 2017), it is anticipated that there will be a gradual shift toward more capability and functionality on the part of older adults, making our efforts in Part V of PDM-2 even more relevant and important.

BIBLIOGRAPHY

Arai, H., Ouchi, Y., Yokode, M., Ito, H., Uematsu, H., Eto, F., . . . Kita, T. (2012). Members of Subcommittee for Aging. Toward the realization of a better aged society: Messages from gerontology and geriatrics. *Geriatrics and Gerontology International, 12*(1), 16–22.

Butler, R. N. (1969). Age-ism: Another form of bigotry. *The Gerontologist, 9*(4, Pt. 1), 243–246.

Butler, R. N. (1975). *Why survive?: Being old in America.* New York: Harper & Row.

Casey, B. J., Craddock, N., Cuthbert, B. N., Hyman, S. E., Lee, F. S., & Ressler, K. J. (2013). DSM-5 and RDoC: Progress in psychiatry research? *Nature Reviews Neuroscience, 14*(11), 810–814.

Erikson, E. H., Erikson, J. M., & Kivnick, H. Q. (1994). *Vital involvement in old age.* New York: Norton.

Institute of Medicine. (2015). *Cognitive aging: Progress in understanding and opportunities for action.* Washington, DC: National Academies Press.

Mungas, D., Beckett, L., Harvey, D., Farias, S. T., Reed, B., Carmichael, O., . . . DeCarli, C. (2010). Heterogeneity of cognitive trajectories in diverse older persons. *Psychology and Aging, 25*(3), 606–619.

Pew Research Center. (2014). Attitudes about aging: A global perspective. Retrieved from *www.pewglobal.org/2014/01/30/attitudes-about-aging-a-global-perspective.*

Reynolds, K., Pietrzak, R. H., El-Gabalawy, R., Mackenzie, C. S., & Sareen, J. (2015). Prevalence of psychiatric disorders in U.S. older adults: Findings from a nationally representative survey. *World Psychiatry, 14*(1), 74–81.

Silverstein, M., & Heap, J. (2015). Sense of coherence changes with aging over the second half of life. *Advances in Life Course Research, 23*, 98–107.

Wang, S., & Nussbaum, A. M. (2017). *DSM-5 pocket guide for elder mental health.* Arlington, VA: American Psychiatric Association Publishing.

Wickrama, K. K., Mancini, J. A., Kwag, K., & Kwon, J. (2013). Heterogeneity in multidimensional health trajectories of late old years and socioeconomic stratification: A latent trajectory class analysis. *Journals of Gerontology: Series B. Psychological Sciences and Social Sciences, 68*(2), 290–297.

CHAPTER 12

Profile of Mental Functioning for the Elderly

ME Axis

CHAPTER EDITORS

Franco Del Corno, MPhyl, DPsych **Daniel Plotkin, MD**

CONSULTANTS

Emanuela Brusadelli, PhD Giuseppe Cafforio, DPsych Alessia Zoppi, PhD

Introduction

There is a general tendency in the literature to delineate a psychological and physical process of development called "typical (normal) aging," which involves a gradual decline of psychophysical and social capabilities, according to a cumulative process of age-specific involution (Allen, Morris, Stark, Fortin, & Stark, 2015; Moran, 2013; Palmore, 1974).

At the same time, many authors have also pointed out that in normal aging, this process of decline is compensated for by several different possible processes of enrichment, integration, and completion of identity and autobiographical narrative. These processes can enable an elderly person to take on the role of "wise old man/woman" (the positive polarity of the archetypical "Senex," according to Jungian psychology, as well as a classic literary figure). So when we talk about the natural development of "senile personality" in the elderly, we must think not only about the decrease in psychophysical resources, with the related changes of behavior, emotions, and attitudes, but also about the emergence of a new way of life, with new habits, new roles (e.g., the grandpa, the grandma, the expert, the wise man/woman), and new relationships. This emergence is best expressed by the concept of "successful aging" (Rowe &

Kahn, 1987, 1997), which is achieved through a set of experiences that protect elderly individuals against melancholy, anxiety, and social isolation, so common in old age. Moreover, the subject of death may be faced in different ways by the elderly, depending on whether a person has attained a healthy self-integration or, conversely, has a terrifying sense of dispersion and loss of hope. The ability to use old skills with new functions can be a sign of the ego's integrative capacity, like the capacity to reorganize the old relationships in more useful ways, according to the needs at the moment (e.g., asking for help from children). In general, it is absolutely normal for the elderly to change their behaviors, with gradual modifications of the ways they experience and manifest emotions, social interests, and cognitive abilities. In fact, although the elderly lose some roles and opportunities for interaction and influence in some macro-level contexts, in parallel they may acquire new roles and identities in micro-level social contexts and within their families. An older relative may become the "memory" of a family or community group and the bearer of wisdom and knowledge—conveying a sense of continuity, coherence, and integration, as well as the awareness of having been the protagonist of a story in which his or her true self was built amid the multiplicity of possible selves. This story can be made available to others, with the awareness that the elder has completed his or her life and doesn't necessarily look to the future with longing or with expectations of change. Consequently, old people may have a meditative and spiritual sense of life that opens them up to a different level of knowledge about themselves and the world.

The assessment of mental functioning in persons over 70 years old requires attention to an intricate interplay of biological, psychological, and social factors. Moreover, although aging does not necessarily involve the presence of illness, the likelihood of falling ill is greater than in other periods of life. It is particularly important to keep in mind that "patients experiencing major medical illnesses may have reduced capacity for symbolic thought due to the physical demands of their illness and stress associated with mortality" (McClintock Greenberg, 2009, p. 37). This aspect is reinforced, of course, by the need for continual medical treatments.

Physical illness in old age is addressed in different ways than in previous stages of life, when falling ill is a more or less fortuitous event against which an individual attempts to react. In older adults, every disease may be seen as something substantially inherent in the aging process; the most common attitude is resignation, in a very similar way to what happens with regard to death, which may be imagined as relatively close.

Another aspect that a clinician should consider in the evaluation of an elderly individual's mental functioning is the balance between mental abilities and demands/requests of the environment. This means that the individual's life context must be taken into account: An old person who lives in a nursing home needs different skills from those required by one who still lives in his or her own home, for example.

The literature indicates that the quality and quantity of environmental stimuli produce differences in brain aging, which involve modifications in functions and mental abilities (Churchill et al., 2002; Fratiglioni, Paillard-Borg, & Winblad, 2004). In other words, a properly stimulating environment can contribute to the maintenance—and sometimes to the improvement—of mental functioning; conversely, a poorly stimulating one can produce possible decline.

Yet another factor in evaluating the elderly is the possible presence of neurocognitive disorders, which involve the presence of a cognitive impairment in one or more domains, according to the *Diagnostic and Statistical Manual of Mental Disorders*, fifth edition (DSM-5; American Psychiatric Association, 2013). An individual with a neurocognitive disorder may be unable to adequately understand events related to him- or herself, as well as to react properly to stimuli. This diagnosis is particularly important in old age because every neurocognitive disorder is in fact a global and pervasive illness (at various levels of impairment), with the capacity to affect emotions and behaviors more or less deeply.

Brain aging and the state of mental functions in older adults are determined both by genetic factors (species-specific and individual) (Caleb, Finch, & Tanzi, 1997; Rodríguez-Rodero et al., 2011) and by past and present environmental conditions (Ryff & Singer, 2005). However, clinicians must remember that "brain is not mind. The physical organ of the brain is not the same as one's mind . . . a person's mind may remain sharp although the speed with which his or her brain functions may decline" (Ilardo, 1998, p. 10).

It is important to mention in this connection the construct of "cognitive aging," proposed in a recent report by the Institute of Medicine (2015) of the U.S. National Academies of Sciences. As noted in the report, cognitive aging is inherent in humans and other animals, and it occurs across the spectrum of elderly individuals, regardless of their initial levels of cognitive functioning. Such functioning in older adults can improve in some areas (such as those related to wisdom and experience) and decline in other areas (such as memory, attention, and speed of processing). In other words, cognitive aging is a lifelong process of gradual, ongoing, yet highly variable changes in cognitive functions that occur as people get older; it is not a disease or a quantifiable level of functioning because its ramifications for internal mental processes in older adults are yet well known or characterized.

To summarize, the assessment of mental functioning in the elderly requires a differential diagnosis of the following:

- Optimal mental abilities, preserved despite aging.
- Mental abilities impaired by aging.
- Impaired or low-level mental abilities that are aspects of the individual's developmental history, and on which aging has not exercised a special influence.

Furthermore, aging itself is a potential stressor (Cesari, Vellas, & Gambassi, 2013) to which an individual can respond either optimally, preserving his or her own capacities to the extent possible, or with a further deterioration of mental functioning (e.g., if confronted by any other stressful situation). According to some authors (Cohen-Sachs, 2006; Desjardins & Warnke, 2012), the capacity to face this kind of stress is strengthened by a significant investment in an urge toward self-realization, which is pursued throughout the life course and helps to assign a sense of meaning and purpose to the physical and emotional difficulties that frequently occur in the last years of life. (The discussion of the capacity for meaning and purpose, toward the end of this chapter, is particularly relevant here.)

In other words, the normal age-related decline is a highly stressful experience for some individuals, but less so for others. Of course, this consideration can be applied also to personality functioning, as discussed in Chapter 13 on the PE Axis.

In the remainder of this chapter, we describe the 12 categories of basic mental functions delineated in Chapter 2 on the M Axis as they apply to older adults. The goal is to encourage clinicians to use these categories as a means of capturing the richness and individuality of older patients, without neglecting to consider the presence of any difficulties and impairments. Although no profile can hope to capture the full panoply of an elderly person's mental life, the 12 ME-Axis categories highlight a number of crucial areas.

As in the other M-Axis chapters, we have also introduced an assessment procedure called the Summary of Basic Mental Functioning (see Table 12.1, pp. 770–771) for the ME Axis, whereby a clinician can indicate on a 5-point scale the level at which each mental function is articulated. Descriptors of key characteristics at levels of functioning 5, 3, and 1 are provided in the chapter text for *each* mental function.

Neuropsychological Tests for General Use with the Elderly

The following neuropsychological tests are helpful in assessing general cognition and other areas of neuropsychological functioning in elderly persons. The tests listed in the discussion of capacity 1, below, are useful in assessing specific areas.

Mini-Mental State Examination

The purpose of the Mini-Mental State Examination (MMSE; Folstein, Folstein, & McHugh, 1975) is to screen briefly for potential mental impairment, particularly in the elderly. The test consists of items that assess orientation to time and place, attention/concentration, language, constructional ability, and immediate and delayed recall. The MMSE can be administered in 5–10 minutes.

Alzheimer's Disease Assessment Scale

The Alzheimer's Disease Assessment Scale (ADAS; Rosen, Mohs, & Davis, 1984) was developed specifically to assess the severity of cognitive and noncognitive behavioral dysfunctions typical of persons with Alzheimer's disease. The scale consists of 11 cognitive items (ADAS-Cog) and 10 noncognitive items (ADAS-Non-Cog), which can be used separately. ADAS-Cog includes performance-based short neuropsychological tests; ADAS-Non-Cog includes observation-based behavioral rating items.

Cambridge Mental Disorders of the Elderly Examination

The standard form of the Cambridge Mental Disorders of the Elderly Examination (CAMDEX; Roth et al., 1986) includes 340 items; the short form (Revised, or CAMDEX-R; Roth, Huppert, Mountjoy, & Tym, 1998) includes 67 items. The time required for administration is approximately 60–90 minutes for the standard form or 20–40 minutes for the short form.

Frontal Assessment Battery

The Frontal Assessment Battery (FAB; Dubois, Slachevsky, Litvan, & Pillon, 2000) is a short cognitive and behavioral six-subtest battery for a bedside mental status examination (which is particularly useful in cases of frontal and subcortical dementia). The time required is approximately 10 minutes.

Dementia Rating Scale

The Dementia Rating Scale (DRS; Mattis, 1988) provides an index of cognitive functioning in individuals with known or suspected dementia. The global measure of dementia is derived from subscores for specific cognitive capacities: attention; initiation and perseveration; construction; conceptualization; and verbal and nonverbal short-term memory. The time required is approximately 10–15 minutes for normal elderly persons or 30–45 minutes for patients with dementia.

MicroCog: Assessment of Cognitive Functioning

The MicroCog (Powell, Kaplan, Whitla, Catlin, & Funkenstein, 1993) is a computer-administered and computer-scored test to screen for mental impairment in individuals ages 18–89 years. The standard form consists of 18 subtests; the short form contains 12 of these subtests, organized into five domains (attention/mental control, memory, reasoning/calculation, spatial processing, and reaction times). The MicroCog is essentially self-administered. The standard form can be administered in 60 minutes; the short form requires about 30 minutes.

Montreal Cognitive Assessment

The Montreal Cognitive Assessment (MoCA; Nasreddine et al., 2005) was designed as a rapid screening instrument for mild cognitive dysfunction. It assesses different cognitive domains: attention/concentration, executive functions, memory, language, visual-constructional skills, conceptual thinking, calculations, and orientation. Administration time is approximately 10 minutes.

1. Capacity for Regulation, Attention, and Learning

For a broader definition of the first capacity, and a fuller listing of related evaluation tools, see the description of this capacity in Chapter 2 on the M Axis (p. 77).

In rating this capacity in individuals 70 years of age and older, it is important to consider possible changes in the neurobiological substrate, such as neurocognitive disorders (see above). Problems in the domain of memory are frequently recognized as leading symptoms of such disorders because such problems (particularly impairments in immediate and recent memory, less frequently those in long-term memory) have an impact on daily functioning in all its aspects and features.

In the elderly, difficulty in learning new tasks seems normative and often is the consequence of a progressive "tightening" of overall mental functioning. Whereas younger people are able to receive and process new stimuli readily, the elderly may often process only stimuli that are very similar to each other; this makes it difficult for them to deal with new inputs.

However, recent findings highlight the possibility that older persons can maintain sufficient learning abilities even in old age. This research indicates strategies (teaching modes and training techniques) that can promote attention (Chaffin & Harlow, 2005; Saczinski, Willis, & Schaie, 2002; Wrenn & Maurer, 2004) and preserve good cognitive functioning.

Rating Scale

For this and each of the other M-Axis capacities, a 5-point rating scale in which each mental function can be assessed from 5 to 1, is provided in Table 12.1 at the end of the chapter, as noted earlier. Descriptions of the anchor points for levels 5, 3, and 1 are provided for each capacity in the text.

5. At this level, the individual's ability to express thoughts, affects, and other inner experiences is not damaged by the process of aging. Memory, attention, executive functions, and learning capacities are maintained and well integrated, given the normal age-related decrease in overall psychological and physical functioning.
3. The individual may be able to express thoughts, affects, and other inner experiences only for relatively short periods and when specifically motivated. In other conditions, and/or under stress, some impairments connected to the process of aging become more evident, and problems in language, information processing, and other more or less specific cognitive abilities may emerge.
1. At this level, the process of aging has damaged the individual's capacity to remain focused, organized, and attentive. This interferes with his or her abilities to learn and to maintain active and adequate behaviors in response to external stimuli.

Most Relevant Assessment Tools

Brief Test of Attention

The Brief Test of Attention (BTA; Schretlen, Bobholz, & Brandt, 1996) is used to assess the ability to divide auditory attention. It consists of two parallel forms that are presented via audio CD. Respondents are administered both forms (each requires 4 minutes).

Visual Pattern Test

The Visual Pattern Test (VPT; Della Sala, Gray, Baddeley, & Wilson, 1999) assesses visual short-term memory in persons between 13 and 92 years of age. As the test distinguishes storage memory from other aspects of visual short-term memory, it is also useful for evaluating attention and mental imagery.

Rey–Osterrieth Complex Figure Test

The Rey–Osterrieth Complex Figure Test (CFT; Corwin & Bylsma, 1993; Osterrieth, 1944) was developed to assess visual–spatial constructional ability and visual memory. The administration involves four tasks: copy of the figure; 3-minute recall (i.e., recall after a 3-minute delay filled with talking or another verbal task); delayed recall (i.e., recall after about 30 minutes); and recognition (the respondent has to circle the figures that were part of the design that was copied). The time required is about 15 minutes.

Rivermead Behavioural Memory Test

The Rivermead Behavioural Memory Test—Third Edition (RBMT-3; Wilson et al., 2008) is discussed under capacity 1 in Chapter 2 on the M Axis (p. 83).

2. Capacity for Affective Range, Communication, and Understanding

For a broader definition of the second capacity, and a listing of related evaluation tools, see the description of this capacity in Chapter 2 (p. 77).

The nature and direction of the emotional changes that affect elderly people depend on "the level of emotional adjustment each person reached during his/her younger years" (Ilardo, 1998, p. 13). This level is, of course, affected by cultural milieu, social norms, and previous experiences. Above all, the type and valence of previous experiences may have a fundamental influence: The capacity to understand and express affective states and emotions may decrease or become constricted if previous experiences have been negative. Conversely, a less rigid adherence to social norms, typical of some older individuals and of their increased sense of freedom, may increase the individuals' disposition to evaluate and share with others their positive and negative feelings (Gross et al., 1997). Many variations on these patterns may be captured in an individual's life narrative.

Rating Scale

5. At this level, the individual's ability to understand a wide range of emotions and to express and communicate them remains untouched by the process of aging, and the resources in this area are consistent with the degree of this capacity achieved in previous periods of life.
3. The individual's range of emotional states is limited, and he or she shows some difficulty in communicating specific types of affects. The normal age-related decline represents a condition of stress, which constricts and impoverishes the expression of emotions and their adequacy to the situation and social expectations.
1. The individual's emotional expression is chaotic, and the incongruence between environmental stimuli and affective responses is evident. At this level of functioning, it is often difficult to distinguish the impact of a more or less severe cognitive decline from a previous low level of resources in this mental area.

3. Capacity for Mentalization and Reflective Functioning

For a broader definition of the third capacity, and a listing of related evaluation tools, see the description of this capacity in Chapter 2 (p. 77).

The age-related reduction of social contacts and the diminished chance to gain experiences—especially new types of experiences—may influence the capacity to reflect upon internal life, as well as to make inferences regarding the mental states of other people. Moreover, older adults sometimes react to difficulties or unpleasant events through somatic impairments, which may be connected to age-related physical vulnerability, and this may constitute a kind of alternative to reflective functioning. As McClintock Greenberg (2009, p. 56) writes, "the imposing threat to the integrity and cohesion of the self, as well as the distressing fear of death, [can] result in reduced access to symbolic thought."

In other cases, if individuals have exhibited good mentalization and reflective functioning skills during previous periods of life, they may experience an increase in the capacity to understand both their own reactions to different experiences and the mental states of others, due to the knowledge and experience they have acquired (Happé, Winner, & Brownell, 1998; Melehin, 2015).

Understanding age-related changes in adult mentalizing capacity is particularly important in order to assess reflective functioning impairments due to neurocognitive decline or mental disorders (see Chapters 13 and 14 on the PE and SE Axes, respectively).

Rating Scale

5. At this level, the individual is able to understand his or her own mental states, as well as to construct representations of the internal experiences underlying others' behaviors and reactions. This capacity is maintained even when the situation is challenging or distressing. The process of aging doesn't have a significant impact on the individual's psychological insight and capacity to identify the mental states of others. Mentalization and reflective functioning are used to modulate impulses and to distinguish inner from outer reality.
3. In the face of conflicts or strong emotions, the individual may show a remarkable decline in his or her usual mentalization and reflective functioning skills. There may be symptoms of somatization and/or increased impulsivity. The diminished availability of physical and psychological resources related to the process of aging may further decrease the individual's ability to reflect on his or her behaviors and feelings, and to pay attention to those of others.
1. The individual's age-related decrease in cognitive flexibility, and/or the need to cope with physical difficulties, may result in inability to pay attention to his or her affective states or to distinguish between internal and external experiences. Reality testing sometimes seems confused, and the person finds it hard to put into words the emotions he or she is experiencing; both of these difficulties tend to decrease the individual's capacity to reflect and choose appropriate behaviors.

4. Capacity for Differentiation and Integration (Identity)

For a broader definition of the fourth capacity, and a listing of related evaluation tools, see the description of this capacity in Chapter 2 (p. 77).

The sense of identity and the integration of self are not acquired in old age; the individual enjoys good functioning in this category only if these qualities were developed in the previous periods of life. The number and nature of previous experiences may indeed result in a stronger sense of self-confidence, based on more established values, beliefs, and habits. However, the process of aging can also weaken the sense of identity because of the reduction of some physical resources, as well as the normal age-related decrease in cognitive capacities, which may increase the need to depend on others.

Rating Scale

5. The flexibility and spontaneity typical of a good sense of identity are maintained from previous periods of life into old age. The person's understanding of his or her motives, wishes, and different affective states allows the individual to cope optimally with the difficulties and experiences related to the aging process.
3. In the face of stressful experiences, the person's normal age-related impairments adversely affect the sense of identity. At this level, the individual may be confused about his or her wishes and needs, and sometimes may be unable to cope with different conditions or to maintain an integrated and stable sense of self.
1. The person's diminished cognitive, psychological, and physical resources have a major impact on the capacity for differentiation and integration. The individual is unable to perceive the continuity between the previous periods of life and the present, and his or her sense of identity is fragmented or rigidly compartmentalized. There are maladaptive defenses (based on splitting mechanisms), and reality testing tends to decline.

5. Capacity for Relationships and Intimacy

For a broader definition of the fifth capacity, and a listing of related evaluation tools, see the description of this capacity in Chapter 2 (p. 78).

In the evaluation of this capacity in an elderly person, it is important to pay attention to the difference between the actual numbers/types of social contacts and the persistence of the person's need to share affects and emotions with significant individuals in the environment. Some sensory impairments common in later life (e.g., hearing and visual deficits) can restrict social contacts and thus can sometimes increase isolation, but the capacity for relatedness may be preserved or even increased.

The concept of dependence itself needs specific evaluation in older adults as their needs and life circumstances change. For example, "older people's relations with family members who must look after them can suffer, as the caretaker and the patient are likely to feel torn between anger and guilt over the new roles" (Zarit, 1980, p. 47). Moreover, "as changes in physical health or cognitive abilities become too daunting for community living, many people move to nursing homes, assisted living facilities, or retirement communities" (Kring, Davison, Neale, & Johnson, 2007, p. 523). The need for various kinds of help from relatives, friends, and others (health care professionals, institutional personnel, etc.) may modify the kinds of relationships an elderly person has with significant others in the environment.

Issues related to sexuality in old age need special consideration. Reductions in the need for sexual intercourse and in the sharing of sexual fantasies and desires are normally related to the process of aging, but may represent specific difficulties for individuals who have previously found sexuality an important part of their identity. In this regard, depressive reactions may sometimes result from the reduction of sexual interest; conversely, there may be a defensive increasing of sexually disinhibited behaviors (not in connection with a manic episode or a neurocognitive disorder; see Chapter 14 on the SE Axis). Of course, an appropriate balance in earlier stages of life between sexuality and other interests and ways of establishing relationships is a useful background for addressing the changes that aging produces in this area.

Rating Scale

5. Despite possible relationship difficulties related to aging (sensory impairments, difficulty in movement, etc.), the individual at this level retains the desire for contact with others and is able to maintain deep and meaningful relationships, even with a possible romantic involvement.
3. The individual retains the capacity to have meaningful contacts with friends, relatives, and possibly romantic partners. However, withdrawal and isolation may emerge in the presence of physical or emotional difficulties; conversely, the demand for care and relationships may become excessive and unrealistic.
1. The individual is unable to maintain meaningful relationships and has little interest in sharing his or her own experiences with others. Indifference and withdrawal may be results of experiences in previous periods of life, or may be linked to physical impairments and/or psychological difficulties related to aging. The capacity to provide support to others or accept help is mostly absent.

6. Capacity for Self-Esteem Regulation and Quality of Internal Experience

For a broader definition of the sixth capacity, and a listing of related evaluation tools, see the description of this capacity in Chapter 2 (p. 78).

Several authors point out that aging is often accompanied by a feeling of mourning, related to an older person's need to change his or her self-image and find new ways to establish relationships (based on capacities and personal characteristics other than those of the past), while preserving at the same time a sense of continuity. This is, in essence, a process of accepting a progressive identity crisis and coping with it (Goswami, 2013; Ploton, 2001). The process may occur at the expense of self-esteem, but it can also strengthen the person's level of confidence and self-regard. The number and nature of previous experiences may be helpful. Of course, age-related physical impairments or reductions in sensory capacities, as well as increasing needs for dependence on children, relatives, and professional helpers, may interfere with the various features of this capacity.

Rating Scale

5. At this level, the individual maintains a stable sense of confidence, vitality, and realistic self-esteem, even when confronted with age-related decline or impairments. The decreasing of some sensory capacities and motor skills does not correspond to a reduction in self-reliance, and the person is able to maintain a positive view of him- or herself, which influences relationships with others and the environment.
3. The person's level of confidence and self-esteem is generally adequate, but may be frequently disrupted by stressful situations and by age-related impairments. The individual expresses inner feelings of inadequacy, based on diminished confidence in his or her sensory and motor resources. The willingness to have relationships with others is damaged by the perception of declines in these skills.
1. The person's perception of vulnerability, based on declines in sensory and motor skills, produces feelings of emptiness, incompleteness, and emotional withdrawal.

There is limited (or even no) capacity for resiliency in responding to the age-related difficulties. As a result, self-confidence and self-esteem are either abnormally low or sometimes too high because of mechanisms of overcompensation, and a balance between these extremes may be lacking. Indeed, the individual may react to the age-related changes by transforming his or her objective weakness into an illusory sense of strength, and thus into various inappropriate behaviors (e.g., underestimation of danger).

7. Capacity for Impulse Control and Regulation

For a broader definition of the seventh capacity, and a listing of related evaluation tools, see the description of this capacity in Chapter 2 (p. 78).

The process of aging may adversely affect this capacity, and some individual features in the previous periods of life may be predictive of the specific kind of dysregulation. A pattern of overcontrol or undercontrol of impulse expression may increase with the passing of time, and the deficiencies in this capacity may become more evident. Furthermore, it is necessary to keep in mind that this capacity may be severely impaired in the presence of a neurocognitive disorder.

Rating Scale

5. The individual at this level is able to control impulses and regulate emotions. Urges and needs are expressed in a modulated and adaptive way, and changes related to age have not adversely affected these capabilities.
3. The person's impulse control and emotion regulation may decrease in the presence of conflicts and tensions. The reduced availability of physical, cognitive, and emotional resources does not allow the individual to govern his or her impulses (e.g., there may be a difficulty in managing anger), or it may produce a defensive withdrawal, together with denial of needs and feelings.
1. The person's experiences and feelings related to old age (intolerance of dependence, decreased self-esteem linked to poor control of sensory and motor skills, and/or lack of cognitive resources) greatly decrease the ability to modulate needs, motivations, and feelings. The individual may also have shown little capacity to control and regulate his or her impulses in previous periods of life; this pattern may be maintained in old age, or may become more severe and obvious.

8. Capacity for Defensive Functioning

For a broader definition of the eighth capacity, and a listing of related evaluation tools, see the description of this capacity in Chapter 2 (p. 78).

The process of aging, and the consequent lower availability of physical resources and cognitive abilities, may affect defensive capacities. Flexibility of behaviors and of reactions to events and interpersonal relationships may decrease. It can happen that an older adult uses preferentially experienced defensive patterns because they are familiar, even if they are not appropriate to the situation.

Some objectively difficult life events (retirement, widowhood, death of relatives and friends, illnesses, and need for hospitalization or for professional help by nurses and/or social workers), as well as general age-related physical and emotional vulnerability, can favor the use of more primitive defensive patterns, in which splitting prevails over more adaptive reactions. In some cases, however, individuals in favorable conditions and with positive past experiences may show higher-level defensive functioning, due to an increased capacity to reflect upon events and their own feelings.

Rating Scale

5. The increasing of age-related impairments has not weakened the individual's defensive structure, in which neurotic-level adaptive defenses (repression, isolation, intellectualization, etc.) predominate. These defenses allow the experience of a wide range of affects, appropriate interactions with others, and the expression of some level of creativity. The individual is aware of the difficulties related to age and behaves accordingly, without resorting to more primitive defenses.
3. The experience of age-related physical and psychological limits favors the use of lower-level defenses such as denial, as well as idealization or devaluation of self and others, particularly when the individual feels threatened or is anxious. Consequently, reality testing is sometimes less effective, and the person may not recognize important aspects of his or her condition.
1. The experience of physical difficulties (especially in the presence of severe diseases or other impairments) may distort reality testing, and the individual may be overwhelmed by anxiety. Defenses based on splitting may become part of delusional ideation (delusional projection). The use of more mature and adaptive defenses is mostly difficult and becomes impossible when stress increases.

9. Capacity for Adaptation, Resiliency, and Strength

For a broader definition of the ninth capacity, and a listing of related evaluation tools, see the description of this capacity in Chapter 2 (p. 78).

The different stages of the process of aging involve a broad array of events and circumstances, which may stress an individual's capacity to cope effectively with occurrences such as losses, changed living conditions, awareness of limited time, and global weakening of physical and/or cognitive resources. Confronted with these new experiences, the elderly person has to exercise whatever capacity he or she has for adaptation in order to react properly.

Some specific points of strength (e.g., the ability to manage a wide range of adverse conditions) can be helpful and should be taken into account in the diagnostic evaluation (Cyrulnik & Ploton, 2014). Moreover, it is necessary to pay attention to a possible impairment of this capacity, due to the presence of a neurocognitive disorder.

A special case is the elderly individual who needs to enter a nursing home. As Ilardo writes (1998, p. 198), "we are territorial creatures, and our environment is our territory." When an older adult loses his or her territory and its usual reference points, it's normal for the person to feel edgy and angry. In such a case, however, it is not only still possible but important to evaluate the individual's capacity for resiliency and adaptation, as well as to plan appropriate support interventions.

Rating Scale

5. Even in the presence of considerable stress, complex social-emotional contexts, and novel events, the individual at this level is able to manage his or her emotional states and maintain a good level of interpersonal functioning, with an adequate expression of cognitive abilities. Reality testing is preserved, with a proper understanding of self and others. Empathy and sensitivity to environmental requests are expressed, together with assertiveness and promotion of positive interactions.
3. There are moderate levels of impairment in thought processes and interpersonal functioning. When the person is confronted with particularly complex and/or stressful situations, the normal age-related physical and emotional impairments are more evident and influence the person's feelings and behavior. The individual is, however, able to maintain a certain degree of adaptation without severe consequences.
1. The need to cope with new situations, difficult emotional states, and unfamiliar types of interpersonal relationships leads the person to rely on primitive defenses and uncontrolled affective states. The decline of cognitive, emotional, and relational capacities is in the foreground; weakness and vulnerability are rapidly spreading. The capacity for adaptation and resiliency is greatly impaired, and the individual needs continual support to relate appropriately with the environment.

10. Self-Observing Capacities (Psychological Mindedness)

For a broader definition of the next set of capacities, and a listing of related evaluation tools, see the description in Chapter 2 on the M Axis (p. 78).

In the process of aging, various types of uncomfortable experiences often take place, as detailed throughout this chapter. All these conditions require a good degree of psychological mindedness—which, like other capacities, a person may have had to a greater or lesser extent in earlier life, and which may be affected by the process of aging. It may be worth emphasizing that sometimes self-observing capacities increase during old age, thanks to an elderly person's previous experiences and positive reactions to other similar events. The person may indeed have developed a deeper awareness of his or her capacities for functional behaviors and adequate emotional responses in different difficult situations.

Rating Scale

5. At this level, the individual has high motivation and capacity to observe and understand his or her feelings, thoughts, and behaviors, as well as their variations in different situations, even under pressure. The person's psychological mindedness is not substantially impaired by the process of aging. The capacity to reflect on previous experiences plays a significant role in helping the person evaluate and organize affective responses and behavioral reactions.
3. The process of aging and its typical features partially impair the individual's degree of insight into his or her own and others' feelings and behaviors. Under pressure, the capacities for self-observing and understanding are not available, but may be recovered when the stress decreases.

1. Self-awareness is lacking, and the individual seems unable to reflect upon his or her feelings, thoughts, and behaviors. There are polarized affect states. The individual is unable to observe mindfully the typical features of old age, both physical and emotional; these may be either over- or underestimated, sometimes with a significant impairment of reality testing.

11. Capacity to Construct and Use Internal Standards and Ideals

For a broader definition of capacity 11, and a listing of related evaluation tools, see the description of this capacity in Chapter 2 (pp. 78–79).

The process of aging may frequently result in a person's developing more rigid moral standards. This may sometimes be a defensive measure against rapid changes in the environment (widespread modifications in areas such as sexual habits, social norms, and relationships between the generations, as well as the tremendously rapid changes in technology, which the elderly may perceive as foreign and difficult to manage). In other cases, it may be a reaction to declining physical and cognitive resources, as well as to a diminishing network of friends and relatives (losses, modified social roles because of retirement, etc.).

On the other hand, sometimes an older adult may feel entitled to express a relative independence from social and cultural customs, in view of his or her diminished expectations of social rewards.

Rating Scale

5. The individual at this level is aware of his or her behavioral standards and moral beliefs, and expresses them in a flexible way, with consideration for the social contexts and capacities of other people; the person tries to understand the reasons behind the others' behaviors, even when these aren't explicit and evident. This allows the person to base moral judgments not on feelings of guilt and punishment, but on a balance of compassion and empathy (toward others as well as him- or herself).

3. The individual is not always able to adapt his or her internal standards and ideals to current norms and values in different social contexts. The person is moderately rigid and inflexible, showing a less realistic understanding of the capacities, values, and ideals of other people. Self-esteem is driven more by feelings of guilt and/or shame than by the responsibility or wish to produce more adequate behaviors.

1. The person is not able to cope with behaviors that are far from his or her moral standards, even when they are acceptable within current social contexts. Expressions of criticism and indictment are frequent. The comparison between the ethical standards of earlier periods of the person's life and current moral habits is always rigid and inflexible. The value of the moral standards of the past is overestimated. There is no place for empathy and positive criticism, and genuine dialogue with others is mostly impossible.

12. Capacity for Meaning and Purpose

For a broader definition of the final capacity, and a listing of related evaluation tools, see the description of this capacity in Chapter 2 (p. 79).

In evaluating this capacity, we can also use the term "engagement." In fact, in the elderly, the capacity for meaning and purpose reflects a sense of belonging to and being an active member of a family, a society, and a community. It also reflects the ability not only to accept but to work with the ongoing processes of change—adapting old projects, or, conversely, creating new projects—according to an individual's new personal status and roles. All of this is able to give meaning to the current stage of the individual's life, regardless of evaluations based only on efficiency and productivity. It is also helpful in dealing with issues such as death, mourning, age-related declines in psychological and physical resources, and more or less profound changes in the conditions of life (e.g., the need for continuous assistance, entrance into a nursing home).

The elderly person who functions at a high level in this capacity typically shows the following:

- The ability and willingness to identify and pursue new interests and activities (reading, travel, volunteering, hobbies, etc.).
- An interest and investment in developing new relationships (and/or, if possible, in maintaining previous ones), as well as the ability to break away from maladaptive behaviors and conflictual relationships.
- The ability to accept and adapt to the realignment of his or her roles within various reference groups.
- The capacity for sharing knowledge that comes from previous experiences with other persons (above all, with young ones).
- The ability to wonder about and appreciate scientific and technological advances, and the willingness to learn the use of new devices in particular.
- The capacity to think about the future of loved ones after his or her death.

Rating Scale

5. The individual may experience and accept a feeling of finiteness, and implements only reasonable behaviors intended to preserve health, to maintain physical appearance, and ultimately to prolong life. The person's slogan could be "I prefer not to live at all costs," or "I agree not to be young forever." The possible role of "old wise person" is appreciated and allows the individual to establish satisfactory relationships within the family and community. In the appraisal of previous periods of life, the person can remember and evaluate mistakes and achievements, successes and failures, without either becoming the victim of guilt/regrets or denigrating the present. If the individual cultivates some form of spirituality or adheres to any specific ideology, he or she doesn't show all-or-none behaviors and attitudes, but uses and expresses adaptively his or her own beliefs.

3. The individual maintains with some difficulty his or her sense of purpose and meaning. The person's awareness of his or her limited time and decreased efficiency and productivity is sometimes a source of stress and worry, as well as of depressive feelings. There is a marked level of discomfort with the physical and aesthetic manifestations of aging, and the search for remedies is sometimes compulsive. The

TABLE 12.1. Summary of Basic Mental Functioning: ME Axis

To obtain a quantitative rating of the patient's overall mental functioning, the clinician should add up the 1–5 point ratings assigned to each of the 12 capacities (Table 12.1a). This yields a single numerical index of overall functioning ranging from 12 to 60, with higher scores reflecting healthier functioning. This numerical index allows the clinician to assign the patient to one of the categories outlined in Table 12.1b, which provides short qualitative descriptions of seven levels of mental functioning.

TABLE 12.1a. ME-Axis Functioning: Total Score

ME-Axis capacities	Rating scale				
1. Capacity for regulation, attention, and learning	5	4	3	2	1
2. Capacity for affective range, communication, and understanding	5	4	3	2	1
3. Capacity for mentalization and reflective functioning	5	4	3	2	1
4. Capacity for differentiation and integration (identity)	5	4	3	2	1
5. Capacity for relationships and intimacy	5	4	3	2	1
6. Capacity for self-esteem regulation and quality of internal experience	5	4	3	2	1
7. Capacity for impulse control and regulation	5	4	3	2	1
8. Capacity for defensive functioning	5	4	3	2	1
9. Capacity for adaptation, resiliency, and strength	5	4	3	2	1
10. Self-observing capacities (psychological mindedness)	5	4	3	2	1
11. Capacity to construct and use internal standards and ideals	5	4	3	2	1
12. Capacity for meaning and purpose	5	4	3	2	1
	Total score = ____				

TABLE 12.1b. Levels of Mental Functioning

ME1. Healthy/optimal mental functioning (range = 54–60)

The individual shows very good functioning in most mental capacities. Possible variations in flexibility and adaptation are related to age-specific vulnerabilities or distressing events, and are transient.

ME2. Good/appropriate mental functioning with some areas of difficulty (range = 47–53)

The individual shows an appropriate level of mental functioning. However, some specific and limited areas of difficulty are present, in relation to specific conditions or events, as well as to some age-related cognitive or emotional impairments.

ME3. Mild impairments in mental functioning (range = 40–46)

The individual shows areas of constriction and inflexibility in some domains of mental functioning. The age-related impairments adversely affect self-esteem regulation and stiffen defensive functioning.

(continued)

TABLE 12.1. *(continued)*

ME4. Moderate impairments in mental functioning (range = 33–39)

The individual shows moderate constriction and alterations in almost all domains of mental functioning. The age-related vulnerabilities produce significantly impaired responses to environmental demands and a poor capacity for adaptation.

ME5. Major impairments in mental functioning (range = 26–32)

The individual shows major alterations in almost all domains of mental functioning. The aging process helps produce severe difficulties of integration and self–object differentiation. Some age-related cognitive deficits and emotional difficulties worsen the (already damaged) mental functioning of previous periods of life, or result directly in a state of impairment.

ME6. Significant defects in basic mental functions (range = 19–25)

The individual shows significant defects in most domains of mental functioning. The stress caused by the aging process greatly worsens the person's ability to react to the difficulties of daily life.

ME7. Major/severe defects in basic mental functions (range = 12–18)

The individual shows severe defects in almost all domains, with impairments in basic mental functions (perception, integration, cognitive and affective regulation, memory, etc.) that either result directly from the aging process or reflect previous deficits. The capacity to face the difficulties of aging is compromised overall, and autonomy is almost completely lost.

recourse to spirituality or the adherence to specific ideologies has a compensatory and utilitarian aim. In regard to previous periods of life, negative memories are more frequent; the past positive events rarely constitute a reason for comfort, and the majority of memories evoke sadness and regret.

1. The individual has lost the sense of purpose and meaning in his or her life. The subjective experiences of decreased energy, greater chances of getting sick, body modifications, restriction of social roles, and so forth, as well as other negative age-related events (losses, retirement, diminished relationships, etc.), may induce a sense of alienation, meaninglessness, and isolation. On the other hand, the individual may resort to primitive (manic/hypomanic) defense mechanisms in order to deny the difficulties of old age. Spirituality and the willingness to transcend the present moment may be absent; conversely, they may be rigid and excessive, to the point of assuming the characteristics of delusional beliefs or compulsive behaviors.

Summary of Basic Mental Functioning

Following the same approach introduced in the other M-Axis chapters, we recommend that clinicians summarize basic mental functioning quantitatively (see Table 12.1).

BIBLIOGRAPHY

General Bibliography

Agronin, M. E. (2004). *Dementia.* Philadelphia: Lippincott Williams & Wilkins.

Allen, A. T., Morris, A. M., Stark, S. M., Fortin, N. J., & Stark, C. E. L. (2015). Memory for sequences of events impaired in typical aging. *Learning and Memory, 22,* 138–148.

American Psychiatric Association. (2013). *Diagnostic and statistical manual of mental disorders* (5th ed.). Arlington, VA: Author.

Baddeley, A. (1996). *Your memory: A user's guide.* London: Prion.

Baltes, M. M., & Carstensen, L. L. (1996). The process of successful ageing. *Ageing and Society, 16*(4), 397–422.

Caleb, E., Finch, C. E., & Tanzi, R. E. (1997). Genetics of aging. *Science, 278,* 407–411.

Cesari, M., Vellas, B., & Gambassi, G. (2013). The stress of aging. *Experimental Gerontology, 48*(4), 451–456.

Churchill, J. D., Galvez, R., Colcombe, S., Swain, R. A, Kramer, A. F., & Greenough, W. T. (2002). Exercise, experience and the aging brain. *Neurobiology of Aging, 23*(5), 941–955.

Cohen-Sachs, B. (2006). Coping with the stress of aging—creatively. *Stress Medicine, 9,* 45–49.

Desjardins, R., & Warnke, A. J. (2012). *Ageing and skills* (OECD Education Working Paper No. 72). Paris: Organisation for Economic Co-operation and Development.

Dubois, B., Slachevsky, A., Litvan, I., & Pillon, B. (2000). The FAB: A frontal assessment battery at bedside. *Neurology, 55,* 1621–1626.

Folstein, M. F., Folstein, S. E., & McHugh, P. R. (1975). Mini-Mental State: A practical method for grading the cognitive state of patients for the clinicians. *Journal of Psychiatric Research, 12,* 189–198.

Fratiglioni, L., Paillard-Borg, S., & Winblad, B. (2004). An active and socially integrated lifestyle in late life might protect against dementia. *Lancet Neurology, 3*(6), 343–353.

Grady, C. (2012). The cognitive neuroscience of ageing. *Nature Reviews Neuroscience, 13,* 491–505.

Hayflick, L. (1994). *How and why we age.* New York: Ballantine Books.

Hertzog, C. (1996). Research design in studies of aging and cognition. In J. E. Birren, K. W. Schaie, R. P. Abeles, M. Gatz, & T. A. Salthouse (Eds.), *Handbook of the psychology of aging* (4th ed., pp. 24–37). San Diego, CA: Academic Press.

Ilardo, J. A. (1998). *As parents age.* Acton, MA: VanderWyck & Turnham.

Institute of Medicine. (2015). *Cognitive aging: Progress in understanding and opportunities for action.* Washington, DC: National Academies Press.

Kunzmann, U., Little, T. D., & Smith, J. (2000). Is age-related stability of subjective well-being a paradox?: Cross-sectional and longitudinal evidence from the Berlin Aging Study. *Psychology and Aging, 15*(3), 511–526.

Mattis, S. (1988). *Dementia Rating Scale: Professional manual.* Odessa, FL: Psychological Assessment Resources.

McClintock Greenberg, T. (2009). *Psychodynamic perspectives on aging and illness.* New York: Springer.

Moran, J. M. (2013). Lifespan development: The effects of typical aging on theory of mind. *Behavioural Brain Research, 15,* 32–40.

Nasreddine, Z. S., Phillips, N. A., Bédirian, V., Charbonneau, S., Whitehead, V., Collin, I., . . . Chertkow, H. (2005). The Montreal Cognitive Assessment, MoCA: A brief screening tool for mild cognitive impairment. *Journal of the American Geriatrics Society, 53*(4), 695–699.

Nussbaum, P. D. (Ed.). (1997). *Handbook of neuropsychology and aging.* New York: Springer.

Palmore, E. B. (1974). *Normal aging II: Reports from the Duke Longitudinal Studies, 1970–1973.* Durham, NC: Duke University Press.

Powell, D. H., Kaplan, E. F., Whitla, D., Catlin, R., & Funkenstein, H. H. (1993). *Manual for MicroCog: Assessment of Cognitive Functioning.* San Antonio, TX: Psychological Corporation.

Ravdin, L. D., & Katzen, H. L. (Eds.). (2013). *Handbook on the neuropsychology of aging and dementia.* New York: Springer.

Rodríguez-Rodero, S., Fernández-Morera, J. L., Menéndez-Torre, E., Calvanese, V., Fernández, A. F., & Fraga, M. F. (2011). Aging genetics and aging. *Aging Diseases, 2*(3), 186–195.

Rosen, W., Mohs, R., & Davis, K. (1984). A new rating scale for Alzheimer's disease. *American Journal of Psychiatry, 141,* 1356–1364.

Roth, M., Huppert, F. A., Mountjoy, C. Q., & Tym, E. (1998). *The Cambridge Examination for Mental Disorders of the Elderly—Revised.* Cambridge, UK: Cambridge University Press.

Roth, M., Tym, E., Mountjoy, C. Q., Huppert, F. A., Hendrie, H., Verma, S., & Goddard, R. (1986). CAMDEX: A standardized instrument for the diagnosis of mental disorders in the elderly with special reference to the early detection of dementia. *British Journal of Psychiatry, 149,* 698–709.

Rowe, J. W., & Kahn, R. L. (1987). Human aging: Usual and successful. *Science, 237,* 143–149.

Rowe, J. W., Kahn, R. L. (1997). Successful aging. *The Gerontologist, 37*(4), 433–440.

Ryff, C. D., & Singer, B. H. (2005). Social environments and the genetics of aging: Advancing knowledge of protective health mechanisms. *Journal of Gerontology, 60B,* 12–23.

Salthouse, T. A. (2009). When does age-related cognitive decline begin? *Neurobiology of Aging, 30*(4), 507–514.

Schaie, K. W., & Willis, S. L. (Eds.). (2011). *Handbook of the psychology of aging* (7th ed.). Burlington, MA: Academic Press.

Siberski, J. (2012). Dementia and DSM-5: Changes, cost, and confusion. Retrieved from *www.agingwellmag.com/archive/110612p12.shtml.*

Storandt, M., & Vandenbos, G. R. (Eds.). (1994). *Neuropsychological assessment of dementia and depression in older adults: A clinician's guide.* Washington, DC: American Psychological Association.

Strawbridge, W. J., Wallhagen, M. I., & Cohen, R. D. (2002). Successful aging and well-being: Self-rated compared with Rowe and Kahn. *The Gerontologist, 42*(6), 727–733.

Stuart-Hamilton, I. (2006). *The psychology of ageing: An introduction.* London: Jessica Kingsley.

Wilcock, G. K., Bucks, R. S., & Rockwood, K. (Eds.). (1999). *Diagnosis and management of dementia.* Oxford, UK: Oxford University Press.

Woodruff-Pak, D. S. (1997). *The neuropsychology of aging.* Malden, MA: Blackwell.

1. Capacity for Regulation, Attention, and Learning

Baltes, P. B. (1993). The aging mind: Potential and limits. *The Gerontologist, 33*(5), 580–594.

Brink, J. L., & McDowd, J. M. (1999). Aging and selective attention: An issue of complexity or ultiple mechanisms? *Journal of Gerontology, 54B*(1), 30–33.

Brummer, L., Stopa, L., & Bucks, R. (2013). The influence of age on emotion regulation strategies and psychological distress, *Behavioural and Cognitive Psychotherapy, 42*(6), 1–14.

Cavanaugh, J. C., & Blanchard-Fields, F. (2002). *Adult development and aging.* Belmont, CA: Wadsworth/Thomson Learning.

Chaffin, A. J., & Harlow, S. D. (2005). Cognitive learning applied to older adult learners and technology. *Educational Gerontology, 31*, 301–329.

Clark, M. C., & Caffarella, R. S. (Eds.). (1999). *An update on adult development theory: New ways of thinking about the life course.* San Francisco: Jossey-Bass.

Corwin, J., & Bylsma, F. W. (1993). Psychological examination of traumatic encephalopathy by A. Rey and "The Complex Figure Copy Test" by P. A. Osterrieth. *The Clinical Neuropsychologist, 7*, 3–21.

Della Sala, S., Gray, C., Baddeley, A., & Wilson, L. (1997). *Visual Patterns Test: A test of short-term visual recall.* Bury St. Edmunds, UK: Thames Valley Test Company.

Hurry, H. L., & Gross, J. J. (2010). Emotion regulation in older age. *Current Directions in Psychological Science, 19*(6), 352–357.

Lowy, L., & O'Connor, D. (1986). *Why education in the later years?* Lexington, MA: D.C. Heath.

Mahoney, J. R., Verghese, J., Goldin, Y., Lipton, R., & Holtzerl, R. (2010). Alerting, orienting, and executive attention in older adults. *Journal of the International Neuropsychological Society, 16*(5), 877–889.

McDowd, J. M., & Birren, J. E. (1990). Aging and attentional processes. In J. E. Birren & K. W. Schaie (Eds.), *Handbook of the psychology of aging* (3rd ed., pp. 222–233). San Diego, CA: Academic Press.

Osterrieth, P. A. (1944). Le test de copie d'une figure complex: Contribution a l'étude de la perception et de la mémoire. *Archives de Psychologie, 30*, 286–356.

Saczynski, J. S., Willis, S. L., & Schaie, K. W. (2002). Strategy use in reasoning raining with older adults. *Aging, Neuropsychology and Cognition, 9*(1), 48–60.

Schretlen, D., Bobholz, J. H., & Brandt, J. (1996). Development and psychometric properties of the Brief Test of Attention. *The Clinical Neuropsychologist, 10*, 80–89.

Trenerry, M. R., Crosson, B., DeBoe, J., & Leber, W. R. (1990). *Visual Search and Attention Test.* Odessa, FL: Psychological Assessment Resources.

Williamson, A. (1997). "You're never too old to learn!": Third-age perspectives on lifelong learning. *International Journal of Lifelong Education, 16*(3), 173–184.

Wilson, B. A., Greenfield, E., Clare, L., Baddeley, A., Cockburn, J., Watson, P., . . . Nannery, R. (2008). *The Rivermead Behavioural Memory Test—Third Edition (RBMT-3).* London: Pearson.

Wrenn, K. A., & Maurer, T. J. (2004). Beliefs about older workers' learning and development behaviour in relation to beliefs about malleability of skills, age-related decline, and control. *Journal of Applied Social Psychology, 34*(2), 223–242.

2. Capacity for Affective Range, Communication, and Understanding

Carstensen, L. L., & Charles, S. T. (1998). Emotion in the second half of life. *Current Directions in Psychological Science, 7*(5), 144–149.

Gross, J. J., Carstensen, L. L., Pasupathi, M., Tsai, J., Skorpen, C. G., & Hsu, A. Y. (1997). Emotion and aging: Experience, expression, and control. *Psychology and Aging, 12*(4), 590–599.

Levenson, R. W., Carstensen, L. L., Friesen, W. V., & Ekman, P. (1991). Emotion, physiology, and expression in old age. *Psychology and Aging, 6*(1), 28–35.

Scheibe, S., & Carstensen, L. L. (2010). Emotional aging: Recent findings and future trends. *Journals of Gerontology: Series B. Psychological Sciences and Social Sciences, 65*(2), 135–144.

Worrall, L. E., & Hickson, L. M. (2003). Theoretical foundations of communication disability in aging. In L. E. Worrall & L. M. Hickson (Eds.), *Communication disability in aging: From prevention to intervention* (pp. 32–33). Clifton Park, NY: Delmar Learning.

3. Capacity for Mentalization and Reflective Functioning

Happé, F., Winner, E., & Brownell, H. (1998). The getting of wisdom: Theory of mind in old age. *Developmental Psychology, 34*, 358–362.

Henry, J. D., Phillips, L. H., Ruffman, T., & Bailey, P. E. (2013). A meta-analytic review of age differences in theory of mind. *Psychology and Aging, 28*(3), 826–839.

Maylor, E. A., Moulson, J. M., Muncer, A. M., & Taylor, L. A. (2002). Does performance on theory of mind tasks decline in old age? *British Journal of Psychology, 93*(4), 465–485.

Melehin, A. I. (2015). Theory of mind in normal aging. *Social Psychology and Society, 1*, 139–150.

Moran, J. M. (2013). Lifespan development: The effects of typical aging on theory of mind. *Behavioural Brain Research, 15*, 32–40.

Pardini, M., & Nichelli, P. F. (2009). Age-related decline in mentalizing skills across adult life span. *Experimental Aging Research, 35*(1), 98–106.

4. Capacity for Differentiation and Integration (Identity)

Biggs, S., & Kimberley, H. (2013). Adult ageing and social policy: New risks to identity. *Social Policy and Society, 12*(2), 287–297.

Coleman, P. G. (1996). Identity management in later life. In R. T. Woods (Ed.), *Handbook of the clinical psychology of ageing* (pp. 93–113). Chichester, UK: Wiley.

Coupland, N., Coupland, J., & Giles, H. (1991). *Language, society and the elderly: Discourse, identity and ageing.* Oxford, UK: Blackwell.

Hubble, N., & Tew, P. (2013). *Ageing, narrative and identity: New qualitative social research.* London: Palgrave Macmillan.

Moen, P., Erickson, M. A., & Dempster-McClain, D. (2000). Social role identities among older adults in a continuing care retirement community. *Research on Aging, 22*(5), 559–579.

5. Capacity for Relationships and Intimacy

Arber, S., Davidson, K., & Ginn, J. (2003). *Gender and ageing: Changing roles and relationships.* Maidenhead, UK: Open University Press.

Davidson, K., & Fennell, G. (2002). New intimate relationships in later life. *Ageing International, 27*(4), 3–10.

Davidson, K., & Fennell, G. (Eds.). (2004). *Intimacy in later life.* New Brunswick, NJ: Transaction.

Kaplan, H. S. (1990). Sex, intimacy, and the aging process. *Journal of the American Academy of Psychoanalysis, 18*(2), 185–205.

Kring, A. M., Davison, G. C., Neale, J. M., & Johnson, S. L. (2007). *Abnormal psychology* (10th ed.). Hoboken, NJ: Wiley.

Zarit, S. H. (1980). *Aging and mental disorders: Psychological approach to assessment and treatment.* New York: Free Press.

6. Capacity for Self-Esteem Regulation and Quality of Internal Experience

Cotter, V. T., & Gonzalez, E. W. (2009). Self-concept in older adults: An integrative review of empirical literature. *Holistic Nursing Practice, 23*(6), 335–348.

Goswami, P. (2013). Ageing and its effect on body-self image, mood and self esteem of middle age women and older women. *Journal of Humanities and Social Sciences, 18*(5), 63–73.

McAuley, E., Elavsky, S., Motl, R. W., Konopack, J. F., Hu, L., & Marquez, D. X. (2005). Physical activity, self-efficacy, and self-esteem: Longitudinal relationships in older adults. *Journals of Gerontology: Series B. Psychological Sciences and Social Sciences, 60*(5), 268–275.

Ploton, L. (2001). *La personne âgée, son accompagnement médical et psychologique et la question de la démence.* Lyon, France: Editions Cronique Sociale.

Pruessner, J. C., Lord, C., Meaney, M., & Lupien, S. (2004). Effects of self-esteem on age-related changes in cognition and the regulation of the hypothalamic–pituitary–adrenal axis. *Annals of the New York Academy of Sciences, 1032*, 186–190.

Sneed, J. R., & Whitbourne, S. K. (2001). Identity processing styles and the need for self-esteem in middle-aged and older adults. *International Journal of Aging and Human Development, 52*(4), 311–321.

7. Capacity for Impulse Control and Regulation

Brummer, L., Stopa, L., & Bucks, R. (2014). The influence of age on emotion regulation strategies and psychological distress. *Behavioural and Cognitive Psychotherapy, 42*(6), 668–681.

Desai, R. A. (2012). Impulse control disorders and older adults. In J. E. Grant & M. N. Potenza (Eds.), *The Oxford handbook of impulse control disorders* (pp. 487–498). Oxford, UK: Oxford University Press.

Hurry, H. L., & Gross, J. J. (2010). Emotion regulation in older age. *Current Directions in Psychological Science, 19*(6), 352–357.

Phillips, L. H., Henry, J. D., Hosie, J. A., & Milne, A. B. (2008). Effective regulation of the experience of negative affect in old age. *Journals of Gerontology: Series B. Psychological Sciences and Social Sciences, 63*, 138–145.

Samanez-Larkin, G. R., Robertson, E. R., Mikels, J. A., Carstensen, L. L., & Gotlib, I. H. (2009). Selective attention to emotion in the aging brain. *Psychology and Aging, 24*, 519–529.

Tamam, L., Bican, M., & Keskin, N. (2014). Impulse control disorders in elderly patients. *Comprehensive Psychiatry, 55*(4), 1022–1028.

8. Capacity for Defensive Functioning

Costa, P. T. Jr., Zonderman, A. B., & McCrae, R. R. (1991). Personality, defense, coping, and adaptation in older adulthood. In E. M. Cummings, A. L. Greene, & K. H. Karraker (Eds.), *Life-span developmental psychology* (pp. 277–293). Mahwah, NJ: Erlbaum.

Labouvie-Vief, G., Hakim-Larson, J., & Hobart, C. J. (1987). Age, ego level, and the life-span development of coping and defense processes. *Psychology of Aging, 2*(3), 286–293.

Segal, D. L., Coolidge, F. L., & Mizuno, H. (2007). Defense mechanism differences between younger and older adults: A cross-sectional investigation. *Aging and Mental Health, 11*(4), 415–422.

Yu, Y., Chamorro-Premuzic, T., & Honjo, S. (2008). Personality and defense mechanisms in late adulthood. *Journal of Aging and Health, 20*(5), 526–544.

9. Capacity for Adaptation, Resiliency, and Strength

Cyrulnik, B., & Ploton, L. (2014). *Vieilissement et resilience.* Paris: Odile Jacob.

Fry, P. S., & Keyes, C. L. M. (Eds.). (2013). *New frontiers in resilient aging.* Cambridge, UK: Cambridge University Press.

Gattuso, S. (2003). Becoming a wise old woman: Resilience and wellness in later life. *Health Sociology Review, 12*(2), 171–177.

Hicks, M. M., & Conner, N. E. (2014). Resilient ageing: A concept analysis. *Journal of Advanced Nursing, 70*(4), 744–755.

Resnick, B., Gwyther, L. P., & Roberto, K. (Eds.). (2011). *Resilience in aging: Concepts, research, and outcomes.* New York: Springer.

Wild, K., Wiles, J. L., & Allen, R. E. S. (2011). Resilience: Thoughts on the value of the concept for critical gerontology. *Ageing and Society, 33*(1), 137–158.

10. Self-Observing Capacities (Psychological Mindedness)

Harty, S., O'Connell, R. G., Hester, R., & Robertson, I. H. (2013). Older adults have diminished awareness of errors in the laboratory and daily life. *Psychology and Aging, 28*(4), 1032–1041.

11. Capacity to Construct and Use Internal Standards and Ideals

Frilund, M., Fagerström, L., Eriksson, K., & Eklund, P. (2013). Assessment of ethical ideals and ethical manners in care of older people. *Nursing Research and Practice, 2013*, 1–11.

Gergen, K. J., & Gergen, M. M. (2000). The new aging: Self construction and social values. In K. W. Schaie & J. Hendricks (Eds.), *The evolution of the aging self* (pp. 281–306). New York: Springer.

Ludwick, R., & Silva, M. (2003). Ethical challenges in the care of elderly persons. *Journal of Issues in Nursing, 9*(1). Retrieved from *www.nursingworld.org/MainMenuCategories ANAMarketplace/ANAPeriodicals/OJIN/TableofContents/Volume92004/No1Jan04/EthicalChallenges.aspx.*

Marinova, D. (2013). Cultural alienation in the ageing person. *Psychological Thought, 6*(2). Retrieved from *http://psyct.psychopen.eu/article/view/63.*

12. Capacity for Meaning and Purpose

Baars, J., Dohmen, J., Grenier, A., & Phillipson, C. (2013). *Ageing, meaning and social structure*. Bristol, UK: Policy Press.

Carr, A., Biggs, S., & Kimberley, H. (2013). *Meanings of a long life*. Melbourne, Australia: Brotherhood of St. Laurence and University of Melbourne Centre for Public Policy.

Dittman-Kohli, F. (1990). The construction of meaning in old age: Possibilities and constraints. *Ageing and Society, 10*, 279–294.

Hedberg, P., Gustafson, Y., & Brulin, C. (2010). Purpose in life among men and women aged 85 years and older. *International Journal of Aging and Human Development, 70*(3), 213–229.

MacKinlay, E. B., & Trevitt, C. (2007). Spiritual care and ageing in a secular society. *Medical Journal of Australia, 186*(10), S74–S76.

McCarthy, V. L., & Bockweg, A. (2013). The role of transcendence in a holistic view of successful aging: A concept analysis and model of transcendence in maturation and aging. *Journal of Holistic Nursing, 31*(2), 84–92.

Mendes de Leon, C. F. (2005). Social engagement and successful aging. *European Journal of Ageing, 2*(1), 64–66.

Moore, S. L., Metcalf, B., & Schow, E. (2006). The quest for meaning in aging. *Geriatric Nursing, 27*(5), 293–299.

Onyx, J., & Warburton, J. (2003). Volunteering and health among older people: A review. *Australasian Journal on Ageing, 22*(2), 65–69.

Pinquart, M. (2002). Creating and maintaining purpose in life in old age: A meta-analysis. *Ageing International, 27*(2), 90–114.

Polivka, L. (2000). Postmodern aging and the loss of meaning. *Journal of Aging and Identity, 5*(4), 225–235.

Steptoe, A., Deaton, A., & Stone, A. A. (2015). Subjective wellbeing, health, and ageing. *Lancet, 385*(9968), 640–648.

Wong, P. T. P. (1989). Successful aging and personal meaning. *Canadian Psychology, 30*, 516–525.

Wong, P. T. P. (1998). Spirituality, meaning, and successful aging. In P. T. P. Wong & P. Fry (Eds.), *The human quest for meaning: A handbook of psychological research and clinical applications* (pp. 359–394). Mahwah, NJ: Erlbaum.

CHAPTER 13

Personality Patterns and Syndromes in the Elderly

PE Axis

CHAPTER EDITORS

Franco Del Corno, MPhyl, DPsych **Daniel Plotkin, MD**

CONSULTANTS

Emanuela Brusadelli, PhD Alessia Zoppi, PhD

Introduction

Like the adult P Axis (see Chapter 1), the PE Axis represents a "map" of personality styles, designed to facilitate clinical understanding—in this case, of older adults. Since older adults have traditionally been excluded from studies of personality, this map remains one of relatively uncharted territory. Thus important questions remain unanswered, such as these: Do personality styles remain stable or change over the life course? How do personality styles interact with the physical, cognitive, and other conditions that are so common in old age? Do diagnosable personality disorders occur for the first time in old age? Are certain personalities more likely to be associated with "successful aging" and/or longevity? Fortunately, as noted by Oldham and Skodol (2013, p. 709), "there is increasing interest in, and an accumulating body of knowledge about, the longitudinal course of personality traits and personality disorders . . . and the interaction of these uniquely defining features of who we are with cognitive functioning, mood states, and patterns of behavior in later life."

Prevalence estimates of personality disorders among the elderly vary by setting, with estimates of 2.8–13% of elderly persons in the community, 5–33% of elderly outpatients, and 7–61.5% of elderly inpatients (van Alphen, Engelen, Kuin, & Derksen,

2006). Findings from the U.S. National Epidemiologic Survey on Alcohol and Related Conditions indicate that approximately 8% of American older adults (65 years of age and older) have at least one personality disorder, with the most common being obsessive–compulsive personality disorder. Some studies find that 17% of elderly patients present with obsessive–compulsive personality disorder and 12% with avoidant personality disorder, as opposed to only 5% with borderline personality disorder (Mordekar & Spence, 2008).

The PDM-2 PE Axis differs from the *Diagnostic and Statistical Manual of Mental Disorders* (DSM) and *International Classification of Diseases* (ICD) systems in focusing on people rather than disorders, and on (1) *level* of personality organization and (2) personality *style* or *pattern*. The level of organization ranges from primitive and psychotic to mature and realistic. Characteristics of wisdom, resilience, and integrity (Eriksonian, as in integrity vs. despair) are particularly relevant in the elderly. The term "personality styles" or "personality patterns" relates to clinically familiar personality types that cross-cut levels of personality organization. Of course, personality assessment is a challenging area, reflecting nuances and complexities of human beings. To complicate the picture further, DSM-5 (American Psychiatric Association, 2013) reflects changes in the diagnostic criteria for personality disorders. Prior versions of DSM have used a categorical perspective, based on the notion that personality disorders are qualitatively distinct clinical syndromes (and DSM-5 still identifies 10 such disorders). However, a dimensional perspective has been favored by most researchers and clinicians, and this perspective is also presented in DSM-5 (albeit in Section III, "Emerging Measures and Models," as opposed to the main diagnostic criteria in Section II), with 6 rather than 10 disorders identified. The result is not particularly relevant or useful for older adults, with phrases such as "personality change due to another medical condition" included and no mention of "late-onset personality disorders" (van Alphen, Rossi, Dierckx, & Oude Voshaar, 2014).

Prior work in the area has tended to refer to DSM personality disorder clusters—Cluster A (odd–eccentric: paranoid, schizoid, schizotypal), Cluster B (dramatic–emotional: antisocial, borderline, histrionic, narcissistic), and Cluster C (anxious–fearful: avoidant, dependent, obsessive–compulsive). Another model of personality with a significant literature is the five-factor model (Costa & McRae, 1992), comprising the domains of (1) extraversion versus introversion, (2) agreeableness versus antagonism, (3) conscientiousness versus impulsivity, (4) neuroticism versus emotional stability, and (5) being open versus closed to experience. It is worth noting that the five-factor model is a dimensional, trait-based model of personality, and that it has been used in older adult populations. For example, some traits, such as neuroticism and extraversion, have been associated with depression, anxiety, and cognitive impairment in older adults (Abrams & Bromberg, 2007; Dar-Nimrod et al., 2012; Debast et al., 2014; Graham & Lachman, 2012; Lautenschlager & Förstl, 2007; Seivewright, Tyrer, & Johnson, 2002; van den Broeck, 2012). At the same time, low neuroticism and high extraversion may be associated with exceptional longevity (Andersen et al., 2013). Conscientiousness is also positively associated with longevity (Hill, Turiano, Hurd, Mroczek, & Roberts, 2011).

Regarding the question of whether personality disorders remain relatively stable or subject to change in older age groups, the concept of "heterotypic continuity" recognizes that mental disorders predict future episodes of other mental disorders (Gutiérrez et al., 2012; Karaklic & Bungener, 2010; Rosowsky, Abrams, & Zweig, 1999). Thus adults may maintain a stable basic core of a disorder, but it may change in its behavioral expression over time. Some traits may be exaggerated and stiffened, while others may diminish. So there would be a latent continuity, expressed through a behavioral discontinuity, according to a logic of "functional equivalence" (Debast et al., 2014).

With regard to personality traits, the presence and intensity of expression of some traits can evolve and change over the course of life (e.g., in old age, extraversion and conscientiousness are reduced), but the avoidance of harm increases. With regard to personality disorders, DSM Cluster A types may increase in older adults, especially the paranoid and schizoid disorders (Gutiérrez et al., 2012; Rosowsky et al., 1999). DSM Cluster B types decrease with aging, including borderline personality disorder and impulsive disorders (Abrams & Horowitz, 1999; Coolidge, Segal, Hook, & Stewart, 2000; Oltmanns & Balsis, 2010, 2011; Seivewright et al., 2002; Singleton, Meltzer, Gatward, Coid, & Deasy, 1998; Stevenson, Meares, & Comerford, 2003; van Alphen et al., 2006). DSM Cluster C types, characterized by anxious–resistant behaviors, tend to worsen in old age.

It is not currently known whether diagnostic criteria and instruments designed for younger adults will be a good match for older adults, but in general it appears that modifications will be necessary. At least one group is currently studying a diagnostic instrument, the Gerontological Personality Disorder Scale (Penders, Rossi, Metsemakers, Duimel-Peeters, & van Alphen, 2015), designed specifically for use with older adults. An important challenge will be to differentiate "normal" aspects of aging from potentially pathological or unhealthy behaviors. For example, an older man who reduces his social life and contacts may appear to have schizoid traits, but may actually prefer to stay alone and reduce his social contacts for many reasons: diminished energy, some physical deficits, and the consequences of specific life events (retirement, widowerhood). In such a case, it would be a mistake to diagnose schizoid personality disorder. Another challenge will be to gather reliable information on an older individual's past life and functioning and relationships.

In conclusion, it is important to acknowledge that personality does not develop in a vacuum, but in a culture and society, so cultural issues are particularly relevant when considering personality and aging. Clearly, there are different sensibilities and expectations in different cultures, and these play an important role in such considerations as whether an aged widowed parent will live in a house with family members or in a residential facility (Caldwell, Low, & Brodaty, 2014). In Western cultures, there is an emphasis on youth, beauty, independence, and productivity. In Eastern cultures, there is more of a sense of duty, harmony, and respect for elders, and dependency is less stigmatized. In Eastern cultures, loss of cognitive skills is not considered as pathological as in Western societies, so there is greater tolerance for cognitively impaired elders (Helman, 2005). Personal growth is more valued by older adults in Eastern cultures than in Western cultures, but a sense of purpose in life is lower in older adults in both Western and Eastern cultures (Karasawa et al., 2011). Older adults tend to be motivated to maximize positivity across cultures, yet Western older adults maximize positivity in a more pronounced way than do Eastern older adults (Grossmann, Karasawa, Kan, & Kitayama, 2014). In general, with urbanization and modernity there is a shift, so that older adults tend to have lower status than they have traditionally had in smaller, rural societies.

In the remainder of this chapter, we describe every personality type according to the structure of the P Axis in adults (see Chapter 1), and we attempt to address the following issues:

- The possible age-related behavioral features that may confound the diagnosis of a personality pattern or disorder.
- The particular expressions of a personality style or disorder which are the results of the process of aging, as opposed to previous pathological personality functioning.
- The specific features of the process of aging in the presence of some personality styles or disorders—that is, the impact of the personality functioning on the life of the individual in old age.

The different levels of personality organization, described in detail in Chapter 1, can be applied also to the elderly and can be useful for clinical assessment. The aging process may increase the severity of certain symptoms and behaviors typical of the various pathological personalities, or, in certain cases, can reduce the extent and the amount of pain subjectively felt or objectively observed. This means that even the elderly may move from less developed to more advanced levels of personality organization (or vice versa) due to life events specific to old age, as well as to age-related physical, psychological, and cognitive modifications. In most cases, however, what changes are the behavioral manifestations and the prevalent emotions connected to the level of personality organization typical of a patient in his or her earlier adulthood.

It is well known that the aging process offers countless changes in an individual's life—certainly more frequent and incisive changes than those that have occurred during middle age—and that these changes may worsen a person's level of personality organization or its manifestations. Conversely, there are also some objective opportunities for disengagement (from social relations, professional commitments, or intimate relationships) that, in certain personalities, encourage better adaptation. This complex interplay between objective variables and personality organization is an important reason for reflecting on the clinical features of different personality styles in old age.

PE-Axis Personality Syndromes

Depressive Personalities, Including Hypomanic Variants

Potential Diagnostic Biases Related to Age

Of course, depressive personalities should not be confused with major depressive disorder or depression associated with dementia (see Chapter 14 on the SE Axis). A correct diagnosis of this class of personality patterns is complicated in the elderly because of the prevalence of depressive disorders and the frequency of stressful events that can lead to overlapping depressive symptoms. Stressful events and circumstances include loss of relationships, declining functional status, declining health status, retirement, moving, and social isolation. Indeed, depressive problems may be overlooked in older adults because of assumptions that depression is "normal" for older adults. Some older adults may also have a genetic constitutional predisposition to depression (Alexopoulos, 2005). It may be particularly difficult to distinguish between chronic depressive illness and depressive personality. Also, older adults may reduce their social networks in what has been termed "relational pruning," which may not be representative of depressive illness. Generally, however, a clinical history of depressive personality increases the risk of depressive reactions to various age-specific events. Often such a person's spouse or other family members have played a compensatory role that cushioned pathological traits, which may emerge when the spouse dies or the children get married (isolation in the moment of the "empty nest"). Even retirement can trigger a depressive response because work can provide a protective context.

The counterpart of depressive traits is hypomanic behavior—that is, an increase and acceleration of activities, amplification of emotions, and increases in the speed and superficiality of thoughts and projects, not justified by toxicological causes or other medical conditions. Exaggerated behaviors may emerge, and they can put a person in vulnerable situations (Segal, Coolidge, & Rosowsky, 2006). Also, inadequate relational patterns and misconduct may be present. All these behaviors are characterized by euphoria and should not be confused with other disorders linked to neurocognitive impairments. Moreover, they may represent a relational style rather than a real mood disorder, and the alternation between the depressive/self-defeating approach and the hypomanic one is different from the cycling seen in a bipolar disorder (see Chapter 14 on the SE Axis).

Masochistic (self-defeating) individuals are less frequent among elderly people. Self-sabotaging behaviors are more easily expressed, for example, in the working environment or within romantic relationships; retirement and the narrowing of opportunities to meet new romantic partners decrease the incidence of this version of the depressive personality.

Features of Depressive Personalities in Older Adults

The central issue of depressive personalities, in the elderly as in younger adults, is the perception of the self as defective, bad, and unlikable. This perception has a significant impact on the imagined judgments of others, whose rejection is strongly feared. A self-fulfilling prophecy can lead to social isolation and feelings of rejection. Alternatively, a very active social calendar can be maintained as a compensation for underlying fears.

In the elderly, the mechanism of negative self-attribution (which is often connected to the self-defeating attitude) emerges in relation to regrets/guilt/missed opportunities of the past. Such individuals talk about themselves through recriminations (e.g., "I have not been able to . . ."). Current loneliness is felt to be a result of past malice or selfishness. Compensations may include religiosity and helping others, to assuage underlying feelings of worthlessness. Failures of these compensatory investments may lead to a profound and catastrophic sense of loneliness that may develop into major depression.

Age-related impairments are difficult to accept. Psychosomatic symptoms or particular anguish may emerge, as well as obsessive thoughts of abandonment, death, or obligatory loneliness (Costa, Weiss, Duberstein, Friedman, & Siegler, 2014; Wongpakaran, Wongpakaran, Boonyanaruthee, Pinyopornpanish, & Intaprasert, 2015). Unwelcome anger and resentment toward others can also emerge in various situations. These feelings appear to be directed toward the environment, but the fundamental belief concerns personal errors, limits, and past mistakes.

Even in old age, it is clinically relevant to make the distinction between two different types of depressive affects, the introjective and the anaclitic (Blatt, 2004, 2008). Their nuclear characteristics are comparable to those found for depressive personalities in adulthood (see Chapter 1 on the P Axis), and they have different effects on the process of aging.

Introjectively depressive individuals, whose clinical history is characterized by feelings of guilt, self-criticism, and perfectionism, fare badly with age-related decreases in physical, psychological, and cognitive resources. Their feelings of inadequacy and emptiness are consequently emphasized, stiffening their depressive mood.

Anaclitically depressive individuals, with a clinical history characterized by feelings of inadequacy, emptiness, and needs for relationships and intimacy, show high reactivity to life events such as loss, separation, and grief, which for them are particularly difficult to elaborate and accept. The main features of their depressive condition are feelings of despair and complaints of hopelessness and loneliness.

Of course, these differences must also be kept in mind in the choice of treatments. More generally, it can be quite useful to understand whether a patient's prevalent psychological orientation, independent of his or her personality style, is anaclitic or introjective (again, see Chapter 1).

Impact of Depressive Personalities on the Process of Aging

Of course, comorbid mental disorders such as generalized anxiety and depression may occur; such disorders in old age have a significant impact on cognitive functioning and can lead to marked slowdown and loss of residual tasks (Alexopoulos, 2005; Fiske, Wetherell, & Gatz, 2009; Vink, Aartsen, & Schoevers, 2008). If there is a previous history of suicidal gestures, the combined condition of aging and depressive personality may provoke the reactivation of this risk, especially if adequate social support is lacking or there is a comorbid ongoing depressive disorder (Alexopoulos, Bruce, Hull, Sirey, & Kakuma, 1999; Chan, Chiu, Lam, Wong, & Conwell, 2014; Harwood, Hawton, Hope, & Jacoby, 2001). There are reports in the literature of concomitant alterations of the immune, endocrinological, and cardiac systems (Alexopoulos, 2005). Anxiety and depression may also speed up the development of markedly disabling neurocognitive disorders.

Suggestions for Treatment

Individuals with depressive personalities often do not receive adequate diagnosis and treatment because of subclinical presentations (depression and hypomanic symptoms are less evident and disabling than in major depressive or bipolar disorder).

The treatment of introjectively depressive patients must take into account the massive presence of negative feelings, which often threaten to affect clinicians as well. These patients often tend either to isolate themselves or to join other individuals who share their pessimism. If their clinicians attempt to counteract their negative feelings, they often react with irritation or drop out of treatment. Every therapeutic intervention with these individuals ends up being a balance between the effort to arouse any hope of change and the acceptance of the patients' difficulty in modifying their negative feelings.

As noted above, anaclitically depressive patients often react painfully to separation or abandonment, both real and imagined. A clinician must develop with such a patient a relationship characterized by attention and acceptance, with the aim of encouraging the recovery of personal resources and reducing dependency needs.

Finally, the main difficulty in treating hypomanic patients is linked to their use of defense mechanisms such as denial and reaction formation. The pervasive fear of experiencing depressive feelings should be both respected and worked through, in order to help these people to develop more adaptive skills and advanced capacities.

The "Key Features" box for adult depressive personalities in Chapter 1 on the P Axis (p. 33), listing patterns, preoccupations, pathogenic beliefs, and ways of defending, is also useful for understanding the core features of these personalities in the elderly. In the following table, we have expanded upon the Chapter 1 listing by adding a more detailed description of functioning in elderly depressive personalities, and comparing it with normal age-related personality functioning in older adults.

Key features	Depressive personality functioning in the elderly	Normal age-related personality functioning
Contributing constitutional–maturational patterns	A genetic predisposition to depression is possible. It is also important to ascertain previous episodes of subclinical mood disorders in the person's clinical history.	
Central tension/ preoccupation: Self-criticism and self-punitiveness or preoccupation with relatedness and loss (or both)	The person's judgments of his or her value are critical and dichotomous. Past episodes are remembered and reviewed, to discover faults and shortcomings, and thus to justify self-criticism; in other cases, an attitude of self-absolution triggers feelings of euphoria. Balanced judgments of either self or others are not frequent.	The aging process can lead to taking stock of past experiences and reflecting on personal worth and identity, but the judgments are generally not dichotomous, and individuals are not constantly preoccupied with their goodness–badness or worth–unworthiness.
Central affects: Sadness, guilt, shame	The age-related physical, emotional, and cognitive impairments, though often minor, trigger feelings of shame and sadness. Hypomanic reactions, if any, are usually short-lived and do not alleviate the suffering.	Feelings of shame or embarrassment are connected to specific physical impairments. The sense of guilt about the past, if any, is proportionate to the entirety of the events in which a person was involved.
Characteristic pathogenic belief about self: "There is something essentially bad or inadequate about me," "Someone or something necessary for well-being has been irretrievably lost"	The age-related decrease in physical and emotional resources reinforces the feeling of fragility and inadequacy. Often the attitude of renunciation is the answer in the face of difficulties, or the person devalues the results when he or she does agree to engage and do something.	The reaction to the difficulties related to age produces only sporadic feelings of sadness and guilt. The mood is generally appropriate to the situation and consistent with its identifiable specific causes.
Characteristic pathogenic belief about others: "People who really get to know me will reject me"	The person views possible adaptation to the environment and relationships, despite some physical or cognitive age-related impairments, as false and reprehensible. The fear of getting caught in his or her own fragility and of being rejected is always present. Others are experienced as intolerant and severe.	Shame and embarrassment may result from physical, emotional, and/or cognitive difficulties characterizing old age, but the sense of self remains undiminished, as does a confidence in the ability of others to appreciate the person's remaining qualities and tolerate deficiencies.
Central ways of defending Introjection, reversal, idealization of others, devaluation of self	Idealization of others' resources and devaluation of self are increased by the age-related decline in physical and cognitive abilities; aggression is directed toward the self.	The comparison with others' resources does not produce a symmetrical devaluation of a person's abilities, which indeed are recognized and utilized.

Dependent Personalities

Potential Diagnostic Biases Related to Age

In elderly people, the problem of dependency in its various behavioral and emotional expressions is central—not only to assessing the evolution of a possible previous dependent personality pattern, but also to understanding "functional and structural dependency" as an indispensable display of the elderly adult's needs (Townsend, 1981). Factors that are associated with the need for support and assistance (and related subjective reactions) are varied: loss of central relationships (e.g., spousal death and other causes of grief); "empty nest syndrome" (the children get married); outbreaks of disease; cognitive deficits; reduced autonomy; the natural age-related decrease of the emotional investment in daily life and in personal responsibilities; and so on.

The subjective tendency to respond with an attitude of dependency to the problems of age seems to correlate with different personality variables: the previous sense of autonomy, the capacity of emotional reactivity, the effectiveness of coping abilities, and the like (Gignac, Cott, & Badley, 2000).

In some cases (conditions of stress, health difficulties, environmental problems, etc.), elderly adults seem to regress to a state of dependency with the aim to survive and to safeguard themselves. This regression may not be indicative of a dependent personality disorder, but may be a natural response related to the manifold interactions between the aging process and living conditions (Segal et al., 2006). In the presence of neurocognitive disorders as well as severe physical limitations, older persons are inevitably and necessarily dependent on others, and the possible effect of a previous personality pattern or disorder is superimposed on real current difficulties (Agüero-Torres et al., 1998; Boström et al., 2014; Gignac et al., 2000; Jones, Wootton, & Vaccaro, 2012; Williamson & Schulz, 1988).

A specific diagnostic problem concerns the responses of dependency "induced" by institutionalization. Sometimes the elderly can benefit from entering a nursing home, in which their needs for physical and psychological support are satisfied by trained personnel. If relationships with children and other relatives are maintained, the elderly adults do not feel isolated and can appreciate the professional help, especially if they have illnesses that require continuous attention.

Of course, old people who have always been very independent and have favored their autonomy and distance from others will have different reactions. These persons may suffer from the unwelcome contact with their peers and may demonstrate closure and isolation, particularly if the institutionalization was partially forced. However, every institutionalization brings out the individual's personality with respect to the problem of dependency.

Sometimes it is difficult for a clinician to recognize a personality pattern or disorder alongside the expected age-related problems. As always, the history of previous periods of life acquires an important meaning in these cases; past manifestations of a dependent personality will help the clinician to properly assess the current psychopathological condition properly. In other words, the clinician has to consider the extent to which the attitude to dependency has been typical and stable over the years or has emerged with age.

Features of Dependent Personalities in Older Adults

Older adults with dependent personalities exhibit clinging behavior related to an excessive need to be taken care of. This is often associated with an internal experience of self as weak, fragile, frightened, and unable to handle the different tasks of life. The need for proximity is at the core of the relational request (Segal et al., 2006). Its starting point is the fear of loneliness, abandonment, death and a vision of the self as unable to stay alone. The features of this personality pattern are particularly marked when an older individual reacts to the death of his or her spouse (on whom the person has often depended in earlier periods of life); when children or grandchildren are less willing to take care of the person; or when other events related to the aging process (e.g., retirement) have produced conditions of greater isolation. Since older adults often have real and realistic physical, cognitive, and social challenges to face, it may be difficult to determine whether a diagnosis of dependent personality is warranted.

The dependent personality pattern may have comorbid depressive or anxious symptoms (Lawton & Oltmanns, 2013); it may also coexist with some specific fears (e.g., fear of falling), and separation anxiety symptoms related to children or grandchildren (Donald & Bulpitt, 1999; Wijeratne & Manicavasagar, 2003; Yur'yev et al., 2010). Separation anxiety is manifested by continuous needs for contacts and daily visits or phone calls for confirmation, support in making decisions, and discussions about fears and doubts. Of course, these symptoms may be worsened by the recent deaths of friends or family members (Wijeratne & Manicavasagar, 2003).

Often there is chronic anxiety in the histories of these individuals, as well as a marked dependency on familiar figures. Dependent persons are particularly submissive to others, and can request contact at the expense of the expression of their own needs, with the omission of important requirements related to health or well-being.

Sometimes dependency is characterized by an evident hostility, which represents the passive–aggressive aspect of the disorder. Oppositional behavior may occur, leading to an angry isolation (being grumpy, declining aid and social support, or self-neglect as in "Diogenes syndrome"), but also to alcohol or drug abuse (Saka, Kaya, Ozturk, Erten, & Karan, 2010; Tomstad, Söderhamn, Espnes, & Söderhamn, 2012).

Impact of Dependent Personalities on the Process of Aging

Dependency in old age, if pervasive enough to constitute a personality disorder, has important consequences for families and caregivers. Sometimes it can increase the risk for neglect/abuse of the "fragile" elderly (Agüero-Torres et al., 1998). Special conditions apply when elderly individuals need to be institutionalized. Various scenarios are possible. Some older adults can openly express to the staff their needs for affection and closeness; others at least initially show submissiveness and acquiescence; there are also request modes that become repetitive and petulant, generating boredom, fatigue, and burnout in caregivers (Baltes, Honn, Barton, Orzach, & Lago, 1983; Cobo, 2014; Segal et al., 2006).

Conversely, it may be very difficult to manage older individuals with a marked intolerance of dependency and an insistent need for autonomy because of their ambivalence and demands. Sometimes the requested autonomy is impossible because of various impairments that a person denies (e.g., the individual doesn't want to be washed, helped to eat, or moved in a wheelchair) (Caljouw, Cools, & Gussekloo, 2014). In such a case, the person may appear gruff and irritable.

In addition, institutionalization often produces a decrease in autonomy and quality of life. This may be due in part to the person's or institution's underestimation of available resources or to a nonfacilitating physical environment (Cobo, 2014). On the other hand, dependency can be regarded either as a loss of autonomy due to age-related impairments (Rodin & Langer, 1977), or as an instrument of control over the environment, to the extent that others respond to the person's requests and support him or her (Baltes et al., 1983). As indicated above, depressive disorders and chronic anxiety or panic attacks may be comorbid with dependent personalities in old age.

Suggestions for Treatment

In taking care of these patients, it is important to note that the attitudes of dependency and passive–aggressive counterdependency may alternate. Often, in the elderly, the frequency of this alternation can be increased by particular life events. For example, the worsening of disease symptoms or the reduction of specific physical and cognitive resources may increase the need for closeness and support; conflicts with spouse or children (or with care staff, if the elder is institutionalized) can accentuate irritability and withdrawal. For the clinician (and generally for the service personnel), the challenge lies in maintaining an adequate balance between addressing the demands of the patient and protecting his or her independence of judgment and autonomy of action.

The "Key Features" box for adult dependent personalities in Chapter 1 on the P Axis (p. 36), listing patterns, preoccupations, pathogenic beliefs, and ways of defending, is also useful for understanding the core features of these personalities in the elderly. In the following table, we have expanded upon the Chapter 1 listing by adding a more detailed description of functioning in elderly dependent personalities and comparing it with normal age-related personality functioning in older adults.

Key features	Dependent personality functioning in the elderly	Normal age-related personality functioning
Contributing constitutional–maturational patterns	Unknown.	
Central tension/ preoccupation: Keeping versus losing relationships.	The person emphasizes physical and psychological age-related difficulties as justified reasons for requesting closeness and support. Fear of abandonment induces the person to show him- or herself as weaker than he or she really is.	A call for help and support is made only when an actual physical or psychological difficulty limits personal autonomy. The individual appreciates the occasions when, despite some impairment, he or she can "go it alone."
Central affects	Feelings of weakness and powerlessness are prominent, increased by age-related difficulties.	The awareness of dependency needs, related to the difficulties associated with the process of aging, can produce requests for aid; however, these are never made at the expense of the autonomy allowed by one's personal resources.

Key features	Dependent personality functioning in the elderly	Normal age-related personality functioning
Characteristic pathogenic belief about self: "I am inadequate, needy, impotent" (including its conscious converse in passive–aggressive and counterdependent individuals).	The age-related difficulties worsen feelings of inadequacy and helplessness, as well as passive–aggressive behavior. Manifestations of excessive need for support and comfort are frequent in the person's previous clinical history.	The calls for help and support are proportional to the objective age-related difficulties. The person is aware of the resources that are not affected by age and uses them to preserve his or her autonomy.
Characteristic pathogenic belief about others: "Others are powerful, and I need (but may resent) their care."	The person continually uses the image of the "poor old man/woman" to compare his or her own weakness to the strength of others. This comparison can produce feelings of anger and resentment.	The person can use the resources of family and friends to make up for the effects of age-related reduced autonomy. Feelings of gratitude for the help received can be openly expressed.
Central ways of defending: Regression, reversal, avoidance, somatization.	Age-related physical, cognitive, and emotional difficulties worsen the regression and avoidance tendencies that are already present in the person's previous clinical history. In the counterdependent/passive–aggressive version of this personality pattern, reaction formations and pseudoindependence may be present.	Marked attitudes of dependency are not present in the person's previous clinical history. Sporadic regressive attitudes and avoidance behaviors are normal responses to age-related decreases in autonomy.

Anxious–Avoidant and Phobic Personalities

Potential Diagnostic Biases Related to Age

Anxiety is common in the elderly (Alwahhabi, 2003) and may be traced back to earlier life experiences, including childhood separation anxiety (Milrod et al., 2014). Indeed, anxiety is a frequent component of a wide range of personality styles (Shedler & Westen, 2004). Generally, however, it is relatively easy to distinguish the characteristics of a clearly pathological anxiety from the emotional strain often related to cognitive and physical challenges of the aging process. In the case of anxious–avoidant and phobic personalities, the differential diagnosis may be more difficult.

In DSM-5 (American Psychiatric Association, 2013), avoidant personality disorder presents some specific features (e.g., being socially inhibited and feeling inadequate, with a resulting diminution in social contacts) that should not be confused with the reduction in the social network commonly seen in normal aging. Moreover, faced with new situations, experiences, and social relations, an elderly person may develop anxious attitudes and, at times, phobic manifestations; again, however, these do not characterize the person's whole relationship with the environment or all activities of everyday life. This category includes cautious attitudes toward situations that the person fears can worsen his or her sometimes already poor health and resources (refusal of certain foods, activities, places, etc.). Also, some difficulties with new technologies and devices may produce specific avoidant behaviors (e.g., when an older adult continues a professional career and is confronted in the workplace with changes requiring technological skills that may be difficult to learn). Resultant withdrawal and avoidance in these situations are not necessarily indicative of avoidant personality. Likewise, we should not forget that some typical concerns of the elderly (e.g., being criticized or marginalized in social situations), as well as some reasons for embarrassment (e.g., decreased sensory abilities or motor skills), cannot be diagnosed as evidence of problematic personality functioning, but must be traced to common physical difficulties associated with aging.

A differential diagnosis must also be made between anxious–avoidant behavior and schizoid personality, as well as social phobia (Gretarsdottir, Woodruff-Borden, Meeks, & Depp, 2004). Individuals with schizoid personality are generally at ease in their state of isolation, while avoidant individuals fear social contacts with others but yearn for closer contact; feelings of shyness and embarrassment about social contacts are much more pervasive and persistent (experienced not only with people, but also in regard to places, situations, etc.) in anxious–avoidant personalities than in social phobia.

Finally, it is worth nothing that some older people are able to enjoy their isolation and deliberately choose it. "Clinicians should assess whether the isolation is due to adventitious circumstances (e.g., losses, illness), choice, or life-long traits of shyness, timidity, and inhibition (the latter being indicative of personality pathology)" (Segal et al., 2006, p. 107).

Features of Anxious–Avoidant and Phobic Personalities in Older Adults

Typically, in adults, the features of an anxious–avoidant personality pattern include social inhibition, shyness, and diffidence, as well as ambivalence between desire and fear of relationships. These feelings may become more intense in old age because of diminished self-confidence, in part due to decreased physical, cognitive, and emotional resources (Coolidge et al., 2000). Sometimes anxiety itself is experienced by an older adult as an unbearable emotion, which can be controlled only by withdrawing from relationships with others and from unknown situations.

The tendency toward isolation makes it more challenging for older adults to receive needed assistance and support from others. This may be particularly problematic when medical/physical conditions become more severe and/or when an older adult needs to be hospitalized or institutionalized.

Impact of Anxious–Avoidant and Phobic Personalities on the Process of Aging

Social isolation and withdrawal may increase the risk of developing depression and anxiety disorders. When events that are common in later life occur (losses, retirement, widowhood, decreased availability of children, etc.), an avoidant attitude makes it more difficult for older adults to receive help and support. Furthermore, avoidant older adults may have relatively few opportunities to establish new relationships that, at least in part, could replace those lost.

As Segal and colleagues (2006, p. 107) write, these older adults are "isolated but desperately lonely, too shy to seek warmth and comfort from others."

Suggestions for Treatment

Even in situations where help is needed (for physical or psychological difficulties), anxiety may be prominent and may induce withdrawal rather than a willingness to engage in relationships. In every contact with nurses, doctors, and other helping professionals, the fear of judgment and the constant embarrassment may be obstacles that are difficult to overcome. An attitude of assertiveness and of empathy with these fears can help such a person to build a relationship with a clinician, which can serve as a starting point to experience more extensive contacts in everyday life (van Alphen, 2011).

In a therapeutic relationship, another attitude must be expected: An anxious older adult can develop an excessive neediness and dependence on a clinician or other health care worker. This development highlights the need for contact and relationship that is hidden behind the avoidance. In such cases, it is challenging to strike a balance between maintaining a therapeutic distance and gratifying the patient's compelling needs.

The "Key Features" box for adult anxious–avoidant and phobic personalities in Chapter 1 on the P Axis (p. 38), listing patterns, preoccupations, pathogenic beliefs, and ways of defending, is also useful for understanding the core features of these personalities in the elderly. In the following table, we have expanded upon the Chapter 1 listing by adding a more detailed description of functioning in elderly anxious–avoidant and phobic personalities and comparing it with normal age-related personality functioning in older adults.

Key features	Anxious–avoidant and phobic personality functioning in the elderly	Normal age-related personality functioning
Contributing constitutional–maturational patterns	The person's clinical history reveals the presence of an anxious temperament and a propensity to withdrawal.	
Central tension/ preoccupation: Safety versus danger.	The issue of safety and the fear of dangers are in the foreground, and almost all behavioral choices are driven by these concerns.	The physical and emotional difficulties related to the aging process increase the need for safety and caution, especially in dealing with unusual situations or new relationships. However, this attitude is not pervasive and gives way to feelings of curiosity and to the need for new experiences.
Central affects	The anxiety dominates behaviors and attitudes, regardless of actual degrees of risk in situations. The age-related impairments increase the feeling of danger associated with diminished self-confidence.	When the interaction with the environment highlights the person's scarcity of resources linked to the aging process, anxiety may be evident, but it will be sporadic and not pervasive.

Key features	Anxious–avoidant and phobic personality functioning in the elderly	Normal age-related personality functioning
Characteristic pathogenic belief about self: "I am in constant danger that I must somehow elude."	Old age is seen as a threat to the person's integrity and capacity to react to challenges and threats. The person's reactions are not realistic requests for help, or attempts to enhance physical and psychological resources. Avoidant behaviors take priority over consideration of the price to be paid for such behaviors (isolation, loneliness, depression, etc.).	Feelings of insecurity linked to the vulnerability of old age are not pervasive. The choice of avoidant behaviors to cope with anxiety-inducing situations is carefully evaluated before it is applied.
Characteristic pathogenic belief about others: "Others are sources of either unimagined dangers or magical protection."	The person has feelings of shame linked to numerous physical and psychological aspects of aging. The judgment of others is feared because it is assumed to be negative and humiliating. Sometimes an attitude of submission is used to ward off anxiety.	The fear of being judged by others is related to situations and events that can be realistic sources of embarrassment (sensory and motor difficulties, impediments to performing normal physiological functions, etc.). The person is, however, still able to distinguish his or her identity from these adverse occurrences, and also has confidence in the capacity of others to understand and support him or her.
Central ways of defending: Symbolization, displacement, avoidance, rationalization; inchoate anxieties may mask more upsetting specific anxieties (i.e., anxiety itself may be defensive).	Avoidance behaviors and phobias are rationalized to justify the withdrawal; denial and other primitive defenses are utilized.	Stiffening of defenses and phobic avoidance are sporadic and related to specific situations that the elderly person perceives as stressful. The suggestions of others to establish relationships and enter new experiences are carefully evaluated and accepted or rejected on the basis of realistic motives.

Obsessive–Compulsive Personalities

Potential Diagnostic Biases Related to Age

Obsessive–compulsive personality applies when an individual is preoccupied with orderliness, control, details, and rules. Its association with rigidity, a quality often associated with aging, leads to diagnostic challenges in older adults who suffer from anxiety-related conditions. Indeed, the negative stereotype of rigidity in old age is a common belief among old people themselves (Levy, 2008). It is further complicated because, in general, the symptoms of obsessive–compulsive personality (like those of other personality patterns, such as paranoid) increase in old age. The obsessive–compulsive personality pattern or disorder is often chronic and stable; it may occur in comorbidity with obsessive–compulsive disorder (OCD) or other conditions involving anxiety or psychosis (Barton, Karner, Salih, Baldwin, & Edwards, 2014; Calamari et al., 2014). It can also appear in old age in the presence of neurocognitive symptoms or disorders (behavioral and psychological symptoms of dementia; frontotemporal syndromes; and "Diogenes syndrome" or hoarding) (Cervellati et al., 2013; Low, Brodaty, & Draper, 2002; Sabbe & Vandenbulcke, 2014). Moreover, patients with Parkinson's disease present with an increased frequency of obsessive–compulsive personality disorder (Nicoletti et al., 2013). In addition, some symptoms associated with OCD and obsessive–compulsive personality (such as those in Tourette syndrome) may reappear in old age, even after reportedly being absent for more than 40 years (Shprecher, Rubenstein, Gannon, Frank, & Kurlan, 2014).

One important issue is the applicability of the DSM-5 diagnostic criteria for obsessive–compulsive personality disorder to the elderly. For example, perfectionism and solipsistic/defensive isolation at work may not be evident in a retired person. Similarly, the criterion involving miserliness and hoarding of money may be of limited use with older individuals, many of whom are financially conservative. The current generation of older adults includes many very frugal individuals who grew up during the Great Depression years (the 1930s), which greatly affected their habits and character. Also, poverty is often a part of aging, and the resulting penurious perspective is not indicative of obsessive–compulsive personality. On the contrary, a history of greed in wealthy individuals throughout life is a major index of obsessive–compulsive personality (Segal et al., 2006). Another issue that cannot be easily applied to the elderly is the preference to act alone rather than with other people; often this preference is due to bereavements and losses or to age-related reduction of social contacts.

The presence of an obsessive–compulsive personality style in a person's previous clinical history generally facilitates the diagnosis in old age. Some constitutional patterns remain stable: These individuals may be irritable, touchy, meticulous, demanding, perfectionist, greedy, stubborn, rigid, orderly, conscientious, and moralizing. The mechanisms of intellectualization and moralization can also remain stable, and are often actually enhanced by the role that older people play in society. One last important diagnostic point is the need to evaluate the level of organization of the subject's personality. In fact, the obsessive style, expressed at a cognitive level with obsessions, may cover different underlying personality organizations: A serious borderline level can facilitate the emergence of marked OCD symptoms up to psychosis; a neurotic level can favor the appearance of anxiety and depression.

Features of Obsessive–Compulsive Personalities in Older Adults

Obsessive and compulsive thoughts and behaviors can change in content over time, but not in their meaning and structure; they can also exhibit a marked resistance to treatment, especially the obsessive aspects. Delusions, anxiety, and depression can also emerge (Ayers et al., 2014; Kichuk et al., 2013). In old age, people with obsessive–compulsive personalities may express traits of control through specific demands related to the management of their space and/or objects at home; they don't want these to be touched, moved, cleaned, or changed. They can also have specific difficulties in discarding worthless objects (old newspapers, envelopes, boxes, etc.), generating phenomena of compulsive hoarding, which is sometimes a significant public health problem (Ayers et al., 2014; Turner, Steketee, & Nauth, 2010). Finally, these individuals may refuse to be compared with others/controlled by others and may manifest childish attitudes, rigidity of thought, intransigence, and refusal to recognize their difficulties or impairments. This means that often they are alone and isolated, and they may respond to this with deep depression. They may also develop delusions, sometimes of a paranoid type (fears of being robbed, cheated, spied on, etc.). Often their life histories indicate a significant intellectual path that has had a protective role with respect to the issue of control, and that recurs in old age in the form of "stiffening of attitudes."

Impact of Obsessive–Compulsive Personalities on the Process of Aging

These individuals often become extremely dependent on family care or others, and this relational need is tackled in a hard and painful way. They hate change and any other form of external demand that breaks their routine. If they need drug therapy, they need to exercise stiff control over prescription and doses (Bloch et al., 2013; Grant, Mancebob, & Weinhandlc, 2013). When they are hospitalized or enter a nursing home, an increase in this rigidity may occur because of the forced increase in dependency. They also find it difficult to change the rhythm of life and of daily tasks, and feel great suffering if they have to move away from their usual structured environment. Sometimes attitudes such as "I am old; I know how things are; I lived things" can emerge; these can be highly demeaning and devaluing not only of younger health care personnel, but also of younger family members who must assume increased care of a person after the death of his or her spouse.

Suggestions for Treatment

These individuals are very resistant to treatment, in old age as in youth. The obsessive–compulsive symptomatology tends to become chronic, and it increases the risk of developing dementia, functional disability, and marginalization (Barton et al., 2014). Considerable time is required to free these patients, even only partially, from the siege of their concerns about control. Their perceived age-related weakness and impairments make this task even more difficult. Interventions designed to ameliorate environmental situations that threaten such a person may prove useful and increase the possibility of forming a therapeutic alliance. For example, practical, tangible help with organizing clothes or other objects and compensating for age-related sensory deficits may lead to decreased agitation and decreased compulsive behavior.

The "Key Features" box for adult obsessive–compulsive personalities in Chapter 1 on the P Axis (p. 40), listing patterns, preoccupations, pathogenic beliefs, and ways of defending, is also useful for understanding the core features of these personalities in the elderly. In the following table, we have expanded upon the Chapter 1 listing by adding a more detailed description of functioning in elderly obsessive–compulsive personalities and comparing it with normal age-related personality functioning in older adults.

Key features	Obsessive–compulsive personality functioning in the elderly	Normal age-related personality functioning
Contributing constitutional–maturational patterns	The clinical history includes rigidity, irritability, and constant preoccupation with orderliness, cleanliness, and control over others/ the environment.	

Key features	Obsessive–compulsive personality functioning in the elderly	Normal age-related personality functioning
Central tension/ preoccupation: Submission to versus rebellion against controlling authority.	The issue of control, over both the self and others, is essential. The aging process is seen as a threat to the ability to exercise control, and this leads to a stiffening of the obsessive concerns and compulsions.	A decrease in the person's control over the self and the environment is part of the difficulties that must be addressed in the process of aging. Elderly people can put in place a series of behaviors in order to reassure themselves about their ability to manage different situations, but adequate flexibility is maintained, and suggestions from others are taken into account to produce changes in attitudes and reactions.
Central affects: Anger, guilt, shame, fear.	Feelings of fear, shame, and anger are addressed through ruminative and intellectualized thoughts or through actions designed to exert control. The person responds angrily to any attempt to interfere with this attitude, and stiffens the repetitive thoughts and behaviors.	Some repetitive concerns and behaviors are meant to reassure the elderly when faced with new situations or unknown environments (such as a hospital or a nursing home). A healthy older adult is still capable of adapting his or her reactions to the situation at hand and is able to accept help from others.
Characteristic pathogenic belief about self: "Most feelings are dangerous and must be controlled."	There is constant fear of losing control, increased by the perception of age-related cognitive, emotional, and physical weaknesses. Emotions and impulses are perceived as dangerous and possibly avoided.	The age-related decreases in control over the self and the environment are mostly accepted. Feelings of sorrow or regret for the resources of the past are not avoided, but can be considered and communicated.
Characteristic pathogenic belief about others: "Others are less precise and in control than I am, so I have to control what they do and resist being controlled by them."	The age-related increased dependence on others directs the person's attention to the accuracy and reliability of the others' behavior. These judgments are mostly negative, and the person tries to increase his or her control to overcome the shortcomings of others.	The need to rely on others (spouse, children, nurses, etc.) leads an elderly person to pay attention to his or her behavior. However, the person is able to recognize when others behave appropriately for his or her needs, and is willing to tolerate some imprecision and delay without feeling forced to rely solely on his or her ability to control everything and everyone.
Central ways of defending: Isolation of affect, reaction formation, intellectualizing, moralizing, undoing.	Several defense mechanisms are utilized to avoid awareness of emotions, urges, and impulses, and to maintain control over one's own and other people's behavior. The need for certainty and precision causes a distortion of thoughts and actions.	The person may express a desire to avoid strong emotions, as well as desires and needs that cannot be satisfied because of age. Defenses such as reaction formation or isolation of affect may be present, but mostly in relation to specific situations of stress; the need for control is adequate to situations, and compulsive behaviors are absent or sporadic.

Schizoid Personalities

Potential Diagnostic Biases Related to Age

The process of aging is often associated with the strengthening of personality traits similar to those of schizoid personalities. For example, older adults may reduce the number and range of their relationships—perhaps as a result of a propensity to emotional detachment (Lang, 2001), but more likely in order to maximize their emotional rewards (Carstensen, Isaacowitz, & Charles, 1999). Moreover, some sensory impairments common in later life (e.g., hearing and vision deficits) can restrict social contacts. Some typical events of old age (retirement, widowhood, and other losses) contribute further to reduced social contacts. Finally, there is diminished interest in sexual experiences, though in older adults it can be related to the lack of suitable partners as well as to the normal age-related decrease in libido.

Thus the challenge is to distinguish between the reduced social network that is sometimes associated with aging and the features of schizoid personality. What makes this distinction less challenging for the clinician is the mental status examination, which reveals the particular and specific kinds of withdrawal, detachment, flattened affectivity, and emotional coldness that characterize schizoid individuals and differentiate them from older adults who may simply be socially isolated.

Furthermore, individuals with schizoid personalities may be placed on a continuum from high-functioning to severely disordered (Badcock & Dragović, 2006; Bora & Arabaci, 2009).

Features of Schizoid Personalities in Older Adults

Some of the changes that are associated with aging (e.g., retirement or widowhood) may actually be better tolerated by older schizoid individuals, who have a reduced need for social contact, than they are by normal older adults (Stevens, 1995; van Tilburg, 1992). For older individuals who may have schizoid personality disorder, an important condition to consider in the differential diagnosis is late-onset schizophrenia (please see Chapter 14 on the SE Axis for a full discussion).

Impact of Schizoid Personalities on the Process of Aging

Individuals with schizoid personalities may find it particularly difficult to cope with some of the events that are common in old age, such as being hospitalized or moving to a retirement home or skilled nursing facility. The increased dependency needs that are usually precursors to such placements may be very difficult for older schizoid individuals to tolerate. In addition, the sensory deficits of old age are associated with an increased need for assistance and with reduced independence, both of which are challenging for these individuals.

Suggestions for Treatment

As in younger patients, the treatment of schizoid older adults must allow both a certain level of emotional intimacy and respect of their needs for adequate interpersonal space. With a seriously disturbed patient with a marked schizoid component, it is necessary to take into account frequent moments of withdrawal and closure; the clinician must not force the person into intimacy, but at the same time must communicate to the patient an attitude of availability.

The "Key Features" box for adult schizoid personalities in Chapter 1 on the P Axis (p. 42), listing patterns, preoccupations, pathogenic beliefs, and ways of defending, is also useful for understanding the core features of these personalities in the elderly. In the following table, we have expanded upon the Chapter 1 listing by adding a more detailed description of functioning in elderly schizoid personalities and comparing it with normal age-related personality functioning in older adults.

Key features	Schizoid personality functioning in the elderly	Normal age-related personality functioning
Contributing constitutional–maturational patterns	Withdrawal from relationships and poor emotional investments are seen. There is a previous history of withdrawal and hypersensitivity to stimuli.	
Central tension/ preoccupation: Fear of closeness versus longing for closeness.	The ambivalent attitude toward relationships and intimacy with others (fear of closeness vs. longing for closeness) continues. Sometimes intellectualization and the use of metaphors, artistic and/or literary references, and the like replace the communication of feelings and emotions.	Overcoming momentary conditions of difficulty coincides with the recovery of motivation toward relationships.
Central affects: General emotional pain when overstimulated; affects so powerful that persons feel they must suppress them.	The presence of others is seen as overly challenging and is usually avoided. There is little expression of interest in the thoughts, emotions, or behaviors of others.	Albeit with moments of retreat (especially as a defense related to stressful situations), there remains a desire for positive stimuli. The decrease in sexual needs does not affect the desire for relationships and emotional intimacy.
Characteristic pathogenic belief about self: "Dependency and love are dangerous."	Self-esteem is preserved only in a state of almost total self-sufficiency. Offers of help produce anxiety, discomfort, and irritation.	The sense of autonomy strengthens self-esteem, and attempts to "go it alone" are rewarding, but offers of help are accepted and used when needed.
Characteristic pathogenic belief about others: "The social world is impinging, dangerously engulfing."	The need to keep others at a distance may produce inappropriate behavior and endanger the person's health or physical integrity. The attentions of others are perceived with annoyance, even when they are needed to make up for shortcomings or difficulties related to age. The refusal to accept help may increase vulnerability to situations of neglect and isolation.	There may be periods of withdrawal in response to decreases in mental and physical resources, or as reactions to changes in activity and quality of life. The avoidance of dependence on others serves to preserve self-esteem, but age-related limitations are generally accepted. Appropriate interpersonal skills and investments can be found in previous personal history.

Key features	Schizoid personality functioning in the elderly	Normal age-related personality functioning
Central ways of defending: Withdrawal, both physically and into fantasy and idiosyncratic preoccupations.	Withdrawal, closure, and justification of behavior are based on idiosyncratic reasons and maintained with considerable rigidity in reaction to different stimuli and conditions.	Defenses of withdrawal and disinvestment are motivated by specific events and justifiable conditions. The inventory of defenses against relational anxiety is quite broad and flexible.

Somatizing Personalities

Potential Diagnostic Biases Related to Age

DSM-5 does not include a diagnosis of somatizing personality disorder, but it does have a new diagnostic category called somatic symptom and related disorders. This new category includes several diagnoses that share the following characteristics: distressing somatic symptoms, accompanied by abnormal thoughts about and preoccupations with the symptoms. Previous editions of DSM emphasized medically unexplained symptoms; this emphasis on the lack of something (i.e., the lack of a satisfactory medical explanation for symptoms) presented unnecessary confusion and complications in making these diagnoses. In the first PDM, a somatizing personality disorder was posited, and it remains on the P Axis in PDM-2, with the caveat that "some scholars see this kind of clinical presentation as outside the personality spectrum" (Chapter 1, p. 42).

Since older adults generally have several chronic medical conditions, and have some symptoms associated with those conditions, it is a challenge to distinguish between a normal concern about these symptoms and an abnormal preoccupation with somatic difficulties. The latter preoccupation characterizes individuals with somatizing personality disorder. Of course, many medical conditions are comorbid with psychological symptoms, and this makes the diagnosis even more complex (Parmelee, Harralson, McPherron, & Ralph Schumacher, 2013).

For a diagnosis of a somatizing personality, the starting point is the individual's medical history, as well as the observation of his or her current behavior. Some indicators of a possible somatizing personality should be considered if the following apply (Mailis-Gagnon, Nicholson, Yegneswaran, & Zurowski, 2008):

- Bodily complaints are not associated with an identified disease or appear to be connected to many different diseases.
- The patient implements avoidance behaviors or social isolation and justifies them with the bodily difficulties.
- The patient enacts a bizarre behavior that is incongruous with the actual disease or not justified by it.
- There is a change in the expression and severity of symptoms in specific situations (e.g., to avoid social relationships) or when specific figures are present (children, spouse, doctors, or other health care professionals, etc.).
- Bodily difficulties seem to correlate with specific life events (retirement, abandonment, grief, etc.).

- There is a suggestion of "secondary gain" related to the physical difficulties (more attention from children, spouse, etc.).
- There is a previous history of multiple medical treatments for poorly identified ailments.

A second relevant aspect to consider for a differential diagnosis is the exclusion of a depressive syndrome with somatic aspects (the so-called "masked depression," which is frequent in elderly persons). In this case, the ongoing depression may overlap with the somatization. In other cases, generalized anxiety disorder characterized by relevant bodily complaints may also be present. In turn, comorbid generalized anxiety or depression may increase the severity of a somatizing personality pattern or disorder (Calleo et al., 2009; Hoedeman, Blankenstein, Krol, Koopmans, & Groothoff, 2010; Maharaj et al., 2013).

Features of Somatizing Personalities in Older Adults

The core of a somatizing personality pattern is an altered representation of disease ("illness representation"), such that somatic symptoms become the expressions of psychological pain. The illness representation is strongly influenced by anxious and depressive states that find somatic rather than verbal expression; the condition in which individuals are not aware of their emotions and are unable to articulate them is sometimes referred to as "alexithymia." In the elderly, the somatic expression may be overdetermined because of the common occurrence of comorbid medical conditions, which have created over time a perception of poor health, low self-esteem, and a damaged sense of self-efficacy (Nützel et al., 2014). The thought of death and the fear of physical and cognitive decline, expressed with excessive anxiety or through a reactive depression, are central themes in these patients. Concerns about the body become repetitive, spiral out of control, and invade the subject's everyday life (Letamendi et al., 2013). Hypochondriacal behaviors can lead to substance use disorders, as well as to unnecessary medical diagnostic and other procedures. Of course, the clinician must consider the possibility that the diagnostic and/or therapeutic interventions that have been applied have been inadequate and failed to identify important underlying "real" conditions and associated suffering (Mailis-Gagnon et al., 2008; Parmelee et al., 2013).

Impact of Somatizing Personalities on the Process of Aging

The impact of somatizing personalities is relevant not only for the affected individuals, but also for their children, spouses, friends, and health care professionals (as well as care providers if the persons are hospitalized or must enter a nursing home). This personality pattern exacerbates all physical and psychological age-related difficulties. Such an individual responds poorly to treatments, may be repeatedly hospitalized (the so-called "revolving door" phenomenon), and has a reduced quality of life. The continuing concern over body illnesses leads to a level of stress that may facilitate the emergence of new symptoms or aggravate existing diseases.

Suggestions for Treatment

The treatment of elderly people with somatizing personality patterns can be particularly challenging because of their difficulty in identifying and acknowledging the underlying emotions associated with the somatic symptoms. Generally, their inability to understand and share the contents of their inner worlds has characterized their whole lives, along with the desire for withdrawal, disinvestment, and refuge in physical ailments. Since relationships with these individuals are often difficult, it is very likely that in old age they may be isolated or marginalized, which may increase the expression of emotional discomfort through the body rather than through explicit verbal communication with others. A clinician has to overcome the temptation of disengagement caused by such a patient's persistent somatic complaints and to acknowledge that the patient's suffering, regardless of its psychological origin, is real.

The "Key Features" box for adult somatizing personalities in Chapter 1 on the P Axis (p. 44), listing patterns, preoccupations, pathogenic beliefs, and ways of defending, is also useful for understanding the core features of these personalities in the elderly. In the following table, we have expanded upon the Chapter 1 listing by adding a more detailed description of functioning in elderly somatizing personalities and comparing it with normal age-related personality functioning in older adults.

Key features	Somatizing personality functioning in the elderly	Normal age-related personality functioning
Contributing constitutional–maturational patterns	Previous physical fragility, early sickliness, and previous episodes of somatization are present in the person's clinical history and can be verified.	
Central tension/ preoccupation: Integrity versus fragmentation of bodily self.	The age-related decline of bodily integrity worsens the fragility of the self and decreases self-esteem and confidence in physical and psychological resources.	The person is aware of age-related physical difficulties and deals with the weakening body with the help of family, friends, and health care professionals. The person is able to recognize improvements in health and does not have excessive anxiety or depressive reactions that produce other somatic symptoms.
Central affects: Global distress; inferred rage; alexithymia, preventing acknowledgment of emotion.	The age-related weakening of cognitive abilities and an unwillingness/inability to deal with emotions worsens a likely previous condition of alexithymia. In particular, emotions such as rage and the suffering related to prolonged stressful situations hinder the verbal expression of discomfort, which is translated into somatic discomfort and preoccupations, with repeated requests for help with bodily impairments.	The subject is aware of stress and malaise related to the difficulties of aging and communicates them to family members, friends, and health care professionals, as well as staff members if he or she is institutionalized. The physical diseases are not means for communicating discomfort, but arise as a result of age-related decreases in diminished somatic resources.

Key features	Somatizing personality functioning in the elderly	Normal age-related personality functioning
Characteristic pathogenic belief about self: "I am fragile, vulnerable, in danger of dying."	Feelings of somatic fragility and vulnerability mark the perception of self and relationships with others.	The person is aware of his or her physical difficulties, but also of resources.
Characteristic pathogenic belief about others: "Others are powerful, healthy, and indifferent."	The repeated requests for help for somatic symptoms seem to be based on the belief that others possess inexhaustible resources of health, vigor, and strength. If others are not available to address these requests, they are viewed as hostile and indifferent.	The requests for help for somatic symptoms may be frequent, but they are appropriate to the severity of the discomfort and a realistic assessment of environmental resources.
Central ways of defending: Somatization, regression.	The majority of psychological, relational problems and distress are expressed through somatic difficulties, which become the individual's primary concern. The normal age-related bodily fragility is the breeding ground for the worsening of the somatic symptoms. The use of regressive defenses is massive.	The person complains of diseases and physical symptoms, but can also express emotions and feelings connected to psychological and relational problems. The use of regressive defenses is possible, but it coexists with a more mature defensive pattern.

Hysteric–Histrionic Personalities

Potential Diagnostic Biases Related to Age

Hysteric–histrionic personalities are characterized by some well-known personality traits: neuroticism and attention seeking. Neuroticism is understood as an intensity of emotions and their instability—anxiety, depression, impulsiveness, vulnerability, suggestibility, affective lability, separation anxiety, hostility, suspiciousness, and perseveration. These traits can be expressed as theatrical and eccentric behavior; these patients may rely on dissociation (expressed in the context of stressful conditions), and may show conversion syndromes as well as hypochondria. Historically, core aspects of the diagnosis have been the sexualization and eroticization of relationships, used as defensive mechanisms in response to a deep sense of inadequacy and humiliation (McWilliams, 2011; see also the discussion of hysteric–histrionic personalities in Chapter 1).

In the elderly, some of these traits remain stable, while others diminish with age. Traits that are maintained include the intensity and instability of emotions, as well as the phenomena of conversion and somatization. Traits that diminish include the use of sexuality to express conflict; this decrease is presumably a result of the aging process, which makes it more difficult to use the body as an instrument of seduction. There is also a reduced frequency of dissociative experiences, although in a clinical evaluation that is preoccupied with cognitive decline, dissociative states may not be identified. It is often difficult to differentiate real physical illnesses from psychological amplifications of them, especially when they overlap, as in cases of physical weakness, lack of energy, decreased vision, apathy, gastrointestinal disturbances, and autonomic symptoms (Wongpakaran & Wongpakaran, 2014). Often in older adults, these somatic symptoms and the social isolation increase, whereas histrionic expressiveness decreases.

Features of Hysteric–Histrionic Personalities in Older Adults

Histrionic symptoms may be tempered by the aging process, perhaps due to the weakening of narcissism, so that there is a different expression of this personality pattern in the face of life changes. However, the trait of "infantilizing" egocentrism generally remains intact, with special attention to the body and hypochondriacal fears (whether or not there are real organic problems), as well as reactive depression and anxiety (Dewsbury, 1973; Dols, Rhebergen, Eikelenboom, & Stek, 2012; Hilderink et al., 2009; Reynolds, 2012).

Sometimes dissociative symptoms present as cognitive impairments or hallucinatory episodes. It is also possible that a continuum can be identified between hysterical symptoms in young adulthood and delusions or hallucinations in the elderly.

Impact of Hysteric–Histrionic Personalities on the Process of Aging

Hysteric–histrionic personalities are often plaintive, act childishly, and feel themselves to be victims. In old age, they try to attract the attention of relatives, friends, and care providers (if institutionalized) through physical complaints and problems of adaptation in the context of life. They can feel abandoned if not adequately cared for and can respond with self-commiseration or anger to real or fantasized difficulties. The aging process is often difficult for them to accept, especially with regard to physical appearance; they may resort to plastic surgery or various "anti-aging" interventions to prevent or correct bodily expressions of old age. The perceived stress related to body limitations and dependency needs can produce symptoms of depression or anxiety. Older hysteric–histrionic individuals may have a faster cognitive decline, mainly due to the presence of depression (reactive to the environment, to the limits imposed by the aging process, to lack of attention [real or perceived] from family members, etc.), anxiety, and a worse response to novel stimuli.

Suggestions for Treatment

In old age, hysteric–histrionic personalities show a poor response to most therapeutic interventions. Individuals with this personality pattern may be unable to accept treatment, including hospitalization/institutionalization. If they enter a nursing home, their relationships with health care personnel and staff members may be difficult because of their incessant demands, the continuous sound of the bell if they are bedridden, their persistent requests for drugs to quell their anxiety, and their plaintive ruminations.

The characteristics of excessive emotionality and attention-seeking behavior are maintained even in old age. In psychotherapy, there may be attempts to eroticize the relationship (see, e.g., Segal et al., 2006). Such a patient tends to perceive his or her relationships (including the one with the therapist) as more intimate than they actually are and often expects to be repaid with equal interest. The therapist must remember that behind this attitude (and often also behind the story of extraordinary social achievements) hide failed or superficial relationships. The patient's seductiveness should not be refused, but understood and interpreted—and, when possible, elaborated to unearth the sense of emptiness and discomfort.

The "Key Features" box for adult hysteric–histrionic personalities in Chapter 1 on the P Axis (p. 46), listing patterns, preoccupations, pathogenic beliefs, and ways of defending, is also useful for understanding the core features of these personalities in the elderly. In the following table, we have expanded upon the Chapter 1 listing by adding a more detailed description of functioning in elderly hysteric–histrionic personalities and comparing it with normal age-related personality functioning in older adults.

Key features	Hysteric–histrionic personality functioning in the elderly	Normal age-related personality functioning
Contributing constitutional–maturational patterns	A low threshold of responsiveness to stimuli is present in the person's clinical history, along with a clear need for attention from others.	
Central tension/ preoccupation: Gender and power; unconscious devaluation of own gender and fear of opposite gender.	In old age, issues of gender and power may be less often identified as the central tension/preoccupation, but the seductiveness remains. Theatricality can relate to present diseases or a history of previous therapeutic interventions (surgical, medical, psychological)—or, conversely, to some current successes, as well as episodes of his or her previous life. However, the core of all interactions remains the trait of egocentrism.	Some typical fears of old age (death, diseases, loss of autonomy, etc.) can produce attitudes of particular concern about themselves, to the detriment of the attention that can be given to others. Also, a certain level of regression toward infantilized behaviors may occur. But these kinds of interactions are relatively temporary and do not represent stable traits in the perception of identity and in relationships with others.
Central affects: Fear, shame, guilt (over competition).	The characteristics of the aging process are faced with fear and shame; the related emotions are amplified and expressed in a largely excessive way.	Needs for attention, complaints about physical and psychological age-related hardships, regrets about the past, and awareness of the little time the person has left can sometimes produce moments of overemphatic affective expression, but these moments are not characteristic of the person's usual narrative.
Characteristic pathogenic belief about self: "There is something problematic with my gender and its meaning."	A sense that the self is weak and of low value is omnipresent. The diminished physical attractiveness connected to the aging process may increase the need for reassurance. Attempts at seduction may occur, sometimes still based on eroticism, but more often on the need to dramatize needs and feelings or on past successes.	The person is aware of his or her decreased seductive skills related to the process of aging, but may maintain a certain level of need for power via sexuality and gender. However, the person does not require excessive attention from others, and the dramatization of needs and feelings is only sporadic.

Key features	Hysteric–histrionic personality functioning in the elderly	Normal age-related personality functioning
Characteristic pathogenic belief about others: "The world is best understood in terms of gender binaries and gender conflicts."	There are simultaneous needs for care from others and fears of being overstimulated in relationships. Self-dramatization is used to maintain some form of control. Conditions of isolation may increase the attention-seeking behaviors and the excessive or impulsive expressions of needs.	The desire to be in the foreground can compensate for the person's diminished physical resources. The search for compliments and assurances is sometimes insistent, but the person is also able to draw upon internal skills, which strengthen identity and autonomy.
Central ways of defending: Repression, regression, conversion, sexualizing, acting out.	Concerns about sexuality, power, and identity are handled by defense mechanisms, among which conversion and regression are particularly important. Such concerns may also be the basis of physical symptoms that are difficult to explain in medical terms. The possible use of eroticization of relationships should not be overlooked, despite the limitations imposed by age.	Conversion/somatizing mechanisms may be present, but the person remains able to get in touch with his or her emotions and to communicate them in a proper narrative.

Narcissistic Personalities

Potential Diagnostic Biases Related to Age

Narcissistic personalities are characterized by grandiosity, need for admiration, and lack of empathy. Sometimes older people may demand attention and/or respect from relatives and from others, and may express their needs with somewhat arrogant attitudes. Some older individuals may require admiration; for example, elderly people frequently communicate with great pride their age or underline the persistence of some intellectual skills (e.g., memory capacity) or physical skills (e.g., strength and resistance).

However, these behaviors and attitudes may not be indicative of a narcissistic personality pattern or disorder—for example, if the individual did not exhibit these characteristics earlier in life. Some features of the aging process may actually increase a person's realistic need for reassurance from the environment about his or her value, identity, and quality of interpersonal relationships (Balsis, Eaton, Uke, Cooper, & Oltmanns, 2011). Moreover, the need for attention may translate into enhanced attachments and reduced loneliness.

Features of Narcissistic Personalities in Older Adults

Generally, the core features of narcissism (grandiose sense of self, need for admiration, poor capacity for empathy, arrogance, interpersonal exploitation) are maintained in old age if they were already present in a person's younger years, but their intensity is decreased (Foster, Campbell, & Twenge, 2003; Twenge, Konrath, Foster,

Keith Campbell, & Bushman, 2008). In particular, it is possible that the core features improve simply as a result of the aging process (Segal et al., 2006).

When the core features persist in old age, they may manifest themselves somewhat differently than in earlier years. For example, the elderly may experience a certain degree of reduction in power and influence, which may diminish their opportunities to exploit others narcissistically, either in family or in work settings. Fantasies of success may decrease, along with fewer occasions to meet others in different social areas (Bressler-Feiner, 1981). Accordingly, some characteristic of narcissistic personalities may find other modes of expression, which must not, however, escape diagnostic observation. Sometimes the arrogance turns into stubbornness; the tendency to exploit others increases depressive symptoms linked to progressive isolation; or the need for admiration can lead to imprudent behavior.

Impact of Narcissistic Personalities on the Process of Aging

The narcissistic personality pattern has a negative effect on the process of aging. During old age, narcissistic individuals are often alone and isolated, and may begin to regret the successes of their earlier lives. The lack of a capacity to maintain persistent and deep relationships, as well as to empathize, may lead to a reduction of supportive relationships and to Eriksonian "despair" and emptiness rather than "integrity" and fulfillment. Moreover, narcissistic individuals find it difficult to manage typical age-related physical changes; physical illnesses and general body deterioration (hair loss, wrinkles, diminished sensory and motor skills, etc.) have a negative impact on their view of themselves, and they cannot tolerate their new appearance. Increased dependency on others is also poorly tolerated, as it is associated with a diminished sense of self, which contrasts with the previous attitude of independence, power, and control (Clark, 1993; Heisel, Links, Conn, van Reekum, & Flett, 2007). All of these situations may lead to depression and suicide risk.

Suggestions for Treatment

Providing therapeutic support to older narcissistic patients is a challenge for clinicians and for the staff of any hospital or nursing home. The main problems are forming a therapeutic alliance (in psychotherapy) and compliance with medical treatments. The patients' requests tend to be excessive; the recognition of benefits is often impossible; and regret for the previous condition of autonomy and power is the dominant content in all relationships. In facilities, this situation may be addressed by repeated changes of the nursing staff, sometimes also in response to demands from a patient's relatives. Actually, health care professionals trained to be attentive to these particular characteristics of older narcissistic patients can identify some options for collaboration and useful support (Garner, 2002).

The "Key Features" box for adult narcissistic personalities in Chapter 1 on the P Axis (p. 48), listing patterns, preoccupations, pathogenic beliefs, and ways of defending, is also useful for understanding the core features of these personalities in the elderly. In the following table, we have expanded upon the Chapter 1 listing by adding a more detailed description of functioning in elderly narcissistic personalities and comparing it with normal age-related personality functioning in older adults.

Key features	Narcissistic personality functioning in the elderly	Normal age-related personality functioning
Contributing constitutional–maturational patterns	No clear data.	
Central tension/ preoccupation: Inflation versus deflation of self-esteem.	The core characteristics of the individual's personality have been the protection of his or her image (physical, social, etc.) and the fear of its devaluation. Consequently, the difficulties related to the aging process (diminished force, energy, autonomy, physical attractiveness, etc.) can exacerbate all the other features of this pattern.	There are concerns about maintaining a good physical appearance, as well as regret over the physical, emotional, and relational difficulties linked to the aging process. However, the person maintains a sense of his or her identity and value in continuity with earlier periods of life, and does not perceive the manifestations of aging as an attack on self-esteem that can induce depressive reactions.
Central affects: Shame, humiliation, contempt, envy.	Comparison of the person's earlier life with the increasing difficulties associated with aging produces feelings of bitterness, shame, and regret. Relationships with younger people can be marked by envy, sometimes expressed in a rancorous way.	The difficulties associated with aging are generally accepted, and feelings related to the loss of the characteristics of youth are present but sporadic. Relationships with younger people can be used as resources for testing new ideas and new perspectives, and they increase vitality and emotional investments.
Characteristic pathogenic belief about self: "I need to be perfect to feel OK."	It is important to check whether in the person's medical/psychological history, the need for attention and praise has been the main guideline of behavior and emotions. Physical, psychological, and cognitive age-related difficulties are more closely linked by the person to the deterioration of his or her image in the opinion of others, than to the normal regret for the reduced availability of resources.	The acquired characteristics due to the aging process are not mainly linked by the person to concerns about his or her image and judgments of others.
Characteristic pathogenic belief about others: "Others enjoy riches, beauty, power, and fame; the more of those I have, the better I will feel."	Bitterness and envy predominate, limiting the person's ability to seek and accept help. Anger, isolation, and regret are frequent.	The person does not deny his or her difficulties and is aware of other people's possibly greater resources, but he or she is mostly able to ask for and get help without feelings of humiliation and envy.
Central ways of defending: Idealization, devaluation.	The fear of self-devaluation and the tendency to idealize others are based on the use of rigid primitive defense mechanisms such as denial, projection, and splitting.	The defense mechanisms are varied and flexible, and allow the person to manage age-related difficulties in a number of different ways, sometimes even by demonstrating creative skills

PE9 Paranoid Personalities

Potential Diagnostic Biases Related to Age

The diagnosis of a paranoid personality pattern or disorder is assigned when distrust, suspiciousness of others, and doubts about the loyalty of friends and relatives (or sometimes suspicions, without justification, regarding the fidelity of a spouse or sexual partner) are recurrent and prominent. A corollary is that the person's lifetime history reveals a lack of lasting friendships and deep relationships because of constant concern about "remaining vigilant" to prevent exploitation and interpersonal deceit.

With aging, a certain amount of distrust or suspicion is common, making the diagnosis of paranoid personality a challenging one. This suspicious attitude may be related to the weakening of sensory, motor, and cognitive capacities, which decreases the feeling of control and mastery. Consequently, an older adult feels him- or herself to be less reactive to the environment and less able to cope with difficulties and dangers.

In evaluating an older adult for possible paranoia, it is crucial to assess for the presence of ongoing or past situations of maltreatment (Wolf, 1998). Indeed, the elderly, because of their fragility (and sometimes because of some characteristics of their personality functioning), may be victims of abuse, with a resultant increase of distrust and suspiciousness (Akaza et al., 2003).

Paranoid feelings intensify isolation and withdrawal from relationships and contacts with others. This behavior should not be confused with the features of schizoid personality, which is founded on the ambivalence between fear of closeness and longing for closeness, not on perceptions of malicious and deceitful intents in others.

Features of Paranoid Personalities in Older Adults

The very nature of paranoid personalities is founded in "the belief that they cannot openly and authentically relate to others because anything that they share can and will be used against them" (Segal et al., 2006, p. 28).

Episodes of manifest hostility toward others and aggressive actions are often present in a person's clinical history. These features of the pattern may of course be less frequent (or even disappear altogether) in old age, owing to the reduced availability of physical energies.

The effects of the process of aging are problematic for the paranoid personality type. Physical illnesses, sensory decline, and increased dependence strengthen the underlying suspiciousness and may worsen pathological traits.

The subjective perception of cognitive decline can often increase the concern about being attacked or humiliated by others (Forsell & Henderson, 1998). In these cases, the development of paranoid attitudes can also occur later in life and may be diagnosed as a result of a neurocognitive disorder.

Impact of Paranoid Personalities on the Process of Aging

The feelings of distrust and the concerns about interpersonal exploitation make the management of difficulties related to the aging process more difficult for paranoid individuals. Offers of help by friends, family members, or health care workers are often not easily accepted. Moreover, increased dependence on others may provoke the fear of losing autonomy and the need for control and caution. If such an individual needs to be hospitalized or to enter a nursing home, agitation and suspiciousness may increase because doctors, nurses, other care providers, and fellow patients are perceived as intrusive, with recurrent doubts about their trustworthiness.

Suggestions for Treatment

Sometimes the elderly suffer real abuse, both within their families and in nursing homes. If an older adult relates difficult relationships within his or her environment, it is important to ascertain the actual living conditions and be cautious about attributing the person's suffering and discomfort to the presence of paranoid fears. As always, a careful investigation of the previous clinical history is helpful in the differential diagnosis.

Even when a patient's fears are paranoid rather than realistic, an attitude of empathy for the patient's concerns is essential to creating even a minimal alliance, which, though often at risk of breakage, is the premise of any therapeutic intervention (Bateman & Fonagy, 2000).

The "Key Features" box for adult paranoid personalities in Chapter 1 on the P Axis (p. 49), listing patterns, preoccupations, pathogenic beliefs, and ways of defending, is also useful for understanding the core features of these personalities in the elderly. In the following table, we have expanded upon the Chapter 1 listing by adding a more detailed description of functioning in elderly paranoid personalities, and comparing it with normal age-related personality functioning in older adults.

Key features	Paranoid personality functioning in the elderly	Normal age-related personality functioning
Contributing constitutional–maturational patterns	In the clinical history there is a pattern of irritability, with possible episodes of manifest aggression or other hostile behavior resulting from felt shame and humiliation.	
Central tension/ preoccupation: Attacking versus being attacked by humiliating others.	The worry about being attacked and mistreated is repeatedly present and is increased by age-related physical, cognitive, and emotional difficulties. Often this concern is not expressed directly, but must be perceived in behaviors and attitudes such as irritability, isolation, and discomfort.	The decreased ability to control one's physical, emotional, and cognitive skills can produce a feeling of insecurity and increase a cautious attitude. Confidence in relatives and friends is maintained, however, and the person is able to build new relations of trust with caregivers outside the family.
Central affects: Fear, rage, shame, contempt.	Feelings of fear, anger, and suspiciousness are excessive and not justified by the awareness of the age-related reduced ability to control.	Caution may be exhibited, especially about strangers and new situations. With the increase of knowledge and familiarity, however, can arise relations of trust and confidence. If the elderly person is institutionalized, these capacities become particularly evident.

Key features	Paranoid personality functioning in the elderly	Normal age-related personality functioning
Characteristic pathogenic belief about self: "I am in constant danger."	The person behaves as if he or she is constantly in danger. Relationships with others are sources of potential maltreatment or deception. Any deficiencies related to caregiving, or to medical interventions in case of physical disease, are believed to be intentional and fuel the person's feeling of being a victim. If the elderly person is institutionalized, these feelings can be particularly intense and can hinder the care.	The older person is aware of his or her difficulties, but has an attitude of substantial confidence and trust. Behavior toward others may be cautious, especially with strangers, but it leaves plenty of room for the development of positive feelings.
Characteristic pathogenic belief about others: "The world is full of potential attackers and users."	All other people are potential attackers, regardless of their degree of intimacy and friendship.	The person's perception of his or her need for help, connected with the age-related decrease in resources, leads him or her to establish relationships cautiously and can motivate some initial attitudes of suspicion. If the elderly person is institutionalized, these attitudes may be more obvious. However, positive experiences of support and caregiving are able to reassure the person and allow him or her to experience greater trust and confidence.
Central ways of defending: Projection, projective identification, denial, reaction formation.	Primitive defenses based on splitting are used.	The use of primitive defenses is only temporary and is mostly linked to the initial period of the relationship with a new person or environment (e.g., when the elderly individual enters a nursing home).

Psychopathic Personalities

Potential Diagnostic Biases Related to Age

Generally, psychopathic (antisocial) personalities are less frequent among older than younger people (Oltmanns & Balsis, 2011), and their numbers decrease with age (Engels, Duijsens, Haringsma, & van Putten, 2003; Grant et al., 2008). Some common features of the psychopathic pattern in younger adults, such as taking pleasure in duping others and manipulating them, are of course less frequent (and maybe less possible) in old age, due to the decline of social relations and to diminished physical, cognitive, and affective resources. However, an individual's need to express power for the sake of doing so (and/or to compensate for a sense of diminished personal power) can persist into old age. Especially in some contexts—for example, the world of business and finance—some charismatic figures in old age can maintain their attitude of manipulation and control over others, as well as of noncompliance with social norms.

A psychopathic personality pattern should not be confused with normal developmental aspects of aging, such as a sense of freedom from societal and occupational demands, together with awareness of a limited lifespan, lessened concern about the opinions of others, and more focus on the self.

Finally, some characteristics of antisocial behavior (e.g., impulsivity, aggressiveness, and lack of consideration for others) may be seen in individuals in the early stages of a neurocognitive disorder.

Features of Psychopathic Personalities in Older Adults

An older adult's attitude of giving priority to his or her own needs may result in a lack of empathy for others and may be associated with antisocial behaviors. Other possible expressions of antisocial behavior in older adults include treatment nonadherence, as well as misuse of prescribed medications and/or recreational substances.

Impact of Psychopathic Personalities on the Process of Aging

Psychopathy can have a significant impact on the process of aging (van Alphen, Nijhuis, & Oei, 2007). The lack of respect for the needs and feeling of others, the frequently challenging attitude, and the residual impulsivity and aggression may induce other people (including family members) to avoid contact with a psychopathic elder, leading to a condition of isolation.

Suggestions for Treatment

As with younger psychopathic (antisocial) individuals, any type of therapeutic intervention is very difficult, owing to difficulty establishing an alliance with a shared purpose. If an elder with psychopathy has to enter a nursing home, management difficulties are likely in relation to other patients, as well as to health care professionals and institutional personnel. Conflicts may emerge frequently—for example, the appropriation of others' belongings or noncompliance with the rules of the institution. Clear and consistent rules and expectations can be helpful with such individuals. It is of course helpful for the treatment team to recognize that behind the adversarial position and frequent transgressions lie the person's need to affirm his or her sense of identity and relative autonomy, both of which have been compromised by the perceived difficulties related to the process of aging.

The "Key Features" box for adult psychopathic personalities in Chapter 1 on the P Axis (p. 51), listing patterns, preoccupations, pathogenic beliefs, and ways of defending, is also useful for understanding the core features of these personalities in the elderly. In the following table, we have expanded upon the Chapter 1 listing by adding a more detailed description of functioning in elderly psychopathic personalities and comparing it with normal age-related personality functioning in older adults.

Key features	Psychopathic personality	Normal age-related personality functioning
Contributing constitutional–maturational patterns	Aggressiveness and high threshold for affective/emotional stimulation can be congenital.	
Central tension/ preoccupation: Manipulating versus fear of being manipulated.	The worry about being exploited/ manipulated causes the person to engage in transgressive behavior and attempts to dominate and subjugate others. This attitude can be particularly noticeable if the person is institutionalized and then forced to close off relationships with support staff or other elderly people. Domination over others produces obvious feelings of reassurance and sometimes sadistic pleasure. The person's clinical history shows that this tension/preoccupation has been constant through the various earlier stages of his or her life.	The awareness of the age-related decline of physical and psychological resources can produce the fear of being manipulated or deceived, but this does not cause symmetrical behaviors of domination or exploitation of others. Systematic violations of the rules of the environment in which the elderly person is living are absent. The medical history does not record previous instances of attacks on others or on social norms.
Central affects: Rage, envy.	Rage and envy are often evident in the person's relations with others, independently of specific situations or special events.	There may be sporadic episodes of anger linked to the awareness of age-related subject's weakness or reduced autonomy. Envy of the greater resources of others may be present, but this envy does not involve exploitative behavior or transgression. The capacity for empathy toward others is well preserved.
Characteristic pathogenic belief about self: "I can do whatever I want."	In the elderly, the transgression of rules and the exploitation of others are sometimes supported by the belief that they have suffered wrongs in previous periods of life or have acquired special merits that have never been recognized. In these persons, old age is a kind of permission to do whatever they want. In the case of an elder with psychopathy, the clinical history shows that this attitude has been constant and that the old age is only another justification for the usual sociopathic/psychopathic behavior.	Any difficulties of the person's past life are recognized, but these are not used as an excuse for disrespect of the needs of others or of rules. If the elder is hospitalized or enters a nursing home, the difficulties of relationships with others can produce attitudes of withdrawal and caution, but not of exploitation. Living with others is safeguarded, and if the rules of the environment are sometimes transgressed, this doesn't involve a sadistic pleasure.

Key features	Psychopathic personality	Normal age-related personality functioning
Characteristic pathogenic belief about others: "Everyone is selfish, manipulative, dishonorable, and/or weak."	In old age, the psychopathic individual feels that because others are selfish and manipulative, they can take advantage of the person's age-related weakness.	The person's awareness of his or her weakness may undermine trust in others. All relationships with persons in new environments can be characterized by mistrust and fear of being mistreated. The reaction to these fears, however, is not to engage in behaviors that disregard the rules and do not respect others.
Central ways of defending: Reaching for omnipotent control.	Domination, omnipotent control, and contempt of others are continually present.	Attitudes of arrogance or dominance over others are sporadic and reactive to specific and identifiable circumstances that have produced feelings of fear for the person's sense of autonomy and identity.

Sadistic Personalities

Potential Diagnostic Biases Related to Age

The nature and frequency of sadistic patterns in the elderly are relatively unknown, as there is no literature on which to develop a complete understanding. Sadistic personalities are related to psychopathy and criminal behavior and do not appear in the DSMs. Given the declines in social network, physical functional status, and cognitive status in older adults, it would be unlikely that they would display the sadistic behaviors typical of younger adults, such as physical violence and cruelty; thus it is possible that older adults with such tendencies would be overlooked by traditional diagnostic classifications. Sometimes, however, difficulties associated with the aging process, or the increase in personal dependency, or even difficult—or simply new—environmental situations (e.g., when an older adult needs hospitalization or enters a skilled nursing facility) can produce feelings of anger, which can be expressed through aggressive or humiliating behavior. This attitude is functional; its purpose is to enable the person to maintain a certain level of power and influence. If the elderly person does not have a previous history of manifest sadism, these episodes tend to be brief and do not constitute a specific characteristic of relationships with others.

Features of Sadistic Personalities in Older Adults

As Segal and colleagues (2006, p. 142) write, "emotional cruelty seems to know no age limits." Consequently, expressions of sadism may remain even in old age: humiliating attitudes or sadistic glee associated with the suffering of others. Manifestations of contempt or continual reproaches addressed to people on whom the older adult depends (family members, nurses, other caregivers) are typical. In some family constellations, when an older adult who has been the primary decision maker and authority in the household develops cognitive and/or physical impairment, the family—instead of shifting the dynamics to accommodate new roles—allows the impaired older adult to continue to "call the shots" and disregard other family members. Sadistic elements may arise in this context.

Impact of Sadistic Personalities on the Process of Aging

Since hatred and contempt are the central affects of sadistic personalities, the aging process, which reduces the possibility of expressing superiority and increases dependency, is tolerated with great difficulty. When hospitalization is required or the older adult enters a care facility, the relationships with doctors, nurses, and other residents can become an opportunity to express sadistic attitudes and behaviors.

Suggestions for Treatment

Individuals with sadistic personalities tend to have limited insight into their own feelings and behaviors, as well as into the consequences or effects they have on others. They believe that their behaviors and feelings are completely normal and acceptable. The treatment of these individuals is therefore particularly difficult and often must be limited to the containment of the most striking behavioral manifestations, as well as to the active defense of targeted people, especially in institutional settings.

The "Key Features" box for adult sadistic personalities in Chapter 1 on the P Axis (p. 52), listing patterns, preoccupations, pathogenic beliefs, and ways of defending, is also useful for understanding the core features of these personalities in the elderly. In the following table, we have expanded upon the Chapter 1 listing by adding a more detailed description of functioning in elderly sadistic personalities and comparing it with normal age-related personality functioning in older adults.

Key features	Sadistic personality functioning in the elderly	Normal age-related personality functioning
Contributing constitutional–maturational patterns	Unknown.	
Central tension/ preoccupation: Suffering indignity versus inflicting such suffering.	The fear of being humiliated produces an anticipatory defense based on the devaluation of others.	Devaluing attitudes and excessive criticism are short-lived, and they signal discomfort that the person is sometimes able to recognize. The person may even be able to implement some reparative actions and attitudes.
Central affects: Cold hatred, contempt, pleasure (sadistic glee).	Hatred and contempt, as well as pleasure associated with the suffering of others, are evident in the person's previous clinical history.	Sometimes the person seems comforted by the fact that others also have difficulties or suffer. However, the ability to empathize is preserved, and the person is willing to help if possible.
Characteristic pathogenic belief about self: "I am entitled to hurt and humiliate others."	The subject continues to feel entitled to humiliate and hurt others on the basis of his or her own superiority.	The subject may attack others to attempt to demonstrate that he or she is still powerful, but these tend to be isolated events, and such events are absent from the previous clinical history.

Key features	Sadistic personality functioning in the elderly	Normal age-related personality functioning
Characteristic pathogenic belief about others: "Others exist as objects for my domination."	There is no respect for others or capacity for empathy. Humiliating attitudes are intentionally acted out.	In stressful situations, the person may humiliate or criticize others, but still retains the ability to empathize and to appreciate the effects he or she has on others.
Central ways of defending: Detachment, omnipotent control, reversal, enactment.	Omnipotent control and emotional detachment are in the foreground.	The capacity to share the experiences of others is preserved, even in difficult situations. Sometimes there may be an attitude of defensive detachment, but not sadistic glee.

Borderline Personalities

Potential Diagnostic Biases Related to Age

The diagnosis of borderline personality in old age is very complex because of the heterogeneous clinical manifestations of this pattern, as well as the presence of multiple comorbid symptoms. The central traits commonly described in the literature—such as impulsivity, labile and hard-to-control emotions, difficulties in feeling a continuity of experience, identity instability, and feelings of an inner "void"—may appear less frequently and with less intensity than in earlier phases of life, making diagnosis difficult.

Features of Borderline Personalities in Older Adults

A persistent inability to mediate emotional changes in response to environmental stressors remains in borderline older adults (Stevenson et al., 2003), but the behavioral expressions of this inability may change with aging (Powers, Gleason, & Oltmanns, 2013). For example, instead of self-harm and suicidal gestures exhibited in response to anxiety and feeling of emptiness, in older adults we may observe eating disorders, sabotage of medical treatments, substance misuse, affect dysregulation, anxiety and somatic syndromes, dissociative phenomena, or psychotic slips (Epstein, Fischer-Elber, & Al-Otaiba, 2007; Galione & Oltmanns, 2013; Landesman, 2003; Sadavoy, 1987).

Zanarini, Frankenburg, Hennen, and Silk (2003) reports that only one-quarter of subjects with borderline personalities maintain the same features of the pattern during older age. For example, the tumultuous and chaotic behavior linked to impulsivity and "acting out" seems to diminish in elderly individuals, possibly due to physical age-related limitations rather than to a real change in core personality functioning. Other core traits remain stable throughout life, such as defensive style, affective responses to changes and to stressful events, feelings of emptiness, and fear of abandonment. It is not known whether the changes in behavioral expression represent a genuine improvement of the underlying condition.

Older adults with this personality structure have difficulty with relationships, and may end up being socially isolated as a result (Landesman, 2003).

Impact of Borderline Personalities on the Process of Aging

The presence of borderline personality functioning in elderly persons has a significant impact on their responses to age-related stressful life events and to the process of aging itself (Powers et al., 2013). A diagnosis of borderline personality disorder at a younger age is associated with greater severity of the physical, psychological, and cognitive symptoms of aging (Ruocco, Lam, & McMain, 2014; Salzbrenner et al., 2009). Also, the previous chronic use of drugs or alcohol increases the risk for development of neurocognitive disorders. Overall, borderline personalities in elderly individuals are associated with poor quality of life, poor response to medical and/or psychological treatments, increased use of psychotropic medications, increased psychiatric hospitalizations, and difficulty adjusting to transitions, such as moving to an assisted living or a skilled nursing facility.

Suggestions for Treatment

As indicated above, the treatment of borderline elderly patients is less likely to involve symptoms such as self-injury, suicidal gestures, or sexual acting out than is the treatment of younger adults. Older adults tend to manifest feelings of emptiness and vague discomfort in treatment, as well as difficulties with identity, perhaps increased by vulnerabilities related to the aging process. Also, dependency needs may be particularly intense to begin with, and may be increased by the social isolation related to a life of tumultuous, chaotic, and unsatisfactory relationships. It may be helpful to enlist a treatment team, in order to provide tangible resources and services for socially isolated older individuals with borderline personalities.

The "Key Features" box for adult borderline personalities in Chapter 1 on the P Axis (pp. 54–55), listing patterns, preoccupations, pathogenic beliefs, and ways of defending, is also useful for understanding the core features of these personalities in the elderly. In the following table, we have expanded upon the Chapter 1 listing by adding a more detailed description of functioning in elderly borderline personalities and comparing it with normal age-related personality functioning in older adults.

Key features	Borderline personality functioning in the elderly	Normal age-related personality functioning
Contributing constitutional–maturational patterns	In earlier periods of life, difficulties with affect regulation, capacity to be soothed, and impulsivity are present. All these personality features may be less obvious in older people.	
Central tension/ preoccupation: Self-cohesion versus fragmentation; engulfing attachment versus abandonment despair.	Intense abandonment despair is not appeased by the proximity of friends and relatives. The feeling of emptiness is deep and causes a sense of fragmentation, to which the person reacts by building engulfing relationships.	The proximity of friends and family soothes the person's momentary feelings of loneliness. The person has good self-cohesion and knows how to keep an appropriate distance in relationships.

Key features	Borderline personality functioining in the elderly	Normal age-related personality functioning
Central affects: Intense affects generally, especially rage, shame, and fear.	The manifestations of feelings of anger, fear, and shame may be less noticeable because of the age-related reduced number of significant relationships. The intensity of needs, however, is excessive. The person's clinical history includes a marked reactivity to different environmental conditions, as well as possible symptoms of mood disorders or psychotic slips.	The intensity of the person's emotional response is commensurate with the characteristics of different situations and environmental conditions. Mood or psychotic disorders are not present in the person's clinical history.
Characteristic pathogenic belief about self: "I don't know who I am; I inhabit dissociated self-states rather than having a sense of continuity."	Dissociative episodes may signal the discontinuity of the self and identity. The reactions to stimuli and the relationship with others are discontinuous, and different states of the self are present, although their expression can be moderated by age-related factors (fewer opportunities for engagement and relationships, fewer emotional resources). It is important in the differential diagnosis to consider possible neurocognitive impairments (memory, attention) that can complicate the personality pattern.	The continuity of the self is maintained. The person knows who he or she is and what he or she wants, even if sometimes the person's responses to environmental stimuli and relationships can be characterized by alternations of emotions and feelings due to decreased reliability of cognitive, physical, and emotional resources.
Characteristic pathogenic belief about others: "Others are one-dimensional and defined by their effects on me, rather than by a sense of their complex individual psychology."	The person remains indifferent to others' emotional lives and to the reasons for their behaviors.	Interest in relationships can normally be reduced by factors related to the aging process (lower sensory abilities, minor relational needs), but the person's judgments of others capture the complexity of their motivations and behaviors.
Central ways of defending: Splitting, projective identification, denial, dissociation, acting out, and other primitive defenses.	Primitive defenses, rigidity of habits, and excessive reactions are present.	Flexibility of reactions and higher-level defense mechanisms are seen, although the possible use of well-known and repetitive behaviors signals the difficulty of addressing new stimuli and situations because of age-related diminished physical and emotional resources.

BIBLIOGRAPHY

Abrams, R. C., & Bromberg, C. E. (2007). Personality disorders in the elderly. *Psychiatric Annals, 37*(2), 123–127.

Abrams, R. C., & Horowitz, S. V. (1999). Personality disorders after age 50: A meta-analytic review of the literature. In E. Rosowsky, R. C. Abrams, & R. A. Zweig (Eds.), *Personality disorders in older adults: Emerging issues in diagnosis and treatment* (pp. 55–68). Mahwah, NJ: Erlbaum.

Agüero-Torres, H., Fratiglioni, L., Guo, Z., Viitanen, M., von Strauss, E., & Winblad, B.(1998). Dementia is the major cause of functional dependency in the elderly: 3-year follow-up data from a population-based study. *American Journal of Public Health, 88*(10), 1452–1456.

Akaza, K., Bunai, Y., Tsujinaka, M., Nakamura, I., Nagai, A., Tsukata, Y., & Ohya, I. (2003). Elder abuse and neglect: Social problems revealed from 15 autopsy cases. *Legal Medicine, 5*(1), 7–14.

Alexopoulos, G. S. (2005). Depression in the elderly. *Lancet, 365,* 1961–1970.

Alexopoulos, G. S., Bruce, M. L., Hull, J., Sirey, J. A., & Kakuma, T. (1999). Clinical determinants of suicidal ideation and behavior in geriatric depression. *Archives of General Psychiatry, 56*(11), 1048–1053.

Alwahhabi, F. (2003). Anxiety symptoms and generalized anxiety disorders in the elderly: A review. *Harvard Review of Psychiatry, 11,* 180–193.

American Psychiatric Association. (2013). *Diagnostic and statistical manual of mental disorders* (5th ed.). Arlington, VA: Author.

Andersen, S. L., Sun, J. X., Sebastiani, P., Huntly, J., Gass, J. D., Feldman, L., . . . Perls, T. T. (2013). Personality factors in the Long Life Family Study. *Journal of Gerontology: Series B. Psychological Sciences and Social Sciences, 68*(5), 739–749.

Ayers, C. R., Ly, P., Howard, I., Mayes, T., Porter, B., & Iqbal, Y. (2014). Hoarding severity predicts functional disability in late-life hoarding disorder patients. *International Journal of Geriatric Psychiatry, 29*(7), 741–746.

Badcock, J. C., & Dragović, M. (2006). Schizotypal personality in mature adults. *Personality and Individual Differences, 40*(1), 77–85.

Balsis, S., Eaton, C. R., Uke, D., Cooper, L. D., & Oltmanns, T. F. (2011). The presentation of narcissistic personality disorder in an octogenarian: Converging evidence from multiple sources. *Clinical Gerontology, 34*(1), 71–87.

Balsis, S., Woods, C. M., Gleason, M. E. J., & Oltmanns, T. F. (2007). Overdiagnosis and underdiagnosis of personality disorders in older adults. *American Journal of Geriatric Psychiatry, 15*(9), 742–753.

Baltes, M. M., Honn, S., Barton, E. M., Orzach, M., & Lago, D. (1983). On the social ecology of dependency and independency in elderly nursing home residents: A replication and extension. *Journal of Gerontology, 38*(5), 556–564.

Barton, S., Karner, C., Salih, F., Baldwin, D. S., & Edwards, S. J. (2014). Clinical effectiveness of interventions for treatment-resistant anxiety in older people: A systematic review. *Health Technology Assessment, 18*(50), 1–59.

Bateman, A. W., & Fonagy, P. (2000). Effectiveness of psychotherapeutic treatment of personality disorder. *British Journal of Psychiatry, 177*(2), 138–143.

Blatt, S. (2004). *Experiences of depression: Theoretical, clinical, and research perspectives.* Washington, DC: American Psychological Association.

Blatt, S. J. (2008). *Polarities of experience: Relatedness and self-definition in personality development, psychopathology, and the therapeutic process.* Washington, DC: American Psychological Association.

Bloch, M. H., Green, C., Kichuk, S. A., Dombrowski, P. A., Wasylink, S., Billingslea, E., . . . Pittenger, C. (2013). Long-term outcome in adults with obsessive–compulsive disorder. *Depression and Anxiety, 30*(8), 716–722.

Bogner, H. R., Shah, P., & de Vries, H. S. (2009). A cross-sectional study of somatic symptoms and the identification of depression among elderly primary care patients. *Journal of Clinical Psychiatry, 11*(6), 285–291.

Bora, E., & Arabaci, L. B. (2009). Effect of age and gender on schizotypal personality traits in the normal population. *Psychiatry and Clinical Neurosciences, 63*(5), 663–669.

Boström, G., Conradsson, M., Rosendahl, E., Nordström, P., Gustafson, Y., & Littbrand, H. (2014). Functional capacity and dependency in transfer and dressing are associated with depressive symptoms in older people. *Clinical Interventions in Aging, 9,* 249–257.

Bressler-Feiner, M. (1981). Narcissism and role loss in older adults. *Journal of Geriatric Psychiatry, 14*(1), 91–109.

Calamari, J. E., Woodard, J. L., Armstrong K. M., Molino, A., Pontarelli, N. K., Socha, J., & Longley, S. L. (2014). Assessing older adults' obsessive–compulsive disorder symptoms: Psychometric characteristics of the obsessive compulsive inventory-revised. *Journal of Obsessive–Compulsive and Related Disorders, 3*(2), 124–131.

Caldwell, L., Low, L. F., & Brodaty, H. (2014). Caregivers' experience of the decision-making process for placing a person with dementia into a nursing home: Comparing caregivers from Chinese ethnic minority with those from English-speaking backgrounds. *International Psychogeriatrics, 26*(3), 413–424.

Caljouw, M. A. A., Cools, H. J. M., & Gussekloo, J. (2014). Natural course of care dependency in residents of long-term care facilities: Prospective follow-up study. *BMC Geriatrics, 14*(67), 1–8.

Calleo, J., Stanley, M. A., Greisinger, A., Wehmanen, O., Johnson, M., Novy, D., . . . Kunik, M. (2009). Generalized anxiety disorder in older medical patients: Diagnostic recognition, mental health management and service utilization. *Journal of Clinical Psychology in Medical Settings, 16*(2), 178–185.

Carstensen, L. L., Isaacowitz, D. M., & Charles, S. T. (1999). Taking time seriously: A theory of socioemotional selectivity. *American Psychologist, 54,* 165–181.

Cervellati, C., Cremonini, E., Bosi, C., Magon, S., Zurlo, A., Bergamini, C. A., & Zuliani, G. (2013) Systemic oxidative stress in older patients with mild cognitive impairment or late onset Alzheimer's disease. *Current Alzheimer Research, 10*(4), 365–372.

Chan, S. M. S., Chiu, F. K. E., Lam, C. W. L., Wong, S. M. C., & Conwell, Y. (2014). A multidimensional risk factor model for suicide attempts in later life. *Neuropsychiatric Disease and Treatment, 10,* 1807–1817.

Clark, D. C. (1993). Narcissistic crises of aging and suicidal despair. *Suicide and Life-Threatening Behavior, 23,* 21–26.

Cobo, C. M. S. (2014). The influence of institutionalization on the perception of autonomy and quality of life in old people. *Revista da Escola de Enfermagem USP, 48*(6), 1011–1017.

Coolidge, F. L., Segal, D. L., Hook, J. N., & Stewart, S. (2000). Personality disorders and coping among anxious older adults. *Journal of Anxiety Disorders, 14*(2), 157–172.

Costa, P. T., Jr., & McCrae, R. R. (1992). *Revised NEO Personality Inventory (NEO PI-R) and NEO Five-Factor Inventory (NEO-FFI) professional manual.* Lutz, FL: Psychological Asssessment Resources.

Costa, P. T., Weiss, A., Duberstein, P. R., Friedman, B., & Siegler, I. C. (2014). Personality facets and all-cause mortality among Medicare patients aged 66 to 102: A follow-on study of Weiss and Costa (2005). *Psychosomatic Medicine, 76*(5), 370–378.

Dar-Nimrod, I., Chapman, B. P., Robbins, J. A., Porsteinsson, A., Mapstone, M., & Duberstein, P. R. (2012). Gene by neuroticism interaction and cognitive function among older adults. *International Journal of Geriatric Psychiatry, 27*(11), 1147–1154.

Debast, I., van Alphen, S. P. J., Tummers, J. H. A., Rossi, G., Bolwerk, N., Derksen, J. L. L., & Rosowsky, E. (2014). Personality traits and personality disorders in late middle and old age: Do they remain stable?: A literature review. *Clinical Gerontologist, 37,* 253–271.

Dewsbury, A. R. (1973). Hypochondriasis and disease-claiming behaviour in general practice. *Journal of the Royal College of General Practitioners, 23,* 379–383.

Dols, A., Rhebergen, D., Eikelenboom, P., & Stek, M. L. (2012). Hypochondriacal delusion in an elderly woman recovers quickly with electroconvulsive therapy. *Clinics and Practice, 2*(11), 21–22.

Donald, I. P., & Bulpitt, C. J. (1999). The prognosis of falls in elderly people living at home. *Age and Ageing, 28,* 121–125.

Engels, G. I., Duijsens, I. J., Haringsma, R., & van Putten, C. M. (2003). Personality disorders in the elderly compared to four younger age groups: A cross-sectional study of community residents and mental health patients. *Journal of Personality Disorders, 17*(5), 447–459.

Epstein, E. E., Fischer-Elber, K., & Al-Otaiba, Z. (2007). Aging, and alcohol use disorders. *Journal of Women and Aging, 19*(1–2), 31–48.

Fiske, A., Wetherell, J. L., & Gatz, M. (2009). Depression in older adults. *Annual Review of Clinical Psychology, 5,* 363–389.

Forsell, Y., & Henderson, A. S. (1998). Epidemiology of paranoid symptoms in an elderly population. *British Journal of Psychiatry, 172*(5), 429–432.

Foster, J. D., Campbell, W. K., & Twenge, J. M. (2003). Individual differences in narcissism: Inflated self-views across the lifespan and around the world. *Journal of Research in Personality, 37*(6), 469–486.

Gadit, A. M., & Smigas, T. (2012). Efficacy of ECT in severe obsessive–compulsive disorder with Parkinson's disease. *BMJ Case Reports,* 1–3.

Galione, J. N., & Oltmanns, T. F. (2013). The relationship between borderline personality disorder and major depression in later life: Acute versus temperamental symptoms. *American Journal of Geriatric Psychiatry, 21*(8), 747–756.

Garner, J. (2002). Psychodynamic work and older adults. *Advances in Psychiatric Treatment, 8*(2), 128–135.

Gignac, M. A. M., Cott, C., & Badley, E. M. (2000). Adaptation to chronic illness and disability and its relationship to perceptions of independence and dependence. *Journals of Gerontology: Series B. Psychological Sciences and Social Sciences, 55*(6), 362–372.

Graham, E. K., & Lachman, M. E. (2012). Personality stability is associated with better cognitive performance in adulthood: Are the stable more able? *Journals of Gerontology: Series B. Psychological Sciences and Social Sciences, 67*(5), 545–554.

Grant, B. F., Chou, S., Goldstein, R., Huang, B., Stinson, F. S., Saha, T. D., . . . Ruan, W. J. (2008). Prevalence, correlates, disability, and comorbidity of DSM-IV borderline personality disorder: Results from the Wave 2 National Epidemiologic

Survey on Alcohol and Related Conditions. *Journal of Clinical Psychiatry, 69*(4), 533–545.

Grant, J. E., Mancebob, M. C., & Weinhandlc, E. (2013). Longitudinal course of pharmacotherapy in obsessive–compulsive disorder. *International Clinical Psychopharmacology, 28*(4), 200–205.

Gretarsdottir, E., Woodruff-Borden, J., Meeks, S., & Depp, C. (2004). Social anxiety in older adults: Phenomenology, prevalence, and measurement. *Behaviour Research and Therapy, 42*(4), 459–475.

Grossmann, I., Karasawa, M., Kan, C., & Kitayama, S. (2014). A cultural perspective on emotional experiences across the life span. *Emotion, 14*(4), 679–692.

Gutiérrez, F., Vall, G., Peri, J. M., Baillés, E., Ferraz, L., Garriz, M., & Caseras, X. (2012). Personality disorder features through the life course. *Journal of Personality Disorder, 26*(5), 763–774.

Harwood, D., Hawton, K., Hope, T., & Jacoby, R. (2001). Psychiatric disorder and personality factors associated with suicide in older people: A descriptive and case- control study. *International Journal of Geriatric Psychiatry, 16,* 155–165.

Heisel, M. J., Links, P. S., Conn, D., van Reekum, D., & Flett, G. L. (2007). Narcissistic personality and vulnerability to late-life suicidality. *American Journal of Geriatric Psychiatry, 15*(9), 734–741.

Helman, C. G. (2005). Cultural aspects of time and ageing. *EMBO Reports, 6*(Suppl. 1), S54–S58.

Hilderink, P. H., Benraad, C. E. M., van Driel, T. J. W., Buitelaar, J. K., Speckens, A. E. M., Olde Rikkert, M. G. M., & Oude Voshaar, R. C. (2009). Medically unexplained physical symptoms in elderly people: A pilot study of psychiatric and geriatric characteristics. *American Journal of Geriatric Psychiatry, 17*(2), 1085–1088.

Hill, P. L., Turiano, N. A., Hurd, M. D., Mroczek, D. K., & Roberts, B. W. (2011). Conscientiousness and longevity: An examination of possible mediators. *Health Psychology, 30*(5), 536–541.

Hoedeman, R., Blankenstein, A. H., Krol, B., Koopmans, P. C., & Groothoff, J. W. (2010). The contribution of high levels of somatic symptom severity to sickness absence duration, disability and discharge. *Journal of Occupational Rehabilitation, 20,* 264–273.

Jones, M. K., Wootton, B. M., & Vaccaro, L. D. (2012). The efficacy of exposure and response prevention for geriatric obsessive compulsive disorder: A clinical case illustration. *Case Reports in Psychiatry, 2012,* 394603.

Karaklic, D., & Bungener, C. (2010). Course of borderline personality disorder: Literature review. *Encephale, 36*(5), 373–379.

Karasawa, M., Curhan, K. B., Markus, H. R., Kitayama, S. S., Love, G. D., Radler, B. T., & Ryff, C. D. (2011). Cultural perspectives on aging and well-being: A comparison of Japan and the United States. *International Journal of Aging and Human Development, 73*(1), 73–98.

Kichuk, S. A., Torres, A. R., Fontenelle, L. F., Rosario, M. C., Shavitt, R. G., Miguel, E. C., . . . Bloch, M. H. (2013). Symptom dimensions are associated with age of onset and clinical course of obsessive–compulsive disorder. *Progress in Neuro-Psychopharmacology and Biological Psychiatry, 44,* 233–239.

Landesman, E. (2003). Mahler's developmental theory: Training the nurse to treat the older adults with borderline personality disorders. *Journal of Gerontological Nursing, 29*(2), 22–28.

Lang, F. (2001). Regulation of social relationships in later adulthood. *Journal of Gerontology: Psychological Sciences, 56*(6), 321–326.

Lautenschlager, N. T., & Förstl, H. (2007). Personality change in old age. *Current Opinion in Psychiatry, 20,* 62–66.

Lawton, E. M., & Oltmanns, T. F. (2013). Personality pathology and mental health treatment seeking in a community sample of older adults. *Personality and Mental Health, 7,* 203–212.

Letamendi, A. M., Ayers, C. R., Ruberg, J. L., Singley, D. B., Wilson, J., Chavira, D., . . . Wetherell, J. L. (2013). Illness conceptualizations among older rural Mexican-Americans with anxiety and depression. *Journal of Cross-Cultural Gerontology, 28*(4), 421–433.

Levy, B. (2008). Rigidity as a predictor of older persons' aging stereotypes and aging self-perceptions. *Social Behavior and Personality, 36*(4), 559–570.

Low, L. F., Brodaty, H., & Draper, B. (2002). A study of premorbid personality in behavioral and psychological symptoms of dementia in nursing home residents. *International Journal of Geriatric Psychiatry, 17,* 779–783.

Magoteaux, A. L., & Bonnivie, J. F. (2009). Distinguishing between personality disorders, stereotypes, and eccentricities in older adults. *Journal of Psychosocial Nursing and Mental Health Services, 47*(7), 19–24.

Maharaj, R. G., Alexander, C., Bridglal, C. H., Edwards, A., Mohammed, H., Rampaul, T., . . . Thomas, K. (2013). Somatoform disorders among patients attending walk-in clinics in Trinidad: Prevalence and association with depression and anxiety. *Mental Health in Family Medicine, 10,* 81–88.

Mailis-Gagnon, A., Nicholson, K., Yegneswaran, B., & Zurowski, M. (2008). Pain characteristics of adults 65 years of age and older referred to a tertiary care pain clinic. *Pain Research and Management, 13*(5), 389–394.

McWilliams, N. (2011). *Psychoanalytic diagnosis* (2nd ed.). New York: Guilford Press.

Milrod, B., Markowitz, J. C., Gerber, A. J., Cyranowski, J., Altemus, M., Shapiro, T., . . . Glatt, C. (2014). Childhood separation anxiety and the pathogenesis and treatment of adult anxiety. *American Journal of Psychiatry, 171*(1), 34–43.

Mordekar, A., & Spence, S. (2008) Personality disorder in older people: How common is it and what can be done? *Advances in Psychiatric Treatment, 14,* 71–77.

Nicoletti, A., Luca, A., Raciti, L., Contrafatto, D., Dibilio, V., . . . Zappia, M. (2013). Obsessive compulsive personality disorder and Parkinson's disease. *PLoS ONE, 8*(1), 1–5.

Nützel, A., Dahlhaus, A., Fuchs, A., Gensichen, J., König, H.-H., Riedel-Heller, S., . . . Bickel, H. (2014). Self-rated health in multimorbid older general practice patients: A cross-sectional study in Germany. *BMC Family Practice, 15,* 1.

Oldham, J. M., & Skodol, A. E. (2013). Personality and personality disorders, and the passage of time. *American Journal of Geriatric Psychiatry, 21,* 709–712.

Oltmanns, T. F., & Balsis, S. (2010). Assessment of personality disorders in older adults. In P. A. Lichtenberg (Ed.), *Handbook of assessment in clinical gerontology* (pp. 101–122). Burlington, MA: Academic Press/Elsevier.

Oltmanns, T. F., & Balsis, S. (2011). Personality disorders in later life: Questions about the measurement, course, and impact of disorders. *Annual Review of Clinical Psychology, 27*(7), 321–349.

Parmelee, P. A., Harralson, T. L., McPherron, J. A., & Ralph Schumacher, H. (2013). The structure of affective symptomatology in older adults with osteoarthritis. *International Journal of Geriatric Psychiatry, 28*(4), 393–401.

Penders, K. A., Rossi, G., Metsemakers, J. F., Duimel-Peeters, I. G., & van Alphen, S. P. (2015). Diagnostic accuracy of the Gerontological Personality Disorder Scale (GPS) in Dutch general practice. *Aging and Mental Health, 16,* 1–11.

Powers, A., Gleason, M. E. J., & Oltmanns, T. F. (2013). Symptoms of borderline personality disorder predict interpersonal (but not independent) stressful life events in a community sample of older adults. *Journal of Abnormal Psychology, 122*(2), 469–474.

Reynolds, E. H. (2012). Hysteria, conversion and functional disorders: A neurological contribution to classification issues. *British Journal of Psychiatry, 201,* 253–254.

Rodin, J., & Langer, E. (1977). Long-term effects of a control-relevant intervention with the institutionalized aged. *Journal of Personality and Social Psychology, 35,* 897–902.

Rosowsky, E., Abrams, R. C., & Zweig, R. A. (Eds.). (1999). *Personality disorders in older adults: Emerging issues in diagnosis and treatment.* Mahwah, NJ: Erlbaum.

Ruocco, A. C., Lam, J., & McMain, S. F. (2014). Subjective cognitive complaints and functional disability in patients with borderline personality disorder and their nonaffected first-degree relatives. *Canadian Journal of Psychiatry, 59*(6), 335–344.

Sabbe, T., & Vandenbulcke, M. (2014). Obsessief-compulsief gedrag bij de rechter temporale variant van frontotemporale dementia. *Tijdschrift voor Psychiatrie, 56*(10), 685–688.

Sadavoy, J. (1987). Character pathology in the elderly. *Journal of Geriatric Psychiatry, 20,* 165–178.

Saka, B., Kaya, O., Ozturk, G. B., Erten, N., & Karan, M. A. (2010). Malnutrition in the elderly and its relationship with other geriatric syndromes. *Clinical Nutrition, 29,* 745–748.

Salzbrenner, S., Brown, J., Hart, G., Dettmer, J., Williams, R., Ormeno, M., . . . Shippy, J. (2009). Frontotemporal dementia complicated by comorbid borderline personality disorder: A case report. *Psychiatry, 6*(4), 28–31.

Schuster, J. P., Hoertel, N., Le Strat, Y., Manetti, A., & Limosin, F. (2013). Personality disorders in older adults: Findings from the National Epidemiologic Survey on Alcohol and Related Conditions. *American Journal of Geriatric Psychiatry, 21,* 757–768.

Segal, D. L., Coolidge, F. L., & Rosowsky E. (2006). *Personality disorders and older adults. Diagnosis, assessment, and treatment.* Hoboken, NJ: Wiley.

Seivewright, H., Tyrer, P., & Johnson, T. (2002). Change in personality status in neurotic disorders. *Lancet, 359,* 2253–2254.

Shedler, J., & Westen, D. (2004). Refining personality disorder diagnoses: Integrating science and practice. *American Journal of Psychiatry, 161,* 1350–1365.

Shprecher, D. R., Rubenstein, L. A., Gannon, K., Frank, S. A., & Kurlan, R. (2014). Temporal course of the Tourette syndrome clinical triad. *Tremor and Other Hyperkinetic Movements, 4,* 243.

Singleton, N., Meltzer, H., Gatward, R., Coid, J., & Deasy, D. (1998). *Psychiatric morbidity among adults in England and Wales.* London: The Stationery Office.

Stevens, N. (1995). Gender and adaptation to widowhood. *Ageing and Society, 15,* 37–58.

Stevenson, J., Meares, R., & Comerford, A. (2003). Diminished impulsivity in older patients with borderline personality disorder. *American Journal of Psychiatry, 160,* 165–166.

Tomstad, S. T., Söderhamn, U., Espnes, G. A., & Söderhamn, O. (2012). Living alone, receiving help, helplessness, and inactivity are strongly related to risk of undernutrition among older home-dwelling people. *International Journal of General Medicine, 5,* 231–240.

Townsend, P. (1981). The structured dependency of the elderly: A creation of social policy in the twentieth century. *Ageing and Society, 1*(1), 5–28.

Turner, K., Steketee, G., & Nauth, L. (2010). Treating elders with compulsive hoarding: A pilot program. *Cognitive and Behavioral Practice, 17*(4), 449–457.

Twenge, J. M., Konrath, S., Foster, J. D., Keith Campbell, W., & Bushman, B. J. (2008). Egos inflating over time: A cross-temporal meta-analysis of the Narcissistic Personality Inventory. *Journal of Personality, 76,* 875–902.

van Alphen, S. P. J. (2011). Psychotherapy of an older adult with an avoidant personality disorder. *International Psychogeriatrics, 23*(4), 662–665.

van Alphen, S. P. J., Engelen, G. J. J. A., Kuin, Y., & Derksen, J. J. L. (2006). Editorial: The relevance of a geriatric sub-classification of personality disorders in DSM-V. *International Journal of Geriatric Psychiatry, 21,* 205–209.

van Alphen, S. P. J., Nijhuis, P. E. P., & Oei, T. I. (2007). Antisocial personality disorder in older adults: A qualitative study of Dutch forensic psychiatrists and forensic psychologists. *International Journal of Geriatric Psychiatry, 22*(8), 813–815.

van Alphen, S. P. J., Rossi, G., Dierckx, E., & Oude Voshaar, R. C. (2014). DSM-5-classificatie van persoonlijkheidsstoornissen bij ouderen [DSM-5 classification of personality disorders in older persons]. *Tijdschrift voor Psychiatrie, 56*(12), 816–820.

van den Broeck, J. (2012). *A trait-based perspective on the assessment of personality and personality pathology in older adults.* Unpublished doctoral dissertation, Vrije Universiteit Brussel, Brussels.

van Tilburg, T. (1992). Support networks before and after retirement. *Journal of Social and Personal Relationships, 9,* 433–445.

Vink, D., Aartsen, M. J., & Schoevers, R. A. (2008). Risk factors for anxiety and depression in the elderly: A review. *Journal of Affective Disorders, 106,* 29–44.

Wijeratne, C., & Manicavasagar, V. (2003). Separation anxiety in the elderly. *Anxiety Disorders, 17,* 695–702.

Williams, J. W., Barrett, J., Oxman, T., Frank, E., Katon, W., Sullivan, M., . . . Sengupta, A. (2000). Treatment of dysthymia and minor depression in primary care: A randomized controlled trial in older adults. *Journal of the American Medical Association, 284*(12), 1519–1526.

Williamson, G. M., & Schulz, R. (1990). Relationship orientation, quality of prior relationship and distress among caregivers of Alzheimer's patients. *Psychology and Aging, 5,* 502–509.

Wolf, R. S. (1998). Domestic elder abuse and neglect. In I. H. Nordhus, G. R. VandenBos, S. Berg, & P. Fromholt (Eds.), *Clinical geropsychology* (pp. 161–165). Washington, DC: American Psychological Association.

Wongpakaran, N., Wongpakaran, T., Boonyanaruthee, V., Pinyopornpanish, M., & Intaprasert, S. (2015). Comorbid personality disorders among patients with depression. *Neuropsychiatric Disease and Treatment, 11,* 1091–1096.

Wongpakaran, T., & Wongpakaran, N. (2014). Personality traits influencing somatization symptoms and social inhibition in the elderly. *Clinical Interventions in Aging, 9,* 157–164.

Yur'yev, A., Leppik, L., Tooding, L. M., Sisask, M., Värnik, P., Wu, J., & Värnik, A. (2010). Social inclusion affects elderly suicide mortality. *International Psychogeriatrics, 22*(8), 1337–1343.

Zanarini, M. C., Frankenburg, F. R., Hennen, J., & Silk, K. R., (2003). The longitudinal course of borderline psychopathology: 6-year prospective follow-up of the phenomenology of borderline personality disorder. *American Journal of Psychiatry, 160*(2), 274–283.

CHAPTER 14

Symptom Patterns in the Elderly: The Subjective Experience

SE Axis

CHAPTER EDITORS

Franco Del Corno, MPhyl, DPsych **Daniel Plotkin, MD**

CONSULTANTS

Emanuela Brusadelli, PhD
Giuseppe Cafforio, DPsych
Salvatore Gullo, PhD
Douglas W. Lane, PhD
Emanuela Mundo, MD
Eleonora Piacentini, PhD

Introduction

This chapter both refers to the diagnoses and categories of the *Diagnostic and Statistical Manual of Mental Disorders,* fifth edition (DSM-5; American Psychiatric Association, 2013), and differentiates PDM-2 diagnoses and categories from them. We follow the PDM-2 format for S-Axis chapters, using categories of affective patterns, cognitive patterns, somatic states, and relationship patterns to describe an older individual's subjective experience of each symptom pattern. Because DSM-5 does not have a section on older adults, and there is a paucity of data on older adults' subjective experience of psychiatric disorders, this chapter is necessarily limited. Still, it should serve as a starting point for further work. Whereas the other PDM-2 S-Axis chapters refer to the *International Classification of Diseases,* 10th revision (ICD-10; World Health Organization, 1992) and DSM-5 classifications for all disorders, the textual discussion in this chapter on the SE Axis is limited to DSM-5 because ICD-10 does not specifically address the elderly. (Table 14.2, pp. 871–876, does include ICD-10 diagnoses corresponding to PDM-2 and DSM-5 diagnoses.) In most cases, psychodynamics of symptoms in elderly patients overlap with those of adults and are not repeated here. For these, readers should refer to the corresponding sections of Chapter 3.

A particularly central and common aspect of the subjective experience of older adults with psychiatric conditions is loneliness (Booth, 2000; Eloranta, Arve, Isoaho, Lehtonen, & Viitanen, 2015; Masi, Chen, Hawkley, & Cacioppo, 2011). Accordingly, this chapter begins with a brief account of the condition. Loneliness is the distressing subjective feeling associated with personal isolation, with the pain of feeling alone. Although there is no diagnostic category of loneliness in DSM-5, this feeling is associated with a wide range of diagnostic categories, particularly with depressive disorders (Cacioppo, Hawkley, & Thisted, 2010). There is a complicated relationship among loneliness, depression, and social isolation (Steptoe, Shankar, Demakakos, & Wardle, 2013; Tilvis, Laitala, Routasalo, & Pitkälä, 2011; Weiss, 1973). Evidence suggests that loneliness and depression are distinct but overlapping conditions. With respect to social isolation, the quality of and the satisfaction derived from relationships are more important determinants of loneliness than the mere number of contacts. Individuals may feel lonely in a marriage or in a crowd (Tornstam, 1992). Among the interventions aimed to ameliorate suffering from loneliness, those that address maladaptive social cognitions appear to be the most effective.

In general, loneliness is a common experience in older individuals, with prevalence ranging from 20 to 40% of a community population. It is associated with poor quality of life, multiple medical conditions, dependency, cognitive impairment, increased use of psychotropic drugs, and even an increase in mortality rate. In general, older individuals with poor self-rated health who live alone are most likely to suffer from loneliness. Older men tend to report loneliness less often than women, but elderly men are psychologically compromised to a greater degree than are women with loneliness.

Table 14.1 provides an overview of the SE Axis, listing the sections and subsections of the various conditions we address.

SE1 Predominantly Psychotic Disorders

DSM-5 defines its category of schizophrenia spectrum and other psychotic disorders as comprising schizophrenia, delusional disorder, schizophreniform disorder, schizoaffective disorder, schizotypal (personality) disorder, psychotic disorder due to another medical condition, and catatonia (see also Chapter 3 on the S Axis). We have provided a concordance (see Table 14.2 at the end of the chapter) between the PDM-2 classification and the ICD-10 and DSM-5 classifications of psychotic disorders in the elderly.

SE15 Late-Onset Psychosis

Late-onset psychosis can be associated with mood disorders, dementia, or late-onset schizophrenia spectrum disorders. The last, which is the subject of this section and is referred to here as "late-onset schizophrenia" (LOS), affects 2–4% of older adults. There is a general paucity of research on the condition, as is true for many geriatric syndromes. In the past it was often called "paraphrenia," particularly when seen in elderly individuals who developed psychosis with predominantly paranoid delusions. In the late 1990s, a panel of international experts concluded that LOS with onset between 40 and 60 years of age should be regarded as a subtype of schizophrenia, whereas LOS with onset after age 60 years should be called "very-late-onset schizophrenia-like-psychosis."

TABLE 14.1. Symptom Patterns in the Elderly: The Subjective Experience—SE Axis

SE1 Predominantly psychotic disorders
- SE15 Late-onset psychosis

SE2 Mood disorders
- SE22 Depressive disorders
- SE23 Cyclothymic disorder
- SE24 Bipolar disorders

SE3 Disorders related primarily to anxiety
- SE31 Anxiety disorders
- SE32 Obsessive–compulsive and related disorders
  - SE32.1 Obsessive–compulsive disorder
  - SE32.2 Body dysmorphic disorder
  - SE32.3 Hoarding disorder
  - SE32.4 Trichotillomania and excoriation disorder

SE4 Event- and stressor-related disorders
- SE41 Trauma- and stressor-related disorders
  - SE41.2 Acute and posttraumatic stress disorders
- SE42 Dissociative disorders
- SE43 Conversion disorder
- SE45 Persistent complex bereavement disorder (complicated grief)

SE5 Somatic symptom and related disorders
- SE51 Somatic symptom disorder
- SE52 Illness anxiety disorder (Hypochondriasis)
- SE53 Factitious disorders
- SE54 Psychological factors affecting other medical conditions

SE6 Specific symptom disorders
- SE61 Feeding and eating disorders
- SE62 Sleep–wake disorders
- SE63 Sexual dysfunctions
- SE64 Paraphilic disorders

SE7 Disorders related to addiction
- SE71 Addictions
  - SE71.1 Substance-related disorders
  - SE71.2 Behavioral addictions
    - SE71.2.1 Gambling disorder
    - SE71.2.2 Sexual addiction

SE13 Neurocognitive disorders
- SE131 Delirium
- SE132 Mild neurocognitive disorder (mild cognitive impairment)
- SE133 Major neurocognitive disorder (dementia)

SEApp Appendix: Psychological experiences that may require clinical attention
- SEApp1 Demographic minority populations (ethnic, cultural, linguistic, religious, political)
- SEApp2 Lesbian, gay, and bisexual populations
- SEApp3 Gender incongruence

LOS shares many core demographic and clinical characteristics with early-onset schizophrenia (EOS), although there are some differences to suggest that LOS may represent a distinct condition. Differences include higher prevalence among females, lower severity of positive symptoms, better performance on a theory-of-mind (ToM) task, and lower antipsychotic medication dose requirements. It is likely that the lower medication requirements may result from age-related metabolic changes rather than changes in core disease characteristics. Meanwhile, the psychological and social needs of older adults with psychotic disorders are often unmet.

Recently, genetic and molecular studies have been conducted to identify the underlying pathophysiology of LOS. So far, however, it remains something of an enigma, with uncertainty as to its relationship to EOS and other psychotic conditions.

The Subjective Experience of Predominantly Psychotic Disorders in the Elderly

Affective Patterns

Individuals with LOS often express a sense of being "different" from others, "not belonging to this world," with accompanying social isolation and a solitary coping style. Like elderly individuals in general, those with psychosis attempt to explain and find meaning in their experiences, but their sense of being different from others often leads to lower overall morale in relation to aging, compared to morale in normal control groups.

Cognitive Patterns

Both LOS and EOS are associated with cognitive deficits, but they are stable over time and do not show trends consistent with dementia or other neurocognitive disorders. While memory and intellect in individuals with LOS are relatively spared, cognition is often characterized by hypervigilence and paranoia. In contrast, their comparatively good ToM performance suggests a protective effect that may modulate age at onset, perhaps delaying development of a psychotic disorder. For information about insight in psychosis, see the discussion in Chapter 3 (pp. 139–141).

Somatic States

Persons with LOS or EOS are prone to develop and complain of idiosyncratic and sometimes frankly delusional somatic symptoms and beliefs. Such experiences can lead to otherwise unnecessary and invasive diagnostic procedures and even to unnecessary treatment interventions, which carry risks of their own.

Relationship Patterns

In general, relationships are stressed, especially if an individual with LOS is demanding and needy, as is often the case. Family members and close friends may be left feeling frustrated and exasperated if they attempt to reason with the psychotic individual. They eventually find that it is usually more effective to sympathize with the genuine distress of the psychotic individual than to try to persuade him or her that the delusional beliefs are not real.

Suggestions for Treatment

The subjective experience of taking antipsychotic medication may be specific in the elderly. First-generation antipsychotics may exert side effects such as flattened emotional reactions and a relative state of indifference to environmental stimuli. Some older adults react negatively to these drugs because they may worsen cognitive functions (attention and concentration) often already affected by age. These effects are generally milder for second-generation antipsychotics.

In a case of LOS, a clinician should search for recent specific life events that may have precipitated its onset. Because emotional vulnerability is a susceptibility factor for LOS, the clinician should also inquire about whether, in previous periods of the patient's life, there were critical events or situations where emotional frailty was evident. The patient's relationships with relatives are often characterized by reciprocal reactions of anxiety and fear that reinforce each other. The clinician can help relatives understand that it is useless to fight the delusional beliefs. This simple intervention often reduces environmental pressure on the patient, who may then achieve some reduction in symptoms or a better adaptation to the disorder.

Clinical Illustration

An 83-year-old married woman who had enjoyed considerable business success developed delusional disorder, associated with her husband's illness and with their aging and declines in functioning. When her husband became bed-bound and required home nursing care, her symptoms worsened. Although her general cognitive functioning remained intact, her delusional beliefs about cleanliness and hygiene caused her to interfere with her husband's medical care, which in turn reinforced her sense of being different and victimized by others. When a geriatric psychiatrist was consulted, she was reluctant to engage in treatment, but she was gradually able to establish a good relationship with the psychiatrist; eventually she had a fairly good response to psychotherapy and antipsychotic medication.

SE2 Mood Disorders

SE22 Depressive Disorders

The DSM-5 classification (American Psychiatric Association, 2013) of depressive disorders includes disruptive mood dysregulation disorder, major depressive disorder, persistent depressive disorder (dysthymia), premenstrual dysphoric disorder, substance/medication-induced depressive disorder, depressive disorder due to another medical condition, other specified/unspecified depressive disorder, and a list of specifiers that apply to various diagnoses. According to DSM-5, depressive disorders are generally characterized by markedly diminished interest or pleasure in activities nearly every day; feeling of worthlessness; excessive or inappropriate guilt; diminished ability to think and concentrate; thoughts of death and/or suicidal ideation; and somatic impairments such as weight loss, insomnia or hypersomnia, and fatigue or loss of energy. It is interesting that the list of specifiers includes psychotic features and anxious distress.

If we exclude premenstrual dysphoric disorder, all of the depressive disorder diagnoses can also be applied to people in old age. A useful general principle is that most people with a psychological disorder in old age, especially depression and related disorders, are experiencing a recurrence of a condition that started earlier in life (Gallo & Lebowitz, 1999). One-year prevalence rates for major depressive episode and unipolar major depression are, respectively, 6.5% and 5.3% in persons ages 18–54, against 3.8% and 3.7% in persons over age 55 (U.S. Department of Health and Human Services, 1999).

Despite this low prevalence rate, almost half of the admissions of older adults to mental health care are due to depressive disorders. More frequently these individuals are women, who also tend to have more depressive episodes than men over the lifespan (Gallo & Lebowitz, 1999). Depression in late life is frequently comorbid with alcohol use disorders, as well as with cognitive symptoms, especially those affecting memory and concentration (Lockwood, Alexoppulos, Kakuma, & van Gorp, 2000).

Differential diagnosis between depression and dementia is a critical task but may present many difficulties (Kring, Davison, Neale, & Johnson, 2007, p. 515). Kiloh (1961) originally used the term "pseudodementia" for cases where cognitive impairment seemed to resolve with treatment of a depression. Alternative terms, such as "depression-related cognitive dysfunction" and "dementia syndrome of depression," have been proposed more recently. Approximately 20% of older depressed patients show cognitive deficits that justify such labels (LaRue, D'Elia, Clark, Spar, & Jarvik, 1986; Storand & VandenBos, 1997). Sometimes even specific neuropsychological tests may not distinguish with certainty between depression and neurocognitive impairments (Swainson et al., 2001). Yet it remains true that treatment of depression in the elderly also produces a significant improvement in cognitive abilities (LaRue, 1992).

Of course, depression and neurocognitive disorders may be present together. Sometimes an older person realizes that his or her progressive cognitive impairment may react with symptoms of depression; conversely, depression in middle age can increase the risk of subsequent Alzheimer's disease (Rosenblatt, Mehta, Romanoski, Eaton, & Lyketsos, 2003; Teri & Reifler, 1987).

Depression, in both elderly and younger people, is the major risk factor for suicide. In people over 65, the suicide rate is three times that in younger adults, and their suicide attempts rarely fail (Butler, Lewis, & Sunderland, 1998). Older adults may find passive ways to commit suicide—for example, by neglecting their medication or diet or by exposing themselves to dangerous behavior in relation to their age. (For a brief overview of suicide risk assessment, see Chapter 3.)

Many causes of depression in old age do not differ from those that trigger the disorder in younger adults. During late life, however, some specific problems may emerge, which must be taken into account with depressed patients. Stroke and other vascular disease are frequent in individuals who develop a first episode of depression in late life. Moreover, depression predicts worse outcomes in the case of cardiovascular diseases (Camus, Kraehenbuhl, Preisig, Bula, & Waeber, 2004).

Other causes of depression in the elderly may include the following:

- Medical illnesses (Marengo & Westermeyer, 1996)
- Physical disabilities, such as trouble walking (Gallo & Lebowitz, 1999)
- Widowhood (Wilcox et al., 2003) and other losses
- Social isolation
- Retirement

Nonetheless, there are also numerous factors that may protect the elderly from the potential depressant effects of such events. For example, in old age a need for a certain kind of "social selectivity" can arise (Kring, Davison, Neale, & Johnson, 2007), which results in a lower number of contacts, but more satisfactory ones. If retirement does not involve a substantial reduction of income, it can be seen as an opportunity to cultivate hobbies, have free time, learn new skills, and enjoy other activities. Kim and Moen (2001) write that high self-efficacy and self-esteem, in addition to resources such as high education and good marital relationships, protect individuals effectively from depression after retirement. Perhaps we can conclude that "adaptation rather than depression is the common reaction to loss and stress in late life" (Kring et al., 2007, p. 516).

Some authors (e.g., Sheikh, 1996) propose paying attention to the specific "language" with which depression is expressed. A depressed elder's complaints may focus on physical elements (e.g., disruption of sleep–wake cycle, change in appetite, constipation, psychomotor agitation or retardation), or on interpersonal or financial difficulties. Physical symptoms may mask a case of persistent depressive disorder (dysthymia). This diagnosis may sometimes be overlooked because there are no unequivocal symptoms as in the case of major depressive disorder. Older patients are often reticent about or detached from their depressive thoughts and sometimes fear medications, hospitalization, and other changes to their routine. The patients' primary care physicians, social workers, and family members may have to unmask the depressive symptoms hidden behind such complaints.

Among depressed elders, problems in self-esteem are not so frequent as in depressed younger adults. Feelings of emptiness are often in the foreground, along with hopelessness and helplessness about the future. Many elders may also describe situations or events related to feelings of uselessness, sometimes because of normal age-related difficulties in concentration, movement, and reaction time, which may be experienced with shame and annoyance.

It is fundamental to assess the general environmental conditions of an elderly patient. Depression may be the answer to family members' inappropriate caregiving (which is not always neglect; sometimes it may consist of excessive attention and control). Stress and conflict with adult children or witnessing of conflict among relatives (especially when it seems to involve the elderly person's estate), may also trigger depression.

The Subjective Experience of Depressive Disorders in the Elderly

Physical, psychological, and cognitive changes, and changes in an individual's context and environment, may produce depressive reactions at any age. Each change potentially creates stress between the affected person and the altered situation. This is particularly true for the elderly, when events such as losses, role changes within family and society, and decreased physical resources compound age-related frailty; "depression may be a by-product of a person's inability to manage these changes" (Sheikh, 1996, p. 6).

Affective States

Ineffective coping strategies applied to age-related changes or painful life events often intensify negative feelings and less adequate reactions. This may be true even for small age-related impairments; mild decliness in attention, concentration, and memory may be experienced in a particularly negative way. The depressive reaction may be accompanied by irritability and agitation. In some cases, subjective perception of lower efficiency and decreased control may engender suspiciousness or thoughts of being exploited and cheated. Sometimes the development of paranoid worries (e.g., "People are following me") can be a defense against the unbearable feeling of passivity linked to diminished physical resources and autonomy. Interventions that promote better acceptance of the difficulties associated with the aging process often resolve or diminish the paranoid ideation. In those who suffered from depression in prior years, the normally difficult experiences of aging can trigger depressive episodes. A comprehensive assessment requires the exploration of feelings and beliefs about aging, disability, illness, and death in elderly patients. The surrounding culture influences their views of the world and their consequent concerns, as well as their attitude toward psychological and practical help in both the past and present.

Cognitive Patterns

Even in the absence of neurocognitive disorders, depression slows cognitive processes, impairs memory and concentration, and makes it difficult to process new information. As previously noted, the differential diagnosis between dementia and depression is inescapable but may be difficult, partly because complaints about memory problems are symptomatic of both normal aging and depressive symptoms. A number of researchers have observed (for a review, see Storand & VandenBos, 1997) that many depressed older adults complain about memory difficulties, even though no memory performance deficits are detectable. As is true of other disorders comorbid with depression, memory complaints decrease when depressive symptomatology improves. Conversely, subjects affected by a genuine neurocognitive disorder (e.g., Alzheimer's disease or vascular dementia) often subjectively overestimate their memory ability, while demonstrating clear memory performance impairment.

Assessment of the cognitive abilities of depressed older adults and differential diagnosis of depressive disorders from neurocognitive disorders are also critical for addressing the elderly persons' needs for assistance and planning for the future. Difficulties with instrumental activities of daily living (managing money, reading, shopping, cooking) are common in depressed older adults, along with challenges in bathing, grooming, and eating, but the resolution or alleviation of depressive symptoms tends to free them to resume a more normal life. In contrast, when symptoms occur in a state of dementia, such deficits tend to worsen and to require continued support.

Somatic States

Some physical illnesses (e.g., cancer, AIDS, thyroid hypofunction) involve somatic symptoms that mimic depression. Conversely, depression itself may produce specific physical disorders: malnutrition, intoxication by medication overdose, or the consequences of some kind of addiction (alcohol, tranquilizers, antidepressants, analgesics, etc.). Therefore, depressed older adults require a complete medical evaluation to identify and treat comorbid physical disorders, as well as a careful assessment of their medications and dosages.

On the other hand, physical illness is the most common trigger of a depression in old age. The severity and duration of a depression are often related to the characteristics of the disease, which may contribute directly to specific impairments, such as immobility, incontinence, and sexual dysfunction; in turn, these impairments may precipitate or exacerbate depression. The management of physical illness and concurrent depression requires support for an older patient's cognitive and emotional capacities to cope, as well as a specific attention to the person's quality of life. In old age, every disease, even when not serious, seems to presage death. The attitudes characteristic of the elderly person's milieu can make a major contribution to the resilience of the sick person or can be an obstacle to handling the symptoms of both physical illness and depression.

Relationship Patterns

Isolation and detachment from friends and social activities are part of the depressive condition. The elderly may be reluctant to allow clinicians to contact family members or friends, and yet relatives and significant others may be very useful informants, especially if an older person's cognitive functioning is impaired. In addition, the therapist may feel frustrated, impotent, excessively sympathetic, and uncertain about the diagnosis, sometimes conflating a depressive state and an adjustment disorder. An interview with the patient's spouse and/or adult relatives (e.g., sons or daughters) may help to identify etiology, development, and triggers of depression, as well as possible comorbid conditions, and may illuminate the therapist about the patient's diagnosis and history of previous treatments.

Tools for Assessment

For the differential diagnosis between dementia and depression, see Storand and VandenBos (1997) for a careful clinician's guide to neuropsychological assessment in older adults. These authors report detailed psychometric data on older adults from the Beck Depression Inventory (BDI) and the Geriatric Depression Scale (GDS), which they recommend; they also review other instruments for assessing presence and severity of depression in older adults, describing their strengths and limitations (cfr. also Korczyn, & Halperin, 2009) .

Suggestions for Treatment

The scholarly literature on late-life depression reports many treatment approaches, including drug therapy and various psychotherapeutic and psychosocial interventions. Because there is not yet any professional consensus on them (particularly on pharmacology), we do not describe in detail these different possibilities (see Kring et al., 2007; Sheikh, 1996). One almost universal conclusion, however, is that despite the fact that the aging process carries with it many physical and psychological difficulties, depression is *not* a normal consequence of growing old (Sheikh, 1996).

SE23 Cyclothymic Disorder

Although rarer than bipolar disorder, cyclothymic disorder may be found in the elderly. It is a persistent mood fluctuation, not severe or persistent enough to be classified as bipolar disorder, but different from the normal recurrence of sadness and moments of relief—a recurrence that is particularly frequent in old age.

The subjective experience of cyclothymic patients may be particularly distressing for the elderly. The mood variations may increase patients' fears of losing stability of self and control of mental capacities. Cyclothymic disorder may also seriously affect the patients' behavior and social relationships. The subjective experience of the therapist resembles the countertransference to patients with bipolar disorder.

SE24 Bipolar Disorders

Bipolar disorders usually present in young adulthood but may persist into old age. Their clinical presentation in older adults are similar to that in younger adults (see Chapter 3, pp. 158–160), except that mania is often less severe (i.e., the DSM-5 diagnosis of bipolar II disorder is more common in the elderly than bipolar I), and there is increased likelihood of cognitive impairment. In general, they evolve into a more complex illness, with somatic comorbidity and critical issues of polypharmacy. This condition implies an increased likelihood of cognitive impairment.

It has long been known that mania can occur for the first time at ages over 50 years, in which case the bipolar disorder is termed "late-onset." Compared to early-onset bipolar disorder, late-onset is more likely to be caused by (or at least associated with) medical/neurological conditions or triggered by medication use. Individuals with late-onset bipolar disorder have better premorbid functioning and less family history of bipolar disorder than those with the early-onset type. In the past, manic episodes of late-onset bipolar disorder associated with neurological conditions and/or medication reaction were referred to as "secondary mania." More recent formulations suggest that late-onset bipolar disorder may represent the outward expression of a long-standing underlying brain condition, perhaps even a multisystem inflammatory disease process. In this scenario, late-onset mania may be considered a kind of "neuroprogression" that is triggered by various medical/neurological conditions in vulnerable individuals. As with most geriatric conditions, there is relatively little research on which to base clear conclusions about these issues.

Most epidemiological studies have been based on psychiatric inpatient samples, where bipolar disorder accounts for 8–10% of late-life psychiatric admissions. Overall prevalence of late-life mania is estimated to be 6.0% in that setting. On average, life expectancy is decreased in individuals with bipolar disorder. Causes include cardiovascular disease, cancer, suicide, and lifestyle factors (e.g., smoking, poor diet, substance abuse). However, older bipolar patients report fewer unmet needs than do older patients with depression, schizophrenia, and dementia.

The Subjective Experience of Bipolar Disorders in the Elderly

Affective States

Affective states correspond to mania/hypomania or depression at other ages. Compared with normal elderly controls, older adults with bipolar disorder may be more passive in their coping styles.

Cognitive Patterns

Cross-sectional studies have demonstrated an association with cognitive impairment, including abnormalities in attention, working memory, executive function, verbal memory, and processing speed, and a significant impact on disability. Longitudinal studies will be necessary to shed light on whether the cognitive impairments are causes or effects of the bipolar states.

Somatic States

Older adults with bipolar disorder generally have multiple chronic medical conditions, sometimes related to metabolic syndromes. The picture is complicated by the fact that older adults with bipolar disorder are likely to have taken psychotropic medications for an extended period, which may contribute to a metabolic syndrome. Thus it is currently difficult to know whether older adults with bipolar disorder have an inherent increased risk of medical problems, or whether at least some of the associated medical problems are due to long-term use of psychotropic medications.

Relationship Patterns

As there are for most persons suffering from serious mental conditions, there are predictable disruptions in significant relationships. The episodic and cyclic longitudinal trend of bipolar disorder adds further complexity and uncertainty, which are stressful both to individuals with bipolar disorder and to their loved ones. There is often a feeling of "waiting for the other shoe to drop" (i.e., waiting for the inevitable manic or depressive episode that will consume thoughts and cause disability).

Suggestions for Treatment

In older adults, manic/hypomanic symptoms may be viewed as defenses against the pervasive fear of experiencing depressive feelings and symptoms. Sometimes anxiety induced by age-related physical, psychological, and cognitive changes and difficulties may worsen this defensive attitude and induce manic-like symptoms and behaviors.

Clinical treatment requires the ability to understand what is happening to the older bipolar patient, as well as to work through massive primitive defense mechanisms to help the patient to keep in touch with feelings and realities and develop more adaptive cognitive attitudes and behaviors.

Clinical Illustration

A 74-year-old married woman with a history of bipolar disorder who had been relatively stable and high functioning for 20 years had a bout of serious respiratory illness necessitating hospitalization and treatment in the intensive care unit. Rehabilitation was slow and difficult, and she developed some relatively mild depressive symptoms. A year later, she developed hypomanic symptoms, with mind racing, preoccupation with events from early life, paranoia, and mild insomnia. Despite treatment with psychotherapy and medications (lamotrigine and quetiapine), her symptoms worsened, and she was eventually hospitalized for psychiatric treatment. Gradually, her symptoms resolved as her chronic marital difficulties were addressed and as important changes were made to increase the quality of her life.

SE3 Disorders Related Primarily to Anxiety

SE31 Anxiety Disorders

In DSM-5, anxiety disorders are characterized by excessive fear in the absence of obvious danger, as well as prominent avoidant behaviors. Associated symptoms include insomnia; trouble sleeping, or sleeping more than normal; irregular heartbeat; muscular tension; and impaired concentration or feeling as though the mind goes blank. To meet diagnostic criteria for disorders, the irrational fears and reactions must also result in interference with social life, work life, or other areas of functioning. Typical worries in younger populations concern job responsibilities or performance, personal health or the health of family members, financial matters, and other everyday life circumstances.

Convergent evidence suggests that that some of these criteria are inadequate for diagnosing anxiety late in life because anxiety is more heterogeneous in older than in younger adults, and is both experienced and expressed in ways that differ from their counterparts in younger populations (Bryant et al., 2013). Anxiety in the elderly is strongly affected by medical conditions common in geriatric patients and by medical comorbidity, cognitive decline, and effects of age-related physiological and psychological changes. A unique feature of anxiety in old age is high comorbidity with depression; the diagnosis of mixed anxiety–depression (or, in DSM-5, a depressive disorder carrying the specifier "with anxious distress") may be particularly useful in late-life conditions. Older anxious adults may also have other symptoms that are not being assessed, or they may describe the same symptoms by different terms. Moreover, anxiety symptoms often overlap with medical conditions (e.g., hyperthyroidism); older patients tend to express anxiety as medical or somatic problems such as pain, with related difficulties for distinguishing psychological from physical symptoms (Wolitzky-Taylor, Castriotta, Lenze, Stanley, & Craske, 2010).

When a medical illness is present, comorbid anxiety can exacerbate functional decline, with a consequent increase in use of health services. Comorbidity with cognitive impairment complicates the picture. For example, the relationship between anxiety and dementia is complex. Anxiety symptoms and cognitive difficulties can emerge concurrently, in which case the anxiety may be part of the disease course giving rise to the cognitive decline, or the anxiety can represent fears or worry related to increasing cognitive difficulties. When the anxiety symptoms predate the cognitive decline, the elderly patient may be diagnosed with a separate anxiety disorder; alternatively, the anxiety may be seen as a prodromal manifestation of dementia (Kogan, Edelstein, & McKee, 2008). Finally, as to the other key DSM-5 criterion for diagnosing anxiety disorders—impairment in work or social relationships, or other areas of functioning—such impairment may not be apparent if the person is retired or socially isolated and thus more able to avoid anxiety-provoking situations. It may be more acceptable for older adults with persistent fears of social situations to avoid them, as stereotypes of aging may foster older people's withdrawal from such situations (Lenze & Loebach Wetherell, 2011).

Late-life anxiety disorders have been underrecognized and underestimated by both clinicians and researchers. Identification of anxiety disorders in older adults may be challenging because elders tend to underreport psychological symptoms of anxiety and to overendorse somatic symptoms. Estimated prevalence for anxiety disorders in adults over age 65 ranges from 3 to 14%. Although rates are slightly higher in younger adults, anxiety disorders remain highly prevalent among older people (Gum,

King-Kallimanis, & Kohn, 2009). Perhaps because of Western stereotypes about beauty and youth, anxieties about aging are notably higher in females. Other social factors, such as chronic medical conditions, level of education, socioeconomic status, and physical limitations in daily activities, also influence the experience of aging.

Some evidence suggests that prevalence and severity may vary among subgroups within the broad category of "older adults," decreasing from middle to old age and increasing again after age 80. Anxiety disorders in the elderly are often associated with traumatic events, such as acute physical illness, falls, or muggings. Later onset is infrequent; anxiety symptoms in elderly patients are more common among those with a lifetime history of any affective disorder. With respect to nature and severity of symptoms and responsiveness to treatment, age of onset explains significant variance in the expression of disorders (Bryant, Jackson, & Ames, 2008). Later onset of generalized anxiety disorder has been associated with less symptom severity, higher prevalence of comorbid mood and other psychiatric disorders, and worse health-related quality of life; late-onset panic disorder seems to be associated with less distress during panic attacks than panic disorder with earlier onset (Le Roux, Gatz, & Wetherell, 2005).

Many who report panic attacks and/or phobias earlier in their lives, especially if inadequately treated, experience these symptoms again in later life. According to Sheikh (1996, p. 80), late-onset panic disorder is relatively infrequent and is characterized by "fewer panic symptoms, less avoidance and lower scores on somatization measures compared to early-onset panic disorder." In the elderly, it is often hard to determine whether avoidance behaviors are due to a phobia or to physical impairments. Phobias and somatic problems are often mutually reinforcing; both must be taken into account.

From a psychodynamic perspective, anxiety is an alerting mechanism that arises when our unconscious motivations conflict with the constraints of our conscious minds. Among the different kinds of anxiety that psychodynamic clinicians have identified (see Chapter 3, pp. 164–167), older individuals seem particularly vulnerable to loneliness, separation, and grief. Different patterns of anxious feeling, intensity, and meanings may be expected among the elderly because (1) sources of aging anxiety and (2) exposure to, and impact of, risk factors vary with age (Beekman, 1998). Life changes associated with old age (losses of mental abilities, physical competence, partner, friends, health, independence, and self-esteem related to employment, along with the approaching reality of death) are associated with increased likelihood of having an anxiety disorder late in life. Consequently, anxieties in elderly patients may be typically experienced as feelings of agitation, dread of impending doom, fear of falling, hoarding, and worries about health, whereas worries about work, physical appearance, and a sense of general apprehension are less characteristic of elderly than of younger patients. In particular, fears of falling and worries about death seem to be the most common experiences of anxiety in the elderly, often exacerbated by feelings of "uncontrollability" (Gagnon, Flint, Naglie, & Devins, 2005). Separation anxiety is common in this population, engendering repeated expressions of concern about the health and safety of loved ones. Ruminations about losing people, efforts to remain close to caregivers, and avoidance of being alone at home are common expressions of separation anxiety in the elderly (Wijeratne & Manicavasagar, 2003).

Anxiety late in life may also be triggered by reminders of past anxiety or trauma. Another common source comprises intense feelings of anger and frustration about unwanted changes in life circumstances. Older people with anxiety diagnoses are more likely than younger ones to reduce drastically the amount of time they spend actively, and thus tend to achieve less than they would like. In some older people, worry about minor issues may serve as a way to avoid thinking about their primary concerns. Although older adults do face unique challenges for which worry and subsequent avoidance behaviors may be adaptive (Diefenbach, Stanley, & Beck, 2001), it is also true that age-related stereotypes sometimes increase avoidance of previously enjoyed activities because eliminating them is seen as an inevitable part of "getting older" rather than as the result of anxiety.

The ability to adapt to changing social, psychological, and physical environments across the age span has been found to reduce anxiety in later life by minimizing the negative effects of stereotypes of aging (Lynch, 2000). Old age includes stressful life events such as the loss of loved ones, progressive health impairment, and disability, any of which can make older people vulnerable to emotional disturbance. Bereavement is a primary cause of loneliness and distress because it usually requires a change in close relationships, loss of social support, and changes in coping strategies. Need for help in this context may trigger increased levels of emotional hyperactivation and anxiety, particularly death anxiety.

Identifying anxiety disorders in older adults may be challenging because older individuals tend to underreport psychiatric or emotional problems and to emphasize somatic symptoms, as noted earlier. Symptoms can be extremely distressing and disabling, and sometimes are misdiagnosed and inappropriately treated. This is understandable because anxiety is very heterogeneous in later life, and a significant proportion of the elderly may express anxiety disorders in a singular way. A clinician's first task should be to assess whether a patient's current level of functioning or impairment warrants a diagnosis of anxiety. After this, the clinician should take a thorough psychological history, with the objective of identifying any medical conditions that are common but underdiagnosed in the elderly or any medications that mimic the symptoms of anxiety. The clinician also needs to be clear, given the realistic difficulties in later life, about the specific content of older adults' worries, to determine with the patient which topics should be addressed in treatment.

The Subjective Experience of Anxiety Disorders in the Elderly

Affective States

Anxious older adults report decreased life satisfaction and increased loneliness. They do not always acknowledge depressed mood; some authors suggest that depression without sadness is characteristic for older adults, although other authors suggest that depression is *not* a normal aspect of old age (see the earlier discussion of depressive disorders). Experiences of anxiety in younger persons include uneasiness, worry, fear, and general apprehension, whereas subjective feelings of agitation and dread of impending doom seem more characteristic of anxiety in the elderly. Some evidence suggests that older adults experience fewer negative emotional states and a lower level of negative affect (depression, anxiety, guilt, hostility, and shame) relative to younger individuals.

Cognitive Patterns

Cognitive patterns include irrational worries, fears that something awful may happen, preoccupations with unpleasant thoughts, memory impairment, poor perceptions of one's own health, and concurrent fears about any physical signs of difficulty. Elderly people may handle death anxiety in different conscious and unconscious ways; for example, they may protect themselves by "immobilizing time and making everything monotonous" (Quinodoz, 2009, p. 775). The same actions are repeated every day, without meanings or links among them, with no new development taking place over time. Typical cognitive patterns in later years are also characterized by the sense of a more external locus of control.

Somatic States

In later life, anxiety often manifests itself in somatic symptoms, such as motor tension and reduced ability to perform daily activities. Although motor tension is listed in DSM-5 as a symptom of anxiety, older people typically endorse other issues, such as pain and sleep disturbance. Other prominent physical symptoms of anxiety include sweating, restlessness, muscle tension, pacing, tachycardia, poor concentration, fatigue, dizziness, paresthesia, dry mouth, gastrointestinal disturbances, facial grimacing and flushing, palpitations, tremor, and body aches and pains.

Relationship Patterns

Anxious geriatric patients are less independent and therefore increase the burden on family and caregivers. They may become overly warm and nurturant, sometimes to the point of intrusiveness, to alleviate separation anxiety. Anxiety symptoms and avoidant behaviors may require responsiveness from family members, enhancing attention to an anxious elder's frailty and helplessness, generating resentment or guilt, and fostering conflicts among members with different solutions to the problems of care for the elderly relative. For example, the drama of whether to insist that an elderly parent relocate from home to a care facility is common, with different family members taking strong positions on different sides of the question.

The subjective experience of the therapist encountering an elderly patient with an anxiety disorder may vary according to the presence or absence of two variables. First, when anxiety is linked to difficulties related to the aging process, the relationship with the patient is easier because it primarily requires reassurance and supportive interventions. Conversely, when the anxiety is free-floating and not linked to identifiable situations, psychological treatment is more difficult and often requires pharmacological support.

Tools for Assessment

Only a few elder-specific measures have been developed to assess anxiety in the elderly. The Adult Manifest Anxiety Scale—Elderly Version (Lowe & Reynolds, 2006) includes three subscales: worry/stress, fear of aging, and physiological symptoms. Other psychogeriatric assessment measures that specifically target anxiety symptoms in the elderly include the Geriatric Anxiety Scale (GAS; Segal, June, Payne, Coolidge, & Yochim, 2010) and the Geriatric Anxiety Inventory (GAI; Byrne & Pachana, 2011).

Clinical Illustrations

A 72-year-old woman had been widowed and was now living alone. A reserved person, she had great difficulty expressing emotions in public, despite her obvious grief.

She described herself as an anxious child who had often returned home soon after being dropped off at school by her mother. In her 20th year, she had suffered from panic attacks when she had to leave for college. She had never sought treatment for such problems. When she was 56, one of her three daughters had a car accident; this event led to constant and severe ruminations about the safety of her other daughters and her grandchildren, whom she continued to contact daily. She reported significant physical symptoms of anxiety, such as palpitations and abdominal discomfort, when family visits ended.

Another patient, a 69-year-old married man, denied having been a particularly anxious child, despite rare occasional anxiety about attending school and being left alone at home. At age 53, he suffered from heart attacks; since then, he had been worrying about his health. He described himself as a chronic worrier, experiencing physical anxiety and catastrophic fantasies whenever he had to leave the house or whenever his wife would leave him alone. The fear of falling while out of the house led him to avoid going out, except in the company of his wife, thus exacerbating his sense of isolation and loneliness.

SE32 Obsessive–Compulsive and Related Disorders

Clinical features of obsessive–compulsive and related disorders in the elderly are consistent with the standards described in DSM-5 (American Psychiatric Association, 2013). This category includes obsessive–compulsive disorder (OCD), body dysmorphic disorder (BDD), hoarding disorder, trichotillomania, excoriation or skin-picking disorder, substance/medication-induced obsessive–compulsive and related disorders, obsessive–compulsive and related disorders due to another medical condition, and other specified or unspecified obsessive–compulsive and related disorders. Several other types of disorders are often comorbid with this group of disorders, such as anxiety and mood disorders, as well as obsessive–compulsive personality disorder. Hoarding disorder in particular is often comorbid with more serious psychiatric pathologies, such as major depression and schizophrenia.

There is very little research on obsessive–compulsive and related disorders in the elderly. If untreated, all these disorders tend to become chronic; or, if they do seem to remit, they can recur more often and for longer periods, depending on stressful events. Events involving age-related losses (retirement, bereavement, separation from children, loss of family home), as well as neurocognitive impairments can exacerbate obsessive–compulsive pathology, particularly if untreated in previous life stages.

The most common features of OCD (concerns about cleanliness and contamination, control over one's own forbidden thoughts or taboos, control over causing harm to oneself or others, etc.) are also found in the elderly population affected by the disorder, but the extent of symptoms, forms of expression, and kinds of internal experiences depend on previous clinical history and any already implemented treatments. Biopsychosocial factors related to advancing age can exacerbate the disorder. Relevant research, although limited, shows that if OCD is not treated on its first occurrence, or at least during the first years of its full manifestation, it will generally become chronic.

SE32.1 *Obsessive—Compulsive Disorder*

After age 35, the onset of OCD is uncommon, and old-age onset of OCD is virtually unknown (Ayers, 2010; Carmin, 2002; Kumar, 2000). But elderly individuals with prior susceptibility to obsessive and compulsive symptoms may find that recurrent preoccupations can fluctuate on the basis of stressful events. Without treatment, recovery rates in adults, particularly in the elderly, are low. The limited research on OCD in the elderly does suggest, however, that a history of negative emotionality and behavioral inhibition are risk factors, and stressful and traumatic events are environmental factors that may exacerbate the disorder. A first-degree blood relationship with someone with the disorder increases its likelihood. Integrated pharmacological and psychological therapies can improve quality of life in older people with OCD, even if rates of complete remission of symptoms are very low (Colvin, 1997; Michel, 2003).

SE32.2 *Body Dysmorphic Disorder*

Elderly individuals with a history of BDD may continue "processing" their own bodies obsessively. Unavoidable old-age bodily aesthetic changes amplify these concerns. Individuals with a more integrated personality organization can sometimes diversify or attenuate the disorder (e.g., obsessive thoughts about one's body recur less often, and criticism for perceived defects becomes less severe). In such people, however, other obsessive priorities can occur; or, more typically, depressive symptoms can partially take the place of the ideational overinvestment in the body. BDD is markedly persistent in elderly individuals with a narcissistic personality structure.

In addition, as younger adults with BDD often do (see Chapter 3, pp. 174–176), elderly subjects may seek cosmetic surgery to minimize or remove physical signs of aging. It can be challenging to discriminate between seeking such surgery to suppress symptoms of BDD and doing so to modify physiological changes of the aging body that the person cannot tolerate. The latter may be related to the personality of the elderly subject, as well as to some psychodynamic issues (e.g., the subjective experience of loss) that are typical of the subject's age.

The subjective experience of a therapist encountering an elderly person with body dysmorphic disorder is similar to that of encountering a younger adult with BDD (again, see the discussion of BDD in Chapter 3).

SE32.3 *Hoarding Disorder*

Hoarding disorder is characterized by a persistent difficulty in disposing of or otherwise parting with one's own things, either bought or collected, regardless of their real value. It differs fundamentally from normal collecting, which has a certain organization and order and is connected to specific classes of objects (see also Chapter 3, p. 176). Onset is usually between age 20 and 30. If untreated, it worsens in old age, especially in connection with age-related typical stressful events (Ayers, 2010; Kim, Steketee, & Frost, 2001). In recent years, researchers have dedicated increasing attention to hoarding disorder in the elderly, and have been looking at the social, political, and health care implications of the problem.

Consequences of pathological hoarding include obstructing living spaces (house, office, car) to the point of preventing their intended use, creating serious problems of personal hygiene, and provoking problems with the neighborhood. In the elderly, the social implications of the disorder appear more significant than the implications for health. People living alone or with weak family ties seem particularly vulnerable to hoarding. In such a case, social and psychiatric service providers need to activate integrated interventions to support the patient in eliminating large quantities of collected material. Hoarding behaviors (e.g., digging through garbage, stealing, and/or hiding small things) are also frequent in patients affected by Alzheimer's, Parkinson's, and Huntington's diseases, or by frontotemporal dementia. Differential diagnosis is thus necessary.

SE32.4 *Trichotillomania and Excoriation Disorder*

DSM-5 now identifies two disorders involving body-focused repetitive behaviors: trichotillomania and excoriation (skin-picking) disorder. The behaviors are often preceded or accompanied by specific emotional states, including boredom and anxiety, or by an increase in tension. They produce temporary satisfaction or subjective relief. The various behaviors are accompanied by different degrees of awareness. There are insufficient research data to allow us to highlight differences between elderly and nonelderly populations affected by these disorders.

The Subjective Experience of Obsessive–Compulsive and Related Disorders in the Elderly

Affective States

Affective states of elderly persons with obsessive–compulsive or related disorders are similar to those of younger individuals. Anxiety is the dominant emotion, often associated with generalized impatience toward the invasiveness of the obsessions (Beekman, 1998); continuous self-criticism over one's inadequacy in ridding oneself of the obsessive thoughts and fears; and, occasionally, social shame for not being able to change. In OCD, anxiety can take on the characteristics of restlessness, and it decreases only after the completion of compulsive behavior that is experienced as ordering or regularizing what has been perceived as intolerable (e.g., untidiness) (Kirmizioglu, 2009).

The elderly may show distinctive characteristics in relation to different variables. Greater physical fragility may create a "relentless tenacity" in the fear of losing control. Intensity of control mechanisms can diminish or vary with health, such that a person cannot invest as much energy in fueling the compulsions as before (e.g., reduced physical agility thwarts exercise of acquired rituals). Sometimes the anxiety may find new expressions more compatible with new physical states, redefinition of roles, and changes in the environmental and socioeconomic situation (e.g., depressive symptoms may occur). Consolidations or adjustments in obsessive–compulsive and related disorders will therefore depend on the subjective personality factors, as well as on the quality of family relations and environmental conditions.

Cognitive Patterns

As noted, the content of obsessions in the elderly can change in conjunction with changes in personal life conditions. The critical faculties of the brain that influence the contents of obsessions and compulsions can weaken, along with the weakening of neurocognitive functions. Specific neurocognitive disorders can substantially affect cognitive patterns.

Somatic States

Somatic states in obsessive–compulsive and related disorders are generally connected to the different levels of anxiety and are mostly expressed at the musculoskeletal and neurovegetative levels. High bodily tension can trigger the obsessive mechanisms. In the elderly, overall physical condition affects possible anxiety-induced impairments—a factor that must be taken into account during any evaluation.

Relationship Patterns

Obsessions and compulsions often involve avoidance of social contacts, particularly in situations that trigger compulsive thoughts such as fear of contamination or aggression. This process may reinforce an elderly person's isolation, which then increases the risk of marginality that old age may bring even in the absence of psychopathology. Elderly patients needing assistance are most likely to let their symptomatology be known by their families or those caring for them. This disclosure can lead to increased interpersonal tensions by introducing new difficulties, especially if an elderly person, now in a different and less influential position than before, tries to ensure that the compulsive rules are respected, and to influence family life in accordance with the obsessions (Cullen, 2008).

In the elderly, subjective meanings of BDD and hoarding disorder have more in common with each other than with what happens in younger adults or adolescents. The key subjective issue is loss (of some aesthetic characteristics of the body or of objects in everyday life). The painful perception of the deteriorating body in BDD is faced via continuous and scrupulous observation, which may lead to attempts to re-establish some form of control. Accumulation of objects in hoarding disorder is as such the opposite of the feeling of loss; moreover, the objects, in their inertia, promote the illusion of exercising power. The angry refusal to throw away collected items is often an assertion of strength (against relatives, clinicians, social workers, etc.). Some conditions associated with aging (e.g., increased isolation, consequences of events such as retirement or widowhood) are common to both BDD and hoarding disorder.

Clinical Illustrations

A retired hotel keeper, 75 years old, had had a few relationships with women, but he had never married and had no children. He had been suffering from OCD from a young age, having finally asked for help from a psychologist at age 45, after his father had granted him management of the hotel and houses owned by the family. He was tormented by doubts and fears that he could say publicly, in a fit of temper, that some villagers and politicians were dishonest persons, thieves, or people taking advantage of public money or illegitimate inheritances. His realistic appraisals, and the normal welcome he received from the people he would have offended in his thoughts, were of no use in countering such doubts. This obsessive worry alternated with, and was exacerbated by, doubts over whether he had hit some pedestrian with his car. It was no use checking the rear-view mirror or going back with the car, as he often did, to assure himself that nothing had happened; nothing could reassure him.

After his initial request for help, he had been in psychotherapy for 2 years for obsessions and compulsions. Fearing negative effects, he had refused any pharmacological support. At age 70, he returned to the psychologist. He was now living through two stressful situations: A small skin cancer was diagnosed on his face that required a simple surgical operation, and two nephews decided to renovate the hotel. He felt excluded from their decisions, unable either to control what was going on or to openly oppose the innovations. As in the past, he worried that he had said derisive things and hit someone with the car. He now also feared he had said things to his nephews that might have hurt them. The new treatment required several months to recover the essence of what he had learned during the previous psychological treatment.

In another case, a 72-year-old woman was referred when social services personnel were notified by her sisters, who were worried by her neglect of herself and her home since her retirement. Her apartment was a chaotic health hazard: Newspapers and books were everywhere; there was excessive food, some rotten or expired; in the bedroom were boxes of cookies; clothes and other belongings were in disorderly piles. She originally approached psychotherapy as a kind of cultural entertainment—a premise that allowed her to be more comfortable in the therapeutic relationship. She gradually expressed shame and acknowledged her own limits and accepted the help of both a psychiatrist and a home attendant. Thanks to the latter, she was able to keep the house more tidy and clean. With pharmacological and psychological support, there was a decrease in her symptoms, allowing her to attain a better quality of life.

SE4 Event- and Stressor-Related Disorders

Exposure to a traumatic or stressful event is newly listed in DSM-5 as an explicit diagnostic criterion for all conditions in this section: posttraumatic stress disorder (PTSD), acute stress disorder, and adjustment disorders. Prior editions of DSM listed PTSD as an anxiety disorder, but it has also been construed as a dissociative disorder, an affective disorder, and a personality disorder. Thus the category itself is something of a moving target. The problem dates back at least to Freud's *Introductory Lectures* (1915–1917) and focuses on a fundamental question: Why do some people develop a mental problem as a result of trauma, while others do not? This question is relevant to all health-related conditions, physical as well as mental. Although there is no definitive answer, it has been addressed in terms of personality factors that may increase vulnerability (Mills, 2008; Verhaeghe & Vanheule, 2005) and by efforts to identify positive and protective factors (i.e., resilience) that are activated in many older individuals (Pietrzak & Cook, 2013).

Another stressor-related category in DSM-5 is persistent complex bereavement disorder, listed in DSM-5 as a "condition for further study."

Of the relatively few studies on these disorders in older adults, most focus on PTSD. There is also some literature on "complicated grief" in older adults. We address both these diagnostic categories here.

SE41 Trauma- and Stressor-Related Disorders

SE41.2 *Acute and Posttraumatic Stress Disorders*

For essential features of acute stress disorder and PTSD according to DSM-5 and related concepts, see Chapter 3—specifically, the "Prefatory Comments" in section S4, "Event- and Stressor-Related Disorders" (pp. 177–180).

Acute stress disorder and PTSD in older adults are even more complicated than in younger ones, for many reasons. One involves the time elapsed since the traumatic experience occurred. Thus it is useful to subcategorize PTSD in the elderly as "de novo," "chronic," "delayed-onset," or "complex" (Charles, Garand, Ducrocq, & Clément, 2005). Advanced age is associated with declining health, retirement, cognitive impairment, dependency, and loss of loved ones (and other events considered stressors and/or sources of trauma). More years of life mean more opportunities for new-onset trauma. Medical diagnoses and treatments can themselves be traumatic for older adults (Moye & Rouse, 2015). In addition, PTSD symptoms can emerge or reemerge late in life (e.g., the so-called *après coup* effect), and cumulative trauma may also be important (Cloitre et al., 2009). Previous trauma experience may have an "inoculating" effect on subsequent coping mechanisms (Palgi, Gelkopf, & Berger, 2015). PTSD may impair the ability of elderly persons to deal with life stress and to negotiate the stages of late life successfully (Weintraub & Ruskin, 1999).

Experiences of traumatic events and subsequent reactions may differ between younger and older adults. A recent study (Konnert & Wong, 2014) reports on age differences in the experiencing and processing of emotion, autobiographical memory, and combat experiences. There is also evidence to suggest that age at trauma exposure (early vs. late life) may play a role in subsequent symptomatology (Böttche, Kuwert, & Knaevelsrud, 2012). Epidemiological studies indicate that in the general population, 70–90% of adults over 65 have been exposed to at least one potentially traumatic event (Norris, 1992). Gender differences exist with respect to trauma exposure; these are perhaps attributable to differences in combat exposure. One study found that approximately 70% of older men reported lifetime exposure to trauma, while only 41% of older women reported this (Creamer & Parslow, 2008).

Compared to the general population, older veterans have higher rates of both lifetime trauma exposure and PTSD symptomatology. One type of interpersonal trauma especially relevant for older women is intimate-partner violence. Middle-aged and older women (ages 45–70) are more likely than younger women to have experienced intimate-partner violence (Wilke & Vinton, 2005). As reported in several community studies, prevalence of PTSD in adults over 60 ranges from 1.5 to 4% (Acierno et al., 2007). A recent study of posttraumatic stress syndrome in primary care settings in Québec reported the 6-month prevalence to be 11% (Lamoureux-Lamarche, Vasiliadis, Préville, & Berbiche, 2015). Lifetime prevalence of PTSD in the general adult population is about 8% (Kessler et al., 2005), with point estimates ranging from 2 to 17% among U.S. military samples (Richardson, Frueh, & Acierno, 2010).

Although many older adults do not meet full criteria for a PTSD diagnosis, they may still show some symptoms. The percentage of older adults with subclinical levels of PTSD symptoms ranges from 7 to 15% (Glaesmer, Gunzelmann, Braehler, Forstmeier, & Maercker, 2010; Schnurr, Spiro, Vielhauer, Findler, & Hamblen, 2002; van Zelst, de Beurs, Beekman, Deeg, & van Dyck, 2003). Given the scarcity of studies and the lower tendency for older adults to report psychic (especially emotional) symptoms, these figures may underestimate the actual prevalence of these symptoms in older adults (Cook & Niederehe, 2007).

A particularly interesting phenomenon is the *après coup* effect (also called *Nachträglichkeit* or deferred retroactive impact; see Chapter 3, p. 184), which involves the complex relationship between a significant event that is not initially experienced as traumatic, and the new meaning that it takes on later, when some other event triggers old memories and gives the initial event new meaning (Fohn & Heenen-Wolff, 2011). The resurgence of the event in one's consciousness can itself be traumatic.

With respect to treatment, there is a paucity of studies on PTSD in older adults, but fortunately recent researchers are taking the issues seriously (Cook & O'Donnell, 2005) and beginning to generate useful findings (Cook et al., 2013). In general, increasing age is associated with reduced utilization of mental health services (Smith, Cook, Pietrzak, Hoff, & Harpaz-Rotem, 2016). Psychotherapy interventions validated in younger and middle-aged populations appear acceptable and efficacious with older adults (Dinnen, Simiola, & Cook, 2014), and older adults who resist negative age stereotypes tend to have better outcomes (Levy, Pilver, Chung, & Slade, 2014).

The Subjective Experience of Trauma- and Stressor-Related Disorders in the Elderly

Older patients may talk about problems or respond to questions differently than younger people do. For example, older individuals (veterans and nonveterans alike) may be more likely to report physical concerns or pain, sleep difficulties, gastrointestinal issues, and cognitive difficulties, or to use a general term like "stress." They are less likely to describe emotional difficulties, such as depression or anxiety, and may describe "issues" or "concerns" rather than report "problems."

Affective States

Affective states include anxiety, anger, and feeling overwhelmed, as well as emotional numbing, with dissociation of affect. Fear of recurrent danger may be prominent. Guilt is often present, focused on the event or its aftermath. There may be associated feelings of shame. Avoidance of reminders of the loss is common. A psychoanalytic self-psychology perspective emphasizes the primacy of affect and the conceptualization of trauma as unbearable affect (Carr, 2011).

Cognitive Patterns

Cognitive patterns include difficulty concentrating, as well as negative, distorted thoughts related to traumatic events. Flashbacks and recurrent images are common, as are sleep disturbances associated with nightmares. PTSD in elderly combat veterans and Holocaust survivors is associated with substantial impairments in learning, recall, and recognition memory, compared to nonexposed elders. PTSD is associated with considerable cognitive burden, increasing with age (Golier, Harvey, Legge, & Yehuda, 2006).

Somatic States

Somatic states include hypochondriacal complaints as well as increased vulnerability to various medical conditions. Compared to younger adults, older adults' declining health, worsening cognitive functioning, and social isolation may exacerbate PTSD symptoms. Indeed, the disorder is associated with negative health perceptions, increased use of primary care, and suicidal ideation. Individuals with PTSD are at increased risk of hypertension, dislipidemia, diabetes, and stroke (Cheng et al., 2015).

Prevalence increases after a transient ischemic attack, along with a subjectively overestimated risk of stroke (Kiphuth et al., 2014). When PTSD extends into older adulthoood, there may be fewer symptoms of hyperarousal, avoidance, negative cognitions, and negative mood than in younger adults with PTSD, but older adults report more avoidance, sleep problems, and hyperarousal (Goenjian et al., 1994).

Relationship Patterns

Relationship patterns include social isolation and loneliness (Kuwert, Knaevelsrud, & Pietrzak, 2014). For the other relationship patterns specific to posttraumatic disorders (including the subjective experience of the therapist), see the discussion in Chapter 3.

SE42 Dissociative Disorders

DSM-5 includes the following syndromes in its section on dissociative disorders: dissociative identity disorder, dissociative amnesia, depersonalization/derealization disorder, and other specified or unspecified dissociative disorder. Dissociative disorders are characterized by disruption in potentially every area of psychological functioning, including the normal integration of consciousness, memory, identity, emotion, perception, body representation, motor control, and behavior. There is almost no literature on dissociative disorders in older adults, perhaps because these conditions are rare in the elderly. At least one study suggested a reduction in dissociative experiences with aging (Walker, Gregory, Oakley, Bloch, & Gardner, 1996). Another study, however, describes dissociative disorders in older women, noting that individual differences dictate different approaches (Kluft, 2007). Given the lack of information on this condition in older adults, a meaningful presentation specific for this age group of affective states, cognitive patterns, somatic states, and relationship patterns is not possible.

SE43 Conversion Disorder

Conversion disorder, which involves a list of functional neurological symptoms, requires special consideration. DSM-5's instruction to specify the presence versus absence of psychological stressors is particularly germane to older adults. In harsh environments (which may include family settings, hospitals, or nursing homes), conversion symptoms may be responses to stress, replacing more appropriate reactions that have become impossible because of diminished age-related resources. Sometimes, particularly in old age, the difference between a persistent conversion episode and an acute one is connected to the possibility of modifying the situation that produced the functional neurological symptom. When the diagnosis of conversion disorder is assessed, the therapist's subjective experience resembles the one the therapist experiences when faced with an adult (see Chapter 3, pp. 206–207).

SE45 Persistent Complex Bereavement Disorder (Complicated Grief)

Persistent complex bereavement disorder is listed in DSM-5 as a "condition for further study." Consensus is currently lacking not only on criteria for this proposed diagnosis

(Shear, 2015; Shear et al., 2011), but also on whether it represents a distinct clinical entity (Holland, Neimeyer, Boelen, & Prigerson, 2009; Zisook et al., 2010a, 2010b). Some controversy focuses on length of time since the loss; the DSM-5 proposed criteria for persistent complex bereavement disorder require that severe grief reactions persist for at least 12 months after the death of the loved object.

Prior to the publication of DSM-III (American Psychiatric Association, 1980), bereavement was not part of psychiatry's official nomenclature. DSM-III introduced the "bereavement exclusion" (i.e., the statement that major depressive symptoms after loss of a loved one do not constitute major depressive disorder). Currently, however, in addition to the DSM-5 diagnosis "for further study," the Working Group on the Classification of Disorders Specifically Associated with Stress is proposing including a diagnosis of prolonged grief disorder in ICD-11 (Prigerson et al., 2009; Shear, 2015).

Regardless of uncertain nomenclature and diagnostic categorization, the syndrome clearly relates to the stress and possible trauma of losing of a loved one—an occurrence more common with advancing age. It is characterized by intense grief lasting longer than would be expected by social norms and causing impairment in daily functioning. Although its natural history is not well understood, clinical experience suggests that without treatment, symptoms of complicated grief diminish slowly but can persist.

Data are lacking for older adults, but epidemiological studies suggest that complicated grief affects 2–3% of the population worldwide (He et al., 2014; Kersting, Brahler, Glaesmer, & Wagner, 2011). Prevalence is approximately 10–20% after the death of a partner, and even higher among parents who have lost children (Meert et al., 2011); it is more likely when a death is sudden or violent (van Denderen, de Keijser, Kleen, & Boelen, 2015; Mitchell, Kim, Prigerson, & Mortimer, 2005; Tal Young et al., 2012) or accidental (Nakajima, Ito, Shirai, & Konishi, 2012). It is less common after the loss of a parent, grandparent, sibling, or close friend. Prevalence of complicated grief is highest among women older than 60 (Kersting, Brahler, Glaesmer, & Wagner, 2011). Views and experiences of grief are influenced to a high degree by cultures (Burton et al., 2012; Tsutsui, Hasegawa, Hiraga, Ishiki, & Asukai, 2014).

As in acute grief, the hallmarks of complicated grief are persistent, intense yearning, longing, and sadness; symptoms are usually accompanied by insistent thoughts or images of the deceased and by a sense of disbelief or inability to accept the painful reality of the person's death. Rumination is common and often focuses on angry or guilty recrimination related to circumstances of the death. Avoidance of situations that remind one of the loss is also common, as is the urge to hold onto the deceased person by constantly reminiscing or by viewing, touching, or smelling the person's belongings. People with complicated grief often feel shocked, stunned, or emotionally numb; they may also become estranged from others because of the belief that their happiness is inextricably tied to the person who died. They may have a diminished sense of self or discomfort with a changed social role and are often confused by their seemingly endless grief. Friends and relatives frustrated by the apparent uselessness of their support may become critical or stop contacting the bereaved person, increasing the individual's feelings of isolation.

Although they may share many symptoms, complicated grief can be distinguished from major depression and PTSD (Miller, 2012). Anhedonia and self-deprecating feelings are not usually present with complicated grief, but are common in depression and PTSD. Seeking proximity to the deceased person is common in complicated grief, but not in depression or PTSD.

Causes of complicated grief are probably multiple. Risk factors include a history of mood or anxiety disorders, alcohol or drug misuse, and multiple losses. Depression in persons who have been caregivers during a loved one's terminal illness (Allen, Haley, Small, Schonwetter, & McMillan, 2013) and depression early in bereavement (Guldin, O'Connor, Sokolowski, Jensen, & Vedsted, 2011) are predictors of complicated grief later in bereavement. Neuropsychological studies suggest that certain abnormalities are associated with complicated grief—including alterations in functioning of the reward system (in response to reminders of the deceased person) (O'Connor et al., 2008), as well as abnormalities in autobiographical memory (Robinaugh & McNally, 2013), in neural systems involved in emotional regulation (Gupta & Bonanno, 2011), and in neurocognitive functioning (Hall et al., 2014; O'Connor & Arizmendi, 2014).

Personal factors such as these may interact with characteristics of the relationship with the deceased or with the circumstances, context, or consequences of the death to increase the risk. Losing someone with whom one has had a close relationship can be especially hard if the bereaved person had a difficult upbringing or if there are unusually stressful consequences of the death, inadequate social supports, serious conflicts with friends or relatives, or major financial problems after the death.

Complicated grief is associated with other health problems, such as sleep disturbance, substance use disorders, suicidal thinking and behavior, and abnormalities in immune functioning; there are also increased risks of cardiovascular disease and cancer (Buckley et al., 2012). Sleep disturbance, in particular, may contribute to other negative health consequences. In addition, complicated grief may interfere with adherence to prescribed therapeutic regimens for a range of diseases.

The Subjective Experience of Complicated Grief in the Elderly

Affective States

Affective states include feelings of sadness and loss, with yearning and longing for the loved one who died. Guilt is not unusual, and it is generally focused on regrets related to the deceased. Anxiety may be present as well, often related to insecurity without the deceased. There may be rumination about troubling aspects of the death. Anhedonia and feelings of worthlessness are not usually present.

Cognitive Patterns

Cognitive patterns include preoccupation with recurring thoughts, images, and memories of the deceased.

Somatic States

Somatic states include disturbed sleep, although nightmares are not common. There may be disturbed eating behaviors, such as avoiding foods or mealtimes associated with memories of the deceased.

Relationship Patterns

Relationship patterns include avoidance of reminders of the loss, which can include avoidance of individuals and relationships associated with the deceased.

Clinical Illustration

Four years after the death of her husband had ended a long and successful marriage, a 78-year-old woman came to her primary physician because of trouble sleeping. She was sleeping on a couch in her den because she could not bear to sleep in the bed she had shared with her spouse. She had renounced many formerly pleasurable activities because they remind her of him and made her miss him too much. She was declining most social invitations and had become socially isolated. She often ruminated about how unfair it was for her husband to die, how she had not expected him to die before her, and how she wished she could "be with him." She was alternately angry and sad, sometimes blaming herself for not recognizing her husband's illness earlier (which, realistically, would not have made much difference in outcome).

SE5 Somatic Symptom and Related Disorders

Some authors (e.g., Frances, 2013) consider the DSM-5 category of somatic symptom and related disorders absurdly hyperinclusive and recommend using it with caution. Even in the case of elderly patients, prudent use is required, but some other reflections are also needed. Old age is not a disease in itself. In this section, we emphasize "successful aging"—that is, the possibility that an elderly person remains active and engaged in social tasks and functions as a valued point of reference for friends and younger family members.

The aging process does involve the need to cope with new stresses, such as the increased likelihood of illness. Moreover, the elderly are more keenly aware than younger people of the finiteness of time and inevitability of death. Although current living conditions in industrialized society allow longer lifespans, and many adults have only minor medical problems in old age, many others develop multiple somatic symptoms and chronic diseases. McClintock Greenberg (2009) notes that aging increases susceptibility to illness. Incidence of heart disease, for example, is 13.6% in adults ages 45–64, 26.8% of adults ages 65–74, and 36.6% of adults age 75 and older (U.S. Department of Health and Human Services, 2006).

SE51 Somatic Symptom Disorder

Frances (2013, p. 175) suggests a diagnostic prototype: frequent visits to doctors, resistance to realistic reassurance about health, and a life centered around health issues. Behaviors of this type occur in every phase of adulthood, but may be particularly common in old age. In the presence of such concerns in the elderly, reactions of health care professionals and family members may be problematic. Believing that illness is inevitable in old age, they may underestimate an older person's complaints and be unwilling to carry out a careful clinical examination or an assessment of other mental conditions, such as bipolar, depressive, anxiety, or psychotic disorders. Or the reverse may occur: Diagnostic evaluations and medical treatments may be scheduled without consideration for whether the symptomatic condition involves unrealistic health concerns. In all these responses, the real disorder is neither recognized nor treated.

Pain (in DSM-5, "with predominant pain" is one of the specifiers of somatic symptom disorder) presents special challenges. Regardless of its etiology (from arthritis to cancer), pain is almost always associated with some depressive feelings. Patients may feel that life is no longer worth living, if living means having to endure chronic pain (Sheikh, 1996). Often the biggest risk for an elderly person is poorly controlled or even untreated pain because the treating doctor fears an overdose with painkillers or focuses on the depressive reaction, mistakenly believing it to be the cause of the pain. Proper treatment of pain ameliorates mood, reduces anxiety, and improves quality of life.

Finally, the cultural context in which the disorder is expressed may be overlooked: "Different cultures have highly varying thresholds of acceptance of somatic symptoms as being normal and everyday versus being a sign of mental disorder" (Frances, 2013, p. 177). This is especially true with older adults. A clinician may be tempted to underestimate or overestimate the symptomatic complaints because of views expressed by an elderly person's family members and friends.

SE52 Illness Anxiety Disorder (Hypochondriasis)

Nussbaum (2013) reminds us of the criteria for an indispensable differential diagnosis of somatic symptom disorder versus illness anxiety disorder. If worry about ongoing somatic symptoms predominates, we are likely in the presence of somatic symptom disorder; if worry about being ill (without symptoms, or with only mild symptoms) predominates, we are probably in the presence of illness anxiety disorder. This second case is common in old age because the older individual fears that having a serious illness could further aggravate age-related diminished autonomy, increased dependency, and the possible need to be hospitalized or to enter a nursing home or similar facility. DSM-5 introduces a distinction of particular significance for the elderly: There are two groups of individuals affected by illness anxiety disorder, those who are "care-seeking" and those who are "care-avoidant." The first group requires reassurance through demands for continuing diagnostic and medical interventions; the second suffers too much anxiety to put in place all the necessary measures to prevent getting really sick. The etiology of these two different attitudes derives from a patient's personality—for example, dependent or hysteric–histrionic versus avoidant or schizoid (see Chapters 1 and 13 on the P and PE Axes, respectively).

SE53 Factitious Disorders

Factitious disorders are not frequent in old age. In the absence of other mental disorders, such as delusions or psychosis, elderly individuals seem rarely to falsify their psychological or physical symptoms or to induce injury or disease with the intent to deceive. Still, the elderly do sometimes emphasize their suffering as a way to seek attention and support. In such instances, global personality functioning is implicated in the behavior. For example, elderly individuals whose personality style is hysteric–histrionic can involve themselves in dramatizing absent or insignificant symptoms, and the boundary between conscious and unconscious falsification may be uncertain.

SE54 Psychological Factors Affecting Other Medical Conditions

Among the disorders in this chapter of DSM-5, the most important for the elderly may be the diagnosis of psychological factors affecting other medical conditions. This diagnosis is assigned if "a person has a documented medical condition other than a mental disorder, but behavioral or psychological factors adversely affect the course of his medical condition by delaying recovery, decreasing adherence, significantly increasing health risks, or influencing the underlying pathophysiology" (Nussbaum, 2013, p. 99). In general, but especially in older people, the occurrence of a disease can trigger psychological reactions that worsen the discomfort and the possibility of healing—again depending on stress level and underlying personality tendencies. With respect to symptoms that may cause embarrassment (e.g., those related to elimination problems), feelings of shame can interfere with the possibilities for help.

Frances (2013) offers examples of individual differences across ages: After a heart attack, depression can increase the risk of a second attack; a passive–aggressive individual may not follow medical prescriptions; a person who resorts to denial may refuse necessary surgery; and so on. In old age, such situations may occur more often, for multiple reasons: Each disease threatens a loss of autonomy even greater than that connected to the aging process; each symptom is a reminder of the closeness of death; and family members, friends, and health care personnel may react to a disease by increasing their control over the elderly patient via diets, drugs, prohibitions, injunctions, and other well-intentioned but intrusive interventions.

The Subjective Experience of Somatic Symptom and Related Disorders in the Elderly

McClintock Greenberg (2009, pp. 45–46) construes medical illness as "adult-onset trauma," noting that "The conceptualization of PTSD and PTSD symptoms can help us begin to make sense of the kind of experiences people with medical illness have. The diagnosis of PTSD is common in medical patients." This reflection allows us to understand why physical illness can arouse such severe emotional reactions, which may be even more important and pervasive in the elderly. They are already having to deal with minor insults of the aging process. These may be felt as attacks on their integrity and identity. In most cases, elderly people cope well with such difficulties. But the discovery of a disease (or the fear of getting sick) can sometimes threaten their psychological equilibrium.

Affective States

Anxiety is in the foreground, but shame may play a large role (McClintock Greenberg, 2009). Sometimes there may also be guilt based on the conviction of having caused the disease or not having taken the necessary steps to avoid it. An elderly person may call all of his or her bad habits (which may have a long history) into question: diet, smoking, sedentary lifestyle, and other vices. Denial and dissociation may be triggered, along with manic defenses that may interfere with compliance with medical prescriptions (Jerant, Chapman, Duberstein, Robbins, & Franks, 2011). Finally, a special case is represented by people who have experienced earlier trauma: Illness and aging may trigger the recall of such painful events, reactivating old feelings of vulnerability, weakness, and impotence.

Cognitive Patterns

Pervasive anxiety can prevent the use of cognitive resources. Faced with somatic symptoms, or even with the mere possibility of getting sick, an elderly person may be unable to implement effective coping strategies. The negative emotional reactions to the stress represented by the illness, in addition to the sources of stress related to the aging process, may prevent the person from taking direct actions to solve the physical problems or to seek information and help.

Somatic States

Anxiety and alarm worsen every ongoing disease, but especially age-related ailments, increasing the level of concern about health and symptoms.

Relationship Patterns

Disproportionate and persistent thoughts about the seriousness of symptoms, along with intense preoccupation about health, may undermine the autonomy of an elderly person and increase the burden on family members and caregivers. Poor adherence to treatment, excessive dependency or counterdependency, and other maladaptive behaviors may irritate relatives, friends, and health care professionals.

Suggestions for Treatment

The hyperinclusiveness of this diagnosis makes it virtually impossible to give general guidance for treatment. One consideration is that aging inevitably produces physical changes—changes in appearance, sensory and cognitive decline, and vulnerability to illness. All this must be integrated into an evolving sense of self. This is not an easy task, of course, but only by accepting such changes can elderly people enjoy the positive aspects of living a long life, such as stable self-esteem, the acquisition of wisdom, and pleasure in witnessing the growth of the next generation. When possible, professional interventions should be aimed at helping elderly individuals reduce denial and omnipotence, minimize narcissistic concerns, and rely on others when necessary. Some favorable alterations, including weakening of previously automatic defenses, can occur with aging (Zinberg, 1964). Older people often feel keenly the urgency, given their limited remaining time, to change as fast as possible. Therapists and others need to appreciate not only their vulnerabilities, but also their strengths and potential resilience.

Clinical Illustration

A 75-year-old widow was referred by her general practitioner, who was tired of prescribing lab tests and specialist visits that she would repeatedly demand but then avoid for various improbable reasons. Despite the absence of symptoms, she was continually worried about having an unspecified serious illness (cancer, heart disease, diabetes, etc.). Her psychologist suggested that her excessive preoccupation made it so frightening to ascertain the truth about her health status that she had to avoid all further investigation. Her behavior triggered a vicious circle: more anxiety, new requests to the GP, more avoidance, and so on. She asked for help with going for the tests, and a sister-in-law agreed to accompany her. She appeared for most of them and submitted the results to the GP. The finding that she was in good health seemed to calm her a bit, but she asked for more tests at a later date.

SE6 Specific Symptom Disorders

In Chapter 3 on the S Axis, disruptive, impulse-control, and conduct disorders are included in section S6, "Specific Symptom Disorders." Since many of these disorders first occur in childhood and adolescence, and most are not particularly relevant for a section on older adults (indeed, only kleptomania and pyromania are discussed in Chapter 3), they are not included here.

Elimination disorders are also usually diagnosed in children or adolescents, and, by DSM definition, are not attributable to a substance (e.g., a medication) or another medical condition. Elimination problems in older adults (e.g., urinary or bowel incontinence) are almost always associated with medical conditions and/or medications. They are not included in section S6 on the S Axis. Therefore, we do not include them here, either.

SE61 Feeding and Eating Disorders

Clinical features of feeding and eating disorders in the elderly are consistent with the DSM-5 criteria for these disorders. Eating disorders have generally been considered conditions of adolescent girls and young women, but emerging evidence suggests that they can occur throughout the lifespan. Reported prevalence of late-life eating disorders is about 2–4% of this population (Mangweth-Matzek et al., 2006; Smink, van Hoeken, & Hoek, 2012). Eating disorders affect both men and women, but societal responses to the aging process put women in a place of increased vulnerability (Peat, Peyerl, & Muehlenkamp, 2008); in fact, women represent 90% of the reported cases of eating disorders in the elderly. There is some evidence, however, that eating disorders are increasing among older men. For elderly women, eating disorders may occur either in those who never recovered from an early-onset eating disorder or in those with a remitting/relapsing pattern throughout life (Scholtz, Hill, & Lacey, 2010). A relatively small percentage of women develop eating disorders for the first time in their 50s, 60s, and 70s.

Interestingly, DSM-5 diagnostic changes could have implications for older populations. DSM-IV-TR criterion D for anorexia nervosa, requiring amenorrhea, has been deleted from DSM-5; criterion B now permits diagnosis in the absence of fear of gaining weight when there are behaviors that interfere with weight gain; criterion C now requires only lack of recognition of the seriousness of current low body weight. In light of some case reports of late-life eating disorders, fear of food and body image problems, the changes in DSM-5 are likely to increase the percentage of older patients with abnormal eating behaviors who are diagnosed as having anorexia nervosa. No definitive data are currently available about the prevalence of bulimia nervosa or binge-eating disorder in older women. Some evidence suggests that nearly half of those with binge-eating disorder begin bingeing as adults, and that compared with the other eating disorders, binge-eating disorder is more frequent among both males and older individuals (Smink et al., 2012).

Although most of the clinical features of eating disorders are similar between elderly and younger populations, there are differences in causes, drives, and underlying psychological mechanisms. In the elderly, the decline in food intake and the loss of motivation to eat may be caused by social, physiological, or psychological factors, or a combination of these (Huffmann, 2002). Poverty, loneliness, and social isolation contribute to decreased food intake in the elderly. Weight loss or gain may be due to medical illnesses or treatments, leading vulnerable older individuals to engage in unhealthy eating behaviors. Depression, often associated with loss or deterioration of social networks, is a common psychological problem in the elderly and a significant cause of loss of appetite. An aging physical appearance (with age-related body and physiological changes) and changes in familial relationships are associated with level of preoccupation with weight, dieting, and exercise (Lewis & Cachelin, 2001).

Typical features of feeding and eating disorders in the elderly are inappropriate self-control around food, distorted body image, and unsuitable eating attitudes. Some older adults may use eating as a control mechanism to regain power in their lives—a consequence of the loss of control in old age (Harris & Cumella, 2006). For others, an eating disorder may be a way to gain control over loved ones through protest and to draw attention to their discontent with their current lives (Duggal & Lawrence, 2001).

The Subjective Experience of Feeding and Eating Disorders in the Elderly

Precipitating events such as personal losses and life changes amplify the sense of loss of control in older adults, and eating disorders may be a method of coping with these stressful events. Restricting and/or bingeing/purging behaviors can become powerful methods for regulating mood and emotion. Postmenopausal women are increasingly encouraged to stay "fit" and appear youthful, despite the natural signs of aging, and these messages may prompt eating-disordered behaviors among some. Among their many other challenges, many bereaved or divorced old people feel pressures to look as youthful as possible as they begin to socialize with new friends and potential dating partners. Again, these pressures may precipitate disordered eating in vulnerable individuals. Some women spend inordinate energy on diets in attempts to preserve a youthful appearance. For others, the role of caregiver has been consistent throughout their adult years; the transition to an "empty nest" (Brandsma, 2007) may instigate attempts to cope by overeating. Finally, eating disorders in older adults may be a form of indirect suicide.

Affective States

Affective states prevalent among persons with late-onset eating disorders include anxiety over the future; fears of losing attractiveness and sexuality; loneliness and sadness linked to bereavement or discouragement; and annoyance or anger at loss or reduction of social and domestic responsibilities, loss of control over others, and increased outside involvement in their lives. Older individuals are often overwhelmed by feelings of frailty. Shame and humiliation can lead them to engage in secretive behaviors to hide their disorder from others.

Cognitive Patterns

Cognitive patterns may include preoccupations with being useless, worthless, and unloved. Some evidence indicates that older patients with eating disorders have less concern about body shape than younger ones, yet a fear of fatness is usually present.

In some individuals, the disorders follow a lifelong preoccupation with weight and dieting. Individuals with anorexia nervosa tend to be perfectionistic, whereas those who binge tend to engage in dichotomous thinking, seeing the world in stark terms of perfection versus failure. Older individuals commonly appear unconcerned about weight loss.

Somatic States

Somatic states may involve patients' confusion about or distorted views of bodily sensations or perceptions of themselves as heavier than they actually are. The feeling of physical emptiness in the stomach may be associated with the sense of an empty, depleted self. A sense of general fatigue and loss of energy is common.

Relationship Patterns

Relationship patterns in the elderly with eating disorders are characterized by loss of independence from others, due to loss of ability to care for themselves. Loss of control can engender family conflicts in which eating behaviors become a way to protest restrictions placed on the elderly persons by family members, caregivers, or care facility personnel. Food refusal may be used to gain control by inducing guilt and drawing attention to the patients' frailty and helplessness. Family members often report the feeling of being manipulated.

Suggestions for Treatment

Eating disorders are often unrecognized in the elderly, who may be at special risk from associated complications. Given the significant morbidity associated with eating disorders in the elderly, early recognition and proper treatment are essential to improving the quality of life for those affected. Addressing eating disorders in elderly patients can be challenging, as symptoms may coexist with medical or psychiatric disorders or may result from medications (Lapid et al., 2010). Elderly patients may be reluctant to discuss psychological issues and eating issues. Some refuse to admit to their problems, demonstrating the largely ego-syntonic nature of their illness. It is critical to take a careful history and to consult with family members to get a complete picture. Empirically supported treatments developed and evaluated with younger women should be used with appropriate modifications with older adults (Brandsma, 2007).

Clinical Illustration

A 75-year-old woman was referred for evaluation of low weight and bingeing approximately twice a day. She had a history of being overweight and attempting ineffective diets, but never losing significant amounts of weight. Shortly after the death of her husband, she moved closer to her only son. She became homesick, missing her old friends and neighborhood. Around her 70th birthday, and shortly after the death of her sister, she became very sensitive to the topics of death and illness; she stopped driving, declaring herself "too old and frail." She began strenuous dieting, but then began binge eating. She attempted to limit her food intake to low-calorie foods such as vegetables, but would then binge, especially late in the evening. She declined treatment, but said she would consider it at a later time.

SE62 Sleep–Wake Disorders

DSM-5 classifies sleep–wake disorders into the following categories: insomnia and hypersomnolence disorders; narcolepsy; breathing-related sleep disorders; circadian rhythm sleep–wake disorders; several types of parasomnias; substance/medication-induced sleep disorder; and six other specified/unspecified diagnoses.

Sleep problems are often unrecognized and undiagnosed. Because coexisting medical conditions are common, it is not surprising that sleep disorders are prevalent in older adults, who have multiple chronic medical conditions. Awakening is the most commonly reported disturbance, with initial insomnia a close second. Discrepancy between subjective and objective measures of sleep increases with age. There is evidence for racial and ethnic differences in sleep in older adults, perhaps related to reporting differences. Interestingly, there may be a psychological mechanism explaining differences in subjective sleep reports, called "repressive coping"; this is perhaps related to older adults' relative positivity and enhanced ability to keep negative emotions from consciousness. In regard to physical/medical aspects, there is some evidence that airway anatomy is more important in older adults (whereas ventilatory control system sensitivity is more important in younger adults). Poor subjective sleep increases the risk of depression, frailty, and death. Sleep apnea and periodic limb movements are, as expected, associated with poor sleep.

Sleep disorders are associated with multiple adverse conditions and outcomes, such as obesity, diabetes, heart disease, cognitive changes, and mood disorders, as well as interpersonal and occupational difficulties. In the daytime, both lethargy and irritability are frequent concomitants of sleep disorders. Use of alcohol before bedtime can increase wakefulness, causing a vicious cycle of seeking alcohol to sleep, then waking more, then drinking more. Sleep–wake disorders also increase the risk of dependence on sleep medications. Some variations in sleep–wake patterns are not related to pathological conditions, but rather to aging itself.

The Subjective Experience of Sleep–Wake Disorders in the Elderly

Affective States

Affective states usually include feelings of distress, frustration, irritability, and anger. There is often a discrepancy between subjective and objective measures of sleep; this tends to increase with age, as noted above.

Cognitive Patterns

Sleep-disordered breathing is associated with impairments of attention and concentration, executive function, and verbal recall. Individuals with insomnia may become preoccupied with sleep—a state of mind that increases tension and anxiety, making sleep even more difficult to achieve.

Somatic States

Daytime fatigue is associated with poor night sleep. As noted above, multiple medical conditions (e.g., obesity, cardiovascular disease) are associated with poor sleep.

Relationship Patterns

Sleep problems often lead to altered sleep arrangements (e.g., separate beds or bedrooms), which affect intimacy and sexual life.

Clinical Illustration

An 80-year-old widowed female with lifelong sleep difficulties had worsening sleep patterns and daytime lethargy. She also had considerable anxiety and had developed a dread of night and of not being able to sleep. Consultation with her primary care physician led to multiple prescriptions for medications, none of which were effective for more than a short time. She was referred for psychotherapy, where important and relevant early life experiences were discussed, with some diminishment of her insomnia. Her remaining insomnia led to a discussion of her sleep habits. Subsequent work on her sleep hygiene, as well as integrating these efforts with her personal history and current psychological experience, resulted in satisfactory resolution of her sleep problems.

SE63 Sexual Dysfunctions

DSM-5 has changed its diagnoses of sexual and gender identity disorders, categorizing these disorders in three new sections: sexual dysfunctions, gender dysphoria, and paraphilic disorders. (Paraphilic disorders are discussed in section SE64. In PDM-2, gender dysphoria is called gender incongruence and is not considered a disorder; see section SEApp3 of the Appendix to the SE Axis, pp. 868–870.) DSM-5 indicates that sexual concerns and disorders can vary with age, implying that some have a normative decrement in strength over a long lifetime, but there are no further comments relevant to the elderly. Despite recent literature on the prevalence of sexual difficulties in men and women in late life (Bauer, McAuliffe, & Nay, 2007), there is still a lack of specific and comprehensive knowledge on sexual disorders in old age.

Sexuality plays an increasingly valuable role in the lives of older men and women (Lemieux, Kaiser, Pereira, & Meadows, 2004). As they age, individuals reconceptualize what "sex" means to them, reprioritizing its role in their lives (Gott & Hinchliff, 2003). Risk factors can complicate this adjustment to such an extent that some older people experience a crisis. The normative aging process and the presence of age-related medical conditions may strongly affect the level of distress in response to modification of sexual habits and changed interpretation of the role of sexual functioning. Societal stereotypes may also have a conditioning effect; older individuals can be overwhelmed by assumptions about sexuality—for example, that it is unimportant or shameful.

Cultural views of elderly sexuality can also be powerful barriers to older people's sexual satisfaction. As for younger individuals, sexual health is not simply the absence of sexual disorder; it includes the sense of a pleasurable activity without shame or coercion. In their sexualities, older people are not homogeneous. Some choose not to engage in sexual intercourse or express their sexuality, even in the absence of illness, impairment, or sexual dysfunction; others consider sexual activity a central aspect of their lives. In later years, attitudes about sexuality seem to converge in men and women toward emphasizing a shared enjoyment of the expression of emotional intimacy via sexual expression (Kleinplatz, 2008). Elderly patients may be more reluctant than younger ones to discuss sexual aspects of their lives and may not spontaneously raise such issues with a clinician.

The Subjective Experience of Sexual Dysfunctions in the Elderly

"Sexual dysfunctions" can be defined as obstacles or impairments to activity leading to orgasm or sexual satisfaction. They include not only erectile dysfunction and orgasmic disorder, but also low sexual desire. Many lines of evidence indicate a prevalence of about 19–21% of periodic or frequent sexual problems in men and women ages 40–80 years (Nicolosi et al., 2006). Older age in men is associated with greater prevalence of delayed ejaculation; increased incidence of erectile disorder; decreases in sexual desire and in the potency of sexual cues; and increased prevalence of early ejaculation. In women, older age is associated with decreased sexual interest and arousal and with increased pain related to vaginal dryness (Laumann et al., 2005). Older people also take longer at each phase of the sexual response cycle. Normative age-related physical changes play a role in sexual dysfunctions; psychological age-related concerns may have an exacerbating effect, building barriers to satisfaction of sexual desires.

Depressed older adults are more likely than the general population to have low interest in sexual activity. Anxiety about performance may lead aging males to withdraw from coital activity rather than risk repeated episodes of sexual inadequacy (Bauer et al., 2007). Anxiety and concerns relating to body image may discourage older women from expressing their sexual desires and pursuing sexual activities in their later years or may be consequences of unsatisfying or painful sexual activity (Gelfand, 2000). An older person's sexual activity and interest may also be limited because of the unavailability of a partner or by boredom with the partner who is available. Older adults with partners have reported feeling that a satisfying sexual relationship is important, whereas those without partners have not described such urgency. Psychological difficulties in forming new sexual partnerships may limit enjoyment of, interest in, and frequency of sexual activities. Factors that affect sexuality in later life also include the internalization of social prescriptions of what a "normal" sex life is for older adults (Camacho & Reyes-Ortiz, 2005). In the context of such assumptions, it is common for older adults to deprioritize sex.

Affective States

Affective states vary widely in relation to sexual dysfunctions. Elderly men with erectile dysfunction may feel shame and fear of poor performance, leading to low self-esteem and annoyance. When desire for sexual intimacy is high, however, sexual relations in the elderly may be satisfying even when dysfunctions are present—perhaps especially for women, who face fewer issues of "performance." Religious and social beliefs can also affect sexual expression and feelings of comfort with sexuality.

Cognitive Patterns

Cognitive patterns in men may include concerns about their health status. In both men and women, there may be preoccupation with being useless, worthless, and unloved. Older patients may still have concerns about their sexual orientation, which, if denied, can have deleterious effects not only on sex itself, but also on their self-image, social relationships, and mental health.

Somatic States

Somatic states include low arousal or feelings of irritation in response to intimate kissing, cuddling, or rubbing. Fatigue may set in when it takes a long time to reach orgasm.

Relationship Patterns

Relationship patterns may include taking care of the partner as a kind of substitute for sexual intimacy or avoidance of sex altogether. In older men, interest in and desire for genital sex often shift to the need and sensation of feeling loved as central to their identity related to sexual activity.

Clinical Illustration

A 68-year-old man was referred to his physician for erectile dysfunction. He had been widowed 3 years previously, after 30 years of marriage. He reported sexual desire, but lacked the ability to achieve and maintain an erection. He noted that he had avoided sexual contact with some women he had recently gotten to know in order to avoid the embarrassment of "not being able to perform." Psychological consultation inferred low mood, concerns about self-image and self-worth, and poor motivation to maintain healthy interpersonal relationships.

SE64 Paraphilic Disorders

"Paraphilic disorders" are defined by DSM-5 as persistent and intense atypical sexual arousal patterns that are accompanied by clinically significant distress or impairment. The manual states that advancing age may be associated with decreases in exhibitionistic sexual preferences and behavior, and with reduced drive preference for sexual masochism and other paraphilic behaviors. The psychodynamic literature on paraphilic disturbance in the elderly is dated and anecdotal. Generally, as primary paraphilic disorders in the elderly have had an early onset, they are seen as phenomena that continue in late life. Alternatively, a paraphilia may be secondary to underlying psychopathology, such as dementia, mania, or depressive illness. In these cases, sexual functioning may be characterized by alteration of desire, leading some older men to seek satisfaction through pornography and paraphilic behaviors. They may engage in sadomasochism, fetishism, and especially voyeurism and exhibitionism. A feasible interpretation for exhibitionism suggests that elderly men may have a history of impotence problems and may seek a socially censured behavior to vent their sexual frustrations (Du Mello Kenyon, 1989).

The subjective experience of therapists encountering elderly persons with paraphilic disorders is quite similar to that of therapists treating younger adults with these disorders (see Chapter 3, pp. 220–223).

SE7 Disorders Related to Addiction

SE71 Addictions

SE71.1 *Substance-Related Disorders*

The DSM-5 classification of substance-related disorders is highly complex; we recommend consulting the manual for details. (Table 14.2 at the end of the chapter gives an abbreviated listing of the ICD-10 classification.)

For many reasons, these disorders are underrecognized and underdiagnosed in older adults. As with younger adults, alcohol is a major problem. Compared to younger adults with alcoholism, older adults tend to have less family history of alcoholism and fewer personality disorders. They drink smaller amounts and have more somatic problems.

For older adults, the situation is complicated because significant numbers are addicted to prescribed medications, including sleeping agents, anxiolytics, and analgesics. These addictions are not identified partly because of prevailing myths and "ageist" attitudes—for example, the view that older persons do not develop addictions or the attitude that it does not matter if they do become addicted because they have only a few years to live. Sometimes the prescribing physicians as well as the patients are in some degree of ignorance and/or denial. Even when the problem is brought to their attention, patients often say such things as "Who cares if I'm addicted? I'm 85 years old!" or "My doctor prescribed it for me." Attempts to discontinue sleep medication are often aborted after a day or two, partly because of predictable discomfort related to reduced amounts of the substance, and partly because of unrealistic expectations and lack of proper support for medication withdrawal. The "baby-boomer" generation, now approaching old age, is more likely to use mood-altering substances and is projected to have increased rates of addiction over the next few decades (Gfroerer, Penne, Pemberton, & Folsom, 2003).

The Subjective Experience of Substance-Related Disorders in the Elderly

Affective States

Experiences will differ with the individual as well as with the substance, but in general the substance will ward off both psychological distress (e.g., feelings of shame, guilt, and anxiety) and physiological withdrawal symptoms. If the distress is predominantly anxiety, insomnia, and/or pain, the drug is likely to be a benzodiazepine, sleeping agent, or pain medication. If the distress is associated with a lack of energy and/or motivation, the drug is likely to include a stimulating agent. For older adults with loneliness, alcohol or a benzodiazepine may offer temporary relief. All these agents are associated with depressed mood and irritability. Individuals who develop physiological dependence tend to experience more negative emotions and more dissatisfaction with their coping than those who do not.

Cognitive Patterns

Alcohol and benzodiazepines increase the risk of cognitive impairment, ranging from problems with attention and concentration to problems with memory impairment that may indicate dementia.

Somatic States

Use of alcohol and/or sedatives/hypnotics increases the risk of falls, with subsequent hip fracture and other medical complications.

Relationship Patterns

Addiction generally presents problems for those who are close to the addicted individual. Self-help groups such as Alcoholics Anonymous (AA) and Al-Anon can provide valuable support and affiliation for both addicted individuals and their families and friends.

If the elderly person has had a substance-related disorder more or less continuously during life, the subjective experience of the therapist is quite similar to that with an adult with the same type of problem. On the other hand, the process of aging generally makes the need for previously misused substances less compulsive. Late-onset addictive disorders are less frequent than earlier-onset addictions, and they mainly serve the function of self-medication. In these cases, the therapist must take account of the most frequent reactions to the disorders by family members and the social environment. Sometimes an addiction is tolerated as an extreme manifestation of the aging process; at other times, it is judged severely because it contradicts the idea of responsibility and wisdom, stereotypically attributed to the elderly.

Clinical Illustrations

A 70-year-old married man, a successful attorney, developed alcoholism. He was able to maintain a fairly high functional level, but his wife and adult sons noticed his excessive drinking at family events. His initial denial eventually gave way to acknowledgment, and he joined AA and soon became a leader. His understanding of the causes of his alcoholism was initially superficial and stereotyped. After falling off the wagon, he engaged in psychotherapy and discovered unwelcome aspects of himself that were clearly related to his drinking. He was gradually able to confront his significant chronic marital problems, and he eventually achieved an amicable divorce. For the first time, he was able to pursue a passionate and meaningful emotional life. He remained sober, and his drinking became almost a nonissue.

In another case, an 85-year-old widowed woman with loneliness, mild cognitive impairment, anxiety, and multiple chronic medical problems was followed by her competent but overly busy internist. At the end of another hurried visit, she asked him for something to help her sleep, and she was prescribed a benzodiazepine without discussion about the proper use of such medications. The medication was helpful and so was continued on a nightly basis, with development of dependence, tolerance, depression, and mild cognitive impairment. The family noticed the decline and brought the reluctant woman for psychiatric consultation. With supportive psychotherapy, sleep hygiene techniques, and careful tapering and discontinuation of medication, the woman improved and returned to her baseline level of functioning.

SE71.2 *Behavioral Addictions*

SE71.2.1 GAMBLING DISORDER

In DSM-5, gambling disorder is included in the new chapter titled "Substance-Related and Addictive Disorders." The rationale for this change is that gambling activates brain reward systems similar to those activated by drugs of abuse, and produces behavioral symptoms that appear comparable to those produced by the substance use disorders. The essential feature of gambling disorder is persistent, recurrent, maladaptive gambling behavior that disrupts personal, family, and/or vocational pursuits.

There has been very little research in this area.According to DSM-5, "in the general population the life-time prevalence rate is about 0.4%–1.0%" (American Psychiatric Association, 2013, p. 587). Prevalence of gambling disorder is higher among younger age groups (of older adults) and among males as compared to females. Those with gambling disorder are more likely to be single, divorced, separated, or widowed. Cross-cultural studies suggest important differences among cultural groups in gambling course, behavior, and personal antecedents.

The Subjective Experience of Gambling Disorder in the Elderly

Affective States

Affective states may include shame, guilt, and irritability related to poor self-control and symptoms of anxiety and depression. Gambling is initially attractive because of the "rush" it provides when the gambler risks a lot and wins. Older adults may gamble in an effort to ameliorate negative emotional states; they may have limited access to other exciting activities; or they may be unable to participate in activities that they previously enjoyed, and may be attempting to fill this gap with gambling.

Cognitive Patterns

Gambling is associated with poor decision-making capabilities.

Somatic Patterns

The psychological literature contains no information on somatic aspects of gambling disorder.

Relationship Patterns

Relationship patterns are similar to those characteristic of substance-related disorders. Relationships suffer as the individual denies problems while spending family funds, lying about money, and persisting in secret activities destructive to self and others.

SE71.2.2 SEXUAL ADDICTION

Although relatively infrequent, sexual addiction may be present in old age. The critical differential diagnosis here involves its organic versus psychological basis. The first is a particular feature of a behavioral variant of frontotemporal dementia; the second is an increase in sexual needs, often associated with stressful situations or symptomatic of some mental disorders (e.g., hypomanic episodes).

Chapter 3 (p. 228) states that sexual addiction does not necessarily have to do with a particularly high level of sexual drive. In other words, the problem is the addiction and not the sexual urge itself. This is particularly true in old age, when a sexual addiction may coexist even with a reduced sexual performance and sometimes with a relatively reduced sexual drive. In cases of only modest desire, compulsive behaviors may be aimed at awakening drives that are feared to be disappearing forever. Thus it is common to rely upon paid sex and to use pornography via magazines or the internet. When level of desire and quality of performance are good, sexual addiction can be motivated by the need to reassure oneself of one's ability to seduce and satisfy a partner, protecting one's sexual self-esteem. It is common for sexually addicted elderly individuals to have dysfunctional behaviors that can threaten their health, safety, or resources. Asking for help, even when the addiction has created difficult problems, is infrequent because of shame and fears of disapproval or blame by the family members. In such cases, two culturally determined feelings of uneasiness merge: one involving sexuality and the other involving aging. This combination may be seen as ugly and unspeakable even when suffering is conspicuous.

SE13 Neurocognitive Disorders

SE131 Delirium

DSM-5 defines "delirium" as a disturbance of inattention and awareness—a change in cognition that is not better accounted for by a preexisting, established, or evolving dementia. The disturbance develops over a short period and tends to fluctuate during the day. There is evidence that a general medical condition, a medication or other substance, or some combination causes the disturbance. Delirium is a complex syndrome, not a discrete disease entity. It manifests itself in different ways, such as with predominant hyper- or hypoactivity, psychotic symptoms (hallucinations and/or delusions and/or misidentifications), or severe alterations of consciousness. Incidence varies, depending on the setting: 15% of older adults develop delirium after some types of elective surgery, and up to 80% in intensive care units show symptoms of delirium. Delirium was not well researched in the past, but more studies have appeared in recent years. It was previously thought to be self-limiting, with expected return to baseline functioning, but it is now understood as often being associated with long-term effects and poor health outcomes.

The Subjective Experience of Delirium in the Elderly

Affective States

Delirium may be associated with fear, anxiety, dread, and a sense of loss of control. Conversely, it is sometimes akin to a dream state and may even involve pleasurable emotions. Sometimes these different affective states coexist or alternate.

Cognitive Patterns

In individuals who already have some degree of cognitive impairment, delirium appears to alter the slope of further cognitive decline. In those who do not have demonstrable cognitive impairment, it is associated with increased risk of decline. Recent findings suggest that markers of cognitive resources that are important for delirium may be different from those important for dementia.

Somatic States

Delirium is by definition associated with coexisting medical or surgical illness. Older adults are thought to have less physiological resources and therefore less capacity to maintain homeostasis in the face of stress than younger adults. There appears to be a role for neuroinflammation in delirium syndrome, perhaps related to changes in the blood–brain barrier.

Relationship Patterns

Relationships are generally stressed and disrupted. It can be particularly distressing for family members and friends to see their loved ones in such an altered state, perhaps expressing ideas that are based on delusions or misidentifications.

Clinical Illustration

An 85-year-old widowed man with mild cognitive impairment underwent elective knee surgery. During postoperative recovery, he developed delirium manifested by agitation and inability to cooperate with hospital staff. His subjective experience shifted dramatically, as he seemed quite frightened and irritable at some times and relatively calm and comfortable at others. With frequent visits from his adult children, reassurance and orienting discussions by the hospital staff, and low-dose antipsychotic medication, the delirium resolved, and he was able to recover psychologically as well as physically.

SE132 Mild Neurocognitive Disorder (Mild Cognitive Impairment)

In DSM-5, the new category of neurocognitive disorders covers both mild and severe forms of dysfunction. Major neurocognitive disorder replaces the term "dementia," and mild neurocognitive disorder replaces the term most often used in the literature, "mild cognitive impairment" (or, in DSM-IV, cognitive disorder not otherwise specified). This confusing set of changes is further complicated by the claim of DSM-5 that neurocognitive disorders "are unique among DSM-5 categories in that these are syndromes for which the underlying pathology, and frequently the etiology as well, can potentially be determined" (American Psychiatric Association, 2013, p. 591). Such a claim is not supported by real-life clinical situations in real time. Indeed, the diagnosis of major or mild neurocognitive disorder remains clinical, as there are no laboratory, genetic, or imaging studies that can allow definitive diagnosis in a living patient. Furthermore, these diagnostic considerations often require longitudinal follow-up. There is currently intense investigation of putative biomarkers, but such an approach is not ready for clinical use.

Regardless of diagnostic nomenclature, the syndrome of mild neurocognitive disorder (mild cognitive impairment) denotes subtle features of impairment that are distinct from aging, but do not interfere with functional status and do not represent dementia. Not surprisingly, there are large numbers of older individuals (young-old as well as old-old) who experience subjective and/or objective mild cognitive impairment, many of whom suffer from fear of developing major neurocognitive disorder (dementia due to Alzheimer's disease or other causes). Prevalence estimates range from 11 to 42%, with an average of 19%. The course of mild neurocognitive disorder is variable: It can stabilize, remit, fluctuate, or develop into major neurocognitive disorder. In primary care settings, about one-quarter of individuals so diagnosed develop major neurocognitive disorder (or dementia) within 3 years. Currently, there is no accepted treatment for mild neurocognitive disorder, although individuals are often counseled to exercise their bodies and minds and are sometimes prescribed medications indicated for treatment of major neurocognitive disorder.

Previous categorizations of mild cognitive impairment into amnestic (i.e., primarily memory) and nonamnestic (executive, language, visual–spatial abilities) types have been of limited value.

Perception of one's own memory is colored by personality and level of insight, as well as by mood symptoms (anxiety and depression). A complicated relationship exists among subjective memory complaints, assessments by observers (e.g., family members), and performance on objective measures of memory and cognition. Changes in subjective memory perceptions are associated with changes in memory performance, but the size of associations between levels of impairment and changes in subjective memory and performance is modulated by personality characteristics and depressive symptoms. Factors other than memory are closely associated with memory perceptions, including overall health status.

The Subjective Experience of Mild Neurocognitive Disorder in the Elderly

Affective States

Symptoms of anxiety, worry, obsessive fears, and dread may accompany mild neurocognitive disorder. The subjective experience is often related to how an individual deals with uncertainty. Denial is common and used to be considered a reliable sign that a true dementing disorder was developing. Although that sign is no longer considered reliable, it can still be a useful barometer. On the other hand, it is common for individuals with apparently mild impairment to portray themselves as having more significant impairment—a tendency that is often experienced by others as exaggeration.

Cognitive Patterns

Cognitive patterns are inherent to the disorder, and are discussed above.

Somatic States

As the syndrome occurs in older adults who tend to have multiple chronic medical problems, there is almost always consideration of interactions and of potential etiological effects.

Relationship Patterns

These problems often cause strain on family and friends, with frustration on both sides. The issues particularly affect close family and friends, especially those with feelings of responsibility toward the individual and/or society (e.g., intense concerns about driving).

Clinical Illustration

An 82-year-old married woman presented with multiple chronic medical conditions and complaints that she was forgetting people's names and could not easily come up with words in casual conversation. She recalled one of her grandparents' becoming "senile" in old age, and she experienced considerable worry that this might happen to her. She was able to function in her usual activities, although they required more effort than previously, and sometimes she needed assistance from a caregiver/assistant. She was taking a dozen medications, some known to have effects on cognition (e.g., a benzodiazepine to help with anxiety and sleep, and an anticholinergic medication for bladder control). Her family vacillated between being dismissive toward what seemed like exaggerated complaints and being (overly) concerned that she was declining quickly. Evaluation and treatment included the patient, her family, and her primary care physician. With close follow-up and careful implementation of only one intervention at a time, the patient's medication regimen was simplified, and a combination of individual and family therapy resulted in stabilization and slight improvement in her cognitive impairment.

SE133 Major Neurocognitive Disorder (Dementia)

The publication of DSM-5 brought significant changes in the conceptualization of dementia. Under the new system, DSM-IV diagnoses, such as dementia of the Alzheimer's type and dementia due to Parkinson's disease, have been replaced by the global diagnosis of major neurocognitive disorder. Major neurocognitive disorder comprises the definitional core of neurocognitive and behavioral symptoms, such as impairment in encoding, recall of information, or executive dysfunction. Once the diagnosis has been established, it is refined by specifying presumed etiology, such as vascular type or frontotemporal type. As noted in the previous section, DSM-5 has further established the new diagnosis of mild neurocognitive disorder, in which cognitive problems are present but are milder than those of major neurocognitive disorder, and do not carry the functional impairments found in major neurocognitive disorder.

The subjective experience of a person with major neurocognitive disorder can vary widely based on premorbid history, etiology of the disorder, and stage of the illness. But the disorder itself often prevents clinicians from developing a substantive sense of the person's unique reality. The person may well have lost the capacity for insight and the language with which to conceptualize inner psychic life. Nonetheless, the person can experience significant emotional and behavioral concerns that warrant intervention. With current clinical and regulatory standards advising against sole reliance on psychotropic medications in these cases, there is a clear need for additional systems of thought with which to conceptualize the person's distress and design complementary interventions. Clinicians need a way of understanding the distress of those who can no longer speak for themselves.

Emotional and behavioral symptoms of major neurocognitive disorder are not merely manifestations of the illness; they also reflect the social and environmental context, as well as the person's intrapsychic perceptions and reactions. Current functions and symptoms need to be understood in the context of that individual's personal narrative. Appreciation of the person's subjective experience can augment more traditional medical evaluation and identify opportunities to intervene therapeutically that might not otherwise be considered.

The Subjective Experience of Major Neurocognitive Disorder in the Elderly

Affective States

Perhaps the greatest of all human fears can be realized in major neurocognitive disorder: disintegration of one's sense of self. In the early stage of the illness, common emotions include anger, depression, and fear. These reactions are often responses to the loss of cognitive abilities, independence, mastery, and sense of control. Frank feelings of panic can emerge, along with guilt over the impact of the illness on loved ones. Frustration and resentment directed at those who are not affected by such illness can occur, as well as loss of self-regard, with the person becoming very sensitive to perceived judgment or correction from others. Taken as a whole, major neurocognitive disorder is a narcissistic wound administered from within, but beyond the control of the self; as such, it represents a violation of our most deeply held human assumptions about self-coherence.

Early in the illness, a person's ego is still present, and the individual is aware of the threat to psychic integrity and connections with relational objects. The person may come under pressure from his or her ego ideal to maintain integrity. Commonly encountered defense in the early stages include anger and projection ("fight") or denial and withdrawal ("flight"). An awkward sense of balance can be maintained for a while. The person retains adequate cognitive functioning to maintain a degree of congruence between ego and ego ideal, and may employ defenses such as those described in order to deal with instances when cognitive errors occur and betray the underlying illness.

For those diagnosed in the early phase, two processes of adjustment can unfold. The first is adaptation to the diagnosis itself; the second is the ever-evolving process of adjusting to the effects of the illness as they emerge. A shift into end-of-life processing can occur at an age earlier than the person ever imagined having to make such a shift. Depending on the type of major neurocognitive disorder, the person may try to resolve the great challenges of Erikson's late-life developmental phase (integrity vs. despair) in ways that would otherwise have been seen as frankly premature. Common to these efforts are complex emotions such as guilt and regret, but also pride, gratitude, and contentment. Although the diagnosis itself must be integrated into the person's life narrative, it need not erase these positive developmental emotional experiences.

Some people with major neurocognitive disorder do "rise to the occasion." That is, they cope through a variety of positive mechanisms, such as activating social supports, gathering information and knowledge, using humor, activating resiliencies gained through managing significant stressors earlier in life, and taking philosophical perspectives. It is not unusual to see individuals alternate between periods of grief over the losses ("loss orientation") and compensatory efforts ("restoration orientation"). Both embracing and avoiding grief can be healthy and adaptive if taken in their own time.

In major neurocognitive disorder, the person's ego gradually becomes weaker as the person moves from early to middle stages. It remains present, however, and thus the person experiences a crisis that has been informally termed "dementia with preserved insight." In other words, the person has some understanding of what is happening but lacks the full ego strength to cope with it. Moreover, the individual's connection with important objects (both external and internal) thins, thereby impairing the natural affect regulation mechanisms these objects represent. With the loss of ability to maintain stable, internal object representations, the sense of a coherent, stable self falters as well. The person becomes more and more reliant on others to maintain a sense of self and to serve as external sources of ego strength.

Even later in the illness, as ego functioning keeps diminishing, the person will lose the ability to engage in reality testing and maintain boundary integrity, thus devolving into primary consciousness. The "autobiographical self" is lost, and existence becomes moment-to-moment. With advancing illness, there is a total loss of object constancy and a reversal of individuation, with increasing dependency. The ability to use mature defenses decays, and regression to more and more primitive defenses takes place.

Cognitive Patterns

Because of neurological changes, the person with major neurocognitive disorder experiences a loss of what have been called "ego functions." These are neurologically mediated and correspond neuropsychologically to frontal executive functions. Among these are the following:

- *Reality testing.* This term refers to the capacity to distinguish what is occurring in one's own mind from what is occurring in the external world. It is perhaps the single most important ego function because it is necessary for negotiating with the outside world. A very common manifestation of impaired reality testing in major neurocognitive disorder is the presence of paranoid delusions.
- *Impulse control.* This is the ability to manage aggressive and/or libidinal wishes without immediate discharge through behavior or symptoms.
- *Affect regulation.* This refers to the ability to modulate feelings without being overwhelmed.
- *Judgment.* This process includes identifying possible courses of action, anticipating and evaluating likely consequences, and making decisions about what is appropriate in certain circumstances.
- *Thought processes.* These are the abilities to engage in logical, coherent, and abstract thoughts.
- *Synthesis.* The synthetic function is the capacity to organize and unify other functions within the personality. It enables the individual to think, feel, and act coherently. It includes the capacity to integrate potentially contradictory experiences, ideas, and feelings; for example, "A girl loves her mother, yet also has angry feelings toward her at times." The ability to synthesize such ideas and feelings is a pivotal developmental achievement.

Somatic States

Although there is no unique pattern of somatic symptoms associated with major neurocognitive disorder, symptoms of other comorbid medical conditions can be frightening for people with cognitive illness. Changes in recall, insight, and self-coherence make individuals unable to understand and cope with symptoms such as pain (e.g., from arthritis). Moreover, they may not be able to remember a medical care provider's explanation of the symptoms or what is being done about them.

Relationship Patterns

Major neurocognitive disorder engenders significant changes of roles in key personal relationships. As the illness advances, a spouse, children, other family members, and friends assume roles that the person with the illness must surrender. These can include instrumental roles (such as holding a job or attending to household duties) and emotional roles (such as serving as a companion for a spouse or parent for a child). Physical intimacy between romantic partners will decline, but may be replaced by renegotiated emotional intimacy. Most fundamentally, boundaries can blur between being a spouse of someone with major neurocognitive disorder and widowhood.

As major neurocognitive disorder progresses, the person becomes more and more dependent on others. Fortunately, the capacity to form attachments, even at a primitive level, can remain intact deep into the illness. With increased dependency comes an increased anxiety about perceived loss of those on whom the person relies (spouse, family, friends, or professional caregivers). For those with premorbid personality pathology or a history of attachment disruptions, such transitions can be especially difficult to complete. Some people with major neurocognitive disorder develop marked apathy as the illness advances, which can be hard for loved ones to understand. Even harder are cases in which the person with major neurocognitive disorder no longer recognizes loved ones or reacts with hostility or suspicion. Caring for someone with major neurocognitive disorder has been described as negotiating a long process of successive transitions and losses or as having to watch a beloved person die at least twice.

Nonetheless, people with major neurocognitive disorder retain the fundamental human needs for connection and nurturance. Vitally, the person's ability to serve as a source of nurturance for others can be preserved as well. In other words, a person with major neurocognitive disorder can remain able to engage in some degree of mutual interaction for a significant time during the illness course. It is a grave error to withdraw interpersonal contact and support from people with major neurocognitive disorder, no matter what stage the illness has reached. Maintenance of connections with others, such as spouses, loved ones, friends, and professionals, can mitigate the loss of selfhood for a considerable time.

SEApp Appendix: Psychological Experiences That May Require Clinical Attention

SEApp1 Demographic Minority Populations (Ethnic, Cultural, Linguistic, Religious, Political)

As stated in Chapter 3 (pp. 232–233), issues related to ethnic, cultural, linguistic, religious, and political diversity are likely to exert influence in an individual's life. Thus demographic minority topics are essential dimensions to be considered in the diagnostic process. The American Psychiatric Association (1994) included sections on cultural formulations and culture-bound syndromes in DSM-IV in response to the increasing awareness of the role of culture in diagnosis. The American Psychological Association developed guidelines for providers of services to ethnic, linguistic, and culturally diverse clients; these were eventually followed by guidelines on multicultural education, training, research, practice, and organizational change (*www.apa.org/pi/oema/resources/policy/multicultural-guidelines.aspx*). To increase psychotherapy's effectiveness, cultural competence and multicultural training need to be emphasized in clinical training programs (Hayes, Owen, & Bieschke, 2015; Tummala-Narra, 2015).

As noted in Chapter 3, an accurate diagnostic assessment must take into account the complex interactions among individual variables and norms, as well as the cultural, social, and family values in relation to which mental disorders are shaped and defined. Especially for elderly patients, it is dangerous to separate aging from ethnic minority issues, since beliefs about aging are grounded in the context of specific societies and specific social practices (Miville & Ferguson, 2014). The ethnic background of an older person is intimately connected to values, roles, affective states, cognitive contents, and relational patterns.

In addition, there are significant ethnicity-related differences in how older adults relate to family members and other social support systems. For example, Miville and Ferguson (2014) reported that older Hispanic Americans occupy a central role in their family and cultural contexts, where there is a focus on interdependence and intergenerational contacts. For older Native Americans, tribal identity, with its high respect for interdependence and connectedness, is central to individual identity, especially in elderly individuals. We note that for Native Americans, the term "elder" denotes a status not necessarily rooted to chronological age; therefore, "older" is not synonymous with "elder."

Ethnicity acts as a filter to the aging process, influencing health, health-related beliefs and behavior, and interaction with health professionals. Many ethnic groups, while identifying and incorporating certain elements of scientifically based understanding of disorder and illness into their lives, nevertheless adhere to more traditional paradigms of health and illness, or associate health-related beliefs and behaviors with specific traditional beliefs that diverge from mainstream (i.e., Western) concepts.

Cultural issues also mark both the shape and content of expression of symptoms. From this perspective, cultural competence is linked with social justice, including ensuring access to appropriate mental health services (Sue, 2001). Researchers estimate that almost two-thirds of older adults with mental disorders do not receive needed services. This problem is particularly acute in such underserved groups as those living in rural areas, those living in poverty, and some ethnic and racial groups (American Psychological Association, 2014; Averill, 2012; Coburn & Bolda, 1999). McClelland, Khanam, and Furnham (2014) examined cultural and age differences in beliefs about depression in a group of British Bangladeshis versus British whites. Older British Bangladeshis viewed depression as an illness that brings shame and loss of dignity to the individual and family. They also favored a lay referral system for sufferers and had more superstitious beliefs about depression than either younger British Bangladeshis or British whites. Older individuals in both groups also tended to feel that depression is not helped by psychological intervention. Attitudes toward depression in the young were similar (and generally positive) in both ethnic groups.

Lawrence and colleagues (2006) explored and compared beliefs about the nature and causes of depression using a multicultural approach incorporating perspectives of black Caribbean, South Asian, and white British older adults. Results showed that depression was often viewed as an illness arising from adverse personal and social circumstances accruing in old age. White British and black Caribbean participants defined depression in terms of low mood and hopelessness; South Asian and black Caribbean participants frequently defined it in terms of worry. These findings underline how cultural beliefs may act to facilitate or deter older people's decisions to seek treatment.

When elderly individuals face life events such as migration from one country to another, the diagnostic process should consider the clinical implications of the complex intersection of different identities, experiences, and membership in different racial and ethnic communities. Space and time are dimensions that strongly qualify the vicissitudes of an elderly person. With respect to life events such as migration, a clinician needs to consider the patient's subjective experiences of the country of origin (which may or may not be the country where the patient grew up), the country where the patient now resides, and the historical period(s) in which the migration(s) occurred. Tummala-Narra (2015) notes that the experience of immigration has been described by psychoanalytic scholars as involving cumulative trauma, disorganization, pain, and frustration (Grinberg & Grinberg, 1989), as well as regression into earlier stages of development, "culture shock," and discontinuity of identity (Akhtar, 2011). Akhtar has used the term "third individuation" to describe changes in identity inherent in the immigration process, while others have focused on interpersonal losses and trauma incurred in immigration and cultural adjustment (Ainslie, 2011; Boulanger, 2004; Foster, 2003). These findings highlight the necessity to provide more culturally sensitive and accessible services for migrant communities and particularly for older individuals in these communities.

Clinical Illustration

A 65-year-old man from a small rural village came to his primary care doctor because of exhaustion, lack of energy, frequent thoughts about death, and loss of appetite. After general medical diagnostic tests, the GP asked whether he had ever consulted a psychologist to examine his mental status and his feelings. The patient stated that he had never even thought that physical well-being could depend on his mind. He wondered what his relatives and his friends would think if he were to go to "a shrink." He believed he did not need such a consultation "because I'm not insane. I've got everything from my life: a wife, beautiful children, and a job. Why shoud I need a psychologist?" Nevertheless, the GP found a sensitive way to appreciate his cultural background and his doubts and beliefs about psychological issues and to evoke his inner feelings. He eventually accepted a referral for counseling.

SEApp2 Lesbian, Gay, and Bisexual Populations

As noted in Chapter 3 (pp. 237–240), lesbians, gay men, and bisexuals living in stigmatizing contexts are subject to minority stress, including internalized homophobia that undermines their psychological and relational well-being. Few studies, however, have focused on lesbian, gay, and bisexual older adults (Fredriksen-Goldsen et al., 2011; for a comprehensive approach, see Harley & Teaster, 2016).

On the basis of prejudice, lesbian, gay, and bisexual older adults may be rejected by other elderly people or by residences for the elderly. Many lesbian, gay, and bisexual older adults are childless and thus less able than their heterosexual cohort to rely on support and assistance from their progeny. The American Psychiatric Association's (2005) "Position Statement on Support of Legal Recognition of Same-Sex Civil Marriage" states that "excluding these adults from civil marriage protections of survivorship and inheritance rights, financial benefits, and legal recognition as a couple in health care settings increases the psychological burden associated with aging."

Specific risk factors for the lesbian, gay, and bisexual elderly concern their health care. Heterosexist attitudes of doctors and paramedics, along with their own fears about discrimination, can increase risk. Many avoid medical checks and treatments (McFarland & Sanders, 2003). The "chosen family"—people considered as family members, although not biologically or legally related—constitutes a critical source of support for sexual minorities. In later life, such "chosen" relationships may be even more important. Nevertheless, they often are not recognized by health care institutions (Institute of Medicine, 2011).

Clinicians may need to take a broader approach than usual—for example, by helping lesbian, gay, and bisexual clients deal with practical issues (asserting their legal rights, identifying social support networks, etc.). It may be useful to retrace the steps of the coming-out process and its success: Individuals with less internalized homophobia and well-integrated sexual identity may have developed a "competence" (Berger, 1980; Kimmel, 1978) relevant to other challenging situations, such as those associated with aging.

Clinical Illustration

A 75-year-old man sought counseling for a depressed mood. He told the examining doctor that a dear friend of his had died 6 months earlier. In the following sessions, feeling more comfortable with the counselor, he clarified that the deceased was his partner. They had been together 15 years, and now he felt very lonely. When he was involved in this relationship, he had had many friends; many of those friends were now dead, several of AIDS. Moreover, the apartment where he lived was owned by his partner, and the partner's heirs wanted him to leave his home of many years. Whereas his partner had had a well-integrated gay identity, the patient had a moderate level of internalized homophobia, which increased after the partner's death. This had several consequences in many areas of everyday life; for example, it prevented him from meeting other gay people and from asserting his rights with his partner's family.

SEApp3 Gender Incongruence

Gender incongruence is characterized by significant distress caused by a discrepancy between an individual's gender identity and the gender assigned at birth. As clarified in Chapter 3 (pp. 240–244), PDM-2 no longer classifies gender incongruence as a disorder, although DSM-5 still includes gender dysphoria as a diagnosis. Late onset (in adulthood) of gender incongruence is quite infrequent; most cases in the elderly originated in childhood or adolescence (Lawrence, 2010). When childhood gender incongruence remains unresolved and continues into adolescence ("persisters"), individuals can feel forced as older people to suppress their transgender identity and live within the confines of gender expectations. The age at which older gender minorities self-identify as transgender, the age at which they come out, their generational cohort, and the age at which they engage in social and/or medical transitions may affect their socialization into gender role behaviors and expectations based on sex assigned at birth (American Psychological Association, 2015). For example, elders who made a gender transition before the 1980s were strongly encouraged by health care providers to "pass" in society as cisgender and heterosexual and to avoid associating with other sexual minorities.

Gender identity concerns may continue to preoccupy such individuals throughout their lives (Stryker, 2008). Old age can represent a phase when it is possible to reflect on one's gender identity and on how one wants to express oneself, sometimes in dramatic ways (van Wagenen, Driskell, & Bradford, 2013). Several factors can converge in late adulthood to reactivate a personal gender identity crisis: Death of a parent, retirement from work, loss of a partner, or the realization of the imminence of one's own death may suddenly provide an opportunity to think about such questions as "Who really am I?", "How have I been conditioned by others until now?", and "How do I want to live my remaining time?"

In this spirit, people can perceive the later stages of life as a chance to explore their gender identity, to find a gender role comfortable for them, and to live and be accepted as a person of the subjectively experienced gender. Changes in the aging body, however, can reduce the possibility of changing to one's preferred gender, causing personal and internal distress. Older people have numerous ways to deal with gender-incongruence-related distress: by partially living in the desired role, by seeking hormone treatment and/or surgery, or by adopting an unconventional gender role (Fabbre, 2015). Elderly people belonging to a gender minority may be more fearful of revealing their identities, despite having had no such problems when younger. Fear of violence and discrimination, as well as actual episodes of violence and discrimination, can increase the risk of refusing medical checks and treatments. They may need supportive social services to deal with current and past discrimination, including housing and employment discrimination. As with lesbian, gay, and bisexual elders, however, transgender older adults may have developed resilient and effective ways of coping with adversities (Fruhauf & Orel, 2015).

Gender surgical reassignment is often the treatment of choice for people with adulthood-onset gender incongruence. Older individuals may be discouraged from seeking sex affirmation surgery, but they may have a smoother gender transition because of age-related decreases in hormone levels (Witten & Eyler, 2012). Although addressing transgender phenomena in the elderly has been facilitated by recent changes in Western countries, these phenomena have not yet been consistently studied in this population (Fredriksen-Goldsen & Muraco, 2010).

The Subjective Experience of Gender Incongruence in the Elderly

Older patients who suffer from gender incongruence report great heterogeneity both in their personal characteristics and in their lifelong gender-related stories (Stoller, 1980). The late recognition that one's gender identity has been externally constrained for many years often comes with depressive feelings and a sense of frustration and failure related to the "years lost" or regrets about how one has lived one's life (Ettner & Wylie, 2013). Achieving awareness and acceptance of one's own gender identity is often a long process, in which older persons set new expectations for themselves and live authentically on their own terms. Although dealing with a "trans identity" in old age may be rather unproblematic for some, others may endure difficult experiences with major consequences, such as high levels of anxiety, anger, tension, and pressure (Hodgkiss, Denman, & Watson, 1991; Kremer & den Daas, 1990; Lothstein, 1979; Siverskog, 2014). In comparison to lesbian, gay, and bisexual elders, transgender and transsexual elders are at higher risk for depression and suicidal ideation (Auldridge, Tamar-Mattis, Kennedy, Ames, & Tobin, 2012; Fredriksen-Goldsen et al., 2011; for a comprehensive discussion, see Harley & Teaster, 2016).

Older patients contemplating a gender transition in late life may feel an urgent sense of time passing; they may feel that identity alteration, especially sex reassignment surgery, must take place quickly. They may see the present as the last chance to express themselves. To attain this new life, patients may become demanding, manipulative, controlling, coercive, and even paranoid.

Affective States

Affective states are characterized by feelings of anxiety, confusion, excitement, and hope linked to what is perceived as the last chance to resolve lifelong gender conflicts. Feelings of shame, ridicule, and self-consciousness may arise when a patient's cross-dressing is treated with derision. Older gender-incongruent patients have been described as depressed, isolated, withdrawn, and subject to profound dependency conflicts.

Cognitive Patterns

Cognitive patterns may include concerns about body appearance, as well as a mix of great expectations and apprehension about what life will be like after hypothetical transgender change. Some older male patients have experienced profound difficulties with their role as fathers.

Somatic States

Physical tension and somatoform symptoms may elicit feelings of irritation, confusion, and anxiety from the gender identity crisis and may sometimes alternate with arousal and excitement about a keenly anticipated new life.

Relationship Patterns

Relationship patterns can be characterized by loneliness and isolation as a consequence of the choice to change gender identity or after a surgery that does not magically provide a lover.

Clinical Illustration

A 73-year-old man came to a gender identity clinic for sex reassignment surgery. Retired from an insurance company, he had had a 28-year-long marriage and two children. Three years after his retirement, he resolved to come out to his family; then he decided to leave his wife and live alone. During the marriage, he had had occasional, unsatisfying experiences of sexual intercourse, as well as recurring and intrusive thoughts about wanting to be female. After the separation, he started a new relationship with a younger woman, but he ended it abruptly 6 months later and fell into a state of deep crisis in which he planned suicide by self-neglect. The crisis ended with his decision to live as a woman. In the psychological consultation, he recalled having had a very restless childhood and adolescence, marked by doubts about his sexual preference. On occasion, he secretly wore women's clothes. The patient reported some lability of mood, apprehension, and a sense of urgency about his "remaining time."

TABLE 14.2. Concordance of PDM-2 and ICD-10/DSM-5 Diagnostic Categories for the Elderly

PDM-2

SE1 Predominantly psychotic disorders
SE15 Late-onset psychosis

ICD-10	DSM-5
F20–29. Schizophrenia, schizotypal, and delusional disorders	Schizophrenia spectrum and other psychotic disorders
F23. Acute and transient psychotic disorder	F23. Brief psychotic disorder
F28/29. Other/unspecified nonorganic psychoses	F28/29. Other specified/unspecified schizophrenia spectrum and other psychotic disorders
	NB: For substance/medication-induced psychotic disorder, see SE71.1. Substance-related disorders.
	For psychotic disorder due to another medical condition, see Table 3.2 (S Axis), S72. Mental disorders due to another medical condition.

PDM-2

SE2 Mood disorders
SE22 Depressive disorders
SE23 Cyclothymic disorder
SE24 Bipolar disorders

ICD-10	DSM-5
F30–39. Mood (affective) disorders	Bipolar and related disorders
F30. Manic episode	F31. Bipolar I disorder
F31. Bipolar affective disorder	Current or most recent episode manic
.0. Current episode hypomanic	.11/.12/.13. Mild/moderate/severe
.1/.2. Current episode manic without/with psychotic symptoms	.2. With psychotic features
	.73/.74. In partial/full remission
.3. Current episode mild/moderate depression	.0. Current or most recent episode hypomanic
.4/.5. Current episode severe depression without/with psychotic symptoms	.73/.74. In partial/full remission
	Current or most recent episode depressed
.6. Current episode mixed	.31/.32. Mild/moderate
.7. Currently in remission	.4. Severe
.8/.9. Other/unspecified bipolar affective disorder	.5. With psychotic features
	.75/.76. In partial/full remission
	F31.81. Bipolar II disorder
	F34.0. Cyclothymic disorder
	F31.89/.9. Other specified/unspecified bipolar and related disorders
	Depressive disorders
F32. Depressive episode	F32. Major depressive disorder (single episode)
.0/.1. Mild/moderate depressive episode	.0/.1/.2. Mild/moderate/severe
.2/.3. Severe depressive episode without/with psychotic symptoms	.3. With psychotic features
	.4/.5. In partial/full remission
.8/.9. Other/unspecified depressive episode	F33. Major depressive disorder (recurrent episode)
F33. Recurrent depressive disorder	.0/.1/.2. Mild/moderate/severe
.0/.1. Current episode mild/moderate	.3. With psychotic features
.2/.3. Current episode severe without/with psychotic symptoms	.41/.42. In partial/full remission
	F34.1. Persistent depressive disorder (dysthymia)

(continued)

TABLE 14.2. *(continued)*

ICD-10	DSM-5
.4. Currently in remission	N94.3. Premenstrual dysphoric disorder
.8/.9. Other/unspecified recurrent depressive disorder	F32.8/.9. Other specified/unspecified depressive disorder
F34. Persistent mood disorders	
.0. Cyclothymia	
.1. Dysthymia	
.8/.9. Other/unspecified persistent mood disorder	
F38/39. Other/unspecified mood disorders	

PDM-2

SE3 Disorders related primarily to anxiety
- SE31 Anxiety disorders
- SE32 Obsessive–compulsive and related disorders
  - SE32.1 Obsessive–compulsive disorder
  - SE32.2 Body dysmorphic disorder
  - SE32.3 Hoarding disorder
  - SE32.4 Trichotillomania and excoriation disorder

ICD-10	DSM-5
F40–48. Neurotic, stress-related, and somatoform disorders	
F40. Phobic anxiety disorders	Anxiety disorders
.0. Agoraphobia (with and without panic)	F40.2x. Specific phobias
.1. Social phobias	F40.1. Social anxiety disorder (social phobia)
.2. Specific (isolated) phobias	F41.0. Panic disorder
F41. Other anxiety disorders	F40.00. Agoraphobia
.0. Panic disorder [episodic paroxysmal anxiety]	F41.1. Generalized anxiety disorder
.1. Generalized anxiety disorder	Substance/medication-induced anxiety disorder
.2. Mixed anxiety and depressive disorder	Specify if: With onset during intoxication. With onset
.3. Other mixed anxiety disorders	during withdrawal, With onset after medication use.
.8./.9. Other specified/unspecified anxiety disorders	F06.4. Anxiety disorder due to another medical condition
	Obsessive–compulsive and related disorders
F42. Obsessive–compulsive disorder	F42. Obsessive–compulsive disorder
.0. Predominantly obsessional thoughts or ruminations	F45.22. Body dysmorphic disoder
	F42. Hoarding disorder (same code as OCD)
.1. Predominantly compulsive acts	F63.3. Trichotillomania
.2. Mixed obsessional thoughts and acts	L98.1. Excoriation (skin-picking) disorder
F63. Habit and impulse disorders	
.3. Trichotillomania	

(continued)

TABLE 14.2. *(continued)*

PDM-2

SE4 Event- and stressor-related disorders
- SE41 Trauma- and stressor-related disorders
  - SE41.2 Acute and posttraumatic stress disorders
- SE42 Dissociative disorders
- SE43 Conversion disorder
- SE45 Persistent complex bereavement disorder (complicated grief)

ICD-10	DSM-5
F40–48. Neurotic, stress-related, and somatoform disorders	
F43. Reaction to severe stress, and adjustment disorders	Trauma- and stressor-related disorders
.0. Acute stress reaction	F43.10. Posttraumatic stress disorder
.1. Posttraumatic stress disorder	F43.0. Acute stress disorder
.2. Adjustment disorders	F43.2. Adjustment disorders
.20. Brief depressive reaction	.21. With depressed mood
.21. Prolonged depressive reaction	.22. With anxiety
.22. Mixed anxiety and depressive reaction	.23. With mixed anxiety and depressed mood
.23. With predominant disturbance of other emotions	.24. With disturbance of conduct
.24. With mixed disturbance of emotions and conduct	.25. With mixed disturbance of emotions and conduct
F48.1. Depersonalization-derealization syndrome	Dissociative disorders
F44. Dissociative (conversion) disorders	F44.81. Dissociative identity disorder
F44.0. Dissociative amnesia	F44.0. Dissociative amnesia. *Specify if:*
F44.1. Dissociative fugue	F44.1. With dissociative fugue
F44.3. Trance and possession disorders	F48.1. Depersonalization/derealization disorder
F44.7. Mixed dissociative (conversion) disorders	F44.88. Other specified dissociative disorder (OSDD)
F44.8. Other dissociative (conversion) disorders	F44.81. OSDD-1, chronic and recurrent syndromes of mixed dissociative symptoms
.80. Ganser's syndrome	F44.88. OSDD-2, identity disturbance due to prolonged and intense coercive persuasion
.81. Multiple personality disorder	F44.88. OSDD-3, acute dissociative reactions to stressful events
.88. Other specified dissociative (conversion) disorders	F44.3. OSDD-4, dissociative trance
F44.9. Dissociative (conversion) disorder, unspecified	
.2. Dissociative stupor	
.4. Dissociative motor disorders	
.5. Dissociative convulsions	Somatic symptom and related disorders
	F44. Conversion disorder
	.4. With weakness or paralysis
	.4. With abnormal movement
	.4. With swallowing symptoms
	.4. With speech symptoms
	.5. With attacks or seizures
	.6. With anesthesia or sensory loss
	.6. With special sensory symptom
	.7. With mixed symptoms

PDM-2

SE5 Somatic symptom and related disorders
- SE51 Somatic symptom disorder
- SE52 Illness anxiety disorder (Hypochondriasis)
- SE53 Factitious disorders
- SE54 Psychological factors affecting other medical conditions

(continued)

TABLE 14.2. *(continued)*

ICD-10	DSM-5
F45. Somatoform disorders .0. Somatization disorder .1. Undifferentiated somatoform disorder .2. Hypochondriacal disorder .3. Somatoform autonomic dysfunction .4. Persistent somatoform pain disorder .8/.9. Other specified/unspecified somatoform disorders F68. Other disorders of adult personality and behavior .1. Intentional production or feigning of symptoms or disabilities, either physical or psychological (factitious disorder)	Somatic symptom and related disorders F45.1. Somatic symptom disorder F45.21. Illness anxiety disorder F68.10. Factitious disorders F45.8/.9. Other specified/unspecified somatic symptom and related disorders

PDM-2

SE6 Specific symptom disorders
- SE61 Feeding and eating disorders
- SE62 Sleep–wake disorders
- SE63 Sexual dysfunctions
- SE64 Paraphilic disorders

ICD-10	DSM-5
F50–59. Behavioral syndromes associated with physiological disturbances and physical factors F50. Eating disorders .0. Anorexia nervosa .2. Bulimia nervosa .8/.9. Other/unspecified eating disorder F51. Nonorganic sleep disorders F51.0. Nonorganic insomnia F51.1. Nonorganic hypersomnia F51.2. Nonorganic disorder of the sleep–wake schedule F51.3. Sleepwalking (somnambulism) F51.4. Sleep terrors F51.5. Nightmares F51.8/.9. Other/unspecified sleep disorders *NB: G codes for DSM-5 disorders at right indicate that these are not considered psychiatric by ICD-10 and are listed elsewhere in ICD-10.*	Feeding and eating disorders F50.01. Anorexia nervosa, restricting type F50.02. Anorexia nervosa, binge-eating/purging type F50.2. Bulimia nervosa F50.8. Binge-eating disorder F50.8/.9. Other specified/unspecified feeding or eating disorders Sleep–wake disorders G47.00. Insomnia disorder G47.10. Hypersomnolence disorder G47.4x. Narcolepsy Breathing-related sleep disorders G47.3x. Obstructive sleep apnea hypopnea, central sleep apnea, sleep-related hypoventilation G47.2x. Circadian rhythm sleep–wake disorders Parasomnias F51.3. Non-REM sleep arousal disorder, sleepwalking type F51.4. Non-REM sleep arousal disorder, sleep terror type F51.5. Nightmare disorder G47.52 . REM sleep behavior disorder G47.8/.9. Other specified/unspecified sleep–wake disorder

(continued)

TABLE 14.2. *(continued)*

ICD-10	DSM-5
F52. Sexual dysfunction, not caused by organic disorder or disease	Sexual dysfunctions
.0. Lack or loss of sexual desire	F52.32. Delayed ejaculation
.1. Sexual aversion and lack of sexual enjoyment	F52.21. Erectile disorder
.2. Failure of genital response	F52.31. Female orgasmic disorder
.3. Orgasmic dysfunction	F52.22. Female sexual interest/arousal disorder
.4. Premature ejaculation	F52.6. Genito-pelvic pain/penetration disorder
.5. Nonorganic vaginismus	F52.0. Male hypoactive sexual desire disorder
.6. Nonorganic dyspareunia	F52.4. Premature ejaculation
.7. Excessive sexual drive	F52.8/.9. Other specified/unspecified sexual dysfunction
.8/9. Other/unspecified sexual dysfunctions	
F65. Disorders of sexual preference	Paraphilic disorders
.0 Fetishism	F65.3. Voyeuristic disorder
.1. Fetishistic transvestism	F65.2. Exhibitionistic disorder
.2. Exhibitionism	F65.81. Frotteuristic disorder
.3. Voyeurism	F65.51. Sexual masochism disorder
.4. Paedophilia	F65.52. Sexual sadism disorder
.5. Sadomasochism	F65.4. Pedophilic disorder
.6. Multiple disorders of sexual preference	F65.0. Fetishistic disorder
.8/9. Other/unspecified disorders of sexual preference	F65.1. Transvestic disorder
	F65.89. Other specified paraphilic disorder
	F65.9. Unspecified paraphilic disorder

PDM-2

SE7 Disorders related to addiction
- SE71 Addictions
  - SE71.1 Substance-related disorders
  - SE71.2 Behavioral addictions
    - S71.2.1 Gambling disorder
    - S71.2.2 Sexual addiction

ICD-10		DSM-5
F10–19. Mental and behavioral disorders due to psychoactive substance use Mental and behavioral disorder due to use of:		Substance-related and addictive disorders
F10. Alcohol	To specify clinical condition:	Substance-related disorders
F11. Opioids	x.0. Acute intoxication	*NB: See abridged ICD-10 listing at left. For a full listing, see pp. 483–585 of DSM-5.*
F12. Cannabinoids	x.1. Harmful use	
F13. Sedatives or hypnotics	x.2. Dependence syndrome	Non-substance-related disorders
F14. Cocaine	x.3. Withdrawal state	F63.0. Gambling disorder
F15. Other stimulants (incl. caffeine)	x.4. Withdrawal state with delirium	*NB: In ICD-10, gambling is in F60–69. Disorders of adult personality and behavior; F63. Habit and impulse disorders, F63.0. Pathological gambling.*
F16. Hallucinogens	x.5. Psychotic disorder	
F17. Tobacco	x.6. Amnesic syndrome	
F18. Volatile solvents	x.7. Residual and late-onset psychotic disorder	
F19. Multiple drug use and use of other psychoactive substances	x.8/.9. Other/unspecified mental and behavioral disorders	
		NB: Sexual addiction per se is not listed in either ICD-10 or DSM-5.

(continued)

TABLE 14.2. *(continued)*

PDM-2

SE13 Neurocognitive disorders
- SE131 Delirium
- SE132 Minor neurocognitive disorder (mild cognitive impairment)
- SE133 Major neurocognitive disorder (dementia)

ICD-10	DSM-5
F00–09. Organic, including symptomatic, mental disorders F00. Dementia in Alzheimer's disease F01. Vascular dementia F02. Dementia in other diseases classified elsewhere F03. Unspecified dementia F04. Organic amnesic syndrome, not induced by alcohol and other psychoactive substances F05. Delirium, not induced by alcohol and other psychoactive substances F06. Other mental disorders due to brain damage and dysfunction and to physical disease .0. Organic hallucinosis .1. Organic catatonic disorder .2. Organic delusional disorder .3. Organic mood disorder .4. Organic anxiety disorder .5. Organic dissociative disorder .6. Organic emotionally labile disorder .7. Mild cognitive disorder .8/9. Other specified/unspecified mental disorder F07. Personality and behavioral disorders due to brain disease, damage, and dysfunction F09. Unspecified organic or symptomatic mental disorder	F06. Mental disorders due to another medical condition (AMC) (each one in its respective diagnostic grouping): .2. Psychotic delusional disorder due to AMC .0. Psychotic hallucinatory disorder due to AMC .1. Catatonia associated with/due to AMC .3. Depressive or bipolar and related disorder due to AMC .4. Anxiety disorder due to AMC .8. Obsessive–compulsive and related disorder due to AMC Neurocognitive disorders Delirium: Substance intoxication Substance withdrawal Medication-induced Due to AMC Major or mild neurocognitive disorder (numerous types, each with its own subtypes): Due to Alzheimer's disease; involving frontotemporal lobes; with Lewy bodies; of vascular origin; due to traumatic brain injury; due to a substance/medication; due to HIV infection; due to prion disease; due to Parkinson's disease; due to Huntington's disease; due to another medical condition; due to multiple etiologies *NB: For a full listing, see pp. 591–643 of DSM-5.*

PDM-2

SEApp Appendix: Psychological experiences that may require clinical attention
- SEApp1 Demographic minority populations (ethnic, cultural, linguistic, religious, political)
- SEApp2 Lesbian, gay, and bisexual populations
- SEApp3 Gender incongruence

ICD-10	DSM-5
F64. Gender identity disorders F64.0. Transsexualism F64.1. Dual-role transvestism F64.8. Other gender identity disorders F64.9. Gender identity disorder, unspecified	F64. Gender dysphoria F64.1. Gender dysphoria in adolescents and adults

ACKNOWLEDGMENTS

The Chapter Editors are grateful to Joan Cook, PhD, New Haven, Connecticut, for her valuable commentary and suggestions regarding PTSD, and to Tamara McClintock Greenberg, PsyD, San Francisco, California, for her suggestions for the SE-Axis depression section.

BIBLIOGRAPHY

General Bibliography

American Psychiatric Association. (2013). *Diagnostic and statistical manual of mental disorders* (5th ed.). Arlington, VA: Author.

Booth, R. (2000). Loneliness as a component of psychiatric disorders. *Medscape General Medicine, 2*(2), 1–7.

Cacioppo, J. T., Hawkley, L. C., & Thisted, R. A. (2010). Perceived social isolation makes me sad: Five year cross-lagged analyses of loneliness and depressive symptomatology in the Chicago Health, Aging, and Social Relations Study. *Psychology and Aging, 25*(2), 453–463.

Eloranta, S., Arve, S., Isoaho, H., Lehtonen, A., & Viitanen, M. (2015). Loneliness of older people aged 70: A comparison of two Finnish cohorts born 20 years apart. *Archives of Gerontology and Geriatrics, 61*(2), 254–260.

Masi, C. M., Chen, H. Y., Hawkley, L. C., & Cacioppo, J. T. (2011). A meta-analysis of interventions to reduce loneliness. *Personality and Social Psychology Review, 15*(3), 219–266.

Sheikh, J. D. (Ed.). (1996). *Treating the elderly.* San Francisco: Jossey-Bass.

Steptoe, A., Shankar, A., Demakakos, P., & Wardle, J. (2013). *Social isolation, loneliness, and all-cause mortality in older men and women. Proceedings of the National Academy of Sciences USA, 110*(15), 5797–5801.

Tilvis, R. S., Laitala, V., Routasalo, P. E., & Pitkälä, K. H. (2011). Suffering from loneliness indicates significant mortality risk of older people. *Journal of Aging Research*, 534–781.

Tornstam, L. (1992). Loneliness in marriage. *Journal of Social and Personal Relationships, 9*(2), 197–217.

Weiss, R. S. (1973). *Loneliness: The experience of emotional and social isolation.* Cambridge, MA: MIT Press.

World Health Organization. (1992). *The ICD-10 classification of mental and behavioural disorders.* Geneva: Author.

SE1 Predominantly Psychotic Disorders

Giblin, S., Clare, L., Livingston, G., & Howard, R. (2004). Psychosocial correlates of late-onset psychosis: Life experiences, cognitive schemas, and attitudes to ageing. *International Journal of Geriatric Psychiatry, 19*(7), 611–623.

Maglione, J. E., Ancoli-Israel, S., Peters, K. W., Paudel, M. L., Yaffe, K., Ensrud, K. E., & Stone, K. L. (2014). Study of Osteoporotic Fractures Research Group: Subjective and objective sleep disturbance and longitudinal risk of depression in a cohort of older women. *Sleep, 37*(7), 1179–1187.

Meesters, P. D., Comijs, H. C., Dröes, R. M., de Haan, L., Smit, J. H., Eikelenboom, P., . . . Stek, M. L. (2013). The care needs of elderly patients with schizophrenia spectrum disorders. *American Journal of Geriatric Psychiatry, 21*(2), 129–137.

Meesters, P. D., de Haan, L., Comijs, H. C., Stek, M. L., Smeets-Janssen, M. M., Weeda, M. R., . . . Beekman, A. T. (2012). Schizophrenia spectrum disorders in later life: Prevalence and distribution of age at onset and sex in a Dutch catchment area. *American Journal of Geriatric Psychiatry, 20*(1), 18–28.

Quin, R. C., Clare, L., Ryan, P., & Jackson, M. (2009). "Not of this world": The subjective experience of late-onset psychosis. *Aging and Mental Health, 13*(6), 779–787.

Smeets-Janssen, M. M., Meesters, P. D., Comijs, H. C., Eikelenboom, P., Smit, J. H., de Haan, L., . . . Stek, M. L. (2013). Theory of mind differences in older patients with early-onset and late-onset paranoid schizophrenia. *International Journal of Geriatric Psychiatry, 28*(11), 1141–1146.

Arts, B., Jabben, N., Krabbendam, L., & van Os, J. (2008). Meta-analyses of cognitive functioning in euthymic bipolar patients and their first-degree relatives. *Psychological Medicine, 38*(6), 771–785.

Azorin, J. M., Kaladjian, A., Adida, M., & Fakra, E. (2012). Late-onset bipolar illness: The geriatric bipolar type VI. *CNS Neuroscience and Therapeutics, 18*(3), 208–213.

Berk, M., Kapczinski, F., Andreazza, A. C., Dean, O., Giorlando, F., Maes, M., . . . Dean, B. (2011). Pathways underlying neuroprogression in bipolar disorder: Focus on inflammation, oxidative stress and neurotrophic factors. *Neuroscience and Biobehavioral Reviews, 35,* 804–817.

Bourne, C., Aydemir, O., Balanza-Martinez, V., Bora, E., Brissos, S., Cavanagh, J. T., . . . Goodwin, G. M. (2013). Neuropsychological testing of cognitive impairment in euthymic bipolar disorder: An individual patient data meta-analysis. *Acta Psychiatrica Scandinavica, 128*(3), 149–162.

Butler, R. N., Lewis, M. I., & Sunderland, T. (1998). *Aging and mental health: Positive psychosocial and biomedical approaches* (5th ed.). Boston: Allyn & Bacon.

Camus, V., Kraehenbuhl, H., Preisig, M., Bula, C. J., & Waeber, G. (2004). Geriatric depression and vascular diseases: What are the links? *Journal of Affective Disorders, 81,* 1–16.

Dautzenberg, G., Lans, L., Meesters, P. D., Kupka, R., Beekman, A., Stek, M. L., & Dols, A. (2015). The care needs of older patients with bipolar disorder. *Aging and Mental Health, 5,* 1–9.

Depp, C. A., & Jeste, D. V. (2004). Bipolar disorder in older adults: A critical review. *Bipolar Disorders, 6*(5), 343–367.

Dols, A., Kupka, R. W., van Lammeren, A., Beekman, A. T., Sajatovic, M., & Stek, M. L. (2014). The prevalence of late-life mania: A review. *Bipolar Disorders, 16*(2), 113–138.

Gallo, J. J., & Lebowitz, B. D. (1999). The epidemiology of common late-life mental disorders in the community: Themes for the new century. *Psychiatric Services, 59,* 1158–1166.

Kessing, L. V., Vradi, E., & Andersen, P. K. (2015). Life expectancy in bipolar disorder. *Bipolar Disorders, 17*(5), 543–548.

Kiloh, L. G. (1961). Pseudo-dementia. *Acta Psychiatrica Scandinavica, 37,* 336–351.

Kim, J. E., & Moen, P. (2001). Is retirement good or bad for subjective well-being? *Current Directions in Psychological Science, 10*(3), 83–86.

Korczyn, A. D., Halperin, I. (2009) Depression and dementia. *Journal of the Neurological Sciences, 283,* 139–142.

Krauthammer, C., & Klerman, G. L. (1978). Secondary mania: Manic syndromes associated with antecedent physical illness or drugs. *Archives of General Psychiatry, 35*(11), 1333–1339.

Kring, A. N., Davison, G. C., Neale, J. M., & Johnson, S. L. (2007). *Abnormal psychology* (10th ed.). Hoboken, NJ: Wiley.

Lala, S. V., & Sajatovic, M. (2012). Medical and psychiatric comorbidities among elderly individuals with bipolar disorder: A literature review. *Journal of Geriatric Psychiatry and Neurology, 25*(1), 20–25.

LaRue, A. (1992). *Aging and neuropsychological assessment.* New York: Plenum Press.

LaRue, A., D'Elia, L. F., Clark, E. O., Spar, J. E., & Jarvik, L. F. (1986). Clinical tests of memory in dementia, depression and healthy aging. *Journal of Psychology and Aging, 1,* 69–77.

Lockwood, K. A., Alexoppulos, G. S., Kakuma, T., & van Gorp, W. G. (2000). Subtypes of cognitive impairment in depressed older adults. *American Journal of Geriatric Psychiatry, 8,* 201–208.

Marengo, J., & Westermeyer, J. F. (1996). Schizophrenia and delusional disorders. In L. L. Carstensen, B. A. Edelstein, & L. Dornbrand (Eds.), *The practical handbook of clinical gerontology* (pp. 255–273). Thousand Oaks, CA: SAGE.

Rosenblatt, A., Mehta, K. M., Romanoski, A., Eaton, W., & Lyketsos, C. (2003). Major depression and cognitive decline after 11.5 years: Findings from the ECA study. *Journal of Nervous and Mental Disease, 191,* 827–830.

Sajatovic, M., Forester, B. P., Gildengers, A., & Mulsant, B. H. (2013). Aging changes and medical complexity in late-life bipolar disorder: Emerging research findings that may help advance care. *Neuropsychiatry, 3*(6), 621–633.

Schouws, S. N., Paans, N. P., Comijs, H. C., Dols, A., & Stek, M. L. (2015). Coping and personality in older patients with bipolar disorder. *Journal of Affective Disorders, 184,* 67–71.

Storand, M., & VandenBos, G. N. (Eds.). (1997). *Neuropsychological assessment of dementia and depression in older adults: A clinician's guide.* Washington, DC: American Psychological Association.

Swainson, R., Hodges, J. R., Galton, C. J., Semple, J., Michael, A., Dunn, B. D., . . . Sahakian, B. J. (2001). Early detection and differential diagnosis of Alzheimer's disease and depression with neuropsychological tasks. *Dementia and Geriatric Cognitive Disorders, 12,* 265–280.

Teri, L., & Reifler, B. V. (1987). Depression and dementia. In L. L. Carstensen & B. A. Edelstein (Eds.), *Handbook of clinical gerontology* (pp. 112–119). New York: Pergamon Press.

Wilcox, S., Evenson, K. R., Aragaki, A. Wassertheil-Smoller, S., Mouton, C. P., & Loevinger, B. L.(2003). The effects of widowhood on physical and mental health, health behavior and health outcomes: The Women's Health Initiative. *Health Psychology, 22,* 513–522.

SE3 Disorders Related Primarily to Anxiety

Ayers, C. L. (2010). Age at onset and clinical features of late life compulsive hoarding. *International Journal of Geriatric Psychiatry, 25*(2), 142–149.

Barrett, A. E., & Robbins, C. (2008). The multiple sources of women's aging anxiety and their relationship with psychological distress. *Journal of Aging and Health, 20*(1), 32–65.

Beekman, A. T. F., de Beurs, E., van Balkom, A. J. L. M., Deeg, D. J. H., van Dyck, R., & van Tilburg, W. (2000). Anxiety and depression in later life: Co-occurrence and communality of risk factors. *American Journal of Psychiatry, 157,* 89–95.

Beekman, A. W. (1998). Anxiety disorders in later life: A report from the Longitudinal Aging Study Amsterdam. *International Journal of Geriatric Psychiatry, 13*(10), 717–726.

Bryant, C., Jackson, H., & Ames, D. (2008). The prevalence of anxiety in older adults: Methodological issues and a review of the literature. *Journal of Affective Disorders, 109,* 233–250.

Bryant, C., Mohlman, J., Gum, A., Stanley, M., Beekman, A. T. F., Loebach Wetherell, J., . . . Lenze, E. J. (2013). Anxiety disorders in older adults: Looking to DSM5 and beyond. *American Journal of Geriatric Psychiatry, 21*(9), 872–876.

Byrne, G. J. & Pachana, N. A. (2011). Development and validation of a short form of the Geriatric Anxiety Inventory—the GAI-SF. *International Psychogeriatrics, 23*(1), 125–131.

Carmin, C. L. (2002). Treatment of late-onset OCD following basal ganglia infarct. *Depression and Anxiety, 15*(2), 87–90.

Colvin, C. A. (1997). Behaviour therapy for obsessive compulsive disorder in a 78-year-old woman. *International Journal of Geriatric Psychiatry, 12*(4), 488–491.

Cullen, B. G. (2008). Demographic and clinical characteristics associated with treatment status in family members with obsessive–compulsive disorder. *Depression and Anxiety, 25*(3), 218–224.

Diefenbach, G. J., Stanley, M. A., & Beck, J. G. (2001). Worry content reported by older adults with and without generalized anxiety disorder. *Aging and Mental Health, 5,* 269–274.

Gagnon, N., Flint, A. J., Naglie, G., & Devins, G. M. (2005) Affective correlates of fear of falling in elderly persons. *American Journal of Geriatric Psychiatry, 13,* 7–14.

Gum, A. M., King-Kallimanis, B., & Kohn, R. (2009). Prevalence of mood, anxiety, and substance-abuse disorders for older Americans in the National Comorbidity Survey-Replication. *American Journal of Geriatric Psychiatry, 17*(9), 769–781.

Kim, H. J., Steketee, G. H., & Frost, R. O. (2001). Hoarding by elderly people. *Health and Social Work, 26*(3), 176–184.

Kirmizioglu, Y. G. (2009). Prevalence of anxiety disorders among elderly people. *International Journal of Geriatric Psychiatry, 24*(9), 1026–1033.

Kogan, J. N., Edelstein, B. A., & McKee, D. R. (2008). Assessment of anxiety in older adults: Current status. *Journal of Anxiety Disorders, 14*(2), 109–132.

Krasucki, C. A. (1998). The relationship between anxiety disorders and age. *International Journal of Geriatric Psychiatry, 13*(2), 79–99.

Kumar, T. S. (2000). Obsessive–compulsive disorder with onset in old age. *Canadian Journal of Psychiatry, 45*(2), 196–197.

Le Roux, H., Gatz, M., & Wetherell, J. L. (2005). Age at onset of generalized anxiety disorder in older adults. *American Journal of Geriatric Psychiatry, 13,* 23–30.

Lenze, E. J., & Loebach Wetherell, J. (2011). Anxiety disorders: New developments in old age. *Journal of Anxiety Disorders, 14*(2), 109–132.

Lowe, P. A., & Reynolds, C. R. (2006). Examination of the psychometric properties of the Adult Manifest Anxiety Scale—Elderly Version scores. *Educational and Psychological Measurement, 66*(1), 93–115.

Lynch, S. (2000). Measurement and prediction of aging anxiety. *Research on Aging, 22,* 533–558.

Michel, B. (2003). Use of paroxetine for the treatment of depression and anxiety disorders in the elderly: A review. *Human Psychopharmacology: Clinical and Experimental, 18*(3), 185.

Quinodoz, D. (2009). Growing old: A psychoanalyst's point of view. *International Journal of Psychoanalysis, 90,* 773–793.

Segal, D. L., June, A., Payne, M., Coolidge, F. L., & Yochim, B. (2010). Development and initial validation of a self-report assessment tool for anxiety among older adults: The Geriatric Anxiety Scale. *Journal of Anxiety Disorders, 24,* 709–714.

Wijeratne, C., & Manicavasagar, V. (2003). Separation anxiety in the elderly. *Anxiety Disorders, 17,* 695–702.

Wolitzky-Taylor, K. B., Castriotta, N., Lenze, E. J., Stanley, M. A., & Craske, M. G. (2010). Anxiety disorders in older adults: A comprehensive review. *Depression and Anxiety, 27,* 190–211.

SE4 Event- and Stressor-Related Disorders

Acierno, R., Lawyer, S. R., Rheingold, A., Kilpatrick, D. G., Resnick, H. S., & Saunders, B. E. (2007). Current psychopathology in previously assaulted older adults. *Journal of Interpersonal Violence, 22,* 250–258.

Allen, J. Y., Haley, W. E., Small, B. J., Schonwetter, R.

S., & McMillan, S. C. (2013). Bereavement among hospice caregivers of cancer patients one year following loss: Predictors of grief, complicated grief, and symptoms of depression. *Journal of Palliative Medicine, 16,* 745–751.

American Psychiatric Association. (1980). *Diagnostic and statistical manual of mental disorders* (3rd ed.). Washington, DC: Author.

Böttche, M., Kuwert, P., & Knaevelsrud, C. (2012). Posttraumatic stress disorder in older adults: An overview of characteristics and treatment approaches. *International Journal of Geriatric Psychiatry, 27*(3), 230–239.

Böttche, M., Pietrzak, R. H., Kuwert, P., & Knaevelsrud, C. (2015). Typologies of posttraumatic stress disorder in treatment-seeking older adults. *International Psychogeriatrics, 27*(3), 501–509.

Buckley, T., Sunari, D., Marshall, A., Bartrop, R., McKinley, S., & Tofler, G. (2012). Physiological correlates of bereavement and the impact of bereavement interventions. *Dialogues in Clinical Neuroscience, 14,* 129–139.

Burton, C. L., Yan, O. H., Pat-Horenczyk, R., Chan, I. S. F, Ho, S., & Bonanno, G. A. (2012). Coping flexibility and complicated grief: A comparison of American and Chinese samples. *Depression and Anxiety, 29*(1), 16–22.

Carr, R. B. (2011). Combat and human existence: Toward an intersubjective approach to combat-related PTSD. *Psychoanalytic Psychology, 28,* 471–496.

Charles, E., Garand, L., Ducrocq, F., & Clément. J. P. (2005). [Post-traumatic stress disorder in the elderly]. *Psychologie et NeuroPsychiatrie du Vieillissement, 3*(4), 291–300.

Cheng, B., Huang, X., Li, S., Hu, S., Luo, Y., Wang, X., . . . Gong, Q. (2015). Gray matter alterations in post-traumatic stress disorder, obsessive–compulsive disorder, and social anxiety disorder. *Frontiers in Behavioral Neuroscience, 9,* 219.

Chu, J. A. (2010). Posttraumatic stress disorder: Beyond DSM-IV. *American Journal of Psychiatry, 167*(6), 615–617.

Cloitre, M., Stolbach, B. C., Herman, J. L., van der Kolk, B., Pynoos, R., Wang, J., & Petkova, E. (2009). A developmental approach to complex PTSD: Childhood and adult cumulative trauma as predictors of symptom complexity. *Journal of Traumatic Stress, 22*(5), 399–408.

Cook, J. M., & Niederehe, G. (2007). Trauma in older adults. In M. J. Friedman, T. M. Keane, & P. A. Resick (Eds.), *Handbook of PTSD: Science and practice* (pp. 252–276). New York: Guilford Press.

Cook, J. M., & O'Donnell, C. (2005). Assessment and psychological treatment of posttraumatic stress disorder in older adults. *Journal of Geriatric Psychiatry and Neurology, 18*(2), 61–71.

Cook, J. M., O'Donnell, C. O., Dinnen, S., Bernardy, N., Rosenheck, R., & Desai, R. (2013). A formative evaluation of two evidence-based psychotherapies for PTSD in VA residential treatment programs. *Journal of Traumatic Stress, 26,* 56–63.

Creamer, M., & Parslow, R. (2008). Trauma exposure and posttraumatic stress disorder in the elderly: A community prevalence study. *American Journal of Geriatric Psychiatry, 16,* 853–856.

Dinnen, S., Simiola, V., & Cook, J. M. (2015). Posttraumatic stress disorder in older adults: A systematic review of the psychotherapy treatment literature. *Aging and Mental Health, 19*(2), 144–150.

Fohn, A., & Heenen-Wolff, S. (2011). The destiny of an unacknowledged trauma: The deferred retroactive effect of apres-coup in the hidden Jewish children of Wartime Belgium. *International Journal of Psychoanalysis, 92,* 5–20.

Freud, S. (1915–1917). Introductory lectures on psychoanalysis. *Standard Edition, 15–16.*

Glaesmer, H., Gunzelmann, T., Braehler, E., Forstmeier, S., & Maercker, A. (2010). Traumatic experiences and post-traumatic stress disorder among elderly Germans: Results of a representative population-based survey. *International Psychogeriatrics, 22*(4), 661–670.

Goenjian, A. K., Najarian, L. M., Pynoos, R. S., Steinberg, A. M., Manoukian, G., Tavosian, A., & Fairbanks, L. A. (1994). Posttraumatic stress disorder in elderly and younger adults after the 1988 earthquake in Armenia. *American Journal of Psychiatry, 151,* 895–901.

Golier, J. A., Harvey, P. D., Legge, J., & Yehuda, R. (2006). Memory performance in older trauma survivors: Implications for the longitudinal course of PTSD. *Annals of the New York Academy of Sciences, 1071,* 54–66.

Guldin, M. B., O'Connor, M., Sokolowski, I., Jensen, A. B., & Vedsted, P. (2011). Identifying bereaved subjects at risk of complicated grief: Predictive value of questionnaire items in a cohort study. *BMC Palliative Care, 10,* 9–9.

Gupta, S., & Bonanno, G. A. (2011). Complicated grief and deficits in emotional expressive flexibility. *Journal of Abnormal Psychology, 120,* 635–643.

Hall, C. A., Reynolds, C. F. III, Butters, M., Zisook, S., Simon, N., Corey-Bloom, J., . . . Shear, M. K. (2014). Cognitive functioning in complicated grief. *Journal of Psychiatric Research, 58,* 20–25.

He, L., Tang, S., Yu, W., Xu, W., Xie, Q., & Wang, J. (2014). The prevalence, comorbidity and risks of prolonged grief disorder among bereaved Chinese adults. *Psychiatry Research, 219,* 347–352.

Herman, J. L. (1992). Complex PTSD: A syndrome in survivors of prolonged and repeated trauma. *Journal of Traumatic Stress, 5,* 377–391.

Holland, J. M, Neimeyer, R. A., Boelen, P. A., & Prigerson, H. G. (2009). The underlying structure of grief: A taxometric investigation of prolonged and normal reactions to loss. *Journal of Psychopathology and Behavioral Assessment, 31,* 190–201.

Kersting, A., Brahler, E., Glaesmer, H., & Wagner, B. (2011). Prevalence of complicated grief in a representative population-based sample. *Journal of Affective Disorders, 131,* 339–343.

Kessler, R. C., Berglund, P. A., Demler, O., Jin, R., Merikangas, K. R., & Walters, E. E. (2005). Lifetime prevalence and age-of-onset distributions of DSM-IV disorders in the National Comorbidity Survey Replication. *Archives of General Psychiatry, 62,* 593–602.

Khouzam, H. R. (2008). Posttraumatic stress disorder and aging. *Postgraduate Medicine, 120*(3), 122–129.

Kiphuth, I. C., Utz, K. S., Noble, A. J., Köhrmann, M., Schenk, T., . . . Schenk, T. (2014). Increased prevalence of posttraumatic stress disorder in patients after transient ischemic attack. *Stroke, 45*(11), 3360–3366.

Kluft, R. P. (2007). The older female patient with a complex chronic dissociative disorder. *Journal of Women Aging, 19*(1–2), 119–137.

Konnert, C., & Wong, M. (2014). Age differences in PTSD among Canadian veterans: Age and health as predictors of PTSD severity. *International Psychogeriatrics, 9,* 1–8.

Kuwert, P., Knaevelsrud, C., & Pietrzak, R. H. (2014). Loneliness among older veterans in the United States: Results from the National Health and Resilience in Veterans Study. *American Journal of Geriatric Psychiatry, 22*(6), 564–569.

Kuwert, P., Pietrzak, R. H., & Glaesmer, H. (2013). Trauma and posttraumatic stress disorder in older adults. *Canadian Medical Association Journal, 185*(8), 685.

Lamoureux-Lamarche, C., Vasiliadis, H. M., Préville, M., & Berbiche, D. (2015). Post-traumatic stress syndrome in a large sample of older adults: Determinants and quality of life. *Aging and Mental Health, 24,* 1–6.

Levy, R. B., Pilver, C., Chung, P. H., & Slade, S. (2014). Subliminal strengthening: Improving older individuals' physical function over time with an implicit-age-stereotype intervention. *Psychological Science, 25,* 2127–2135.

Lunney, C. A., Schnurr, P. P., & Cook, J. M. (2014). Comparison of clinician- and self-assessments of posttraumatic stress symptoms in older versus younger veterans. *Journal of Traumatic Stress, 27*(2), 1444–1451.

Meert, K. L., Shear, K., Newth, C. J. L., Harrison, R., Berger, J., Zimmerman, J., . . . Nicholson, C. (2011). Follow-up study of complicated grief among parents eighteen months after a child's death in the pediatric intensive care unit. *Journal of Palliative Medicine, 14,* 207–214.

Miller, M. D. (2012). Complicated grief in late life. *Dialogues in Clinical Neuroscience, 14*(2), 195–202.

Mills, J. (2008). Attachment deficits, personality structure, and PTSD. *Psychoanalytic Psychology, 25,* 380–385.

Mitchell, A. M., Kim, Y., Prigerson, H. G., & Mortimer. M. K. (2005). Complicated grief and suicidal ideation in adult survivors of suicide. *Suicide and Life-Threatening Behavior, 35,* 498–506.

Moye, J., & Rouse, S. J. (2015). Posttraumatic stress in older adults: When medical diagnoses or treatments cause traumatic stress. *Psychiatric Clinics of North America, 38*(1), 45–57.

Nakajima, S., Ito, M., Shirai, A., & Konishi, T. (2012). Complicated grief in those bereaved by violent death: The effects of post-traumatic stress disorder on complicated grief. *Dialogues in Clinical Neuroscience, 14,* 210–214.

Norris, F. H. (1992). Epidemiology of trauma: Frequency and impact of different potentially traumatic events on different demographic groups. *Journal of Consulting and Clinical Psychology, 60*(3), 409–418.

O'Connor, M. F., & Arizmendi, B. J. (2014). Neuropsychological correlates of complicated grief in older spousally bereaved adults. *Journals of Gerontology: Series B. Psychological Sciences and Social Sciences, 69,* 12–18.

O'Connor, M. F., Wellisch, D. K., Stanton, A. L., Eisenberger, N. I., Irwin, M. R., & Lieberman, M. D. (2008). Craving love?: Enduring grief activates brain's reward center. *NeuroImage, 42,* 969–972.

Palgi, Y., Gelkopf, M., & Berger, R. (2015). The inoculating role of previous exposure to potentially traumatic life events on coping with prolonged exposure to rocket attacks: A lifespan perspective. *Psychiatry Research, 227*(2–3), 296–301.

Pietrzak, R. H., & Cook J. M. (2013). Psychological resilience in older U.S. veterans: Results from the National Health and Resilience in Veterans Study. *Depression and Anxiety, 30*(5), 432–443.

Prigerson, H. G., Horowitz, M. J., Jacobs, S. C., Parkes, C. M., Aslan, M., Goodkin, K., . . . Maciejewski, P. K. (2009). Prolonged grief disorder: Psychometric validation of criteria proposed for DSM-V and ICD-11. *PLoS Medicine, 6*(8), e1000121.

Richardson, L., Frueh, C., & Acierno, R. (2010). Prevalence estimates of combat-related post-traumatic stress disorder: Critical review. *Australian and New Zealand Journal of Psychiatry, 44,* 4–19.

Robinaugh, D. J., & McNally, R. J. (2013). Remembering the past and envisioning the future in bereaved adults with and without complicated grief. *Clinical Psychological Science, 1,* 290–290.

Rosellini, A. J., Stein, M. B., Colpe, L. J., Heeringa, S. G., Petukhova, M. V., Sampson, N. A., . . . Army STARRS Collaborators. (2015). Approximating a DSM-5 diagnosis of PTSD using DSM-IV criteria. *Depression and Anxiety, 32*(7), 493–501.

Schnurr, P. P., Spiro, A., Vielhauer, M. J., Findler, M. N., & Hamblen, J. L. (2002). Trauma in the

lives of older men: Findings from the Normative Aging Study. *Journal of Clinical Geropsychology, 8,* 175–187.
Shear, M. K. (2015). Complicated grief. *New England Journal of Medicine, 372,* 153–160.
Shear, M. K., Simon, N., Wall, M., Zisook, S., Neimeyer, R., Duan, N., . . . Keshaviah, A. (2011). Complicated grief and related bereavement issues for DSM-5. *Depression and Anxiety, 28,* 103–117.
Smith, N. B., Cook, J. M., Pietrzak, R., Hoff, R., & Harpaz-Rotem I. (2016). Mental health treatment for older veterans newly diagnosed with PTSD: A national investigation. *American Journal of Geriatric Psychiatry, 24*(3), 201–212.
Tal Young, I., Iglewicz, A., Glorioso, D., Lanouette, N., Seay, K., Ilapakurti, M., & Zisook, S. (2012). Suicide bereavement and complicated grief. *Dialogues in Clinical Neuroscience, 14*(2), 177–186.
Tsutsui, T., Hasegawa, Y., Hiraga, M., Ishiki, M., & Asukai, N. (2014). Distinctiveness of prolonged grief disorder symptoms among survivors of the great east Japan earthquake and tsunami. *Psychiatry Research, 217*(1–2), 67–71.
van Denderen, M., de Keijser, J., Kleen, M., & Boelen, P. A. (2015). Psychopathology among homicidally bereaved individuals: A systematic review. *Trauma, Violence and Abuse, 16*(1), 70–80.
van Zelst, W. H., de Beurs, E., Beekman, A. T. F., Deeg, D. J. H., & van Dyck, R. (2003). Prevalence and risk factors of posttraumatic stress disorder in older adults. *Psychotherapy and Psychosomatics, 72,* 333–342.
Verhaeghe, P., & Vanheule, S. (2005). Actual neurosis and PTSD: The impact of the other. *Psychoanalytic Psychology, 22,* 493–507.
Walker, R., Gregory, J., Oakley, S., Jr, Bloch, R., & Gardner, M. (1996). Reduction in dissociation due to aging and cognitive deficit. *Comprensive Psychiatry, 37*(1), 31–36.
Weintraub, D., & Ruskin, P. E. (1999). Posttraumatic stress disorder in the elderly: A review. *Harvard Review of Psychiatry, 7*(3), 144–152.
Wilke, D. J., & Vinton, L. (2005). The nature and impact of domestic violence across age cohorts. *Affilia, 20,* 316–328.
Zisook, S., Reynolds, C. F., Pies, R., Simon, N., Lebowitz, B., Madowitz, J., . . . Shear, M. K. (2010a). Bereavement, complicated grief, and DSM: Part 1. Depression. *Journal of Clinical Psychiatry, 71*(7), 955–956.
Zisook, S., Simon, N. M., Reynolds, C. F., Pies, R., Lebowitz, B., Young, I. T., Madowitz, J., & Shear, M. K. (2010b). Bereavement, complicated grief, and DSM: Part 2. Complicated grief. *Journal of Clinical Psychiatry, 71*(8), 1097–1098.

SE5 Somatic Symptom and Related Disorders

Frances, A. (2013). *Essentials of psychiatric diagnosis.* New York: Guilford Press.
Jerant, A., Chapman, B., Duberstein, P., Robbins, J., & Franks, P. (2011). Personality and medication non-adherence among older adults enrolled in a six-year trial. *British Journal of Health Psychology, 16*(1), 151–169.
McClintock Greenberg, T. (2009). *Psychodynamic perspectives on aging and illness.* New York: Springer.
Nussbaum, A. M. (2013). *The pocket guide to the DSM-5 diagnostic exam.* Arlington, VA: American Psychiatric Publishing.
U.S. Department of Health and Human Services. (2006). *Summary health statistics for U.S. adults, National Health Interview Survey, 2005* (Series 10, No. 232). Hyattsville, MD: Author.
Zinberg, N. E. (1964). Psychoanalytic consideration of aging. *Journal of the American Psychoanalytic Association, 12,* 151–159.

SE6 Specific Symptom Disorders

Bauer, M., McAuliffe, L., & Nay, R. (2007). Sexuality, health care and the older person: An overview of the literature. *International Journal of Older People Nursing, 2,* 63–68.
Brandsma, L. (2007). Eating disorders across the lifespan. *Journal of Women and Aging, 19*(1–2), 155–172.
Camacho, M. E., & Reyes-Ortiz, C. A., (2005). Sexual dysfunction in the elderly: Age or disease? *International Journal of Impotence Research, 17,* S52–S56.
Du Mello Kenyon, M. (1989). The management of exhibitionism in the elderly: A case study. *Sexual and Marital Therapy, 4*(1), 93–100.
Duggal, A., & Lawrence, R. M. (2001). Aspects of food refusal in the elderly: The "hunger strike." *International Journal of Eating Disorders, 30*(2), 213–216.
Edwards, B. A., Wellman, A., Sands, S. A., Owens, R. L., Eckert, D. J., White, D. P., & Malhotra, A. (2014). Obstructive sleep apnea in older adults is a distinctly different physiological phenotype. *Sleep, 37*(7), 1227–1236.
Gelfand, M. M. (2000). Sexuality among older women. *Journal of Women's Health and Gender-Based Medicine, 9*(Suppl. 1), S15–S20.
Gott, M., & Hinchliff, S. (2003). How important is

sex in later life?: The views of older people. *Social Science and Medicine, 56,* 1617–1628.

Harris, M., & Cumella, E. J. (2006). Eating disorders across the life span. *Journal of Psychosocial Nursing, 44,* 21–26.

Huffmann, G. B. (2002). Evaluating and treating unintentional weight loss in the elderly. *American Family Physician, 65*(4), 640–651.

Kay, D. B., Buysse, D. J., Germain, A., Hall, M., & Monk, T. H. (2015). Subjective–objective sleep discrepancy among older adults: Associations with insomnia diagnosis and insomnia treatment. *Journal of Sleep Research, 24*(1), 32–39.

Kleinplatz, P. J. (2008). Editorial: Sexuality and older people: Doctors should ask patients, regardless of age, about sexuality. *British Medical Journal, 337,* 121–122.

Lapid, M., Prom, M., Burton, M., McAlpine, D., Sutor, B., & Rummans, T. (2010). Eating disorders in the elderly. *International Psychogeriatrics, 22*(4), 523–536.

Laumann, E. O., Nicolosi, A., Glasser, D. B., Gingell, C., Moreira, E., Wang, T., & GSSAB Investigators' Group. (2005). Sexual problems among women and men aged 40–80 y: Prevalence and correlates identified in the Global Study of Sexual Attitudes and Behaviors. *International Journal of Impotence Research, 17,* 39–57.

Leblanc, M. F., Desjardins, S., & Desgagné, A. (2015). Sleep problems in anxious and depressive older adults. *Psychology Research and Behavior Management, 11*(8), 161–169.

Lemieux, L., Kaiser, S., Pereira, J. & Meadows, L. M. (2004). Sexuality in palliative care: Patient perspectives. *Palliative Medicine, 18,* 630–637.

Lewis, D., & Cachelin, F. (2001). Body image, body dissatisfaction, and eating attitudes in midlife and elderly women. *Eating Disorders, 9,* 29–39.

Maglione, J. E., Thomas, S. E., & Jeste, D. V. (2014). Late-onset schizophrenia: Do recent studies support categorizing LOS as a subtype of schizophrenia? *Current Opinion in Psychiatry, 7*(3), 173–178.

Mangweth-Matzek, B., Rupp, C. I., Hausmann, A., Assmayr, K., Mariacher, E., Kemmler, G., . . . Biebl, W. (2006). Never too old for eating disorders or body dissatisfaction: A community study of elderly women. *International Journal of Eating Disorders, 39,* 583–586.

Nicolosi, A., Buvat, J., Glasser, D. B., Hartmann, U., Laumann, E. O., Gingell, C., & GSSAB Investigators' Group. (2006). Sexual behaviour, sexual dysfunctions and related help seeking patterns in middle-aged and elderly Europeans: The Global Study of Sexual Attitudes and Behaviors. *World Journal of Urology, 24,* 423–428.

Peat, C. M., Peyerl, N. L., & Muehlenkamp, J. J. (2008). Body image and eating disorders in older adults: A review. *Journal of General Psychology, 135,* 343–358.

Rodriguez, J. C., Dzierzewski, J. M., & Alessi, C. A. (2015). Sleep problems in the elderly. *Medical Clinics of North America, 99*(2), 431–439.

Scholtz, S., Hill, L. S., & Lacey, H. (2010). Eating disorders in older women: Does late onset anorexia nervosa exist? *International Journal of Eating Disorders, 43,* 393–397.

Smink, F. R., van Hoeken, D., & Hoek, H. W. (2012). Epidemiology of eating disorders: Incidence, prevalence and mortality rates. *Current Psychiatry Reports, 14,* 406–414.

Zimmerman, M. E., & Aloia M. S. (2012). Sleep-disordered breathing and cognition in older adults. *Current Neurology and Neuroscience Reports, 12*(5), 537–546.

SE7 Disorders Related to Addiction

Folkman, S., Bernstein, L., & Lazarus, R. S. (1987). Stress processes and the misuse of drugs in older adults. *Psychological Aging, 4,* 366–374.

Gfroerer, J., Penne, M., Pemberton, M., Folsom, R. (2003). Substance abuse treatment need among older adults in 2020: The impact of the aging baby-boom cohort. *Drug and Alcohol Dependence, 69*(2), 127–135.

Kuerbis, A., Sacco, P., Blazer, D. G., & Moore, A. A. (2014). Substance abuse among older adults. *Clinics in Geriatric Medicine, 30*(3), 629–654.

Medeiros, G. C., Leppink, E., Yaemi, A., Mariani, M., Tavares, H., & Grant, J. (2015). Gambling disorder in older adults: A cross-cultural perspective. *Comprensive Psychiatry, 58,* 116–121.

Mendez, M. F., & Shapira, J. S. (2013). Hypersexual behavior in frontotemporal dementia: A comparison with early-onset Alzheimer's disease. *Archives of Sexual Behavior, 42*(3), 501–509.

Pilver, C. E., Libby, D. J., Hoff, R. A., & Potenza, M. N. (2013). Problem gambling severity and the incidence of Axis I psychopathology among older adults in the general population. *Journal of Psychiatric Research, 47*(4), 534–541.

Shahpesandy, H., Pristásová, J., Janíková, Z., Mojzisová, R., Kasanická, V., & Supalová, O. (2006). Alcoholism in the elderly: A study of elderly alcoholics compared with healthy elderly and young alcoholics. *Neuroendocrinology Letters, 27*(5), 651–657.

Subramaniam, M., Wang, P., Soh, P., Vaingankar, J. A., Chong, S. A., Browning, C. J., & Thomas, S. A.

(2015). Prevalence and determinants of gambling disorder among older adults: A systematic review. *Addictive Behaviors, 41,* 199–209.

Tse, S., Hong, S. I., Wang, C. W., & Cunningham-Williams, R. M. (2012). Gambling behavior and problems among older adults: A systematic review of empirical studies. *Journals of Gerontology: Series B. Psychological Sciences and Social Sciences, 67*(5), 639–652.

Vaillant, G. E. (2003). A 60-year follow-up of alcoholic men. *Addiction, 98*(8), 1043–1051.

SE13 Neurocognitive Disorders

AGS/NIA Delirium Conference Writing Group, Planning Committee and Faculty. (2015). The American Geriatrics Society/National Institute on Aging Bedside-to-Bench Conference: Research agenda on delirium in older adults. *Journal of the American Geriatrics Society, 63,* 843–852.

Crammer, J. L. (2002). Subjective experience of a confusional state. *British Journal of Psychiatry, 180,* 71–75.

Evans, D., & Lee, E. (2014). Impact of dementia on marriage: A qualitative systematic review. *Dementia, 13*(3), 330–349.

Evans, S. (2008). Beyond forgetfulness: How psychoanalytic ideas can help us to understand the experience of patients with dementia. *Psychoanalytic Psychotherapy, 22*(3), 155–176.

Fang, M. L., Coatta, K., Badger, M., Wu, S., Easton, M., Nygård, L., . . . Sixsmith, A. (2015). Informing understandings of mild cognitive impairment for older adults: Implications from a scoping review. *Journal of Applied Gerontology.* [Epub ahead of print]

Feinberg, T. E., & Keenan, J. P. (Eds.). (2005). *The lost self: Pathologies of the brain and identity.* New York: Oxford University Press.

Hülür, G., & Gerstorf, D. (2015). Editorial: Subjective perceptions of memory functioning in old age—nature, correlates, and developmental trajectories. *Gerontology, 61*(3), 218–222.

Hülür, G., Hertzog, C., Pearman, A. M., & Gerstorf, D. (2015). Correlates and moderators of change in subjective memory and memory performance: Findings from the Health and Retirement Study. *Gerontology, 61*(3), 232–240.

Kaduszkiewicz, H., Eisele, M., Wiese, B., Prokein, J., Luppa, M., Luck, T., . . . The Study on Aging, Cognition, and Dementia in Primary Care Patients (AgeCoDe) Study Group. (2014). Prognosis of mild cognitive impairment in general practice: Results of the German AgeCoDe Study. *Annals of Family Medicine, 12*(2), 158–165.

Kasl-Godley, J., & Gatz, M. (2000). Psychosocial interventions for individuals with dementia: An integration of theory, therapy, and a clinical understanding of dementia. *Clinical Psychology Review, 20*(6), 755–782.

Langa, K. M., & Levine, D. A. (2014). The diagnosis and management of mild cognitive impairment: A clinical review. *Journal of the American Medical Association, 312*(23), 2551–2561.

Lee, S. M., Roen, K., & Thornton, A. (2014). The psychological impact of a diagnosis of Alzheimer's disease. *Dementia, 13*(3), 289–305.

Loboprabhu, S., Molinari, V., & Lomax, J. (2007). The transitional object in dementia: Clinical implications. *International Journal of Applied Psychoanalytic Studies, 4*(2), 144–169.

Luszcz, M. A., Anstey, K. J., & Ghisletta, P. (2015). Subjective beliefs, memory and functional health: Change and associations over 12 years in the Australian Longitudinal Study of Ageing. *Gerontology, 61*(3), 241–250.

Petersen, R. C. (2004). Mild cognitive impairment as a diagnostic entity. *Journal of Internal Medicine, 256,* 183–194.

Petersen, R. C., Caracciolo, B., Brayne, C., Gauthier, S., Jelic, V., & Fratiglioni, L. (2014). Mild cognitive impairment: A concept in evolution. *Journal of Internal Medicine, 275*(3), 214–228.

Sachs-Ericsson, N., & Blazer, D. G. (2015). The new DSM-5 diagnosis of mild neurocognitive disorder and its relation to research in mild cognitive impairment. *Aging and Mental Health, 19*(1), 2–12.

Saczynski, J. S., Inouye, S. K., Kosar, C., Tommet, D., Marcantonio, E. R., Fong, T., . . . Jones, R. N. (2014). Cognitive and brain reserve and the risk of postoperative delirium in older patients. *Lancet Psychiatry, 1*(6), 437–443.

Simpson, J. R. (2014). DSM-5 and neurocognitive disorders. *Journal of the American Academy of Psychiatry and Law, 42*(2), 159–164.

Thompson, C. L., Henry, J. D., Rendell, P. G., Withall, A., & Brodaty, H. (2015). How valid are subjective ratings of prospective memory in mild cognitive impairment and early dementia? *Gerontology, 61*(3), 251–257.

Westhoff, D., Witlox, J., Koenderman, L., Kalisvaart, K. J., de Jonghem, J. F., van Stijn, M. F., . . . van Gool, W. A. (2013). Preoperative cerebrospinal fluid cytokine levels and the risk of postoperative delirium in elderly hip fracture patients. *Journal of Neuroinflammation, 10,* 122.

Winblad, B., Palmer, K., Kivipelto, M., Jelic, V., Fratiglioni, L., Wahlund, L. O., . . . Petersen, R. C. (2004). Mild cognitive impairment—beyond controversies, towards a consensus: Report of the International Working Group on Mild Cognitive Impairment. *Journal of Internal Medicine, 256*(3), 240–246.

SEApp Appendix: Psychological Experiences That May Require Clinical Attention

Ainslie, R. C. (2011). Immigration and the psychodynamics of class. *Psychoanalytic Psychology, 28,* 560–568.

Akhtar, S. (2011). *Immigration and acculturation: Mourning, adaptation, and the next generation.* Lanham, MD: Aronson.

American Psychiatric Association. (1994). *Diagnostic and statistical manual of mental disorders* (4th ed.). Washington, DC: Author.

American Psychiatric Association. (2005, May). Position statement on support of legal recognition of same-sex civil marriage. Available at *www.psych.org/public_info/libr_publ/resource.cfm:1-3.*

American Psychological Association. (2003). Multicultural guidelines: Education, research, and practice. *American Psychologist, 58,* 377–402.

American Psychological Association. (2014). Guidelines for psychological practice with older adults. Retrieved from *www.apa.org/practice/guidelines/older-adults.pdf.*

American Psychological Association. (2015). Guidelines for psychological practice with transgender and gender nonconforming people. Retrieved from *www.apa.org/practice/guidelines/transgender.pdf.*

Auldridge, A., Tamar-Mattis, A., Kennedy, S., Ames, E., & Tobin, H. J. (2012). *Improving the lives of transgender older adults: Services and advocacy.* New York: Services and Advocacy for LGBT Elders/Washington, DC: National Center for Transgender Equality. Retrieved from *www.lgbtagingcenter.org/resources/resource.cfm?r=520.*

Averill, J. B. (2012). Priorities for action in a rural older adults study. *Family and Community Health, 35*(4), 358–372.

Berger, R. M. (1980). Psychological adaptation of the older homosexual male. *Journal of Homosexuality, 5*(3), 161–175.

Boulanger, G. (2004). Lot's wife, Cary Grant, and the American dream: Psychoanalysis with immigrants. *Contemporary Psychoanalysis, 40,* 353–372.

Coburn, A., & Bolda, E. (1999). The rural elderly and long-term care. In T. C. Ricketts (Ed.), *Rural health in the United States* (pp. 179–189). New York: Oxford University Press.

Ettner, R., & Wylie, K. (2013). Psychological and social adjustment in older transsexual people. *Maturitas, 74,* 226–229.

Fabbre, V. D. (2015). Gender transitions in later life: A queer perspective on successful aging. *The Gerontologist, 55*(1), 144–153.

Foster, R. P. (2003). Considering a multicultural perspective for psychoanalysis. In A. Roland, B. Ulanov, & C. Barbre (Eds.), *Creative dissent: Psychoanalysis in evolution* (pp. 173–185). Westport, CT: Praeger.

Fredriksen-Goldsen, K. I., Kim, H. J., Emlet, C. A., Muraco, A., Erosheva, E. A., Hoy-Ellis, C. P., . . . Petry, H. (2011). *The aging and health report: Disparities and resilience among lesbian, gay, bisexual, and transgender older adults.* Seattle, WA: Institute for Multigenerational Health.

Fredriksen-Goldsen, K. I., & Muraco, A. (2010). Aging and sexual orientation: A 25-year review of the literature. *Research on Aging, 32*(3), 372–413.

Fruhauf, C. A., & Orel, N. A. (2015). Fostering resilience in LGBT aging individuals and families. In N. A. Orel & C. A. Fruhauf (Eds.), *The lives of LGBT older adults: Understanding challenges and resilience* (pp. 217–227). Washington, DC: American Psychological Association.

Grinberg, L., & Grinberg, R. (1989). *Psychoanalytic perspectives on migration and exile.* New Haven, CT: Yale University Press.

Harley, D. A., & Teaster, P. B. (Eds.). (2016). *Handbook of LGBT elders: An interdisciplinary approach to principles, practices, and policies.* Cham, Switzerland: Springer International.

Hayes, J. A., Owen, J., & Bieschke, K. J. (2015), Therapist differences in symptom change with racial/ethnic minority clients. *Psychotherapy, 52*(3), 308–314.

Hodgkiss, A., Denman, C., & Watson, J. P. (1991). Gender dysphoria in old age: A single case study. *International Journal of Geriatric Psychiatry, 6,* 819–822.

Institute of Medicine. (2011). *The health of lesbian, gay, bisexual, and transgender people: Building a foundation for better understanding.* Washington, DC: National Academies Press.

Jenkins, D., Walker, C., Cohen, H., & Curry L. (2010). A lesbian older adult managing identity disclosure: A case study. *Journal of Gerontological Social Work, 53,* 402–420.

Kimmel, D. C. (1978). Adult development and aging: A gay perspective. *Journal of Social Issues, 34*(3), 113–130.

Kremer, J., & den Daas, H. P. (1990). Case report: A man with breast dysphoria. *Archives of Sexual Behavior, 19*(2), 179–181.

Lawrence, A. A. (2010). Sexual orientation versus age of onset as bases for typologies (subtypes) for gender identity disorder in adolescents and adults. *Archives of Sexual Behavior, 39,* 514–545.

Lawrence, V., Murray, J., Banerjee, S., Turner, S., Sangha, K., Byng, R., . . . Macdonald, A. (2006). Concepts and causation of depression: A cross-cultural study of the beliefs of older adults. *Gerontologist, 1,* 23–32.

Lothstein, L. M. (1979) The aging gender dysphoria (transsexual) patient. *Archives of Sexual Behavior, 8,* 431–444.

McClelland, A., Khanam, S., & Furnham, A. (2014). Cultural and age differences in beliefs about depression: British Bangladeshis vs. British whites. *Mental Health, Religion and Culture, 17*(3), 225–238.

McFarland, P. L., & Sanders, S. (2003). A pilot study about the needs of older gays and lesbians: What social workers need to know. *Journal of Gerontological Social Work, 40*(3), 67–80.

Miville, M. L., & Ferguson, A. D. (2014). *Handbook of race–ethnicity and gender in psychology.* New York: Springer.

Orel, N. A. (2004). Gay, lesbian, and bisexual elders: Expressed needs and concerns across focus groups. *Journal of Gerontological Social Work, 43*(2–3), 57–77.

Siverskog, A. (2014). "They just don't have a clue": Transgender aging and implications for social work. *Journal of Gerontological Social Work, 57,* 386–406.

Stoller, R. J. (1980). Gender identity disorders. In H. I. Kaplan, A. M. Freedman, & B. J. Sadock (Eds.), *Comprehensive textbook of psychiatry* (3rd ed., Vol. 2, pp. 1695–1705). Baltimore: Williams & Wilkins.

Stryker, S. (2008). Transgender history, homonormativity, and disciplinarity. *Radical History Review, 100,* 144–157.

Sue, D. W. (2001). Multidimensional facets of cultural competence. *The Counseling Psychologist, 29,* 790–821.

Tummala-Narra, P. (2015). Cultural competence as a core emphasis of psychoanalytic psychotherapy. *Psychoanalytic Psychology, 32*(2), 275–292.

van Wagenen, A., Driskell, J., & Bradford, J. (2013). "I'm still raring to go": Successful aging among lesbian, gay, bisexual, and transgender older adults. *Journal of Aging Studies, 27,* 1–14.

Witten, T. M., & Eyler, A. E. (2012). *Gay, lesbian, bisexual, and transgender aging: Challenges in research, practice, and policy.* Baltimore: Johns Hopkins University Press.

PART VI

Assessment and Clinical Illustrations

CHAPTER **15**

Assessment within the PDM-2 Framework

CHAPTER EDITORS

Sherwood Waldron, MD **Robert M. Gordon, PhD, ABPP** **Francesco Gazzillo, PhD**

CONSULTANTS

Allan Abbass, MD
John S. Auerbach, PhD
Jacques Barber, PhD
Mark Blais, PsyD
Robert F. Bornstein, PhD
Anthony Bram, PhD, ABAP
Manfred Cierpka, MD
John F. Clarkin, PhD
Franco Del Corno, MPhyl, DPsych
Kathryn DeWitt, PhD
Diana Diamond, PhD
Federica Genova, PhD
Carol George, PhD
Mark J. Hilsenroth, PhD
Per Høglend, MD
Steven K. Huprich, PhD
Lawrence Josephs, PhD
Horst Kächele, MD, PhD
Guenther Klug, MD
Michael J. Lambert, PhD
Patrick Luyten, PhD
Marianne Leuzinger-Bohleber, PhD
Seymour Moscovitz, PhD
John C. Norcross, PhD
J. Christopher Perry, MPH, MD
John H. Porcerelli, PhD
Piero Porcelli, PhD
Jeremy D. Safran, PhD
George Silberschatz, PhD
Anna Maria Speranza, PhD
Michelle Stein, PhD
William Stiles, PhD
Karl Stukenberg, PhD
Annalisa Tanzilli, PhD

Introduction

The aim of this chapter is to introduce tools that we have specifically developed for PDM-2 assessment and to survey a broad range of empirically validated assessment tools that may enhance clinicians' use of PDM-2 for diagnostic formulations, clinical reports, treatment planning, or research. We also describe several ways that these various measures have already led to findings relevant to psychopathology and psychotherapy.

First, we introduce specific PDM-2-derived assessment tools: the Psychodiagnostic Chart–2 (PDC-2) and the PDCs for all the PDM-2 age groups; and the Psychodynamic Diagnostic Prototypes–2 (PDP-2). The PDC-2 is aimed at guiding the clinician through the entire PDM-2 diagnostic formulation: personality organization, personality syndromes or disorders, mental functioning, subjective experience of symptoms, manifest symptoms and complaints, and cultural, contextual and other relevant considerations. The original Psychodiagnostic Chart (PDC; Gordon & Bornstein, 2012) was derived from the first edition of PDM and has been used and validated in both public and private settings in the United States and Europe.

The original Psychodynamic Diagnostic Prototypes (PDP; Gazzillo, Lingiardi, & Del Corno, 2012) provided prototypical examples of the various personality styles or disorders listed on the P Axis (adult) of the first PDM. The PDP-2 (Gazzillo, Genova, & Lingiardi, 2016) allows more precise assessment of patients according to the P-Axis dimensions, together with prototypical descriptions of the different levels of personality organization and the main features of the anaclitic and introjective psychologies and personality disorders.

After introducing these specific PDM-2 tools, we describe additional instruments that can enhance the assessment of patients according to the PDM-2 classification (personality organization, personality patterns or disorders, and mental functions). We generally do not describe tests of specific symptoms or syndromes outside the context of personality dynamics.

Some of these clinician-rated instruments have directly influenced the construction of both PDMs. These include the Shedler–Westen Assessment Procedure (SWAP; Westen & Shedler, 1999a, 1999b; Westen, Shedler, Bradley, & DeFife, 2012; Westen, Shedler, Durrett, Glass, & Martens, 2003; Westen, DeFife, Malone, & DiLallo, 2014); the Structural Interview for Personality Organization (STIPO; Stern et al., 2010); the Karolinska Psychodynamic Profile (KAPP; Weinryb, Rossel, & Asberg, 1991a, 1991b); the Defense Mechanism Rating Scales (DMRS; Perry, 1990); the Social Cognition and Object Relations Scale (SCORS; Stein, Hilsenroth, Slaven-Mulford, & Pinsker, 2011; Westen, 1991a, 1991b); and the Object Relations Inventory (ORI; Blatt & Auerbach, 2001).

The other instruments reviewed in this chapter, such as self-reports (e.g., the Minnesota Multiphasic Personality Inventory–2 [MMPI-2; Butcher, Dahlstrom, Graham, Tellegen, & Kaemmer, 1989]) and performance-based assessment tools (e.g., the Rorschach Inkblot Test [Rorschach, 1921/1942] or the Thematic Apperception Test [TAT; Murray, 1943]), are widely used both in assessment practice (Bram & Peebles, 2014) and in psychodynamic research (Bornstein, 2010). They can be useful aids in a PDM-2 formulation for describing and understanding the psychological capacities and personality features of patients and their overall level of functioning and well-being. We also briefly describe assessment tools that can help clinicians to assess patients' functioning as directly observed in treatment—a source of direct information that also has relevance for overall assessment. Finally, we provide a clinical illustration with a detailed description of the application of many instruments described in the chapter, in order to demonstrate their utility.

General Considerations

Personality assessment can be considered from different perspectives. One of these is the point of view from which data are derived: (1) the clinician's report (e.g., the SWAP and STIPO); (2) the patient's self-report (e.g., the MMPI-2); (3) significant others' reports of the patient; (4) reports by independent judges or observers of the patient; and (5) observations of the patients' performance, often on unstructured or minimally structured tasks that were formerly described as "projective."

Another perspective on assessment is the content or focus of the assessment: (1) the patient's internal personality structure; (2) the patient's external observable behavior in daily interactions, the patient's ideas about his or her personality features, level of perceived wellness, and capacity for functioning; and (3) the patient's observable behavior within the consulting office. We would add still another: (4) the patient's contributions to the psychotherapeutic process.

Research has shown considerable divergence among these points of view and methodologies (Bornstein, 2002, 2009; Hunsley & Mash, 2014). Similarities and differences between the results of assessments developed from the different points of view and methods (clinician report, self-report, other-report, or performance-based) may be quite informative from a clinical perspective (Bram & Peebles, 2014; Bram & Yalof, 2014), with respect both to diagnostic formulation and to conceptualization of personality dynamics and interpersonal functioning (Bornstein, 2010). For example, a large divergence between a patient's self-report and the patient's results on a performance-based test may indicate the influence of difficulty in mentalizing, defensive processes blocking self-awareness, or dissimulation on the patient's part. It is well known that unconscious motivations, more easily assessable with performance-based instruments, are more predictive of long-term life choices than are conscious motivations assessable through self-reports (Shedler, Mayman, & Manis, 1993; Westen, 1999).

Clinicians observe patients and interact with them; ask them to describe themselves, their lives, their relationships, and what brings them to assessment or treatment; and are sensitive to the emotions that patients stir up in them. These are unique data that need a clinician's perspective to interpret, even though such interpretation tends to be highly variable (e.g., Seitz, 1966). The variability is decreased when these descriptions are systematized with sound empirical tools, as described below. Validated clinician report instruments help a clinician to perform this task by supporting, amplifying, or modifying clinical impressions and self-report or performance-based data in a reciprocally enriching process (Meehl, 1996; Westen & Weinberger, 2004). Both assessment validity and clinical utility are improved by using a battery of assessment instruments from different points of view (Bornstein, 2010; Hopwood & Bornstein, 2014). Instruments with contrasting methodologies should be employed, if feasible, to illuminate convergences and divergences between different perspectives and methods (Bornstein, 2009; Cogswell, 2008; De Fife, Drill, Nakash, & Westen, 2010).

Some of the tools we describe are also time-consuming, and this feature may discourage their use in routine clinical practice. Nevertheless, their richness of information and their methodological and theoretical soundness can prove valuable to clinicians at all levels of experience; therefore, especially when complex clinical questions are being addressed, implementation of more time-consuming, labor-intensive assessments may be warranted.

Bram and Yaloff (2014) discuss three particularly useful clinical issues that benefit from testing: (1) assessment of suitability for treatment; (2) evaluation of treatments that are not proceeding well; and (3) modification of treatment to take account of aspects of personality (including limitations) that influence, positively or negatively, the likelihood of treatment success.

Most of the measures we have chosen are aimed at the assessment of personality organization, fundamental mental functions, and global adjustment and well-being—not simply at symptom patterns or symptom severity. We have made these choices because symptoms such as alterations in sleep and eating, depressed mood, inexplicable pain, sexual difficulties, phobias, or panic attacks are easily observable by clinicians or explicitly reported by patients (or both). In contrast, personality features and implicit or unconscious mental processes are not. In addition, from a psychodynamic perspective, the assessment of personality organization and features is relevant for understanding the meaning, function, etiology, and prognosis of the different syndromes and symptoms (Gazzillo et al., 2013; Thompson-Brenner, Eddy, Satir, Boisseau, & Westen, 2008; Thompson-Brenner & Westen, 2005a, 2005b; Westen, Gabbard, & Blagov, 2006; Westen & Harnden-Fisher, 2001).

Part One of this chapter (below) covers clinician report measures that assist in PDM-2 diagnosis of personality organization and mental functioning and are easiest for clinicians to use. We begin by discussing the PDM-2-derived tools mentioned briefly above. Then we discuss additional tools that require more training for the clinician or clinician-researcher, but that are important for clinicians to know about because of the richness of empirical findings relevant to clinical work. We have arranged Part Two of the chapter, on self-reports, so that the order in which the tools are described corresponds with the PDM-2 tasks of first determining level of personality structure, then personality patterns, and finally mental functioning.

Part One. Instruments for PDM-2 Diagnostic Formulations

We start with the tools specifically developed for PDM/PDM-2 and then review other assessments that can be helpful in the process of PDM-2 diagnostic formulation.

A. PDM-2-Derived Assessment Tools

Psychodiagnostic Charts

In 2011, Robert M. Gordon and Robert F. Bornstein agreed that the first PDM needed a short, user-friendly tool that would (1) guide practitioners through all sections of the PDM taxonomy; (2) be idiographic, flexible, and useful for clinicians of any theoretical orientation; and (3) integrate PDM with the symptom classifications of the *Diagnostic and Statistical Manual of Mental Disorders* (DSM) or *International Classification of Diseases* (ICD). Gordon and Bornstein developed the PDC with this in mind.

The PDC-2 is an updated version of the PDC that is compatible with PDM-2 and incorporates the changes introduced during the PDM revision process. The modifications are not expected to affect the reliability and validity of the PDC-2.

The goal of the PDC-2 is to offer a person-based nosology that may be used for teaching PDM-2, supervision, diagnoses, treatment formulations, progress reports, and outcome assessment, as well as for empirical research on personality, psychopathology, and treatment. The overarching aim is to make psychodiagnostic formulation more useful to practitioners by combining the symptom-focused ICD and DSM with the full range and depth of human mental functioning addressed by PDM and PDM-2 (see, e.g., Bornstein, 2011; Lingiardi, McWilliams, Bornstein, Gazzillo, & Gordon, 2015a).

The PDC-2 is for use with adult clients, but the basic format and research for the PDC-2 have been adapted for Psychodiagnostic Charts for the different age groups addressed in PDM-2: the Psychodiagnostic Chart—Adolescent (PDC-A), Psychodiagnostic Chart—Childhood (PDC-C), Psychodiagnostic Chart—Infancy and Early Childhood (PDC-IEC), and Psychodiagnostic Chart—Elderly (PDC-E). However, the PDCs for these age groups will need to undergo their own validity and reliability studies.

The PDC-2 requires some familiarity with PDM-2. The clinician must perform (or have access to) diagnostic interview data and psychological assessment data to derive optimal PDC-2 ratings. We recognize that this is not always feasible and that in many instances a clinician will code an initial impression, then reassess as additional information accrues. If the PDC-2 is used for progress notes, there will be opportunities to reassess and revise the person's diagnosis as well. The validity of this chart can be enhanced with the integration of relevant psychological tests as suggested in this chapter. Blank copies of all five versions of the PDC are available in the Appendix to this manual, and purchasers can also download enlarged versions of these forms for use in clinical practice (see the box at the end of the table of contents).

Qianna Snooks helped to format the PDC-2 Version 8.1, as well as a digital form for computers that has a reset button for repeated uses, that has a drop-down menu for dominant personality patterns, that automatically totals the individual M-Axis scores, and that has a large dialogue box for further contextual information. The digital form also allows the ratings to be exported to Excel for data collection and statistical analysis for research purposes.

Psychodiagnostic Chart–2

The PDC-2 starts with Section I: Level of Personality Organization. First, the practitioner rates four mental functions on a scale from 1 (severely impaired) to 10 (healthy): (1) identity, or the ability to view the self in complex, stable, and accurate ways; (2) object relations, or the ability to maintain intimate, stable, and satisfying relationships; (3) level of defenses; and (4) reality testing, or the ability to appreciate conventional notions of what is realistic. Then the practitioner rates the patient's overall personality organization (psychotic, borderline, neurotic, or healthy) on the basis of his or her ratings of the four component scales and overall clinical judgment.

Section II: Personality Syndromes (P Axis) asks the practitioner to determine the patient's personality patterns or disorders by checking as many relevant personality patterns as apply; then the practitioner notes the one or two most dominant patterns. For research purposes, each pattern can be given a rating from 1 (severe) to 5 (high functioning).

Section III: Mental Functioning (M Axis) is a detailed consideration of the patient's various strengths and limitations along 12 dimensions that are subsumed in four main domains: cognitive and affective processes; identity and relationships; defense and coping; and self-awareness and self-direction. The 12 mental functions are summed to derive a score for overall level of personality severity. The digital form of the PDC-2 automatically derives these scores.

Section IV: Symptom Patterns (S Axis) asks the practitioner to describe the patient's main symptom patterns from those that are related to predominantly psychotic disorders, mood disorders, disorders primarily related to anxiety, event- and stressor-related disorders, and so forth. If required, the practitioner may use DSM or ICD symptoms and codes here. The dominant symptoms are rated on a 5-point scale from 1 (severe) to 5 (mild).

In Section V, Cultural, Contextual, and Other Relevant Considerations, the practitioner may choose to add relevant information about the client's environment or circumstances. The digital form of the PDC-2 has a dialogue box allowing for more narrative space.

Finally, the practitioner integrates all the sections into a cohesive clinical picture that provides a nuanced understanding of the whole person.

Psychodiagnostic Chart—Infancy and Early Childhood

Anna Maria Speranza, a Chapter Editor of Chapter 10 (the Infancy and Early Childhood chapter), has developed the PDC-IEC on the basis of the adult PDC-2 as a user-friendly tool to guide clinicians in the assessment of infants and young children as proposed in Chapter 10. Specifically, the PDC-IEC requires a clinician to assess an infant or young child's presenting problems and symptomatology; functional emotional developmental capacities; constitutional and maturational variations in regulatory–sensory processing; relational patterns and disorders; and other medical and neurological diagnoses. Each of these dimensions not only contributes to an overall view of the child's functioning, but also indicates the role each area may play in pathogenesis. The sections of the PDC-IEC are as follows:

- Section I: Primary Diagnoses (corresponding to Axis I of the IEC classification). The main IEC diagnoses are indicated, and each diagnosis can be given a rating of 1 (severe) to 5 (mild).
- Section II: Functional Emotional Developmental Capacities (corresponding to Axis II of the classification). These capacities are rated in terms of six expected emotional functions from 1 (severe deficits) to 5 (healthy).
- Section III: Regulatory–Sensory Processing Capacities (corresponding to Axis III of the classification). Aspects of the child's sensory modulation, sensory discrimination, and sensory-based motor functioning are rated from 1 (severe problem or almost always a problem) to 4 (no indication; never or rarely a problem). An overall regulatory sensory profile is rated from 1 (severe deficits) to 5 (healthy).
- Section IV: Relational Patterns and Disorders (corresponding to Axis IV of the classification). Aspects of the infant/child's relationship with each of two significant caregivers are rated on eight dimensions. The overall level of relational pattern and the attachment pattern for each caregiver are then evaluated.
- Section V: Other Medical and Neurological Diagnoses (corresponding to Axis V of the classification). This section permits the clinician to record any relevant information about a child's diagnoses in these areas.

Psychodiagnostic Chart—Child

Norka Malberg, Larry Rosenberg, and Johanna C. Malone, Chapter Editors of the chapters in Part III (Childhood), have developed the PDC-C on the basis of the adult PDC-2 as a user-friendly tool to guide clinicians in the assessment of children as described in Part III. The PDC-C starts with Section I: Mental Functioning (MC Axis), which asks the practitioner to rate the patient's level of strength or weakness on each of 11 mental functions on a scale from 1 (severe deficits) to 5 (healthy), and then to provide a rating for overall level of personality severity as the sum of these 11 ratings. Section II: Emerging Level of Personality Pattern and Difficulties calls for ratings of identity, object relations, and reality testing similar to these ratings in the PDC-2, and also calls for the clinician to provide an overall rating of emerging personality pattern as either "normal" (healthy), mildly dysfunctional (neurotic), dysfunctional (borderline), or severely dysfunctional (psychotic). Section III: Symptom Patterns (SC Axis) allows the clinician to rate symptoms or concerns on a scale from 1 (severe) to 5 (mild). Finally, Section IV: Influencing Factors and Relevant Clinical Observations Informing Diagnosis allows the clinician to record other information as relevant.

Psychodiagnostic Chart—Adolescent (PDC-A)

Norka Malberg, Johanna C. Malone, Nick Midgley, and Mario Speranza, Chapter Editors of the chapters in Part II (Adolescence), have developed the PDC-A on the basis of the adult PDC-2 as a user-friendly tool to guide clinicians in the assessment of adolescents as described in Part II. The PDC-A starts with Section I: Mental Functioning (MA Axis), which asks the practitioner to rate the patient's level of strength or weakness on each of 12 mental functions on a scale from 1 (severe deficits) to 5 (healthy), and then to provide an overall rating for level of personality severity as the sum of these 12 ratings. Section II: Level of Personality Organization calls for ratings of identity, object relations, level of defenses, and reality testing similar to these ratings in the PDC-2, and also calls for the clinician to provide an overall rating of emerging personality pattern as either "normal" (healthy), mildly dysfunctional (neurotic), dysfunctional (borderline), or severely dysfunctional emerging personality patterns (psychotic). Section III: Emerging Adolescent Personality Styles/Syndromes (PA Axis) asks the practitioner to determine the patient's emerging personality patterns by checking as many relevant patterns as apply; then the practitioner notes the one or two most dominant patterns. For research purposes, each pattern can be given a rating from 1 (severe) to 5 (high functioning). Section IV: Symptom Patterns (SA Axis) and Section V: Cultural, Contextual, and Other Relevant Considerations are similar to their counterparts in the PDC-2.

Psychodiagnostic Chart—Elderly

Franco Del Corno and Daniel Plotkin, Chapter Editors of the chapters in Part V (Later Life) of PDM-2, have developed the PDC-E on the basis of the adult PDC-2 as a user-friendly tool to guide clinicians in the assessment of elderly persons as described in Part V. It starts with Section I: Mental Functioning (ME Axis), which asks the practitioner to rate the patient's level of strength or weakness on each of 12 mental functions, on a scale from 1 (severe deficits) to 5 (healthy), and then to provide an overall rating for level of personality severity as the sum of these 12 ratings. Although most older adults do not have significant cognitive impairment, it is important to assess for presence of cognitive impairment or neurocognitive disorders that may affect mental functioning. Similarly, in Section II: Level of Personality Organization, the clinician is instructed: "Consider your patient's mental functions in determining the level of personality organization." As the PDC-2 does, the PDC-E uses ratings of identity, object relations, level of defenses, and reality testing (1 = severe, 10 = healthy) to efficiently capture the level of personality organization; it also notes, " . . . don't forget you are evaluating an older person who falls into one of these age groups: young-old (55–64 years of age), middle-old (65–74 years of age), old-old (75–84 years of age), and oldest-old (85 years of age and older)." Section III: Personality Syndromes (PE Axis); Section IV: Symptom Patterns (SE Axis); and Section V: Cultural, Contextual, and Other Relevant Considerations are all similar to their counterparts in the PDC-2.

Strengths of the PDCs

The PDC for adults has good reliability and validity. It guides the practitioner through a PDM-2 formulation using all the axes. It is only three pages long and user-friendly. It provides a broad summary of the PDM-2 adult axes and can be integrated with ICD and DSM diagnoses. Preliminary results lend strong support for the original PDM taxonomy and the usefulness of the original PDC with experts, as well as with "typical" practitioners of various theoretical orientations (Bornstein & Gordon, 2012; Gordon & Stoffey, 2014; Gordon, Blake, et al., 2016). The PDC has also been shown to be a valuable instrument for personality research (Gordon, Stoffey, & Perkins, 2013; Huprich et al., 2015). All these results are generalizable to the PDC-2. As noted earlier, the four PDCs derived from the PDC-2 will need to undergo their own validity and reliability studies.

Limitations of the PDCs

The PDCs are not tests in that they do not produce data independent of a clinician's insight. Rather, they are guides to assist practitioners in organizing, charting, and contextualizing complete PDM-2 formulations. That is, they are methods for describing patients along multiple domains to aid in diagnostic formulation and treatment planning.

Psychodynamic Diagnostic Prototypes–2

The original Psychodynamic Diagnostic Prototypes (PDP; Gazzillo, Lingiardi, & Del Corno, 2012) is a clinician report instrument developed by Francesco Gazzillo and Vittorio Lingiardi from Sapienza University of Rome, together with Franco Del Corno, past-president of the Italy Area Group of the Society for Psychotherapy Research. It is composed of 19 prototypic descriptions of personality disorders, one for each disorder on the P Axis in the first PDM.

The PDP was developed to help clinicians and researchers complete the P Axis, even without a previous knowledge of PDM. For this reason, Gazzillo and colleagues (2012) took the PDM descriptions of all the P-Axis patterns/disorders, deleted the references presented in the manual, and simplified the PDM personality descriptions, which were more complex or inferential than needed in evaluating a patient. The descriptions were also enriched by a careful study of the descriptions in other well-validated dynamic assessments.

In order to use the PDP, the clinician or rater assesses on a 5-point scale to what degree the patient resembles one or more PDP prototypes. A score of 1 means no resemblance, while a score of 5 means a complete match between the patient's clinical presentation and the prototype. A categorical diagnosis of the disorder is indicated when the score is 4 or 5. Three to five sessions are usually required to provide the clinician with sufficient knowledge of the patient to make an accurate assessment.

The second edition of the PDP, the PDP-2 (Gazzillo, Genova, & Lingiardi, 2016), is an adaptation of the PDP to the P Axis of PDM-2. The basic structure of the instrument is the same, but the PDP-2 takes into account the personality patterns described in the PDM-2 P Axis; it also assists the clinician also in the assessment of the level of personality organization of the patient and of the relevance of anaclitic or introjective themes in her/his personality.

For the assessment of the level of personality organization, the clinician or rater has to read a prototypical description of each level of personality organization (healthy, neurotic, borderline, psychotic) derived from the P Axis of PDM-2 and then rate his or her patient on an 8-point Likert scale.

For identifying the prevalence of an anaclitic or introjective orientation, the clinician or rater takes into account both the personality pattern identified as more representative of the patient and a brief description of the main features of the two psychological orientations and then assesses the patient on two 5-point Likert scales.

Strengths of the PDP and PDP-2

Most of the PDP personality patterns or disorders show good interrater reliability, concurrent and discriminant validity, and construct validity (Gazzillo et al., 2012). The PDP descriptions are easy to use. Common emotional reactions to a patient with a given disorder are also described because these can assist in the assessment of the patient. This provides an educational value as well.

Limitations of the PDP and PDP-2

Like all clinician report assessments, the PDP and PDP-2 are only as accurate as a clinician's judgment, supported by clear descriptions of levels of personality organization and personality patterns. It was not possible to assess the convergent and discriminant validity of some of the PDP disorders because there were no empirical instruments assessing the same disorders as described by a different diagnostic manual.

B. Other Clinician-Rated Tools for PDM-2 Assessment

This section provides descriptions of other instruments available for clinician-based ratings of core dimensions of personality functioning.

Structured Interview for Personality Organization

Otto Kernberg and his group at the Personality Disorders Institute in White Plains, New York, developed the Structured Interview for Personality Organization (STIPO) to operationalize the structural interview developed by Kernberg (1984). The STIPO comprises a structured interview of 97 questions that are used to assess the following domains of personality functioning: identity, object relations, defenses, reality testing, coping and rigidity, aggression, and moral values. The clinician's reply to each of the questions is scored on a 3-point Likert scale, from 0 (absence of pathology) to 3 (presence of pathology), with descriptive scoring anchors for each item. Moreover, the rater makes an overall estimation for each of the seven domains on a 5-point scale from 1 (healthy) to 5 (pathological).

A group of researchers from Italy and America has developed an adolescent version of the STIPO, the Interview of Personality Organization Processes in Adolescence (IPOP-A), and its initial validation data are promising (Ammaniti et al., 2014).

Strengths of the STIPO

The STIPO and the IPOP-A may prove useful for assessing the level of personality organization according to the P and PA Axes of PDM-2, respectively. Five of the domains are highly similar: identity, object relations, moral values/superego integration, reality testing, and coping and rigidity/resilience. The STIPO also assesses the domain of aggression, whereas the P and M Axes of PDM-2 assess more general emotional and relational capacities.

The internal consistency of the two most important STIPO domains (identity and object relations) is high, but it is just acceptable for the reality testing domain and unknown for the other domains. The interrater reliability is acceptable, and the convergent and discriminant validity, compared to those values for other measures of similar constructs, is promising for the major domains of the STIPO.

Limitations of the STIPO

For evaluators to achieve acceptable reliability, the STIPO and the IPOP-A require specific training, as well as a good knowledge of psychodynamic theory and of Kernberg's model of personality organization. It is also time-consuming (3–4 hours on average for the STIPO and 2 hours for the IPOP-A).

Karolinska Psychodynamic Profile

The Karolinska Psychodynamic Profile (KAPP) is a rating instrument founded upon psychoanalytic theory and developed in Sweden over 25 years ago by Weinryb, Rössel, and Åsberg (1991a, 1991b) at the Karolinska Institute. The clinician uses the material of a structured diagnostic interview such as the STIPO (see above) for the KAPP assessment. Clinician ratings are made on the basis of a detailed scoring system kept close to clinically observable phenomena. The scoring system generates 5-point scores (1, 1.5, 2, 2.5, 3) on 18 subscales.

The KAPP assesses relatively stable features of personality and mental functions, such as object relationships (intimacy and reciprocity, dependency and separation); ego strengths and flexibility (frustration tolerance, impulse control, capacity for regression in the service of the ego, coping with aggressive affects); body image and conceptions of body appearance and functioning; sexual life (sexual functioning and sexual satisfaction); social support (sense of belonging, sense of being needed, access to advice and help); alexithymic, normopathic, and controlling personality traits; and the overall level of personality organization.

Strengths of the KAPP

Like the STIPO, the KAPP may be useful for the assessment of the level of personality organization and its core functions (P Axis) and of several aspects of mental functioning (M Axis), such as the capacities for relationship and intimacy, for impulse control and regulation, and for adaptation, resiliency, and strength. The KAPP makes possible an assessment of personality and mental functioning from a psychoanalytic perspective that is psychometrically sound and that requires minimal training. KAPP scales show good validity and high reliability with minimal to modest training. They can be used to identify personality features differentiating patients with different clinical disorders, to differentiate personality subtypes of patients with the same clinical disorder, and to assess the personality changes of patients in the course of psychoanalysis and psychotherapy (Charitat, 1996; Turrina et al., 1996; Weinryb, Gustavsson, & Barber, 2003; Weinryb & Rössel, 1991; Weinryb et al., 1991a, 1991b; Weinryb, Rössel, Gustavsson, Åsberg, & Barber 1997; Wilczek, Barber, Gustavsson, Asberg, & Weinryb, 2004).

Limitations of the KAPP

A reliable assessment with the KAPP requires familiarity with the underlying psychodynamic concepts. No empirically derived norms are yet available.

Shedler–Westen Assessment Procedure

The first version of the SWAP, the SWAP-200 (Shedler, 2015; Westen & Shedler, 1999a, 1999b; Shedler, Westen, & Lingiardi, 2014), is a clinician-rated instrument that uses a Q-sort method (explained below) to evaluate personality styles and disorders. The SWAP-200 items were developed from a U.S. nationwide survey of clinicians experienced in the treatment of personality disorders. After numerous iterations, a pool of 200 items was developed to organize clinical observations and inferences about a patient's personality and to provide an in-depth portrait of a patient's psychological functioning.

The SWAP provides three score profile graphs that assess (1) DSM-IV and DSM-5 personality disorder diagnoses; (2) an alternative set of empirically identified personality syndromes (called the Q factors), designed to be more clinically accurate and informative than DSM personality disorder diagnoses; and (3) 12 trait dimensions that highlight specific areas of personality functioning (this requires a specific informatic procedure).

A revised version of the SWAP, the SWAP-II, was developed for research use (Westen et al., 2012; Westen & Shedler, 2007). The SWAP-II differs from the SWAP-200 in three respects. First, the SWAP-II has a slightly modified item set. Second, the newer edition possesses a different, empirically derived taxonomy of adult personality disorders subdivided into four spectra: (1) internalizing (depressive, anxious–avoidant, dependent–victimized, and schizoid–schizotypal disorders); (2) externalizing (antisocial–psychopathic, narcissistic, paranoid); (3) borderline–dysregulated (borderline–dysregulated disorder); and (4) neurotic (obsessional and hysteric–histrionic disorder). Third, the SWAP-II was validated on a larger sample, more representative of the population ordinarily found in clinical practice, whereas the SWAP-200 validation sample contained only personality-disordered patients.

There is also an adolescent version of the SWAP-II, the Shedler–Westen Assessment Procedure for Adolescents (SWAP-II-A; Westen, Dutra, & Shedler, 2005); it follows a format similar to that of the adult versions of the SWAP (see Chapter 5 on the PA Axis). It uses a modified item set and an empirically derived taxonomy of adolescent personalities articulated in two personality styles (healthy functioning and inhibited–self-critical) and five personality disorders (avoidant–constricted, antisocial–psychopathic, histrionic, narcissistic, and emotionally dysregulated). Reliability and validity are impressive (DeFife, Malone, DiLallo, & Westen, 2013).

On any version of the SWAP, the rater assigns a score from 0 (not descriptive) to 7 (most descriptive) to each of the 200 items according to their descriptiveness of a patient's personality and functioning. All versions of the SWAP require the clinician to use a fixed-score distribution (i.e., assessors must assign each score a prespecified number of items). Use of a fixed-score distribution minimizes rater bias and maximizes reliability and validity (Block, 1961/1978).

The SWAP items are most conveniently sorted by using a web-based scoring program (available at *www.swapassessment.org*). Users can select three diagnostic reports, including a Clinical Interpretive Report that features a comprehensive interpretation of all test scores, as well as personality diagnoses, clinical case formulations, and treatment recommendations.

Other than a description of pathological personality features, the SWAP also provides descriptors of positive mental health, represented in 24 of the 200 items, and generates a profile of a healthy, high-functioning individual.

The 200 items of the SWAP, and the seven degrees of salience assigned to each item, generate nearly innumerable permutations that permit the capture of complex personality patterns (Shedler, 2015). Further studies (Lingiardi, Shedler, & Gazzillo, 2006; Waldron et al., 2011) have shown that the 30 items receiving the highest scores provide a useful summary of patient functioning, such that they can be used as the core of a case formulation.

To improve the SWAP's utility for evaluating a patient's level of health–sickness, and the patient's areas of health and sickness, two supplemental score indices were developed by a group of researchers in New York and have been described, along with evidence for their validity (Waldron et al., 2011). The first index, the Personality Health Index (PHI), provides a global assessment of personality health using the 200 SWAP item scores, which are then converted into a percentile score for mental health compared to psychoanalytic patients in treatment (Cogan & Porcerelli, 2004, 2005). The percentile standing provides a ready and understandable metric of overall psychological health or illness.

The second index derived from the SWAP, the RADIO, delineates an individual's particular strengths and difficulties within five central domains of personality functioning: Reality testing, Affect regulation and tolerance, Defensive organization, Identity integration, and Object relations (hence the acronym RADIO), in five separate charts. These domains are similar to those used in PDM-2 to describe levels of personality functioning.

Two published case examples demonstrate how the SWAP indices may prove useful clinically. While these indices have obvious applications for psychotherapeutic and psychoanalytic research, they comprise a useful resource for clinical work and training as well (Gazzillo et al., 2014; Waldron, Gazzillo, Genova, & Lingiardi, 2013).

Strengths of the SWAP

The SWAP, in its different versions, can be useful in assessment of the PDM-2 P and PA Axes, while the PHI and RADIO may help in assessment of the M and MA Axes. The SWAP also provides systematic personality diagnoses and case formulations by allowing clinicians to record their clinical observations systematically, and then applying statistical and psychometric methods to the resulting data to optimize diagnosis and clinical case description (Lingiardi, Gazzillo, & Waldron, 2010; Lingiardi et al., 2006). The information is useful to treating clinicians in developing clinically rich case formulations that can guide effective intervention. It shows excellent validity and reliability (Shedler, 2015). Clinicians and researchers can use the SWAP to compare a patient's overall health–sickness at different points in treatment, providing a valuable method for demonstrating change over the course of psychotherapy (Gazzillo et al., 2014; Waldron et al., 2013). The items are straightforward, jargon-free clinical statements about the individual being rated. The SWAP's reliability and validity have been reported and extended over the past 10 years (Shedler, 2015; Shedler & Westen, 2006; Westen & Muderrisoglu, 2006).

Limitations of the SWAP

The SWAP requires between 40 and 120 minutes to score (depending on the assessor's familiarity with the instrument); this amount of time is not readily available in many clinical settings. Moreover, for a reliable SWAP assessment, the clinician or rater should know the patient well. The SWAP authors recommend a minimum of six clinical sessions for patients in treatment—or, for individuals being seen for assessment only, a systematic interview for personality assessment, the Clinical Diagnostic Interview, which can be administered in approximately 2½ hours.

Operationalized Psychodynamic Diagnosis

The Operationalized Psychodynamic Diagnosis (OPD) Task Force was founded in 1992 in Germany by a group of psychoanalysts, specialists in psychosomatic medicine, and psychiatrists with a background in psychotherapy research. The goal of the group was to broaden the descriptive and symptom-oriented ICD-10 classification system to include fundamental psychodynamic dimensions. This task force developed a diagnostic inventory and a handbook designed for training and clinical purposes for experienced therapists (Arbeitskreis OPD, 1996). Since then, the manual has been translated into 11 languages. Further translations are in preparation.

A second version, the OPD-2 (Arbeitskreis OPD, 2006; OPD Task Force, 2008), includes a textbook that manualizes how to select the focus for individual treatment planning. On the basis of therapeutic foci, it is possible to evaluate the treatment outcome and follow-up. In addition, the Heidelberg Structure Change Scale allows the evaluation of clinical changes (Grande, Rudolf, Oberbracht, & Pauli-Magnus, 2003).

Recently, the second version of the German-language manual of the OPD for child and adolescent psychotherapists was published (Arbeitskreis OPD-KJ, 2014). A self-report instrument to measure the patient's level of structural integration is also available (Ehrenthal et al., 2012). Additional resources, such as modules for substance abuse, forensic patients and trauma, are under development.

The OPD requires the clinician to complete five axes:

- *Axis I: Experience of illness and prerequisites for treatment.* The clinician characterizes the severity of illness; degree of suffering; subjective illness attributions (the patient's understanding of the cause of his or her illness); models of change (the patient's ideas about how treatment may help); and resources (personal resources such as ego strengths, humor, intellect, and psychosocial support from family, friends, and companions).

- *Axis II: Interpersonal relations.* The clinician characterizes the patient's dysfunctional habitual relationship experiences and describes the patient's relationship to the therapist as well.
- *Axis III: Conflict.* The clinician describes the patient according to seven inner conflicts: individuation versus dependency; dependence versus self-sufficiency; control versus submission; valuing self versus valuing others; guilt conflict; oedipal conflict; and identity conflict.
- *Axis IV: Structure.* The clinician rates eight dimensions, each with three facets: (a) self-perception (related to the patient's capacity for self-reflection and sense of identity); (b) object perception (related to the patient's capacity to differentiate self from object); (c) self-regulation (e.g. impulse control); (d) regulation of object relationships and interests; (e) internal communication (fantasies, body awareness); (f) communication with others (being in contact, empathy); (g) attachment capacity to internal objects (use of introjects, variability of introjects); and (h) attachment capacity to others (including the capacity to separate). Ratings are combined in a global score.
- *Axis V: Mental disorders, personality disorders, and psychosomatic disorders* (in conjunction with Chapter V (F) of ICD-10 or with DSM-IV/DSM-5).

After an initial 1- to 2-hour interview, the clinician (or a clinical observer) evaluates the patient's psychodynamic profile on the basis of the OPD-2 axes and categories. The OPD interview technique alternates between relatively unstructured phases of free exploration and more structured questions. The interviews are designed to elicit all relevant information for assessing an interviewee's maladaptive relationship patterns, enduring motivational conflicts, and structural capabilities. Guidelines on how to conduct the interview are sufficiently flexible that the interview can still be conducted as an open psychodynamic interview.

The OPD can be applied by experienced raters with relatively good reliability and can be recommended for teaching.

Strengths of the OPD

The OPD can be a very useful aid in the assessment of PDM-2's P, M, S, PA, MA, and SA Axes. Trained and experienced clinicians can reliably apply the OPD rating to clinical interview material (Cierpka, Rudolf, Grande, & Stasch, 2007), and its validity is well supported in 17 samples, including data from more than 2,000 participants (Zimmermann et al., 2012). An OPD expert consensus study confirmed that OPD Axis IV (the structure axis) is highly similar to the proposed Level of Personality Functioning Scale for the alternative DSM-5 model for personality disorders (Zimmermann et al., 2012).

The OPD fulfills Strupp's recommendation of the need for "problem–treatment–outcome congruence" in psychodynamic psychotherapy (Strupp, Schacht, & Henry, 1988). The system is also applicable for pre–post–follow-up evaluations of psychoanalytic therapies (Rudolf et al., 2002).

Limitations of the OPD

The OPD system is a comprehensive approach. Learning the basic use of this tool requires at least 60 hours of training. Completion of the evaluation sheets for all five OPD axes takes approximatively 30 minutes. Moreover, the OPD is limited thus far to therapy planning, with no attempt to manualize intervention processes. However, operationalized psychodynamic therapies for different disorders are currently being developed by the OPD group.

Psychodynamic Functioning Scales

Per Høglend and his colleagues, primarily in Norway, have carried out extensive systematic studies of processes and outcomes of dynamic psychotherapies. Recognizing the need for better outcome studies, they started more than 25 years ago to develop instruments to respond to this imperative (Høglend, 1995; Høglend et al., 2000).

The Psychodynamic Functioning Scales (PFS) instrument uses six scales, with the same 0–100 format as the DSM-IV Global Assessment of Functioning (GAF), to measure psychological functioning over the previous 3 months. Three of the scales measure interpersonal aspects: quality of family relationships, quality of friendships, and quality of romantic/sexual relationships. The other three scales measure intrapersonal functioning: tolerance for affects, insight, and problem-solving capacity. The evaluation is based on interview data (the interview takes 1–2 hours). The scales have been translated into German, French, and Portuguese.

Strengths of the PFS

The PFS can be a useful aid in the assessment of PDM-2 M-Axis functions (e.g., capacities for relationships and intimacy; affective range, communication, and understanding; and psychological mindedness) and overall mental functioning. Aspects of content validity, internal domain construct validity, discriminant validity from symptom measures, and sensitivity for change in dynamic therapy have been established in different samples of patients and evaluators (Bøgwald & Dahlbender, 2004; Hagtvet & Høglend, 2008; Høglend, 2004; Høglend et al., 2000). The instrument is brief, and there are many levels, to increase sensitivity to change. Findings about the role of transference and transference interpretations have added to clinical understanding (Høglend et al., 2008, 2011).

Limitations of the PFS

So far, reliability has only been tested with clinicians who have several years of dynamic training.

Scales of Psychological Capacities

The Scales of Psychological Capacities (SPC) measure is an interview-based instrument developed by Robert S. Wallerstein and colleagues at the University of California, San Francisco. The instrument was designed to reflect treatment-related changes in underlying personality organization.

The SPC comprises 36 Likert-type scales, measuring 17 positive "capacities," that are applied by trained raters to semistructured clinical interviews or recorded treatment sessions. A "capacity" is defined as a psychological resource needed to achieve adaptive functioning and life satisfaction. The healthy end of each of the 17 dimensions is anchored by a title and definition. The dimensions are self-coherence; self-esteem; zest for life; hope; flexibility; responsibility; persistence; standards and values; affect regulation; impulse regulation; regulation of sexuality; assertion; empathy; trust; reliance on others; relationship commitment; and reciprocity. Each dimension has between one and three unhealthy opposites (e.g., self-esteem vs. grandiosity and self-depreciation), yielding 36 subdimensions, each of which is rated on a 4-point Likert scale from fully adaptive functioning (0) to seriously or obviously compromised (3). Definitions and clinical examples anchor each scale point.

Wallerstein enlisted the help of clinicians from many countries and theoretical orientations in developing the capacity set. The scales are designed to be theoretically neutral so as to increase their applicability to a wide range of treatments and patient populations. The SPC is written in plain English in order to minimize ambiguity and optimize its ease of use and its translatability into other languages. A manual that includes semistructured "probe questions" is available, along with Spanish and Hebrew translations and an adolescent version.

Strengths of the SPC

The SPC taps areas (beyond symptom changes) that are important to an individual's general positive functioning and areas that are typical of impairments seen in psychiatric outpatients. The measure may assist in the assessment of PDM-2 M- and MA-Axis capacities (especially the capacities for differentiation and integration [identity]; self-esteem regulation and quality of internal experience; adaptation, resiliency, and strength; and relationships and intimacy). The instrument has demonstrated good interrater and test–retest reliability, content and construct validity, and ability to reflect treatment-related change in studies by groups in California (DeWitt, Milbrath, & Wallerstein, 1999) and in Germany (Huber, Henrich, & Klug, 2013; Leuzinger-Bohleber & Fischmann, 2007).

Limitations of the SPC

Training requires 4–6 hours for evaluators to achieve reliability. The assessment tool has not been applied to sufficient numbers of patients to fully evaluate its potential to reflect treatment-related change.

Social Cognition and Object Relations Scale

The Social Cognition and Object Relations Scale (SCORS) was originally created by Westen (1991a, 1991b) to systematically assess (via free-response data) multiple dimensions of cognitive and affective processes that mediate interpersonal functioning beyond the patient's overt presentation. It integrates clinically based object relations theories with experimentally generated theories of social cognition (Stein, Slavin-Mulford, Sinclair, Siefert, & Blais, 2012). There are three versions of the SCORS. This discussion focuses on the SCORS Global Rating Method (SCORS-G; Westen, 1995).

The SCORS-G consists of eight variables that are scored on 7-point anchored scales; lower scores indicate more pathological responses, and higher scores indicate healthier and more mature aspects of object relations. The eight variables are as follows:

1. Complexity of representations of people (COM), which assesses presence, degree, and differentiation of internal states and relational boundaries.
2. Affective quality of representations (AFF), which examines the emotional lens through which a person views his or her environment.
3. Emotional investment in relationships (EIR), which assesses the level of intimacy and emotional sharing.
4. Emotional investment in moral standards (EIM), which measures how a person views others and acts in relation to morality and compassion for others.
5. Understanding of social causality (SC), which evaluates the extent to which the person understands human behavior, as well as the narrative's coherence, logic, and reasoning.
6. Experience and management of aggressive impulses (AGG), which explores the person's ability to tolerate and manage aggression.
7. Self-esteem (SE).
8. Identity and coherence of self (ICS), which is the degree to which a person has an integrated sense of who he or she is.

The SCORS-G can be applied to numerous forms of narrative data, such as psychotherapy sessions, TAT data, early memory narratives, the Relationship Anecdotes Paradigm (RAP) interview, and clinical interviews.

The SCORS-G discriminates between aspects of psychopathology and personality (Ackerman, Clemence, Weatherill, & Hilsenroth, 1999; DeFife, Goldberg, & Westen, 2015; Stein et al., 2012). Other studies have explored the SCORS-G as it relates to aspects of attachment and trauma (Calabrese, Farber, & Westen, 2005; Ortigo, Westen, DeFife, & Bradley, 2013). Numerous studies have used the SCORS-G in the context of process and outcome research in psychotherapy (see Fowler et al., 2004).

Strengths of the SCORS

The SCORS-G can be a very useful aid for the assessment of several capacities on PDM-2's M and MA Axes, such as the capacities for differentiation and integration, self-esteem regulation and quality of internal experience, and relationships and intimacy, as well as the capacity to construct and use internal standards and values. The SCORS-G is one of the most common psychodynamic measures used to rate narrative data. Anchor points are worded in an experience-near way, useful to clinicians from various orientations. Interrater reliability and convergent and discriminant validity have been consistently demonstrated in previous research (Stein et al., 2014).

Limitations of the SCORS

The most significant weakness of the SCORS-G is its limited normative data. Also, there are medium to high intercorrelations between the eight variables (Stein et al., 2012).

Psychodynamic Conflict Rating Scales

The first version of the Psychodynamic Conflict Rating Scales (PCRS), which J. Christopher Perry developed in 1980, was derived from the tradition of understanding intrapsychic or psychological conflict; it was then broadened to include more recent developments in both self psychology and object relations. Each scale consists of a series of statements reflecting some aspect of conflict among motives (wishes and fears), internal states, external events (especially interpersonal interactions), and defensive functioning. The results of conflict may lead to either symptom formation or compromise formations, which are also noted. However, because conflict is internal and partly or wholly unconscious, it can only be inferred indirectly through what can be observed as anomalies or disturbances.

The PCRS assesses 14 defined conflicts. These are divided into 7 focal conflicts (presumed to be developmentally later in origin and to be largely synonymous with oedipal-level conflicts) and 7 global conflicts (presumed to have earlier developmental origins and to be largely synonymous with oral-level conflicts).

The focal conflicts include (1) dominant other, (2) dominant goal, (3) counterdependency, (4) ingratiation–disappointment, (5) ambition–achievement, (6) competition–hostility, and (7) sexual pleasure versus guilt. The global conflicts include (8) overall gratification inhibition, (9) separation–abandonment, (10) experience and expression of emotional needs and anger, (11) object-hunger, (12) fear of fusion, (13) rejection of others, and (14) resentment over being thwarted by others. The PCRS also has 14 companion scales that assess healthy adaptation to each conflict, so that pathology and healthy adaptation are represented separately (Perry, 1997, 2006; Perry & Cooper, 1986).

For clinical use, a thorough history in the context of dynamic interviewing or therapy sessions is sufficient. For research purposes, two data sources are suggested: (1) a dynamic intake or follow-up type interview and (2) an interview that focuses on relationship stories, such as the RAP interview (Beck & Perry, 2008).

The original version of the PCRS consisted of a definition of each conflict and a section on discriminating it from near-neighbor conflicts. The rater then filled out a 4-point pattern identification score that was readily used. The current version improved upon this psychometrically by assessing each conflict with a series of 8–15 items, each of which is a low-inferential statement of some aspect of the conflict, scored as (0) absent, (1) somewhat true, or (2) definitely present or true. Statements represent affective, behavioral, or cognitive facets of the conflict and are generally worded in nontechnical English. Scores for each conflict are converted to reflect the proportion of the maximum score (scaled from 0 to 1.00).

Interrater reliability determined on an early version was adequate to good (Perry & Cooper, 1986; Perry & Perry, 2004); more recent studies have generally found good to excellent internal consistency and interrater reliability (Perry, Constantinides, & Simmons, 2017). Cutoffs define the definite presence or absence of a conflict or the presence of healthy adaptation. Additional separate scales summarize the (1) affective, (2) behavioral, and (3) cognitive features of each conflict. Mean summary scores are then calculated for the scales assessing focal conflicts, global conflicts, overall pathological conflict, and adaptation to conflict. Two studies examining change with short-term or longer-term treatments have demonstarated convergent and discriminant validity (Perry et al., 2017).

Strengths of the PCRS

The PCRS can give useful data for the assessment of PDM-2's P and PA Axes and for assessing the capacity for relationships and intimacy on the M and MA Axes. Clinicians can use the original pattern recognition version, with minimal time required for rating. The conflicts are intuitively understandable, and the statements readily reflect clinical observation, as well as conflict issues to which clinicians attend. The method has demonstrated usefulness for measuring change over time and can determine when individuals are dynamically recovered.

Limitations of the PCRS

Training requires rating about three to five training cases and intermittent calibration by doing consensus ratings. Although the PCRS can be rated after a single dynamic interview, several interviews are preferable to ensure adequate coverage of data. Research use requires recorded interviews. Ratings require about 90–120 minutes per session rated.

Object Relations Inventory

The Object Relations Inventory (ORI) is an unstructured method developed by Blatt and colleagues for assessing a person's representations of self and significant figures—that is, a person's object world. It derives originally from work on the use of parental descriptions as a method for assessing object representations (Blatt, Wein, Chevron, & Quinlan, 1979); this work in turn was based on cognitive developmental theory and developmental object relations theories current in psychoanalysis in the 1970s (e.g., the work of Fraiberg, Anna Freud, Jacobson, Kernberg, Kohut, Mahler, and Winnicott). Since the 1980s, with the influence of further developmental theories (e.g., those of Stern, Beebe, and Lachmann) as well as of intersubjectivity theory rooted in Hegelian philosophy (e.g., the work of Aron, Benjamin, Fonagy, and colleagues), the ORI has come to use an individual's descriptions of significant figures to assess the person's ability to understand both the self and his or her intersubjective interpersonal matrix.

The ORI in its current format, as an interview, was developed by Sugarman (personal communication to J. S. Auerbach, August 29, 2014). A respondent is asked to describe parents, significant others (including pets), self, and therapist, with inquiry by the interviewer.

The content and cognitive structural organization of the descriptions are evaluated, and several methods for doing so have been developed. The best-known of these are (1) the conceptual level (CL) scale (Blatt, Chevron, Quinlan, Schaffer, & Wein, 1988), which describes a Piagetian developmental progression, including sensorimotor, perceptual, external iconic, internal iconic, and conceptual levels; and (2) the differentation–relatedness (D-R) scale (Diamond, Blatt, Stayner, & Kaslow, 1991; Diamond, Kaslow, Coonerty, & Blatt, 1990), which, influenced by modern relational theory, delineates a 10-level progression from boundary collapse through polarization to object constancy and eventually to intersubjectivity. In addition, Blatt and colleagues (Blatt et al., 1979, 1988; Quinlan, Blatt, Chevron, & Wein, 1992) evaluated the CL descriptions for three qualitative or thematic factors: benevolence, punitiveness, and striving. Later factor-analytic studies (e.g., Heck & Pincus, 2001; Huprich,

Auerbach, Porcerelli, & Bupp, 2016a) developed factors of agency, communion, and punitiveness.

Blatt and colleagues (Blatt, Bers, & Schaffer, 1993) also developed a rating manual to capture the structural complexities involved in the description of self. Eighteen reliable dimensions, including CL, were resolved into five factors: agency, reflectivity, differentiation, relatedness, and relatedness to the examiner.

Reviews of research findings with the various ORI methods (e.g., Bender, Morey, & Skodol, 2011; Blatt, 2008; Blatt & Auerbach, 2001; Huprich et al., 2016a; Priel, 2005) suggest that variables like CL and D-R can be considered structural dimensions, reflective of a person's underlying level of organization, regardless of whether significant figures are described in predominantly positive or predominantly negative terms on the qualitative–thematic factors. For example, a description of a significant figure can be very negative in content and yet still organized at a high developmental level.

Strengths of the ORI

The ORI can be useful in assessing the prevalence of an introjective or anaclitic orientation on PDM-2's P Axis, as well as in assessing several M-Axis capacities (such as those for differentiation and integration, self-esteem regulation and quality of internal experience, and relationships and intimacy). The ORI is easy to administer. It collects information about how a person understands the significant figures in his or her life. At the same time, it permits the assessment of structural dimensions of object relations that are not immediately evident and that reflect underlying levels of personality organization. Some raters without a psychodynamic or psychoanalytic background have been successfully trained to reliability in 2 days, both in Belgium and in Israel (Luyten, personal communication to J. S. Auerbach, November 14, 2014). However, Diamond (personal communication to J. S. Auerbach, May 3, 2015) believes that a master's degree, clinical experience with psychodynamic theory, and a 2-day training session are necessary for competence in coding D-R.

Limitations of the ORI

ORI scales are strongly tied to psychoanalytic object relations theories, and these ties may limit the measures' generalizability and understandability for clinicians not conversant with these theories. In addition, the historical evolution and the scoring complexity of the ORI do not favor busy practitioners. For scoring, the 30- to 60-minute interview must be transcribed verbatim and then rated by a reliable coder—methods that are rare in routine practice. Clinical understanding of the findings requires understanding of the value of differentiating between the affective content of a significant-figure description and its level of psychological organization.

Adult Attachment Interview

The Adult Attachment Interview (AAI) classification system developed by Mary Main and colleagues (George, Kaplan, & Main, 1984, 1985, 1996; Main, Hesse, & Goldwyn, 2008) examines the structural and discourse characteristics of adult autobiographical narratives about attachment experiences and relationships. The AAI is a semistructured clinical interview designed to elicit thoughts, feelings, and memories about early attachment experiences, in order to elucidate an individual's attachment representations (i.e., internalized object relations) and current state of mind with respect to early attachment relationships and experiences.

The interview consists of 20 questions asked in a set order with standardized probes. Individuals are asked to give five words that reflect their childhood relationships with each parent, and then to provide episodic memories that support their semantic descriptions. They are also asked about how their parents responded to them when they were in physical or emotional distress and about experiences of rejection. In addition, there are questions about loss and physical and sexual abuse or other overwhelming or threatening experiences. Other questions encourage individuals to reflect on how their childhood experiences with their parents have affected their adult personalities. The technique has been described as having the effect of "surprising the unconscious" (George et al., 1985) and allowing numerous opportunities for the interviewee to elaborate upon, contradict, or fail to support previous statements.

The AAI is transcribed verbatim, and trained coders score the transcripts to assess the nature of the experiences and relationships described. Coders use subscales that assess the rater's inferences about the individual's experiences of parents in childhood; the individual's style of discourse and overall state of mind with respect to attachment; and the extent to which the individual is unresolved with regard to loss or trauma (Main & Goldwyn, 1998). Subscales are rated from 1 (absent or very low) to 9 (high) for the dimension in question.

The patterns of ratings are then used to assign individuals to one of five primary attachment classifications, the first three of which are considered "organized" and the last two "disorganized":

1. *Secure–autonomous,* characterized by ready access to attachment-related memories that are expressed in a coherent, well-organized, fresh, and spontaneous manner, and with internally consistent and integrated portrayal of attachment relationships.
2. *Dismissing,* characterized by devaluing or idealizing states of mind with respect to attachment, with little corroborating evidence or with loss of recall of attachment-related memories and experiences.
3. *Preoccupied,* characterized by current involving anger, and/or by oscillation between positive and negative valuations of an attachment figure with whom the individual remains emotionally entangled.
4. *Unresolved for loss and abuse,* characterized by lapses in the monitoring of reasoning and discourse (e.g., highly implausible statements regarding the causes and consequences of traumatic attachment-related events; loss of memory for attachment-related traumas; or lapses into confusion and silence in response to specific questions about early attachment traumas and losses).
5. *Cannot classify,* when there are oscillations between two or more opposing attachment states of mind (such as dismissing and preoccupied) or shifts in attachment strategy midway through the interview or in regard to different attachment figures (Main & Goldwyn, 1998).

The first three categories of adult attachment (secure, dismissing, and preoccupied) correspond to attachment patterns first identified in 1-year-old children by Ainsworth, Blehar, Waters, and Wall (1978) through observation of caregiver–infant transactions in the Ainsworth Strange Situation. After the interviewer has met mother and child, the mother leaves the infant alone with the interviewer for a brief time, and on the basis of the reactions of the child both during the separation and upon reunion with the mother, the infant is classified as secure, avoidant, or anxious in response to this stress. These infant categories have been found to correspond to the adult attachment classifications, in that both involve specific identifiable and consistent strategies for regulating emotion in the context of attachment relationships. By contrast, the two disorganized classificiations (unresolved and cannot classify)—both of which were identified later by Main and her colleagues (see, e.g., Hesse, 2008) as a result of failure to classify a significant proportion of interviews in the organized categories—are characterized by lack of integration in the attachment system and have been associated with disorganized/disoriented infant attachment behaviors in the Ainsworth Strange Situation.

Main and colleagues (2008) have noted that the AAI interview and classification system parallel the process of analytic listening, in that they involve paying attention to what individuals say, how they say it, and what they omit. The AAI classification system also provides linguistic markers to track defensive processes and modes of expressing and regulating affect, which are useful to clinicians even if they do not have formal AAI training.

Strengths of the AAI

The AAI can be a useful aid in the assessment of several relevant capacities on PDM-2's M Axis, such as the capacities for relationships and intimacy and for self-observing (psychological mindedness). Previous research has shown remarkable stability and predictive validity of the AAI (Hesse, 2008; Waters & Hamilton, 2000). Parents' mental representations of attachment both before and after the birth of their children have been found to predict later infant attachment status in over 18 international studies in a meta-analysis (van IJzendoorn, 1995). Thus the patterns of attachment revealed on the AAI appear to provide a window on the nature of early parent–child relationships and to tap into behavioral manifestations of normal and disturbed internalization of object relations (internal working models) that strongly predict adjustment many years later.

The AAI classification may substantially affect therapeutic discourse and process, and has been found to be associated with treatment alliance, transference–countertransference, and outcome (see Slade, 2008, for a review), as well as with different types of psychopathology. For example, in a number of studies, borderline personality disorder has been associated primarily with the preoccupied and unresolved (disorganized) attachment categories (Bakersman-Kranenburg & van IJzendoorn, 2009; Diamond, Stovall-McClough, Clarkin, & Levy, 2003; Fonagy et al., 1996; Levy et al., 2006). In addition, the AAI is a useful instrument to assess change in attachment representational states from insecure to secure and disorganized to organized attachment status in borderline patients over the course of psychoanalytically oriented psychotherapy (e.g., Diamond et al., 2003; Levy et al., 2006).

Limitations of the AAI

Formal training to become an AAI coder is a lengthy process. The interviews must be audio-recorded and carefully transcribed according to a set of rules that capture both verbal utterances and breaks in the flow. AAI training requires a 2-week-long workshop with a certified AAI trainer; this workshop involves learning to administer the interview and to understand the fundamentals of the coding system and its research and theoretical underpinnings, followed by independent coding of several sets of AAI transcripts in order to achieve reliability. There are also limitations to the coding system, in that it provides one overall attachment classification and does not take into account differences in the attachment representations of different figures (e.g., mother and father). Finally, the AAI classification system does not provide a dimensional measure of security or insecurity.

Adult Attachment Projective Picture System

The Adult Attachment Projective (AAP) Picture System (George & West, 2012) is a free-response assessment of adult attachment status. The assessment is based on the analysis of "story" responses to a set of seven drawings depicting attachment scenes (four scenes of individuals alone and three of individuals in attachment dyads). Individuals tell a story for each stimulus, guided by a standard set of prompts to elicit events as well as characters' thoughts and feelings. Coding examines narrative-based representational integration and attachment relationship sensitivity, based on content and defensive processing strategies. The content of responses to the drawings of persons alone is used to evaluate "agency of self" and "connectedness." The content of responses to the dyadic drawings is used to evaluate relationship "synchrony."

Defensive processes are coded for all responses. This coding feature provides insight into differences among classification groups. Attachment theory delineates three forms of defense (Bowlby, 1980; George & West, 2012) that are also evaluated in the AAP: "deactivation," "cognitive disconnection," and "segregated systems." Deactivation shifts attention away from events, individuals, or emotion (e.g., rejection). Cognitive disconnection fractures attention to attachment details and affect resulting in confusion or contradiction. Segregated systems block attention from pain, fear, and helplessness. Finally, responses are evaluated for "personal experience"; this evaluation assesses whether individuals are able to maintain self–other boundaries, and whether there is evidence of absorption with distress or trauma.

The AAP designates four standard adult attachment groups (secure, dismissing, preoccupied, and unresolved), as well as pathological mourning. Secure attachment is characterized by substantial evidence of representational integration and value of attachment relationships. Dismissing and preoccupied attachments are characterized by defensive interference with integration; however, these representations help individuals maintain daily activities and relationships. Unresolved attachment represents failures of integrative function in the presence of evident attachment trauma. Pathological mourning is evaluated from the presence of traumatic indicators in AAP responses and demonstrates risk for failure to complete the mourning process; such failure is associated with heightened psychological and relationship distress (Bowlby, 1980).

The AAP has established concurrent validity and reliability with the AAI (see, e.g., George & West, 2012), as well as research and clinical utility. It has also been shown to be a useful resource for examining the neurophysiological attachment underpinnings of adult disorders (e.g., Buchheim et al., 2009), and to be valid for use with adolescents 13 years of age and older (e.g., Aikins, Howes, & Hamilton, 2009).

Strengths of the AAP

The AAP can be useful for assessing several PDM-2 M- and MA-Axis functions, particularly those connected to defensive functioning and relational capacities. The AAP is a validated, user-friendly, and economical measure that identifies developmental attachment patterns. It can be used clinically to evaluate treatment progress and change over the course of time. The nonbiographical nature of the task may make it more trauma-sensitive than interviews, in which trauma themes may be uncomfortable or otherwise problematic (Spieker, Nelson, DeKlyen, Jolley, & Mennet, 2011). The free-response methodology is straightforward, and administration is easy to learn. Administrators do not need to be reliable coders. The AAP is easily used with non-English-speaking interviewees, as has been demonstrated to date in European samples. Work examining use of the AAP with speakers of Asian and African languages is underway.

Limitations of the AAP

The AAP requires about 30–45 minutes and needs to be administered in an individualized (i.e., private) setting. Stimuli are only available in the course of training in coding and classification. The time it takes to achieve reliability is offset by making available reliable master judges who can code and classify cases.

Reflective Functioning Scale

Integrating contributions from attachment theory, psychoanalysis, philosophy, and developmental affective neuroscience, the concept of "reflective functioning" or "mentalization" refers to the capacity to reflect on the self and others in terms of intentional mental states such as thoughts, feelings, and desires (Allen, Fonagy, & Bateman, 2008; Fonagy, Gergely, Jurist, & Target, 2002). The capacity to mentalize is conceptualized as developing from secure attachment experiences characterized by affective contingency and marked mirroring with caregivers; it has critical implications for the maturation of adaptive relational capacities and affect regulation (Fonagy et al., 2002). Clinician-researchers in the United Kingdom have developed this concept and an instrument to measure it, the Reflective Functioning Scale (RFS), over the past 20 years (Fonagy, Target, Steele, & Steele, 1998).

Mentalizing has been predominantly assessed with the RFS as applied to the AAI or the Parent Development Interview (PDI; Slade, Aber, Bresgi, Berger, & Kaplan, 2004). The RFS is applied to transcripts of different sections of the AAI or PDI that specifically relate to interactions with attachment figures. Coders assess the extent to which the interviewee understands attachment-associated experiences in terms of mental states. The process of coding relies on distinguishing between "demand" and "permit" questions, with demand questions weighted more heavily. Demand questions directly probe for reflective functioning, whereas permit questions do not.

Answers to each question from the AAI are rated on an 11-point scale from –1 (systematic dismissal, derogation, or hostility at any attempts at reflection; active avoidance of mentalization) to 9 (exceptional sophistication in the understanding of complex mental states; exceptional mentalization). A score of 5 is proposed as a normal level of mentalization and is given when convincing indications of a coherent model of the mind are shown. A global score is obtained by individually weighting and totaling the ratings of the demand questions and permit questions, and allowing for a consideration of the interview as a whole.

A comprehensive review (Taubner et al., 2013) showed that the global RFS score can be determined with good interrater reliability and has good stability across time. Studies with the RFS have shown that the measure is related to infant and adult attachment status. Furthermore, the RFS has been associated with a wide range of psychopathology, including borderline personality disorder, depression, eating disorders, panic disorder, and psychosis. The RFS has also been related to trauma (deprivation in particular) and to posttraumatic stress disorder. Finally, studies also suggest that reflective functioning as measured with the RFS may moderate or mediate treatment outcome in various types of psychotherapy (for reviews, see Katznelson, 2014; Luyten, Fonagy, Lowyck, & Vermote, 2012).

Strengths of the RFS

The RFS can aid both in assessing the capacities for mentalization/reflective functioning and self-observing on PDM-2's M and MA Axes, and in assessing basic personality functions. Over the past two decades, perhaps the most generative new concept in psychoanalysis has been that of mentalizing. For example, reflective functioning has been shown to have a direct effect on results of treatment (Gullestad et al., 2013). Studies with the RFS and other measures of reflective functioning (Luyten et al., 2012) promise to shed light on a key factor in personality development and the therapeutic process. The research base on the RFS is well established and growing rapidly.

Limitations of the RFS

The training program to score the RFS reliably is extensive and takes considerable time and practice. As a result, the RFS has not been much used in routine clinical applications.

Quality of Object Relations

The Quality of Object Relations (QOR) scale was created by Piper and colleagues (Azim, Piper, Segal, Nixon, & Duncan, 1991; Piper, McCallum, & Joyce, 1993) and modified by Høglend (1993). From a single assessment interview, the quality of object relations is rated on a spectrum from primitive to mature. It is largely psychodynamic in its focus, with emphasis on recurring interpersonal patterns in development and current life.

The QOR assessment is standardized and is based on a 1- to 2-hour interview in which the rater first asks for a history of the significant relationships of the client, reported in a spontaneous way, and then assesses the quality of object relations on an 8-point scale. The scale points are described as follows (Høglend, 1993):

8–7: A history of most relationships characterized by stability, gratification, and mutuality. Others are seen as whole, autonomous persons.

6–5: Recent interpersonal functioning may be poorer, but the patient can give detailed examples from at least one earlier important high-quality relationship, in adulthood, adolescence, or childhood. Conflictual feelings may be seen toward same-sex persons, and fears of loss may be present toward opposite-sex persons.

4–3: Stability, but less gratification and mutuality, in most important relations. Passivity, dependency, need to control others, or separation anxiety may be predominant. Difficulty describing others as unique individuals.

2–1: Mostly unstable relations with little-valued persons. Others are seen as need-gratifying objects. Stable, overly dependent relations only with parental objects.

Two additional scales of the QOR, with points defined as above, assess the history of intimate sexual relationships and history of friendships.

Validation of the QOR has been reported by Piper and Duncan (1999). A recent study showed the modifying impact of the quality of object relations on the results of treatment in regard to self-concept (Lindfors, Knekt, & Virtala, 2013). This finding converges with the findings of Høglend and colleagues (2011) about differences in the impact of transference interpretations, depending on level of object relations (see the discussion of the PFS, above).

Strengths of the QOR

The QOR can be useful in assessing the capacity for relationships and intimacy on PDM-2's M Axis and can also give useful information for the assessment of the P Axis. As may be seen in the description of the scale points above, there are many overlaps among the QOR, the SCORS, and the ORI (see the discussions of the latter two instruments above). The SCORS and the ORI are more precisely developed; however, the QOR has the great advantage of being based on a single semistructured clinical interview and not requiring specific training for clinician-raters beyond careful study of the manual.

Limitations of the QOR

The QOR's emphasis on interpersonal and object relations functioning often needs to be integrated with other aspects of psychodynamic understanding, such as defensive operations, identity, reflective functioning, and values. Moreover, other instruments are better developed and researched. Studies of convergent validity with other measures of interpersonal relations would be valuable.

Plan Formulation Method

The Plan Formulation Method (PFM; Curtis & Silberschatz, 2005, 2007; Curtis, Silberschatz, Sampson, & Weiss, 1994) is a psychodynamic formulation method based on Sampson and Weiss's control–mastery theory. There are five interrelated components in the plan formulation:

- The patient's adaptive conscious and unconscious short-term and long-term goals.
- The unconscious pathogenic beliefs or schemas (developed as a consequence of shock and strain trauma) that impede goal attainment.

- The adverse or traumatic childhood experiences that led to the pathogenic beliefs or schemas.
- The patient's unconscious tests of the therapist in order to disconfirm pathogenic beliefs and expectations.
- New information or insight that might help the patient to overcome her or his pathogenic beliefs or schemas and their consequences.

Excellent reliability and validity data have been reported for the PFM. Trained clinicians show a high level of interrater reliability with regard to dimensions of the model such as the patient's unconscious goals and pathogenic beliefs (Curtis & Silberschatz, 2005, 2007). Research on detailed study of audio recordings has also shown that plan formulations can be used to predict which therapist responses and interventions are helpful to patients and which are not (e.g., Silberschatz & Curtis, 1993; for a review, see Silberschatz, 2005).

Strengths of the PFM

The PFM may be a useful aid for assessing pathogenic beliefs on PDM-2's P Axis, and for assessing the capacity for relationships and intimacy on the M Axis. This method provides systematic measures for creating a dynamic formulation. The major strength of the PFM is its high degree of reliability and validity. The method has yielded strong reliability data for psychoanalytic cases, brief dynamic psychotherapy, cognitive therapy, and crisis intervention (Silberschatz, 2005). Research has also shown that the formulations derived from the PFM can be used to assess the suitability or responsiveness of therapist interventions (Silberschatz, 2005).

Limitations of the PFM

As with any complex approach to formulation, mastery of the PFM requires some investment of time and supervision. Most practitioners and many investigators may not have the resources to learn this method, and this problem has undoubtedly limited its widespread use for research or for training purposes.

Core Conflictual Relationship Theme

Luborsky and Crits-Christoph (1990) defined the Core Conflictual Relationship Theme (CCRT) measure as a method of understanding an individual's way of relating to others and how this manner of interaction plays out in the relationship with the psychotherapist. The method requires first identifying, in recorded text, "relationship episodes" (REs). Luborsky noted that patients' narratives showed a considerable redundancy in the expression of a core wish (W), occasionally more than one; a typical anticipated or actual "response from other persons" (RO) in the narrative; and then a subsequent "response from the self" (RS) to the RO.

Initially, Luborsky identified these three components for a given relationship episode by clinical inspection. The specifications of W, RO, and RS were idiographic—that is, described by raters in words they thought most appropriate, without reference to any established categories. When multiple judges were used, there were difficulties in assessing the degree of agreement between them. To solve this, agreement judges were used. With these procedures, it was possible to establish consensus formulations.

Such formulations suffered, however, from both the complexity of the procedures and the difficulty in estimating the reliability of the results. Therefore, Luborsky's research group developed standard categories (about 30) for each of the three components (W, RO, and RS). Later, a German-speaking research group developed a different categorization of the CCRT components, the Core Conflictual Relational Theme—Leipzig/Ulm (CCRT-LU; Albani et al., 2002).

Typically, two or three early sessions from early in a treatment are recorded, and REs are identified until 10 have been obtained. Each RE is subdivided into thought units, which are essentially sentences, and each sentence is classified as a W, an RO, or an RS. The most frequent W, RO, and RS (if any) for each RE is designated and counted for each of the 10 REs. The CCRT for the patient is defined as simply the sum of the most frequent W, RO, and RS, across the 10 REs.

Luborsky and Crits-Christoph (1990) classify RO and RS as to whether the response is positive or negative. This is relevant because psychological conflict is initiated by wishes that threaten to provoke negative responses from others or from the self. Furthermore, the degree to which people are able to arrange for positive responses to their wishes directly reflects their adequacy in handling life. In studying the Penn Psychotherapy sample of 33 cases, the authors found that early in treatment, negative attitudes of others and of self (RO and RS) tended to be much more frequent than positive ones. In the course of good-outcome treatments, judged by two independent measures of improvement, the negative attitudes substantially decreased and the positive ones substantially increased, but there was no significant change in wishes.

Strengths of the CCRT

The CCRT may be useful in PDM-2 assessment of pathogenic beliefs about oneself and other people on the P Axis, and of the capacity for relationships and intimacy on the M Axis. The assessment of positive and negative responses provides a method of systematically assessing what patients experience and what kinds of changes occur over the course of treatment. The accuracy of interpretations has also been assessed on the basis of how much the Ws, ROs, and RSs are characterized in the interventions. Changes in the patients' self-awareness may be reflected in their awareness of the CCRT components as well. These indices constitute a rough grid that can be applied to therapy recordings and thereby can permit systematic assessment.

Limitations of the CCRT

First, the CCRT requires considerable time and training to score. Second, Luborksy and collaborators conceived of the CCRT in terms of a sequenced pattern of reactions by the patient (or other person). Yet the CCRT as operationally defined does not necessarily reflect the patterns of the patient's concerns (see the example in Waldron, 1995, p. 400).

Defense Mechanism Rating Scales

J. Christopher Perry, with his colleagues, came to the description of defense mechanisms as a product of his efforts to develop systematic methods of case formulation and to determine the differences between the functioning of borderline patients and others. By classifying defenses according to function and level of general adaptiveness,

Perry was able to develop an index of overall defensive functioning, the Defense Mechanisms Rating Scales (DMRS; see Chapter 2 on the M Axis).

The DMRS manual (Perry, 1990) describes how to identify 30 individual defense mechanisms in video- or audio-recorded sessions or transcripts. The manual presents a definition of each defense, a description of how the defense functions, a guide for the differential diagnosis of each defense, and a 3-point scale. Each scale is clearly identified, with specific examples of (0) no use, (1) probable use, and (2) definite use of the defense. The examples provide prototypical instances of the defense that expand and complement the formal definitions.

In the DMRS, there are seven defense levels arranged hierarchically, with each defense assigned to a particular level. The defense levels are characterized as follows, in descending order of health:

7. *High adaptive level* (also called *mature*): Affiliation, altruism, anticipation, humor, self-assertion, self-observation, sublimation, suppression.
6. *Obsessional*: Isolation, intellectualization, undoing.
5. *Other neurotic*: Repression, dissociation, reaction formation, displacement.
4. *Minor image-distorting* (also called *narcissistic*): Omnipotence, idealization (of self and of other people), devaluation (of self and of other people).
3. *Disavowal*: Denial, projection, rationalization, autistic fantasy.
2. *Major-image-distorting* (also called *borderline*): Splitting of others' images, splitting of self-images, projective identification.
1. *Action*: Acting out, passive aggression, help-rejecting complaining.

This ordering is based on a series of empirical studies. Not included in the manual, but included in an appendix, are the psychotic defenses.

The rater identifies each use of the defense as it occurs, bracketing the part of the text in which it operates. After the completion of the ratings, the number of times each defense was identified in the text is divided by the total instances of all defenses to produce a percentage score for each defense. Then the total percentage of defenses at each level forms the basis for a "defense profile," which represents the nature of the patient's functioning and which can be compared with earlier or later functioning in the course of treatment.

All of the defense scores are summarized by an "overall defensive functioning" (ODF) score (Perry, 2014), an average of the scores for all scored defenses. In clinical samples based on whole interviews, scores usually range between 2.5 and 6.5. Approximate reference scores for ODF are as follows:

1. Scores below 5.0 are associated with personality disorders, severe depression, or borderline conditions.
2. Scores between 5.0 and about 5.5 are associated with neurotic character and symptom disorders.
3. Scores from 5.5 to 6.0 are associated with average healthy–neurotic functioning.
4. Scores above 6.0 are associated with superior functioning.

A Q-sort version of the instrument has been recently developed and validated (Di Giuseppe, Perry, Petraglia, Janzen, & Lingiardi, 2014).

The DMRS served as the basis for the DSM-IV Defensive Functioning Scale (DFS; American Psychiatric Association, 1994; Porcerelli, Kogan, Kamoo, & Miller, 2010). Reliability and validity of the DFS have been reported in several studies (see Perry & Bond, 2012, for a review). It has been implemented in large studies on personality, psychopathology, and defense mechanisms, as well as on changes in defense mechanisms during psychotherapy.

Strengths of the DMRS

The DMRS serves well to assess defensive functioning according to PDM-2's M and MA Axes and is also useful in assessing the level of personality organization (P Axis). The psychometric reliability of the DMRS and its capacity to discriminate different disorders and levels of functioning make it an excellent instrument for the assessment of patients in psychodynamic psychotherapy (Perry, 2014; Perry & Bond, 2012). It also provides a general measure of health–sickness and can reflect changes in this dimension during the course of therapy. Several such studies have shown interesting results supporting the beneficial effects of the work on defenses in psychotherapy (Perry & Bond, 2012).

Limitations of the DMRS

The DMRS requires several days of specific training to achieve reliability, and the assessment is time-consuming (approximately 2–3 hours for a 50-minute session), although the amount of time needed for the assessment can be substantially reduced with the Q-sort version. Moreover, there is no complete agreement on the definition and the categorization of some defenses (e.g., dissociation). The DFS gives a less detailed, precise, and reliable picture of patients' functioning than does the DMRS.

Defense Mechanisms Manual

The Defense Mechanisms Manual (DMM) assesses three developmentally anchored defenses—denial, projection, and identification—applied to TAT stories (Cramer, 1991, 2006). The defenses are represented by seven facets that are coded each time they occur within a story. Total scores or relative scores can be used clinically and for research purposes.

Interrater reliability of .80 has been reported for the DMM (Meyer, 2004) and has shown adequate stability over a 3-year period (Cramer, 1998). The validity of the DMM has been supported through cross-sectional and longitudinal studies of child, adolescent, and young adult development, with these studies showing differentiation of diagnostic groups, of levels of personality organization, and of change following psychodynamic treatment. The impact of stress on defense use has also been studied (Cramer, 2006; Porcerelli et al., 2010).

Strengths of the DMM

The DMM can be a useful aid for the assessment of defensive functioning on the MC Axis when TAT materials are available. The DMM is a reliable measure, and its validity is supported by cross-sectional, longitudinal, and experimental studies.

Limitations of the DMM

The DMM includes only three defense mechanisms, and the defense of identification may be less useful than are other defenses in the assessment of adults because its use diminishes after late adolescence. Administration of the TAT, creation of a transcript from the TAT stories, and use of the DMM rating system may take several hours in routine practice.

Part Two. Additional Instruments Useful for the PDM-2 Evaluation Process

A. Self-Reports

Minnesota Multiphasic Personality Inventory–2

Hathaway and McKinley (1943) developed the Minnesota Multiphasic Personality Inventory (MMPI) as an empirically based self-report instrument from a pool of statements found in patient records and other sources. It has had various improvements over the years, including a variety of scales based on the differing scores of various categories of patients. In 1989, the MMPI-2 (Butcher et al., 1989) was released; it was based on the same empirical methodology used for the construction of the original MMPI, but used a more representative normative sample than the 1930s Minnesota medical outpatients who constituted most of the nonclinical participants in the initial control samples. There is also an adolescent version of the test, the MMPI-A (Butcher et al., 1992), which was normed for persons between the ages of 14 and 18.

Hathaway and McKinley (1943) developed scales on the basis of which items reliably differentiated clinical or criterion groups from a nonclinical group. For example, items that differentiated people diagnosed with hypochondriasis from both medical patients and nonclinical individuals became the items in the hypochondriasis scale (scale 1). Similarly, scales were developed for depression (scale 2), hysteria (scale 3), psychopathic deviance (scale 4), masculinity–femininity (scale 5), paranoia (scale 6), psychasthenia (scale 7), schizophrenia (scale 8), and hypomania (scale 9). Scales were also developed to measure validity and bias: the lie scale (L); the infrequency scale (F), measuring rare psychopathology and exaggeration; and, with Meehl, the correction scale (K). The K scale measures claims of high functioning, which can be a sign of defensiveness; it is added, in whole or in part, to particular scales of psychological tendencies likely to be underreported (e.g., scale 8). Later, Drake (1946) developed a social introversion scale (scale 0).

Although the MMPI-2 was not developed as a psychodynamically oriented test, it can be useful in helping to determine PDM-2 diagnoses. The L scale can indicate primitive defenses such as denial and splitting (Gordon, Stoffey, & Bottinelli, 2008), which are relevant to borderline personality and psychotic personality organizations. The MMPI-2 basic clinical scales can measure traits to help in the assessment of the PDM-2 personality syndromes: For example, scale 2 (depression) may suggest a depressive personality, scale 3 (hysteria) a hysterical (histrionic) personality, and so on. It is best to interpret the clinical scales as two- and three-point code configurations. For example, elevations on scales 1 and 3 are considered a "1–3/3–1" profile, indicative of a high degree of somatic concern; in conjunction with a low score on scale 2, they constitute a profile often found in conversion disorder or classical hysteria.

Strengths of the MMPI-2

The MMPI-2 basic clinical scales measure traits that help in the assessment of the PDM-2 personality syndromes. The instrument is used in many settings around the world. It is 80–90% accurate in assessing personality traits and defensiveness (Butcher et al., 1989, p. 102). Bram and Peebles (2014) consider the MMPI-2, TAT, Rorschach, and Wechsler Adult Intelligence Scale (WAIS) as constituting the core battery of personality assessment. Anyone with at least a sixth-grade reading ability can take the MMPI-2.

The MMPI-2 measures rather stable psychopathology. Because it is insensitive to low-dose treatments, it is rarely used as a dependent measure in treatment outcome research. However, Gordon (2001) found that after an average of 3 years of psychoanalytic treatment, scores on most of the clinical scales were significantly reduced, and the score on the ego strength (Es) scale (Barron, 1953) was significantly increased.

Limitations of the MMPI-2

The MMPI-2 is limited by its methodology—specifically, its dependence on an individual's "true" or "false" responses to written questions. It does not probe further on a hint of a symptom or a defense or use branching logic to rule out certain diagnoses by obtaining relevant information. For example, it does not ask questions such as "How long have you been depressed?" or "Did some bad things happen to you before you became depressed?" or "Do you have periods of feeling very energetic after feeling depressed?" Such follow-up questions are often valuable in differentiating major depression from dysthymia, posttraumatic stress disorder, or bipolar disorder.

Moreover, the MMPI is a long test: About 45–60 minutes are required to complete the 370-item form and 60–90 minutes to complete the 567-item form. Finally, it must be administered and interpreted by a psychologist with appropriate training.

Personality Assessment Inventory

The Personality Assessment Inventory (PAI) is a 344-item self-report measure of psychopathology, developed to provide measures of constructs that are central in treatment planning, implementation, and evaluation (Morey, 1991, 1996). Items are rated on a 4-point Likert scale (from "false" to "very true"). There is an adolescent version as well, the PAI-A. Both versions require a fourth-grade reading level.

Twenty-two nonoverlapping scales measure a broad range of psychological constructs: 4 validity scales (inconsistency, infrequency, negative impression management, and positive impression management); 11 clinical scales (somatization, anxiety, anxiety-related disorders, depression, mania, paranoia, schizophrenia, borderline features, antisocial features, alcohol use, and drug use); 5 treatment consideration scales (aggression, suicidal ideation, stress, nonsupport, and treatment rejection); and 2 interpersonal scales (dominance and warmth). Ten of the full scales contain "conceptually derived subscales" (Morey, 1996, p. 3).

There are also supplemental indices, some of which include mean clinical elevation (general psychiatric distress), suicide and violence potential, and a treatment process index (composite score predicting treatment amenability).

Computer scoring offers an interpretative report and diagnostic considerations. Normative data include 1,000 nonpatients age-distributed according to census data, a large mixed sample of inpatients and outpatients, and a large college student sample. Results are profiled as *T* scores relative to the census sample. The PAI profile includes indications of unusual elevations on the basis of data from the reference sample of patients. Extensive reliability and validity data are available in the literature, much of which is summarized in the revised edition of the test manual (Morey, 2007) and in two other interpretive and summarizing books (Blais, Baity, & Hopwood, 2010; Morey, 1996).

Strengths of the PAI

The PAI is easy to administer and requires a relatively low reading level. It "differs from other well-known self-report multi-scale inventories in several important ways that are largely a consequence of the construct validation approach to test construction" (Hopwood, Blais, & Baity, 2010, p. 1). It has a dimensional response scale (4-point Likert) rather than a categorical one (true–false). Items are nonoverlapping. There are normative data for specialty populations, including personnel selection and forensics. It has a high degree of internal consistency across samples; results are stable over periods of 2–4 weeks. Validity studies demonstrate convergent and discriminant validity with more than 50 other measures of psychopathology. It includes a short form, calculating 20 of the 22 full scales, that is based on the first 160 items for patients who fatigue easily or if the clinician wishes a quick overview. The short form has adequate to strong psychometric properties (Morey, 1991; Siefert et al., 2012; Sinclair et al., 2009, 2010).

The PAI assesses both state (i.e., depression, anxiety, mania, etc.) and trait (i.e., borderline and antisocial features) phenomena; it is thus useful in assessing PDM-2 personality features (P Axis) and overt or manifest symptoms (S Axis). The PAI can also assist in the assessment of the M Axis (Blais & Hopwood, 2010).

Limitations of the PAI

The PAI is a widely used broad-band measure of psychological functioning, but, as with any self-report measure, it is based purely on the patient's perspective. Also, because of its breadth and depth, even its shorter version is long.

Millon Clinical Multiaxial Inventory and Other Millon Inventories

The various versions of the Millon Clinical Multiaxial Inventory (MCMI) are anchored in Theodore Millon's (2011) evolutionary theory of personality and psychopathology. The original MCMI was designed to assess both Axis I and Axis II disorders in DSM-III and to assist clinicians in formulating diagnoses and in developing a treatment plan that takes into account the patient's personality style and coping behavior. The MCMI-III was first published in 1994 (a revised version appeared later; Millon, Millon, Davis, & Grossman, 2006a) and reflected the changes in DSM-IV. It has 175 true–false questions and usually takes about 30 minutes to complete. It can be used by clients 18 years of age or older and requires an eighth-grade reading level. It also uses combined gender norms. The MCMI-IV (Millon, Grossman, & Millon, 2015) is renormed, and some of the scales are better constructed; there is only one new clinical scale.

The MCMI-III assesses 14 personality styles and subtypes: retiring/schizoid, shy/avoidant, pessimistic/melancholic, cooperative/dependent, sociable/histrionic, confident/narcissistic, nonconforming/antisocial, assertive/sadistic, conscientious/

compulsive, skeptical/negativistic, aggrieved/masochistic, eccentric/schizotypal, capricious/borderline, and suspicious/paranoid. The MCMI-IV also includes a turbulence scale.

The 10 clinical syndrome scales (which, in the MCMI-III, coincide with DSM-IV Axis I disorders) are anxiety, somatoform, bipolar manic, dysthymia, alcohol dependence, drug dependence, posttraumatic stress disorder, thought disorder, major depression, and delusional disorder. There are 5 validity and bias scales.

For both the MCMI-III and -IV, after scales were rationally constructed (which means that items had face validity), individuals diagnosed with each of the disorders in the scale were administered the test, and cutoffs for the various levels of each scale were determined in accordance with the number of individuals in the pool with the particular disorder. The MCMI is the second most frequently used self-report instrument after the MMPI; this popularity may be due in part to the quality of the computer-generated narrative descriptions, which are readable, clinically applicable, and descriptive of the patient in plain English. Another asset is the use not of conventional percentile or standardized scores, but of base rate scores (BRs), which are based on the probabilities of each disorder's meeting diagnostic thresholds.

The MCMI has been adapted for assessment of adolescents as the Millon Adolescent Clinical Inventory (MACI; Millon, Millon, Davis, & Grossman, 2006b). Construction of the MACI has involved changes in items, age-appropriate norms, and name revisions for the scales. The interpretive strategies are different as well. For instance, there is more emphasis on interpreting individual scales than on configurations of scales. Similarly, the MCMI has been adapted for preadolescents as the Millon Pre-Adolescent Clinical Inventory (M-PACI; Millon, Tringone, Millon, & Grossman, 2005).

Strengths of the Millon Inventories

The MCMI, MACI, and M-PACI can be useful aids in the assessment of virtually all PDM-2 axes for adults, adolescents, and children. One of the strengths of the MCMI is that it is normed on a pathological population, and the BR scores indicate the probability or confidence of the diagnosis. Each Millon inventory has good validity and reliability. The ability of some of the self-report scales (e.g., borderline) to identify personality pathology reliably is impressive.

Limitations of the Millon Inventories

The Millon inventories are highly stable over a short period of time; however, no long-term data are available. As with the MMPI and the PAI, the MCMI-III is a self-report measure and can be affected by lack of insight, and it does not have as many or as well-researched validity scales as the MMPI. The MCMI-III is based on clinical samples and thus is applicable only to individuals who evidence problematic emotional and interpersonal symptoms or who are undergoing treatment or a psychodiagnostic evaluation.

Severity Indices of Personality Problems–118

The Severity Indices of Personality Problems–118 (SIPP-118; Verheul et al., 2008) is a self-report questionnaire covering core components of personality functioning. The assumption upon which the SIPP-118 is founded is that personality pathology can be understood as a consequence of alterations in human adaptive capacities, and the instrument's aim is to assess these capacities.

The 118 items are each answered on a 4-point Likert scale from 1 (fully disagree) to 4 (fully agree), for 16 domains: emotion regulation, effortful control, stable self-image, self-reflective functioning, aggression regulation, frustration tolerance, self-respect, purposefulness, enjoyment, feeling recognized, intimacy, enduring relationships, responsible industry, trustworthiness, respect, and cooperation. These domains constitute homogeneous item clusters (i.e., the clusters are unidimensional and internally consistent) that fit well into five clinically relevant higher-order domains: self-control, identity integration, relational capacities, social concordance, and responsibility. The domains appeared to have good concurrent validity across various populations, good convergent validity in terms of associations with interview ratings of the severity of personality pathology, and good discriminant validity in terms of associations with trait-based personality disorder dimensions.

The domain scores were stable over a time interval of 14–21 days in a student sample, but were sensitive to change over a 2-year follow-up interval in a treated patient population. The SIPP-118 thus provides a set of five reliable, valid, and efficient indices of the core components of (mal)adaptive personality functioning. Initial research has shown cross-national validity of this tool (Arnevik, Wilberg, Monsen, Andrea, & Karterud, 2009).

Strengths of the SIPP-118

The SIPP-118 can be a useful aid for the PDM-2 assessment of basic mental capacities in both adolescents and adults (M and MA Axes). It is a clinically relevant, psychometrically sound, and user-friendly tool. Available in seven different languages, it can be used both for clinical assessment and for research in psychotherapy.

Limitations of the SIPP-118

The SIPP-118 does not provide a personality or clinical diagnosis of a patient. Research conducted with this tool thus far has been limited. The instrument is less well known and used than other self-report instruments reviewed in this section of the chapter. To date, its degree of overlap with other interpersonal measures, such as the Inventory of Interpersonal Problems (see below), is unknown.

Inventory of Interpersonal Problems

The Inventory of Interpersonal Problems (IIP) is a self-report inventory designed to identify problematic areas of relational functioning (Horowitz, Alden, Wiggins, & Pincus, 2000; Horowitz, Rosenberg, Baer, Ureño, & Villaseñor, 1988). It is based on a circumplex model of interpersonal behavior that draws from a rich theoretical and empirical literature (see Alden, Wiggins, & Pincus, 1990, for a review). This model is a two-dimensional circumplex defined by two orthogonal and bipolar axes of interpersonal style: dominance versus submission and love versus hate. The circumplex space is divided into eight octants that form a circular array of blends of the dominance and love dimensions and can reflect various interpersonal problems.

The original IIP (Horowitz et al., 1988) consisted of 127 items, but the most widely used version of this instrument is the Inventory of Interpersonal Problems—Circumplex

(IIP-C; Alden et al., 1990; Horowitz et al., 2000), comprising 64 items. Many additional short forms (see, e.g., the IIP-32; Barkham, Hardy, & Startup, 1996) and derivative tools containing item sets have been developed to accomplish specific purposes (e.g., screening for personality disorders). Also, various methods for scoring the IIP are available (Hughes & Barkham, 2005; Gurtman, 2006). In this discussion, we focus on the IIP-C.

The 64 items of the IIP-C assess the interpersonal behaviors that an individual shows in excess (e.g., "I fight with other people too much") or areas of difficulty (e.g., "It is hard for me to join in groups"). Each item is rated on a 7-point Likert scale ranging from 1 (not at all) to 7 (extremely). The overall score of the IIP-C is used as an indicator of general interpersonal problems, but the IIP-C also yields scores on eight subscales indicating specific difficulties: domineering, vindictive, cold, socially inhibited, nonassertive, exploitable, overly nurturant, and intrusive.

The IIP-C has strong psychometric properties. Internal consistency alpha coefficients for the subscales range from .76 to .88, and test–retest reliabilities for scales range from .58 to .84 (Horowitz et al., 2000). Subscales of the IIP-C converge with measures tapping similar constructs in clinical (Gurtman, 2006; Haggerty, Hilsenroth, & Vala-Stewart, 2009) and nonclinical (Alden et al., 1990; Horowitz et al., 2000) samples. This measure is also sensitive to change and, for this reason, is frequently employed in psychotherapy outcome research (e.g., Ruiz et al., 2004).

Strengths of the IIP

The IIP may be useful in PDM-2 assessment of some personality features (P Axis) and of the capacity for relationships and intimacy on the M Axis. It is easy to administer and requires minimal training. It has good psychometric properties; in particular, it is reliable over time, sensitive to change, convergent with similar tools, and predictive of treatment outcome. It can be effectively employed with clinical and nonclinical samples. Finally, it provides an overall assessment of interpersonal functioning, as well as of specific relational domains.

Limitations of the IIP

The IIP-C suffers from the same biases as other self-report measures: It can be faked and is affected by a patient's limitations in acknowledging, mentalizing, or communicating difficulties. Moreover, this measure does not include any validity scales. The normative data and clinical cutoffs are not clearly established on large, representative samples.

Central Relationship Questionnaire

In 1998, Barber, Foltz, and Weinryb constructed the original Central Relationship Questionnaire (CRQ) to measure interpersonal patterns. The 101-item Central Relationship Questionnaire—Revised (CRQ-R; McCarthy, Connolly Gibbons, & Barber, 2008) is a self-report version of the CCRT measure described above (Luborsky & Crits-Christoph, 1990). It involves revisions of the original CRQ to increase the interpersonal dimensions it captures, reduce its length, and model a higher-order factor structure (McCarthy et al., 2008).

The CRQ-R is used to assess representations of patients' wishes in interpersonal relationships, their perceptions of the responses of others to their wishes, and their own responses to the other. Participants are instructed to rate each of their four central relationships (relationships with romantic partner, mother, father, and best friend) in terms of the three main relationship themes: wishes (W), responses from others (RO), and responses of self (RS). Participants rate the likelihood that a particular interpersonal theme is present in each of their central relationships on a 7-point Likert scale. Scores for each interpersonal theme can be aggregated across relationships, such that each patient will have one score on each of the 16 themes representing the patient's general representations of interpersonal relationships: five types of Ws (be independent, be intimate, be hurtful, be sexual, be submissive); five types of ROs (is hurtful, is independent, is loving, is sexual, is submissive); and six types of RSs (am autonomous, am avoidant, am domineering, am intimate, am nonconfrontational, am sexual).

Strengths of the CRQ

Either version of the CRQ can be a useful aid for PDM-2 assessment of object relationships on both the P and M Axes. The psychometric properties of the original CRQ were found to be adequate (Barber et al., 1998). Several studies have demonstrated the relevance and contributions of the CRQ-R to psychotherapy research. For example, greater rigidity across interpersonal relationships was related to fewer symptoms and interpersonal problems (McCarthy et al., 2008). Moreover, patients' pretreatment representations of significant others predicted a substantial part of the therapeutic alliance throughout the course of treatment (Zilcha-Mano, McCarthy, Dinger, & Barber, 2014).

Limitations of the CRQ

Although the CRQ-R is shorter than the original CRQ, it is still time-consuming, especially when a patient needs to rate 101 items for each of several significant others in his or her life. Neither version of the instrument has received much research or clinical use beyond that of the developers.

Toronto Alexithymia Scale–20

Alexithymia is a multifaceted personality construct representing a deficit in the cognitive processing of emotions. It is composed of two higher-order factors: deficits in affect awareness (difficulty identifying and describing feelings) and in operatory thinking (externally oriented thinking and poor imaginal processes) (Taylor & Bagby, 2012). It is strongly influenced by early interactions with caregivers because inadequate responses to a child's emotions have a major influence on the ability to self-regulate both emotional and neurobiological states in adulthood (Taylor, Bagby, & Parker, 1997). The construct is most widely assessed with the self-reported 20-item version of the Toronto Alexithymia Scale (TAS-20; Bagby, Parker, & Taylor, 1994a, 1994b), a self-report questionnaire that assesses three facets of alexithymia: difficulty identifying feelings, difficulty describing feelings, and externally oriented thinking. Although alexithymia is a dimensional construct, an empirically derived score of >60 identifies respondents in the higher-alexithymia range.

Strengths of the TAS-20

The TAS-20 can be a useful aid in PDM-2 assessment of affect regulation, deficits in mentalizing affective states, inability to use symbolic expressions, and emotional arousal dissociated from psychological meanings (Taylor, 2010) on both the P and M Axes. Extensive validation, replication of the factor structure in several languages and countries, short administration time, and ease of use have been among the reasons why the TAS-20 has become the reference standard for measuring alexithymia in several psychiatric and medical settings (Lumley, Neely, & Burger, 2007).

Limitations of the TAS-20

There are doubts that alexithymia can be validly assessed by a self-report scale because it is, by definition, the inability to report individual psychological states. Therefore, the need for measures of alexithymia using other methods has been repeatedly highlighted in recent years.

Clinical Outcomes in Routine Evaluation

The Clinical Outcomes in Routine Evaluation (CORE) self-report measure (also known as the CORE Outcome Measure, or CORE-OM) was developed from a pantheoretical perspective by Chris Evans, Michael Barkham, and colleagues in Britain. Thirty-four items all address the previous 7 days, covering domains of well-being, problems, functioning, and risk. Each item is rated on a 5-point frequency scale from 0 (not at all) to 5 (most or all of the time). Eight items are reverse-scored to ensure some variety across the items.

An extensive survey of psychotherapists and counselors of different modalities, different core professions (psychology, psychiatry, etc.), and different employment settings identified the CORE items. Initial psychometric exploration showed acceptability and usability; good internal reliability and test–retest reliability; small effects of age and gender; good convergent validity with established self-report measures of depression; good sensitivity to change; and discrimination between clinical and nonclinical groups (Evans et al., 2002). These psychometric properties have been replicated in clinical samples in the original English and in an increasing number of translations into other languages. Jacobson and Truax's (1991) reliable change index and cutting points for clinically significant change were given for the English version and are becoming available for translations.

The self-report version is complemented by a practitioner-completed CORE Assessment (CORE-A), comprising the Therapy Assessment Form (TAF) and the End of Therapy (EoT) form. The TAF asks about social situation, focal problems, past mental health care, medication, and diagnosis (optional), and about the therapy planned. The EoT covers details about the therapy actually given.

A short form of the CORE is designed to be used in general population, nonclinical survey work (CORE-GP). An even shorter form, the CORE-10, has been produced, and there are several other versions for special purposes.

Recent developments include scoring that uses scores on six CORE-OM items to give economic "quality equivalence," expressing changes as gains in quality-adjusted life years (Mavranezouli, Brazier, Rowen, & Barkham, 2013); the YP-CORE for young people (ages 11–17; Twigg et al., 2009); and the Systemic CORE (SCORE), a self-report evaluation of families (not the individuals in them) for family-systemic therapies. A summary (Evans, 2012) is free to download, as is all the information at the CORE website (*www.coresystemtrust.org.uk*).

Strengths of the CORE

All CORE instruments are completely free. The CORE-OM has shown good psychometric properties in all evaluations, including in translations, and has been used with a very wide diversity of therapies. Shortened measures exist. Adaptations and extensions have been constructed for evaluations of people with learning disabilities, young people, and families. The website also hosts a growing collection of information about the system and an index of publications using CORE instruments or elements of the CORE system.

Limitations of the CORE

The CORE system does not provide a complete picture of change in therapy, and all self-report measures are open to manipulation.

Outcome Questionnaire–45

The Outcome Questionnaire–45 (OQ-45; Lambert et al., 1996a, 1996b; Lambert, Kahler, Harmon, Burlingame, & Shimokawa, 2013) is a 45-item self-report scale used to estimate a patient's degree of disturbance at the outset and over the course of treatment. It provides an index of mental and interpersonal health or well-being for adults 18 years of age or older. A person who takes the measure is compared to inpatient, outpatient, and nonclinical populations. Scores on the measure are referenced against expected treatment responses, based on the progress of 11,000 treated individuals across the United States. These data provide a benchmark of success in order to identify treatment nonresponders and persons at risk for negative outcomes. The OQ-45 also provides cutoff scores for reliable change and recovery as markers for gauging treatment success and possible termination of services. It has been translated into more than 30 languages other than English. It requires reading ability at the sixth-grade level.

Because almost all adults who enter treatment experience symptoms of anxiety and depression, half of the items of the OQ-45 measure core aspects of symptomatic distress or subjective discomfort. Because a satisfactory quality of life and sense of well-being depend on positive interpersonal functioning, a quarter of the items assess disturbance in interpersonal relationships with intimate others. The final quarter of the items assess functioning in social roles, such as work, school, homemaking, and leisure activities.

The OQ-45 can be used regardless of the type of psychotherapy, mode of psychotherapy, or medication intervention. It is atheoretical in nature and serves as a mental health vital sign or lab test to be used by clinicians to manage illness by quantifying patients' current mental health functioning. In contrast to purely symptom-based measures, the OQ-45 attempts to assess quality-of-life factors that are particularly important to patients, and that are goals of clinicians with a psychodynamic orientation—interpersonal relations and social role functioning.

Nowadays, and ideally, the OQ-45 is administered online, via a hand-held device or via a personal computer (it can be administered and scored on hard copy as well). It takes about 5–10 minutes of patient time to rate all of the 45 items, typically prior to a treatment session. Each item (e.g.,"I feel hopeless about the future") is answered on a 5-point scale according to the patient's recollection of the preceding week, on a scale from "almost always" to "never." Software (OQ-Analyst) scores the measure and then graphs the results both in relation to earlier administrations, and in relation to normative functioning and expected treatment response from other individuals who have the same initial level of disturbance.

The OQ-45 is part of a larger outcome measurement system called the OQ-Analyst, which includes measures of child functioning, the Brief Psychiatric Rating Scale, and the Assessment for Signal Clients (a clinical support tool used to guide problem solving with difficult cases). The OQ-Analyst can be set up to provide clinical information to members of interdisciplinary teams who are also working with each specific patient. This shared information enables all team members to be aware of an absent or negative treatment response and to settle on coordinated efforts to turn the course of treatment in a positive direction.

Dozens of studies have been published on the psychometric properties of the OQ-45. It has high internal consistency; good test–retest reliability; and concurrent validity with scales such as the Symptom Checklist–90 and the Beck Depression Inventory. Factor-analytic studies support the presence of an overall distress factor, with three subordinate factors consistent with the subscales. Most items, the subscales, and the total score are sensitive to the effects of interventions while remaining stable in untreated individuals.

The OQ-45 correlates significantly with the Schwartz Outcome Scale–10 (Blais et al., 1999; see below), a brief measure developed to monitor outcomes, at both the individual and group levels.

Strengths of the OQ-45

The OQ-45 can be a useful aid in PDM-2 assessment of overall level of mental functioning on the M Axis, particularly of a patient's level of subjective well-being and adjustment. It assesses general psychological distress, interpersonal functioning, and role functioning. Versions are available for youth, adults, and even patients in group therapy.

The OQ-45 is supported by extensive published evidence of the degree to which providing feedback to clinicians and patients based on the OQ-45 alert system maximizes patient outcomes and reduces treatment failures. Eleven randomized controlled trials have been completed showing that the feedback and problem-solving tools delivered to therapists work in a variety of routine care settings. The OQ-45 has been judged by the U.S. National Registry of Evidence-Based Programs and Practices as an evidence-based practice.

Limitations of the OQ-45

The OQ-45 is a self-report measure that suffers from the same limitations as other self-report measures: It is easy to manipulate the scores one way or another if a patient is motivated to do so. It can be used by patients to test what their therapists will do if they answer in a particular way (e.g., exaggerating their scores to punish the therapists). The instrument and the scoring are expensive and typically require computer use. In addition, because the measure was not developed from psychodynamic theories, it has not shed light on constructs of special importance to psychodynamic psychotherapists; neither does it lend itself to the task of diagnosis. Finally, most of the research supporting its use is based on short-term treatments lasting no more than 20 sessions.

Schwartz Outcome Scale–10 (SOS-10)

The Schwartz Outcome Scale–10 (SOS-10; Blais et al., 1999) is a distinctive, low-burden measure developed to monitor outcomes at both the individual and group levels. Construction of the SOS-10 was guided by insights obtained from a diverse group of senior clinicians and patients. Interviews conducted with senior psychologists, psychiatrists, and a neurosurgeon, as well as with patient focus groups, were used to discover the changes that occurred (excluding symptoms) with successful treatment. The interviews and focus group discussions were transcribed and reviewed for common themes. Common themes were used to generate an initial item pool. Empirical evaluation and refinement identified 20 well-performing items, and Rasch analysis was employed to reduce the scale to its final 10-item version (Blais et al., 1999). Although the scale was initially developed for use with adults (ages 17 and up), recent research has extended its utility to adolescent populations.

The SOS-10 has 10 items rated on a scale of 0 (never) to 6 (all or nearly all the time). Higher scores represent greater psychological health and well-being; lower scores indicate emotional distress and poorer psychological health. The SOS-10 can be administered in traditional paper-and-pencil format or electronically. It is recommended that a patient complete the scale prior to a treatment appointment. This way, the clinician can make sure that the SOS-10 is completed and can review the total score for clinical implications before the session.

Owen and Imel (2010) outline a rationale and a practice-friendly procedure for incorporating the SOS-10 into ongoing clinical care. The availability of nonpatient reference data allows for calculation of both a reliable change index and clinically significant improvement (Blais et al., 2011). The ability to apply more sophisticated treatment effectiveness analyses enhances the information obtained from treatment-as-usual outcome-monitoring programs and increases the comparability of findings across studies.

Scores on the SOS-10 can also be used to identify a patient's level of emotional distress or psychological dysfunction. The following distress ranges, which draw on data from over 10,000 outpatients, may prove helpful markers: minimal (59–40), mild (39–33), moderate (32–23), and severe (22–1). Accurately identifying a patient's level of distress at the outset of treatment can help clarify the intensity of services needed (e.g., weekly individual psychotherapy, multiple sessions per week, or multiple forms of treatments). Lastly, because SOS-10 items are *not* directly related to psychiatric symptoms, reviewing responses to individual items with patients can afford a non-threatening avenue for discussing personal strengths and weaknesses.

The SOS-10 has solid psychometric properties, with strong internal consistency and test–retest reliability. Multiple studies both of the original English version and of translations have found the SOS-10 to be unifactorial. The accumulated research also supports the construct validity of the SOS-10 as a broad measure of psychological functioning (Blais et al., 1999; Haggerty, Blake, Naraine, Siefert, & Blais, 2010; Young et al., 2003). The SOS-10 correlates significantly with the OQ-45, discussed above (Lambert et al., 1996a, 1996b).

Strengths of the SOS-10

The SOS-10 may help clinicians to assess patients on the M, MC, and MA Axes of PDM-2—in particular, the impact of global mental health on patients' subjective well-being. It reliably and quickly assesses a patient's conscious distress level. The SOS-10 has also demonstrated sensitivity to change for a wide variety of treatment modalities, including early treatment change (Hilsenroth, Ackerman, & Blagys, 2001). The SOS-10 has been employed as an outcome measure in studies of psychodynamic psychotherapy, dialectical behavior therapy, residential treatment for refractory obsessive–compulsive disorder, inpatient psychiatric treatment as usual, and inpatient substance abuse treatment as usual (Blais et al., 2011, 2013). Although the SOS-10 is a proprietary instrument, the scale is made available free of charge for practitioners, researchers, and nonprofit health care organizations.

Limitations of the SOS-10

The SOS-10 is a brief self-report instrument with no measures of personality disorders or interpersonal functioning. It suffers from all the response style manipulation concerns associated with such tools and does not contain validity scales to identify such response styles. Although the instrument is easier to complete than the OQ-45 (see above), it does not have the same breadth of development.

B. Performance-Based Tools

Rorschach Inkblot Test

The Rorschach Inkblot Test involves the serial presentation of a set of 10 inkblot cards composed of ambiguous and evocative stimuli. A participant is seated beside the examiner and is instructed to describe what he or she sees in each card ("What might this be?"). Each response, freely given by the respondent, is scored after appropriate inquiry, according to the features selected by the subject as relevant. These main features are related to perceptual organization and integration (location, developmental quality, and integrative process); characteristics that are actually contained in the card (e.g., form, color, and shading); or characteristics that are subjectively added to it (e.g., perception of movement). Evaluations are also made of the perceptual adequacy of the responses given to the stimuli (form quality); contents of the representation (animal, human figure, anatomical perception, sexual aspects, etc.); and ideation (thought processes in giving the response). Reliable scoring criteria are provided for coding each separate aspect.

Although Hermann Rorschach (1921/1942) initially developed his inkblots to assess personality dynamics and refine psychiatric diagnoses, he conceptualized these stimuli primarily as measures of perceptual style and cognitive organization—that is, as means of assessing people's characteristic ways of perceiving and processing information.

The range of constructs measured by the Rorschach expanded following Rorschach's death in 1922. Beck (1937) adhered closely to Rorschach's initial emphasis on perceptual and cognitive processes, but added various perceptual and information-processing scores to the measure. Klopfer (1937), emphasizing the idiographic and psychodynamic aspects of inkblot responses, developed rules for scoring and interpreting thematic content (e.g. dependency, aggression, preoccupation with control). Rapaport,

Gill, and Schafer (1945–1946, 1968) formulated a systematic psychoanalytic approach to the test and developed a method of analyzing test verbalizations for indications of thought disorder. In this same period, Frank (1939) offered his now-famous "projective hypothesis," wherein he speculated that unstructured procedures like the Rorschach compel the respondent to reveal hidden wishes, needs, fears, and motives by projecting these private concerns onto ambiguous stimuli (hence the term "projective test"). Given its early history, it is not surprising that over the years the Rorschach has come to be seen in multiple ways—as a perceptual task, a problem-solving task, an index of associational patterns, an interpersonal task (because responses must be given to an examiner), and a measure of personality dynamics.

Multiple Rorschach scoring and interpretation systems evolved during subsequent decades. By the late 1960s, the considerable variability in the validity and clinical utility of scores derived from different scoring methods prompted Exner (1969, 2003) to review the literature in this area, identify those Rorschach variables with the strongest empirical support, and combine these variables into a single overarching scoring and interpretation system that he termed the Comprehensive System (CS). For the next several decades, the CS became the most widely used and studied Rorschach scoring and interpretation system, having a far-reaching impact on the assessment of personality and psychopathology and becoming a standard part of psychological test batteries (Bornstein, 2010).

Although many clinicians and researchers continue to use the CS, in 2011 an alternative Rorschach scoring and interpretation system was created, in response to some of the criticisms that had been leveled at the CS (e.g., Wood, Nezworski, Lilienfeld, & Garb, 2003), to strengthen the psychometric underpinnings of the Rorschach. The Rorschach Performance Assessment System (RPAS; Meyer, Viglione, Mihura, Erard, & Erdberg, 2011) was based in part on the results of a comprehensive meta-analysis of CS variables that identified those scores with the greatest predictive power (Mihura, Meyer, Dumitrascu, & Bombel, 2013). Although the CS and RPAS represent the two most influential omnibus scoring and interpretation systems for the Rorschach, a number of other well-validated, clinically useful methods exist that allow for the derivation of narrower Rorschach indices (e.g., thought disorder, defense style, primary-process thinking, object relations; Bornstein & Masling, 2005; Huprich, 2006).

Rorschach variables have sometimes been grouped into two broad categories: thematic (content) variables (e.g., the proportion of oral-dependent imagery in a protocol) and structural (perceptual) variables (e.g., the degree to which the respondent emphasizes common vs. unusual details when interpreting the inkblots). However, distinctions between these two categories are less sharp than once thought, and clinical and forensic predictions typically draw on both types of scores (Exner & Erdberg, 2005; Hilsenroth & Stricker, 2004). In both the CS and RPAS, these variables are summarized in a standardized summary sheet often referred to as a "structural summary"; most Rorschach interpretations are based on the analysis of combinations of scores from a CS or RPAS structural summary sheet.

Rorschach scoring and interpretation are complex, requiring considerable formal training and experience. In addition to individual scores, various ratios, percentages, and other derivations are used in Rorschach interpretation. The particular outcome variables of greatest interest in a given assessment situation are determined by the patient's characteristics, the purpose of the assessment, and the referral question.

Because the Rorschach requires a respondent to engage in an unfamiliar task during the testing session, with little guidance and minimal feedback regarding the purpose of the test or the types of outputs produced, the method has long been considered a useful means of assessing aspects of the patient's personality and functioning that might not be accessible to conscious awareness and deliberate self-report. With this in mind, optimal use of the Rorschach in psychological assessment requires that scores be interpreted in the context of the patient's performance on tests from other modalities. Exploration of divergences between information that is accessible via introspection and information that shapes behavior unconsciously, implicitly, or reflexively can yield important information regarding underlying personality structure, coping, and defenses.

Strengths of the Rorschach

The Rorschach can be a useful aid in the PDM-2 assessment of M- and MA-Axis capacities. When administered and scored properly, the Rorschach yields information on a broad array of psychological domains relevant to personality functioning, unconscious conflicts, and treatment planning. It is useful for assessing children, adolescents, adults, and older adults. It is also sensitive to change in psychotherapy. Substantial clinical and meta-analytical evidence (Mihura et al., 2013; Weiner, 2003) supports the use of Rorschach variables to assess the following M-Axis functions:

- Cognitive and affective processes: Organizational processing of stimuli (Z scores), reality testing (XA% and WDA%), ideational process (WSum6), psychotic features (PTI), depressive features (DEPI, MOR), and mentalizing activity (M).
- Identity and relationships: Dependency traits (ROD), object representations (GHR:PHR), interpersonal relationships (CDI, SumH, COP, AG), and intimacy needs (SumT).
- Defense and coping: Stable and situational stress control and tolerance (D scores), adaptation resources (EA), dysphoric feelings (SumShading), some defensive functioning (Lambda index and hypochondriacal concerns), impulse and emotional modulation (WSumC, color ratio, Afr), and ego functions (EII-2).
- Self-awareness and self-direction: Narcissistic-like sense of entitlement (Reflection responses) and mature versus immature identifications (H ratio).

Evidence indicates that the Rorschach can be of tremendous value in rendering predictions within the clinical setting (Meyer & Handler, 1997), especially for those areas that center on psychological processes largely inaccessible to verbal report (e.g., reality testing, stress tolerance, impulse control). Thus Rorschach scores have been shown to add incremental validity (unique predictive value) in diagnostic and therapeutic settings (Bram & Peebles, 2014; Meyer, 2000; Perry, Minassian, Cadenhead, & Braff, 2003). Moreover, the psychometric properties of scores derived from the Rorschach are quite strong (Bornstein, 2012): Meta-analytic procedures to estimate retest reliability for a broad array of CS and non-CS Rorschach scores revealed that both short- and long-term retest reliability for Rorschach scores were good (Grønnerød, 2003, 2006). Other studies have documented the convergent and discriminant validity of Rorschach scores (Mihura et al., 2013).

Limitations of the Rorschach

Becoming competent in Rorschach administration, scoring, and interpretation requires considerable supervised training (at least 100 hours) and experience. Moreover, the Rorschach is usually lengthy to administer; it is labor-intensive for the patient as well as the examiner. The Rorschach also may not be suitable for very low-functioning patients or those who are dysregulated at the time of testing. For these reasons, as well as because of the complexity of test scoring and interpretation and the method's strong historical links to psychodynamic theory, the Rorschach has been less widely used in recent years. Surveys demonstrate that it is also less widely taught in graduate training programs than in the past.

An additional limitation of the method concerns Rorschach interpretation and the ways in which it has occasionally been misused and mislabeled. Contrary to the assertions of critics (e.g., Wood et al., 2003), the Rorschach is not a diagnostic tool: Its scores tap underlying psychological processes that are only indirectly related to PDM/PDM-2 and DSM symptoms and diagnoses. Rorschach scores can be used to refine differential diagnoses because certain superficially similar disorders have contrasting underlying dynamics. However, the scores constitute (at best) an adjunct to more traditional diagnostic screening instruments, and by themselves they are not appropriate for making diagnostic classification decisions.

Thematic Apperception Test

The Thematic Apperception Test (TAT) was the creation of artist Christiana Morgan and psychiatrist Henry Murray (Morgan & Murray, 1935). Murray (1943, p. 3) described the TAT as "a method of revealing some of the dominant drives, emotions, sentiments, complexes, and conflicts of personality." The TAT consists of 31 stimulus cards, originally meant to be selected according to a respondent's gender and age. However, since its development, there has been increased flexibility regarding the choice of both the type and number of cards. The selection of cards can vary in response to the clinical question about a patient, whereas some clinicians maintain a standard set of TAT cards across patients. The lack of a specific set of rules regarding the construction of a TAT protocol creates a challenge for researchers who seek to validate scores derived from the TAT and to document its clinical utility empirically.

The cards consist of single to multiple figures in various interpersonal situations, all of which evoke a mixture of self and interpersonal themes and are "differently arousing" (Ehrenreich, 1990). Individuals are asked to make up a story based on each picture, with a beginning, middle, and ending. Also, individuals are asked to indicate what the character(s) may be thinking and feeling.

There are two methods of TAT interpretation: nomothetic (using an empirically validated scoring system and comparing responses to normative data) and idiographic (examining individual responses and discerning meaning about what these responses express about underlying personality structure). Clinicians are encouraged to use a combination of both approaches when interpreting TAT protocols (Aronow, Weiss, & Reznikoff, 2001).

The two most common measures used to rate TAT narratives are the SCORS (Westen, 1991a, 1991b, 1995; see above) and the DMM (Cramer, 1991, 2006; see above). Historical accounts of the TAT by major contributors to its literature can be found in Gieser and Stein (1999). Jenkins (2008) created a comprehensive handbook of TAT scales that have been used in the literature.

Clinicians focus more on the thematic content (see, e.g., Schafer, 1958) than on a specific scoring system to code narrative data; they usually focus on dominant themes, as well as on how responses deviate from the stimulus pull of the card (Stein et al., 2014). The more idiosyncratic the responses, the more TAT narratives may reflect aspects of psychopathology or personality. Also, the way a patient approaches the TAT (i.e., responding to ambiguous, emotionally arousing interpersonal situations) and the patient's behavior during testing can be helpful in understanding the patient's internal world (Aronow et al., 2001).

Strengths of the TAT

The TAT can be a useful measure in assessing implicit processes that are not readily observed or explicitly stated, such as thought process, interpersonal and object relational themes, dominant affects or emotions, defensive functioning, and psychological conflicts. Many of the PDM-2's M- and MA-Axis capacities can be evaluated with the TAT; however, some of these capacities are easier to assess than others. For example, SCORS-G ratings of TAT narratives can provide information regarding most mental functions that are captured in the M and MA Axes (with the exception of defensive functioning). The capacity for defensive functioning can be formally assessed with the DMM (see above) or freely by a clinician familiar with such functioning. Evaluating the capacity for affective range, communication, and understanding is relatively easy to accomplish, and does not require a formal coding system. Identification of themes permits ready comparison with other test data. There have been numerous studies demonstrating the TAT's clinical utility and value in the psychotherapy process and outcome literature (e.g., Fowler et al., 2004), particularly in psychodynamic treatment.

Research has demonstrated the utility of the TAT in assessing defense mechanisms across diagnostic groups (Cramer & Kelly, 2004), between genders (Cramer, 2002), in longitudinal contexts (Cramer, 2012), and in the context of therapeutic change (Cramer & Blatt, 1990).

Limitations of the TAT

Administration of the TAT takes much time and can often be complex, especially with participants who have difficulty in constructing and telling stories based on its pictures. The lack of a standard set of TAT cards to administer limits generalizability in clinical research, as does the lack of a widely accepted TAT scoring system. The vast majority of clinicians using and interpreting the TAT rely on their clinical judgment, with all of its attendant strengths and established limitations. When comprehensive scoring systems are used to interpret the TAT, they are time-consuming and require considerable training. There have also been questions regarding cultural sensitivity and the dated content of cards. For all of these reasons, as well as because projective techniques are so strongly linked to psychodynamic theory, surveys show that psychologists are using the TAT less frequently than in the past, and graduate training programs are teaching it less frequently as well.

Table 15.1 summarizes the applicability to PDM-2 assessment of the tools described to this point in this chapter.

TABLE 15.1. Applicability of Various Tools to PDM-2 Assessment

Clinician report tools	Self-report tools	Performance-based tools
	P Axis	
PDC-2 and other PDCs PDP-2 SWAP KAPP OPD-2 (P-Axis functions and level of personality organization) PCRS CCRT (conflict/relationship aspects of personality patterns)	MMPI-2 (personality organization and personality pattern facets) PAI MCMI (personality patterns) CRQ (P-Axis functions and level of personality organization)	
	M Axis	
PDC-2 and other PDCs SWAP (PHI and RADIO) PFS SPC SCORS ORI AAI AAP RFS QOR PCRS CCRT DMRS DMM (All the instruments above may be useful for assessing several M-Axis capacities.)	SIPP-118 IIP TAS-20 (specific M-Axis capacities) CORE-OM OQ-45 SOS-10 (overall M-Axis level)	Rorschach TAT

C. Instruments for Evaluating Patients in Treatment

The following instruments have utility for assessing treatments, for determining how a patient is functioning with a particular therapist, and for evaluating the patient's psychological functioning and health directly in a particular setting. Furthermore, changes in the way the patient and therapist are functioning over the course of treatment are likely to reflect changes in psychological health and to constitute a measure of interpersonal functioning. Of course, the functioning of the therapeutic dyad also reflects the skill and relational capacity of the therapist in general and with that individual patient in particular. Nevertheless, many studies have provided evidence that patient characteristics play an important role in variation in the therapy relationship and in outcome (Norcross, 2011).

Working Alliance Inventory

The Working Alliance Inventory (WAI; Horvath, 1982; Horvath & Greenberg, 1986, 1989, 1994) is a widely used instrument for assessing the therapeutic alliance. It is based on a pan-theoretical model of this alliance as involving a mutual agreement between client and clinician on the goals of treatment and the tasks necessary to achieve them, together with the establishment of a relational bond that maintains the collaboration between participants (patient and therapist) in the therapeutic work. It consists of 36 items rated on a 7-point, Likert-type scale ranging from 1 (never) to 7 (always). The inventory generates three 12-item subscales for (1) the goal, (2) the task, and (3) the bond.

Horvath and his colleagues developed three versions of the WAI: a client form (WAI-P), a therapist form (WAI-T), and an observer form (WAI-O). Although the WAI-P and WAI-T are administered at the end of a therapy session, the WAI-O is used for rating psychotherapy session transcripts. Several briefer forms have been developed as well. A short form, the WAI-S (Tracey & Kokotovic, 1989), comprises 12 items and is available in two versions (client and therapist). A short version of the WAI was also developed and validated by Hatcher and Gillapsy (2006) and is widely used.

Internal consistency of the three subscales of the WAI-P and WAI-T are high, as are internal consistency and interrater reliability values of the WAI-O's subscales (Horvath & Greenberg, 1986, 1989, 1994). In general, the three dimensions (bond, task, goal) are strongly correlated (Horvath & Greenberg, 1989, 1994). Despite the high correlations, they are distinct but overlapping dimensions (Tracey & Kokotovic, 1989).

Strengths of the WAI

The WAI is a valid and reliable measure of the working alliance that can be administered easily and completed rapidly, whether by a client, a therapist, or a nonparticipant observer. It has been used by researchers and practitioners of all theoretical orientations interested in exploring how the alliance interacts with and affects treatment process and outcome. Many studies have shown a strong relationship between working alliance and benefit from treatment (e.g., Horvath & Bedi, 2002; Norcross, 2011); indeed, the alliance as viewed by the patient and as measured at an early session is a robust predictor of and contributor to treatment outcome in all forms of psychotherapy evaluated.

Limitations of the WAI

All versions of the WAI measure the quality of the therapeutic alliance at a macro level and thus may not prove useful for assessing in-session therapeutic alliance fluctuations (e.g., alliance ruptures and resolutions) through a microanalytic investigation of the way patient and therapist co-construct their relationship. WAI scores, like self-report measures in general, can also be easily manipulated or faked by the patient.

Therapist Response Questionnaire

The Therapist Response Questionnaire (TRQ; Betan, Heim, Zittel Conklin, & Westen, 2005), previously called the Countertransference Questionnaire, is a 79-item clinician report designed to assess the clinician's emotional reactions to a patient in psychotherapy.

The items measure a wide spectrum of thoughts, feelings, and behaviors expressed by therapists toward their patients, ranging from relatively specific feelings (e.g., "I feel bored in sessions with him/her") to more complex constructs (e.g., "More than with most patients, I feel like I've been pulled into things that I didn't realize until after the session was over"). They were derived by reviewing the clinical, theoretical, and empirical literature on countertransference and related variables, and are written in straightforward jargon-free terms close to clinical experience, so that clinicians of any theoretical orientation can easily understand them. A therapist is asked to assess each item on a 5-point Likert scale ranging from 1 (not true) to 5 (very true).

The TRQ's factor structure comprises eight emotional dimensions that are clinically sensitive and conceptually coherent: overwhelmed/disorganized, helpless/inadequate, positive, special/overinvolved, sexualized, disengaged, parental/protective, and criticized/mistreated. These scales showed excellent internal consistency and good criterion validity. Several studies (see, e.g., Colli, Tanzilli, Dimaggio, & Lingiardi, 2014; Gazzillo et al., 2015; Tanzilli, Colli, Del Corno, & Lingiardi, 2016) showed that therapists' emotional response patterns are related in predictable ways to patients' personality pathology across therapeutic approaches, and that clinicians, regardless of therapeutic orientation, can make diagnostic and therapeutic use of their own emotional responses to patients.

The adolescent version of the TRQ (Satir, Thompson-Brenner, Boisseau, & Crisafulli, 2009) consists of 86 items, and its factor structure comprises six emotional response dimensions similar to those of the TRQ for adults: angry/frustrated, warm/competent, aggressive/sexual, failing/incompetent, bored/angry at parents, and overinvested/worried.

Strengths of the TRQ

The TRQ may be a useful aid for PDM-2 assessment of the P and PA Axes. It is a valid and reliable instrument for the assessment of clinicians' emotional responses. It is easy to score and can be used for both clinical and research purposes.

Limitations of the TRQ

The main limitation of the TRQ is the possible influence of social desirability bias or implicit defensive processes affecting all self-report measures. Empirical investigations of clinicians' emotional responses could benefit from research designs including other methods of measurement and different perspectives (e.g., those of external observers or supervisors).

Psychotherapy Relationship Questionnaire

The Psychotherapy Relationship Questionnaire (PRQ; Bradley, Heim, & Westen, 2005) is a 90-item clinician questionnaire that assesses a patient's interpersonal patterns in the relationship with his or her therapist. The PRQ items measure a wide range of thoughts, feelings, motives, conflicts, and behaviors expressed by patients toward their therapists. They were derived by a review of the clinical, theoretical, and empirical literature on transference, therapeutic or working alliance, and related constructs and are written in everyday language, without jargon, so that the instrument can be used by clinicians of any theoretical approach. A therapist assesses each item on a 5-point Likert scale, ranging from 1 (not true) to 5 (very true).

The PRQ's factor structure comprises five transference dimensions that are clinically and theoretically coherent: angry/entitled, anxious/preoccupied, secure/engaged, avoidant/counterdependent, and sexualized. The PRQ's scales have shown excellent internal consistency and good criterion validity (i.e., they are systematically related to personality pathology). In addition, four of the five relational patterns of the PRQ are similar to the adult attachment styles identified with the AAI (see the discussion of the AAI, above).

Strengths of the PRQ

The PRQ can be a useful aid in PDM-2 assessment of the P, PA, M, and MA Axes (in particular, the capacity for relationships and intimacy on the M and MA Axes). It is a psychometrically robust instrument for the assessment of patients' relational patterns emerging in the therapeutic relationship; it provides a window on patients' personality and relational capacities in general that is based on direct observation. It is easy to administer and relatively brief.

Limitations of the PRQ

The PRQ is subject to any inherent biases (countertransference) of the clinician. Therefore, any findings would be strengthened by obtaining ratings from an external observer as well.

Assimilation of Problematic Experiences Scale

The Assimilation of Problematic Experiences Scale (APES) summarizes a developmental progression that patients experience as they overcome problems in successful psychotherapy, according to the assimilation model (Stiles, 2005, 2011; Stiles et al., 1991). Specifically, it describes the assimilation of problematic experiences, such as traumas or dysfunctional relationships, into the patient's normal schemas. After the experiences are assimilated, they are no longer problematic but become resources, available as called upon to meet life's challenges and opportunities. For example, uncontrolled verbal outbursts may become assimilated as a capacity for assertiveness (Stiles, 1999).

The APES is construed as a continuum anchored by eight stages, numbered 0–7, that characterize the changing relation of an initially problematic experience to the rest of the self: (0) warded off/dissociated, (1) unwanted thoughts/active avoidance, (2) vague awareness/emergence, (3) problem statement/clarification, (4) understanding/insight, (5) application/working through, (6) resourcefulness/problem solution, and (7) integration/mastery. In successful psychotherapy, problematic experiences move through some portion of this sequence.

Stages of the APES can be rated from any clinical material, including audio or video recordings, transcripts, session summaries, or patient-produced materials. Rater selection and training procedures have varied a good deal across studies, and there exist several versions of this tool, both qualitative and quantitative (for one example, see Tikkanen, Stiles, & Leiman, 2013).

The relation of the APES to symptom intensity measures has been studied. Theoretically, distress and symptom intensity vary systematically across APES stages, but the relation is not linear (Stiles, Osatuke, Glick, & Mackay, 2004). Patients who enter therapy with problematic experiences that are warded off or avoided (APES stages 0 or 1) are likely to feel worse before they feel better, as these experiences emerge and are acknowledged and confronted. The most intense and sustained emotional pain is expected at APES stage 2 (vague awareness/emergence). Progress though APES stages 2–6 is characterized by decreasing distress (stages 2–4) and then increasing positive affect (stages 4–6). The most rapid change occurs across stages 3–5, as the patient identifies, labels, and formulates the problem; works toward an understanding; and explores applications of the understanding in everyday life. The consolidation at APES stages 6–7 is expected to involve integrating and normalizing, and may involve decreases in the euphoric feeling associated with solving a problem.

As recognized not only in psychodynamic therapies but across many theoretical approaches, insight and understanding are intimately linked with psychotherapy outcome, assessed as symptom intensity reduction (Castonguay & Hill, 2007). Understanding of conventional outcome criteria via the assimilation model thus suggests that APES stage 4 (understanding/insight) represents the point of greatest reduction in distress and symptom intensity. Consistent with this analysis, APES stage 4 appears pivotal in distinguishing conventionally assessed good-outcome cases from poor-outcome cases (Detert, Llewelyn, Hardy, Barkham, & Stiles, 2006).

Strengths of the APES

The APES can be useful for PDM-2 assessment of such M, MA, and MC dimensions as the capacities for mentalization and reflective functioning; self-observing (psychological mindedness); and adaptation, resiliency, and strength. It is applicable to a broad range of patient populations and treatment settings. The APES goes beyond conventional symptom-intensity-based outcome measures to assess the internal dynamics of psychological change, sometimes described as structural change, as viewed by the OPD group (see the earlier discussion of the OPD and OPD-2; see also Grande, Rudolf, Oberbracht, & Jakobsen, 2001; Grande, Rudolf, Oberbracht, & Pauli-Magnus, 2003). It links to an evolving description of the process of psychological change and can be applied to a broad range of clinical material. There are many overlaps of potential interest between the APES and measures of personality described earlier in this chapter, such as the SCORS, ORI, and RFS. The APES also overlaps with the Analytic Process Scales measures of patient functioning in the therapeutic hour (see below).

Limitations of the APES

Considerable clinician time is required to rate the clinical material according to the APES, which has rarely been used for routine clinical use. Indeed, the APES is not a psychological test or an instrument per se. Most of the research on it consists of smaller, qualitative studies. The APES is an evolving tool, and there are many versions of procedures for applying it. Although all aim at describing the same developmental sequence, there is not a single standard procedure.

Psychotherapy Process Q-Set

The Psychotherapy Process Q-Set (PQS; Jones, 2000) consists of 100 items assessed through a Q-sort method (Block, 1961/1978). PQS items cover a wide range of dimensions of the psychotherapy process, including both relational and technical aspects. Moreover, the PQS items describe patient contributions to the psychotherapy process (e.g., Q97: Patient is introspective, readily explores inner thoughts and feelings); therapist contributions (e.g., Q50: Therapist draws attention to feelings regarded by the patient as unacceptable, such as anger, envy, or excitement); and patient–therapist interactions (e.g., Q39: There is a competitive quality to the relationship).

The PQS provides a description of the psychotherapy process in both adult and adolescent treatment, suitable for comparison and quantitative analysis (Jones, 2000). After studying the transcripts of a therapy hour, clinical judges proceed to the ordering of the 100 items. These were originally printed separately on cards to permit easy arrangement and rearrangement, and are sorted into nine piles on a continuum from least (category 1) to most (category 9) characteristic. This sort is now more readily accomplished with a computer program. PQS ratings, like other Q-sort measures, are based on forced choice, so that the number of items scored at each level is fixed (ranging from 5 items required at the extremes to 18 in the middle category) and conforms approximately to a normal distribution.

The reliability of the instrument was found to be strong with evaluators of different theoretical orientations (Jones, Hall, & Parke, 1991; Jones & Pulos, 1993). PQS results were reliable in the evaluation of session transcripts from treatments of different orientations and were successful in differentiating between types of therapies. An early fruit of this labor was the demonstration that in samples of both psychodynamic and cognitive-behavioral treatments, better results were associated with the psychodynamic aspects of treatment than with the cognitive-behavioral aspects (Ablon & Jones, 1998).

Strengths of the PQS

The portrayal of the patient–therapist relationship emerging from the PQS assesses the patient's capacities for relatedness; this can aid in PDM-2 assessment of the P and PA Axes, and more particularly of the capacity for relationships and intimacy on the M and MA Axes. The PQS enables a qualitative and quantitative assessment of psychotherapy process and leads to both a global and a detailed picture of a session and a period of therapy.

Like other Q-sort procedures, the PQS prevents scores from being biased upward or downward by temperament and is based on the assessment of several different dimensions of patient and therapist contributions to the therapeutic process.

The PQS can be useful in capturing the richness and complexity of psychotherapy, as well as the particular nature of the patient and therapist relationship. Careful recognition and understanding of these repetitive interactions are useful in clinical practice because these patterns can be linked to positive or negative therapy outcomes (Josephs, Sanders, & Gorman, 2014).

Limitations of the PQS

The PQS requires recorded sessions, from which transcripts are made, in order to evaluate the treatment systematically. The PQS assessment is also time-consuming (in general, 90 minutes are needed to assess a 50-minute session, with reading the transcript and listening to the session included) and requires lengthy training (an average of 25 hours). Also, some of the profiles of types of treatment are now regarded as reflecting certain outdated psychoanalytic concepts, such as neutrality, abstinence, and avoiding expression of one's own subjectivity, As a consequence, findings about the efficacy of different profiles of practice using the PQS can be misleading.

Analytic Process Scales

The Analytic Process Scales (APS; Waldron et al., 2004a) instrument was developed by a research group of experienced psychoanalysts who began this work in 1985. There are 32 scales (scored 0–4) aimed at the assessment of different dimensions of the therapeutic process on the basis of audio-recorded and transcribed sessions of psychotherapy. The patient's contribution to the therapy is assessed via 14 scales, and the therapist's contribution via 18 scales. Definitions and examples of each of these scales are assembled into an 81-page coding manual (Scharf, Waldron, Firestein, Goldberger, & Burton, 2010). The anchoring made possible by the APS coding manual facilitates reliable measurements; it has also been useful to students of psychotherapy because it combines definitions of core psychoanalytic constructs with clinical examples.

The patient scales assess the degree to which the patient is able to convey his or her experiences, self-reflect on them, and convey his or her feelings, both in regard to the therapist and therapeutic relationship and in regard to other relationships; the extensiveness of his or her communications about romantic and sexual themes, assertiveness, aggressiveness, hostility, self-esteem, and developmental experiences; the degree to which the patient is able to respond to the therapist in a useful manner; and the overall productivity of his or her communications. That is, these scales focus on the degree to which the patient's communications show a deepening in self-awareness, contact with his or her own feelings, and cooperation with the therapist.

The therapist scales assess different kinds of interventions (encouraging elaboration, clarification, interpretation, and support); different targets of these interventions (defenses or resistances, transference, and conflicts); and different domains addressed (romantic and sexual life, self-esteem, and development). These scales also enable the assessment of the degree to which the therapist's communications are shaped by his or her feelings and are confrontational, amicable, or hostile. Finally, a scale assesses the overall goodness of therapist interventions—that is, their aptness in kind, content, language, and timing.

The APS variables were originally applied to segments of each session, but the procedure has been expanded to apply to each session in its entirety, so that a much larger number of sessions can be studied in a given time. Reliability has been demonstrated in ratings of segments (Lingiardi et al., 2010; Waldron, Scharf, Hurst, Firestein, & Burton, 2004b) and whole sessions (Waldron et al., 2013). In the whole-session assessment procedure, the scorer estimates both an average and the highest level reached in that session on any given variable.

A replicated finding has been that the rated overall quality of therapist communications is the most powerful element in predicting benefit, regardless of the particular nature of the communication (Gazzillo et al., 2014; Lingiardi et al., 2010; Waldron et al., 2004a; Waldron & Helm, 2004).

Strengths of the APS

The APS provides measures of a patient's ability to form a productive relationship with a therapist and to be thoughtful about his or her mental life; in this way, it can assist in PDM-2 assessment of a patient's capacities on the M Axes, such as the capacities for affective range, communication, and understanding and for self-observing (psychological mindedness). The APS assesses core dimensions of a patient's and therapist's contributions to the dynamic processes of psychotherapy, particularly the *quality* of the therapist's contributions (a rare feature in instruments applied to psychotherapies).

Assessing the segments of each session permits exploration of the moment-to-moment impact of the therapist's communications on the patient and vice versa. It most directly addresses psychodynamic activities of the therapist (encouraging elaboration, clarifying, interpreting, addressing defenses, etc.), so the ratings facilitate exploring connections between therapeutic activity and patient changes. The APS therapist scales can thus help answer questions about the relative contribution of technique and the relationship to treatment outcomes (Waldron et al., 2013).

Limitations of the APS

The segmental assessment of the APS is time-consuming (for a 50-minute session, the segmental coding takes about 4 hours) and therefore is a procedure to be reserved for intensive study. The whole-session assessment is less time-consuming (60 minutes to assess a 50-minute session, including listening while reading the transcript), but does not permit the same level of detailed exploration of the relationship between therapist communication and responses from the patient. The APS has not so far been used nearly as widely as the PQS.

Dynamic Interaction Scales

The Dynamic Interaction Scales (DIS; Waldron et al., 2013) instrument comprises 12 Likert scales (each rated 0–4) for assessing global interactional aspects of the therapeutic process on the basis of audio-recorded and transcribed sessions. The scales were developed to address more global and relational aspects than those explored by the APS (see above) because the field has shifted in a more relational direction in the years since the APS was first conceived, and because an important finding of research using the APS has been the powerful role of therapist communication quality in contributing to short-term benefit. The items are accompanied by a manual describing them.

The DIS is divided into therapist scales, patient scales, and interaction scales. The therapist scales assess the degree to which the therapist is straightforward; is warmly responsive; is responsive to moment-to-moment shifts in the patient's communications or emotional state; conveys aspects of his or her subjective experience to the patient; and is working well with, and helping the patient work with, his or her typical patterns of relating and feeling. The patient scales assess to what degree the patient flexibly shifts to and from experiencing and reflecting; shows a flexible interplay between conscious waking life and dreams; and works well with his or her typical patterns of relating and feelings. The interaction scales assess the degree to which the patient experiences the therapist as empathic; to which the therapist's contribution leads to the further development of the patient's awareness; to which there is an integration of understanding of the relationship with the therapist to other relationships; and to which the engagement in the therapeutic relationship by the two parties is brought forward or experienced in an emotionally meaningful way.

Strengths of the DIS

The DIS makes possible a reliable assessment of some relevant interactional and relational aspects of psychotherapy. It addresses questions relevant to PDM-2 assessment of both the M Axis and the P Axis (e.g., the degree to which the patient is able to oscillate between experiencing and reflecting and to engage in a close working relationship that leads to greater self-understanding). The instrument has the advantage of evaluating several different aspects of the working relationship between patient and therapist, thus broadening what may be learned from the WAI (see above). Measures of these kinds of variables have been infrequent, although there is much clinical evidence to suggest their importance. The DIS is easy to apply; assessment of a 50-minute session takes about 55 minutes (listening to and reading the transcript included).

Limitations of the DIS

The DIS is a new instrument and will benefit from more extensive reliability testing and studies of convergent validity, with use by other investigators. Like other instruments based on transcripts, it is time-consuming and requires training to achieve reliable ratings.

Comparative Psychotherapy Process Scales

The Comparative Psychotherapy Process Scales (CPPS; Hilsenroth, Blagys, Ackerman, Bonge, & Blais, 2005) consists of 20 items, 10 psychodynamic–interpersonal and 10 cognitive-behavioral, that have been found to distinguish empirically between the two general treatment styles. Therapists or researchers rate each item on a 7-point Likert scale from 0 (not characteristic) to 6 (extremely characteristic) on the basis of transcriptions and audio or video recordings of therapy sessions.

Strengths of the CPPS

The CPPS is a reliable and easy-to-use tool for differentiating different treatment modalities and for assessing several technical interventions that are used in psychotherapy.

Weaknesses of the CPPS

The CPPS does not assess the patient's contribution to the therapeutic process, and ad hoc training is needed to apply it reliably.

Part Three. A Clinical Illustration: Tool-Based Assessment[1]

Background Information and Referral Questions

Charlotte is a 19-year-old college freshman on leave from school following a severe depressive episode in which she lapsed in basic self-care and hygiene, was unable to attend classes, retreated to her dorm room, and made minimal connection with peers. It appeared that this episode was triggered by being away from home for an extended period for the first time while facing unfamiliar academic and social pressures. She also was unable or unwilling to seek necessary supports on campus. At the end of the

[1]Contributed by Anthony Bram. Identifying information is disguised in accordance with contemporary standards for published case material. Dr. Bram acknowledges the scoring contributions to this clinical illustration by Drs. Michelle Stein (SCORS-G), Kevin Meehan (ORI), and Joseph Reynoso (ORI), as well as Kiley Gottschalk and Oren Lee-Parritz.

semester—when her failing and incomplete grades became apparent to her family, and when the school administration alerted the family to the severity of her emotional crisis (which she had masked and minimized in weekly phone calls)—she was assisted to take a medical leave of absence and return home for treatment.

Treatment involved trials of various antidepressant and antianxiety medications plus once- or twice-weekly cognitive-behavioral therapy (CBT) aiming at behavioral activation (e.g., creating a routine of structure and activity to counter the depressive cycle created by interpersonal isolation) and at challenges to the maladaptive thought patterns that were leading to Charlotte's feelings of hopelessness and helplessness. Despite nearly 6 months of this outpatient plan, her symptoms and poor functioning largely persisted. Charlotte reported that she could not tolerate different medications because of discomfiting side effects; when side effects were absent, her conviction was that the medications were not helping. Similarly, she continually asserted that therapy was "pointless . . . a waste of time," and that the therapist (a respected, well-trained senior clinician with expertise in CBT) was "useless." She frequently overslept and missed or was late to sessions (even though they were not scheduled early in the morning); was typically uncommunicative with her therapist; and rarely completed between-session homework assignments, even if she had reluctantly agreed to do so. With the treatment mired in impasse, an evaluation with psychological testing was requested by both her psychiatrist and therapist, with her parents' support. The aim of the evaluation was to understand more fully the factors underlying and driving Charlotte's symptoms, as well as the factors impeding her ability to form a productive alliance with her treaters.

The older of two sisters, Charlotte grew up with her biological parents, both successful professionals with advanced degrees. There was a family history of depression, anxiety (including panic disorder), and alcoholism. Charlotte suffered mild developmental delays in fine motor skills and had unusual sensory sensitivities (tactile and auditory in particular). The delays were addressed with occupational therapy during preschool and early elementary school years. She did not have cognitive, speech, or other language delays, and there was no reported history of trauma. Temperamentally, from an early age she was viewed as shy, introverted, inhibited, anxious, and easily overstimulated. Charlotte's parents recall that when she was about age 3—after the birth of her sister, who had a more easygoing temperament and was better able to engage her parents and others in playful, affectionate interaction—Charlotte became less "cuddly" and less inclined to express and seek out affection. Though not overtly hostile and rejecting toward her baby sister, her parents recall that Charlotte was "lukewarm" to her presence in her life. In retrospect, they wondered whether it was around that time that Charlotte had become more interpersonally withdrawn and emotionally shut down.

As a school-age child and adolescent, Charlotte had a small group of friends who shared similar interests, but she did not seek out or make new friends readily. She excelled in and enjoyed dance and gymnastics. Charlotte was viewed as a strong but not highly motivated student until middle school, when she appeared more disorganized and had trouble completing and handing in work on time, often refusing to do so. Neuropsychological and psychoeducational testing conducted at the time revealed her to have overall superior, albeit uneven, intellectual capacities (Wechsler Intelligence Scale for Children [WISC-IV] general ability index at the 95th percentile, with more average-level working memory and processing speed). Weaknesses in executive functioning, and anxiety/avoidance associated with perfectionism, were found to be contributing to her difficulties in staying organized and completing schoolwork. Against her protests, her parents decided to place Charlotte in a small private school for the remainder of middle and high school. At the new school, there was less academic and athletic pressure; the social demands were more manageable; and better supports and accommodations were available for her executive functioning. Her parents report that Charlotte continues to "bristle" when the topics of her cognitive weaknesses and needs for support are explicitly broached.

Multiple efforts to help Charlotte psychotherapeutically with her anxiety during her high school years did not get far. She dreaded and often refused to attend sessions, saying she hated "all the touchy-feely crap." When her parents encouraged her to try a different therapist or modality, Charlotte had a similar response. Ultimately, her parents relented and decided not to push this further. She was completing her schoolwork, receiving solid grades, and participating in dance and gymnastics; she also had a couple of friends in high school. These facts did not create urgency regarding her need for treatment.

As noted earlier, the present evaluation was recommended to obtain a better understanding of the factors associated with Charlotte's failure to adapt to the academic and social requirements of college. Treatments conceptualized and based on her seemingly accurate DSM-5 diagnoses—major depressive disorder and social anxiety disorder—had not been engaging her, ameliorating her symptoms, or improving her functioning. Thus, for the evaluation, it was important to shift diagnostic vantage points to complement the extant DSM-5 symptom-based perspective. Specifically, valuable alternative, complementary frameworks were offered by the combination of the PDM-2 approach and a treatment-centered diagnostic approach (Bram & Peebles, 2014; Peebles, 2012). Such approaches shifted the diagnostic focus toward clarifying the underlying, implicit factors creating and driving Charlotte's manifest symptoms—that is, the roles of personality style and structure, ego functioning (i.e., areas of structural weakness and strength), and possible areas of intrapsychic conflict. The task was also to understand the factors that affected Charlotte's ability to form a therapeutic alliance.

Measures and Methods

The evaluation comprised a combination of performance-based, self-report, and collateral report measures.

- *Performance-based measures*: Selected subtests of the Wechsler Adult Intelligence Scale—Third Edition (WAIS-III); the Rorschach (administered and scored with the Comprehensive System); the Thematic Apperception Test (TAT, scored with the Social Cognition and Object Relations Scale Global Rating Method [SCORS-G] and Symons, Peterson, Slaughter, Roche, and Doyle's [2005] mental state discourse measure); and the Object Relations Inventory (ORI, scored on the differentiation–relatedness scale).
- *Self-report measures*: The Minnesota Multiphasic Personality Inventory–2 (MMPI-2); the Toronto Alexithymia Scale–20 (TAS-20); the Trauma History Questionnaire (Hooper, Stockton, Krupnick, & Green, 2011); the Beck Depression Inventory–II (BDI-II; Beck, Steer, & Brown, 1996); and the Depressive Experiences Questionnaire (DEQ; Blatt, D'Afflitti, & Quinlan, 1976).
- *Collateral report measures*: Developmental questionnaire (completed by parents); the Shedler–Westen Assessment Procedure–200 (SWAP-200; completed by referring therapist).

Diagnostic Summary Based on the Evaluation

Structural Weaknesses and Defenses

Because Charlotte can present herself as a healthy, bright, athletic young woman who does not report or show great vulnerability or distress, it has probably been perplexing for her family and treaters to make sense of the severity and nature of her challenges in functioning that have necessitated her leave of absence from school. The evaluation data indicate that her emotional and behavioral difficulties are attributable to an underlying constellation of certain underdeveloped psychological capacities (i.e., structural weaknesses or deficits), and to her having learned to compensate for and cope with them in ways that have become part of a maladaptive character style.

Charlotte's most significant domain of structural weakness involves *affect regulation*. This is marked by her becoming easily flooded by feelings experienced as intolerable, in a way that leaves her cognitively stymied and helpless. This intensity of emotional reaction must seem confusing and alien to a young woman who is so competent, both intellectually and physically/athletically. Importantly, the findings suggest that her weaknesses in affect regulation are less about her being emotionally unaware and not having the words to communicate feelings, and more about her ability to sit with feelings, tolerate them, and know what to do to manage them. She views thinking and talking about feelings not as potential ways to cope with and regulate them (e.g., by contextualizing them, gaining new perspectives on them, and signaling to others how they can help), but as unnecessarily risking reevoking her noxious experiences of flooding and helplessness. Despite her persistent efforts to shut out and minimize emotions, the present data show that she continues to struggle with anxiety, anger, and variable moods.

The other key area of psychological weakness identified involves underdevelopment of a *basic sense of trust in interpersonal relationships*. She has not yet internalized a stable sense that relationships and interactions with others will be sources of satisfaction and sustenance. She is leery about getting close to others, vigilant about others' potentially hostile intent, and somewhat prone to misperceive or misinterpret others' words and actions in this direction. It is reasonable to speculate that she also is guarded against interpersonal closeness because of its association with sharing of emotional vulnerability, which, as described above, she experiences as threatening.

Data from the evaluation indicate that Charlotte has developed entrenched, habitual ways of managing these areas of structural weakness. These entail her ongoing and automatic/reflexive efforts to (1) keep emotions out of her awareness and discourse to minimize her experience of herself as vulnerable and (2) carefully guard her personal boundaries to maintain what seems to her a safe interpersonal distance. Specifically, she has developed a *defense style* marked by constriction, minimization, rationalization ("I don't feel it's necessary" to consider and discuss emotions), externalizing (viewing distress as existing in or being caused by others), and dismissing/devaluing others viewed as potentially threatening (perhaps because she experiences them as holding the possibility of greater emotional involvement, positive or negative). Such a style is aimed at self-protection, preserving some sense of competence, control, and safety. It is nevertheless also maladaptive, because, among other things, it limits engagement of her creativity, spontaneity, problem-solving options, communication of needs, and satisfactions that come with deeper interpersonal/emotional engagement.

Emotional Regulation

The present data indicate that Charlotte's emotional constriction and uncommunicativeness can be conceptualized as a complex combination of (1) underdevelopment/weakness in the core capacity of emotional regulation and (2) an ingrained character pattern that probably developed out of compensatory efforts at self-protection. The former is marked by Charlotte's tendency to become internally flooded by intense or complex emotions. That is, when her feelings are stirred, she has difficulty accessing her superior cognitive abilities in the service of coping and problem solving, is vulnerable to more confused and illogical thinking, and is more apt to misperceive situations and people (see "Reasoning and Reality Testing," below). Anger, whether she is aware of it or not, is the source of anxiety and is particularly disruptive to such cognitive abilities. Significantly, Charlotte has little internalized sense that anxiety and states of distress and unease can be constructively resolved. During the evaluation, this was most evident in her TAT narratives, where she had difficulty bringing emotional tension states to resolution; she ended stories instead with characters' declarations of futility, helplessness, indecision, or shutting down: " . . . 'Why am I even trying?' ", " 'What should I do now?' ", " . . . wondering what she should do next," and "She's going to go to bed."

Although there is some evidence that at times Charlotte is not aware of and thus may have difficulties naming the feelings that are affecting her, an encouraging finding is that she actually has developed a much richer emotional vocabulary than might be expected from her history. Most notably, through her TAT responses (mostly offered spontaneously and not requiring additional prompting), she demonstrated an ability to articulate a range of pleasant emotional states (e.g., happiness, enjoyment, love, satisfaction) as well as distressing ones (e.g., sadness, frustration, disappointment, fear, loneliness). This is consistent with her response to inquiry on the TAS-20, when she surprisingly endorsed the item "I am able to describe my feelings easily." She elaborated: "I am *able to*. I just *may not want to* . . . in many situations . . . because I don't feel it's necessary." These are crucial findings: They clarify that her difficulty with emotional regulation is *not* predominantly that she is oblivious about feeling states and cannot identify them (although doing so may be more challenging in moments of heightened emotional intensity). It is more that, in spite of this ability, she is frightened by emotions ("affect phobia," in the terms of McCullough et al., 2003), which can acutely flood and destabilize her.

Given Charlotte's vulnerability to the destabilizing impact of emotions, understandably she has developed strong, habitual ways of keeping feelings out of her awareness and discourse. The test data corroborate that when she *is* able to evade emotion, she actually does function better cognitively. Thus it makes psychological sense for her to have developed this style aimed at extruding emotional awareness and expression through constriction, minimization, rationalization, externalizing, and dismissing/devaluing. Striving to keep emotions out enables her to experience a greater sense of control, competence, and safe interpersonal distance. The downside, however, is that this entrenched self-protective pattern is also maladaptive, insofar as it works at the expense of her creativity, spontaneity, ability to see the big picture, communication of her needs, and depth of interpersonal engagement.

Experiences of Self and Others

This young woman's Rorschach percepts of "a mask," "armor," "helmet," and "shield" indicate the premium she places on self-protection and on obscuring from others her inner experience and vulnerability. Although she is certainly not uninterested in other people, Charlotte is highly cautious about emotional closeness with others. When there is a topic that engages her, she believes there to be a "point" to a specific interaction. At such times, she does not feel pressured or threatened and is able to show some reciprocal communication, perspective taking, pleasure in sharing her ideas, and sense of humor. But she is vigilant about whom she really lets in and trusts. Charlotte has a low threshold for experiencing others as intrusive, and she carefully guards her interpersonal boundaries. This vigilance is central to her difficulties in making use of a therapist, as well as to her hesitation in seeking out necessary support for her academic and executive functioning at college.

Reasoning and Reality Testing

Testing does not reveal severe or pervasive weaknesses in Charlotte's capacities to reason logically and perceive situations accurately. Her reasoning and sense of reality are on more solid ground when situations are more highly structured (i.e., expectations are clear and predictable, external monitoring and feedback are provided, and she is less on her own to make sense of and organize things), are less emotionally demanding and intense, and have less of an interpersonal component. As suggested above (see "Emotional Regulation"), when situations are more complex or emotionally loaded—especially if she is angry, anxious, or feeling threatened in some way—these psychological capacities can momentarily deteriorate. Specifically, under such conditions, her reasoning can become more confused and illogical, such that she is more vulnerable to reading undue hostile meaning into the situation or to connecting her ideas in ways that do not make sense and lead to shaky conclusions. Under similar conditions, her perceptions and experiences of situations and people can become more distorted, often in the direction of finding threats that others in the same situation would not.

Treatment Implications

The central therapeutic tasks for Charlotte are to assist her (1) to develop her capacity to tolerate and communicate her feelings, and learn that there are things that she can do (cognitively, behaviorally, interpersonally) to diminish their intensity and handle them more successfully; (2) to internalize a greater sense of trust and comfort with closeness; and (3) to recognize the costs of and modify her constricted, mistrustful, and avoidant defense style.

A therapeutic alliance centering around these aims will not be easily attained and will take time. Because of her previous difficulty in accessing outpatient therapy—likely attributable to her underlying mistrust and affect phobia—she will initially require a residential treatment that will mitigate against her proclivity to emotional avoidance and interpersonal withdrawal. It is hoped that living and participating in a therapeutic milieu will offer her a level of validation, support, and feedback that would be difficult for her to access and accept from a single professional on an outpatient basis.

As regards psychotherapeutic modalities within a residential treatment program and subsequently as an outpatient, the present evaluation points to several options (not mutually exclusive) to be considered by Charlotte, her family, and her treatment team. One possibility is that a therapy including biofeedback could help her to link physical states of tension with particular feelings and themes, and then show her concrete strategies to regulate and resolve the tension. The idea would be to make her feelings more tolerable, so that she can experience mastery over them that she currently lacks. Another option would be a psychotherapy group with a stable membership and balance between a skills- and process-oriented focus, run by a well-trained therapist who would be attuned to Charlotte's vulnerabilities and could play an active role in helping regulate the expectations and pace of her engagement. As in the recommendation for a residential milieu, the group modality would offer opportunities for peer modeling of emotional disclosure and problem solving, as well as for feedback and confrontation about the effects of her interpersonal style on others. Finally, and probably most difficult for her to accept, would be a long-term, multiple-times-per-week, relationally focused psychotherapy or psychoanalysis. This too would need to be carefully paced and would necessarily move slowly for some time, especially with the therapist's recognizing and respecting her needs for constriction and guardedness. The task would be to avoid pressuring Charlotte prematurely for emotional disclosure, but instead gradually to build trust; recognize, discuss, and affirm her strengths and interests; and model and cultivate playfulness, comfort with vulnerability, curiosity, and self-awareness. With the frequency over time, and growing safety in the relationship, there would be increasing opportunities for the here-and-now emotional interaction (positive or negative) between Charlotte and the therapist to be tolerated, reflected on, and discussed. In other words, this would be a more implicit, *in vivo* way for her to learn how to manage and express emotions, as well as to assist her to grapple with her misgivings about trust and closeness.

Evidence for Case Formulation from the PDC-2 and Other Tools

A completed PDC-2 for Charlotte, revealing her full PDM-2 profile, is provided in Figure 15.1. The following description shows how scores from the other test data are integrated with some sections of the PDC-2. It thus illustrates how the PDC-2 can be supplemented by several of the other tools described in this chapter, which provide a deeper and richer portrayal of Charlotte's inner life, conflicts, and defenses.

Section I: Level of Personality Organization

1. **Identity:** Ability to view self in complex, stable, and accurate ways <u>7</u>

   - ORI, differentiation–relatedness, self-description = 7 on 10-point scale: Thoughts, feelings, and needs are differentiated and modulated. Increasing tolerance for and integration of disparate aspects of self.
   - SCORS-G, identity and self-coherence = 4.9 on 7-point scale (above mean for college students): Identity and self-definition are not major preoccupations.

(text resumes on page 954)

Psychodiagnostic Chart–2 (PDC-2)

Psychodiagnostic Chart–2, Adult Version 8.1

Name: *Charlotte* Age: *19* Gender: *Female* Ethnicity: *White North American*

Date of evaluation: *XX / XX / XX* Evaluator: *Psychologist*

Section I: Level of Personality Organization

Consider your client's mental functions in determining the level of personality organization. Use these four mental functions to efficiently capture the level of personality organization. Rate each mental function on a scale from 1 (Severely impaired) to 10 (Healthy).

Severe				Moderate				Healthy	
1	2	3	4	5	6	7	8	9	10

1. **Identity:** Ability to view self in complex, stable, and accurate ways *7*
2. **Object relations:** Ability to maintain intimate, stable, and satisfying relationships *3*
3. **Level of defenses** (using the guide below, select a single number): *4*
   - 1–2: Psychotic level (delusional projection, psychotic denial, psychotic distortion)
   - 3–5: Borderline level (splitting, projective identification, idealization/devaluation, denial, acting out)
   - 6–8: Neurotic level (repression, reaction formation, intellectualization, displacement, undoing)
   - 9–10: Healthy level (anticipation, self-assertion, sublimation, suppression, altruism, and humor)
4. **Reality testing:** Ability to appreciate conventional notions of what is realistic *7*

Overall Personality Organization

Considering the ratings and your clinical judgment, circle your client's overall personality organization.

Psychotic			Borderline			Neurotic		Healthy	
1	2	3	4	(5)	6	7	8	9	10

(continued)

FIGURE 15.1. A completed PDC-2 for Charlotte.

Healthy personality: Characterized by mostly 9–10 scores; life problems rarely get out of hand, and enough flexibility to accommodate to challenging realities. (Use 9 for people at the high-functioning neurotic level.)

Neurotic level: Characterized by mostly 6–8 scores; basically a good sense of identity, good reality testing, mostly good intimacies; fair resiliency, fair affect tolerance and regulation; rigidity and limited range of defenses and coping mechanisms; favors defenses such as repression, reaction formation, intellectualization, displacement, and undoing. (Use 6 for people who go between borderline and neurotic levels.)

Borderline level: Characterized by mostly 3–5 scores; recurrent relational problems; difficulty with affect tolerance and regulation; poor impulse control, poor sense of identity, poor resiliency; favors defenses such as splitting, projective identification, idealization/devaluation, denial, omnipotent control, and acting out.

Psychotic level: Characterized by mostly 1–2 scores; delusional thinking; poor reality testing and mood regulation; extreme difficulty functioning in work and relationships; favors defenses such as delusional projection, psychotic denial, and psychotic distortion. (Use 3 for people who go between psychotic and borderline levels.)

(There are no sharp cutoffs between categories. Use your clinical judgment.)

Section II: Personality Syndromes (P Axis)

These are relatively stable patterns of thinking, feeling, behaving, and relating to others. Normal-level personality patterns do not involve impairment, while personality syndromes or disorders involve impairment at the neurotic, borderline, or psychotic level.

Check off as many personality syndromes as apply from the list below; then circle the one or two personality styles that are most dominant. Leave blank if none.

(For research purposes, you may also rate the level of severity for all styles, using a 1–5 scale: 1 = Severe level; 3 = Moderate severity; and 5 = High-functioning.)

Level of severity

☐ **Depressive** ___

Subtypes:
- Introjective
- Anaclitic
- Converse manifestation: Hypomanic

☐ **Dependent** ___

Subtypes:
- Passive–aggressive
- Converse manifestation: Counterdependent

(continued)

FIGURE 15.1. *(continued)*

	Level of severity
☐ **Anxious–avoidant and phobic** Subtype: • Converse manifestation: Counterphobic	___
☐ **Obsessive–compulsive**	___
☑ **Schizoid**	4
☐ **Somatizing**	___
☐ **Hysteric–histrionic** Subtypes: • Inhibited • Demonstrative	___
☐ **Narcissistic** Subtypes: • Overt • Covert • Malignant	___
☑ **Paranoid**	3
☐ **Psychopathic** Subtypes: • Passive–parasitic, "con artist" • Aggressive	___
☐ **Sadistic**	___
☐ **Borderline**	___

Section III: Mental Functioning (M Axis)

Rate your client's level of strength or weakness on each of the 12 mental functions below, on a scale from 1 to 5 (1 = Severe deficits; 5 = Healthy). Then sum the 12 ratings for a level-of-severity score.

Severe deficits	Major impairments	Moderate impairments	Mild impairments	Healthy
1	2	3	4	5

(continued)

FIGURE 15.1. *(continued)*

- **Cognitive and affective processes**
  1. Capacity for regulation, attention, and learning 3
  2. Capacity for affective range, communication, and understanding 2
  3. Capacity for mentalization and reflective functioning 3
- **Identity and relationships**
  4. Capacity for differentiation and integration (identity) 4
  5. Capacity for relationships and intimacy 2
  6. Self-esteem regulation and quality of internal experience 3
- **Defense and coping**
  7. Impulse control and regulation 4
  8. Defensive functioning 2
  9. Adaptation, resiliency, and strength 3
- **Self-awareness and self-direction**
  10. Self-observing capacities (psychological mindedness) 2
  11. Capacity to construct and use internal standards and ideals 3
  12. Meaning and purpose 3

Overall level of personality severity (Sum of 12 mental functions): 34

[Healthy/optimal mental functioning, 54–60; Appropriate mental functioning with some areas of difficulty, 47–53; Mild impairments in mental functioning, 40–46; Moderate impairments in mental functioning, 33–39; Major impairments in mental functioning, 26–32; Significant defects in basic mental functions, 19–25; Major/severe defects in basic mental functions, 12–18]

Section IV: Symptom Patterns (S Axis)

List the main PDM-2 symptom patterns (those that are predominantly related to psychotic disorders, mood disorders, disorders related primarily to anxiety, event- and stressor-related disorders, etc.).

(If required, you may use the DSM or ICD symptoms and codes here.)

Severe — Moderate — Healthy

1 2 3 4 5

Symptom/concern: *Depression* Level: 2

Symptom/concern: *Social anxiety* Level: 2

Symptom/concern: ___ Level: ___

(continued)

FIGURE 15.1. *(continued)*

Section V: Cultural, Contextual, and Other Relevant Considerations

History of weaknesses in executive function; high-achieving family members; competitiveness with younger sibling.

FIGURE 15.1. *(continued)*

2. **Object relations:** Ability to maintain intimate, stable, and satisfying relationships 3
   - SWAP-200: Elevated on passive–aggressive, paranoid, and schizoid scales. Examples of heavily weighted items include "quick to assume others wish to harm or take advantage of her," "feels misunderstood, mistreated, or victimized," "lacks social skills." SWAP trait dimensions: Elevated on hostility scale.
3. **Level of defenses** (using the guide below, select a single number): 4
   - SWAP-200: Elevated on paranoid scale. Heavily weighted items include "tends to believe her problems are caused by external factors," "tends to become irrational when strong emotions are stirred up; may show a noticeable decline from customary level of functioning."
   - SWAP-200: Also includes heavily weighted items such as "tends to express aggression in passive and indirect ways," "has difficulty acknowledging and expressing anger," "prefers to operate as if emotions were irrelevant or inconsequential," "tends to be inhibited or constricted; has difficulty allowing self to acknowledge or express wishes and impulses."
   - ORI, differentiation–relatedness, descriptions of mother and father = 5 on 10-point scale: "Semidifferentiated, tenuous consolidation of representations through splitting . . . marked oscillation between dramatically opposite qualities."
   - Rorschach and TAT: Devaluation (e.g., "no point to this").

4. **Reality testing:** Ability to appreciate conventional notions of what is realistic 7

   - Rorschach: Form quality ratios are all within standard deviation of mean, but there is evidence that reality testing can lapse under conditions of heightened affect; some vulnerability to distort perceptions of others, viewing them as more malevolent.

Section II: Personality Syndromes (P Axis)

- Endorsements of the schizoid and paranoid personality styles in this section of Charlotte's PDC-2 reflect elevations on corresponding SWAP-200 scales. These categories capture the patient's characterological mistrust, proneness to externalize distress, emotional constriction, and interpersonal distancing.

Section III: Mental Functioning (M Axis)

- **Cognitive and affective processes**

  1. Capacity for regulation, attention, and learning 3

     - Previously documented weaknesses in attention and executive functioning.

  2. Capacity for affective range, communication, and understanding 2

     - SWAP-200: Heavily weighted items include "tends to be angry and hostile," "tends to avoid confiding in others for fear of betrayal," "tends to be irrational when strong emotions are stirred up," "tends to feel shamed or embarrassed," "tends to be anxious," "tends to be inhibited and constricted; has difficulty allowing self to acknowledge or express wishes and impulses."
     - Rorschach: Indicators of affective constriction.
     - TAT: Difficulty resolving characters' emotional tension.

  3. Capacity for mentalization and reflective functioning 3

     - TAT: Able to identity and label mental states. Mental state discourse measure = .35 (within one standard deviation of college-age norms).
     - Rorschach and TAT: Pacing of discourse attuned to examiner.
     - SWAP-200: Heavily weighted items include "has little psychological insight into own motives, behavior, etc.; is unable to consider alternate interpretations of her experience," "tends to perceive malevolent intentions in others' words and actions," "has difficulty acknowledging or expressing anger."

- **Identity and relationships**

  4. Capacity for differentiation and integration (identity) 4

     - See under "Identity" in Section I, above.

  5. Capacity for relationships and intimacy 2

     - See under "Object relations" in Section I, above.

6. Self-esteem regulation and quality of internal experience 3

- SCORS-G, self-esteem = 3.9 (4 ="Self-esteem is bland, absent, or limited").
- SWAP-200: Heavily weighted items include "tends to be self-critical; sets unrealistically high standards for self and is intolerant of own human defects."
- Rorschach: No structural indicators of grandiosity.

- **Defense and coping**

7. Impulse control and regulation 4

- SWAP-200: No heavily weighted items associated with impulsivity.
- Rorschach and TAT: Indicators of inhibition, constriction, and avoidance rather than impulsivity.

8. Defensive functioning 2

- See under "Level of defenses" in Section I, above.

9. Adaptation, resiliency, and strength 3

- Rorschach: Indicators that she is able to recover from moments of emotional destabilization through constriction and avoidance, but at the cost of spontaneity and creativity.
- TAT: Characters flustered, unable to resolve emotional tension.

- **Self-awareness and self-direction**

10. Self-observing capacities (psychological mindedness) 2

- Limited curiosity and reflectiveness during evaluation.

11. Capacity to construct and use internal standards and ideals 3

- SCORS-G, capacity for emotional investments in values and moral standards = 4.1 (within one standard deviation of the mean); no moral concerns raised.
- SWAP-200: Heavily weighted items include "tends to be self-critical; sets unrealistically high standards for self and is intolerant of own human defects," "tends to be critical of others," and "tends to be conflicted about authority"

12. Meaning and purpose 3

- Rorschach and TAT: Multiple indicators of emotional and interpersonal constriction.

ACKNOWLEDGMENTS

The Consultants' contributions have been invaluable. The Chapter Editors wish to give particular thanks to John S. Auerbach for his extensive contributions to the whole chapter.

BIBLIOGRAPHY

Ablon, S., & Jones, E. E. (1998). How expert clinicians' prototypes of an ideal treatment correlate with outcome in psychodynamic and cognitive-behavioral therapy. *Psychotherapy Research, 8,* 71–83.

Ablon, S., & Jones, E. E. (2002). Validity of controlled clinical trials of psychotherapy: Findings from the NIMH Treatment of Depression Collaborative Research Program. *American Journal of Psychiatry, 159,* 775–783.

Ablon, S. J., & Jones, E. E. (2005). On analytic process. *Journal of the American Psychoanalytic Association, 53,* 541–568.

Ablon, J. S., Levy, R. A., & Katzenstein, T. (2006). Beyond brand names of psychotherapy: Identifying empirically supported change processes. *Psychotherapy: Theory, Research, Practice, Training, 43,* 216–231.

Ackerman, S., Clemence, A., Weatherill, R., & Hilsenroth, M. (1999). Use of the TAT in the assessment of DSM-IV Cluster B personality disorders. *Journal of Personality Assessment, 73,* 422–448.

Ackerman, S., Hilsenroth, M., Clemence, A., Weatherill, R., & Fowler, C. (2000). The effects of social cognition and object representation on psychotherapy continuation. *Bulletin of the Menninger Clinic, 64,* 386–408.

Aikins, J. W., Howes, C., & Hamilton, C. (2009). Attachment stability and the emergence of unresolved representations during adolescence. *Attachment and Human Development, 11,* 491–512.

Ainsworth, M. S., Blehar, M. C., Waters, E., & Wall, S. (1978). *Patterns of attachment: A psychological study of the Strange Situation.* Hillsdale, NJ: Erlbaum.

Albani, C., Benninghofen, D., Blaser, G., Cierpka, M., Dahlbender, R. W., Geyer, M., & Kächele, H. (1999). On the connection between affective evaluation of recollected relationship experiences and the severity of psychic impairment. *Psychotherapy Research, 9*(4), 452–467.

Albani, C., Pokorny, D., Blaser, G., Gruninger, S., Konig, S., Marschke, F., . . . Geyer, M. (2002). Reformulation of the Core Conflictual Relationship Theme (CCRT) categories: The CCRT-LU category system. *Psychotherapy Research, 12,* 319–338.

Alden, L. E., Wiggins, J. S., & Pincus, A. L. (1990). Construction of circumplex scales for the Inventory of Interpersonal Problems. *Journal of Personality Assessment, 55,* 521–536.

Allen, J., Fonagy, P., & Bateman, A. (2008). *Mentalizing in clinical practice.* Washington, DC: American Psychiatric Press.

American Psychiatric Association. (1994). *Diagnostic and statistical manual of mental disorders* (4th ed.). Washington, DC: Author.

Ammaniti, M., Fontana, A., Clarkin, A., Clarkin, J. F., Nicolais, G., & Kernberg, O. F. (2014). Assessment of adolescent personality disorders through the Interview of Personality Organization Processes in Adolescence (IPOP-A): Clinical and theoretical implications. *Adolescent Psychiatry, 2,* 36–45.

Arbeitskreis OPD (Hrsg.). (1996). *Operationalisierte Psychodynamische Diagnostik: Grundlagen und Manual.* Bern, Switzerland: Huber.

Arbeitskreis OPD (Hrsg.). (2006). *Operationalisierte Psychodynamische Diagnostik OPD-2: Das Manual für Diagnostik und Therapieplanung.* Bern, Switzerland: Huber.

Arbeitskreis OPD-KJ (Hrsg.). (2014). *Operationalisierte Psychodynamische Diagnostik im Kindes- und Jugendalter (OPD-KJ-2): Grundlagen und Manual.* Bern, Switzerland: Huber.

Archer, R. P., & Krishnamurthy, R. (1993a). Combining the Rorschach and MMPI in the assessment of adolescents. *Journal of Personality Assessment, 60,* 132–140.

Archer, R. P., & Krishnamurthy, R. (1993b). A review of MMPI and Rorschach interrelationships in adult samples. *Journal of Personality Assessment, 61,* 277–293.

Arnevik, E., Wilberg, T., Monsen, J. T., Andrea, H., & Karterud, S. (2009). A cross-national validity study of the Severity Indices of Personality Problems (SIPP-118). *Personality and Mental Health, 3,* 41–55.

Aronow, E., Weiss, K. A., & Reznikoff, M. (2001). *A practical guide to the Thematic Apperception Test: The TAT in clinical practice.* New York: Routledge.

Azim, H., Piper, W., Segal, P., Nixon, G., & Duncan, S. (1991). The Quality of Object Relations scale. *Bulletin of the Menninger Clinic, 55,* 323–343.

Bagby, R. M., Parker, J. D. A., & Taylor, G. J. (1994a). The twenty-item Toronto Alexithymia Scale: I. Item selection and cross-validation of the factor structure. *Journal of Psychosomatic Research, 38,* 23–32.

Bagby, R. M., Parker, J. D. A., & Taylor, G. J. (1994b). The twenty-item Toronto Alexithymia Scale: II. Convergent, discriminant, and concurrent validity. *Journal of Psychosomatic Research, 38,* 33–40.

Bagby, R. M., Taylor, G. J., Parker, J. D., & Dickens, S. E. (2006). The development of the Toronto Structured Interview for Alexithymia: Item selection, factor structure, reliability and concurrent validity. *Psychotherapy and Psychosomatics, 75,* 25–39.

Bakermans-Kranenburg, M. J., & van IJzendoorn, M. (2009). The first 10,000 Adult Attachment Interviews: Distributions of adult attachment representations in clinical and non-clinical groups.

Attachment and Human Development, 11, 223–263.

Barber, J. P., Foltz, C., & Weinryb, R. M. (1998). The Central Relationship Questionnaire: Initial report. *Journal of Counseling Psychology, 45,* 131–142.

Barkham, M., Hardy, G. E., & Startup, M. (1996). The IIP-32: A short version of the Inventory of Interpersonal Problems. *British Journal of Clinical Psychology, 35*(Pt. 1), 21–35.

Barkham, M., Rees, A., Stiles, W. B., Hardy, G. E., & Shapiro, D. A. (2002). Dose–effect relations for psychotherapy of mild depression: A quasi-experimental comparison of effects of 2, 8, and 16 sessions. *Psychotherapy Research, 12,* 263–274.

Barron, F. (1953). An ego-strength scale which predicts response to psychotherapy. *Journal of Consulting Psychology, 17,* 327–333.

Beck, A. T., Steer, R. A., & Brown, G. K. (1996). *Beck Depression Inventory–II (BDI-II).* San Antonio, TX: Psychological Corporation.

Beck, S., & Perry, J. C. (2008). The measurement of interview structure in five types of psychiatric and psychotherapeutic interviews. *Psychiatry: Interpersonal and Biological Processes, 71,* 219–233.

Beck, S. J. (1937). *Introduction to the Rorschach method: A manual of personality study.* New York: American Orthopsychiatric Association.

Bender, D. S., Morey, L. C., & Skodol, A. E. (2011). Toward a model for assessing level of personality functioning in DSM-5: Part I. A review of theory and methods. *Journal of Personality Assessment, 93,* 332–346.

Benecke, C., Bock, A., Wieser, E., Tschiesner, R., Lockmann, M. Kuspert, F., . . . Steinmayr-Gensluckner, M. (2011). Reliabilität und Validität der OPD-KJ-Achsen Struktur und Konflikt. *Praxis der Kinderpsychologie und Kinderpsychiatrie, 60,* 60–73.

Berant, E., Newborn, M., & Orgler, S. (2008). Convergence of Rorschach scales and self-report indexes of psychological distress: The moderating role of self-disclosure. *Journal of Personality Assessment, 90,* 36–743.

Bernecker, S. L., Levy, H. K., & Ellison, W. D. (2014). A meta-analysis of the relation between adult attachment style and the working alliance. *Psychotherapy Research, 24,* 12–24.

Berney, S., de Roten, Y., Beretta, V., Kramer, U., & Despland, J. N. (2014). Identifying psychotic defenses in a clinical interview. *Journal of Clinical Psychology, 70,* 428–439.

Besser, A., & Blatt, S. J. (2007). Identity consolidation and internalizing and externalizing problem behaviors in early adolescence. *Psychoanalytic Psychology, 24,* 126–149.

Betan, E., Heim, A. K., Zittel Conklin, C., & Westen, D. (2005). Countertransference phenomena and personality pathology in clinical practice: An empirical investigation. *American Journal of Psychiatry, 5,* 890–898.

Blagov, P. S., Bi, W., Shedler, J., & Westen, D. (2012). The Shedler–Westen Assessment Procedure (SWAP): Evaluating psychometric questions about its reliability, validity, and impact of its fixed score distribution. *Assessment, 19,* 370–382.

Blais, M. A., Baity, M. R., & Hopwood, C. J. (Eds.). (2010). *Clinical applications of the Personality Assessment Inventory.* New York: Routledge.

Blais, M. A., Conboy, C. A., Wilcox, N., & Norman, D. K. (1996). An empirical study of the DSM-IV Defensive Functioning Scale in personality disordered patients. *Comprehensive Psychiatry, 37,* 435–440.

Blais, M. A., & Hopwood, C. J. (2010). Personality focused assessment with the PAI. In M. A. Blais, M. R. Baity, & C. J. Hopwood (Eds.), *Clinical applications of the Personality Assessment Inventory* (pp. 195–210). New York: Routledge.

Blais, M. A., Lenderking, W. R., Baer, L., deLorell, A., Peets, K., Leahy, L., & Burns, C. (1999). Development and initial validation of a brief mental health outcome measure. *Journal of Personality Assessment, 73,* 359–373.

Blais, M. A., Malone, J., Stein, M., Slavin-Mulford, J., Renna, M., & Sinclair, S. J. (2013). Treatment as usual (TAU) for depression: A comparison of psychotherapy, pharmacotherapy and combined treatment at a large academic medical center. *Journal of Psychotherapy, 50,* 110–118.

Blais, M. A., Sinclair, S., Baity, M., Worth, J., Weiss, A., Ball, L., & Herman, J. (2011). Measuring outcomes in adult outpatient psychiatry, *Clinical Psychology and Psychotherapy, 19*(3), 203–213.

Blatt, S. J. (1974). Levels of object representation in anaclitic and introjective depression. *Psychoanalytic Study of the Child, 29,* 107–157.

Blatt, S. J. (2008). *Polarities of experience: Relatedness and self-definition in personality development, psychopathology, and the therapeutic process.* Washington, DC: American Psychological Association.

Blatt, S. J., & Auerbach, J. S. (2001). Mental representation, severe psychopathology, and the therapeutic process: Affect and self-reflexivity in borderline and schizophrenic patients. *Journal of the American Psychoanalytic Association, 49,* 113–159.

Blatt, S. J., Auerbach, J. S., & Aryan, M. (1998). Representational structures and the therapeutic process. In R. F. Bornstein & J. M. Masling (Eds.), *Empirical studies of psychoanalytic theories: Vol. 8. Empirical investigations of the therapeutic hour* (pp. 63–107). Washington, DC: American Psychological Association.

Blatt, S. J., Bers, S. A., & Schaffer, C. E. (1993). *The assessment of self.* Unpublished research manual, Yale University.

Blatt, S. J., & Blass, R. (1996). Relatedness and self definition: A dialectic model of personality development. In G. G. Noam & K. W. Fischer (Eds.), *Development and vulnerabilities in close relationships* (pp. 309–338). Hillsdale, NJ: Erlbaum.

Blatt, S. J., Chevron, E. S., Quinlan, D. M., Schaffer, C. E., & Wein, S. (1988). *The assessment of qualitative and structural dimensions of object representations* (rev. ed.). Unpublished research manual, Yale University.

Blatt, S. J., D'Afflitti, J. P., & Quinlan, D. M. (1976). Experiences of depression in normal young adults. *Journal of Personality Assessment, 85,* 383–389.

Blatt, S. J., & Shichman, S. (1983). Two primary configurations of psychopathology. *Psychoanalysis and Contemporary Thought, 6,* 187–254.

Blatt, S. J., Wein, S. J., Chevron, E. S., & Quinlan, D. M. (1979). Parental representations and depression in normal young adults. *Journal of Abnormal Psychology, 88,* 388–397.

Block, J. (1978). *The Q-sort method in personality assessment and psychiatric research.* Palo Alto, CA: Consulting Psychologists Press. (Original work published 1961)

Bøgwald, K.-P., & Dahlbender, R. W. (2004). Procedures for testing some aspects of the content validity of the Psychodynamic Functioning Scale and the Global Assessment of Functioning Scale. *Psychotherapy Research, 14,* 453–468.

Bond, M., & Perry, C. J. (2004). Long-term changes in defense styles with psychodynamic psychotherapy for depressive, anxiety, and personality disorders. *American Journal of Psychiatry, 161,* 1665–1671.

Bornstein, R. F. (2002). A process dissociation approach to objective–projective test score interrelationships. *Journal of Personality Assessment, 78,* 47–68.

Bornstein, R. F. (2009). Heisenberg, Kandinsky, and the heteromethod convergence problem: Lessons from within and beyond psychology. *Journal of Personality Assessment, 91,* 1–8.

Bornstein, R. F. (2010). Psychoanalytic theory as a unifying framework for 21st century personality assessment. *Psychoanalytic Psychology, 27,* 133–152.

Bornstein, R. F. (2011). From symptom to process: How the PDM alters goals and strategies in psychological assessment. *Journal of Personality Assessment, 93,* 142–150.

Bornstein, R. F. (2012). Rorschach score validation as a model for 21st century personality assessment. *Journal of Personality Assessment, 94,* 26–38.

Bornstein, R. F., & Gordon, R. M. (2012). What do practitioners want in a diagnostic taxonomy?: Comparing the PDM with DSM and ICD. *Division/Review: Quarterly Psychoanalytic Forum, 6,* 35.

Bornstein, R. F., & Masling, J. M. (Eds.). (2005). *Scoring the Rorschach: Seven validated systems.* Mahwah, NJ: Erlbaum.

Bowlby, J. (1977). The making and breaking of affectional bonds: I. Aetiology and psychopathology in the light of attachment theory. *British Journal of Psychiatry, 130,* 201–210.

Bowlby, J. (1980). *Attachment and loss: Vol. 3. Loss: Sadness and depression.* New York: Basic Books.

Bradley, R., Heim, A. K., & Westen, D. (2005). Transference patterns in the psychotherapy of personality disorders: empirical investigation. *British Journal of Psychiatry, 186,* 342–349.

Bram, A. D., & Peebles, M. J. (2014). *Psychological testing that matters: Creating a road map for effective treatment.* Washington, DC: American Psychological Association.

Bram, A. D., & Yalof, J. (2014). Quantifying complexity: Personality assessment and its relationship with psychoanalysis. *Psychoanalytic Inquiry, 35,* 74–97.

Buchheim, A., Erk, S., George, C., Kaechele, H., Ruchsow, M., Spitzer, M., & Walter, H. (2006). Measuring attachment representation in an fMRI environment: A pilot study. *Psychopathology, 39,* 144–152.

Buchheim, A., & George, C. (2011). Attachment disorganization in borderline personality disorder and anxiety disorder. In J. Solomon & C. George (Eds.), *Disorganized attachment and caregiving* (pp. 343–382). New York: Guilford Press.

Buchheim, A., George, C., Gündel, H., Heinrichs, M., Koops, E., O'Connor, M.-F., & Pokorny, D. (2009). Oxytocin enhances the experience of attachment security. *Psychoneuroendochronology, 34,* 1417–1422.

Buchheim, A., Labek, K., Walter, S., & Viviani, R. (2013). A clinical case study of a psychoanalytic psychotherapy monitored with functional neuroimaging. *Frontiers in Human Neuroscience, 7,* 677.

Butcher, J. N., Dahlstrom, W. G., Graham, J. R., Tellegen, A., & Kaemmer, B. (1989). *MMPI-2: Manual for administration and scoring.* Minneapolis: University of Minnesota Press.

Butcher, J. N., & Williams, C. L. (2009). Personality assessment with the MMPI-2: Historical roots, international adaptations, and current challenges. *Applied Psychology: Health and Well-Being, 1*(1), 105–135.

Butcher, J. N., Williams, C. L., Graham, J. R., Tellegen, A., Ben-Porath, Y. S., Archer, R. P., & Kaemmer, B. (1992). *Manual for administration, scoring, and interpretation of the Minnesota Multiphasic Personality Inventory for Adolescents: MMPI-A.* Minneapolis: University of Minnesota Press.

Calabrese, M. L., Farber, B. A., & Westen, D. (2005). The relationship of adult attachment constructs to object relational patterns of representing the self and others. *Journal of the American Academy of Psychoanalysis and Dynamic Psychiatry, 33,* 513–530.

Castonguay, L. G., & Hill, C. E. (Eds.). (2007). *Insight in psychotherapy.* Washington, DC: American Psychological Association.

Charitat, H. (1996). *Evaluation de lapersonnalite. Traduction et validation du KAPP: Profd Psychodynamique de Karolinska.* Unpublished doctoral dissertation, Universite Paul Sabatier, Toulouse, France.

Cierpka, M., Rudolf, G., Grande, T., & Stasch, M. (2007). Operationalized Psychodynamic Diagnostics (OPD): Clinical relevance, reliability and validity. *Psychopathology, 40,* 209–220.

Cogan, R., & Porcerelli, J. H. (2004). Personality pathology, adaptive functioning, and strengths at the beginning and end of psychoanalysis. *Journal of the American Psychoanalytic Association, 52,* 1229–1230.

Cogan, R., & Porcerelli, J. H. (2005). Clinician reports of personality pathology of patients beginning and patients ending psychoanalysis. *Psychology and Psychotherapy: Theory, Research and Practice, 78,* 235–248.

Cogswell, A. (2008). Explicitly rejecting an implicit dichotomy: Integrating two approaches to assessing dependency. *Journal of Personality Assessment, 90,* 26–35.

Colli, A., & Lingiardi, V. (2009). The Collaborative Interactions Scale: A new transcript-based method for the assessment of therapeutic alliance ruptures and resolutions in psychotherapy. *Psychotherapy Research, 19*(6), 718–734.

Colli, A., Tanzilli, A., Dimaggio, G., & Lingiardi, V. (2014). Patient personality and therapist response: An empirical investigation. *American Journal of Psychiatry, 171,* 102–108.

Colli, A., Tanzilli, A., Gualco, I., & Lingiardi, V. (2016). Empirically derived relational pattern prototypes in the treatment of personality disorders. *Psychopathology, 49*(5), 364–373.

Connolly, M. B., & Strupp, H. H. (1996). Cluster analysis of patient reported psychotherapy outcomes. *Psychotherapy Research, 6,* 30–42.

Cramer, P. (1991). *The development of defense mechanisms: Theory, research, and assessment.* New York: Springer-Verlag.

Cramer, P. (1998). Freshman to senior year: A follow up study of identity, narcissism and defense mechanisms. *Journal of Research in Personality, 32,* 156–172.

Cramer, P. (2000). Defense mechanisms in psychology today: Mechanisms for adaptation. *American Psychologist, 55,* 637–646.

Cramer, P. (2002). The study of defense mechanisms: Gender implications. In R. F. Bornstein & J. M. E. Masling (Eds.), *The psychodynamics of gender and gender role* (pp. 81–127). Washington, DC: American Psychological Association.

Cramer, P. (2006). *Protecting the self: Defense mechanisms in action.* New York: Guilford Press.

Cramer, P. (2012). Psychological maturity and change in adult defense mechanisms. *Journal of Research in Personality, 46,* 306–316.

Cramer, P., & Blatt, S. J. (1990). Use of the TAT to measure change in defense mechanisms following intensive psychotherapy. *Journal of Personality Assessment, 54,* 236–251.

Cramer, P., & Kelly, F. D. (2004). Defense mechanisms in adolescent conduct disorder and adjustment reaction. *Journal of Nervous and Mental Disease, 192*(2), 139–145.

Curtis, J. T., & Silberschatz, G. (2005). The assessment of pathogenic beliefs. In G. Silberschatz (Ed.), *Transformative relationships* (pp. 69–92). New York: Routledge.

Curtis, J. T., & Silberschatz, G. (2007). Plan Formulation Method. In T. D. Eells (Ed.), *Handbook of psychotherapy case formulation* (2nd ed., pp. 198–220). New York: Guilford Press.

Curtis, J. T., Silberschatz, G., Sampson, H., & Weiss, J. (1994). The Plan Formulation Method. *Psychotherapy Research, 4,* 197–207.

Cogswell, A. (2008). Explicitly rejecting an implicit dichotomy: Integrating two approaches to assessing dependency. *Journal of Personality Assessment, 90,* 26–35.

DeFife, J. A., Drill, R., Nakash, O., & Westen, D. (2010). Agreement between clinician and patient ratings of adaptive functioning and developmental history. *American Journal of Psychiatry, 167,* 1472–1478.

DeFife, J. A., Goldberg, M., & Westen, D. (2015). Dimensional assessment of self- and interpersonal functioning in adolescents: Implications for DSM-5's general definition of personality disorder. *Journal of Personality Disorders, 29*(2), 248–260.

DeFife, J. A., & Hilsenroth, M. J. (2005). Clinical utility of the Defensive Functioning Scale in the assessment of depression. *Journal of Nervous and Mental Disease, 193,* 176–182.

DeFife, J. A., Malone, J. C., DiLallo, J., & Westen, D. (2013). Assessing adolescent personality disorders with the Shedler–Westen Assessment Procedure for Adolescents. *Clinical Psychology: Science and Practice, 20,* 393–407.

Detert, N. B., Llewelyn, S. P., Hardy, G. E., Barkham, M., & Stiles, W. B. (2006). Assimilation in good- and poor-outcome cases of very brief psychotherapy for mild depression: An initial comparison. *Psychotherapy Research, 16,* 393–407.

DeWitt, K. N., Hartley, D. E., Rosenberg, S. E., Zilberg, N. J., & Wallerstein, R. S. (1991). Scales of Psychological Capacities: Development of an assessment approach. *Psychoanalysis and Contemporary Thought, 14,* 343–361.

DeWitt, K. N., Milbrath, C., & Wallerstein, R. S. (1999). Scales of Psychological Capacities: Support for a measure of structural change. *Psychoanalysis and Contemporary Thought, 22,* 453–480.

Di Giuseppe, M. G., Perry, J. C., Petraglia, J., Janzen, J., & Lingiardi, V. (2014). Development of a Q-sort version of the Defense Mechanism Rating Scales (DMRS-Q) for clinical use. *Journal of Clinical Psychology, 70,* 452–465.

Diamond, D., Blatt, S. J., Stayner, D., & Kaslow, N. (1991). *Self–other differentiation of object representations.* Unpublished research manual, Yale University.

Diamond, D., Clarkin, J. F., Levine, H., Levy, K., Foelsch, P., & Yeomans, F. (1999). Borderline conditions and attachment: A preliminary report. *Psychoanalytic Inquiry, 19,* 831–884.

Diamond, D., & Dozier, M. (1990). Attachment organization and treatment use for adults with serious psychopathological disorders. *Development and Psychopathology, 2,* 47–60.

Diamond, D., Kaslow, N., Coonerty, S. & Blatt, S. J. (1990). Change in separation–individuation and intersubjectivity in long-term treatment. *Psychoanalytic Psychology, 7,* 363–397.

Diamond, D., Stovall-McClough, C., Clarkin, J., & Levy, K. N. (2003). Patient–therapist attachment in the treatment of borderline personality disorder. *Bulletin of the Menninger Clinic, 67,* 227–259.

Doering, S., Burgmer, M., Heuft, G., Menke, D., Bäumer, B., Lübking, M., . . . Schneider, G. (2014) Diagnosing personality functioning: Validity of the Operationalized Psychodynamic Diagnosis (OPD-2) Axis IV: Structure. *Psychopathology, 47,* 185–193.

Dozier, M., Cue, K. L., & Barnett, L. (1994). Clinicians as caregivers: The role of attachment organization in treatment. *Journal of Consulting and Clinical Psychology, 62,* 793–800.

Drake, L. E. (1946). A social I.E. scale for the MMPI. *Journal of Applied Psychology, 30,* 51–54.

Drapeau, M., & Perry, J. C. (2009). The Core Conflictual Relationship Themes (CCRT) in borderline personality disorder. *Journal of Personality Disorders, 23,* 425–431.

Eagle, M. (2003). Clinical implications of attachment theory. *Psychoanalytic Inquiry, 23,* 12–27.

Eames, V., & Roth, A. (2000). Patient attachment orientation and the early working alliance: A study of patient and therapist reports of alliance quality and ruptures. *Psychotherapy Research, 10,* 421–434.

Eells, T. D. (Ed.). (2007). *Handbook of psychotherapy case formulation* (2nd ed.). New York: Guilford Press.

Eells, T. D. (2009). Contemporary themes in case formulation. In P. Sturmey (Ed.), *Clinical case formulation: Varieties of approaches* (pp. 293–315). Hoboken, NJ: Wiley.

Ehrenreich, J. H. (1990). Quantitative studies of responses elicited by selected TAT cards. *Psychological Reports, 67,* 15–18.

Ehrenthal, J. C., Dinger, U., Horsch, L., Komo-Lang, M., Klinkerfuß, M., Grande, T., & Schauenburg, H. (2012). Der OPD-Strukturfragebogen (OPD-SF): Erste Ergebnisse zu Reliabilität und Validität. *Psychotherapie Psychosomatik Medizinische Psychologie, 62,* 25–32.

Erdelyi, M. H. (2006). The unified theory of repression. *Behavioral and Brain Sciences, 29,* 499–511.

Evans, C. (2012). The CORE-OM (Clinical Outcomes in Routine Evaluation) and its derivatives. *Integrating Science and Practice, 2*(2). Retrieved from *www.ordrepsy.qc.ca/pdf/2012_11_01_Integrating_SandP_Dossier_02_Evans_En.pdf.*

Evans, C., Connel, J., Barkham, M., Margison, F., McGrath, G., Mellor-Clark, J., & Audin, K. (2002). Towards a standardised brief outcome measure: Psychometric properties and utility of the CORE-OM. *British Journal of Psychiatry, 180,* 51–60.

Exner, J. E. (1969). *The Rorschach systems.* New York: Grune & Stratton.

Exner, J. E. (2003). *The Rorschach: A comprehensive system: Vol. 1. Basic foundations and principles of interpretation* (4th ed.). New York: Wiley.

Exner, J. E., & Erdberg, P. (2005). *The Rorschach: A comprehensive system: Vol. 2. Advanced interpretation* (3rd ed.). Hoboken, NJ: Wiley.

Falkenstrom, F., Solbakken, O. A., Moller, C., Lech, B., Sandell, R., & Holmqvist, R. (2014). Reflective functioning, affect consciousness, and mindfulness: Are these different functions? *Psychoanalytic Psychology, 31,* 26–40.

Feenstra, D. J., Hutsebaut, J., Verheul, R., & Busschbach, J. J. V. (2011). Severity Index of Personality Problems (SIPP-118) in adolescents: Reliability and validity. *Psychological Assessment, 23,* 646–655.

Finn, S. (2011). Use of the Adult Attachment Projective Picture System (AAP) in the middle of a long-term psychotherapy. *Journal of Personality Assessment, 93,* 427–433.

Fonagy, P., Gergely, G., Jurist, E. L., & Target, M. (2002). *Affect regulation, mentalization, and the development of the self.* New York: Other Press.

Fonagy, P., Gergely, G., & Target, M. (2007). The parent–infant dyad and the construction of the subjective self. *Journal of Child Psychology and Psychiatry, 48,* 288–328.

Fonagy, P., Leigh, T., Steele, M., Steele, H., Kennedy, R., Mattoon, G., . . . Gerber, A. (1996). The relation of attachment status, psychiatric classification, and response to psychotherapy. *Journal of Consulting and Clinical Psychology, 64,* 22–31.

Fonagy, P., Target, M., Steele, H., & Steele, M. (1998). *Reflective-functioning manual: Version 5 for application to the Adult Attachment Interview.* Unpublished manual, University College London.

Fowler, C., Ackerman, S., Speanburg, S., Bailey, A., Blagys, M., & Conklin, A. C. (2004). Personality and symptom change in treatment-refractory inpatients: Evaluation of the phase model of change using the phase model of change using Rorschach, TAT and DSM-IV Axis V. *Journal of Personality Assessment, 83*, 306–322.

Fowler, J. C., & DeFife, J. A. (2012). Quality of object representations related to service utilization in a long-term residential treatment center. *Psychotherapy, 49*(3), 418–422.

Frank, L. K. (1939). Projective methods for the study of personality. *Journal of Psychology, 8*, 389–413.

Gazzillo, F., Genova, F., & Lingiardi, V. (2016). *Psychodynamic Diagnostic Prototypes–2 (PDP-2)*. Unpublished manuscript, Sapienza University of Rome.

Gazzillo, F., Lingiardi, V., & Del Corno, F. (2012). Towards the validation of three assessment instruments derived from the PDM Axis P: The Psychodynamic Diagnostic Prototypes, the Core Preoccupations Questionnaire and the Pathogenic Beliefs Questionnaire. *Bollettino di Psicologia Applicata, 265*, 1–16.

Gazzillo, F., Lingiardi, V., Del Corno, F., Genova, F., Bornstein, R., Gordon, R., & McWilliams, N. (2015). Clinicians' emotional responses and PDM2 personality disorders: A clinically relevant empirical study. *Psychotherapy, 52*(2), 238–246.

Gazzillo, F., Lingiardi, V., Peloso, A., Giordani, S., Vesco, S., Zanna V., Filippucci, L., & Vicari, S. (2013). Personality subtypes in adolescents with eating disorders. *Comprehensive Psychiatry, 54*, 702–712.

Gazzillo, F., Waldron, S., Genova, F., Angeloni, F., Ristucci, C. & Lingiardi, V. (2014). An empirical investigation of analytic process: Contrasting a good and poor outcome case. *Psychotherapy, 51*, 270–282.

George, C., & Buchheim, A. (2014). Use of the Adult Attachment Projective Picture System with a severely traumatized patient: A psychodynamic perspective. *Frontiers in Psychology, 5*. 865.

George, C., Kaplan, N., & Main, M. (1984, 1985, 1996). *The Adult Attachment Interview*. Unpublished manual, University of California, Berkeley.

George, C., & West, M. (2001). The development and preliminary validation of a new measure of adult attachment: The Adult Attachment Projective. *Attachment and Human Development, 3*, 30–61.

George, C., & West, M. (2012). *The Adult Attachment Projective Picture System: Attachment theory and assessment in adults*. New York: Guilford Press.

Gieser, L., & Stein, M. I. (Eds.). (1999). *Evocative images: The Thematic Apperception Test and the art of projection*. Washington, DC: American Psychological Association.

Goldberg, L. R. (1965). Diagnosticians versus diagnostic signs: The diagnosis of psychosis versus neurosis from the MMPI. *Psychological Monographs, 79*, 1–28.

Gordon, R. M. (2001). MMPI/MMPI-2 changes in long-term psychoanalytic psychotherapy. *Issues in Psychoanalytic Psychology, 23*(1–2), 59–79.

Gordon, R. M. (2006). False assumptions about psychopathology, hysteria and the MMPI-2 restructured clinical scales. *Psychological Reports, 98*, 870–872.

Gordon, R. M. (2007, Spring). The powerful combination of the MMPI-2 and the Psychodynamic Diagnostic Manual. *Independent Practitioner*, pp. 84–85.

Gordon, R. M. (n.d.). Brief manual for the Psychodiagnostic Chart–2 (PDC-2). Available at *https://sites.google.com/site/psychodiagnosticchart*.

Gordon, R. M., Blake, A., Bornstein, R. F., Gazzillo, F., Etzi, J., Lingiardi, V., . . . Tasso, A. F. (2016). What do practitioners consider the most helpful personality taxa in understanding their patients? *Division Review: Quarterly Psychoanalytic Forum*. Retrieved from *https://divisionreview.com/uncategorized/what-do-practitioners-consider-the-most-helpful-personality-taxa-in-understanding-their-patients*.

Gordon, R. M., & Bornstein, R. F. (2012). The Psychodiagnostic Chart (PDC): A practical tool to integrate and operationalize the PDM with the ICD or DSM. Retrieved from *www.mmpi-info.com/pdm-blog/78/the-psychodiagnostic-chart-pdc-free-download*.

Gordon, R. M., Gazzillo, F., Blake, A., Bornstein, R. F., Etzi, J., Lingiardi, V., . . . Tasso, A. F. (2016). The relationship between theoretical orientation and countertransference awareness: Implications for ethical dilemmas and risk management. *Clinical Psychology and Psychotherapy, 23*(3), 236–245.

Gordon, R. M., & Stoffey, R. W. (2014). Operationalizing the Psychodynamic Diagnostic Manual: A preliminary study of the Psychodiagnostic Chart (PDC). *Bulletin of the Menninger Clinic, 78*, 1–15.

Gordon, R. M., Stoffey, R., & Bottinelli, J. (2008). MMPI-2 findings of primitive defenses in alienating parents. *American Journal of Family Therapy, 36*(3), 211–228.

Gordon, R. M., Stoffey, R. W., & Perkins, B. L. (2013). Comparing the sensitivity of the MMPI-2 clinical scales and the MMPI-RC scales to clients rated as psychotic, borderline or neurotic on the Psychodiagnostic Chart. *Psychology, 4*, 12–16.

Graham, J. R., Ben-Porath, Y. S., & McNulty, J. (1999). *Using the MMPI-2 in outpatient mental health settings*. Minneapolis: University of Minnesota Press.

Grande, T., Rudolf, G., Oberbracht, C., & Jakobsen,

T. (2001). Therapeutic changes beyond the symptoms: Effects of inpatient treatment in the view of the Heidelberg Structural Change Scale. *Zeitschrift für Psychosomatische Medizin und Psychotherapie, 47,* 213–233.

Grande, T., Rudolf, G., Oberbracht, C., & Pauli-Magnus, C. (2003). Progressive changes in patients' lives after psychotherapy: Which treatment effects support them? *Psychotherapy Research, 13*(1), 43–58.

Grønnerød, C. (2003). Temporal stability in the Rorschach method: A meta-analytic review. *Journal of Personality Assessment, 80*(3), 272–293.

Grønnerød, C. (2006). Reanalysis of the Grønnerød (2003) Rorschach temporal stability meta-analysis data set. *Journal of Personality Assessment, 86*(2), 222–225.

Gullestad, F. S., Johansen, M. S., Høglend, P., Karterud, S., & Wilberg, T. (2013). Mentalization as a moderator of treatment effects: Findings from a randomized clinical trial for personality disorders. *Psychotherapy Research, 23,* 674–689.

Gurtman, M. B. (2006). Interpersonal problems and the psychotherapy context: The construct validity of the Inventory of Interpersonal Problems. *Psychological Assessment, 8,* 241–255.

Gynther, M. D. (1979). Aging and personality. In J. N. Butcher (Ed.), *New developments in the use of the MMPI* (pp. 39–68). Minneapolis: University of Minnesota Press.

Haggerty, G., Blake, M., Naraine, M., Siefert, C., & Blais, M. (2010). Construct validity of the Schwartz Outcome Scale–10: Comparisons to interpersonal distress, adult attachment, alexithymia, the five factor model, romantic relationship length and ratings of childhood memories. *Clinical Psychology and Psychotherapy, 17*(1), 44–50.

Haggerty, G., Hilsenroth, M. J., & Vala-Stewart, R. (2009). Attachment and interpersonal distress: Examining the relationship between attachment styles and interpersonal problems in a clinical population. *Clinical Psychology and Psychotherapy, 16,* 1–9.

Hagtvet, K. A., & Høglend, P. (2008). Assessing precision of change scores in psychodynamic psychotherapy: A generalizability theory approach. *Measurement and Evaluation in Counseling and Development, 41,* 162–177.

Hannan, C., Lambert, M. J., Harmon, C., Nielsen, S. L., Smart, D. M., Shimokawa, K., & Sutton, S. W. (2005). A lab test and algorithms for identifying patients at risk for treatment failure. *Journal of Clinical Psychology, 61*(2), 155–163.

Hatcher, R. L., & Gillaspy, J. A. (2006). Development and validation of a revised short version of the Working Alliance Inventory (WAI-SR). *Psychotherapy Research, 16,* 12–25.

Hathaway, J. C., & McKinley, S. R. (1943). *Manual for the Minnesota Multiphasic Personality Inventory.* New York: Psychological Corporation.

Haviland, M. G., Warren, W. L., & Riggs, M. L. (2000). An observer scale to measure alexithymia. *Psychosomatics, 41,* 385–392.

Heck, S. A., & Pincus, A. L. (2001). Agency and communion in the structure of parental representations. *Journal of Personality Assessment, 76,* 180–184.

Hersoug, A. G., Ulberg, R., & Høglend, P. (2014). When is transference work useful in psychodynamic psychotherapy?: Main results of the First Experimental Study of Transference (FEST). *Contemporary Psychoanalysis, 50,* 156–174.

Hesse, E. (1996). Discourse, memory, and the Adult Attachment Interview: A note with emphasis on the emerging cannot classify category. *Infant Mental Health Journal, 17,* 4–11.

Hesse, E. (2008). The Adult Attachment Interview: Protocol, methods of analysis, and empirical studies. In J. Cassidy & P. R. Shaver (Eds.), *Handbook of attachment: Theory, research, and clinical applications* (2nd ed., pp. 552–598). New York: Guilford Press.

Hilsenroth, M. J., Ackerman, S., & Blagys, M. (2001). Evaluating the phase model of change during short-term psychodynamic psychotherapy. *Psychotherapy Research, 11,* 29–47.

Hilsenroth, M. J., Blagys, M. D., Ackerman, S. J., Bonge, D. R., & Blais, M. D. (2005). Measuring psychodynamic-interpersonal and cognitive-behavioral techniques: Development of a comparative psychotherapy process scale. *Psychotherapy: Theory, Research, Practice, Training, 42,* 340–356.

Hilsenroth, M. J., & Stricker, G. (2004). A consideration of challenges to psychological assessment instruments used in forensic settings: Rorschach as exemplar. *Journal of Personality Assessment, 83,* 141–152.

Høglend, P. (1993). Transference interpretations and long-term change after dynamic psychotherapy of brief to moderate length. *American Journal of Psychotherapy, 47,* 494–507.

Høglend, P. (1995). *Dynamic Scales: Manual.* Oslo: Department of Psychiatry, University of Oslo.

Høglend, P. (2004). Analysis of transference in dynamic psychotherapy: A review of empirical research. *Canadian Journal of Psychoanalysis, 12,* 280–300.

Høglend, P., Amlo, S., Marble, A., Bøgwald, K. P., Sorbye, O., Sjaastad, M. C., & Heyerdahl, O. (2006). Analysis of the patient–therapist relationship in dynamic psychotherapy: An experimental study of transference interpretations. *American Journal of Psychiatry, 163,* 1739–1746.

Høglend, P., Bøgwald, K. P., Amlo, S., Heyerdahl, O., Sørbye, Ø., Marble, A., . . . Bentsen, H. (2000).

Assessment of change in dynamic psychotherapy. *Journal of Psychotherapy Practice and Research, 9,* 190–199.

Høglend, P., Bøgwald, K. P., Amlo, S., Marble, A., Sjaastad, M. C., Sørbye, Ø., . . . Ulberg, R. (2008). Transference interpretations in dynamic psychotherapy: Do they really yield sustained effects? *American Journal of Psychiatry, 165,* 763–771.

Høglend, P., Hersoug, A. G., Bøgwald, K. P., Amlo, S., Marble, A., Sørbye, Ø., . . . Crits-Christoph, P. (2011). Effects of transference work in the context of therapeutic alliance and quality of object relations. *Journal of Consulting and Clinical Psychology, 79,* 697–706.

Honos-Webb, L., Stiles, W. B., & Greenberg, L. S. (2003). A method of rating assimilation in psychotherapy based on markers of change. *Journal of Counseling Psychology, 50,* 189–198.

Hooper, L., Stockton, P., Krupnick, J., & Green, B. (2011). Development, use, and psychometric properties of the Trauma History Questionnaire. *Journal of Loss and Trauma, 16,* 258–283.

Hopwood, C. J., Blais, M. A., & Baity, M. R. (2010). Introduction. In M. A. Blais, M. R. Baity, & C. J. Hopwood (Eds.), *Clinical applications of the Personality Assessment Inventory* (pp. 1–12). New York: Routledge.

Hopwood, C. J., & Bornstein, R. F. (Eds.). (2014). *Multimethod clinical assessment.* New York: Guilford Press.

Horowitz, L. M., Alden, L. E., Wiggins, J. S., & Pincus, A. L. (2000). *Inventory of Interpersonal Problems manual.* San Antonio, TX: Psychological Corporation.

Horowitz, L. M., Rosenberg, S. E., Baer, B. A., Ureño, G., & Villaseñor, V.S. (1988). Inventory of Interpersonal Problems: Psychometric properties and clinical applications. *Journal of Consulting and Clinical Psychology, 56,* 885–892.

Horvath, A. O. (1982). *Working Alliance Inventory (Revised).* Unpublished manuscript, Simon Fraser University, Burnaby, British Columbia, Canada.

Horvath, A. O., & Bedi, R. P. (2002). The alliance. In J. Norcross (Ed.), *Psychotherapy relations that work.* Oxford, UK: Oxford University Press.

Horvath, A. O., & Greenberg, L. S. (1989). Development and validation of the Working Alliance Inventory. *Journal of Counseling Psychology, 36,* 223–233.

Horvath, A. O., & Greenberg, L. S. (1986). Development of the Working Alliance Inventory. In L. S. Greenberg & W. M. Pinsoff (Eds.), *The psychotherapeutic process: A research handbook* (pp. 529–556). New York: Guilford Press.

Horvath, A. O., & Greenberg, L. S. (Eds.). (1994). *The working alliance: Theory, research, and practice.* New York: Wiley.

Horvath, A. O., & Symonds, B. D. (1991). Relation between working alliance and outcome in psychotherapy: A meta-analysis. *Journal of Counseling Psychology, 38,* 139–149.

Hörz, S., Clarkin, J. F., Stern, B. L., & Caligor, E. (2012). The Structured Interview of Personality Organisation (STIPO): An instrument to assess severity and change of personality pathology. In R. Levy, S. Ablon, & H. Kächele (Eds.), *Psychodynamic psychotherapy research* (pp. 571–592). New York: Humana Press.

Huber, D., Brandl, T., & Klug, G. (2004). The Scales of Psychological Capacities (SPC): Measuring beyond symptoms. *Psychotherapy Research, 14,* 89–106.

Huber, D., Henrich, G., & Klug, G. (2005). The Scales of Psychological Capacities: Measuring change in psychic structure. *Psychotherapy Research, 15,* 445–456.

Huber, D., Henrich, G., & Klug, G. (2013). Moderators of change in psychoanalytic, psychodynamic and cognitive behavioral therapy. *Journal of the American Psychoanalytic Association, 61*(3), 585–589.

Hughes, J., & Barkham, M. (2005). Scoping the inventory of interpersonal problems, its derivatives and short forms: 1988–2004. *Clinical Psychology and Psychotherapy, 12,* 475–496.

Hunsley, J., & Mash, E. J. (2008). *A guide to assessments that work.* New York: Oxford University Press.

Hunsley, J., & Mash, E. J. (2014). Evidence based assessment. In D. H. Barlow (Ed.), *The Oxford handbook of clinical psychology* (pp. 76–97). New York: Oxford University Press.

Huprich, S. K. (Ed.). (2006). *Rorschach assessment of the personality disorders.* Mahwah, NJ: Erlbaum.

Huprich, S. K., Auerbach, J. S., Porcerelli, J. H., & Bupp, L. L. (2016a). Sidney Blatt's Object Relations Inventory: Contributions and future directions. *Journal of Personality Assessment, 98,* 30–43.

Huprich, S. K., & Greenberg, R. P. (2003). Advances in the assessment of object relations in the 1990s. *Clinical Psychology Review, 23,* 665–698.

Huprich, S., Lingiardi, V., McWilliams, N., Bornstein, R. F., Gazzillo, F., & Gordon, R. M. (2015). The *Psychodynamic Diagnostic Manual (PDM)* and the *PDM-2*: Opportunities to significantly affect the profession. *Psychoanalytic Inquiry, 35,* 60–73.

Huprich, S. K., Pouliot, G. S., Nelson, S. M., Pouliot, S. K., Porcerelli, J. H., Cawood, C. D., & Albright, J. J. (2016b). Factor structure of the Assessment of Qualitative and Structural Dimensions of Object Representations (AOR) scale. *Journal of Personality Assessment. 97,* 605–615.

Jacobson, N. S., & Truax, P. (1991). Clinical significance: A statistical approach to defining meaningful change in psychotherapy research. *Journal of Consulting and Clinical Psychology, 59,* 12–19.

Jenkins, S. R. (2008). *A handbook of clinical scoring*

systems for the thematic apperceptive techniques. New York: Taylor & Francis.

Jones, E. E. (2000). *Therapeutic action: A guide to psychoanalytic therapy.* Northvale, NJ: Aronson.

Jones, E. E., Hall, S. A., & Parke, L. A. (1991). The process of change: The Berkeley psychotherapy research group. In L. Beutler & M. Crago (Eds.), *Psychotherapy research: An international review of programmatic studies* (pp. 98–107). Washington, DC: American Psychological Association.

Jones, E. E., & Pulos, S. M. (1993). Comparing the process in psychodynamic and cognitive-behavioral therapies. *Journal of Consulting and Clinical Psychology, 61*(2), 306–316.

Jones, E. E., & Windholz, M. (1990). The psychoanalytic case study: Toward a method for systematic inquiry. *Journal of the American Psychoanalytic Association, 39,* 985–1016.

Josephs, L., Sanders, A., & Gorman, B. S. (2014). Therapeutic interaction with an older personality disordered patient. *Psychodynamic Psychiatry, 42,* 151–172.

Katznelson, H. (2014). Reflective functioning: A review. *Clinical Psychology Review, 34*(2), 107–117.

Kernberg, O. F. (1984). *Severe personality disorders: Psychotherapeutic strategies.* New Haven, CT: Yale University Press.

Klopfer, B. (1937). The present status of the theoretical developments of the Rorschach method. *Rorschach Research Exchange, 1,* 142–147.

Kopta, S. M., Howard, K. I., Lowry, J. L., & Beutler, L. E. (1994). Patterns of symptomatic recovery in psychotherapy. *Journal of Consulting and Clinical Psychology, 62,* 1009–1016.

Lambert, M. J. (2010). *Prevention of treatment failure: The use of measuring, monitoring, and feedback in clinical practice.* Washington, DC: American Psychological Association.

Lambert, M. J., Burlingame, G. M., Umphress, V., Hansen, N. B., Vermeersch, D. A., Clouse, G. C., & Yanchar, S. C. (1996a). The reliability and validity of the Outcome Questionnaire. *Clinical Psychology and Psychotherapy, 3,* 249–258.

Lambert, M. J., Hansen, N. B., & Harmon, S. C. (2010). The OQ-45 system: Development and practical applications in health care settings. In M. Barkham, G. Hardy, & J. Mellor-Clark (Eds.), *Developing and delivering practice-based evidence: A guide for the psychological therapies* (pp. 141–154). Chichester, UK: Wiley-Blackwell.

Lambert, M., Hansen, N., Umphress, V., Lunnen, K., Okiishi, J., Burlingame, G., . . . Reisinger, C. (1996b). *Administration and scoring manual for the Outcome Questionnaire (OQ-45.2).* Wilmington, DE: American Professional Credentialing Services.

Lambert, M. J., Kahler, M., Harmon, C., Burlingame, G. M., & Shimokawa, K. (2013). *Administration and scoring manual for the Outcome Questionnaire–45.2.* Salt Lake City, UT: OQMeasures.

Leuzinger-Bohleber, M., & Fischmann, T. (2007). Application of the Scales of Psychological Capacities in a multiperspective, representative follow-up. In W. Bucci & N. Freedman (Eds.), *From impression to inquiry: A tribute to the work of Robert Wallerstein* (pp. 82–96). London: International Psychoanalytic Association.

Levy, K. N., Meehan, K. B., Kelly, K. M., Reynoso, J. S., Weber, M., Clarkin, J. F., & Kernberg, O. F. (2006). Change in attachment patterns and reflective function in a randomized control trial of transference focused psychotherapy for borderline personality disorder. *Journal of Consulting and Clinical Psychology, 74,* 1027–1040.

Levy, R., Ablon, J., Thomä, H., Kächele, H., Ackerman, J., Erhardt, I., & Seybert, C. (2012). A specimen session of psychoanalytic therapy under the lens of the Psychotherapy Process Q-Set. In R. Levy, S. Ablon, & H. Kächele (Eds.), *Psychodynamic psychotherapy research* (pp. 509–528). New York: Humana Press.

Lindfors, O., Knekt, P., & Virtala, E. (2013). Quality of object relations modifies the effectiveness of short- and long-term psychotherapy on self-concept. *Open Journal of Psychiatry, 3,* 345–350.

Lingiardi, V., Gazzillo, F., & Waldron, S. (2010). An empirically supported psychoanalysis: The case of Giovanna. *Psychoanalytic Psychology, 27,* 190–218.

Lingiardi, V., Lonati, C., Delucchi, F., Fossati, A., Vanzulli, L., & Maffei, C. (1999). Defense mechanisms and personality disorders. *Journal of Nervous and Mental Disease, 187,* 224–228.

Lingiardi, V., McWilliams, N., Bornstein, R. F., Gazzillo, F., & Gordon, R. M. (2015a). The *Psychodynamic Diagnostic Manual* Version 2 (PDM-2): Assessing patients for improved clinical practice and research. *Psychoanalytic Psychology, 32,* 94–115.

Lingiardi, V., Shedler, J., & Gazzillo, F. (2006). Assessing personality change in psychotherapy with the SWAP-200: A case study. *Journal of Personality Assessment, 86,* 23–32.

Lingiardi, V., Tanzilli, A., & Colli, A. (2015b). Does the severity of psychopathological symptoms mediate the relationship between patient personality and therapist response? *Psychotherapy, 52*(2), 228–237.

Lowyck, B., Luyten, P., Verhaest, Y., Vandeneede, B., & Vermote, R. (2013). Levels of personality functioning and their association with clinical features and interpersonal functioning in patients with personality disorders. *Journal of Personality Disorders, 27,* 320–336.

Luborsky, L., & Crits-Christoph, P. (1990). *Understanding transference: The CCRT method.* New York: Basic Books.

Luborsky, L., Crits-Christoph, P., Mintz, J., & Auerbach, A. (1988). *Who will benefit from psychotherapy?: Predicting therapeutic outcomes.* New York: Basic Books.

Lumley, M. A., Gustavson, B. J., Partridge, R. T., & Labouvie-Vief, G. (2005). Assessing alexithymia and related emotional ability constructs using multiple methods: Interrelationships among measures. *Emotion, 5,* 329–342.

Lumley, M. A., Neely, L. C., & Burger, A. J. (2007). The assessment of alexithymia in medical settings: Implications for understanding and treating health problems. *Journal of Personality Assessment, 89,* 230–246.

Luyten, P., Fonagy, P., Lowyck, B., & Vermote, R. (2012). The assessment of mentalization. In A. Bateman & P. Fonagy (Eds.), *Handbook of mentalizing in mental health practice* (pp. 43–65). Washington, DC: American Psychiatric Association.

Main, M., & Goldwyn, R. (1998). *Adult attachment scoring and classification system.* Unpublished scoring manual, University of California, Berkeley.

Main, M., Goldwyn, R., & Hesse, E. (2003). *Adult attachment scoring and classification system* (Version 7.2). Unpublished scoring manual, University of California, Berkeley.

Main, M., Hesse, E., & Goldwyn, R. (2008). Studying differences in language usage in recounting attachment history: An introduction to the AAI. In H. Steele & M. Steele (Eds.), *Clinical applications of the Adult Attachment Interview* (pp. 31–68). New York: Guilford Press.

Main, M., Kaplan, N., & Cassidy, J. (1985). Security in infancy, childhood, and adulthood: A move to the level of representation. In I. Bretherton & E. Waters (Eds.), Growing points of attachment theory and research. *Monographs of the Society for Research in Child Development, 50*(1–2, Serial No. 209), 66–104.

Main, M., & Weston, D. R. (1981). The quality of the toddler's relationship to mother and to father: Related to conflict behavior and the readiness to establish new relationships. *Child Development, 52,* 932–940.

Mavranezouli, I., Brazier, J. E., Rowen, D., & Barkham, M. (2013). Estimating a preference-based index from the Clinical Outcomes in Routine Evaluation—Outcome Measure (CORE-OM): Valuation of CORE-6D. *Medical Decision Making, 33*(3), 321–333.

Mavranezouli, I., Brazier, J. E., Young, T. A., & Barkham, M. (2011). Using Rasch analysis to form plausible health states amenable to valuation: The development of CORE-6D from a measure of common mental health problems (CORE-OM). *Quality of Life Research, 20*(3), 321–333.

McCann, J. T. (1999). *Assessing adolescents with the MACI: Using the Millon Adolescent Clinical Inventory.* New York: Wiley.

McCarthy, K. S., Connolly Gibbons, M. B., & Barber, J. P. (2008). The relation of consistency in interpersonal patterns to symptoms and functioning: An investigation using the Central Relationship Questionnaire. *Journal of Counseling Psychology, 55,* 346–358.

McClelland, D. C., Koestner, R., & Weinberger, J. (1989). How do self-attributed and implicit motives differ? *Psychological Review, 96,* 690–702.

McCullough, L., Kuhn, N., Andrews, S., Kaplan, A., Wolf, J., & Hurley, C. L. (2003). *Treating affect phobia: A manual of short-term dynamic psychotherapy.* New York: Guilford Press.

McKinley, J. C., Hathaway, S. R., & Meehl, P. E. (1948). The Minnesota Multiphasic Personality Inventory: VI. The K scale. *Journal of Consulting Psychology, 12,* 20–31.

Meehl, P. E. (1996). Comparative efficiency of informal (subjective, impressionistic) and formal (mechanical, algorithmic) prediction procedures: The clinical–statistical controversy. *Psychology, Public Policy, and Law, 2,* 293–323.

Meyer, G. J. (2000). The incremental validity of the Rorschach Prognostic Rating Scale over the MMPI Ego Strength Scale and IQ. *Journal of Personality Assessment, 74,* 356–370.

Meyer, G. J. (2004). The reliability of the Rorschach and TAT compared to other psychological and medical procedures: An analysis of systematically gathered evidence. In M. Hersen (Series Ed.) & M. J. Hilsenroth & D. L. Segal (Vol. Eds.), *Comprehensive handbook of psychological assessment: Vol. 2. Personality assessment* (pp. 315–342). Hoboken, NJ: Wiley.

Meyer, G. J., & Handler, L. (1997). The ability of the Rorschach to predict subsequent outcome: A meta-analysis of the Rorschach Prognostic Rating Scale. *Journal of Personality Assessment, 69,* 1–38.

Meyer, G. J., Viglione, D. J., Mihura, J. L., Erard, R. E., & Erdberg, P. (2011). *Rorschach Performance Assessment System: Administration, coding, interpretation, and technical manual.* Toledo, OH: Rorschach Performance Assessment System.

Mihura, J. L., Meyer, G. J., Dumitrascu, N., & Bombel, G. (2013). The validity of individual Rorschach variables: Systematic reviews and meta-analyses of the Comprehensive System. *Psychological Bulletin, 139,* 548–605.

Millon, T. (2011). *Disorders of personality: Introducing a DSM/ICD spectrum from normal to abnormal* (3rd ed.). Hoboken, NJ: Wiley.

Millon, T., Grossman, S., & Millon, C. (2015). *Millon Clinical Multiaxial Inventory–IV (MCMI-IV).* Minneapolis, MN: Pearson Assessments.

Millon, T., Millon, C., Davis, R., & Grossman, S. (2006a). *MCMI-III manual* (rev. ed.). Minneapolis, MN: Pearson Assesments.

Millon, T., Millon, C., Davis, R., & Grossman, S. (2006b). The Millon Adolescent Clinical Inventory (MACI). Minneapolis, MN: Pearson Assessments.

Millon, T., Tringone, R., Millon, C., & Grossman, S. (2005). *Millon Pre-Adolescent Clinical Inventory manual.* Minneapolis, MN: Pearson Assessments.

Morey, L. C. (1991, 1996). *An interpretive guide to the Personality Assessment Inventory (PAI).* Odessa, FL: Psychological Assessment Resources.

Morey, L. C. (2007). *The Personality Assessment Inventory professional manual.* Lutz, FL: Psychological Assessment Resources.

Morey, L. C., & Ambwani, S. (2008). The Personality Assessment Inventory. In G. Boyle, G. Matthews, & D. H. Saklofske (Eds.), *The Sage handbook of personality theory and assessment: Vol. 2. Personality measurement and testing* (pp. 626–645). Thousand Oaks, CA: SAGE.

Morey, L. C., & Hopwood, C. J. (2007). *Casebook for the Personality Assessment Inventory.* Lutz, FL: Psychological Assessment Resources.

Morgan, C. D., & Murray, H. A. (1935). A method of investigating fantasies: The Thematic Apperception Test. *Archives of Neurology and Psychiatry, 34,* 289–306.

Murray, H. A. (1943). *Thematic Apperception Test.* Cambridge, MA: Harvard University Press.

Norcross, J. C. (2011). *Psychotherapy relationships that work: Evidence-based responsiveness* (2nd ed.). New York: Oxford University Press.

Okiishi, J., Lambert, M. J., Eggett, D., Nielsen, S. L., Dayton, D. D., & Vermeersch, D. A. (2006). An analysis of therapist treatment effects: Toward providing feedback to individual therapists on their clients' psychotherapy outcome. *Journal of Clinical Psychology, 62,* 1157–1172.

OPD Task Force. (Ed.). (2008). *Operationalized Psychodynamic Diagnosis (OPD-2): Manual of diagnostics and treatment planning.* Göttingen, Germany: Hogrefe & Huber.

Ortigo, K. M., Westen, D., DeFife, J. A., & Bradley, B. (2013). Attachment, social cognition, and posttraumatic stress symptoms in a traumatized, urban population: Evidence for the mediating role of object relations. *Journal of Traumatic Stress, 26,* 361–368.

Owen, J., & Imel, Z. (2010). Rating scales in psychotherapy practice. In L. Baer & M. Blais (Eds.), *Handbook of clinical rating scales and assessment in psychiatry and mental health* (pp. 257–270). New York: Humana Press.

Paul, L. K., Schieffer, B., & Brown, W. S. (2004). Social processing deficits in agenesis of the corpus callosum: Narratives from the Thematic Apperception Test. *Archives of Clinical Neuropsychology, 19,* 215–225.

Peebles, M. J. (2012). *Beginnings: The art and science of planning psychotherapy* (2nd ed.). New York: Routledge.

Perry, J. C. (1990). *Defense Mechanism Rating Scales (DMRS)* (5th ed.). Cambridge, MA: Author.

Perry, J. C. (1994). Assessing psychodynamic patterns using the Idiographic Conflict Formulation Method. *Psychotherapy Research, 4,* 239–252.

Perry, J. C. (1997). The idiographic conflict formulation method. In T. D. Eells (Ed.), *Handbook of psychotherapy case formulation* (pp. 137–165). New York: Guilford Press.

Perry, J. C. (2006). *The Psychodynamic Conflict Rating Scales (PCRS)* (3rd ed.). Available from the author.

Perry, J. C. (2014). Anomalies and specific functions in the clinical identification of defense mechanisms. *Journal of Clinical Psychology, 70,* 406–418.

Perry, J. C., & Bond, M. (2012). Change in defense mechanisms during long-term dynamic psychotherapy and five-year outcome. *American Journal of Psychiatry, 169,* 916–925.

Perry, J. C., Constantinides, P., & Simmonds, J. (2017). Psychoanalytic dynamic conflicts in recurrent major depression: Does combined short-term psychotherapy and medications lead to healthy dynamic functioning? *Psychology, 34*(1), 3–12.

Perry, J. C., & Cooper, S. H. (1986). A preliminary report on defenses and conflicts associated with borderline personality disorder. *Journal of the American Psychoanalytic Association, 34,* 865–895.

Perry, J. C., & Høglend, P. (1998). Convergent and discriminant validity of overall defensive functioning. *Journal of Nervous and Mental Disease, 186,* 529–535.

Perry, J. C., Høglend, P., Shear, K., Vaillant, G. E., Horowitz, M., Kardos, M. E., & Kagen, D. (1998). Field trial of a diagnostic axis for defense mechanisms for DSM-IV. *Journal of Personality Disorders, 12,* 56–68.

Perry, J. C., Metzger, J., & Sigal, J. J. (2015). Defensive functioning in women with breast cancer and community controls. *Psychiatry: Interpersonal and Biological Processes, 78,* 156–169.

Perry, J. D., & Perry, J. C. (2004). Conflicts, defenses and the stability of narcissistic personality features. *Psychiatry, 67,* 310–330.

Perry, W., Minassian, A., Cadenhead, K., & Braff, D. (2003). Use of the Ego Impairment Index across the schizophrenia spectrum. *Journal of Personality Disorders, 80,* 50–57.

Piper, W. E., & Duncan, S. C. (1999). Object relations theory and short-term dynamic psychotherapy: Findings from the Quality of Object Relations scale. *Clinical Psychology Review, 19,* 669–685.

Piper, W. E., McCallum, M., & Joyce, A. S. (1993). *Manual for assessment of quality of object relations.* Unpublished manuscript.

Porcelli, P., & De Carne, M. (2001). Criterion-related validity of the Diagnostic Criteria for Psychosomatic Research for alexithymia in patients with functional gastrointestinal disorders. *Psychotherapy and Psychosomatics, 70,* 184–188.

Porcelli, P., & Mihura, J. L. (2010). Assessment of alexithymia with the Rorschach Comprehensive System: The Rorschach Alexithymia Scale (RAS). *Journal of Personality Assessment, 92,* 128–136.

Porcerelli, J. H., Cogan, R., Kamoo, R., & Miller, K. (2010). Convergent validity of the Defense Mechanisms Manual and the Defensive Functioning Scale. *Journal of Personality Assessment, 92*(5), 432–438.

Porcerelli, J. H., Cogan, R., Markova, T., Miller, K., & Mickens, L. (2011). The *Diagnostic and Statistical Manual of Mental Disorders,* fourth edition Defensive Functioning Scale: A validity study. *Comprehensive Psychiatry, 52,* 225–230.

Porcerelli, J. H., Huth-Bocks, A., Huprich, S. K., & Richardson, L. (2016). Defense mechanisms of pregnant mothers predict attachment-security, social-emotional competence, and behavior problems in their toddlers. *American Journal of Psychiatry, 73*(2), 138–146.

Priel, B. (2005). Representations in childhood: A dialogical perspective. In J. S. Auerbach, K. N. Levy, & C. E. Schaffer (Eds.), *Relatedness, self-definition, and mental representation: Essays in honor of Sidney J. Blatt* (pp. 43–57). London: Routledge.

Quinlan, D. M., Blatt, S. J., Chevron, E. S., & Wein, S. J. (1992). The analysis of descriptions of parents: Identification of a more differentiated factor structure. *Journal of Personality Assessment, 59,* 340–351.

Rapaport, D., Gill, M. M., & Schafer, R. (1945–1946). *Diagnostic psychological testing.* Chicago: Year Book Medical.

Rapaport, D., Gill, M. M., & Schafer, R. (1968). *Diagnostic psychological testing* (2nd ed., R. R. Holt, Ed.). New York: International Universities Press.

Reid, M., & Osatuke, K. (2006) Acknowledging problematic voices: Processes occurring at early stages of conflict assimilation in patients with functional somatic disorder. *Psychology and Psychotherapy: Theory, Research and Practice, 79,* 539–555.

Rorschach, H. (1942). *Psychodiagnostics: A diagnostic test based on perception* (P. Lemkau & B. Kronenberg, Trans.). Bern: Huber. (Original work published 1921)

Rudolf, G., Grande, T., Dilg, R., Jakobsen, T., Keller, W., Oberbracht, C., . . . Wilke, S. (2002). Structural changes in psychoanalytic therapies: The Heidelberg–Berlin study on long-term psychoanalytic therapies (PAL). In M. Leuzinger-Bohleber & M. Target (Eds.), *Outcomes of psychoanalytic treatment: Perspectives for therapists and researchers* (pp. 201–222). London: Whurr.

Rudolf, G., Grande, T., & Oberbracht, C. (2000). The Heidelberg Restructuring Scale: A model of changes in psychoanalytic therapies and its operationalization on an estimating scale. *Psychotherapeut, 45,* 237–246.

Ruiz, M. A., Pincus, A. L., Borkovec, T. D., Echemendia, R. J., Castonguay, L. G., & Ragusea, S. A. (2004). Validity of the Inventory of Interpersonal Problems for predicting treatment outcome: An investigation with the Pennsylvania Practice Research Network. *Journal of Personality Assessment, 83*(3), 213–222.

Satir, D. A., Thompson-Brenner, H., Boisseau, C. L., & Crisafulli, M. A. (2009). Countertransference reactions to adolescents with eating disorders: Relationships to clinician and patient factors. *International Journal of Eating Disorders, 42*(6), 511–521.

Schafer, R. (1958). How was this story told? *Journal of Projective Techniques, 22,* 181–210.

Scharf, R. D., Waldron, S., Firestein, S. K., Goldberger, M., & Burton, A. (2010). *The Analytic Process Scales (APS) coding manual.* Unpublished manual. Available from *woodywald@earthlink.net.*

Seitz, P. (1966). The consensus problem in psychoanalytic research. In L. A. Gottschalk & A. H. Auerbach (Eds.), *Methods of research in psychotherapy* (pp. 209–225). New York: Appleton-Century-Crofts.

Shedler, J. (2000). A new language for psychoanalytic diagnosis. *Psychologist–Psychoanalyst, 20,* 30–37.

Shedler, J. (2015). Integrating clinical and empirical perspectives on personality: The Shedler–Westen Assessment Procedure (SWAP). In S. K. Huprich (Ed.), *Personality disorders: Toward theoretical and empirical integration in diagnosis and assessment* (pp. 225–252). Washington, DC: American Psychological Association.

Shedler, J., Mayman, M., & Manis, M. (1993). The illusion of mental health. *American Psychologist, 48,* 1117–1131.

Shedler, J., & Westen, D. (2006). Personality diagnosis with the Shedler–Westen Assessment Procedure (SWAP): Bridging the gulf between science and practice. In *Psychodynamic diagnostic manual (PDM)* (pp. 573–613). Silver Spring, MD: Alliance of Psychoanalytic Organizations.

Shedler, J., & Westen, D. (2007). The Shedler-Westen Assessment Procedure (SWAP): Making personality diagnosis clinically meaningful. *Journal of Personality Assessment, 89*(1), 41–55.

Shedler, J., Westen, D., & Lingiardi, V. (2014). *La valutazione della personalità con la SWAP-200.* Milan, Italy: Raffaello Cortina.

Shimokawa, K., Lambert, M. J., & Smart, D. (2010). Enhancing treatment outcome of patients at risk of treatment failure: Meta-analytic and mega-analytic review of a psychotherapy quality assurance program. *Journal of Consulting and Clinical Psychology, 78,* 298–311.

Siefert, C. J., Stein, M., Sinclair, S. J., Antonius, D., Shiva, A., & Blais, M. A. (2012). Development and initial validation of a scale for detecting inconsistent responding on the Personality Assessment Inventory—Short Form. *Journal of Personality Assessment, 94*(6), 601–606.

Silberschatz, G. (2005). An overview of research on control–mastery theory. In G. Silberschatz (Ed.), *Transformative relationships* (pp. 189–218). New York: Routledge.

Silberschatz, G., & Curtis, J. T. (1993). Measuring the therapist's impact on the patient's therapeutic progress. *Journal of Consulting and Clinical Psychology, 61,* 403–411.

Silberschatz, G., Fretter, P. B., & Curtis, J. T. (1986). How do interpretations influence the process of psychotherapy? *Journal of Consulting and Clinical Psychology, 54,* 646–652.

Sinclair, S. J., Antonius, D., Shiva, A., Siefert, C. J., Kehl-Fie, K., Lama, S., & Blais, M. A. (2010). The psychometric properties of the Personality Assessment Inventory—Short Form (PAI-SF) in inpatient forensic and civil samples. *Journal of Psychopathology and Behavioral Assessment, 32,* 406–415.

Sinclair, S. J., Siefert, C. J., Shorey, H., Antonius, D., Shiva, A., Kehl-Fie, K., & Blais, M. A. (2009). A psychometric evaluation of the Personality Assessment Inventory—Short Form (PAI-SF) clinical scales in an inpatient psychiatric sample. *Psychiatry Research, 170,* 262–266.

Slade, A. (2008). The implications of attachment theory and research for adult psychotherapy: Research and clinical perspectives. In J. Cassidy & P. R. Shaver (Eds.), *Handbook of attachment: Theory, research, and clinical applications* (2nd ed., pp. 762–783). New York: Guilford Press.

Slade, A., Aber, J. L., Bresgi, I., Berger, B., & Kaplan, C. A. (2004). *The Parent Development Interview—Revised.* Unpublished protocol, City University of New York.

Smith, J. D., & George, C. (2012). Therapeutic assessment case study: Treatment of a woman diagnosed with metastatic cancer and attachment trauma. *Journal of Personality Assessment, 94,* 1–14.

Spieker, S., Nelson, E. M., DeKlyen, M., Jolley, S. N., & Mennet, L. (2011). Continuity and change in unresolved classifications of Adult Attachment Interviews with low-income mothers. In J. Solomon & C. George (Eds.), *Disorganized attachment and caregiving* (pp. 80–109). New York: Guilford Press.

Spiro, A., III, Butcher, J. N., Levenson, R. M., Aldwin, C. M., & Bosse, R. (2000). Change and stability in personality: A five year study of the MMPI-2 in older men. In J. E. Butcher (Ed.), *Basic sources on the MMPI-2* (pp. 443–462). Minneapolis: University of Minnesota Press.

Steele, H., & Steele. M. (2008). Ten clinical uses of the Adult Attachment Interview. In H. Steele & M. Steele (Eds.), *Clinical applications of the Adult Attachment Interview* (pp. 3–30). New York: Guilford Press.

Stein, M. B., Hilsenroth, M., Slavin-Mulford, J., & Pinsker, J. (2011). *Social Cognition and Object Relations Scale: Global Rating Method* (4th ed.). Unpublished manuscript, Massachusetts General Hospital and Harvard Medical School.

Stein, M. B., Slavin-Mulford, J., Siefert, C. J., Sinclair, S. J., Renna, M., Malone, J., . . . Blais, M. A. (2014). SCORS-G stimulus characteristics of select Thematic Apperception Test cards. *Journal of Personality Assessment, 96*(3), 339–349.

Stein, M. B., Slavin-Mulford, J., Siefert, C. J., Sinclair, S. J., Smith, M., Chung, W. J., . . . Blais, M. A. (2015). External validity of SCORS-G ratings of Thematic Apperception Test narratives in a sample of outpatients and inpatients. *Rorschachiana, 36,* 58–81.

Stein, M. B., Slavin-Mulford, J., Sinclair, S. J., Siefert, C. J., & Blais, M. A. (2012). Exploring the construct validity of the Social Cognition and Object Relations Scale in a clinical sample. *Journal of Personality Assessment, 94*(5), 533–540.

Stern, B. L., Caligor, E., Clarkin, J. F., Critchfield, K. L., MacCornack, V., Lenzenweger, M. F., & Kernberg, O. F. (2010). The Structured Interview of Personality Organization (STIPO): Preliminary psychometrics in a clinical sample. *Journal of Psychological Assessment, 91,* 35–44.

Stiles, W. B. (1999). *Signs, voices, meaning bridges, and shared experience: How talking helps* (Visiting Scholar Series No. 10). Palmerston North, New Zealand: School of Psychology, Massey University.

Stiles, W. B. (2002). Assimilation of problematic experiences. In J. C. Norcross (Ed.), *Psychotherapy relationships that work: Therapist contributions and responsiveness to patients* (pp. 357–365). New York: Oxford University Press.

Stiles, W. B. (2005). Extending the Assimilation of Problematic Experiences Scale: Commentary on the special issue. *Counselling Psychology Quarterly, 18,* 85–93.

Stiles, W. B. (2011). Coming to terms. *Psychotherapy Research, 21,* 367–384.

Stiles, W. B., Morrison, L. A., Haw, S. K., Harper, H., Shapiro, D. A., & Firth-Cozens, J. (1991). Longitudinal study of assimilation in exploratory psychotherapy. *Psychotherapy, 28,* 195–206.

Stiles, W. B., Osatuke, K., Glick, M. J., & Mackay, H. C. (2004). Encounters between internal voices generate emotion: An elaboration of the assimilation model. In H. H. Hermans & G. Dimaggio (Eds.), *The dialogical self in psychotherapy* (pp. 91–107). New York: Brunner-Routledge.

Stratton, P., Lask, J., Bland, J., & Janes, E. (2010). Developing an indicator of family function and a practicable outcome measure for systemic family and couple therapy: The SCORE. *Journal of Family Therapy, 32*(3), 232–258.

Stratton, P., Lask, J., Bland, J., Nowotny, E., Evans, C., Singh, R., . . . Peppiatt, A. (2014). Detecting therapeutic improvement early in therapy: Validation of the SCORE-15 index of family functioning and change. *Journal of Family Therapy, 36*(1), 3–19.

Strupp, H. H., Schacht, T. E., & Henry, W. P. (1988). Problem–treatment–outcome congruence: A principle whose time has come. In H. Dahl, H. Kächele, & H. Thomä (Eds.), *Psychoanalytic process research strategies* (pp. 1–14). New York: Springer.

Symons, D., Peterson, C., Slaughter, V., Roche, J., & Doyle, E. (2005). Theory of mind and mental state discourse during book reading and story-telling tasks. *British Journal of Developmental Psychology, 23,* 81–102.

Tanzilli, A., Colli, A., Del Corno, F., & Lingiardi, V. (2016). Factor structure, reliability, and validity of the Therapist Response Questionnaire. *Personality Disorders: Theory, Research, and Treatment, 7*(2), 147–158.

Tanzilli, A., Colli, A., Gualco, I., & Lingiardi, V. (in press). Patient personality and relational patterns in psychotherapy: Factor structure, reliability, and validity of the Psychotherapy Relationship Questionnaire. *Journal of Personality Assessment.*

Taubner, S., Horz, S., Fischer-Kern, M., Doering, S., Buchheim, A., & Zimmermann, J. (2013). Internal structure of the Reflective Functioning Scale. *Psychological Assessment, 25*(1), 127–135.

Taylor, G. J. (2010). Affects, trauma, and mechanisms of symptom formation: A tribute to John C. Nemiah, MD (1918–2009). *Psychotherapy and Psychosomatics, 79,* 339–349.

Taylor, G. J., & Bagby, R. M. (2012). The alexithymia personality dimension. In T. A. Widiger (Ed.), *The Oxford handbook of personality disorders* (pp. 648–676). New York: Oxford University Press.

Taylor, G. J., Bagby, R. M., & Parker, J. D. A. (1997). *Disorders of affect regulation.* Cambridge, UK: Cambridge University Press.

Tellegen, A., Ben-Porath, Y. S., McNulty, J. L., Arbisi, P. A., Graham, J. R., & Kaemmer, B. (2003). *The MMPI-2 restructured clinical scales: Development, validation, and interpretation.* Minneapolis: University of Minnesota Press.

Thompson-Brenner, H., Eddy, K. T., Satir, D. A., Boisseau, C. L., & Westen, D. A. (2008). Personality subtypes in adolescents with eating disorders: Validation of a classification approach. *Journal of Child Psychology and Psychiatry. 49,* 170–180.

Thompson-Brenner, H., & Westen, D. A. (2005a). A naturalistic study of psychotherapy for bulimia nervosa. *Journal of Nervous and Mental Disease, 193,* 573–595.

Thompson-Brenner, H., & Westen, D. A. (2005b). Personality subtypes in eating disorders: Validation of a classification in a naturalistic sample. *British Journal of Psychiatry, 186,* 516–524.

Tikkanen, S., Stiles, W. B., & Leiman, M. (2013). Achieving an empathic stance: Dialogical sequence analysis of a change episode. *Psychotherapy Research, 23,* 178–189.

Tracey, T. J., & Kokotovic, A. M. (1989). Factor structure of the Working Alliance Inventory. *Psychological Assessment: Journal of Consulting and Clinical Psychology, 1,* 207–210.

Turrina, C., Siani, R., Regini, C., Campana, A., Bologna, R., & Siciliani, O. (1996). Inter-observer and test–retest reliability of the Italian version of the Karolinska Psychodynamic Profile (KAPP) in two groups of psychiatric patients. *Acta Psychiatrica Scandinavica, 93,* 292–287.

Twigg, E., Barkham, M., Bewick, B. M., Mulhern, B., Connell, J., & Cooper, M. (2009). The Young Person's CORE: Development of a brief outcome measure for young people. *Counselling and Psychotherapy Research, 9,* 160–168.

Tyrrell, C. L., Dozier, M., Teague, G. B., & Fallot, R. D. (1999). Effective treatment relationships for persons with serious psychiatric disorders: The importance of attachment states of mind. *Journal of Consulting and Clinical Psychology, 67,* 725–733.

van IJzendoorn, M. H. (1995). Adult attachment representations, parental responsiveness, and infant attachment: A meta-analysis on the predictive validity of the Adult Attachment Interview. *Psychological Bulletin, 117,* 387–403.

van IJzendoorn, M. H., & Bakersman-Kranenburg, M. J. (2008). The distribution of Adult Attachment representations in clinical groups: A meta-analytic search for patterns of attachment in 105 AAI studies. In H. Steele & M. Steele (Eds.), *Clinical applications of the Adult Attachment Interview* (pp. 399–426). New York: Guilford Press.

Varvin, S. (2003). *Mental survival strategies after extreme traumatisation.* Copenhagen: Multivers APS.

Verheul, R., Berghout, C. C., Busschbach, J. J. V., Bateman, A., Helene, A., Dolan, C., . . . Fonagy, P. (2008). Severity Indices of Personality Problems (SIPP-118): Development, factor structure, reliability, and validity. *Psychologic al Assessment, 20,* 23–34.

Vermeersch, D. A., Whipple, J. L., Lambert, M. J., Hawkins, E. J., Burchfield, C. M., & Okiishi, J. C. (2004). Outcome Questionnaire: Item sensitivity to changes in counseling center clients. *Journal of Counseling Psychology, 51,* 38–49.

Vermote, R., Lowyck, B., Luyten, P., Verhaest, Y., Vertommen, H., Vandeneede, B., . . . Peuskens, J. (2011). Patterns of inner change and their relation with patient characteristics and outcome in a psychoanalytic hospitalization-based treatment for personality disordered patients. *Clinical Psychology and Psychotherapy, 18,* 303–313.

Waldron, S. (1995). [Book review: *Understanding Transference: The CCRT Method* by Lester

Luborsky and Paul Crits-Christoph. New York, Basic Books, 1990.] *Psychoanalytic Quarterly, 64,* 398–402.

Waldron, S., Gazzillo, F., Genova, F., & Lingiardi, V. (2013). Relational and classical elements in psychoanalyses: An empirical study with case illustrations. *Psychoanalytic Psychology, 30,* 567–600.

Waldron, S., & Helm, F. (2004). Psychodynamic features of two cognitive/behavioural and one psychodynamic treatment compared using the Analytic Process Scales. *Canadian Journal of Psychoanalysis, 12,* 346–368.

Waldron, S., Moscovitz, S., Lundin, J., Helm, F. L., Jemerin, J., & Gorman, B. (2011). Evaluating the outcome of psychotherapies: The Personality Health Index. *Psychoanalytic Psychology, 28,* 363–388.

Waldron, S., Scharf, R. D., Crouse, J., Firestein, S. K., Burton, A., & Hurst, D. (2004a). Saying the right thing at the right time: A view through the lens of the Analytic Process Scales (APS). *Psychoanalytic Quarterly, 73,* 1079–1125.

Waldron, S., Scharf, R. D., Hurst, D., Firestein, S. K., & Burton, A. (2004b). What happens in a psychoanalysis: A view through the lens of the Analytic Process Scales (APS). *International Journal of Psychoanalysis, 85,* 443–466.

Wallerstein, R. S., DeWitt, K., Hartley, D., Rosenberg, S. E., & Zilberg, N. (1996). *The Scales of Psychological Capacities (Version 1).* Unpublished manuscript.

Waters, E., & Hamilton, C. E. (2000). The stability of attachment security from infancy to adolescence and early adulthood: General introduction. *Child Development, 71,* 678–683.

Waters, E., Treboux, D., Fyffe, C., & Crowell, J. (2001). *Secure versus insecure and dismissing versus preoccupied attachment representation scored as continuous variables from AAI state of mind scales.* Unpublished manuscript, Stony Brook University, State University of New York.

Watkins, R., Cheston, R., Jones, K., & Gilliard, J. (2006). "Coming out" with Alzheimer's disease: Changes in awareness during a psychotherapy group for people with dementia. *Aging and Mental Health, 10,* 166–176.

Webster, L., & Hackett, R. K. (2007). A comparison of unresolved and resolved status and its relationship to behavior in maltreated adolescents. *School Psychology International, 28,* 365–378.

Weiner, I. B. (2000). Making Rorschach interpretation as good as it can be. *Journal of Personality Assessment, 74,* 164–174.

Weiner, I. B. (2003). *Principles of Rorschach interpretation* (2nd ed.). Mahwah, NJ: Erlbaum.

Weinryb, R. M., Gustavsson, J. P., & Barber, J. P. (2003). Personality traits predicting long-term adjustment after surgery for ulcerative colitis. *Journal of Clinical Psychology, 59,* 1015–1029.

Weinryb, R. M., & Rössel, R. J. (1991). Karolinska Psychodynamic Profile—KAPP. *Acta Psychiatrica Scandinavica, 85,* 153–162.

Weinryb, R. M., Rössel, R. J., & Åsberg, M. (1991a). The Karolinska Psychodynamic Profile: I. Validity and dimensionality. *Acta Psychiatrica Scandinavica, 83,* 64–72.

Weinryb, R. M., Rössel, R. J., & Åsberg, M. (1991b). The Karolinska Psychodynamic Profile: II. Interdisciplinary and cross-cultural reliability. *Acta Psychiatrica Scandinavica, 83,* 73–76.

Weinryb, R. M., Rössel, R. J., Gustavsson, J., Åsberg, M., & Barber, J. P. (1997). The Karolinska Psychodynamic Profile (KAPP): Studies of character and well-being. *Psychoanalytic Psychology, 14*(4), 495–515.

Weiss, J., Sampson, H., & the Mount Zion Psychotherapy Research Group. (1986). *The psychoanalytic process.* New York: Guilford Press.

Westen, D. (1991a). Clinical assessment of object relations using the TAT. *Journal of Personality Assessment, 56,* 56–74.

Westen, D. (1991b). Social cognition and object relations. *Psychological Bulletin, 109,* 429–455.

Westen, D. (1995). *Social Cognition and Object Relations Scale: Q-sort for Projective Stories (SCORS-Q).* Unpublished manuscript, Cambridge Hospital and Harvard Medical School, Cambridge, MA.

Westen, D. (1999). The scientific status of unconscious processes: Is Freud really dead? *Journal of the American Psychoanalytic Association, 47,* 1061–1106.

Westen, D., DeFife, J. A., Malone, J. C., & DiLallo, J. (2014). An empirically derived classification of adolescent personality disorders. *Journal of the American Academy of Child and Adolescent Psychiatry, 53,* 528–549.

Westen, D., Dutra, L., & Shedler, J. (2005). Assessing adolescent personality pathology. *British Journal of Psychiatry, 186,* 227–238.

Westen, D., Gabbard, G. O., & Blagov, P. (2006). Back to the future: Personality structure as a context for psychopathology. In R. F. Krueger & J. L. Tackett (Eds.), *Personality and psychopathology* (pp. 335–384). New York: Guilford Press.

Westen, D., & Harnden-Fischer, J. (2001). Personality profiles in eating disorders. In M. R. Leary & J. P. Tangney (Eds.), *Handbook of self and identity* (pp. 643–664). New York: Guilford Press.

Westen, D., & Muderrisoglu, S. (2006). Clinical assessment of pathological personality traits. *American Journal of Psychiatry, 163,* 1285–1287.

Westen, D., & Shedler, J. (1999a). Revising and assessing Axis II: Part I. Developing a clinically and empirically valid assessment method. *American Journal of Psychiatry, 156,* 258–272.

Westen, D., & Shedler, J. (1999b). Revising and assessing Axis II: Part II. Toward an empirically based and clinically useful classification of personality disorders. *American Journal of Psychiatry, 156,* 273–285.

Westen, D., Shedler, J., Bradley, B., & DeFife, J. A. (2012). An empirically derived taxonomy for personality diagnosis: Bridging science and practice in conceptualizing personality. *American Journal of Psychiatry, 169,* 273–284.

Westen, D., Shedler, J., Durrett, C., Glass, S., & Martens, A. (2003). Personality diagnosis in adolescence: DSM-IV Axis II diagnoses and an empirically derived alternative. *American Journal of Psychiatry, 160,* 952–966.

Westen, D., & Weinberger, J. (2004). When clinical description becomes statistical prediction. *American Psychologist, 59,* 595–613.

Wilczek, A., Barber, J. P., Gustavsson, J. P., Asberg, M., & Weinryb, R. M. (2004). Change after long-term psychoanalytic psychotherapy. *Journal of the American Psychoanalytic Association, 52,* 1163–1184.

Wilczek, A., Weinryb, R. M., Gustavsson, P. J., Barber, J. P., Schubert, J., & Asberg, M. (1998). Symptoms and character traits in patients selected for long-term psychodynamic psychotherapy. *Journal of Psychotherapy Practice and Research, 7,* 23–34.

Wood, J. M., Nezworski, M. T., Lilienfeld, S. O., & Garb, H. N. (2003). *What's wrong with the Rorschach?* San Francisco: Jossey-Bass.

Young, J. L., Waehler, C. A., Laux, J. M., McDaniel, P. S., & Hilsenroth, M. J. (2003). Four studies extending the utility of the Schwartz Outcome Scale (SOS-10). *Journal of Personality Assessment, 80,* 130–138.

Zilberg, N. J., Wallerstein, R. S., DeWitt, K. N., Hartley, D. E., & Rosenberg, S. E. (1991). A conceptual analysis and strategy for assessing structural change. *Psychoanalysis and Contemporary Thought, 14,* 317–342.

Zilcha-Mano, S., Chui, H., McCarthy, K., Dinger, D., & Barber, J. P. (2016). *Examining mechanisms underlying the dodo bird effect in depression: Changes in general attributions and relationship representations.* Manuscript in preparation.

Zilcha-Mano, S., McCarthy, K. S., Dinger, U., & Barber, J. P. (2014). To what extent is the alliance affected by transference?: Some empirical findings. *Psychotherapy, 51,* 424–433.

Zimmermann, J., Ehrenthal, J. C., Cierpka, M., Schauenburg, H., Doering, S., & Benecke, C. (2012). Assessing the level of structural integration using Operationalized Psychodynamic Diagnosis (OPD): Implications for DSM-5. *Journal of Personality Assessment, 94*(5), 522–532.

CHAPTER 16

Clinical Illustrations and PDM-2 Profiles

CHAPTER EDITORS

Franco Del Corno, MPhyl, DPsych **Vittorio Lingiardi, MD** **Nancy McWilliams, PhD**

CONSULTANTS

Giuseppe Cafforio, DPsych
Sara Francavilla, DPsych
Mark J. Hilsenroth, PhD
Henriette Loeffler-Stastka, MD
Eleonora Piacentini, PhD
Anna Maria Speranza, PhD
Guido Taidelli, MD

Introduction

This chapter consists of clinical illustrations taken from applied practice in naturalistic settings. One case is provided for each age group covered in PDM-2: adulthood, adolescence, childhood, infancy/early childhood, and later life. Some were contributed by clinicians in Italy, others by clinicians in the United States. Personal details in all clinical illustrations are disguised in accordance with contemporary standards for published case material. Additional PDM-2 clinical illustrations can be found online (see the box at the end of the table of contents).

Our purposes include promoting understanding of the functioning of the whole patient via the PDM-2 classification system; encouraging more thorough explications of various kinds of pathological functioning; and also promoting the eventual development of more adequate research designs, grounded in clearer descriptions of the multiple features of different kinds of mental and emotional suffering.

Each clinical illustration is organized as follows (with some variations):

- Presenting problem.
- Demographic and personal data (age, gender, sexual orientation, education, job, social condition, and marital status, as well as family history and specific features of relationships with caregivers and siblings).
- Information about the history of the problem, along with any prior psychological and/or biological treatments.
- Other important information, such as life events possibly relevant to the problem, and factors such as cultural, ethnic, and religious contexts.
- Psychopathological features, such as relevant affects, defenses, main concerns, and pathogenic beliefs.
- Strengths and resources.
- The clinician's subjective reactions to the patient (i.e., countertransference reactions).
- Therapeutic hypotheses and treatment implications.

The aggregate of these elements distinguishes the clinical illustrations in this chapter from the brief vignettes provided in other chapters, which are designed to highlight particular characteristics of specific disorders or personality patterns. Given that they include contributions from several different clinicians, they are written in somewhat different styles.

Congruent with PDM-2's self-description as a "taxonomy of people" rather than a "taxonomy of diseases," these cases are intended as holistic descriptions. To promote an integration between nomothetic and idiographic knowledge, the cases are integrated with DSM-5 and ICD-10 diagnoses. Each patient is evaluated with the Psychodiagnostic Chart (PDC) for the relevant age range. Blank versions of the PDCs are provided in the Appendix to this manual, and enlarged versions of the forms can also be downloaded (again, see the box at the end of the table of contents).

Adulthood

Martin

Personal Data, Family History, and Specific Features of Relationships with Family Members

Martin is a 39-year-old heterosexual single man of normal size and attractiveness, who sought medical consultation 12 years ago at the recommendation of the psychologist with whom he had been in once-weekly psychotherapy for 4 years, who believed it would be useful to add psychopharmacological therapy.

Martin was the first-born child, with a sister 2 years younger, in a family of high socioeconomic status. His father was a successful lawyer, well read, strong-willed, and rational, who saw his role toward his children as that of providing a model and giving advice, even in contexts of play. The mother was described as attentive, active, pragmatic, aligned with her husband's opinions, and not very good at true emotional connection.

Martin described himself as an even-tempered, adaptable child, closely attached to his mother and maternal grandfather, sociable but not particularly curious. He recalled with some pain his emotional instability and identity problems in adolescence, his feelings of loneliness, and the sense that his parents did not understand him. He tended to prefer intellectual activities such as reading and taking part in cultural or political initiatives, though he often withdrew from them because of the malaise he felt in interacting with other people, whose judgment he feared. He reported difficult romantic experiences, and described a profound lack of self-esteem that clashed with his sexual desire and longing for success. His capacity for emotional investment was checked by the fear of losing control. His performance at school was average, propelled by a sense of duty and of inevitable submission to his teachers. He reported a tendency not to express the emotional aspects of his experiences, but instead to relive them in his mind, with ego-syntonic rumination.

History of the Problem

In late adolescence, Martin suffered from anxiety in connection with important events such as his impending high school exit exam. He described tension, feelings of inadequacy and failure, difficulty concentrating, and perspiration with mild tremors. He also experienced involuntary visualization of scenes from a recently seen horror movie, as well as "obsessive thoughts" about his future. No treatment was undertaken, and the symptoms decreased a month and a half later, once he had passed the exam. About 2 years later, he entered into a major, lasting relationship with a young woman. About a year into this relationship, "after an argument," he experienced a panic attack while on a train (with intense feelings of anguish, confusion, fear of losing his mind, tachycardia, asthenia, and general physical malaise) lasting 20–30 minutes. After this, he developed agoraphobic tendencies about public transport and enclosed spaces, other avoidance behavior, and anticipatory anxiety with obsessive ideation centered on how to protect himself from further attacks. These symptoms resolved in 2–3 months.

The anticipatory anxiety returned 6 months before he was to finish his undergraduate degree in political science, with ruminative ideation centered solely on inadequacy-related themes, such as the fear of not being prepared or of "seizing up" during the exam. These symptoms improved after his graduation but remained at a level that led his psychotherapist to decide he should be sent to a psychiatrist. The latter identified obsessive ideation (in the form of pervasive doubt, constant rethinking, explaining and trying to control emotions considered to be wrong and destabilizing), initial social withdrawal, anxiety, and insomnia. Aside from the hyperemotionality, Martin did not sufficiently acknowledge these tendencies as problems; he also showed firm resistance to the use of tranquilizers, which he criticized as having an overly sedative effect, but which he also feared as potentially diminishing his self-control.

After the therapist explained the need to reduce the anxious ideation, fluvoxamine was prescribed in increasing dosages up to a medium to high level that was maintained for 9–10 months. Martin recognized a positive outcome at the symptomatic level, stating that his head was clearer and his level of anxiety considerably reduced. However, his persisting tendency toward intellectualization and doubt as an approach to the world, "in order to understand things," prompted his spontaneous decision 10 years ago to enter psychoanalysis (three couch sessions a week), while continuing pharmacological treatment at a maintenance level and reducing checkups with the psychiatrist to once or twice per year. Eventually he chose to discontinue the medication, saying that it had negative side effects on his sex life and that "only analysis would help."

Five years ago, he informed the psychiatrist of a noticeable resumption of the ruminative thinking, with feelings of powerlessness that he had difficulty handling, especially since he had expected analysis to be sufficient to control them. He was also withdrawing from various aspects of life, such as seeking a job suited to his skills, seeing his friends frequently, and dating. An attitude of self-pity rather than malaise could be noted in regard to these aspects of his behavior. The psychiatrist suggested that he resume his previous medication treatment at a lower dosage; Martin accepted this suggestion with ambivalence, "because it seemed like a step backward, toward how it was before." After this, he made only rare telephone contact with the psychiatrist, showing that he wanted to conduct the therapy his own way, and breaking it off 3 years ago.

Martin resumed contact with the psychiatrist a year ago, in a condition of "anguish and doubt about everything." He had withdrawn into his home and almost ceased contact with the outside world, with uncontrollable obsessional thinking about sometimes bizarre themes (such as an obsession with the letter A, which was perceived as being negative, and which he thus had to avoid reading) and self-referential interpretations (such as the idea that he might have offended a neighbor, whom he thus had to avoid by going out as little as possible). He also expressed fear of mental confusion and alarm about "not having any touchstones" even among his family. It emerged that for several months the patient had felt more and more that his analysis had reached a deadlock and that there was no longer any prospect of improvement; specifically, he no longer believed in his ability "to understand more," and he began to realize that he had seen psychoanalytic therapy as his sole tool for dealing with life, even at the practical level. He became increasingly incapable of initiative and increasingly discouraged.

The therapist noted the state of existential crisis underlying the return of Martin's symptoms, but also the patient's tendency to assign to him (the therapist) the role of savior, with delegation of total therapeutic responsibility to him, yet with some degree of ambivalence. He therefore suggested to Martin that they jointly examine the problems and possibilities of action, pharmacological and otherwise. Having at least partially achieved this diagnostic alliance, he proposed a pharmacological therapy aimed at reducing the anxiety and obsessive ideation, as well as a psychotherapeutic supportive treatment (two to three sessions per month) oriented toward Martin's gradually resuming contact with the outside world.

Sometimes the therapist reported feeling invested in a powerful role, as a savior responsible for the whole progress of the therapy. He also reported feeling helpless at other times because Martin's intellectualization and limited access to symbolic states often made it impossible to access his inner functioning and forced a focus on simple practicality.

Despite the severity of his symptoms, Martin seemed to make good use of his cognitive resources, which allowed him to continue his studies (not yet completed). Even though his capacities for intimacy and relationship remained at a low level, he began to be capable of reciprocity and mutuality.

Current Situation

Martin has continued with drug therapy, although it has now been reduced to a maintenance dose. He is also continuing with supportive treatment (now at a weekly frequency), and he is actively experimenting with his own emotional reactions, increasing his opportunities to meet other people and to deal with different situations.

DSM-5/ICD-10 Diagnosis

Obsessive–compulsive disorder (ICD-10-CM code: F42)

PDM-2 Diagnosis

P Axis

The central tension in Martin's life seems to be about safety versus danger. Other persons are seen as the sources of unimagined perils that he must somehow elude. In addition to avoidance, his central defenses are symbolization, displacement, intellectualization, and rationalization. Severe anxiety is present. Obsessions and compulsions (see the S Axis) may be viewed as efforts to reduce this anxiety through the establishment of some forms of symbolic control over the outside world.

Personality syndromes: Anxious–avoidant and phobic personality (predominant); obsessive–compulsive personality

M Axis

Martin shows significant defects in most areas of mental functioning, along with difficulties in self–object differentiation and integration.

M6. Significant defects in basic mental functions (range = 19–25)

S Axis

S32.1. Obsessive–compulsive disorder

PDM-2 Profile on the PDC-2

A completed PDC-2 for Martin, revealing his full PDM-2 profile, is provided in Figure 16.1 on the next page.

Adolescence

Michelle

Presenting Problem

Michelle was 17 when she arrived at a local clinic without her parents. When the psychologist asked why she had requested a consultation, she reported having seen a TV story about a girl who suffered from eating disorders and that the story had made her wonder about herself. She felt unsure about what was happening to her and decided to ask for help from someone who might understand. Michelle reported suffering from what she described as "a swing of emotions that makes me feel like a roller coaster: I feel depressed one moment, and the next moment I feel I can conquer the world." She made the appointment after searching for help on the Internet.

Michelle was of slender build, but not excessively thin. She spoke without slang words, in a way that was calm and appropriate. She was well dressed, and overall presented in an age-appropriate manner. About 2 years ago, she had started a weight loss program with her mother, whom she described as a "serial dieter." She lost 35 pounds in about 40 days. She struggled to lose weight, she said, because her body had always

(text resumes on page 982)

Psychodiagnostic Chart–2 (PDC-2)

Psychodiagnostic Chart–2, Adult Version 8.1

Name: *Martin* Age: *39* Gender: *Male* Ethnicity: *White North American*

Date of evaluation: *XX / XX / XX* Evaluator: *Psychotherapist*

Section I: Level of Personality Organization

Consider your client's mental functions in determining the level of personality organization. Use these four mental functions to efficiently capture the level of personality organization. Rate each mental function on a scale from 1 (Severely impaired) to 10 (Healthy).

Severe				Moderate				Healthy	
1	2	3	4	5	6	7	8	9	10

1. **Identity:** Ability to view self in complex, stable, and accurate ways *3*
2. **Object relations:** Ability to maintain intimate, stable, and satisfying relationships *5*
3. **Level of defenses** (using the guide below, select a single number): *6*
   - 1–2: Psychotic level (delusional projection, psychotic denial, psychotic distortion)
   - 3–5: Borderline level (splitting, projective identification, idealization/devaluation, denial, acting out)
   - 6–8: Neurotic level (repression, reaction formation, intellectualization, displacement, undoing)
   - 9–10: Healthy level (anticipation, self-assertion, sublimation, suppression, altruism, and humor)
4. **Reality testing:** Ability to appreciate conventional notions of what is realistic *7*

Overall Personality Organization

Considering the ratings and your clinical judgment, circle your client's overall personality organization.

Psychotic		Borderline			Neurotic			Healthy	
1	2	3	4	5	(6)	7	8	9	10

(continued)

FIGURE 16.1. A completed PDC-2 for Martin.

Healthy personality: Characterized by mostly 9–10 scores; life problems rarely get out of hand, and enough flexibility to accommodate to challenging realities. (Use 9 for people at the high-functioning neurotic level.)

Neurotic level: Characterized by mostly 6–8 scores; basically a good sense of identity, good reality testing, mostly good intimacies; fair resiliency, fair affect tolerance and regulation; rigidity and limited range of defenses and coping mechanisms; favors defenses such as repression, reaction formation, intellectualization, displacement, and undoing. (Use 6 for people who go between borderline and neurotic levels.)

Borderline level: Characterized by mostly 3–5 scores; recurrent relational problems; difficulty with affect tolerance and regulation; poor impulse control, poor sense of identity, poor resiliency; favors defenses such as splitting, projective identification, idealization/devaluation, denial, omnipotent control, and acting out.

Psychotic level: Characterized by mostly 1–2 scores; delusional thinking; poor reality testing and mood regulation; extreme difficulty functioning in work and relationships; favors defenses such as delusional projection, psychotic denial, and psychotic distortion. (Use 3 for people who go between psychotic and borderline levels.)

(There are no sharp cutoffs between categories. Use your clinical judgment.)

Section II: Personality Syndromes (P Axis)

These are relatively stable patterns of thinking, feeling, behaving, and relating to others. Normal-level personality patterns do not involve impairment, while personality syndromes or disorders involve impairment at the neurotic, borderline, or psychotic level.

Check off as many personality syndromes as apply from the list below; then circle the one or two personality styles that are most dominant. Leave blank if none.

(For research purposes, you may also rate the level of severity for all styles, using a 1–5 scale: 1 = Severe level; 3 = Moderate severity; and 5 = High-functioning.)

	Level of severity
☐ **Depressive** Subtypes: • Introjective • Aanaclitic • Converse manifestation: Hypomanic	___
☐ **Dependent** Subtypes: • Passive–aggressive • Converse manifestation: Counterdependent	___

(continued)

FIGURE 16.1. *(continued)*

Level of severity

☑ **Anxious–avoidant and phobic** 3
Subtype:
- Converse manifestation: Counterphobic

☑ **Obsessive–compulsive** 2

☐ **Schizoid** ___

☐ **Somatizing** ___

☐ **Hysteric–histrionic** ___
Subtypes:
- Inhibited
- Demonstrative

☐ **Narcissistic** ___
Subtypes:
- Overt
- Covert
- Malignant

☐ **Paranoid** ___

☐ **Psychopathic** ___
Subtypes:
- Passive–parasitic, "con artist"
- Aggressive

☐ **Sadistic** ___

☐ **Borderline** ___

Section III: Mental Functioning (M Axis)

Rate your client's level of strength or weakness on each of the 12 mental functions below, on a scale from 1 to 5 (1 = Severe deficits; 5 = Healthy). Then sum the 12 ratings for a level-of-severity score.

Severe deficits	Major impairments	Moderate impairments	Mild impairments	Healthy
1	2	3	4	5

(continued)

FIGURE 16.1. *(continued)*

- **Cognitive and affective processes**
  1. Capacity for regulation, attention, and learning 2
  2. Capacity for affective range, communication, and understanding 2
  3. Capacity for mentalization and reflective functioning 2
- **Identity and relationships**
  4. Capacity for differentiation and integration (identity) 2
  5. Capacity for relationships and intimacy 2
  6. Self-esteem regulation and quality of internal experience 2
- **Defense and coping**
  7. Impulse control and regulation 2
  8. Defensive functioning 2
  9. Adaptation, resiliency and strength 2
- **Self-awareness and self-direction**
  10. Self-observing capacities (psychological mindedness) 2
  11. Capacity to construct and use internal standards and ideals 2
  12. Meaning and purpose 2

Overall level of personality severity (Sum of 12 mental functions): 24

[Healthy/optimal mental functioning, 54–60; Appropriate mental functioning with some areas of difficulty, 47–53; Mild impairments in mental functioning, 40–46; Moderate impairments in mental functioning, 33–39; Major impairments in mental functioning, 26–32; Significant defects in basic mental functions, 19–25; Major/severe defects in basic mental functions, 12–18]

Section IV: Symptom Patterns (S Axis)

List the main PDM-2 symptom patterns (those that are predominantly related to psychotic disorders, mood disorders, disorders related primarily to anxiety, event- and stressor-related disorders, etc.).

(If required, you may use the DSM or ICD symptoms and codes here.)

Severe — Moderate — Healthy

1 2 3 4 5

Symptom/concern: *Obsessive–compulsive disorder* Level: 2

Symptom/concern: ______ Level: ___

Symptom/concern: ______ Level: ___

(continued)

FIGURE 16.1. *(continued)*

Section V: Cultural, Contextual, and Other Relevant Considerations

Martin is a white, heterosexual male from a privileged family, from whom high levels of success were expected. His internal experience is in stark contrast to the image of conventional power and achievement expected by his professionally oriented family. Like many people born into higher-status families, he may feel that he has "nothing to complain about," given his level of privilege; this may make it harder for him to access feelings that acknowledge the emotional poverty of his family of origin.

FIGURE 16.1. *(continued)*

been curvy. But she came to the point of hating her body, especially after the changes that occurred with menses. Her breasts had grown, her hips were swelling, and she felt ugly and unworthy of love. She had had just one boyfriend, who was now engaged to one of her friends "because she is more beautiful than me." Sad and depressed about this abandonment, she ascribed his rejection to her inadequate body.

History of the Problem

After she lost weight, Michelle struggled to keep this weight off. She would have liked to be even thinner, but she seemed unable to lose more. She described periods of eating very little (sometimes only a single piece of fruit per day), and said that seeing the scale pointer going down had been highly motivating. She reported "never feeling hungry," even when sensing an acute physical need to eat. She started to look at the scale more than three times a day, and her daily thoughts began to center around issues related to food. She thought of what she was going to eat during the day every morning as soon as she woke up. She especially thought about what *not* to eat. During the day, she drank plenty of water. When she went to bed, she thought immediately about what she should or should not eat the next day. These thoughts were unrelenting and took over her mind. She talked about how unworthy and ineffective she would feel if she could not adhere to her plan for eating.

After about 2 months of dieting, Michelle's weight plateaued, and she stopped menstruating. She began to get depressed over what she called her "failure." She enrolled in a gym, which she then attended twice every day, doing aerobic exercises. The gym became another obsession, along with her weight and food consumption (or lack of it). One day, tired and weary, Michelle came home after the gym and decided to weigh herself, only to find that her weight had increased. Discouraged and angered, she started to eat large amounts of food. The psychologist asked what she ate, but Michelle was not able to remember. She then described the beginning of a period of bingeing. After this first act of bingeing, she followed the same pattern: She would force herself to eat very little, but then, as she perceived herself falling short of her goal of total abstinence, she would start to eat ravenously. When bingeing, she seemed to lose control of the situation; she did not remember what or how much food she had eaten. She alternated sweet and savory foods without any criterion of taste.

Michelle gave some examples of her eating routines. Before a night out with friends, she would not eat all day, "because I can go out only if I have a flat stomach," but when she was out with them, she had persistent thoughts of wanting to go home to eat and eat. Once she returned home, she would spend the evening eating everything that had been forbidden during the day.

At the time of referral, Michelle was still obsessed with fitness and weight; she continued going to the gym every day, and used daily laxatives to evacuate the food. Occasionally she induced vomiting.

Personal Data, Family History, and Specific Features of Relationships with Family Members

Michelle was very good at school, had above-average academic performance, and never caused problems. When the psychologist asked her why she had come to the appointment alone, Michelle said that her parents would "go mad" if they knew that she was hurting herself. They did not suspect anything about her disorder. Michelle described herself as the perfect daughter, who did not want to worry her parents; they were away on business a lot, and she tried in every possible way to hide her suffering. She tried to be seen as always smiling and happy, talented, and diligent. She said, "I've got it all in my life—a high-level school, holidays abroad, fancy clothes—and if they saw me so wasted, they would be disappointed. I'm feeling guilty."

When Michelle spoke about herself, she tended to do so in a depreciative fashion: She described herself as a "weak idiot, so stupidly frail," but she realized she needed help because "I tried everything to feel better, but maybe the problem is in my head." She said that she had a good relationship with her mother, but that sometimes this relationship was difficult to manage. Her mother told Michelle that she was her "best friend, the only one I can confide in." Michelle, by contrast, kept some issues hidden because of her mother's anxiety and because she feared that her mother would be surprised at any sign of weakness in her daughter. Michelle recalled, "When I was little, I used to see my mother cry, and I would try to console her. I don't know why she was crying, but I remember I spent a lot of time trying to cheer her up." Michelle had heard her mother describing her as "a strong, overachieving girl." Her relationship with her father was "neither good nor bad, simply absent." He was often away on business, and when he was home, he inquired only about her studies—"nothing more, nothing less. For example, I'm sure my father doesn't know any of the names of my closer friends." Michelle described a strict and authoritarian man, irascible about little things and always serious. When the psychologist asked her what her parents would think of her if they were listening to their current conversation, Michelle said, "If my parents would listen to my words, they would wonder about me and would think I suck." She said they could feel failure and extreme shame. She seemed starved for care and affection and expressed a longing to be protected and cherished.

Michelle had a brother 4 years older, with whom she did not have a good relationship. They were constantly competitive in several areas: They attended the same school, belonged to the same circle of friends, and were constantly encouraged by their parents to demonstrate "who is the better of the two."

Michelle stated that she had not been able to choose anything relevant to her life: Her schools (prestigious) and friends (wealthy) always seemed to have been chosen for her by her parents. Michelle said, "I'm confused over what I want. I do not know which university to choose, and I feel very scared because I know that my parents have already chosen one for me, but I still don't know if I want to attend the one they will propose to me." She was concerned about being inadequate, incompetent, and unloved. "When I think they have already chosen my university, I feel so angry that I want to scream, but I'll never be able to express it. I'm scared about their reaction, and about a feeling so strong that it could lead me to being out of control."

There was evidence of psychiatric illness in the family history: Michelle's aunt, her mother's sister, suffered from a form of paranoid schizophrenia with adult onset.

Further Observations

Relevant Affects

The main affects Michelle experienced, and examples of how she expressed these, were as follows:

- Sadness (depressive mood): "If in the morning I see that I didn't lose weight, I can stay lying in bed even for the rest of the day. I feel really, really bad, as if I didn't have any energy."
- Despair (low self-esteem): "I'm unworthy and I can't do anything in my life; I'm not even able to lose a pound of my weight."
- Fear of being abandoned: Looking at the psychologist, Michelle asked, "If I come here and I don't have anything special to say, will you still continue to be my therapist?"
- Shame: "I look at my body and shape, and I feel I'm really, really nasty. Don't you think?"
- Fear of weakness and failure: "I can't conceive of failing at school; just thinking about this possibility, I feel bad. No, I can't, I can't, I can't."
- Fear of loss of control over anger and aggression: "This morning my mom came into my room to confide in me about a family problem, but I felt really, really exhausted and tired. I didn't want to listen to her problems, but I had to. I felt really, really angry inside, but I tried to hide that from her. I felt angry enough to scream out loud, but I can't. Sometimes when I feel angry, I'm afraid that if I vent my anger, I could lose control and go crazy."
- Feelings of being unworthy and ineffective: "Are university exams difficult? If I get rejected what happens? I cannot think. I'll meet a lot of girls who are prettier than me."

Defenses

Michelle seemed to feel stuck between her wishes to grow up (yet to be discovered and investigated) and her perceived parental expectations. She had many friends with whom she often went out. She seemed to have good social functioning, despite being continually anxious about her status in the group: She wondered ruminatively whether she was "nice enough" to deserve her friendships. With friends, because she feared disappointing them, she was zealous and eager to please. She tried to be always ready to help others, while fearing that any disappointment they might have in her would lead to withdrawal of their love and then rejection. She commented, "No love is for free. Every love asks something in return."

Michelle was a highly intellectual, gifted girl who excelled in her work, even when she was studying something she did not like. Her ability to wonder about her suffering and her degree of self-awareness constituted strong resources.

Before contacting the clinician, Michelle had not consulted any other specialist. She said she had always been a "good girl." When she was a child, she often did not want to go to school because of somatic problems that arose early in the morning: She suffered from asthma and severe headaches. She remembered that when she was in kindergarten, she struggled a lot over separating from her mother, and when her mother went away, she cried inconsolably. When the psychologist asked her how she reacted to the reappearance of her mother, Michelle said she did not remember.

Main Concerns and Pathogenic Beliefs

Michelle's self-representation seemed to be informed by pathogenic beliefs such as these: "There is something deeply bad or incomplete about me," "I don't deserve the other's love because I'm not perfect," "I feel guilt and shame about myself," and "People who really are close to me sooner or later will discover how unworthy I am and then will reject me." Such beliefs, along with her conflicts about pleasurable emotions and achievements, seemed to weaken her resources despite her cognitive gifts and to compromise her capacity to value the whole development of her personality and identity.

Therapist's Reactions to the Patient

When Michelle spoke and answered questions, the clinician felt as if she was not hearing her "true voice," and experienced her as giving socially acceptable answers rather than genuine responses. Her evident effort to keep her real thoughts hidden caused the psychologist to feel a sense of despair and worry that real intimacy with Michelle might be difficult. She felt as if she was being "fed" a version of Michelle that would distract her from the more authentic feelings she did not want to share because of her fear of rejection.

Treatment Indications

A recommendation was made for twice-weekly psychodynamic psychotherapy, focused on helping Michelle develop the capacity to manage her anxiety by verbalizing it and thinking about her feelings instead of acting them out. It was felt that more intensive psychodynamic work might get in the way of Michelle's existing social relationships and functioning and might reinforce her view of herself as damaged. The hope was that Michelle could work within a therapeutic relationship in which she could feel safe enough to explore new ways of being with others, and to identify the failed strategies that were exhausting her and driving her to compulsive and self-destructive behavior. Medical monitoring of her physical functioning was recommended—ideally, a multidisciplinary, collaborative approach that would ensure both physical and psychological safety (e.g., a team including a nutritionist, primary care doctor, and cognitive-behavioral therapist). In time, it was hoped that Michelle might be persuaded to integrate her parents into her treatment; this would depend, however, on her capacity to develop a sense of trust and safety in the context of a strong therapeutic relationship.

DSM-5/ICD-10 Diagnosis

Bulimia nervosa (ICD-10-CM code: F50.2)

PDM-2 Diagnosis

MA Axis

MA4. Moderate impairments in mental functioning (range = 33–39)

PA Axis

Level of functioning: Borderline
Emerging personality style: Depressive

SA Axis

SA81. Feeding and eating disorders

PDM-2 Profile on the PDC-A

A completed PDC-A for Michelle, revealing her full PDM-2 profile, is provided in Figure 16.2.

Childhood

Alice

Alice is a 7-year-old girl attending second grade. She is the first-born of a long-married couple and has two younger brothers, ages 1 and 2. Her parents are worried about "peculiar behaviors," such as her obsessive concentration on some activities (i.e., listing numbers and playing mathematical games); her extreme sensitivity, leading her to cry or scream exaggeratedly; her social isolation; and some difficulties with affect regulation.

As part of the diagnostic process, a session with the parents, a session with the whole family, and individual sessions with Alice are scheduled.

(text resumes on page 991)

Psychodiagnostic Chart—Adolescent (PDC-A)

Name: Michelle Age: 17 Gender: Female Ethnicity: White North American

Date of evaluation: XX / XX / XX Evaluator: Psychotherapist

Section I: Mental Functioning (MA Axis)

Rate your patient's level of strength or weakness on each of the 12 mental functions below, on a scale from 1 to 5 (1 = Severe deficits; 5 = Healthy). Then sum the 12 ratings for a level-of-severity score.

Severe deficits	Major impairments	Moderate impairments	Mild impairments	Healthy
1	2	3	4	5

- **Cognitive and affective processes**
  1. Capacity for regulation, attention, and learning — 4
  2. Capacity for affective range, communication, and understanding — 4
  3. Capacity for mentalization and reflective functioning — 3
- **Identity and relationships**
  4. Capacity for differentiation and integration (identity) — 3
  5. Capacity for relationships and intimacy — 3
  6. Capacity for self-esteem regulation and quality of internal experience — 2
- **Defense and coping**
  7. Capacity for impulse control and regulation — 2
  8. Capacity for defensive functioning — 3
  9. Capacity for adaptation, resiliency, and strength — 3
- **Self-awareness and self-direction**
  10. Self-observing capacities (psychological mindedness) — 4
  11. Capacity to construct and use internal standards and ideals — 3
  12. Capacity for meaning and purpose — 3

Overall level of personality severity (Sum of 12 mental functions): 37

[Healthy/optimal mental functioning 54–60; Good/appropriate mental functioning with some areas of difficulty, 47–53; Mild impairments in mental functioning, 40–46; Moderate impairments in mental functioning, 33–39; Major impairments in mental functioning, 26–32; Significant defects in basic mental functions, 19–25; Major/severe defects in basic mental functions, 12–18]

(continued)

FIGURE 16.2. A completed PDC-A for Michelle.

Section II: Level of Personality Organization

Consider your patient's mental functions in determining the level of personality organization. Use these four mental functions to efficiently capture the level of personality organization. The clinician should keep in mind the stage of adolescence presented by the patient: early adolescence (approximately 12–14 years old), middle adolescence (approximately 15–16 years old), or late adolescence (17–19 years old). Rate each mental function on a scale from 1 (Severely impaired) to 10 (Healthy).

Severe				Moderate				Healthy	
1	2	3	4	5	6	7	8	9	10

1. **Identity:** Ability to view self in complex, stable, and accurate ways 3
2. **Object relations:** Ability to maintain intimate, stable, and satisfying relationships 4
3. **Level of defenses** (using the guide below, select a single number): 5
   - 1–2: Psychotic level (delusional projection, psychotic denial, psychotic distortion)
   - 3–5: Borderline level (splitting, projective identification, idealization/devaluation, denial, acting out)
   - 6–8: Neurotic level (repression, reaction formation, intellectualization, displacement, undoing)
   - 9–10: Healthy level (anticipation, self-assertion, sublimation, suppression, altruism, and humor)
4. **Reality testing:** Ability to appreciate conventional notions of what is realistic 7

Overall Personality Organization

Considering the ratings and your clinical judgment, circle your client's overall personality organization.

Psychotic		Borderline			Neurotic			Healthy	
1	2	3	4	(5)	6	7	8	9	10

"Normal" emerging personality patterns (Healthy): Characterized by mostly 9–10 scores. These adolescents demonstrate a cohesive emerging personality organization in which their biological endowments, including their temperamental vulnerabilities, are managed adaptively within developmentally appropriate relationships with families, peers, and others. In relation to their stage of adolescent development, they have an increasingly organized sense of self, comprising age-appropriate coping skills and empathic, conscientious ways of dealing with feelings about self and others.

Mildly dysfunctional emerging personality patterns (Neurotic): Characterized by mostly 6–8 scores. These adolescents demonstrate a less cohesive emerging personality

(continued)

FIGURE 16.2. *(continued)*

organization in which their biological endowments, including their temperamental vulnerabilities, are managed less adaptively. Early in life, their primary caregivers may have had trouble helping them manage these constitutional dispositions. Thus relationships with families, peers, and others are more fraught with problems. Such adolescents do not navigate the various developmental levels as successfully as those with less problematic endowments and/or more responsive caregivers. However, their sense of self and their sense of reality are pretty solid. As development proceeds, their adaptive mechanisms may be apparent in moderately rigid defensive patterns, and their reactions to adversities may be somewhat dysfunctional.

Dysfunctional emerging personality patterns (Borderline): Characterized by mostly 3–5 scores. These adolescents demonstrate vulnerabilities in reality testing and sense of self. Such problems may be manifested by maladaptive ways of dealing with feelings about self and others. Their defensive operations may distort reality (e.g., their own feelings may be perceived in others, rather than in themselves; the intentions of others may be misperceived).

Severely dysfunctional emerging personality patterns (Psychotic): Characterized by mostly 1–2 scores. These adolescents demonstrate significant deficits in their capacity for reality testing and forming a sense of self, manifested by consistently maladaptive ways of dealing with feelings about self and others. Their defensive operations interfere with basic capacities to relate to others and to separate their own feelings and wishes from those of others. (Use 3 for adolescents who go between psychotic and borderline levels.)

(There are no sharp cutoffs between categories. Use your clinical judgment.)

Section III: Emerging Adolescent Personality Styles/Syndromes (PA Axis)

In addition to considering level of organization, adolescent patients begin to demonstrate an emerging personality style. Rather than thinking of these styles as categorical diagnoses, it is more useful for clinicians to think of the relative degree to which the patient might be exhibiting an emerging style.

Check off as many personality syndromes as apply from the list below; then circle the one or two personality styles that are most dominant. Leave blank if none.

(For research purposes, you may also rate the level of severity for all styles, using a 1–5 scale: 1 = Severe level; 3 = Moderate severity; and 5 = High-functioning.)

	Level of severity
☑ **Depressive**	2
☐ **Anxious–avoidant**	___
☐ **Schizoid**	___

(continued)

FIGURE 16.2. *(continued)*

Level of severity

☐ **Psychopathic–antisocial** ___

☐ **Narcissistic** ___

☐ **Paranoid** ___

☐ **Impulsive–histrionic** ___

☐ **Borderline** ___

☐ **Dependent–victimized** ___

☐ **Obsessive–compulsive** ___

Section IV: Symptom Patterns (SA Axis)

List the main PDM symptom patterns (those that are related to predominantly psychotic disorders, mood disorders, disorders related primarily to anxiety, event- and stressor-related disorders, etc.).

(If required, you may use the DSM or ICD symptoms and codes here.)

Severe		Moderate		Healthy
1	2	3	4	5

Symptom/concern: *Feeding and eating disorders* Level: *1*

Symptom/concern: ___ Level: ___

Symptom/concern: ___ Level: ___

Section V: Cultural, Contextual, and Other Relevant Considerations

Michelle comes from a wealthy social context, with a self-made father and a mother completely devoted to the family. Family background seems to be more oriented to the expression of educational performances and work skills rather than to the inner worlds of its members, so that any emotional expression has not been permitted, welcomed, or deeply understood.

FIGURE 16.2. *(continued)*

Personal Data, Family History, and Specific Features of Relationships with Family Members

Alice's parents are both working professionals who describe themselves as active in sports. They both depict their marriage as conflictual; the family atmosphere is characterized by recurrent quarrels, in which the parents often shout, curse at each other, and reach the point of slapping or kicking. They both are extremely involved in their working lives, and they report to the psychologist that they put their jobs and personal interests ahead of their family. Their views about the education of children are diametrically opposed: Alice's mother is concerned about school performance and would like Alice to devote her free time to sports; her father would like their children to grow up "free-spirited" and serene, without too many rules. Alice's father is especially concerned about her relationships with peers, and often organizes parties and events. He worries when he sees that the social integration of his children is compromised or put at risk.

It seems that the parents are repeating their own respective backgrounds with their children: severity and rules in the mother's family; freedom and lack of rules in the father's. They have been in couple therapy, and they express their concerns about their children during the consultation.

During the first meeting, Alice's parents describe her as a wanted child who met all her developmental milestones on time or ahead of time without difficulties. She has been characteristically untalkative since an early age, although her vocabulary is impressive. Alice has a strong interest in playing soccer and cards, which take most of her free time; she plays soccer well but does not want to cooperate with the coach. Furthermore, she seems more interested in "male" games than in female ones. Alice does not like to do her homework. She needs her parents to be present, but this often triggers conflicts between them.

The parents started to notice Alice's "peculiar behaviors" a year ago, when she was 6. During the consultation, they state that Alice has no friends; she seeks contact with her peers, but she is not able to cooperate in groups because she wants to determine what games are played. She gets easily angry if she cannot choose the game, provoking frequent fights with her peers. As a result, she is often excluded by her school friends and not invited to their birthday parties.

Further Observations

Family Observation

While the family is in the waiting room, there is an audible, intense conversation between the three children and the parents.

During the session, the parents freely express their anxiety: On the one hand, they want to show off their children's capabilities; on the other, they complain about their children's excessive liveliness and failure to observe rules. The parents' expectations of their children's behavior appear excessively high, given the youngsters' ages.

Relations are fluid, and communication appears spontaneous and lively, especially from children to parents. In particular, Alice's brothers seem to have their "own little club," sometimes excluding others as sources of unwanted interference.

Alice's brothers appear bright and extraverted. Alice is more reflective and introverted, but seems similarly capable of independent initiative. She remains inhibited and constricted, however, throughout most of the family session.

Sometimes Alice shows an oppositional stance by not responding to adults' questions. Moreover, when she is asked to do something, she often accepts the request but then fails to do the task, either with her parents or at school. Often she behaves as if she does not hear the requests, ignoring the adults who are talking to her.

A relatively high amount of mutual emotional investment is immediately visible in the interactions between the parents and their children. When Alice feels welcomed, understood, and "safe" from the parents' fights, it seems easier to approach her. She is more communicative and able to maintain eye contact, she can relate more authentically, and she is able to explain why she does not want to do a certain thing or to express her authentic difficulties with certain activities.

Individual Diagnostic Sessions with Alice

Alice appears to be a curious and lively girl. She enters the consulting room with her mother. She is familiar with the environment from the family observation, and she moves freely in it.

She is able to remain alone in the room with the psychologist, after being reassured by the mother. In the first moments, she shows a forced smile and tries to hide her discomfort.

When she feels sufficiently at ease, she talks like a raging river about whatever she likes. She speaks uninterruptedly about her favorite games, showing, for example, that she knows the names of the various characters in video games. She also shows off her academic skills by mentioning, in great detail, specific concepts about her favorite subject. It seems that Alice wants to make a good impression on the psychologist.

During this first session, at the invitation of the psychologist, Alice draws some pictures: a free drawing, four about emotions (anger, sadness, fear, happiness), and the Koch's Tree Test (tree drawing), for a total of six pictures. She comments on the pictures carefully. The psychologist is impressed by the design of the tree; it is a bare birch that looks more like the leafless skeleton of a birch tree.

The emotion drawings are challenging for Alice. She expresses her immediate difficulty, saying that she does not know what she has to draw. But later she uses some "smiley" emoticons, showing impressive ability as a cartoonist. All drawings are done with a black marker in a very concise manner. After drawing anger, Alice mentions that she gets angry several times a day, and then asks, "Why do I get angry when I don't know the reason? Why do I get angry when I don't know how to do something?" The drawing of sadness looks similar to the previous one, except for the eyebrow tilt of the "smiley." She notes, "It seems to me more worried than sad. I'm sad once a day before I get angry." Alice's sensitivity and the rich complexity and emotional nuance of her internal world are definitively confirmed in her drawing of fear: "This face is afraid of the fear it feels. It happens almost always." Finally, the drawing of happiness is represented by a neutral "smiley": When the psychologist looks at the drawing, she makes a personal association to the popular saying, "Put a good face on a bad game."

During the individual session, the psychologist takes particular note of the following:

- Alice often arranges her underpants and frequently tends to touch her bottom.
- Alice's speech is fast and polished, but her communication alternates between moments of great loquacity and moments of total silence, which exclude the other from any conversation.
- Anger and fear seem central matters for Alice, who appears unable to express them without resorting to defenses that weaken her communicative capacities. Alice's mother wonders about her daughter's reactions when she witnesses the parents' quarrels. The mother states that in those cases, Alice runs to her room and stays there silently for hours and hours.
- Alice sometimes alternates between restless states and states of deep depression and fatigue.

Relevant Affects

Alice is a fearful child, who lives always on the alert and ends up feeling tired and depressed. She is able to respond appropriately to context, but only if emotions or stress are absent, or if she is supported by her parents.

She reacts to her feelings of fear, shame, and unworthiness with anger and aggressive manifestations. The parents are experiencing difficulties with these behaviors and are not able to manage them—either because they do not know what to do or because they are overwhelmed by their own shame and guilt. As a result, Alice lacks support in regulating her emotions and often has to deal with them alone, feeling defeat and frustration.

Both parents are very demanding and limiting of her free expressiveness, and Alice seems to be caught in the conflict between her growing needs and the needs of her parents. Interactions with others are characterized by a remarkable introversion. She lacks support in developing her capacity for mentalization and social-emotional regulation.

Defenses

Alice's isolation and aggressive behaviors toward others are her main defensive strategies. She alternates between states of withdrawal and states of excitement. For example, she tends to take refuge in the world of thought, and then explodes in overly intense or apparently out-of-context angry demonstrations. There is evidence of both somatization and acting out. As her parents say, Alice spends a lot of time in "paper folding" and in mathematics problems—isolating herself with repetitive activities and staying in silence and concentration. When she cannot calm herself, and when the environment has not helped her to contain her feelings, she has crying spells.

Alice also seems to use obsessive defenses when she describes something with excessive details, repeatedly fills lists of numbers and records, proposes logic games with mathematical operations, and so on.

Main Concerns and Pathogenic Beliefs

Alice feels herself to be different from, and superior to, others: "Unlike my friends, I know everything about that game," or "I'm the best in learning things by heart," or "I don't like doing things that other kids like." Such beliefs seem to strengthen her tendency to stay isolated and to disguise her desire to be recognized by family and friends.

It seems that Alice's sense of being different and special covers a sense of insecurity that blocks her own sense of cohesion and development.

Different Levels of Functioning

Alice is organized and focused, able to learn when she is not overstimulated (e.g., in noisy or frantic environments), anxious, or stressed. She presents two levels of functioning: On the one hand, she adapts to people's expectations (Alice tries to be what others want her to be and to behave like an adult); on the other, she appears immature and emotionally troubled (e.g., when she gets tired of doing homework, she starts inconsolably crying; when she tries to play with a peer, she responds to rejection by getting quickly angry, screaming, crying, or throwing herself on the floor). This way of functioning has a profound negative impact on her growing sense of self and agency in the context of relationships.

Strengths and Resources

Alice is an intelligent and sensitive child. She is capable of good verbal expression, and she can focus and spend energy on activities of interest. In dyadic interactions, her emotions are much better regulated than when she is in a group. She loves her parents and wants to talk to them about her problems.

Patient's Opinions about Herself

Alice experiences her emotions in an excessive way and would like to be helped to have more regulated behaviors. She wants to talk about this with her mother and father.

During one session after the assessment, Alice draws a space ship, equipped with a wide range of electronic controls to defend herself and to attack in case of need. The ship is ready to embark on a journey that begins passing through a space–time tunnel, where "everything is pending." Alice can't return to a stable sense of self; it is as if she considers her activities uninteresting in the eyes of others and does not feel lovable. In the context of a safe therapeutic space and after reaching a treatment alliance, Alice seems to accept the help of the psychologist.

Therapist's Reaction to the Patient

Alice's therapist reports a state of some confusion. This may be due to Alice's alternating states of calm and excitement, as well as a bit of impatience the therapist feels while witnessing some of her obsessive behavior.

Alice's creativity across a range of activities (e.g., sports, drawing) raises the therapist's curiosity. Alice seems connected with her and interested in impressing her, while simultaneously reluctant to seek support for what she is struggling with. The psychologist feels a sense of interest and empathy in this context.

Treatment Indications

Child–parent psychotherapy on a weekly basis is recommended. Individual sessions with Alice, as well as sessions with Alice and her parents, are needed. The primary aims of the therapy are as follows:

1. To support Alice in finding adequate, age-appropriate emotional regulatory strategies that will help her to express the variety and complexity of her feelings in more appropriate ways. In turn, this should sustain her capacity to create and maintain relationships with others.
2. To help her parents manage their own aggressive behaviors and Alice's emotional crises, in order to support them in maintaining high levels of warmth, responsiveness, sensitivity, and consistency. Meetings with the parents are needed to address in particular their difficulties with reflective functioning, their lack of realistic developmental expectations, and their lack of curiosity about their child's experience.

DSM-5/ICD-10 Diagnosis

Generalized anxiety disorder (ICD-10-CM code: F41.1)

PDM-2 Diagnosis

MC Axis

Alice shows moderate constriction in some domains of mental functioning, with some specific areas of difficulty. These have a negative impact on the quality and stability of her relationships, her sense of identity, and her ability to tolerate affects.

MC4. Moderate impairments in mental functioning (range = 30–36)

PC Axis

Profile of emerging personality patterns and difficulties: Neurotic level of personality organization

SC Axis

SC31. Anxiety disorders

PDM-2 Profile on the PDC-C

A completed PDC-C for Alice, revealing her full PDM-2 profile, is provided in Figure 16.3 on the next page.

(text resumes on page 999)

Psychodiagnostic Chart—Child (PDC-C)

Name: *Alice* Age: *7* Gender: *Female* Ethnicity: *European*

Date of evaluation: *XX / XX / XX* Evaluator: *Psychotherapist*

Section I: Mental Functioning (MC Axis)

Rate your patient's level of strength or weakness on each of the 11 mental functions below, on a scale from 1 to 5 (1 = Severe deficits; 5 = Healthy). Then sum the 11 ratings for a level-of-severity score.

Severe deficits	Major impairments	Moderate impairments	Mild impairments	Healthy
1	2	3	4	5

- **Cognitive and affective processes**
  1. Capacity for regulation, attention, and learning *4*
  2. Capacity for affective range, communication, and understanding *3*
  3. Capacity for mentalization and reflective functioning *3*
- **Identity and relationships**
  4. Capacity for differentiation and integration (identity) *3*
  5. Capacity for relationships and intimacy *2*
  6. Capacity for self-esteem regulation and quality of internal experience *3*
- **Defense and coping**
  7. Capacity for impulse control and regulation *2*
  8. Capacity for defensive functioning *2*
  9. Capacity for adaptation, resiliency, and strength *4*
- **Self-awareness and self-direction**
  10. Self-observing capacities (psychological mindedness) *3*
  11. Capacity to construct and use internal standards and ideals *3*

Overall level of personality severity (Sum of 11 mental functions): *32*

[Healthy/optimal mental functioning, 50–55; Good/appropriate mental functioning with some areas of difficulty, 43–49; Mild impairments in mental functioning, 37–42; Moderate impairments in mental functioning, 30–36; Major impairments in mental functioning, 24–29; Significant defects in basic mental functions, 17–23; Major/severe defects in basic mental functions, 11–16]

(continued)

FIGURE 16.3. A completed PDC-C for Alice.

Section II: Emerging Level of Personality Patterns and Difficulties

Consider your patient's mental functions in determining the level of personality organization. Use these four mental functions to efficiently capture the current personality patterns and difficulties leading to an emerging level of personality organization. Age-specific characteristics, as well as the high level of fluidity in symptomatology during this stage of development, should be considered—as should other specific external factors influencing current clinical presentation. Rate each mental function on a scale from 1 (Severely impaired) to 10 (Healthy).

Severe				Moderate				Healthy	
1	2	3	4	5	6	7	8	9	10

1. **Identity:** Emerging ability to view self in age-appropriate, stable, and accurate ways — 5
2. **Object relations:** Emerging ability to maintain intimate, stable, and satisfying relationships — 5
3. **Emerging personality pattern** (using the guide below, select a single number): — 7
   - 1–2: Psychotic level
   - 3–5: Borderline level
   - 6–8: Neurotic level
   - 9–10: Healthy level
4. **Reality testing:** Ability to appreciate conventional notions of what is realistic — 7

Overall Emerging Personality Organization

Considering the ratings and your clinical judgment, circle your client's overall emerging personality organization.

Psychotic		Borderline			Neurotic			Healthy	
1	2	3	4	5	6	(7)	8	9	10

"Normal" emerging personality patterns (Healthy): Characterized by mostly 9–10 scores. These children demonstrate a cohesive emerging personality organization in which their biological endowments, including their temperamental vulnerabilities, are managed adaptively within developmentally appropriate relationships with families, peers, and others. In relation to their stage of development, they have an increasingly organized sense of self, comprising age-appropriate coping skills and empathic, conscientious ways of dealing with feelings about self and others.

Mildly dysfunctional emerging personality patterns (Neurotic): Characterized by mostly 6–8 scores. These children demonstrate a less cohesive emerging personality organization in which their biological endowments, including their temperamental

(continued)

FIGURE 16.3. *(continued)*

vulnerabilities, are managed less adaptively. Early in life, their primary caregivers may have had trouble helping them manage these constitutional dispositions. Thus relationships with families, peers, and others are more fraught with problems. Such children do not navigate the various developmental levels as successfully as those with less problematic endowments and/or more responsive caregivers. However, their sense of self and their sense of reality are progressing in an age-appropriate manner. As development proceeds, their adaptive mechanisms may be apparent in moderately rigid defensive patterns, and their reactions to adversities may be somewhat dysfunctional.

Dysfunctional emerging personality patterns (Borderline): Characterized by mostly 3–5 scores. These children demonstrate vulnerabilities in reality testing and sense of self. Such problems may be manifested by maladaptive ways of dealing with feelings about self and others. Their defensive operations may distort reality (e.g., their own feelings may be perceived in others, rather than in themselves; the intentions of others may be misperceived).

Severely dysfunctional emerging personality patterns (Psychotic): Characterized by mostly 1–2 scores. These children demonstrate significant deficits in their capacity for reality testing and forming a sense of self, manifested by consistently maladaptive ways of dealing with feelings about self and others. Their defensive operations interfere with basic capacities to relate to others and to separate their own feelings and wishes from those of others.

(There are no sharp cutoffs between categories. Use your clinical judgment.)

Section III: Symptom Patterns (SC Axis)

List the main PDM symptom patterns (those that are related to predominantly psychotic disorders, mood disorders, disorders related primarily to anxiety, event- and stressor-related disorders, etc.).

(If required, you may use the DSM or ICD symptoms and codes here.)

Severe		Moderate		Healthy
1	2	3	4	5

Symptom/concern: *Anxiety disorder* Level: *2*

Symptom/concern: ______ Level: ___

Symptom/concern: ______ Level: ___

(continued)

FIGURE 16.3. *(continued)*

Section IV: Influencing Factors and Relevant Clinical Observations Informing Diagnosis

1. Epigenetics: *Family history not revealed in exhaustive detail; probable parental anxiety.*
2. Temperament: *Lively girl; limited ability to tolerate frustration.*
3. Neuropsychology: *Developmental milestones on time; no sensory issues; normative verbal abilities when anxiety is low.*
4. Attachment style *Separation and reunion moments during the diagnostic process suggest the hypothesis that Alice may have insecure–avoidant attachment style, as characterized by the fluctuation in proximity–avoidance. Some basic sense of safety is present.*
5. Sociocultural influences: *Upper-middle-class family.*
6. Countertransference–transference manifestations: *The therapist reports a state of some confusion, maybe due to Alice's alternating states of calm and excitement, as well as a bit of impatience in witnessing some of her obsessive behavior. Otherwise, Alice's creativity across a range of activities raises the therapist's curiosity, interest, and empathy in this context.*

FIGURE 16.3. *(continued)*

Infancy and Early Childhood

Paul

Paul is almost 4 years old. He is the first child in his family, the sibling of an 18-month-old brother. His parents, both in their 30s, have sought psychological consultation because of Paul's temper and aggressive behaviors over the past year. Violent outbursts such as bites, punches, and slaps aimed at both parents and at peers have become quite alarming to them. The parents are also worried because Paul continually refuses to comply with requests from authority figures or with rules. He has become an overbearing child, and the parents do not know how to deal with such behaviors.

The assessment process includes two meetings with his parents, a meeting with Paul, and two family observations that do not include his younger brother. The goal of the evaluations is to gauge the quality of relationships in Paul's life and the interaction patterns with his parents.

Personal Data, Family History, and Specific Features of Relationships with Family Members

The parents say that Paul was born at full term after a normal pregnancy. They did not have any particular problems in dealing with him during the first 2 years of his development. Paul's sleep–wake rhythms were quite regular. This was a relief to the mother because both parents worked and needed time to rest and sleep well. He was breast-fed for 9 months, and weaning was an easy process. He still eats everything cooked for him; however, eating time becomes complicated if he becomes angry (he may throw food, stand up on his chair, annoy his brother, and generally disregard rules or orders).

His parents both describe him as very active and full of energy, although he is a bit clumsy and reckless. Often he breaks things or gets hurt.

During his mother's pregnancy with his younger brother, Paul suffered from night terrors and began having oppositional and aggressive behaviors. Both parents describe this period as extremely trying. They think that Paul has been jealous of his younger brother since before the brother was born. During that pregnancy, the mother was hospitalized three times for periods ranging from 4 to 15 days. The father says that Paul reacted to the mother's absence by protesting, seeking attention, and constantly asking for her. The mother remembers that when she arrived home after the longest separation from Paul, he was indifferent to her and withdrawn. Both parents agree that in the mother's absence, he became closer to his father and still asks for him most of the time whenever he needs something (e.g., when he wakes up at night). This causes the mother to feel guilt over her previous absences.

The mother says that Paul is an intelligent boy who is able to speak and comprehend well. However, she is frustrated by the fact that he always wants to do things his own way and does not listen to her. When he cannot get what he wants, he becomes easily frustrated, as demonstrated by crying and outward protesting that cannot be soothed easily. He also becomes angry and aggressive when he is not permitted to do something or when he is not capable of completing things.

Paul frequently has difficulties at preschool and with other children. The mother reports that in the morning, he cries and insists that he does not want to go to preschool. Once he is there, he is often irritable and constantly argues or fights with his peers. His mother says that he is also fragile and demanding. He fears nighttime. Finally, she has sometimes seen him slapping or insulting himself, especially after he has done something wrong or prohibited.

During the first meeting, the parents appear exhausted and frustrated; they complain a lot about Paul's behaviors, and their level of anxiety and preoccupation is very high. Whereas the father tends to minimize the problems and thinks that there is no need for psychological support, the mother has a lot of fears for Paul's future as an adult.

Functional Emotional Developmental Capacities

During the family observation, Paul appears curious, extraverted, and dynamic. He explores autonomously, moving quickly around the office while exploring his immediate surroundings. He rapidly alternates between various forms of play.

Paul is able to experience a full range of age-expected emotions, but his feelings can quickly become intense; he is particularly quick to anger, especially when he fails at doing something. He often rebels against limits and rules imposed by the parents or the therapist. He wants to do things on his own. If he is not allowed to do so, he becomes disorganized and behaviorally aggressive (e.g., he throws things or acts in an undisciplined way).

When the family is seated around a small table, engaging in a more structured play scenario, Paul exhibits a higher-level mastery of his emotional functioning. He plays pleasantly and engages himself in happy interactions with both parents. He is able to initiate and participate actively in a shared game while maintaining adequate levels of attention and concentration. He also utilizes symbolic communication and pretend play, and he shows good ability to understand his own affective states and those of others. Evidence of shame and guilt over his actions appears during the play interactions as well.

Paul is very demanding toward his parents. If they are distracted, he becomes irritable and tends to cry, shout, or hit, despite the fact that he demonstrates a good repertoire of gesture-based expression and communication that permits the expression of his needs and emotions. His expressive language is quite delayed.

Regulatory–Sensory Processing Capacities

Paul shows attentional and observational competencies, curiosity, and capacity for understanding and learning. His regulatory–sensory processing profile is characterized by overresponsiveness, especially in situations of stress, in which he becomes impulsive. Overall, he shows limited ability to tolerate frustration and high levels of reactivity and irritability.

He is active and strong and moves rapidly around the room, showing little impairment in fine motor skills.

Paul's ability to modulate anxiety is still limited, and his capacity for self-regulation is in need of stable support. His difficulties and aggressive behaviors diminish when a good scaffolding is offered by his parents; in such instances, he is able to find more appropriate ways to express his feelings of anger and better ways of tolerating frustration.

Relational Patterns and Disorders

During the observations, Paul interacts positively with both parents and the psychologist. When he is alone with the psychologist, he is initially cautious, but soon becomes comfortable and explores and interacts easily.

Paul's parents appear mostly tense, worried, and apprehensive. They both have negative representations of their child, and they overtly criticize him and often express disapproval.

The mother frequently rebukes Paul verbally and appears excessively worried about rules and limits. Both parents say they are exhausted by his oppositional behaviors and are now adopting an overly punitive parenting style.

The father appears to have a more positive engagement style with Paul. He is able to manage Paul's negative emotional states and behaviors quite well. However, he is not always available and active, and sometimes he displays a tendency to retreat from interaction.

The mother is more unpredictable. She alternates between moments of enthusiastic and aligned positive engagement and periods of emotional unavailability. She often expresses high levels of anxiety and preoccupations that distract her from shared interaction. These moments deeply affect her child, who quickly becomes nervous and irritable. The mother's anxious state also interferes with her reflective capacities. She has trouble managing Paul's aggressive behaviors and negative emotions, especially anger and protest. In particular, when oppositional or disruptive behaviors occur, she is much more concerned about cleaning up any mess Paul makes than about addressing him.

She is extremely concerned about her son's aggressive behaviors because she is familiar with violence in her family of origin. She worries that Paul could became an aggressive and disruptive individual like her father and brother.

Treatment Indications

In this situation, it is important to consider an intervention program focused on Paul's emotional regulatory ability as well as on the patterns of interaction between him and his parents. Given that Paul's emotional regulatory vulnerability can be exacerbated or mitigated in the context of the relationship with his parents, a course of parent–child therapy aimed at improving interpersonal and intrapersonal dyadic emotional regulation is recommended.

The therapy should focus on helping both Paul and his parents to find activities that allow them to share positive affective states, while supporting developmental maturation of implicit emotional regulation processes. Paul needs help in regulating his emotional state and his involvement in dyadic interactions with caregivers, especially in moments of stress.

The therapist should also help the parents find better solutions to, and strategies for handling, Paul's disruptive behaviors. These should include discouraging an overly punitive style of parenting, while supporting more effective ways (such as positive reinforcements) to build his tolerance of limits and rules and to increase periods of shared affection. They also need to be encouraged to welcome his thoughts, feelings, and fantasies about the absences of his mother at a critical time in his development, so that he can rework his evident belief that she left him because there was something wrong with him and then replaced him with a better child.

PDM-2 Diagnosis

Primary Diagnoses

IEC12. Disruptive behavior and oppositional disorder (level 3)

PDM-2 Profile on the PDC-IEC

A completed PDC-IEC for Paul, revealing his full PDM-2 profile, is provided in Figure 16.4.

(text resumes on page 1007)

— Psychodiagnostic Chart—Infancy and Early Childhood (PDC-IEC) —

Name: *Paul* Age: *3y, 10m* Gender: *Male* Ethnicity: *European*

Date of evaluation: XX / XX / XX Evaluator: *Psychotherapist*

Section I: Primary Diagnoses

List the main IEC diagnoses and rate the level of severity for each, using a 1–5 scale. If necessary, you may use the DC: 0–3R, DC: 0–5, or DSM diagnosis here.

Severe		Moderate		Mild
1	2	3	4	5

Principal diagnosis: *Disruptive behavior and oppositional disorder* Level: *3*

Other diagnosis: *Hypersensitive/overresponsive: Negative, stubborn* Level: *4*

Other diagnosis: ______ Level: ______

Section II: Functional Emotional Developmental Capacities

Circle the child's level of strengths or deficits on each of the six emotional functions below, on a scale from 1 to 5 (1 = Severe deficits; 5 = Healthy).

Level	Expected emotional function	Rating scale				
1	Shared attention and regulation	5	(4)	3	2	1
2	Engagement and relating	5	(4)	3	2	1
3	Two-way purposeful emotional interactions	(5)	4	3	2	1
4	Shared social problem solving	(5)	4	3	2	1
5	Creating symbols and ideas	5	(4)	3	2	1
6	Building logical bridges between ideas: Logical thinking	5	(4)	3	2	1

Section III: Regulatory–Sensory Processing Capacities

Axis III describes the child's regulatory–sensory processing profile. There are a number of constitutional–maturational differences in the way in which infants and young children respond to and comprehend sensory experiences and then plan actions. The different observed patterns exist on a continuum from relatively normal variations to disorders.

(continued)

FIGURE 16.4. A completed PDC-IEC for Paul.

Circle the child's level of regulatory–sensory processing capacities in each of the categories below, on a scale from 1 to 4 (1 = Severe problem; 4 = No indication).

Category	Subtype	Challenge in this area: No indication; never or rarely a problem	Mild problem or only occasionally a problem	Moderate problem or frequently a problem	Severe problem or almost always a problem
Sensory modulation	Sensory underresponsivity	(4)	3	2	1
	Sensory overresponsive	4	(3)	2	1
	Sensory seeking	4	(3)	2	1
Sensory discrimination	Tactile	4	(3)	2	1
	Auditory	(4)	3	2	1
	Visual	(4)	3	2	1
	Taste/smell	4	(3)	2	1
	Vestibular/ Propriocep.	(4)	3	2	1
Sensory-based motor functioning	Postural challenges	(4)	3	2	1
	Dyspraxis challenges	4	(3)	2	1

Overall Regulatory–Sensory Profile

Considering the ratings and your clinical judgment, circle the degree to which each regulatory–sensory pattern represents normal variation versus disorder. For scores 1–2, consider a regulatory–sensory processing disorder as a primary diagnosis; for scores 3–4, consider that the disordered regulatory–sensory processing can be associated with other primary diagnoses.

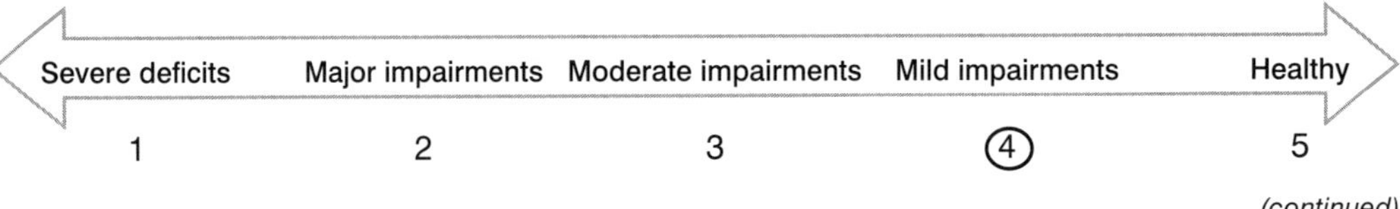

(continued)

FIGURE 16.4. *(continued)*

Section IV: Relational Patterns and Disorders

Each child's relationship with a significant caregiver (mother or father but, if appropriate custodial parent, grandparent, etc.) should be evaluated in this section. Rate the caregiver–child relationship on each of the eight descriptions below, on a scale from 1 to 5 (1 = Severely impaired; 5 = Healthy). Then sum the eight ratings for the degree to which the pattern represents healthy/adapted relationship versus relational disorder.

Caregiver 1: *Mother* (please specify)

Infant/child–caregiver relationship	***Rating scale***				
Quality and flexibility of caregiver's representation of the child	5	4	(3)	2	1
Quality of caregiver's reflective functioning	5	4	(3)	2	1
Quality of caregiver and child's nonverbal engagement	5	(4)	3	2	1
Quality of interactional patterns (reciprocity, synchrony, interactive repair)	5	4	(3)	2	1
Affective tone of the caregiver–infant relationship	5	4	(3)	2	1
Quality of caregiver's behavior (sensitivity vs. threatening and/or frightening behaviors)	5	4	(3)	2	1
Quality of caregiving patterns (comfort, stimulation, response to infant emotional signals, encouragement vs. withdrawal, overstimulation, controlling behavior, insensitivity)	5	4	(3)	2	1
Infant/child's ability to engage and form a significant relationship (vs. specific difficulties that impair this ability)	5	(4)	3	2	1
	Total score = *26*				

Overall Level of Relational Pattern (Caregiver 1)

[Healthy/adapted relational patterns, 36–40; Adapted relational patterns with some areas of difficulty, 29–35; Moderate perturbation or disturbance in relational patterns, 22–28; Significant disturbance in relational patterns, 15–21; Major impairments in relational pattern or relational disorders, 8–14]

Attachment Pattern (Caregiver 1)

Rate the caregiver–child relationship as regards attachment patterns on a scale from 1 (no correspondence) to 5 (high correspondence) for each of the four prototypes.

Secure	*3*
Insecure–avoidant	*2*
Insecure–ambivalent/resistant	*1*
Disorganized/disoriented	*1*

(continued)

FIGURE 16.4. *(continued)*

Caregiver 2: Father (please specify)

Infant/child–caregiver relationship	***Rating scale***				
Quality and flexibility of caregiver's representation of the child	5	(4)	3	2	1
Quality of caregiver's reflective functioning	5	(4)	3	2	1
Quality of caregiver and child's nonverbal engagement	5	(4)	3	2	1
Quality of interactional patterns (reciprocity, synchrony, interactive repair)	5	(4)	3	2	1
Affective tone of the caregiver–infant relationship	(5)	4	3	2	1
Quality of caregiver's behavior (sensitivity vs. threatening and/or frightening behaviors)	5	(4)	3	2	1
Quality of caregiving patterns (comfort, stimulation, response to infant emotional signals, encouragement vs. withdrawal, overstimulation, controlling, insensitivity)	5	(4)	3	2	1
Infant/child's ability to engage and form a significant relationship (vs. specific difficulties that impair this ability)	5	(4)	3	2	1
	Total score = 33				

Overall Level of Relational Pattern (Caregiver 2)

[Healthy/adapted relational patterns, 36–40; Adapted relational patterns with some areas of difficulty, 29–35; Moderate perturbation or disturbance in relational patterns, 22–28; Significant disturbance in relational patterns, 15–21; Major impairments in relational pattern or relational disorders, 8–14]

Attachment Pattern (Caregiver 2)

Rate the caregiver–child relationship as regards attachment patterns on a scale from 1 (no correspondence) to 5 (high correspondence) for each of the four prototypes.

Secure 4

Insecure–avoidant 2

Insecure–ambivalent/resistant 1

Disorganized/disoriented 1

Section V: Other Medical and Neurological Diagnoses

____

____

____

____

FIGURE 16.4. *(continued)*

Later Life

Emilia

Presenting Problem

Some years ago, Emilia was directed to the local psychological center by her general practitioner because she was worried about losing her memory and other mental faculties, and she feared becoming unable to live independently. Her GP did not see a basis for such fears, but urged her to see a psychologist.

Personal Data, Family History, and Specific Features of Relationships with Family Members

Emilia was an 84-year-old woman, kind, good-natured, and well dressed. Her features showed that she had been a beautiful woman when young. She was slightly overweight and walked slowly, leaning on a cane. It was hard to tell whether she did so because she lacked self-confidence or had a real need for the cane.

She had a good level of education and spoke articulately but deliberately. She was slow in her movements as well as in her talking. Her way of thinking showed consistency, although some uncertainties occurred. She liked talking about her life, and was almost surprised by the episodes that she could easily recall. She looked interested in the connections and rewordings that the psychologist offered in connection with the events she related. She asked for suggestions and thanked him for what she initially called "good advice."

Emilia was continuing to read books and do crossword puzzles, although she complained about not being able to remember what she had read only a little earlier. In the waiting room before the session, she was working on a crossword puzzle so as "not to become too stupid."

Emilia was heterosexual and had been a widow for 15 years. Her husband, Giovanni, had died at 70 of a heart attack. She was living on her own and was fairly independent. The people in her neighborhood were helping her with harder tasks.

Her only daughter, Angela, who was turning 60 at the time Emilia came for evaluation, was a housewife married to a retired accountant. Her grandson was 31 and had a child. Her granddaughter, a university researcher, was 27 and single. Emilia was very proud of her grandchildren.

Emilia was the elder of two daughters. Her sister, Barbara, was 10 years younger. There had reportedly always been a good relationship between them, and they were still meeting with their friends once a week to play cards. Her parents were married at the beginning of the 20th century. They belonged to the lower middle class, in which it was common to express criticism toward the authoritarian regime at the time in Italy; for the sake of safety and convenience, however, they did not take an openly hostile attitude.

Emilia looked back nostalgically to her childhood. It seems that her parents were reasonably happy together. She described her mother as a tender woman, devoted to the family and able to manage with care the income of her husband, who was a municipal employee. Emilia maintained a special admiration toward her father. She remembered him as a strict man, stern but right and responsible with his family. His behavior was consistent with his values—in particular, the conjugal fidelity and the sense of responsibility he taught to his daughters. Emilia's parents died not long after the end of the Second World War. After her parents' deaths, Emilia continued to look after her sister, as she had done since she was a child.

Encouraged by her father, Emilia obtained a secretarial diploma. She had pleasant memories of those years in school. At the time, it was uncommon for women to study, and for this reason she was grateful to her parents. She found a job in a factory, where she met Giovanni, a charming man with progressive political views who had fought with the partisans for the liberation of Italy from the Nazis. They fell in love, and soon afterward they decided to live together, even though Giovanni was married to a girl from polite society. Giovanni left the marital home, which involved onerous economic costs and the heavy pressure of his wife's powerful family. This choice, in deep opposition to the morals of that time, forced them to move to another town and seek different work. After many years of life in common, they had their only daughter, Angela. Giovanni struggled in vain for years to invalidate his marriage through the ecclesiastical tribunal. But only the passage of the divorce law in Italy allowed him finally to marry the woman he had fallen in love with, and to realize their dream.

By that time, though, the dream had already begun to be strained by the concrete difficulties of everyday reality—above all, the discovery of the weaknesses, contradictions, and different expectations of each party to the marriage.

Their first important conflict started when Emilia decided to open a bookshop in a working-class neighborhood in the town where they had moved. That was the realization of a long-held wish—one that likely came from the love of culture that her father had passed on to her and that suited her need for emancipation as a woman, certainly ahead of her time and in advance of the Italian feminist movement. Emilia wished to spread the pleasure of reading and to promote culture in a working-class neighborhood. Her bookshop would have been among the first in the area to include a section for children, for whom she had a particular fondness.

The bookshop was successful, but this success was never acknowledged openly in the family; her earnings were good from the start, and her income soon became higher than her husband's. This difference in their earnings accentuated the conflicts already existing between them. Emilia recalled that in the evenings, "As the bookshop shutters were lowered, silence fell in the house, [and] I was in low spirits."

Despite Giovanni's progressive views, his public role in the association of former partisans, and his failure to object overtly, her husband was not happy about his wife's activity. Over the years he would constantly criticize it, blaming many of their problems on this choice. The heaviest accusation he threw at his wife was that she was not a loving mother and that she cared more for the business than for her daughter. This accusation remained an open wound for Emilia.

The distance separating Emilia and Giovanni grew larger and larger; Emilia felt that Angela was affected by the climate of disagreement in the family. Angela also obtained a diploma, but unlike her mother, once she got married and became the mother of two children, she chose to be a housewife. Although the relationship with her husband was difficult, Emilia continued to find fulfillment in her work, where she developed meaningful relationships with the customers. Among these was a friendship she established with the nuns of a foundling hospital, which allowed her to donate money for the children, often doing so without telling her husband. Once, at Christmas, she bought some cloth, which her trusty dressmaker used to make a winter overcoat for each child.

Every now and then, Emilia bought herself some small pieces of jewelry, as if to make up for the lack of recognition from her husband.

In a particularly critical moment with her husband, Emilia made a suicide attempt. She swallowed some tablets and was hospitalized for a few days. The chief psychiatrist, who already knew her as the "generous lady" of the bookshop, gave her special consideration. He was trusted with her confidences, expressed for the first time, about the disappointment and suffering in her marriage, which she had strongly wanted nevertheless. The doctor talked to her husband; he advised him to be nicer to his wife and to recognize her personal qualities more openly. Giovanni changed, as he tried hard to do what the doctor had suggested. Afterward, the couple never talked about what had happened. Their communication was less conflictual, but remained limited to the concrete aspects of everyday life.

Because of her advancing age, and at the urging of her husband, Emilia felt forced to close the bookshop. The grief she felt over the closure of the business had never been quite dealt with. The way she talked about it in the session with the psychologist revealed a painful nostalgia, counteracted to some extent by the solace she drew from encounters with parents living in the neighborhood, who would introduce her to their children as the "bookseller" of their own childhoods. This made her feel happy.

In addition to the closure of the bookshop, Emilia was mourning the loss of her husband, who had died suddenly 15 years ago. Emilia remembered his death vividly. At the time, he was putting documents and writings on the partisans' role in the war in order, with the intention of publishing a book for his association. His work was well advanced when he was stricken by a heart attack in his study. Emilia felt she had to continue the work her husband had begun, but gradually, almost without realizing it, she gave up. This made her feel guilty, and yet she justified her decision defensively—sometimes by reference to her cultural limits, sometimes in terms of the resentment she still bore against him. She remained hurt by his old accusation of her not having been a good mother, and by the privileged bond between father and daughter from which she felt excluded. Emilia was still blaming herself for having been "more for the books than for bodily contact, . . . than for cuddles," agreeing in this way with her husband.

Further Observations

Psychological Intervention

Emilia evidently had not had any particular physical health issues. It was not clear whether in the first part of her life there was any psychological trouble. The suicide attempt was the most serious event—the mark of a personal and family crisis that had been going on for a long time. Though she received support and help, she continued to be unhappy, restless, and silently angry at her husband, but also overwrought with guilt because she thought she should feel satisfied with the realization of her dreams: the "impossible" marriage, the bookshop, and motherhood. Instead, she had to learn to live with her discomfort and with the part of her life that was giving her satisfaction (namely, the commercial activity). But she never found a space for the acknowledgment and release of her personal feelings. It was almost impossible to see a psychologist in the sociocultural and institutional context in which she lived. Only in advanced age did she gain access to a public psychological service, thanks to her GP, who hypothesized an anxiety–depressive disorder and the need for psychological treatment. He had excluded a pharmacological one, putting off that option, if necessary, until after a consultation.

Her propensity toward introspection and her intact cognitive abilities allowed Emilia to make good use of brief psychological support. Paradoxically, rather than being caused by mnemonic weaknesses, her real problems were caused by the very memories she was worried about losing, together with their associated affects: anger, guilt, disappointment, jealousy, and shame. Like her husband, Emilia had the compulsion to reread and relate her "memoirs," which were at risk of remaining "dead letters." During the support sessions, she dealt with her anger, her disappointments, and the blame her life partner had put on her, especially the accusation of having been a bad mother. She also finally confronted how her own self-accusations had joined those of her husband. It was her failings, she believed, that accounted for the daughter's privileged relationship with the father; in her view, "the two of them" had excluded her. For the same reason, her daughter was putatively still angry at her, did not love her, and preferred her mother-in-law, who lived with Angela and who was older, sicker, and less able than Emilia was.

At the beginning of treatment, Emilia's relationship with her daughter appeared full of ambivalence. One the one hand, Angela was insisting that her mother as well as her mother-in-law live with her, so as to be able to have Angela's help in case of illness; on the other hand, the frequent arguments between them prevented real closeness. In addition, Emilia felt that her daughter's proposal was offensive because it meant her giving up her independence, her house, and the relationships she had developed in the neighborhood. However, during the sessions, Emilia gradually succeeded in acknowledging both her jealousy of her daughter's mother-in-law and the fact that her daughter was not (any more) angry at her; otherwise, she would certainly not have wanted her to live in her home.

At a certain point in the support process, Emilia let the psychologist talk to her daughter, who sometimes took Emilia to the local social assistance facility. Angela understood well the guilt her mother felt, but she considered it irrational. As a matter of fact, she stated that Emilia had been a good mother, tender and affectionate with her daughter ("I remember the cuddles, indeed . . .").

In addition, Angela was conscious of the conflict between her parents. She recognized that her father was a charming man, to whom she was very attached. In spite of the mistakes she realized both parents had made, she insisted that "they both made sure I lacked for nothing, either materially or emotionally." Toward her mother, as a result, she expressed deep affection and true protectiveness, even though she had difficulty in accepting her refusal to live with her.

After the meeting between Angela and the psychologist, Emilia seemed much relieved. The subject of her losing her memory or becoming "stupid" had receded. The choice of her independence still remained her bulwark. She reached agreements to see her daughter and her son-in-law almost every day.

After 6 months of weekly psychological support, Emilia and the psychologist agreed that the treatment had been successful and planned follow-up sessions to take place every 3 months. During the follow-ups, Emilia accepted her daughter's suggestion to hire a caregiver. This allowed her both a certain degree of independence and some help in climbing the stairs and moving around the neighborhood.

When she was about 86, 2 years after her first access to the psychology service, Emilia had a stroke that took away her powers of speech and movement, but not her smile and sense of humor. She recovered her faculties only partially in rehabilitation, and therefore her independence was compromised. When the rehabilitative treatment was over, and after a short stay at her daughter's, she obstinately decided to go back home with the caregiver. She met with the psychologist two more times. Then some physical complications required her daughter to take Emilia into her house, where she died some months later.

Despite her suffering and the sad events in her life, Emilia's persistence in seeking help, strength of mind, and ability to keep hope of change for the future were valuable resources. Psychotherapy was able to strengthen her capacity for flexibility and adaptation. The sense of warm emotional closeness that she evoked in the psychologist contributed to the strength of the therapeutic alliance.

DSM-5/ICD-10 Diagnosis

Generalized anxiety disorder (ICD-10-CM code: F41.1)

PDM-2 Diagnosis

ME Axis

Despite Emilia's age, her general cognitive faculties were well preserved. Her capabilities for comprehension and exposition were good. She preserved an overall degree of health that had been strengthened over time by her work. No pathology was found in her mnemonic faculties, only age-related physiological hesitations and slowdowns. However, Emilia did show mild constrictions and areas of inflexibility in some domains of mental functioning, such as self-esteem regulation, defensive functioning, and psychological mindedness.

ME3. Mild impairments in mental functioning (range = 40–46)

PE Axis

Emilia's life was characterized by persistent feelings of sadness, guilt, jealousy, anger, and shame, which she handled through the defenses of repression, introjection, devaluation of herself, idealization of others, humor, and unselfishness.

Emilia's main concerns and pathogenic beliefs were about the dichotomy between goodness and wickedness; for example, "The others [the nuns, the bookshop customers, etc.] believed I was a nice person," versus "I have been a bad mother." As a result, Emilia persistently believed that there was something intrinsically evil or inadequate in herself, and that if people had known her better, she would have been rejected.

Personality syndrome: Depressive personality

Level of personality organization: Neurotic

SE Axis

SE31. Anxiety disorders

PDM-2 Profile on the PDC-E

A completed PDC-E for Emilia, revealing her full PDM-2 profile, is provided in Figure 16.5.

Psychodiagnostic Chart—Elderly (PDC-E)

Name: *Emilia* Age: *84* Gender: *Female* Ethnicity: *European*

Date of evaluation: *XX / XX / XX* Evaluator: *Psychotherapist*

Section I: Mental Functioning (ME Axis)

Rate your patient's level of strength or weakness on each of the 12 mental functions below, on a scale from 1 to 5 (1 = Severe deficits; 5 = Healthy). Then sum the 12 ratings for a level-of-severity score.

Although most older adults do not have significant cognitive impairment, it is important to assess for presence of cognitive impairment or neurocognitive disorders that may affect mental functioning.

Severe deficits	Major impairments	Moderate impairments	Mild impairments	Healthy
1	2	3	4	5

- **Cognitive and affective processes**
  1. Capacity for regulation, attention, and learning *4*
  2. Capacity for affective range, communication, and understanding *4*
  3. Capacity for mentalization and reflective functioning *4*
- **Identity and relationships**
  4. Capacity for differentiation and integration (identity) *4*
  5. Capacity for relationships and intimacy *3*
  6. Capacity for self-esteem regulation and quality of internal experience *3*
- **Defense and coping**
  7. Capacity for impulse control and regulation *4*
  8. Capacity for defensive functioning *3*
  9. Capacity for adaptation, resiliency, and strength *4*
- **Self-awareness and self-direction**
  10. Self-observing capacities (psychological mindedness) *3*
  11. Capacity to construct and use internal standards and ideals *4*
  12. Capacity for meaning and purpose *4*

Overall level of personality severity (Sum of 12 mental functions): *44*

[Healthy/optimal mental functioning, 54–60; Good/appropriate mental functioning with some areas of difficulty, 47–53; Mild impairments in mental functioning, 40–46; Moderate impairments in mental functioning, 33–39; Major Impairments in mental functioning, 26–32; Significant defects in basic mental functions, 19–25; Major/severe defects in basic mental functions, 12–18]

(continued)

FIGURE 16.5. A completed PDC-E for Emilia.

Section II: Level of Personality Organization

Consider your patient's mental functions in determining the level of personality organization. Use these four mental functions to efficiently capture the level of personality organization, and don't forget you are evaluating an older person who falls into one of these age groups: young-old (55–64 years of age), middle-old (65–74 years of age), old–old (75–84 years of age), and oldest–old (85 years of age or older). Rate each mental function on a scale from 1 (Severely impaired) to 10 (Healthy).

Severe				Moderate				Healthy	
1	2	3	4	5	6	7	8	9	10

1. **Identity**: Ability to view self in complex, stable, and accurate ways 7
2. **Object relations**: Ability to maintain intimate, stable, and satisfying relationships 7
3. **Level of defenses** (using the guide below, select a single number): 7
   - 1–2: Psychotic level (delusional projection, psychotic denial, psychotic distortion)
   - 3–5: Borderline level (splitting, projective identification, idealization/devaluation, denial, acting out)
   - 6–8: Neurotic level (repression, reaction formation, intellectualization, displacement, undoing)
   - 9–10: Healthy level (anticipation, self-assertion, sublimation, suppression, altruism, and humor)
4. **Reality testing**: Ability to appreciate conventional notions of what is realistic 8

Overall Personality Organization

Considering the ratings and your clinical judgment, circle your client's overall personality organization.

Psychotic		Borderline			Neurotic			Healthy	
1	2	3	4	5	6	7	(8)	9	10

Healthy personality: Characterized by mostly 9–10 scores; life problems rarely get out of hand, and enough flexibility to accommodate to challenging realities. (Use 9 for people at the high-functioning neurotic level.)

Neurotic level: Characterized by mostly 6–8 scores; basically a good sense of identity, good reality testing, mostly good intimacies, fair resiliency, fair affect tolerance and regulation; rigidity and limited range of defenses and coping mechanisms; favors defenses such as repression, reaction formation, intellectualization, displacement, and undoing. (Use 6 for people who go between borderline and neurotic levels.)

(continued)

FIGURE 16.5. *(continued)*

Borderline level: Characterized by mostly 3–5 scores; recurrent relational problems; difficulty with affect tolerance and regulation; poor impulse control, poor sense of identity, poor resiliency; favors defenses such as splitting, projective identification, idealization/devaluation, denial, omnipotent control, and acting out.

Psychotic level: Characterized by mostly 1–2 scores; delusional thinking; poor reality testing and mood regulation; extreme difficulty functioning in work and relationships; favors defenses such as delusional projection, psychotic denial, and psychotic distortion. (Use 3 for people who go between psychotic and borderline levels.)

(There are no sharp cutoffs between categories. Use your clinical judgment.)

Section III: Personality Syndromes (PE Axis)

These are relatively stable patterns of thinking, feeling, behaving, and relating to others. Normal-level personality patterns do not involve impairment, while personality syndromes or disorders involve impairment at the neurotic, borderline, or psychotic level. Don't forget you are evaluating an older person, so take into consideration:

- Possible age-related behavioral features that may confound the diagnosis of a personality syndrome or disorder
- Possible effects of the aging process on previous personality symptoms
- Possible effects of personality syndromes on the aging process

Check off as many personality syndromes as apply from the list below; then circle the one or two personality styles that are most dominant. Leave blank if none.

(For research purposes, you may also rate the level of severity for all styles, using a 1–5 scale: 1 = Severe level; 3 = Moderate severity; and 5 = High-functioning.)

	Level of severity
☑ **Depressive** Subtypes: • Introjective • Anaclitic • Converse manifestation: Hypomanic	3
☐ **Dependent** Subtypes: • Passive–aggressive • Converse manifestation: Counterdependent	___
☐ **Anxious–avoidant and phobic**	___
☐ **Obsessive–compulsive**	___
☐ **Schizoid**	___

(continued)

FIGURE 16.5. *(continued)*

Level of severity

☐ **Somatizing** ___
☐ **Hysteric–histrionic** ___
☐ **Narcissistic** ___
☐ **Paranoid** ___
☐ **Psychopathic** ___
☐ **Sadistic** ___
☐ **Borderline** ___

Section IV: Symptom Patterns (SE Axis)

List the main PDM symptom patterns (those that are related to predominantly psychotic disorders, mood disorders, disorders related primarily to anxiety, event- and stressor-related disorders, etc.).

(If required, you may use the DSM or ICD symptoms and codes here.)

Severe — Moderate — Healthy
1 2 3 4 5

Symptom/concern: *Anxiety disorders* Level: *3*
Symptom/concern: ______ Level: ___
Symptom/concern: ______ Level: ___

Section V: Cultural, Contextual, and Other Relevant Considerations

Emilia belonged to the lower middle class, obtained a secretarial diploma, and expended her resources to fulfill her wish to marry a beloved man and devote her life to her love for culture (which her father had passed on to her) by opening her own bookshop in a working-class neighborhood. Given the period and context of her life, her determination to work toward self-realization is notable.

FIGURE 16.5. *(continued)*

APPENDIX

Psychodiagnostic Charts (PDCs)

This appendix contains blank versions of the different Psychodiagnostic Chart (PDC) assessment scales described in Chapter 15. The cases in Chapter 16 and in the online supplement (see the box at the end of the table of contents) illustrate how the various PDCs can be used for the various age groups covered in PDM-2.

Purchasers of this book can photocopy these forms for use with clients. Enlarged versions of the forms can also be downloaded (again, see the box at the end of the table of contents).

The PDC-2 (the version for use with adults) is a revision of the original PDC, which was developed by Robert M. Gordon and Robert F. Bornstein. Using Gordon and Bornstein's initial framework, the following colleagues created these variations on the PDC-2 for each of the age groups covered in PDM-2:

- Adolescent version (PDC-A): Norka Malberg, Johanna C. Malone, Nick Midgley, and Mario Speranza
- Child version (PDC-C): Norka Malberg, Larry Rosenberg, and Johanna C. Malone
- Infancy and Early Childhood version (PDC-IEC): Anna Maria Speranza
- Elderly version (PDC-E): Franco Del Corno and Daniel Plotkin

As explained in the Introduction, the order of the axes varies by PDCs. In the PDC-2 (Adults), personality is evaluated before mental functioning, whereas PDC-C, PDC-A, and PDC-E start with the assessment of mental functioning. Our rationale for this inconsistency is that by adulthood, personality (Axis P) has become quite stable and usually requires primary clinical focus, whereas in children and adolescents, developmental issues (Axis M) typically take precedence in clinical evaluations over emerging personality patterns. Late in the life cycle, adaptation to various aspects of aging (Axis M) may again be more important to assess than personality trends. The multiaxial approach for the Infancy and Early Childhood assessment makes the PDC-IEC a special case with its own unique structure.

Psychodiagnostic Chart–2 (PDC-2)

Psychodiagnostic Chart–2, Adult Version 8.1

Name: ______________ Age: ___ Gender: ______ Ethnicity: __________________

Date of evaluation: ___/___/___ Evaluator: ______________________________________

Section I: Level of Personality Organization

Consider your client's mental functions in determining the level of personality organization. Use these four mental functions to efficiently capture the level of personality organization. Rate each mental function on a scale from 1 (Severely impaired) to 10 (Healthy).

Severe				Moderate				Healthy	
1	2	3	4	5	6	7	8	9	10

1. **Identity:** Ability to view self in complex, stable, and accurate ways ___
2. **Object relations:** Ability to maintain intimate, stable, and satisfying relationships ___
3. **Level of defenses** (using the guide below, select a single number): ___
   - 1–2: Psychotic level (delusional projection, psychotic denial, psychotic distortion)
   - 3–5: Borderline level (splitting, projective identification, idealization/devaluation, denial, acting out)
   - 6–8: Neurotic level (repression, reaction formation, intellectualization, displacement, undoing)
   - 9–10: Healthy level (anticipation, self-assertion, sublimation, suppression, altruism, and humor)
4. **Reality testing:** Ability to appreciate conventional notions of what is realistic ___

Overall Personality Organization

Considering the ratings and your clinical judgment, circle your client's overall personality organization.

Psychotic		Borderline			Neurotic			Healthy	
1	2	3	4	5	6	7	8	9	10

(continued)

Healthy personality: Characterized by mostly 9–10 scores; life problems rarely get out of hand, and enough flexibility to accommodate to challenging realities. (Use 9 for people at the high-functioning neurotic level.)

Neurotic level: Characterized by mostly 6–8 scores; basically a good sense of identity, good reality testing, mostly good intimacies; fair resiliency, fair affect tolerance and regulation; rigidity and limited range of defenses and coping mechanisms; favors defenses such as repression, reaction formation, intellectualization, displacement, and undoing. (Use 6 for people who go between borderline and neurotic levels.)

Borderline level: Characterized by mostly 3–5 scores; recurrent relational problems; difficulty with affect tolerance and regulation; poor impulse control, poor sense of identity, poor resiliency; favors defenses such as splitting, projective identification, idealization/devaluation, denial, omnipotent control, and acting out.

Psychotic level: Characterized by mostly 1–2 scores; delusional thinking; poor reality testing and mood regulation; extreme difficulty functioning in work and relationships; favors defenses such as delusional projection, psychotic denial, and psychotic distortion. (Use 3 for people who go between psychotic and borderline levels.)

(There are no sharp cutoffs between categories. Use your clinical judgment.)

Section II: Personality Syndromes (P Axis)

These are relatively stable patterns of thinking, feeling, behaving, and relating to others. Normal-level personality patterns do not involve impairment, while personality syndromes or disorders involve impairment at the neurotic, borderline, or psychotic level.

Check off as many personality syndromes as apply from the list below; then circle the one or two personality styles that are most dominant. Leave blank if none.

(For research purposes, you may also rate the level of severity for all styles, using a 1–5 scale: 1 = Severe level; 3 = Moderate severity; and 5 = High-functioning.)

	Level of severity
☐ **Depressive** Subtypes: • Introjective • Anaclitic • Converse manifestation: Hypomanic	___
☐ **Dependent** Subtypes: • Passive–aggressive • Converse manifestation: Counterdependent	___

(continued)

Level of severity

☐ **Anxious–avoidant and phobic** ___
Subtype:
- Converse manifestation: Counterphobic

☐ **Obsessive–compulsive** ___

☐ **Schizoid** ___

☐ **Somatizing** ___

☐ **Hysteric–histrionic** ___
Subtypes:
- Inhibited
- Demonstrative

☐ **Narcissistic** ___
Subtypes:
- Overt
- Covert
- Malignant

☐ **Paranoid** ___

☐ **Psychopathic** ___
Subtypes:
- Passive–parasitic, "con artist"
- Aggressive

☐ **Sadistic** ___

☐ **Borderline** ___

Section III: Mental Functioning (M Axis)

Rate your client's level of strength or weakness on each of the 12 mental functions below, on a scale from 1 to 5 (1 = Severe deficits; 5 = Healthy). Then sum the 12 ratings for a level-of-severity score.

Severe deficits	Major impairments	Moderate impairments	Mild impairments	Healthy
1	2	3	4	5

(continued)

- **Cognitive and affective processes**
  1. Capacity for regulation, attention, and learning ___
  2. Capacity for affective range, communication, and understanding ___
  3. Capacity for mentalization and reflective functioning ___
- **Identity and relationships**
  4. Capacity for differentiation and integration (identity) ___
  5. Capacity for relationships and intimacy ___
  6. Self-esteem regulation and quality of internal experience ___
- **Defense and coping**
  7. Impulse control and regulation ___
  8. Defensive functioning ___
  9. Adaptation, resiliency, and strength ___
- **Self-awareness and self-direction**
  10. Self-observing capacities (psychological mindedness) ___
  11. Capacity to construct and use internal standards and ideals ___
  12. Meaning and purpose ___

Overall level of personality severity (Sum of 12 mental functions): ___

[Healthy/optimal mental functioning, 54–60; Appropriate mental functioning with some areas of difficulty, 47–53; Mild impairments in mental functioning, 40–46; Moderate impairments in mental functioning, 33–39; Major impairments in mental functioning, 26–32; Significant defects in basic mental functions, 19–25; Major/severe defects in basic mental functions, 12–18]

Section IV: Symptom Patterns (S Axis)

List the main PDM-2 symptom patterns (those that are predominantly related to psychotic disorders, mood disorders, disorders related primarily to anxiety, event- and stressor-related disorders, etc.).

(If required, you may use the DSM or ICD symptoms and codes here.)

Severe		Moderate		Healthy
1	2	3	4	5

Symptom/concern: ______________________________ Level: ___

Symptom/concern: ______________________________ Level: ___

Symptom/concern: ______________________________ Level: ___

(continued)

Section V: Cultural, Contextual, and Other Relevant Considerations

Psychodiagnostic Chart—Adolescent (PDC-A)

Name: ______________ Age: ___ Gender: ______ Ethnicity: __________________

Date of evaluation: ___/___/___ Evaluator: ______________________________

Section I: Mental Functioning (MA Axis)

Rate your patient's level of strength or weakness on each of the 12 mental functions below, on a scale from 1 to 5 (1 = Severe deficits; 5 = Healthy). Then sum the 12 ratings for a level-of-severity score.

Severe deficits	Major impairments	Moderate impairments	Mild impairments	Healthy
1	2	3	4	5

- **Cognitive and affective processes**
  1. Capacity for regulation, attention, and learning ___
  2. Capacity for affective range, communication, and understanding ___
  3. Capacity for mentalization and reflective functioning ___
- **Identity and relationships**
  4. Capacity for differentiation and integration (identity) ___
  5. Capacity for relationships and intimacy ___
  6. Capacity for self-esteem regulation and quality of internal experience ___
- **Defense and coping**
  7. Capacity for impulse control and regulation ___
  8. Capacity for defensive functioning ___
  9. Capacity for adaptation, resiliency, and strength ___
- **Self-awareness and self-direction**
  10. Self-observing capacities (psychological mindedness) ___
  11. Capacity to construct and use internal standards and ideals ___
  12. Capacity for meaning and purpose ___

Overall level of personality severity (Sum of 12 mental functions): ___

[Healthy/optimal mental functioning 54–60; Good/appropriate mental functioning with some areas of difficulty, 47–53; Mild impairments in mental functioning, 40–46; Moderate impairments in mental functioning, 33–39; Major impairments in mental functioning, 26–32; Significant defects in basic mental functions, 19–25; Major/severe defects in basic mental functions, 12–18]

(continued)

Section II: Level of Personality Organization

Consider your patient's mental functions in determining the level of personality organization. Use these four mental functions to efficiently capture the level of personality organization. The clinician should keep in mind the stage of adolescence presented by the patient: early adolescence (approximately 12–14 years old), middle adolescence (approximately 15–16 years old), or late adolescence (17–19 years old). Rate each mental function on a scale from 1 (Severely impaired) to 10 (Healthy).

Severe				Moderate				Healthy	
1	2	3	4	5	6	7	8	9	10

1. **Identity:** Ability to view self in complex, stable, and accurate ways ___
2. **Object relations:** Ability to maintain intimate, stable, and satisfying relationships ___
3. **Level of defenses** (using the guide below, select a single number): ___
   - 1–2: Psychotic level (delusional projection, psychotic denial, psychotic distortion)
   - 3–5: Borderline level (splitting, projective identification, idealization/devaluation, denial, acting out)
   - 6–8: Neurotic level (repression, reaction formation, intellectualization, displacement, undoing)
   - 9–10: Healthy level (anticipation, self-assertion, sublimation, suppression, altruism, and humor)
4. **Reality testing:** Ability to appreciate conventional notions of what is realistic ___

Overall Personality Organization

Considering the ratings and your clinical judgment, circle your client's overall personality organization.

Psychotic		Borderline			Neurotic			Healthy	
1	2	3	4	5	6	7	8	9	10

"Normal" emerging personality patterns (Healthy): Characterized by mostly 9–10 scores. These adolescents demonstrate a cohesive emerging personality organization in which their biological endowments, including their temperamental vulnerabilities, are managed adaptively within developmentally appropriate relationships with families, peers, and others. In relation to their stage of adolescent development, they have an increasingly organized sense of self, comprising age-appropriate coping skills and empathic, conscientious ways of dealing with feelings about self and others.

Mildly dysfunctional emerging personality patterns (Neurotic): Characterized by mostly 6–8 scores. These adolescents demonstrate a less cohesive emerging personality

(continued)

organization in which their biological endowments, including their temperamental vulnerabilities, are managed less adaptively. Early in life, their primary caregivers may have had trouble helping them manage these constitutional dispositions. Thus relationships with families, peers, and others are more fraught with problems. Such adolescents do not navigate the various developmental levels as successfully as those with less problematic endowments and/or more responsive caregivers. However, their sense of self and their sense of reality are pretty solid. As development proceeds, their adaptive mechanisms may be apparent in moderately rigid defensive patterns, and their reactions to adversities may be somewhat dysfunctional.

Dysfunctional emerging personality patterns (Borderline): Characterized by mostly 3–5 scores. These adolescents demonstrate vulnerabilities in reality testing and sense of self. Such problems may be manifested by maladaptive ways of dealing with feelings about self and others. Their defensive operations may distort reality (e.g., their own feelings may be perceived in others, rather than in themselves; the intentions of others may be misperceived).

Severely dysfunctional emerging personality patterns (Psychotic): Characterized by mostly 1–2 scores. These adolescents demonstrate significant deficits in their capacity for reality testing and forming a sense of self, manifested by consistently maladaptive ways of dealing with feelings about self and others. Their defensive operations interfere with basic capacities to relate to others and to separate their own feelings and wishes from those of others. (Use 3 for adolescents who go between psychotic and borderline levels.)

(There are no sharp cutoffs between categories. Use your clinical judgment.)

Section III: Emerging Adolescent Personality Styles/Syndromes (PA Axis)

In addition to considering level of organization, adolescent patients begin to demonstrate an emerging personality style. Rather than thinking of these styles as categorical diagnoses, it is more useful for clinicians to think of the relative degree to which the patient might be exhibiting an emerging style.

Check off as many personality syndromes as apply from the list below; then circle the one or two personality styles that are most dominant. Leave blank if none.

(For research purposes, you may also rate the level of severity for all styles, using a 1–5 scale: 1 = Severe level; 3 = Moderate severity; and 5 = High-functioning.)

	Level of severity
☐ **Depressive**	___
☐ **Anxious–avoidant**	___
☐ **Schizoid**	___

(continued)

Level of severity

- ☐ **Psychopathic–antisocial** ___
- ☐ **Narcissistic** ___
- ☐ **Paranoid** ___

- ☐ **Impulsive–histrionic** ___
- ☐ **Borderline** ___
- ☐ **Dependent–victimized** ___

- ☐ **Obsessive–compulsive** ___

Section IV: Symptom Patterns (SA Axis)

List the main PDM symptom patterns (those that are related to predominantly psychotic disorders, mood disorders, disorders related primarily to anxiety, event- and stressor-related disorders, etc.).

(If required, you may use the DSM or ICD symptoms and codes here.)

Severe		Moderate		Healthy
1	2	3	4	5

Symptom/concern: ______________________________ Level: ___

Symptom/concern: ______________________________ Level: ___

Symptom/concern: ______________________________ Level: ___

Section V: Cultural, Contextual, and Other Relevant Considerations

____

____

____

____

____

____

____

____

____

Psychodiagnostic Chart—Child (PDC-C)

Name: ______________ Age: ___ Gender: ______ Ethnicity: __________________

Date of evaluation: ___/___/___ Evaluator: ________________________________

Section I: Mental Functioning (MC Axis)

Rate your patient's level of strength or weakness on each of the 11 mental functions below, on a scale from 1 to 5 (1 = Severe deficits; 5 = Healthy). Then sum the 11 ratings for a level-of-severity score.

Severe deficits	Major impairments	Moderate impairments	Mild impairments	Healthy
1	2	3	4	5

- **Cognitive and affective processes**
  1. Capacity for regulation, attention, and learning ___
  2. Capacity for affective range, communication, and understanding ___
  3. Capacity for mentalization and reflective functioning ___
- **Identity and relationships**
  4. Capacity for differentiation and integration (identity) ___
  5. Capacity for relationships and intimacy ___
  6. Capacity for self-esteem regulation and quality of internal experience ___
- **Defense and coping**
  7. Capacity for impulse control and regulation ___
  8. Capacity for defensive functioning ___
  9. Capacity for adaptation, resiliency, and strength ___
- **Self-awareness and self-direction**
  10. Self-observing capacities (psychological mindedness) ___
  11. Capacity to construct and use internal standards and ideals ___

Overall level of personality severity (Sum of 11 mental functions): ___

[Healthy/optimal mental functioning, 50–55; Good/appropriate mental functioning with some areas of difficulty, 43–49; Mild impairments in mental functioning, 37–42; Moderate impairments in mental functioning, 30–36; Major impairments in mental functioning, 24–29; Significant defects in basic mental functions, 17–23; Major/severe defects in basic mental functions, 11–16]

(continued)

Section II: Emerging Level of Personality Patterns and Difficulties

Consider your patient's mental functions in determining the level of personality organization. Use these four mental functions to efficiently capture the current personality patterns and difficulties leading to an emerging level of personality organization. Age-specific characteristics, as well as the high level of fluidity in symptomatology during this stage of development, should be considered—as should other specific external factors influencing current clinical presentation. Rate each mental function on a scale from 1 (Severely impaired) to 10 (Healthy).

Severe				Moderate				Healthy	
1	2	3	4	5	6	7	8	9	10

1. **Identity:** Emerging ability to view self in age-appropriate, stable, and accurate ways ___
2. **Object relations:** Emerging ability to maintain intimate, stable, and satisfying relationships ___
3. **Emerging personality pattern** (using the guide below, select a single number): ___
   1–2: Psychotic level
   3–5: Borderline level
   6–8: Neurotic level
   9–10: Healthy level
4. **Reality testing:** Ability to appreciate conventional notions of what is realistic ___

Overall Emerging Personality Organization

Considering the ratings and your clinical judgment, circle your client's overall emerging personality organization.

Psychotic		Borderline			Neurotic			Healthy	
1	2	3	4	5	6	7	8	9	10

"Normal" emerging personality patterns (Healthy): Characterized by mostly 9–10 scores. These children demonstrate a cohesive emerging personality organization in which their biological endowments, including their temperamental vulnerabilities, are managed adaptively within developmentally appropriate relationships with families, peers, and others. In relation to their stage of development, they have an increasingly organized sense of self, comprising age-appropriate coping skills and empathic, conscientious ways of dealing with feelings about self and others.

Mildly dysfunctional emerging personality patterns (Neurotic): Characterized by mostly 6–8 scores. These children demonstrate a less cohesive emerging personality organization in which their biological endowments, including their temperamental

(continued)

vulnerabilities, are managed less adaptively. Early in life, their primary caregivers may have had trouble helping them manage these constitutional dispositions. Thus relationships with families, peers, and others are more fraught with problems. Such children do not navigate the various developmental levels as successfully as those with less problematic endowments and/or more responsive caregivers. However, their sense of self and their sense of reality are progressing in an age-appropriate manner. As development proceeds, their adaptive mechanisms may be apparent in moderately rigid defensive patterns, and their reactions to adversities may be somewhat dysfunctional.

Dysfunctional emerging personality patterns (Borderline): Characterized by mostly 3–5 scores. These children demonstrate vulnerabilities in reality testing and sense of self. Such problems may be manifested by maladaptive ways of dealing with feelings about self and others. Their defensive operations may distort reality (e.g., their own feelings may be perceived in others, rather than in themselves; the intentions of others may be misperceived).

Severely dysfunctional emerging personality patterns (Psychotic): Characterized by mostly 1–2 scores. These children demonstrate significant deficits in their capacity for reality testing and forming a sense of self, manifested by consistently maladaptive ways of dealing with feelings about self and others. Their defensive operations interfere with basic capacities to relate to others and to separate their own feelings and wishes from those of others.

(There are no sharp cutoffs between categories. Use your clinical judgment.)

Section III: Symptom Patterns (SC Axis)

List the main PDM symptom patterns (those that are related to predominantly psychotic disorders, mood disorders, disorders related primarily to anxiety, event- and stressor-related disorders, etc.).

(If required, you may use the DSM or ICD symptoms and codes here.)

Severe		Moderate		Healthy
1	2	3	4	5

Symptom/concern: ____________________ Level: ___

Symptom/concern: ____________________ Level: ___

Symptom/concern: ____________________ Level: ___

(continued)

Section IV: Influencing Factors and Relevant Clinical Observations Informing Diagnosis

1. Epigenetics: ____________________

____

2. Temperament: ____________________

____

3. Neuropsychology: ____________________

____

4. Attachment style ____________________

____

5. Sociocultural influences: ____________________

____

6. Countertransference–transference manifestations: ____________________

____

— Psychodiagnostic Chart—Infancy and Early Childhood (PDC-IEC) —

Name: ______________ Age: ___ Gender: _______ Ethnicity: ____________________

Date of evaluation: ___/___/___ Evaluator: ______________________________________

Section I: Primary Diagnoses

List the main IEC diagnoses and rate the level of severity for each, using a 1–5 scale. If necessary, you may use the DC: 0–3R, DC: 0–5, or DSM diagnosis here.

Severe ← Moderate → Mild

1 2 3 4 5

Principal diagnosis: ____ Level: ______

Other diagnosis: ____ Level: ______

Other diagnosis: ____ Level: ______

Section II: Functional Emotional Developmental Capacities

Circle the child's level of strengths or deficits on each of the six emotional functions below, on a scale from 1 to 5 (1 = Severe deficits; 5 = Healthy).

Level	Expected emotional function	Rating scale				
1	Shared attention and regulation	5	4	3	2	1
2	Engagement and relating	5	4	3	2	1
3	Two-way purposeful emotional interactions	5	4	3	2	1
4	Shared social problem solving	5	4	3	2	1
5	Creating symbols and ideas	5	4	3	2	1
6	Building logical bridges between ideas: Logical thinking	5	4	3	2	1

Section III: Regulatory–Sensory Processing Capacities

Axis III describes the child's regulatory–sensory processing profile. There are a number of constitutional–maturational differences in the way in which infants and young children respond to and comprehend sensory experiences and then plan actions. The different observed patterns exist on a continuum from relatively normal variations to disorders.

(continued)

Circle the child's level of regulatory–sensory processing capacities in each of the categories below, on a scale from 1 to 4 (1 = Severe problem; 4 = No indication).

Category	Subtype	Challenge in this area			
		No indication; never or rarely a problem	Mild problem or only occasionally a problem	Moderate problem or frequently a problem	Severe problem or almost always a problem
Sensory modulation	Sensory underresponsivity	4	3	2	1
	Sensory overresponsive	4	3	2	1
	Sensory seeking	4	3	2	1
Sensory discrimination	Tactile	4	3	2	1
	Auditory	4	3	2	1
	Visual	4	3	2	1
	Taste/smell	4	3	2	1
	Vestibular/ Propriocep.	4	3	2	1
Sensory-based motor functioning	Postural challenges	4	3	2	1
	Dyspraxis challenges	4	3	2	1

Overall Regulatory–Sensory Profile

Considering the ratings and your clinical judgment, circle the degree to which each regulatory–sensory pattern represents normal variation versus disorder. For scores 1–2, consider a regulatory–sensory processing disorder as a primary diagnosis; for scores 3–4, consider that the disordered regulatory–sensory processing can be associated with other primary diagnoses.

Severe deficits	Major impairments	Moderate impairments	Mild impairments	Healthy
1	2	3	4	5

(continued)

Section IV: Relational Patterns and Disorders

Each child's relationship with a significant caregiver (mother or father but, if appropriate custodial parent, grandparent, etc.) should be evaluated in this section. Rate the caregiver–child relationship on each of the eight descriptions below, on a scale from 1 to 5 (1 = Severely impaired; 5 = Healthy). Then sum the eight ratings for the degree to which the pattern represents healthy/adapted relationship versus relational disorder.

Caregiver 1: ____ (please specify)

Infant/child–caregiver relationship	***Rating scale***				
Quality and flexibility of caregiver's representation of the child	5	4	3	2	1
Quality of caregiver's reflective functioning	5	4	3	2	1
Quality of caregiver and child's nonverbal engagement	5	4	3	2	1
Quality of interactional patterns (reciprocity, synchrony, interactive repair)	5	4	3	2	1
Affective tone of the caregiver–infant relationship	5	4	3	2	1
Quality of caregiver's behavior (sensitivity vs. threatening and/or frightening behaviors)	5	4	3	2	1
Quality of caregiving patterns (comfort, stimulation, response to infant emotional signals, encouragement vs. withdrawal, overstimulation, controlling behavior, insensitivity)	5	4	3	2	1
Infant/child's ability to engage and form a significant relationship (vs. specific difficulties that impair this ability)	5	4	3	2	1
	Total score = ___				

Overall Level of Relational Pattern (Caregiver 1)

[Healthy/adapted relational patterns, 36–40; Adapted relational patterns with some areas of difficulty, 29–35; Moderate perturbation or disturbance in relational patterns, 22–28; Significant disturbance in relational patterns, 15–21; Major impairments in relational pattern or relational disorders, 8–14]

Attachment Pattern (Caregiver 1)

Rate the caregiver–child relationship as regards attachment patterns on a scale from 1 (no correspondence) to 5 (high correspondence) for each of the four prototypes.

Secure ________

Insecure–avoidant ________

Insecure–ambivalent/resistant ________

Disorganized/disoriented ________

(continued)

Caregiver 2: ____ (please specify)

Infant/child–caregiver relationship	***Rating scale***				
Quality and flexibility of caregiver's representation of the child	5	4	3	2	1
Quality of caregiver's reflective functioning	5	4	3	2	1
Quality of caregiver and child's nonverbal engagement	5	4	3	2	1
Quality of interactional patterns (reciprocity, synchrony, interactive repair)	5	4	3	2	1
Affective tone of the caregiver–infant relationship	5	4	3	2	1
Quality of caregiver's behavior (sensitivity vs. threatening and/or frightening behaviors)	5	4	3	2	1
Quality of caregiving patterns (comfort, stimulation, response to infant emotional signals, encouragement vs. withdrawal, overstimulation, controlling, insensitivity)	5	4	3	2	1
Infant/child's ability to engage and form a significant relationship (vs. specific difficulties that impair this ability)	5	4	3	2	1
	Total score = ___				

Overall Level of Relational Pattern (Caregiver 2)

[Healthy/adapted relational patterns, 36–40; Adapted relational patterns with some areas of difficulty, 29–35; Moderate perturbation or disturbance in relational patterns, 22–28; Significant disturbance in relational patterns, 15–21; Major impairments in relational pattern or relational disorders, 8–14]

Attachment Pattern (Caregiver 2)

Rate the caregiver–child relationship as regards attachment patterns on a scale from 1 (no correspondence) to 5 (high correspondence) for each of the four prototypes.

Secure ________

Insecure–avoidant ________

Insecure–ambivalent/resistant ________

Disorganized/disoriented ________

Section V: Other Medical and Neurological Diagnoses

____

____

____

____

Psychodiagnostic Chart—Elderly (PDC-E)

Name: ______________ Age: ___ Gender: _______ Ethnicity: __________________

Date of evaluation: ___/___/___ Evaluator: ______________________________________

Section I: Mental Functioning (ME Axis)

Rate your patient's level of strength or weakness on each of the 12 mental functions below, on a scale from 1 to 5 (1 = Severe deficits; 5 = Healthy). Then sum the 12 ratings for a level-of-severity score.

Although most older adults do not have significant cognitive impairment, it is important to assess for presence of cognitive impairment or neurocognitive disorders that may affect mental functioning.

Severe deficits	Major impairments	Moderate impairments	Mild impairments	Healthy
1	2	3	4	5

- **Cognitive and affective processes**
  1. Capacity for regulation, attention, and learning ___
  2. Capacity for affective range, communication, and understanding ___
  3. Capacity for mentalization and reflective functioning ___
- **Identity and relationships**
  4. Capacity for differentiation and integration (identity) ___
  5. Capacity for relationships and intimacy ___
  6. Capacity for self-esteem regulation and quality of internal experience ___
- **Defense and coping**
  7. Capacity for impulse control and regulation ___
  8. Capacity for defensive functioning ___
  9. Capacity for adaptation, resiliency, and strength ___
- **Self-awareness and self-direction**
  10. Self-observing capacities (psychological mindedness) ___
  11. Capacity to construct and use internal standards and ideals ___
  12. Capacity for meaning and purpose ___

Overall level of personality severity (Sum of 12 mental functions): ___

[Healthy/optimal mental functioning, 54–60; Good/appropriate mental functioning with some areas of difficulty, 47–53; Mild impairments in mental functioning, 40–46; Moderate impairments in mental functioning, 33–39; Major Impairments in mental functioning, 26–32; Significant defects in basic mental functions, 19–25; Major/severe defects in basic mental functions, 12–18]

(continued)

Section II: Level of Personality Organization

Consider your patient's mental functions in determining the level of personality organization. Use these four mental functions to efficiently capture the level of personality organization, and don't forget you are evaluating an older person who falls into one of these age groups: young-old (55–64 years of age), middle-old (65–74 years of age), old–old (75–84 years of age), and oldest–old (85 years of age or older). Rate each mental function on a scale from 1 (Severely impaired) to 10 (Healthy).

Severe				Moderate				Healthy	
1	2	3	4	5	6	7	8	9	10

1. **Identity**: Ability to view self in complex, stable, and accurate ways ___
2. **Object relations**: Ability to maintain intimate, stable, and satisfying relationships ___
3. **Level of defenses** (using the guide below, select a single number): ___
   - 1–2: Psychotic level (delusional projection, psychotic denial, psychotic distortion)
   - 3–5: Borderline level (splitting, projective identification, idealization/devaluation, denial, acting out)
   - 6–8: Neurotic level (repression, reaction formation, intellectualization, displacement, undoing)
   - 9–10: Healthy level (anticipation, self-assertion, sublimation, suppression, altruism, and humor)
4. **Reality testing**: Ability to appreciate conventional notions of what is realistic ___

Overall Personality Organization

Considering the ratings and your clinical judgment, circle your client's overall personality organization.

Psychotic		Borderline			Neurotic			Healthy	
1	2	3	4	5	6	7	8	9	10

Healthy personality: Characterized by mostly 9–10 scores; life problems rarely get out of hand, and enough flexibility to accommodate to challenging realities. (Use 9 for people at the high-functioning neurotic level.)

Neurotic level: Characterized by mostly 6–8 scores; basically a good sense of identity, good reality testing, mostly good intimacies, fair resiliency, fair affect tolerance and regulation; rigidity and limited range of defenses and coping mechanisms; favors defenses such as repression, reaction formation, intellectualization, displacement, and undoing. (Use 6 for people who go between borderline and neurotic levels.)

(continued)

Borderline level: Characterized by mostly 3–5 scores; recurrent relational problems; difficulty with affect tolerance and regulation; poor impulse control, poor sense of identity, poor resiliency; favors defenses such as splitting, projective identification, idealization/devaluation, denial, omnipotent control, and acting out.

Psychotic level: Characterized by mostly 1–2 scores; delusional thinking; poor reality testing and mood regulation; extreme difficulty functioning in work and relationships; favors defenses such as delusional projection, psychotic denial, and psychotic distortion. (Use 3 for people who go between psychotic and borderline levels.)

(There are no sharp cutoffs between categories. Use your clinical judgment.)

Section III: Personality Syndromes (PE Axis)

These are relatively stable patterns of thinking, feeling, behaving, and relating to others. Normal-level personality patterns do not involve impairment, while personality syndromes or disorders involve impairment at the neurotic, borderline, or psychotic level. Don't forget you are evaluating an older person, so take into consideration:

- Possible age-related behavioral features that may confound the diagnosis of a personality syndrome or disorder
- Possible effects of the aging process on previous personality syndromes
- Possible effects of personaity syndromes on the aging process

Check off as many personality syndromes as apply from the list below; then circle the one or two personality styles that are most dominant. Leave blank if none.

(For research purposes, you may also rate the level of severity for all styles, using a 1–5 scale: 1 = Severe level; 3 = Moderate severity; and 5 = High-functioning.)

	Level of severity
☐ **Depressive** Subtypes: • Introjective • Anaclitic • Converse manifestation: Hypomanic	___
☐ **Dependent** Subtypes: • Passive–aggressive • Converse manifestation: Counterdependent	___
☐ **Anxious–avoidant and phobic**	___
☐ **Obsessive–compulsive**	___
☐ **Schizoid**	___

(continued)

Level of severity

☐ **Somatizing** ___

☐ **Hysteric–histrionic** ___

☐ **Narcissistic** ___

☐ **Paranoid** ___

☐ **Psychopathic** ___

☐ **Sadistic** ___

☐ **Borderline** ___

Section IV: Symptom Patterns (SE Axis)

List the main PDM symptom patterns (those that are related to predominantly psychotic disorders, mood disorders, disorders related primarily to anxiety, event- and stressor-related disorders, etc.).

(If required, you may use the DSM or ICD symptoms and codes here.)

Severe		Moderate		Healthy
1	2	3	4	5

Symptom/concern: ______________________________ Level: ___

Symptom/concern: ______________________________ Level: ___

Symptom/concern: ______________________________ Level: ___

Section V: Cultural, Contextual, and Other Relevant Considerations

____

____

____

____

____

____

____

____

____

____

Index

Page numbers followed by *f* indicate figure, *t* indicate table